Brain Injury and Mental Retardation: Psychopharmacology and Neuropsychiatry

Brain Injury and Mental Retardation: Psychopharmacology and Neuropsychiatry

C. THOMAS GUALTIERI, M.D.
Medical Director
North Carolina Neuropsychiatry
Chapel Hill, North Carolina

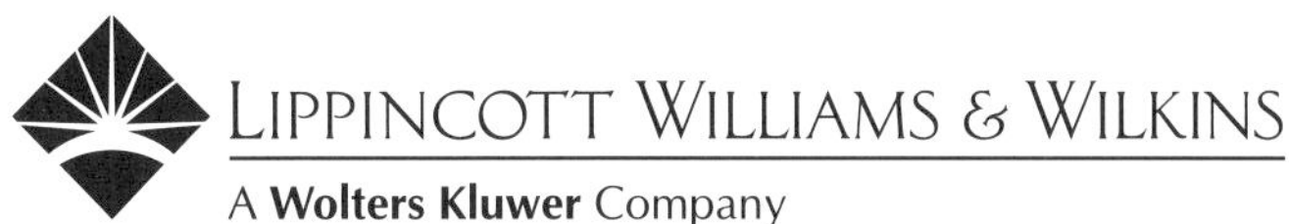

Acquisitions Editor: Charles W. Mitchell
Developmental Editor: Lisa Consoli
Production Editor: Melanie Bennitt
Manufacturing Manager: Colin Warnock
Cover Designer: Jeane Norton
Compositor: Lippincott Williams & Wilkins Desktop Division
Printer: Data Reproductions Corporation

530 Walnut Street
Philadelphia, PA 19106 USA
LWW.com

Printed in the USA

Library of Congress Cataloging-in-Publication Data

Gualtieri, C. Thomas.
Brain injury and mental retardation : psychopharmacology and neuropsychiatry / C. Thomas Gualtieri.
p. ; cm
Includes bibliographical references and index.
ISBN 0-7817-3473-8
1. Brain damage. 2. Mental retardation. I. Title.
[DNLM: 1. Brain Injuries—complications. 2. Mental Retardation—complications. 3. Mental Disorders—drug therapy. 4. Mental Disorders—etiology. 5. Mentally Disabled Persons—psychology. WL 354 G912b 2002]
RC387.5.G83 2002
617.4′810443—dc21

2002016182

---

10 9 8 7 6 5 4 3 2 1

Contents

Preface

Traumatic brain injury and mental retardation are two of the most common conditions in neuropsychiatry. Yet they account for only a small fraction of the published reports, chapters, and monographs in the field. They generate little attention (relative, at least, to their clinical importance) among the sources of research funding and in the academic centers. Physicians and psychologists who are interested in learning about the behavioral and emotional problems that are so common in these patients have never had a single source to which they might refer. The needed information is out there, but it is scattered in the specialized literature of several disciplines.

As a practicing psychiatrist for over twenty-five years, I have always had a special interest in patients with brain injuries and developmental handicaps. They have been the focus of the research my colleagues and I have done over the years, and the subject of our consultations around the country. They are the patients we see every day. Since I had already written a good deal about them for the medical journals, it was only a short jump to collect my thoughts and experience into a summary text. It should be a good starting-place for clinicians who want to understand the psychiatric problems of these unique and sometimes perplexing patients.

Like many physicians who doggedly pursue a special interest, my attachment to these conditions was stimulated, early on, by personal experience with a severely afflicted family member. It happens, sometimes, that a child's experience of tragedy etches a path one follows for a lifetime. So it was for me. But if my initial interest was aroused by personal experience, it has been sustained by the intellectual challenges that are inherent to these extraordinary conditions. It has always been a challenge to contend with clinical problems that were novel and largely uncharted. My work has also been sustained by the reward of working, every day, with the patients and their families, whose gratitude always seems to exceed the value of my prescriptions. It has been supported by the interest of my colleagues, from various disciplines in medicine and psychology, who have been interested in the things I've learned and written about over the years. (Well, at least they seemed interested.)

Whenever I would lecture about the obscure subjects that are the meat of this book, listeners would ask if there were a source I could refer them to. There isn't a single place you can go, I'd have to say, to reach all of the different dimensions of the topic. The information is here and there, in the literature of psychiatry and neurology, genetics and developmental medicine, neuropsychology, behavioral psychology, and neuropharmacology. You have to keep your eye on what is happening in a number of broad and diverse fields.

With this publication, there is a single source to address the problems of psychiatric practice in patients with congenital or acquired injuries of the brain; a primer, if you will. The assiduous student will still have to keep his or her eye on all of those daunting fields, of course, because they are changing rapidly, and no monograph can hope to cover every salient aspect. I have tried to give readers a frame of reference to guide their further reading as well as their clinical practice.

My goal is to present a framework for understanding the psychiatric conditions that arise in these patient groups. So the problems of brain injury patients are presented as the Transient Neurobehavioral Syndromes, the Static or Structural Syndromes, and the Delayed Neurobehavioral Sequelae. Similar problems, arising in mentally handicapped patients, are conceptualized as expressions of the so-called Pathobehavioral Syndromes, or as atypical presentations of the conventional psychiatric disorders, or as almost pure disorders of behavior. The idea is to present taxonomy of the clinical conditions based not only on overt clinical manifestations but also on their etiological and pathophysiological dimensions.

This is a book of clinical descriptions. Occasionally, I will venture into theoretical discussions, and some are admittedly speculative. Theory is introduced to flesh out the clinical, to give it a foundation. In virtually all of the conditions that I discuss, it is possible to link brain systems and functions to issues of diagnosis and treatment. Sometimes the links are tenuous, but they never fail to be interesting. When the discussion turns to "complex functional systems" or "diaschisis" or "non-synaptic diffusion neurotransmission," it will be, one hopes, in the service of clinical understanding. Clinicians are practical-minded people, but they like to know that their practice has a scientific basis, of some sort, at least.

This is also a book about drug treatment. Pharmacological approaches to the problems of brain-injured and mentally handicapped individuals are sufficiently different to warrant a discussion of psychopharmacology addressed specifically to their unique conditions. Neuropsychiatric patients are often resistant to the pharmacological approaches that are common to the day-to-day practice of psychiatry and neurology. They have a lower threshold to drug-induced neurotoxicity. Drugs have to be selected with a careful eye to their effects on cognition; not infrequently, drugs are prescribed to enhance cognition or to prevent cognitive decline. The important issue of drug effects on brain plasticity and cortical recovery following severe injury is central to our discussions; it is dealt with nowhere else that I know.

Drug treatment for individuals with brain injuries has a venerable history. Two generations ago, the Russian neurologist Luria wrote about galanthamine, an acetylcholinesterase inhibitor, for brain-injured veterans of the Great Patriotic War. It is only recently that drugs of that class have been available in North America and Western Europe. The anti-viral drug amantadine was discovered to be effective for patients with Parkinson's disease in 1967; a generation later, it began to be used, with striking success, in brain injury patients. "Megavitamin" treatments for mentally retarded and autistic children have been around since the 1950s. The salience of vitamin therapy and of "nutraceuticals" has only recently won the attention of serious investigators. We shall have a good deal to say about novel treatments, as well as conventional treatments; as it happens, the "novel" treatments are not so new at all.

Finally, this is a book that describes a clinical method. Drug treatment for brain-injured and mentally handicapped patients does not always obey the "practice guidelines" that are proposed, with unnerving regularity, for the various categories in the Diagnostic and Statistical Manual. Indeed, the diagnostic categories themselves are only imperfectly applied to patients with these conditions. Drug treatment for these patients is not so much diagnosis-driven as it is brain-based or, at least, system-based. We propose to relate the cognitive, behavioral, and emotional symptoms of these patients to complex brain systems that have been damaged by brain injury or, in the case of the retarded patient, to developing systems that have failed, or have gone awry.

I can't propose that we have achieved a thorough understanding of complex brain systems or developmental processes. Even with the extraordinary advances in dynamic brain imaging and other technologies, our level of understanding remains imperfect, and achieving a synthesis of brain and behavior is still beyond our grasp. But in patients with certain kinds of brain injuries, lesion analysis permits the clinician to understand the cerebral basis for behavioral aberration. In a few of the mental retardation syndromes, like the Lesch-Nyhan syndrome and the fragile X syndrome, we are able to trace the pathology of behavior from its genetic roots. These are extraordinary accomplishments for medical science. Their impact on the day-to-day practice of neuropsychiatry merits careful attention.

But genetic studies and lesion analysis enlighten only a small proportion of the clinical problems we shall meet within this book, and in most cases we can do no better than offer enlightened guesses. The clinical method we shall propose, therefore, operates on the basis of what sociologists call a "stochastic model," that is, one where uncertainty is the rule. "Fuzzy logic" is another term that can be applied to what we do. Effective clinicians cannot rely on "diagnoses," which may sometimes obfuscate treatment decisions. Rather, they have to generate hypotheses about the nature of the clinical problems with which they are confronted, about their origins in the brain, and about the environmental circumstances that have evoked them. Treatment, then, is not the end, but a means to test one's hypotheses. It is an empirical process or, as the sociologists say, a stochastic process; in other words, trial-and-error.

And so this is what we have: clinical descriptions of the conditions, organized rationally or, at least, organized; psychopharmacology, as it specifically relates to the clinical conditions; and a method for putting the two together. If I have succeeded in enlightening or enlivening this obscure branch of medicine, your patients will be the better for it. For even the small chance of success, then, your author is profoundly grateful.

C. Thomas Gualtieri
Chapel Hill, North Carolina

Acknowledgments

It is appropriate to recognize my research colleagues and co-authors who worked with me on the projects that contributed to this book: Paul Bach-y-Rita, Jarrett Barnhill, George Breese, Mark Chandler, Randy Evans, Lyn Johnson, John Ratey, Steve Schroeder, and Robert Sprague. Especially two who are gone from us and sorely missed: Robert Hicks and Morrie Lipton. Most of the good ideas in this book are theirs; all of the wrong-headed ones are my own.

I also acknowledge my wife and our children, who never complained when I absented myself from family business to bang away at this manuscript. For their understanding and encouragement, I am deeply grateful. They seem to understand that the old man is a perpetual student, just one more of his eccentricities that they abide with grace and good humor. In fact, just as this manuscript is completed, my wife and I will travel to China to adopt another little girl. I have the feeling that Nora will be as gentle and forbearing with her father as her sister and brothers have been.

It is indeed a blessing to spend my life as a student. How fortunate I am to live in this time, in this fair and prosperous country, and to possess the freedom to follow such an inclination. In the Talmud, remember, they say that scholars grow wiser as they age. This scholar is aging, to be sure. If I am wiser at all, it is only for having learned that I am surrounded by good and generous teachers. My unruly and undisciplined mind was a source of vexation, I am sure, to the good Brothers at my high school in Brooklyn and my professors at Columbia and McGill. I wish I could attend to them, again, with the intellectual curiosity and love of learning I have now. It grows stronger with each passing year.

I continue to be surrounded by good and generous teachers, and chief among them these days are my many patients and their families. The word "doctor" means "teacher," but I think that a good doctor is really just a student, learning every day from his or her patients, from their suffering and their successes. If some tribute is due, it is to them, for having guided my studies patiently, and respectfully, and for keeping my spirits high. They have been with me for more than thirty years, and they keep coming. They must believe that someday I'm going to learn to do this job right. *The lyf so short, the crafte so long to lerne.*

My first and best teacher was my father. He taught me how to think clearly and how to write good. He was an exemplary physician, a skillful and intelligent surgeon. He used to say, "You have a moral responsibility to be intelligent." I think he got that from one of his professors at Columbia, John Erskine. My father was an eternal student himself, and I think he enjoyed helping me with this book. His spirit has never been far from my own, and I offer this book in tribute to him.

C. Thomas Gualtieri

Brain Injury and Mental Retardation: Psychopharmacology and Neuropsychiatry

1

Brain Injury

SUMMARY

Brain injury (BI) is a broad topic. The most important types are addressed here, from traumatic brain injury (TBI), by far the most common, to *Pfiesteria* encephalopathy, a rare condition but one that is bound to increase in importance as our estuarine waters are corrupted by development and intensive agriculture.

There are more than two million TBIs in the United States each year. Most are closed head injuries (CHIs) owing to motor vehicle accidents, falls, assaults, and sporting accidents. During wartime, penetrating brain injuries (PBIs) predominate. PBIs give rise to focal symptoms; historically, studies of combat veterans were the impetus for major advances in neuropsychology and lesion analysis. The pathophysiology of CHI, however, is quite different, characterized not only by focal damage but also diffuse axonal injury. As a result, the clinical presentation and pattern of recovery are quite different.

Hypoxic encephalopathy results from drowning, hanging, cardiopulmonary arrest, surgical errors, and other causes. Carbon monoxide is a special case of pure hypoxic injury without ischemia. Hypoxic-ischemic injuries tend to be diffuse, whereas carbon monoxide and hypoglycemia are associated with patterns that are both diffuse and focal.

Electrocution from atmospheric or technical sources can have catastrophic effects on the brain. Less severe cases can raise formidable challenges to proper diagnosis, especially for psychiatrists. Posttraumatic stress disorder and conversion disorder are commonly found in electrocution victims. The risks posed by electromagnetic radiation have probably been overstated. Radiation necrosis, conversely, is a grave condition that leads to progressive degeneration of the central nervous system (CNS).

In all these conditions, one point stands out: the potential neurobehavioral sequelae of BI are generally more disabling than the motor, sensory, or cognitive deficits normally taken to be their defining characteristics.

BRAIN INJURY

People with BI, congenital or acquired, are the largest and the fastest growing population of neuropsychiatric patients in the developed world. Even as some important causes of BI recede in importance, other new ones take their place. After the major wars of this century, there were epidemics of PBIs. Then, with the postwar increase in vehicular transportation, there was a "silent epidemic" of CHIs (1). As public health improves, the old infectious encephalopathies decline in importance, but new ones appear, such as Lyme borreliosis and acquired immunodeficiency syndrome; people worry about postimmunization encephalopathy, even as the incidence of infectious encephalitis declines precipitously. Football helmets are now more protective against head injury than they were in the past, but "heading" the ball in soccer is not entirely benign, at least in the long term. Emergency transport and intensive care have improved dramatically, as has the survival rate of patients with severe TBIs and of very low birth weight babies. Even the genetic conditions may be more troublesome. Down's syndrome is less common, but people with this syndrome live longer than they used to, and their problem now is Alzheimer's disease. It is possible that amplification syndromes like fragile X are prone to increase.

In the winter, we are vulnerable to carbon monoxide poisoning from leaky furnaces; in the summer, there are lightning strikes to worry about. It is a wonder any of us make it at all. We humans are so proud of our big brains and intelligent faces; we relish the accomplishments of intelligence and culture, but it is all so very fragile. There are almost as many ways to damage the brain as there are to realize its extraordinary potential.

Once, when I was about eight, I fell down and bumped my head. I ran back to the summer house with an enormous goose egg on my forehead. My Uncle Jack was mowing the grass, but he stopped to inspect the wound. Then he said: "It's a good thing you hit your head; otherwise you might have hurt yourself." (He had that kind of sense of humor, my Uncle.) Looking back, though, I think he was right. The brain, for all its fragility, is capable of remarkable improvement, even recovery, from the injuries and malformations that affect it.

TRAUMATIC BRAIN INJURY

There are more than two million cases of TBI in the United States each year, and 500,000 cases require hospital admission. Every year, 100,000 people experience lifelong debilitating loss of function from TBI (1,2). Even relatively mild head injuries can lead to permanent encephalopathic changes and prolonged disability (3).

The numbers are formidable and reason enough for beginning this monograph with a discussion of BI, but not the only reason. The clinical manifestations of TBI are protean; virtually every neuropsychiatric disorder is amply represented among patients with TBI. The mechanisms of injury and the principles of treatment of BI are relevant to the other areas of neuropsychiatry discussed here. TBI is, therefore, a prototypical condition.

Many of the behavioral and cognitive disabilities that stem from TBI are amenable to correction or at least to substantial improvement. Sequelae such as amnesia, inattention, depression, psychosis, and personality change may be treated with an appropriate rehabilitation program or timely pharmacologic intervention. A well-directed psychiatric treatment can mean the difference between a productive life and one of chronic disability (4). Indeed, neuropsychiatric deficits contribute disproportionately to chronic disability caused by TBI (63% of cases), accounting for more disability overall than do motor and sensory deficits (5,6). Yet of all the deficits incurred by TBI, neuropsychiatric problems are the most amenable to correction.

The study of TBI during the first part of the past century was confined to hospitals for veterans where physicians and psychologists worked with the victims of battlefield injuries. There was a spate of new head injury research after every war. Although this research became the foundation of much of what we know today, the nature of the problem of BI has changed. Wartime injuries tend to be PBIs from high-speed missiles that penetrate a circumscribed area of the brain, especially the frontal lobes. Such injuries cause focal damage, especially to cortex, but not necessarily diffuse damage. In contrast, CHIs are most common today, from motor vehicle accidents, assaults, falls, and sporting contests. The epidemic of TBI (1) is attributable entirely to the extraordinary growth in the numbers of CHI victims and survivors. Because CHIs are acceleration-deceleration injuries, they entail much more extensive subcortical damage than PBIs do. The pathophysiology of a CHI is very different from that of a PBI. As a result, the cognitive and neurobehavioral sequelae are different.

Epidemiology

CHI is the most prevalent form of BI (2). The more general term TBI refers to CHI and to PBI and open head injuries. The term TBI can also be used to refer to diffuse encephalopathic injury caused by anoxia (diffuse anoxic injury), thermal, electrical, or radiation injury.

Patients with TBI tend to be young. The peak incidence is from 15 to 24 years of age (2). There are secondary peaks for infants, children, and the elderly (2). At every age, males are twice as likely as females to be victims of TBI (7).

The most common causes of TBI are transport-related accidents (motor vehicles, bicycles), falls, interpersonal assaults, especially gunshot wounds, and sports injuries (2,7). In the inner city, the most common cause of TBI is assault; everywhere else in the United States, TBIs are mostly motor vehicle–related. Falls are a common cause of TBI in children and the most common cause of TBI in the elderly.

Factors that predispose to the occurrence of TBI may also complicate the process of diagnosis and treatment. Alcoholism, drug abuse, and risk-taking behavior are obvious elements in TBI related to vehicular accidents (2). Elderly people who are most prone to injury from falling frequently have premorbid evidence of degenerative brain disease (8). Approximately one-third of children who have TBIs were hyperactive before the event (attention deficit hyperactivity disorder). The likelihood of TBI is higher in people who have had a previous TBI, an association that may be mediated by behavioral characteristics (e.g., risk taking, substance abuse) or by deficits in attention, perception, and response time that are attributable to the initial TBI (9). This is important because the neurobehavioral effects of more than one BI may be more than simply additive (10). It also speaks to an important issue in treatment, namely, to warn a patient with TBI of the increased risk of a second injury.

Traumatic Brain Injury and Alcohol

Substance abuse, particularly of alcohol, is strongly implicated as the cause of many head injuries (11). Between 29% and 58% of patients with TBI with positive blood alcohol levels taken on admission to the emergency department are legally intoxicated, and there is evidence of alcohol addiction in 25% to 68% of these cases (11–13). Rimel et al. (14) reported that no fewer than 34% of patients with moderate head injury were problem drinkers before the injury.

There also is evidence that alcohol aggravates the cascade of pathologic events that transpire immediately after TBI. As a result, TBI victims with positive blood alcohol levels at the time of injury have longer duration of coma and a lower level of consciousness during the acute stage of recovery (15) and a longer hospital stay (12). There is even evidence to suggest that high blood alcohol levels at the time of injury have a detrimental effect on the patient's ultimate recovery of neuropsychological function (e.g., memory) (16). Excessive alcohol users have a higher mortality rate after TBI than nonusers or moderate users; they have a higher rate of mass lesions on computed tomography (CT) scan and a lower rate of good outcomes after TBI (17). It is not entirely clear whether these data indicate a direct neurotoxic effect of alcohol felt at the time of acute injury or a premorbid weakness in the alcoholic patient that renders him or her more vulnerable to the direct effects of the injury. Studies of patients who are alcoholics but who have negative blood levels at the time of injury are contradictory (11).

There is also evidence that resumption of alcohol abuse retards cognitive recovery (18). This is important because approximately 50% of patients with TBI return to preinjury levels of alcohol consumption within a year of their injury (12). Patients with physical disabilities as the consequence of TBI are likely to turn to alcohol as a way of alleviating emotional distress (19,20). Furthermore, patients with TBI seem to be more sensitive to the intoxicating effects of alcohol than they were before the injury (21). Alcohol may also interact with medications that are prescribed to patients with TBI (4).

The treatment of the alcoholic patient with TBI is problematic because there is consensus among rehabilitation professionals that traditional approaches to alcoholism treatment usually are inappropriate for patients with TBI with cognitive impairment, particularly those with lack of insight (anosognosia), poor judgment, and poor safety awareness. Many rehabilitation centers have developed special programs for the patient with a dual diagnosis, but there is little in the way of systematic research to allow the physician to recommend any particular approach (11).

Pathology

The pathology of TBI includes a number of events, including skull fracture, epidural, subdural, and intracerebral hemorrhage, and cerebral contusions; these are addressed in Chapter 4. The unique pathology of CHI is discussed here. Motor vehicle accidents or falls cause most of the TBI cases in developed countries. They are, therefore, acceleration-deceleration injuries. Most are CHIs, characterized by a unique pattern of neuropathologic changes that influence the ensuing behavioral pathology. On the subcellular level, the micropathology of TBI and CHI is characterized by a cascade of secondary pathologic events that have a bearing on the development of new treatments.

In CHI, the brain is injured by contusion as a result of direct and contrecoup impact. The cortical lesions that derive from such an impact are more extensive, as a rule, than the lesions of a PBI but are qualitatively similar. In addition, CHI also produces diffuse, microscopic damage to the brain, especially to the subcortical white matter (7). Cortical impact injury is transmitted with particular vehemence to axial structures in the brainstem, generating shear forces that cause scattered multifocal subcortical and brainstem axonal damage (diffuse axonal injury) (7). The combination of cortical, subcortical, and brainstem injury is characteristic of CHI.

The axonal tracts that are disrupted in CHI include monoaminergic projections from the brainstem to cortical and subcortical structures. Experimental studies in laboratory animals and clinical experiments have been consistent in demonstrating persistent deficits in monoamine neurotransmission after CHI (4,22).

Cortical regions that are particularly vulnerable to contusive damage in an acceleration-deceleration injury are the rostral poles and inferior surfaces of the frontal and temporal lobes. They are damaged by impact against the frontal, sphenoid, or temporal bones or by movement along the irregular surface of the cribriform plate. Therefore, the behavioral characteristics of frontal and temporal lobe lesions are common among CHI victims.

The anatomic description of a patient with a CHI comprises the cortical and subcortical lesions that may be demonstrable in the neurologic examination, by brain imaging, or by neuropsychological testing. Diffuse microscopic damage is difficult if not impossible to demonstrate in the living patient. However, if the cortical lesions are extensive or if there has been a prolonged period of unconsciousness, the occurrence of diffuse axonal injury may be inferred. Sometimes, magnetic resonance imaging (MRI) will demonstrate multiple small areas of increased T2 signal in subcortical or brainstem white matter; computed axial tomography scans rarely show these white matter abnormalities (23). Even in patients who have had relatively mild CHIs with no demonstrable signs of a brain lesion, there may still be microscopic hemorrhages, especially in the frontal and temporal lobes, and shear injury to axons throughout the white matter and the brainstem (24).

The irony of a CHI, as well as a dilemma to many patients, is that encephalopathic injury may occur, even with a mild injury, with only a few moments of loss of consciousness (LOC) or none at all (3,25). It is even possible for brain trauma to occur in acceleration-deceleration injuries (e.g., cervical whiplash) where the head itself never strikes a rigid surface (26). Psychiatrists are especially likely to see patients in whom BI has occurred in relatively minor accidents. Notwithstanding such clinically important exceptions, the duration of LOC and the depth of coma, defined by the Glasgow Coma Scale (5), are the most important elements in predicting the extent of encephalopathic damage (27).

Recovery and Outcome

The outcome of any given TBI is determined by four elements:

- The extent and location of gross brain damage,
- The extent of diffuse microscopic brain damage,
- The patient's premorbid status and level of functioning,
- The nature and extent of therapeutic and rehabilitative efforts.

The topography of the specific cortical and subcortical lesions is determined directly by anatomic brain imaging techniques such as CT and MRI. MRI is more sensitive than CT and is the test of choice, if feasible and not contraindicated. Because TBI-related cortical lesions most frequently occur adjacent to bone, the transparency of bone to magnetism gives MRI a substantial advantage over CT. Indirect evidence of brain lesions can be acquired from positron emission tomography, single photon emission computed tomography, electroencephalographic brain mapping, or neuropsychological testing.

The extent of diffuse microscopic brain damage is difficult to assess by imaging procedures. It can be inferred from the duration of LOC, posttraumatic amnesia, posttraumatic confusion, or the severity of the patient's postconcussive symptoms.

The most relevant dimensions of premorbid state are age, IQ, and preexisting neuropsychiatric conditions. The effects of TBI are less devastating to a young person, for example; older patients take longer to recover, even from a mild BI. TBI in an elderly person may unmask or accelerate the development of dementia. The possibility of grossly normal cognitive development despite significant early BI is consistent with theories of "brain plasticity" (28).

High IQ is predictive of good recovery, and low IQ is not (2,29,30). Preexisting psychiatric conditions are almost invariably aggravated by TBI (29), although there are occasional reports of a psychiatric "cure" in patients after TBI (31).

The final determinants of outcome after TBI are therapeutic and rehabilitative efforts. Although there has been continuing skepticism in the medical community about the value of some aspects of TBI rehabilitation (32,33), an attitude of therapeutic nihilism is hardly appropriate. Most people agree that the proper treatment of patients with TBI by professionals who understand the unique requirements of this class of patients has at least some degree of success. Everyone agrees that inappropriate treatment by inexperienced practitioners can have unfortunate consequences. Skepticism about the success of TBI rehabilitation often arises simply because the course of TBI recovery is prolonged and complicated.

Proper treatment for the patient with TBI requires an appreciation of the time required for recovery to occur. Several months may be required for a patient to recover from the postconcussion syndrome. A severely injured patient is capable of functional gains for years after the event, as long as he or she stays healthy and properly engaged (34). That old maxim that 90% of functional recovery after TBI occurs in the first year will always be with us. A healthy brain never stops recovering from BI.

The trajectory of recovery from TBI (4) describes the dynamic thrust of the patient's condition over months and years. It is not a linear process; rather, it is like the process of development and maturation, given to fits and starts. Periods of rapid recovery alternate with plateaux, during which little change may occur. There are times when one should respect a plateau, as if it were a necessary period of stabilization and retrenchment. During such a period, the thrust of rehabilitation should be oriented toward maintenance. If a patient remains, however, on a prolonged plateau, intensive rehabilitation or drug treatment can be directed to move the patient off dead center and to veer the trajectory of recovery back onto the incline.

During the recovery process, it may become clear that some functions are lost completely or are severely impaired and that the damage is irreversible. The orientation of treatment then is directed toward acceptance, compensation, and maintenance. The goal is to maintain the status quo, to make the best of it, and to prevent secondary deterioration.

The trajectory of recovery from TBI can also take a downward turn. Some patients experience secondary deterioration months or years after the injury itself. Delayed deterioration is encountered in other forms of BI, including hypoxic injury and viral encephalitis; the mechanisms are still obscure (see Chapter 8).

HYPOXIC ENCEPHALOPATHY

The common causes of hypoxic injuries to brain are cardiac or respiratory arrest, circulatory collapse, carbon monoxide poisoning, anaphylaxis, suffocation, drowning, anesthesia accidents, and hanging. Like every other form of BI, there is a continuum of severity. Reduced to its simplest formulation, a deficient supply of oxygen to the brain is owing either to the failure of cerebral perfusion (ischemia) or to a reduced amount of circulating arterial oxygen, the result of diminished oxygen saturation or insufficiency of hemoglobin (hypoxia). The most severe cases are sometimes referred to as diffuse anoxic injuries.

Ischemic injury from systemic hypotension leads to focal damage in the border zones between the major cerebral arteries (watershed infarction). Particular brain regions, i.e., parts of the hippocampus and the deep folia of the cerebellum, are most vulnerable to watershed infarction. In severe cases of ischemia or hypoxia, there is first selective damage to cortical tissue, then generalized damage, depending on the basal level of metabolic activity of the particular region. The gray matter of the brain has a higher metabolic rate than the white matter, and hypoxia initially damages the cerebral neurons. The frontal lobes are most vulnerable because of their high metabolism, then the rest of the cerebral cortex, the basal ganglia and deep nuclei, and the cerebellum. Brainstem nuclei are comparatively resistant to anoxic injury.

Some patients who seem to recover from anoxic coma undergo a delayed deterioration in their neurologic state. Delayed postanoxic encephalopathy is predominantly a disorder of the white matter and is characterized by widespread demyelination of the cerebral hemispheres.

When cerebral neurons are deprived of oxygen, there is a remarkable increase of extracellular excitatory neurotransmitters like glutamate and aspartate, which opens calcium channels and leads to a massive calcium influx into the neuron. This unregulated increase in calcium leads to the activation of intracellular enzymes and the consumption of cellular adenosine 5′-triphosphate. The neurons begin to catabolize themselves to maintain activity and in so doing are damaged to a degree that does not permit their survival (35,36) (see Chapter 4).

Outcome

Patients who survive the anoxic episode have a spectrum of outcomes, depending on the severity and duration of the episode. Patients may recover completely, survive with varying degrees of neurologic deficit, or deteriorate further as a result of delayed anoxic encephalopathy.

Even small deviations in the oxygen supply to the brain can result in significant and enduring neurobehavioral sequelae. Damage may even occur when the brain receives physiologically suboptimal levels of oxygen over an extended period of time as a result of congenital heart defects in children, for example, or of chronic obstructive pulmonary disease in adults.

After hypoxic injury, patients can present with subtle symptoms, cognitive slowing, and mild personality changes, similar to frontal lobe patients, or they may be profoundly compromised, with diffuse cognitive and motor impairment. PBIs have the best outcome of all traumatic events, diffuse anoxic injuries the worst prognosis (37,38), and CHIs are in between.

The "continuum of casualty" after diffuse anoxic injury begins with relatively mild executive and memory deficits and includes apperceptive agnosia and visual deficits related to cortical injury and other deficits related to injury to the frontal lobes, hippocampus, and cerebellum. Some typical sequelae of cerebral anoxia include learning impairment, memory deficits, concrete thinking, impaired attention and concentration, and reduced ability to plan, initiate, and carry out mental activities (39). Many patients are described as passive in their general behavior, but generalizations are difficult in this large and diverse group of patients.

Patients with severe hypoxic injuries (diffuse anoxic injury) and patients with delayed postanoxic encephalopathy are severely impaired, with psychomotor slowing, stupor, akinetic mutism, or a persistent vegetative state (40). Basal ganglia symptoms, like rigidity, dystonia, tremor, and bradykinesia are not uncommon.

The cognitive and behavioral deficits that follow hypoxic injury are not necessarily related to the cause of anoxia (40). Survivors of attempted hanging may have persistent anterograde amnesia similar to Korsakoff's syndrome. BI as the result of hanging may be the result of arterial interruption (arterial flow ceases with a 16-kg pull on the noose) or of asphyxiation. Prominent amnestic syndromes have also been reported after cardiac arrest during anesthesia when the patient is intubated and ventilated (pure ischemia) and carbon monoxide poisoning without circulatory collapse (pure hypoxia) (41). Exposure to high altitude without supplemental oxygen can cause residual and lasting deficits in attention, memory, cognitive flexibility, and fine motor skills. In patients with chronic obstructive pulmonary disease, similar deficits have been reported, but verbal ability and memory are relatively spared (42). Subtle neurocognitive deficits have been reported in patients who have undergone coronary artery bypass grafting.

Kriel et al. (43) reported a follow-up study of 25 children who had had anoxic or ischemic BIs at age 2 months to14 years of age. All had been unconscious for at least 24 hours. Eleven children were left in persistent vegetative states, seven were profoundly impaired with little more than a social smile, and seven recovered ambulation but were developmentally impaired. The children who recovered language or ambulation had been in coma less than 60 days. Dystonic rigidity was observed in all the patients who were not ambulatory. Outcome was related to the duration of coma, and the worst outcomes occurred in the near-drowning victims.

Other typical neurologic sequelae of hypoxic injury include choreoathetosis, cerebellar ataxia, myoclonus, and visual agnosia.

Severe anoxic injury to the CNS can have delayed consequences to the extrapyramidal system. Over a span of several months, children can develop postanoxic dystonia, whereas adults are more likely to develop an akinetic-rigid syndrome. It is interesting that this pattern reflects precisely the age-related neurotoxicity of neuroleptic drugs; young patients are more likely to develop dystonia and older patients pseudo-parkinsonism. The postanoxic akinetic-rigid syndrome is more likely to be related to a lesion of the globus pallidus and postanoxic dystonia, a lesion in the putamen (44).

Hysterical symptoms, or bizarre and seemingly nonphysiologic symptoms that are interpreted as hysterical, are sometimes met with in patients who have had hypoxic injuries.

The principles of treatment are the same as they are for other patients with TBI. Symptoms like psychomotor slowing, lack of initiative, abulia, and inattention should be expected to respond to treatment with psychostimulants, amantadine, or the dopamine agonists (45). Sometimes they do, but, in my experience, they work less well in patients with posthypoxia than in patients with TBI.

Carbon Monoxide Encephalopathy

Carbon monoxide (CO) poisoning is a classic example of pure hypoxic injury to brain. CO is a colorless, odorless gas with a much stronger affinity than oxygen for hemoglobin; CO binds to hemoglobin to form carboxyhemoglobin (COHb); as a result, the oxygen-carrying capacity of the blood is drastically reduced. Not only does CO compete successfully with oxygen for hemoglobin binding, but the presence of CO increases the stability of the hemoglobin-O_2 molecule, thus preventing the release of O_2 in the body tissues. (When one of its four heme sites is occupied by a CO molecule, the steric structure of the hemoglobin molecule is changed and the remaining heme sites hold on to their O_2 more tightly.)

The proportion of COHb in the blood is a direct measure of the severity of CO exposure. Normal, healthy human beings living in an environment with the lowest possible levels of CO in the ambient air have levels of 0.5% to 1% COHb. (That is because

CO is a normal catabolic product of the hemoglobin molecule.) Most nonsmoking urban dwellers have COHb levels of 1% to 3%, primarily the result of vehicular emissions, and persons who smoke 20 cigarettes per day have 5% to 6% of hemoglobin saturated with CO. Garage attendants and people who work in tunnels can have a level as high as 15%. At equilibrium, atmospheric CO levels of 50 ppm, 100 ppm, and 200 ppm produce average COHb levels of 8%, 16%, and 30%, respectively. Measurable clinical effects may be noted with exposure for 2 hours to concentrations as low as 100 ppm (46,47) (Table 1.1).

CO is the leading cause of poisoning deaths in the United States, with more than 4,000 casualties annually; unintentional CO poisoning is responsible for approximately one-half of the fatalities (48). It is estimated that 10,000 people seek medical attention for CO intoxication every year. Because CO is a product of incomplete combustion or organic substances, the most common causes of acute and chronic CO poisoning are motor vehicle exhaust fumes, smoke from fires, and fumes from poorly ventilated heating systems. Other sources are the paint stripper methylene chloride and, of course, tobacco smoke.

People are more susceptible to CO poisoning at high altitudes or if they have premorbid cardiovascular or pulmonary disease. Organisms with a high metabolic rate, such as children and household pets, are more vulnerable to CO poisoning. The fetus is particularly vulnerable because fetal hemoglobin has a dissociation curve to the left of adult hemoglobin and binds CO more avidly (49).

CO toxicity results from impaired oxygen delivery and utilization, which leads to cellular hypoxia. Thus, its effects are felt most strongly in tissues with the highest rates of O_2 consumption—the CNS and the myocardium. In the CNS, the histopathologic changes are similar to other causes of hypoxia, to hypoglycemia, heroin overdose, and cyanide poisoning. Acute CO poisoning leads to edema, hemorrhagic focal necrosis, and perivascular infarcts. Bilateral necrosis of the globus pallidus is the characteristic lesion. The substantia nigra, frontal cortex, hippocampus, and cerebellum are particularly vulnerable sites. Delayed anoxic leukoencephalopathy involving the white matter occurs 10 to 40 days after recovery from the acute insult. The white matter is less vulnerable than gray matter to hypoxic injury, so the evolution of delayed leukoencephalopathy suggests that an additional mechanism may be at play.

The signs and symptoms of acute CO poisoning are rather dramatic and not hard to diagnose, although the cherry red color of the mucous membranes that we all learned about in medical school is actually rather uncommon. Subacute or chronic CO poisoning is a more challenging diagnostic problem because patients present to general physicians with relatively nonspecific symptoms like headache, fatigue, dizziness, and mild cognitive impairment. Patients are not likely to suspect that they have a defective furnace or a faulty muffler in the car. One clue to the diagnosis is if their children have similar symptoms.

The clinical outcome of severe poisoning is similar to that of other hypoxic injuries. Approximately 30% of cases of severe poisoning are fatal, 11% have severe neuropsychiatric deficits, and 3% have delayed encephalopathy. At least one-third has enduring problems with memory or attention or personality changes. CO is particularly toxic to the basal ganglia, and extrapyramidal motor deficits after CO poisoning are well known in the literature. A behavioral manifestation of anoxic damage to the basal ganglia is called psychic akinesia, blunting of affect, and loss of

TABLE 1.1. *Carbon monoxide poisoning*

CO in air (%)	Exposure duration	COHb in blood (%)	Symptoms
<0.01%	Indefinite	<10	None
0.01–0.02%	indefinite	10–20	SOB with vigorous exercise, tightness across forehead, headache, cutaneous vasodilatation
0.02–0.03%	5–6 h	20–30	SOB with moderate exercise; throbbing headache
0.04–0.06%	4–5 h	30–40	Severe headache, nausea and vomiting, dim vision, irritability, fatigue, weakness, dizziness, poor judgment; cherry red color
0.07–0.1%	3–4 h	40–50	Syncope, tachycardia, tachypnea headache, confusion
0.11–0.15%	1.5–3 h	50–60	Tachycardia, tachypnea, syncope, coma, convulsions
0.16–0.30%	1–1.5 h	60–70	Coma, convulsions, depressed heart action, respiratory failure
0.50–1.0%	1–2 min	>70	Cardiovascular collapse, death

CO, carbon monoxide; COHb, carboxyhemoglobin; SOB, shortness of breath.

internal motivational drive without motor disturbances or intellectual deterioration. Calcification of the anoxic lesions in the brain may occur very early after CO poisoning (49,50).

The consequences of delayed encephalopathy are quite striking. The development of neuropsychiatric symptoms weeks after an apparent recovery can give rise to diagnostic uncertainty, especially in the context of a medicolegal event, and patients may be thought to be hysterical or worse. In one study of patients who survived severe CO poisoning, only 2% had obvious neuropsychiatric deficits at the time of discharge from hospital. When followed up 3 years later, however, no fewer than 11% had gross neuropsychiatric deficits, 28% had obvious personality change, and 37% had some loss of memory function (51,52). Parkinsonian symptoms are especially prominent in patients with delayed encephalopathy (41,53).

The various symptoms reported in the medical literature are summarized in Table 1.2. Some are readily interpretable in terms of frontal, parietal, hippocampal, or striatal damage. Others, like the hysterical symptoms (e.g., astasia-abasia) are harder to interpret neuroanatomically or physiologically. Patients with hypoxic injuries and electrocution victims, are more prone to bizarre and seemingly hysterical symptoms than any other group of patients with BI (50,51,54–57).

In contrast to the acute symptoms of CO poisoning, the development of persistent neuropsychiatric problems has not been correlated, either clinically or in animal experiments, with the amount or length of exposure to CO or to the COHb level. There remains a strong need for an objective measurement that can predict the severity of outcome after CO poisoning; to date, there is none. What is clear is that hypoxia alone is insufficient to predict the severity of outcome, especially with respect to delayed leukoencephalopathy. It has been suggested that CO may exercise an independent toxic effect on the CNS or, alternatively, an indirect effect by depressing myocardial function (58). It is possible that single photon emission computed tomography can detect early changes in the white matter that will presage delayed encephalopathy and poor outcome (59).

The significance of this problem is amplified by the problem of subacute or chronic low level CO exposure. Agencies concerned with occupational health have set minimum permissible levels of CO exposure, at one time 100 ppm and now even lower. There have been reports of workers exposed chronically to low levels of CO who have reported subjective symptoms such as headache, dizziness, and memory impairment. There have even been reports of subtle neuropsychological deficits (60,61). On the other hand, controlled studies have not confirmed these reports; it should be remembered that heavy cigarette smoking can generate rather high levels of COHb, with no indication of neurocognitive deficit resulting from it (62).

TABLE 1.2. *Neuropsychiatric consequences of CO intoxication*

Amnesia
Akinetic Mutism
Apathy, Indifference
Aphasia
Apraxia
Bradykinesia
Choreoathetosis
Depression and Emotional Incontinence
Dysgraphia, Dysnomia, Dyscalculia
Executive Deficits
Inattention
Irritability, Aggression
Manic-Depressive Psychosis
Manipulative and Hysterical Behavior
Parkinsonian Symptoms
Peripheral Neuritis
Perseverative Speech
Personality Change
Sleep Disturbance
Visual Agnosia

Hypoglycemic Encephalopathy

The brain and the heart are the only two organs that undergo severe functional and structural damage under conditions of hypoglycemia. Hypoglycemia reduces O_2 uptake and reduces cerebral blood flow. Like hypoxic damage, it can provoke an excitotoxic response and permanent injury to neurons (36).

Hypoglycemic injury appears to be a more serious problem for children compared with adults, but not for neonates who are relatively spared, perhaps because of the diminished metabolic requirements of the neonatal brain. Although hypoglycemia occurs frequently in association with hypoxic ischemic injury at term, no additional increment of histopathologic change occurs in babies who are hypoglycemic beyond what occurs simply as a result of hypoxia (63). In children, however, hypoglycemic injury can have enduring effects. In the recent past, aggressive glycemic control among pediatric diabetologists was practiced, a therapeutic stance that soon abated after significant neurocognitive deficits were demonstrated to occur in the children. Specific deficits have been demonstrated in memory, attention, motor speed, and visuospatial ability (64,65). Children with hypoglycemic BI have been found to be impulsive, socially inappropriate, and hyperphagic.

Diffuse encephalopathy can follow hypoglycemic shock, for example, from hyperinsulinism. The condition was especially amenable to study two generations ago, when psychiatrists used insulin shock to treat refractory psychosis. The encephalopathy causes varying degrees of dementia. As a rule, the phylogenetically newer regions of brain are most likely to be affected, and diffuse neuronal degeneration is seen in the frontal, parietal, and occipital cortices, especially in the most superficial layers, to a lesser degree in the basal ganglia, and still less in the lower brainstem (66).

Diabetes mellitus is associated with encephalopathic and neuropathic events including an increased risk of stroke and dementia in adults with diabetes. These events are related to the vascular complications of the disease. Mild neuropsychological deficits are found in adults and children with diabetes, and these have been attributed to the same mechanism that causes peripheral neuropathy, but, in fact, they are probably related to the occurrence of severe hypoglycemic episodes (67,68). Conversely, neurodevelopmental delays in children born to mothers with diabetes do not seem to be related to the degree of glycemic control but to some other mechanism (69).

ORGANIC SOLVENTS

Organic solvents have a special affinity for lipid-rich tissue, especially the brain. They are able to penetrate the CNS quite easily, and the acute behavioral effects are rapid in onset and readily detectable. Prolonged exposure to low levels of organic solvents can have subtle effects that may go undetected or may be misdiagnosed as psychiatric disorders. Exposure is by inhalation or skin contact. Solvent exposure is most often work related, but recreational exposure is not uncommon (70,71).

The extent of CNS damage owing to solvent exposure and its functional reversibility depends on the solvent in question, the dose, and duration of exposure. Pathologic events from solvent poisoning include diffuse demyelination, as would be expected from exposure to a highly lipophilic toxin, and diffuse cortical atrophy. Dynamic imaging studies indicate diffuse cortical damage.

Acute solvent intoxication causes severe effects, such as seizures, toxic psychosis, LOC, ataxia, parkinsonism, and optic neuropathy, but termination of exposure often results in rapid and complete recovery. Chronic exposure, however, can lead to deficits that are different from the effects of acute intoxication and persistent if not irreversible and can lead to continued deterioration even after cessation of exposure. In Sweden, where much relevant research has been done, it is generally accepted that 10 years of exposure to painting with solvent-based paints is sufficient to cause lasting damage (72). The incidence of presenile dementia is high in painters.

Disruptions of memory, attention, and visuospatial skills are the most common neuropsychological sequelae of toxic exposure. Symptoms of mild exposure, such as fatigue, somnolence, impaired concentration, and loss of initiative, are usually reversible. The more advanced symptoms, e.g., personality changes, instability of mood, and subtle neurologic signs, may signal the development of an irreversible process (71). Severe exposure can lead to intellectual deterioration and frank dementia. Frontal/executive impairments have been reported, not surprisingly because they are the least overlearned of all cortical activities, are complex, and involve the integration of numerous complex functional systems. Diffuse damage, therefore, should be expected to affect them first and foremost (72,73).

That solvent exposure can cause severe psychiatric symptoms has been known since the nineteenth century (74). Various psychiatric symptoms have been reported: decreased or increased anxiety, emotional lability, neuroticism, fatigue, somatic complaints, mania, paranoia, and psychosis (72,74).

That chronic exposure to low levels of organic solvents leads to persistent neuropsychiatric abnormalities is widely (but not universally) accepted, especially in the Scandinavian countries, where the chronic painter's syndrome was first described (75). The problems included general intellectual decline, attention and memory impairment, motor incoordination, depression, anxiety, and personality change (71, 75–77).

The cognitive and neurobehavioral consequences of solvent exposure are difficult to summarize, except in the most general terms, because the toxins do not share the same physical or chemical characteristics and exposure often involves exposure to several different chemicals. Neuronal loci, specific damage, cells attacked, and physiologic consequences vary across toxins. Candidate mechanisms include neuronal damage from prolonged depolarization when toxins act as false neurotransmitters, disruption of normal anabolism, axonal breakdown, myelin loss, and damage to the neural vasculature resulting in vascular leakage (72). Solvent effects have been demonstrated in cortical and subcortical regions. Single photon emission computed tomography studies indicate that the temporal and frontal lobes, basal ganglia, and thalamus are the most vulnerable areas (71). Olfactory disturbance has been described with long-term exposure to industrial solvents (78).

Occupational exposure to organic solvents during pregnancy is associated with an increased risk of major fetal malformations (79). More remarkable, however, is recreational solvent inhalation by pregnant women, of which there are more than 100 cases reported in the medical literature. Many of the children were small at birth, with craniofacial abnormalities not unlike those seen in children with fetal alcohol syndrome. Residual cognitive, speech, and motor deficits have been described in these children. Animal studies also indicate low birth weight, skeletal abnormalities, and developmental delay (80).

Recreational use of solvents is usually confined to young adolescents, many of whom have emotional problems or learning disabilities before they ever get into "huffing." Solvent exposure can aggravate the hepatotoxicity of concurrent medications, such as retinoic acid, antidepressants, and anticonvulsants. Drunken behavior, listlessness, anorexia, and moodiness are symptoms of volatile substance abuse, and high doses can lead to convulsions and death. Chronic abuse of organic solvents can produce severe organ damage, especially to the liver, kidney, and brain. The neuropsychiatric sequelae are not insignificant, although it is not easy to disentangle the specific effects of solvents from the effects of other drugs that may also be consumed or of the child's premorbid state (81–83).

ELECTRICAL INJURY

Electrical injuries have widespread manifestations involving almost all the organ systems. Of all the tissues, nerve is most susceptible (84). Electrical actions that are capable of injuring humans are differentiated into atmospheric (i.e., lightning), technical (i.e., household and industrial), and biologic electricity (i.e., electric fish). The actions of electromagnetic radiation represent an entirely different form of injury with a different pattern of possible outcomes.

Epidemiology

Electrocution deaths claim as many as 700 lives annually in the United States—1% to 2% of all accidental deaths (85). Accidental electrocution occurs more frequently at the job site than in other situations, and high-voltage electricity is responsible for most deaths. Issues over workers' compensation often aggravate the already complicated problem of neuropsychiatric diagnosis after electrical injury.

Lightning accidents account for only approximately 150 deaths in the United States each year, but among natural disasters, only floods cause more deaths (86). Florida and the Gulf states have the most lightning fatalities, followed by Colorado and the Rocky Mountain states (87).

Neuropathology

Physical Characteristics

Ohm's law (amperes = volts/ohms) describes the essential physical characteristics of electricity, in which amperes represent current flow, volts measure the force of the current (tension), and ohms reflect the resistance of the object to the passage of the current. Voltage is typically a fixed entity, ranging from the low household standard of 110 V to industrial high voltage lines of 12,000 V. In contrast, resistance is highly variable, measuring 100,000 Ω for dry skin but decreasing to 1,000 Ω for wet skin. The higher the voltage and the lower the resistance, the more current will flow into a person's body. The injury sustained is directly related to amperage (85). Current flow of 0.0001 A causes a barely perceptible tingle, whereas 0.016 A is the "let go" threshold (for alternating current), and 0.100 A is sufficient to cause ventricular fibrillation (85).

The amount of current flow, exposure time, and skin resistance are all important in determining the lethality of an electrical event. To determine whether the patient dies or survives, with or without permanent neurologic sequelae, the essential element is whether the brain or spinal cord lies within the current pathway (86).

Biologic Characteristics

The neuropathology of electrical injury arises from four elements: thermal injury (similar to heat stroke and malignant hyperthermia), anoxic injury (from cardiac arrest or arrhythmia), and direct electrolytic injury. The fourth traumatic element arises from the possibility of TBI if the patient falls from a high place, is thrown by the force of the electrical impact, or is struck by a falling object. In cases of lightning injury, it is particularly difficult to distinguish between the effects of electrodynamic, electrothermic, and electromechanical damage (88).

As current (amperage) passes through high-resistance tissues, electrical energy is converted to heat, producing coagulative necrosis of muscle, nerve, and skin and causing thrombosis of blood vessels (84). The neuropathologic findings in electrical and lightning injuries were first described by MacDonald Critchley in 1934 (86):

- Focal petechial hemorrhages in the brain, especially the medulla, and in the anterior horn cell gray matter when the spinal cord is involved,
- Patchy chromatolysis of pyramidal cells, neurons in the medulla, anterior horn cells, and Purkinje cells of the cerebellum,
- Wide dilation of the perivascular spaces,
- Fragmentation and tortuosity of peripheral nerve axons with myelin breakdown,
- Spiral-like deformities of muscle fibers,
- Softening and edema of brain and parts of the spinal cord.

The effects of lightning on the peripheral nervous system are less well understood, although Critchley described striking myelin ballooning, and there have been individual case reports of mononeuropathies and polyneuropathies after lightning strike (86). The cerebellum can be selectively affected in patients struck by lightning, just as cerebellar degeneration is often found after heat stroke, suggesting that cerebellum may be selectively vulnerable to thermal injury (89). Basal ganglia hemorrhage is the most common brain imaging finding that can be attributed to a lightning strike (90).

Electrical burns are seen only in one-half of low-voltage electrical deaths (91), and even high-voltage deaths are not necessarily associated with external signs. This is particularly true if the area of contact is large (e.g., the flat of the hand) or when contact is made via wet clothing (88).

There is no evidence that electroconvulsive therapy results in structural BI from electrolytic damage (the current is not very strong), thermal damage (negligible), disruption of the blood-brain barrier (does not occur), or the seizure itself. Several well-controlled studies have demonstrated that neuronal loss occurs only after 1.5 to 2.0 hours of continuous seizure activity in primates, and adequate muscle paralysis and oxygenation diminish the effect significantly (92).

Clinical Findings

Atmospheric Electricity

The Empire State Building is one of those places that gets hit by lightning all the time. Measurements of lightning made on the Empire State Building indicate a maximum current strength as high as 220,000 A. Lightning strikes that have been survived must necessarily have involved appreciably smaller amounts of current in small collateral or branch discharges.

Lightning may also lead to a stride potential in which electricity courses through the ground and enters the body from below (88). A direct lightning strike to the head represents a catastrophic event, and death is the result of electrothermal and electromechanical injury. The spectrum of neurologic lesions associated with lightning includes the entire neuraxis from the cerebral hemispheres to the peripheral nerves (87).

Cherington et al. (87) classified the clinical sequelae of lightning injury to the CNS as (i) immediate and transient, (ii) immediate and prolonged or permanent, and (iii) delayed and progressive.

Lightning injury is much more likely to cause LOC than technical electricity, and some degree of clouding of consciousness almost always occurs. Lightning paralysis is pathognomonic. Typical sequelae of lightning injury include mental state changes, transient sensory and motor disturbances of single or multiple limbs, autonomic dysfunction such as hypertension, and then psychological and psychiatric reactions. The latter are quite diverse, and their presentation is said to be determined by predisposing factors in the victim (88). The immediate features tend to be transient.

LOC occurs in 72% of lightning victims (87). Retrograde amnesia is also common but does not always occur. Patients often retain some memory of events immediately preceding and even during the strike. The memory of such an extraordinary event, with paralysis, sensory peculiarities, burning skin and clothes, may provoke a rather malignant form of posttraumatic stress disorder.

The sensory and motor derangements clear after a few hours, as a rule, although paresthesias can persist and vasomotor disorders such as cyanosis and edema can ensue. Damage to the auditory apparatus is not uncommon. Mental state changes can persist or can develop over days or weeks after the injury. These include mental dullness, a sense of oppression, disorientation, slowing of reaction times, withdrawal, and negativism. Rarely, agitation, delirium, and frank psychosis may develop. Other symptoms described in the literature are restlessness, anxiety, misidentification, emotional lability, fluctuating consciousness, pain, and ataxia (88).

Permanent neurologic sequelae to lightning injury are polysymptomatic. A striatal syndrome may occur with bradykinesia, hypokinesia, lack of initiative, tremor, chorea, athetosis, and rigidity. The symptoms may begin as late as 6 months after injury. Hemiparesis, aphasia, and dementia have been described after lightning injuries but not seizures. Psychiatric sequelae include paranoid psychosis and mania (88). Deafness, ataxia, muscle wasting, and abnormal reflexes are sometimes seen.

The delayed features, such as myelopathy, parkinsonism, and motor system disease, tend to be progressive and persistent (89). The latency between trauma and the delayed clinical manifestation can be as long as 10 years. The association is putative, and some authors have maintained that it is illusory. Others have speculated on possible mechanisms, including structural changes to proteins and other macromolecules, to cell membranes, or to blood vessels (87).

Lightning injury may be mediated by a telephone line. Ninety percent of such patients have transient symptoms lasting a week or so (40%) or approximately 3 months (50%). The remaining 10% are said to have persistent symptoms that last for months or years (93), but this is doubtful. A telephone line can carry only so much power.

Surviving a lightning strike has been associated, in popular lore, with a number of positive outcomes, including cures from serious handicaps or illnesses, increased sexuality, improved intelligence, and psychic powers (94). St. Paul may have been struck by lightning on the road to Damascus (95) and seemed to have made a turn for the better as a result.

Technical Electricity

A few special features complicate the diagnosis of cerebral dysfunction after technical electric injury. LOC or amnesia does not necessarily occur. Burns may not be evident. Cerebral symptoms can develop even if the brain was not an obvious part of the electrical pathway. Neurologic disorders can develop that are quite different from the initial sequelae, and these, as with lightning injuries, are quite diverse: striatal and thalamic syndromes, cortical encephalopathy, and brainstem dysfunction. Psychological symptoms and neurologic complications, especially those involving the spinal cord, can develop after a latency period of weeks or months (96). Even the cardiovascular complications of electrical injury can be atypical, delayed in onset, or obscured by other trauma (97).

The largest studies of neurologic sequelae to electrical injury are retrospective and involve patients admitted to the hospital for electrical burns. In one study of 64 patients, CNS complications occurred in 13%, including seizures, obtundation, blindness, quadriparesis, and peripheral neuropathies (98). In a review of 28 patients, 29% sustained peripheral nerve injury (99). In a review of 85 patients, 34 had neurologic damage, and the onset of symptoms tended to be delayed (100). In a review of 90 electrocution cases, 11 of 22 patients who had had low-voltage injuries (Long-term follow-up of 16 electrical injury patients by Hooshmand et al. (106) indicated a stereotyped clinical picture comprising LOC at the time of injury, followed by late complications of depression, seizures, dizziness, and tinnitus. Others have questioned the association of electrical injury with posttraumatic epilepsy, however (88). It has been said that the emotional reactions of some patients resemble conversion reactions (106).

Electricity victims can present, after months or years, with a clinical picture that is primarily subjective: total disability from work and a dramatic change in personality in the absence of overt neurologic abnormalities; vague physical symptoms such as pain, fatigue, tinnitus, and paresthesias; and depression, negativism, and withdrawal alternating with emotional instability, anxiety, angry outbursts, and even paranoia. The neuropsychological findings are nonspecific, similar to postconcussive changes. The original injury may have been associated with relatively low tension, no LOC or amnesia, and a normal examination immediately after the accident. No external burns have ever been apparent, and the course of the electrical current was hand-to-hand or hand to foot. The difficulty arises when such a patient presents in the context of an adversarial proceeding. It may be hard, if not impossible, to say for sure that these problems were or were not caused by electrical trauma. The usual method for evaluating the veracity of a TBI claim may not be relevant here. Even hysterical symptoms or "faking bad" may be symptoms of a bona fide injury, to a degree that is seen, in my opinion, in no other neuropathic condition. In such cases, one may have to base one's diagnosis on the nature and intensity of the electrical event.

Reflex Sympathetic Dystrophy

Although the published literature is largely comprised of case reports, it is believed that reflex sympathetic dystrophy is the most common autonomic disorder after electrical injuries (96). It also occurs in association with other types of injury, such as TBI and various kinds of spinal shock (e.g., cervical whiplash). It may involve severe pain and disability and may be longstanding and difficult to treat. It may also be progressive.

Reflex sympathetic dystrophy is a complex of symptoms causing pain, edema, hyperemia, hyperesthesia, hyperhidrosis, skin atrophy, and limitation in the range of motor movements. It can be caused by physical trauma, even trivial injury, and the severity of the symptoms may be entirely out of proportion to the severity of the injury. Psychological or emotional factors may aggravate the symptom picture.

Reflex sympathetic dystrophy comprises three spontaneous stages:

- The acute stage lasts several weeks and is characterized by burning pain with hyperpathia, allodynia, and hyperalgesia. The skin may be warm and red, then later cold and cyanotic. There are excessive sweating and swelling.
- The dystrophic stage begins after 3 to 6 months, with the spread of swelling and edema and trophic changes, including muscle atrophy, hair and nail loss, joint contracture, and osteoporosis.
- The atrophic stage begins after 6 to 12 months, when the skin is cool, pale and cyanotic, smooth or glossy, pain and hyperpathia increase, and there is diffuse joint stiffness. The changes may be permanent and disabling (107).

Reflex sympathetic dystrophy is presumably related to an abnormal reflex mediated by the sympathetic nervous system. The syndrome becomes noticeable a few weeks after the accident. It may be more prominent after low-voltage injuries because it may be the only residual disorder. Treatment is difficult and the prognosis is uncertain. Treatment begins with nonsteroidal anti-inflammatory drugs but then may proceed to anticonvulsants, antidepressants, or corticosteroids. Sympatholytics and calcium channel blockers have been used. Transcutaneous electrical nerve stimulation (TENS) and physical therapy have been suggested but not splinting or casting (107). Successful treatment has also been described with hydroxyl radical scavengers and intravenous regional guanethidine blockade (96). More recently, gabapentin and mecamylamine have been used with some success.

Electric Fish

The electric ray, or torpedo fish, lives in temperate and tropical waters. Divers commonly encounter them because they reside in shallow depths and are often hidden on the bottom by mud or sand.

The electrical discharge of the torpedo fish ranges from 8 to 220 V, and the ray can deliver a succession of discharges, albeit of diminishing intensity. One has to touch the fish to get a shock.

The electrical discharge may stun or paralyze a person, but the real danger is drowning or aspiration. In the absence of those catastrophic outcomes, recovery is uneventful (108). The therapeutic value of electric fish is discussed in Chapter 24.

Treatment

Patients with electrical injury are as frustrating to treat as they are to diagnose. They often come to clinical attention after countless evaluations, expert opinions that are wildly disparate, psychiatric symptoms far more prominent than neurologic symptoms, and clear indications of hysterical symptoms, exaggeration, and hostility. Quite naturally, the patient's latent paranoia has not been alleviated by the inconsistency of prior recommendations, especially if he or she has had to contend with an adversarial approach to compensation. Many lightning victims are so socially isolated that they are completely misanthropic. They are not easily reassured, and a therapeutic alliance is not easy to build.

Psychopharmacology tends to be complicated. Many of them need a mood-stabilizing drug and/or antidepressant, something for sleep (e.g., trazodone) or for nightmares (e.g., clonidine), something for flashbacks or anxiety attacks (e.g., clonazepam), and something for headache or chest pain (usually more than a nonsteroidal anti-inflammatory drug). Stimulants may help attention and memory problems, but the stimulant response is not nearly so gratifying as it is in other classes of brain trauma. Patients with electrical injury are often treated with multiple medications, and the result may still be imperfect.

PFIESTERIA

In addition to the electric fish previously mentioned, there is *Pfiesteria piscicida*, a dinoflagellate that lives in the estuarine waters of the western Atlantic and Gulf coasts. It is cause for concern in our part of the world because it has killed billions of fish in the Neuse River, the Pamlico Sound, and the Chesapeake Bay (109) and because it has the potential to cause a toxic encephalopathy in humans. *Pfiesteria* has at least two dozen life forms, the most toxic of which is a small, vegetative, flagellated form that produces large amounts of exotoxin in the presence of living fish (110). Toxic zoospores of *P. piscicida* subdue fish by releasing lethal neurotoxins that narcotize the prey, disrupt its osmoregulatory system, and attack its nervous system (111).

Mammalian tissue is an alternative prey for this singularly nasty protozoan, and numerous people have developed symptoms after contact with water, aerosols, or water droplets containing toxins from *P. piscicida*. Human exposure has been associated with bronchospasm, skin rash, severe stomach cramping with nausea and vomiting, secretory diarrhea, and conjunctivitis. The effects of acute exposure include autonomic dysfunction (diaphoresis and cardioarrhythmias), CNS effects (headache, narcosis, confusion, personality change with rage attacks, memory impairment, inattention, and fatigue), and sensory symptoms (tingling and numbness in the lips, hands, and feet) (109). The clinical symptoms usually resolve within days or weeks, although chronic asthma-like symptoms, fatigue, and sensory symptoms can persist for months or years (112). Rats injected with *Pfiesteria* develop persistent learning impairment (113).

There was a study of 24 people exposed to affected waters or to fish with lesions, who reported experiencing headache, confusion, forgetfulness, burning skin, and skin lesions. Significant neuropsychological deficits were detected on standardized tests. The skin lesions cleared rapidly, but the cognitive problems persisted, returning to baseline only after several months had passed. More serious and seemingly permanent cognitive deficits have been reported anecdotally and have been documented in two of our patients who were exposed to *Pfiesteria* toxin in the laboratory for extended periods (114).

Other toxins that are generated by fish parasites (e.g., ciguatoxin, domoic acid) may cause persistent neurologic symptoms similar to those of *Pfiesteria* human illness syndrome (110). Generally, CNS icthyotoxicity is mild and self-limited, although ciguatera fish poisoning (from finfish consumption) and domoic acid intoxication (from shellfish) can produce severe, permanent neuropathology (115–117). The clinical dimensions of the problem are small thus far. If, however, estuarine "blooms" of toxic microorganisms arise from an imbalance in the coastal ecology, as may have occurred in Bengal in 1972 and more recently in Baja, we may see more of this. There are no reports of *Pfiesteria* human illness from eating fish, but that is not true of ciguatera or domoic acid.

ELECTROMAGNETIC RADIATION

A series of epidemiologic investigations since 1979 have suggested that exposure to low-frequency electromagnetic fields (EMFs) is associated with a small increase in the occurrence of cancers (lymphoma, leukemia, brain tumors). In adults, exposure is usually related to occupational exposure and in children to domestic EMF exposures. The evidence is strongest for brain and CNS cancers (118). The association is entirely phenomenal, divorced from a clear hypothesis of molecular damage and cellular EMF transduction mechanisms, although several biochemical effects have been attributed to EMFs in laboratory preparations. The observations, however, are preliminary. Although the epidemiologic studies have gained attention, the purported mechanisms have failed to galvanize scientific opinion (119).

The idea that magnetic flux is capable of exercising constitutional effects and inducing neuropsychiatric disorders is an old one. The converse, magnetic healing, is even older. It achieved prominence in nineteenth-century medicine or, at least, in the alternative medicine of the time, but before very long, animal magnetism and magnetic clothing were abandoned as quackery. Research at Edison's laboratories proved that EMFs of enormous intensity had no physiologic effects. As a result, the electrification of the industrial world during the twentieth century was attended by a long period of medical silence, for better or worse, concerning the health effects of EMFs (119).

Now the world is glowing with electromagnetic energy emissions at most frequencies of the nonionizing portion of the spectrum, from power lines, radio waves, microwaves, household wiring, appliances, and cell phones. The suggestion, therefore, of a possible association between EMFs and cancer has at last led biologists to reflect whether biologic organisms, having evolved in an environment with a much lower level of background EMFs, are suitably equipped to adapt to this new ambiance (120).

The EMFs generated by power distribution and transmission lines, household wiring, and associated appliances have a power frequency of 60 Hz. The energy that is carried by photons of 60-Hz electromagnetic radiation is too meager to break chemical bonds, as x-rays do, or even to heat up things that lie in their path, as microwaves do. The search for a biologic transducer of the electromagnetic force has discovered that low-frequency EMFs are capable of inducing weak electric fields within the body. The recent discovery of intracellular crystals of magnetite (Fe304) in the human brain, if confirmed, may indicate another mechanism of interaction. In any event, the biologic outcome could involve influences on cell-cell signaling, membrane effects, protein expression patterns, calcium homeostasis, inflammatory and immune system function, and DNA synthesis (119,120).

In the CNS, it has been proposed that EMF might influence the integrity of the blood-brain barrier (121) or cause disturbance in the circadian responsiveness of the pineal gland, a magnetosensitive organ (122,123). One study suggested that nocturnal secretion of melatonin from the pineal gland was reduced in humans and in experimental animals by exposure to EMFs (124).

If the association between EMFs and cancer is still controversial, the association between EMFs and neuropsychiatric disorders is totally speculative. However, it has been suggested that EMF exposure may be associated with depression, fatigue, irritability, headache, hyposexuality, disruption of normal sleep/wake patterns, and reduced performance and reaction time (125,126). It is even conceivable that these behavioral events are attributable to something like a low melatonin syndrome. Experimental studies in humans and in animals have indicated that the performance decrements may be real (127,128), although their mediation by melatonin or the pineal gland is unproven. It has been proposed that opioid and dopaminergic systems mediate the effects of EMF exposure on the brain (129,130).

Recent studies have failed to support an association between cell-phone use or occupational radiofrequency exposure and brain tumors or other malignancies, although the possibility of an association has not been completely rejected (131,132).

So-called environmental illness appears to have different manifestations in different countries. In the United States, people seem to be afflicted with multiple chemical sensitivity, whereas in Sweden, it is hypersensitivity to electricity. Victims of this purported malady are said to be "electrosensitive" (133).

RADIATION NECROSIS

Acute radiation injury to the brain occurring during radiotherapy is attributed to the effects of local edema and is usually transient. Delayed cerebral radiation necrosis, the major hazard of therapeutic doses of radiation, is a catastrophic event. The onset of neurologic symptoms can be months or years after exposure. The illness typically runs a stepwise course, with fits and stroke-like episodes occurring against a background of progressive dementia and somnolence. Death occurs after a few years, or the patients can linger on in a severely debilitated state (134).

The symptoms are dependent on the area and volume of brain irradiated. Clinically, radiation necrosis is manifested as a space-occupying lesion, which leads to diagnostic confusion with recurrent tumor or an inflammatory process. Brain biopsy or positron emission tomography may be necessary to make the diagnosis (135). Cortical atrophy and diffuse white matter injury are seen in the later stages. The prior use of chemotherapeutic agents can aggravate the severity of radiation necrosis (136). Neurocognitive deficits may be apparent, especially in children, after radiation doses that are relatively low and that do not cause overt white matter injury (136).

The lesions are thought to result from endothelial injury. Irradiation of the CNS leads to disruption of the tight junctions of the blood-brain barrier. Discrete leakage occurs within 2 weeks after irradiation and may have transient or reversible effects. At 6 months, the results of delayed injury indicate diffuse leakage from the vasculature, severe loss of the capillary network, cortical atrophy, and white matter necrosis (137). The parenchyma shows diffuse infiltration with T cells and activated macrophages that express cytokines (138). It is possible that delayed cerebral radiation necrosis is caused by the same kind of inflammatory reaction that is related to delayed-onset problems after TBI (Chapter 8).

Radiation necrosis can produce symptomatic deficits remote from the original lesion, possibly from changes in the vascular epithelium in the field of the beam (135).

Chemotherapeutic agents for the treatment of cancer are not infrequently associated with neurotoxicity, including seizures, ototoxicity, learning deficits, peripheral neuropathy, Lhermitte's sign, autonomic neuropathy, retrobulbar neuritis, and cerebral herniation (139–141).

REFERENCES

1. Goldstein M. Traumatic brain injury: a silent epidemic. *Ann Neurol* 1990;27:327.
2. Kraus JF. Epidemiology of head injury. In: Cooper PR, ed. *Head injury*, 2nd ed. Baltimore: Williams & Wilkins, 1987:1–19.
3. Marshall LF, Marshall SB. Current clinical head injury research in the United States. In: Becker D, Polishock J, eds. *CNS trauma status report, 1985*. Bethesda, MD: NINCDS, 1985:45–51.
4. Gualtieri CT. The neuropharmacology of inadvertent drug effects in patients with traumatic brain injuries. *J Head Trauma Rehabil* 1990;5:32–40.
5. Jennett B, Teasdale G. *Management of head injuries*. Philadelphia: FA Davis, 1981.
6. Levine MJ, Gueramy M, Friedrich D. Psychophysiological responses to closed head injury. *Brain Inj* 1987; 1:171–181.
7. Bourke RS. *Head injury*. Bethesda, MD: NINCDS, 1988.
8. Masdeu JC, Wolfson L, Lantos G, et al. Brain white-matter changes in the elderly prone to falling. *Arch Neurol* 1989;46:1292–1296.
9. Annegers JF, Grabow JD, Groover RD, et al. Seizures after head trauma: a population study. *Neurology* 1980;30:683–689.

10. Carlsson GS. Long-term effects of head injuries sustained during life in three male populations. *J Neurosurg* 1987;67:197–205.
11. Sparadeo FR, Strauss D, Barth JT. The incidence, impact and treatment of substance abuse in head trauma rehabilitation. *J Head Trauma Rehabil* 1990;5:1–8.
12. Sparadeo F, Gill D. Effects of prior alcohol use on head injury recovery. *J Head Trauma Rehabil* 1989;4: 75–82.
13. Brismar B, Engstrom A, Rydberg U. Head injury and intoxication: a diagnostic and therapeutic dilemma. *Acta Chir Scand* 1982;149:11–14.
14. Rimcl RW, Giordani B, Barth JT, et al. Moderate head injury: completing the clinical spectrum of brain trauma. *Neurosurgery* 1982;11:344–351.
15. Edna T. Alcohol influence and head injury. *Acta Chir Scand* 1982;148:209–212.
16. Brooks N, Symington C, Beattie A, et al. Alcohol and other predictors of cognitive recovery after severe head injury. *Brain Inj* 1989;3:235–246.
17. Ruff RM, Marshall LF, Klauber MR, et al. Alcohol abuse and neurological outcome of the severely head injured. *J Head Trauma Rehabil* 1990;5:21–31.
18. Parsons O. Do neuropsychological deficits predict alcoholics' treatment course and posttreatment recovery? In: Parsons O, Butters N, Nathan P, eds. *Neuropsychology of alcoholism: implications for diagnosis and treatment.* New York: Guilford, 1987, 132–145.
19. Greer BG. Substance abuse among people with disabilities: a problem of too much accessibility. *J Disabil* 1986;14:34–38.
20. Hackler E, Tobis JS. Re-integration into the community. In: Rosenthal MT, Griffith E, Bond M, et al., eds. *Rehabilitation of the head injured adult.* Philadelphia: FA Davis, 1983, 421–434.
21. Oddy M, Coughlan T, Tyerman A. Social adjustment after closed head injury: a further follow-up seven years after injury. *J Neurol Neurosurg Psychiatry* 1985; 48:564–568.
22. Silver JM, Yodofsky SC, Hales RE. Depression in traumatic brain injury. *Neuropsychiatry Neuropsychol Behav Neurol* 1991;4:12–23.
23. Levin HS, Amparo E, Eisenberg HM, et al. Magnetic resonance imaging and computerized tomography in relation to the neurobehavioral sequelae of mild and moderate head injury. *J Neurosurg* 1987;66:706–713.
24. Gennarelli TA, Thibault LE, Adams JH, et al. Diffuse axonal injury and traumatic coma in the primate. *Ann Neurol* 1982;12:564–575.
25. Barth JT, Macciochi SN, Giordani B, et al. Neuropsychological sequelae of minor head injury. *Neurosurgery* 1983;13:529–533.
26. Yarnell PR, Rossie GV. Minor whiplash head injury with major debilitation. *Brain Inj* 1988;2:255–258.
27. Levin HS, Eisenberg HM, Benton AL. *Mild head injury.* New York: Oxford University Press, 1989.
28. Lenneberg E. *Biological foundations of language.* New York: Wiley, 1967.
29. Alves W, Macciocchi SN, Barth JT. Postconcussive symptoms after mild head injury. *J Head Trauma Rehabil* 1993;8:48–59.
30. Levin HS. Neurobehavioral sequelae of head injury. In: Cooper PR, ed. *Head injury*, 2nd ed. Baltimore: Williams & Wilkins, 1987:442–463.
31. Lewis SW, Harvey I, Ron M, et al. Can brain damage protect against schizophrenia? A case report of twins. *Br J Psychiatry* 1990;157:600–603.
32. Berrol S. Issues in cognitive rehabilitation. *Arch Neurol* 1990;47:219–220.
33. Volpe BT, McDowell FH. The efficacy of cognitive rehabilitation in patients with traumatic brain injury. *Arch Neurol* 1990;47:220–222.
34. Gualtieri CT, Nygard NK. Rehabilitation for head injury, five years after the event. *Rebound Q Res Rep* 1988;1:16–26.
35. Abe K, Aoki M, Kawagoe J, et al. Ischemic delayed neuronal death: a mitochondrial hypothesis. *Stroke* 1995;26:1478–1489.
36. Viola J, Ditzler T, Batzer W, et al. Pharmacological management of post-traumatic stress disorder: clinical summary of a five-year retrospective study, 1990–1995. *Mil Med* 1997;162:616–619.
37. Groswasser Z, Cohen M, Costeff H. Rehabilitation outcome after anoxic brain damage. *Arch Phys Med Rehabil* 1989;70:186–188.
38. Heindl UT, Laub MC. Outcome of persistent vegetative state following hypoxic or traumatic brain injury in children and adolescents. *Neuropediatrics* 1996;27:94–100.
39. Roine RO, Kajaste S, Kaste M. Neuropsychological sequelae of cardiac arrest. *JAMA* 1993;269:237–242.
40. Wilson BA. Cognitive functioning of adult survivors of cerebral hypoxia. *Brain Inj* 1996;10:863–874.
41. Medalia AA, Merriam AE, Ehrenreich JH. The neuropsychological sequelae of attempted hanging. *Neurol Neurosurg Psychiatry* 1991;54:546–548.
42. Rourke SB, Adams KM. The neuropsychological correlates of acute and chronic hypoxemia. In: Grant I, Adams KM, eds. *Neuropsychological assessment of neuropsychiatric disorders.* New York: Oxford University Press, 1996:379–402.
43. Kriel RI, Krach LE, Luxenberg MG, et al. Outcome of severe anoxic/ischemic brain injury in children. *Pediatr Neurol* 1994;10:207–212.
44. Bhatt MH, Obeso JA, Marsden CD. Time course of postanoxic akinetic-rigid and dystonic syndromes. *Neurology* 1993;43:314–317.
45. Edby K, Larsson J, Eek M, et al. Amantadine treatment of a patient with anoxic brain injury. *Childs Nerv Syst* 1995;11:607–609.
46. Dreisbach RH. Handbook of poisoning: prevention diagnosis & treatment. Los Altos, CA: Lange Medical Publications, 1983.
47. Ellenhorn MJ, Barceloux DG. Diagnosis and treatment of human poisoning. *Med Toxicol* 1984;827.
48. Yoon SS, Macdonald SC, Parrish G. Deaths from unintentional carbon monoxide poisoning and potential for prevention with carbon monoxide detectors. *JAMA* 1998;279:685–687.
49. Sadovnikoff N, Varon J, Sternbach G. Carbon monoxide poisoning an occult epidemic. *Postgrad Med* 1992; 92:86–96.
50. Lugaresi A, Montagna P, Morreale A, et al. 'Psychic akinesia' following carbon monoxide poisoning. *Eur Neurol* 1990;30:167–169.
51. Smith JS, Brandon S. Morbidity from acute carbon monoxide poisoning at three-year follow-up. *BMJ* 1973;1:318–321.
52. Gorman D, Runciman W. Carbon monoxide poisoning. *Anaesth Intensive Care* 1991;19:506–511.
53. Perry G. What are the potential delayed health effects

of high-level carbon monoxide exposure? *J Med* 1994; 36:595–596.
54. Ginsburg R, Romano J. Carbon monoxide encephalopathy: need for appropriate treatment. *Am J Psychiatry* 1976;133:317–320.
55. Remick R, Miles J. Carbon monoxide poisoning: neurologic and psychiatric sequelae. CMAJ 1977;117: 654–657.
56. Meucci G, Rossi G, Mazzoni M. A case of transient choreoathetosis with amnesic syndrome after acute monoxide poisoning. *Ital J Neurol Sci* 1989;10: 513–517.
57. Deckel AW. Carbon monoxide poisoning and frontal lobe pathology: two case reports and a discussion of the literature. *Brain Inj* 1994;8:345–356.
58. Hardy KR, Thom SR. Pathophysiology and treatment of carbon monoxide poisoning. *Clin Toxicol* 1994;32: 613–629.
59. Sesay M, Bidabe AM, Guyot M, et al. Regional cerebral blood flow measurements with xenon-CT in the prediction of delayed encephalopathy after carbon monoxide intoxication. *Acta Neurol Scand Suppl* 1996;166:22–27.
60. Hartman DE. *Neuropsychological toxicology: identification and assessment of human neurotoxic syndromes*, 2nd ed. New York/London: Plenum Press, 1995.
61. Tvedt B, Kjuus H. Chronic CO poisoning. Use of generator gas during the second world war and recent research. *Tidsskr Nor Laegeforen* 1997;117:2454–2457.
62. Benignus V, Muller K, Malott C. Dose-effects functions for carboxyhemoglobin and behavior. *Neurotoxicol Teratol* 1990;12:111–118.
63. Griffiths AD, Laurence KM. The effect of hypoxia and hypoglycaemia on the brain of the newborn human infant. *Dev Med Child Neurol* 1974;16:308–319.
64. Hershey T, Bhargava N, Sadler M, et al. Conventional versus intensive diabetes therapy in children with type 1 diabetes: effects on memory and motor speed. *Diabetes Care* 1999;22:1318–1324.
65. Rovet JF, Ehrlich RM. The effect of hypoglycemic seizures on cognitive function in children with diabetes: a 7-year prospective study. *J Pediatr* 1999;134: 503–506.
66. Spencer AM. Post-hypoglycemic encephalopathy in Sakel's insulin treatment. *J Med Sci* 1948;94:535–554.
67. Hershey T, Craft S, Bhargava N, et al. Memory and insulin dependent diabetes mellitus (IDDM): effects of childhood onset and severe hypoglycemia. *J Int Neuropsychol Soc* 1997;3:509–520.
68. Biessels GJ. Cerebral complications of diabetes: clinical findings and pathogenetic mechanisms. *Neth J Med* 1999;54:35–45.
69. Ornoy A, Cohen E. Outcome of children born to epileptic mothers treated with carbamazepine during pregnancy. *Arch Dis Child* 1996;75:517–520.
70. Glowa JR. Behavioral toxicology of solvents. *Drug Dev Res* 1990;20:411–428.
71. Morrow LA, Steinhauer SR, Modgson MJ. Delay in P300 Latency in patients with organic solvent exposure. *Arch Neurol* 1992;49:315–320.
72. Hawkins KA. Occupational neurotoxicology: some neuropsychological issues and challenges. *J Clin Exp Neuropsychol* 1990;12:664–680.
73. White RF, Proctor SP. Solvents and neurotoxicity. *Lancet* 1997;349:1239–1243.
74. White DM, Daniell WE, Maxwell JK, et al. Psychosis following styrene exposure: a case report of neuropsychological sequelae. *J Clin Exp Neuropsychol* 1990; 12:798–806.
75. Gade A, Mortensen EL, Bruhn P. "Chronic painter's syndrome." A reanalysis of psychological test data in a group of diagnosed cases, based on comparisons with matched controls. *Acta Neurol Scand* 1988;77: 293–306.
76. Lindstrom K, Riihimaki H, Hanninen K. Occupational solvent exposure and neuropsychiatric disorders. *Scand J Work Environ Health* 1984;10:321–323.
77. Damsgaard MT, Klausen H, Iversen L. Late effects of occupational organic brain damage in painters 6–8 years after diagnosis. Occurrence of mental and psychosomatic health problems and utilization of health services. *Ugeskr Laeger* 1995;157:4027–4031.
78. Schwartz BS, Ford DP, Bolla KI, et al. Solvent-associated olfactory dysfunction: not a predictor of deficits in learning and memory. *Am J Psychiatry* 1991;148: 751–756.
79. Khattak S, K-Moghtader G, McMartin K, et al. Pregnancy outcome following gestational exposure to organic solvents. *JAMA* 1999;281:1106–1109.
80. Jones HE, Balster RL. Inhalant abuse in pregnancy. *Obstet Gynecol Clin North Am* 1998;25:153–167.
81. Chadwick OFD, Anderson HR. Neuropsychological consequences of volatile substance abuse: a review. *Hum Toxicol* 1989;8:307–312.
82. Ikeda M, Tsukagoshi H. Encephalopathy due to toluene sniffing. *Eur Neurol* 1990;30:347–349.
83. Flanagan RJ, Ives RJ. Volatile substance abuse. *Bull Narc* 1994;46:49–78.
84. Grover S, Goodwin J. Lightning and electrical injuries: neuro-ophthalmologic aspects. *Semin Neurol* 1995;15: 335–341.
85. Jumbelic MI. Forensic perspectives of electrical and lightning injuries. *Semin Neurol* 1995;15:342–350.
86. Kleinschmidt-DeMasters BK. Neuropathology of lightning-strike injuries. *Semin Neurol* 1995;15:323–328.
87. Cherington M, Yarnell PR, London SF. Neurologic complications of lightning injuries. *West J Med* 1995; 162:413–417.
88. Panse F. Electrical lesions of the nervous system. In: Vinker PJ, Bruyn GW, eds. *Handbook of clinical neurology, volume 7*. New York: Elsevier, 1970:344–387.
89. Cherington M, Yarnell P, Hallmark D. MRI in lightning encephalopathy. *Neurology* 1993;43:1437–1438.
90. Ozgun B, Castillo M. Basal ganglia hemorrhage related to lightening strike. *Am J Neuroradiol* 1995;16: 1370–1371.
91. Jumbelic MI. Forensic perspectives of electrical and lightning injuries. *Semin Neurol* 1995;15:342–350.
92. Devanand DP, Dwork AJ, Hutchinson ER, et al. Does ECT alter brain structure? *Am J Psychiatry* 1994;151: 957–970.
93. Primeau M, Engelstetter G, Bares K. Behavioral consequences of lightning and electrical injury. *Semin Neurol* 1995;15:279–285.
94. Cooper MA. Myths, miracles and mirages. *Semin Neurol* 1995;15:358–361.
95. Bullock J. Was Saint Paul struck blind and converted by lightning? *Surv Ophthalmol* 1994;39:151–160.
96. ten Duis HJ. Acute electrical burns. *Semin Neurol* 1995;15:381–387.

97. Carleton SC. Cardiac problems associated with electrical injury. *Cardiol Clin* 1995;13:263–266.
98. Solem L, Fischer RP, Strate RG. The natural history of electrical injury. *J Trauma* 1977;17:487–492.
99. Wilkinson C, Wood M. High-voltage electrical injury. *Am J Surg* 1978;136:693–696.
100. Varghese T, Mari MM, Redford JB. Spinal cord injuries following electrical accidents. *Paraplegia* 1986; 24:159–166.
101. Grube BJ, Heimbach DM. Neurological sequelae of electrical injury. In: Lee RC, Cravalho EG, Burke JF, eds. *Electrical trauma: the pathophysiology, manifestations and clinical management*. Cambridge: Cambridge University Press,1992:133–152.
102. Cheng PT, Lee CE, Yang JY. Electrical injury—clinical report of 67 cases. *Chang Keng I Hseuh* 1994;17: 220–225.
103. Hopewell CA. Serial neuropsychological assessment in a case of reversible electrocution encephalopathy. *Clin Neuropsychol* 1983;5:61–65.
104. Jack RA, Daniel DG. Possible interaction between phenelzine and amantadine. *Arch Gen Psychiatry* 1984;41:726.
105. ten Duis HJ. Acute electrical burns. *Semin Neurol* 1995;15:381–387.
106. Hooshmand H, Radfar F, Beckner E. The neurophysiological aspects of electrical injuries. *Clin Electroencephalogr* 1989;20:111–120.
107. Cohen J. Autonomic nervous system disorders and reflex sympathetic dystrophy in lightning and electrical injuries. *Semin Neurol* 1995;15:387–390.
108. Edmonds C. Marine animal injuries. In: Bove AA, Davis JC, eds. *Diving medicine*. Philadelphia: WB Saunders, 1990:115–137.
109. Shoemaker RC. Diagnosis of *Pfiesteria*-human illness syndrome. *Md Med J* 1997;46:521–523.
110. Matuszak DL, Sanders M, Taylor JL. Toxic *Pfiesteria* and human health. *Md Med J* 1997;46:515–520.
111. Burkholder JM, Glasgow HBJ. Tropic controls on stage transformations of a toxic ambush-predator dinoflagellate. *J Eukaryot Microbiol* 1997;44:200–205.
112. Glasgow HB, Burkholder JM, Schmechel DE. Insidious effects of a toxic estuarine dinoflagellate on fish survival and human health. *J Toxicol Environ Health* 1995;46:501–522.
113. Ewing-Cobbs L, Fletcher JM, Levin HS, et al. Longitudinal neuropsychological outcome in infants and preschoolers with traumatic brain injury. *J Int Neuropsychol Soc* 1997;3:581–591.
114. Swinker M, Koltai D, Wilkins J, et al. Is there an estuary associated syndrome in North Carolina? Findings in a series of hotline callers. *N C Med J* 2001;62: 126–132.
115. Lange WR. Ciguatera fish poisoning. *Am Fam Physician* 1994;50:579–584.
116. Cendes F. Temporal lobe epilepsy caused by domoic acid intoxication: evidence for glutamate receptor-mediated excitotoxicity in humans. *Ann Neurol* 1995;37: 123–126.
117. Scallet AC, Ye X. Excitotoxic mechanisms of neurodegeneration in transmissible spongiform encephalopathies. *Ann N Y Acad Sci* 1997;825:194–205.
118. Bates MN. Extremely low frequency electromagnetic fields and cancer: the epidemiologic evidence. *Environ Health Perspect* 1991;95:147–156.
119. Macklis RM. Magnetic healing, quackery, and the debate about the health effects of electromagnetic fields. *Ann Intern Med* 1993;118:376–383.
120. Frey AH. Electromagnetic field interactions with biological systems. *FASEB J* 1993;7:272–281.
121. Salford LG, Brun A, Eberhardt JL, et al. Permeability of the blood-brain barrier induced by various levels of electromagnetic radiation. In: Persson BRR, Sweden L, eds. *Abstracts, First World Congress for Electricity and Magnetism in Biology and Medicine*. Lake Buena Vista, FL: World Congress for Electricity & Magnetism in Biology & Medicine, 1992:1–5.
122. Medalia A, Isaacs-Glaberman K, Scheinberg H. Neuropsychological impairment in Wilson's disease. *Arch Neurol* 1988;45:502–504.
123. Sandyk R, Anninos PA, Tsagas N. Magnetic fields and seasonality of affective illness: implications for therapy. *Int J Neurosci* 1991;58:261–267.
124. Grota LJ, Reiter RJ, Keng P, et al. Electric field exposure alters serum melatonin but not pineal melatonin synthesis in male rats. *Bioelectromagnetics* 1994;15: 427–437.
125. Wilson BW. Chronic exposure to ELF fields may induce depression. *Bioelectromagnetics* 1988;9:195–205.
126. Randall W. The solar wind and affective disorders: a possible relationship due to magnetic disturbances. *J Interdisciplin Cycle Res* 1989;20 no 4:265–272.
127. Salzinger K, Freimark S, McCullough M, et al. Altered operant behavior of adult rats after perinatal exposure to a 60-Hz electromagnetic field. *Bioelectromagnetics* 1990;11:105–116.
128. Graham C, Cook MR, Cohen HD, et al. Dose response study of human exposure to 60 Hz electric and magnetic fields. *Bioelectromagnetics* 1994;15:105–116.
129. Frey AH, Wesler LS. Interaction of psychoactive drugs with exposure to electromagnetic fields. *J Bioelectricity* 1990;9:187–196.
130. Kavaliers M, Ossenkopp K, Tysdale D. Evidence for the involvement of protein kinase C in the modulation of morphine-induced 'analgesia' and the inhibitory effects of exposure to 60-Hz magnetic fields in the snail, Cep. *Brain Res* 1991;554:65–71.
131. Morgan RW, Kelsh MA, Zhao K, et al. Radiofrequency exposure and mortality from cancer of the brain and lymphatic/hematopoietic systems. *Epidemiology* 2000; 11:118–127.
132. Inskip PD, Tarone RE, Hatch EE, et al. Cellular-telephone use and brain tumors. *N Engl J Med* 2001;344: 79–86.
133. Hillert L, Kolmodin-Hedman B, Eneroth P, et al. The effect of supplementary antioxidant therapy in patients who report hypersensitivity to electricity: a randomized controlled trial. *Gen Med* 2001;3:1–12.
134. Morris JG, Grattan-Smith P, Panegyres PK, et al. Delayed cerebral radiation necrosis. *Quant J Med* 1994; 87:119–129.
135. Kaufman MJD, Swartz BE, Mandelkern M, et al. Diagnosis of delayed cerebral radiation necrosis following proton beam therapy. *Arch Neurol* 1990;47:474–476.
136. Schultheiss TE, Kun LE, Ang KK, et al. Radiation response of the central nervous system. *Int J Radiat Oncol Biol Phys* 1995;31:1093–1112.
137. Rubin P, Gash DM, Hansen JT, et al. Disruption of blood-brain barrier as the primary effect of CNS irradiation. *Radiother Oncol* 1994;31:51–60.

138. Kureshi SA, Hofman FM, Schneider JH, et al. Cytokine expression in radiation-induced delayed cerebral injury. *Neurosurgery* 1995;35:822–829.
139. Vassal G, Deroussent A, Hartmann O, et al. Dose-dependent neurotoxicity of high-dose busulfan in children: a clinical pharmacological study. *Cancer Res* 1990;50:6203–6207.
140. Ochs J, Mulhern R, Fairclough D, et al. Comparison of neuropsychologic functioning and clinical indicators of neurotoxicity in long-term survivors of childhood leukemia given cranial radiation or parenteral methotrexate: a prospective study. *J Clin Oncol* 1991;9:145–151.
141. Hamers FPT, Gispen WH, Neijt JP. Neurotoxic side-effects of cisplatin. *Eur J Cancer* 1991;27:372–376.

2

Perinatal and Pediatric Brain Injury

SUMMARY

Here the reader is introduced to the important topic of brain plasticity.

Several mechanisms exist to protect the infant from the trauma of birth and its many complications. Nevertheless, traumatic birth injury and perinatal asphyxia can have severe and enduring effects. The preterm infant can sustain lasting damage as a consequence of periventricular hemorrhage. The association between perinatal injury and later outcome is expressed in terms of a continuum of reproductive casualty, a useful principle in developmental medicine and also in neuropsychiatry. The cognitive deficits resulting from perinatal injury are diffuse rather than specific.

Brain injuries in childhood are usually traumatic and accident related. The neurocognitive sequelae of pediatric brain injury are also diffuse in nature and are manifest, like perinatal injuries, as general intellectual deficit. Even focal injuries in children lead to general rather than specific neurocognitive deficits. That is usually explained in terms of the equipotentiality of the young child's brain. After focal injuries, key functions such as language can be redistributed to undamaged areas that are as yet uncommitted. The equipotentiality of the child's brain, however, is limited. Therefore, specific neuropsychological deficits can also occur after pediatric brain injury.

The young child's brain is said to be relatively "plastic," that is, better able to compensate for the effects of injury. That is true, at least to a point. Brain plasticity is a relevant issue in the study of perinatal injury and of brain injuries occurring in later childhood. But if the child's brain is plastic, it is also vulnerable to certain kinds of injury, and there are circumstances under which the young brain, compared with the mature brain, can be more damaged by a given insult.

Injuries during the perinatal period and infancy are superimposed on an organ system that is undergoing an extraordinary period of growth and development. During this period, exposure to drugs, toxins, and viral infections can have devastating consequences. Fetal alcohol syndrome (FAS) and lead encephalopathy have been studied in great detail and illustrate a number of useful principles. The reader may be more interested in the potential teratogenicity of psychotropic drugs and antiepileptic drugs (AEDs).

Biologic mechanisms of brain plasticity, such as vicariation, collateral sprouting, and neurononeogenesis can have both positive and negative effects on brain recovery from perinatal/pediatric injury. These mechanisms are examined in some detail. Psychosocial influences on brain plasticity are not unimportant and have been the subject of the most elaborate research undertakings in the history of neuropsychiatry. The results point to behavioral compensation as one of the strongest mechanisms of brain plasticity.

PERINATAL BRAIN INJURY

Perinatal brain injury accounts for a small, but significant, proportion of people with mental retardation (MR) and developmental disabilities in general. Chromosomal abnormalities, metabolic and infectious disease, and sociofamilial factors account for a much larger number. The long-term impact of trauma on the early, developing brain, however, resembles more closely the results of other MR etiologic factors than it does the results of late childhood or adult brain injuries. Specific motor deficits are associated with perinatal brain injury, but cognitive deficits tend to be diffuse. For this reason, children whose impairments are the consequence of perinatal trauma have been treated medically and programmatically along with their developmental peers, and the treatment is largely irrespective of etiologic factors. It is only in recent years that neuropsychological research has indicated that perinatal brain injury can cause specific as well as diffuse cognitive deficits and that specialized interventions on behalf of such patients have been undertaken.

The effects of brain injury during the perinatal period and infancy are superimposed on an organ system that is undergoing an extraordinary period of growth and development. Early in fetal development, the growth of the central nervous system (CNS) is dominated by the processes of neuronal proliferation and migration. Fetal brain injury during the first 20 weeks of embryonic life, usually the result of infectious or toxic insults, has devastating consequences and results in a profound degree of developmental arrest. Because this is also the period of organogenesis, major physical anomalies and dysmorphic features characterize such injuries.

By birth, these fundamental processes are complete, whereas the next phase of development, characterized by neuronal differentiation, axonal growth, and synaptogenesis, is still quite active. The vigor of these processes, the extraordinary redundancy of the embryonic neural elements and their resilience confer on the perinatal brain a degree of plasticity that protects against the effects of trauma. It allows a degree of recovery that is, by later standards, quite remarkable. Not every flower flourishes in this garden, however, and there are limits to brain plasticity in early life, as will be seen.

Birth Injury

Everything about the head of the term fetus has been designed to protect it against trauma. A reasonable analogy is the ship in a bottle. As every old tar knows, you don't built the ship in the bottle; you build it on the workbench, designed to flex and bend. When it is finished, you push it gingerly through the neck of the bottle. So it is with the skull of the term infant, which nature has designed to bend and flex as it makes its way through the pelvic canal.

The evolutionary consequence of a large-brained human infant has been called the "obstetric dilemma." To support bipedal locomotion, the human pelvis has become progressively narrower, compared with that of our anthropoid ancestors. At the same time, however, fetuses evolved with larger brains and larger heads—thus, the dilemma of a larger head traversing a smaller pelvis. To solve this dilemma, the human neonate has to enter the pelvic inlet facing sideways because the larger diameter of the inlet is side to side. Then the baby's head has to rotate 90 degrees to accommodate the pelvic outlet, whose largest diameter is front to back. Apes, which have wider pelvises and smaller brained babies, have little difficulty with birthing; however, for humans, both mother and infant, it is an ordeal.

To protect the neonatal brain during this ordeal, it is encased in a skull that is thin and pliable, with sutures unfused and fontanels open. The orbital roof and floor of the middle fossa are smooth and offer little encumbrance to the shifting brain. The brain itself has a high water content; the subarachnoid space is small and close to the dura mater. In addition to these mechanical accommodations, the immature brain is metabolically less active, and cerebral blood flow is much less. It is less well myelinated, which mitigates the "packing" problem; it is also believed that neuronal plasticity is inversely related to the degree of myelination. When injured, edema is less likely to occur. Thus, the immature brain tolerates trauma, reduced blood flow, and anoxia much better than the mature brain (1).

Nature has had to compromise to advance the evolution of bipedalism and intelligence, and no compromise is perfect. Thus, in the days before modern obstetric care, mothers and babies died during childbirth, and not infrequently. Even today, with extraordinary advances in fetal monitoring and obstetric technique, passing through the birth canal is a traumatic event. Uterine and abdominal contractions generate tremendous forces that are compounded by the shearing effects produced by the resistant pelvic bones, and there are limits to the extent to which the brain can be safely deformed. The consequences are skull fractures, subarachnoid hemorrhage, intracranial hematomas, ischemia, and hypoxia.

Premature infants are less prone to birth trauma, of course, because their braincases are smaller, but they are vulnerable to subependymal and intraventricular hemorrhage by virtue of the immaturity of their tissues. As a result, the cerebral lesions that occur in premature newborns tend to be deep (e.g., periventricular leukomalacia); in contrast, perinatal brain damage in term infants tends to be cortical.

Consequences of Perinatal Injury

The clinical consequences of perinatal injury have been the subject of intensive study, extending back to 1861 when Little published a classic monograph *On the influence of Abnormal Parturition, Difficult Labour, Premature Birth and Asphyxia Neonatorum on the Mental and Physical Condition of the Child.* Sigmund Freud began his career as a pediatric neurologist studying children with cerebral palsy at a clinic in Vienna. They both were aware that perinatal brain injury was associated with a tetrad of pathologic outcomes: MR, cerebral palsy, epilepsy, and psychopathology.

For a long time, medical scientists tried to exact a lawful relationship between perinatal brain injury and clinical outcome. The most famous contribution was made by Passamanick and Knobloch in 1959, who coined the phrase "continuum of reproductive casualty," and wrote "There is a lethal component of cerebral damage which results in fetal and neonatal deaths and a sublethal component which gives rise to a series of clinical neuropsychiatric consequences depending on the degree and location of the damage (p.1384)."

This was a straightforward point of view, to be sure, and stated succinctly. It suggests a quantitative, dose-response relationship between the severity of the offending event and the severity of outcome. It is rather like the direct relationship that exists between the outcome of closed head injury and the duration of coma. Yes, there is a direct correlation, but is it possible to be more specific? For example, considering the different kinds of trauma that may occur during the perinatal period, is it possible to predict specific outcomes? What factors, external to trauma, are protective, and what factors are counterproductive? On both the cellular and molecular levels, are there events that can be manipulated or amended to mitigate the effects of injury and thus to improve the clinical outcome?

Modern research has supported a relationship between the severity of perinatal brain injury and the severity of developmental impairment that ensues. The relationship, however, is not entirely linear; there is a threshold of ischemia-hypoxia below which the neonate is protected and above which pathologic sequelae are seen. There are circumstances, as will be seen, where even severe damage can be compensated for, and there are events external to the child and his or her brain that can aggravate the pathologic consequences of even a minor birth injury. There is, indeed, a continuum of casualty, but it is curvilinear, not a straight line.

Hypoxic-Ischemic Injury

The brain of the neonate is relatively protected against hypoxic-ischemic brain injury (HII), and this is satisfactorily explained by its decreased metabolic rate secondary to incomplete elaboration of the dendritic complex (2). Nevertheless, ischemia and hypoxia are the most important causes of cerebral damage in the fetus and newborn. The incidence of perinatal asphyxia is inversely related to gestational age and birth weight: 30% of babies born at 28 weeks' gestation are damaged, compared with 2% to 3% of term infants. Nevertheless, HII is the most important cause of long-term morbidity even in term infants (3).

HII can only be measured indirectly at the time of birth; the absence of objective measures of asphyxial damage makes it difficult to relate its effects to long-term outcome. A persistently depressed Apgar score is suggestive of HII, but other pathologic events can also depress the score. (The causes of low Apgar scores are asphyxia, drugs, trauma, hypovolemia, infection, and anomalies.) Significant neurologic dysfunction during the newborn period is the most useful clinical indicator that a HII has occurred and is predictive of long-term sequelae. The consequences of mild HII are not necessarily clinically manifest early on. The child's neurologic status may appear normal, and the sequelae may only be apparent as mild developmental disabilities emerge during later childhood. Neuroimaging, evoked potentials, and other investigative techniques have been used to clarify the nature and extent of neonatal damage, especially with mild or moderate HII (4).

The areas of the brain that are most vulnerable to HII are those with the highest degree of cerebrovascular and neuronal immaturity at the time that the insult occurs. Hypoxia or anoxia at the time of birth leads to diffuse cortical damage in term babies or subcortical/periventricular damage in preterm babies. Watershed necrotic infarctions occur in watershed areas of the cerebral cortex and subcortical white matter—boundary zones at the margins of the outlying branches of the cerebral arteries. The deep temporal/limbic pathology that may be related to autism is, theoretically at least, the consequence of watershed infarction. Status marmoratus refers to basal ganglia infarction and is related to extrapyramidal symptoms such as athetosis and rigidity. HII of the cerebellum is less common, and the consequences are not usually apparent until the child is much older. Perinatal asphyxia is also associated with visual impairment, damage to cranial nerve nuclei leading to strabismus, sensorineural hearing loss, and, of course, cognitive and learning disabilities. Mild HII, insufficient to cause overt neurologic dysfunction, can cause hippocampal atrophy and memory impairment that is not evident until a child begins school. MR is common in severely asphyxiated infants, especially when the damaged areas include the parasagittal cortex and the thalamus (3,5,6).

Prematurity

The most common variety of neonatal hemorrhage is periventricular/intraventricular hemorrhage (IVH), which typically occurs in the premature infant. The subependymal germinal matrix is a cellular region ventrolateral to the lateral ventricles, containing a rich supply of thin-walled blood vessels that are ready sources of bleeding in response to the metabolic, respiratory, and hemodynamic aberrations that arise in connection with premature birth. IVH can lead to periventricular venous congestion and then to periventricular ischemia and parenchymal infarction. Systemic hypoxia, by itself, can cause IVH. The degree of IVH is directly related to the degree of tissue necrosis that ensues, and the pattern of periventricular leukomalacia is characteristic (7,8).

The outcome of IVH represents a continuum of casualty, ranging from no disability at all to death. Two characteristic outcomes are posthemorrhagic hydrocephalus and spastic diplegia. The most important determinant of hydrocephalus is the quantity of intraventricular blood, and the most important determinant of neurologic deficit is the extent of parenchymal infarction (9).

The developmental outcome of babies with IVH is hard to disentangle from the effects of prematurity, which, by itself, is often associated with respiratory insufficiency, hypoxia, and hypoglycemia, or from the effects of maternal conditions that increase the risk of prematurity, such as maternal age and parity, weight gain, smoking, alcohol or other drug use (e.g., cocaine), family income and education, and the quality of prenatal care. Longitudinal studies, then, to investigate the prognosis of IVH in particular, or of prematurity in general, have found it more fruitful to relate outcome to a risk index of some sort that takes into consideration all the potential noxious influences on development rather than any single element.

Clinical Elements External to Trauma That Influence Outcome

The association between early infant status and later intellectual outcome is complicated by the mediating effects of the environment on growth and development. Except in cases of gross damage to brain structures in infancy, these mediating factors are potent and sometimes control the outcome (5).

The study of premature birth has been an extraordinary opportunity to evaluate the relative contributions of biologic and nonbiologic issues on the developmental outcome of the brain-injured baby. It is an experiment of nature, and nature has contrived an elegant design. Birth weight is strongly correlated with gestational age; birth weight and gestational age are, themselves, positively correlated with the incidence and severity of IVH and HII. Thus, it is possible to investigate a dose-response relationship between one datum (birth weight) and a spectrum of developmental outcomes, which can also be expressed in numerical terms, for example, IQ scores or neuropsychological tests, or in terms of the need for special services in school. With such a design, the dependent and independent variables can be stated in numerical terms, and quantitative relationships are measurable.

This natural experiment, however, is not without confounds. Prematurity and low birth weight are influenced by factors such as maternal age and socioeconomic status (SES), and maternal behavior, such as smoking, drinking, and using drugs—elements that may speak to the postnatal environment of the child and possibly also to his or her genetic endowment. A tendency to premature birth is something that runs in families. Blacks are twice as likely to have premature babies than whites, even when SES is controlled. The incidence of congenital anomalies is twice as high in low birth weight babies compared with full-term babies, suggesting that pathology may be the cause, and not necessarily the result, of prematurity.

During the 1950s, medical scientists documented what had been known for centuries—that small babies were more prone to medical and developmental complications. There was little question in people's minds that low birth weight (less than 2,500 g and especially less than 2,000 g) had a deleterious effect on later intellectual development (10). To refine the understanding of this relationship, the National Institutes of Health sponsored a massive epidemiologic study of birth weight relative to developmental outcome, a longitudinal study known as the Collaborative Perinatal Project that involved the offspring of no fewer than 55,908 pregnancies.

The results of this massive undertaking did, indeed, confirm the expected relationship between birth weight and intellectual performance on standard tests at several points during childhood, but the correlations were not high. For example, at age 4 years, birth weight was discovered to account for only 5% to 6% of the variance in intelligence scores, a much lower percentage than was accounted for by familial and cultural variables. Perinatal anoxia contributed only approximately 1% of the variance in scores. On a statistical level it seemed, then, that prematurity and perinatal anoxia were not quite as deleterious as people had believed (11).

The problem with conclusions drawn from data of this sort is that the deleterious impact of severe prematurity and of severe anoxia occurring in a relatively small number of babies was obscured by the far larger numbers of babies with only a small degree of prematurity, a transiently depressed Apgar score, or a few brief apneic episodes. Most premature infants compare favorably in terms of their neurodevelopmental status to normal term infants; as a group, however, their status is marginally lower because of a small number of infants with severe impairment (12). Modern studies investigating the impact of prematurity are mainly concentrated on the problems of very low birth weight babies, that is, less than 1,500 g at the time of birth. In these studies, the incidence of motor impairment, sensorineural impairment, MR, and other developmental disabilities is quite high indeed.

Further, the relationship between birth weight and developmental outcome is probably not linear but exponential. If the base rate of MR in term infants is 2%, the rate for babies weighing 750 to 1,500 g is 8%, and for babies weighing less than 750 g, it is 21% (13).

What emerges from this cursory examination of the problem of perinatal brain injury is a remarkable consistency with principles already established with respect to brain injuries in general. Infants, even very small infants, are able to endure a mild-to-moderate degree of injury and maintain a sound developmental trajectory. The concept of cerebral reserve is not inappropriate to apply, even to the very young brain. The effects of brain injury are minimized in young children from healthy families with a favorable genetic endowment, good postnatal care, and freedom from other noxious influences pre- or postpartum. Conversely, the effects of perinatal injury interact in a negative way with unfavorable genetic or experiential variables. As the number of unfavorable variables increases, the severity of the developmental outcome increases exponentially.

Mechanisms of Perinatal Brain Injury

The cellular and molecular events that attend perinatal brain injury are not dissimilar to the events that follow traumatic injury or stroke in adults: neuronal excitotoxicity, for example, by excessive activation of glutamate receptors; the generation of highly reactive oxygen free radicals such as superoxide, hydrogen peroxide, and the hydroxyl radical; adenosine 5′-triphosphate depletion and enhanced apoptosis; and the generation of proinflammatory cytokines. In fact, abnormalities in cerebral energy metabolism and cell death can persist for weeks or months after a hypoxic insult to the neonatal brain. A moderate or severe HII at birth gives rise to a cascade of toxic events that exercises a continuing effect on brain development and aggravates the child's developmental outcome.

Conversely, this enduring pathologic environment might be amenable to therapeutic intervention. Glutamate activity at the *N*-methyl-D-aspartate receptor, for example, might be attenuated by an *N*-methyl-D-aspartate antagonist drug. Free-radical scavengers or drugs that reduce the production of reactive oxygen species represent another promising intervention. Other possible interventions might be nitric oxide inhibitors, antiapoptotic agents, and growth factors (14,15).

PEDIATRIC HEAD INJURY

In developed countries, accidents are the number one cause of death of children and adolescents; head injury accounts for approximately half of the fatalities. Traumatic brain injury (TBI) is the largest cause of acquired disability in childhood. There are more than 100,000 TBIs in children each year: 84% are mild, 6% moderate, 5% severe, and 5% fatal. The annual incidence in the United States is 200 per 100,000, and the cumulative incidence of head injury by 14 years of age is 4.1% for boys and 2.4% for girls. Falls account for the majority of head injuries in children, especially younger than 4 years of age, followed by motor vehicle accidents (MVAs) (including MVA-pedestrian and MVA-bicycle injuries), sports and recreation-related injuries, and then assaults. Head injury is the most common cause of death by child abuse; approximately 25% of head injuries in children younger than 2 years of age are inflicted injuries (16,17).

There are some nightmare scenarios. No fewer than 12% of MVA-pedestrian injuries happen to children who are run over in the driveway, usually in the late afternoon and when the car is backing up. One in 200 pediatric injuries to children under 7 years of age occurs when a TV set topples onto them. Falling out of bed, especially an upper bunk, sometimes causes serious injury, including head injury; falling out of windows is almost as common in suburban settings as it is in large cities (18–22). In the Solomon Islands, the most common cause of skull fracture is coconuts falling out of a tree (23). It is a miracle that any of us make it past the age of 20.

In early childhood, some of the same mechanisms that protect the neonate are still operative: the thinness and pliancy of the immature skull, the unfused suture lines, open fontanels, and the smoothness of the cribriform plate. These advantages, and other properties mentioned previously, are mostly lost by middle childhood. Some mechanical advantages persist; for example, the pliant cranial bones are better able to absorb more of the forces of an impact, which reduces the child's vulnerability to cerebral contusion and intracranial hematomas. At the same time, however, their pliancy amplifies forces that lead to shearing injury (16,18). For that reason, the effects of concussion may be more severe in children. They have a lower physiologic threshold for losing consciousness than adults do. This implies that for every increment of transient loss of consciousness, the adult patient has sustained a greater degree of acceleration-deceleration injury compared with a child (24). (Therefore, in a serious rear-end MVA, a grown-up and a child are sitting next to one another, both suitably restrained. The impact velocity is 25 mph. The child is more likely to experience loss of consciousness than the adult. This fact may be useful in medicolegal evaluations.)

Consequences of Pediatric Head Injury

Rutter (25) in Great Britain undertook the first systematic studies of the sequelae of pediatric brain injuries 30 years ago. Many of his conclusions are still valid, although others have been refined and amplified, especially as more sophisticated neurocognitive measures have been brought to bear on the subject. In keeping with the thrust of this chapter, Rutter stated that most of his general conclusions about children with head injuries were also applicable to children with perinatal brain injuries. In accord with the venerable principles of a continuum of casualty and the long-held beliefs concerning adult TBI, he underscored a relationship between the severity of brain injury, as measured by the duration of posttraumatic amnesia (PTA), and the degree of cognitive impairment that ensued. There were, however, some special aspects to pediatric TBI. The cognitive patterns that developed in children with TBI were remarkably similar, regardless of the locus of the injury, and no strong laterality effect could be detected. Brain damage in childhood, like perinatal brain damage, seemed to exercise its main effect on general intelligence rather than on specific neuropsychological functions; what Rutter referred to as the "nonspecificity of localized brain lesions in childhood" (25). It is this last finding that has been expanded on by more recent investigators (26–30).

The observation that brain trauma in neonates and children is most commonly associated with general cognitive impairment, as measured by an IQ test, is supportive of the principle of equipotentiality, that is, that cerebral tissue in the very young is less committed to specific functions. The resilience with which the young brain can reassign functions to uncommitted space has been thought of as a mechanism of brain plasticity.

Focal injuries are less likely to result in focal neuropsychological deficits in children than they are in adults. The classic example, of course, is focal injury to regions of the left hemisphere that would ordinarily result in aphasia in an adult patient. In young children, the outcome is not aphasia but rather speech delay. Ultimately, however, language develops as the child grows up, and more or less normally. Neuropsychological tests usually indicate normal levels of performance on tests of verbal ability, as if the language function were somehow reassigned to other cortical regions, especially in the right hemisphere. The ability of the young brain to relocate this essential function suggests that other cortical regions are equipotential with respect to language. The reassignment does not come without its price, however, and the children often have deficits in visuospatial abilities, as if these functions were "crowded out" by the intrusion of language development.

This is a relatively straightforward cortical space model: that there is only so much capacity in the undeveloped cortex for intellectual development and that subtracting capacity by injuring an area of cortex necessarily results in crowding or inadequate development of later developing skills. Crowding is said to occur when one brain region is damaged and another part of the brain takes over the functions of the damaged area. The intact brain region, in turn, has diminished capacity to subserve the functions for which it was originally intended (18). A simple example of this model is delayed reading in bilingual children; devoting an expanded space to language acquisition at an early age interferes with the child's ability to develop representational language, in the form of reading. (Ultimately, bilingual children develop normal reading ability, but it takes longer.) The equipotentiality of the child's brain confers a degree of protection against injury, but, theoretically at least, the price is crowding.

Neuropsychological investigations in recent years have supported the effect of severe brain injuries in early life on general cognitive impairment (26–30). Although they have not contradicted earlier observations on the diffuse cognitive effects of focal brain injuries, they have demonstrated that specific areas of neurocognitive ability may also be affected by pediatric brain injury.

For example, nonverbal learning disability appears to be the most common specific cognitive deficit in children with any kind of brain injury, focal or diffuse, perinatal or pediatric. Nonverbal disabilities are described in children with periventricular leukomalacia, closed head injuries, meningitis, seizure disorders, and cranial irradiation (26). Attention is another casualty of severe TBI in children; whereas adult TBI causes a more general disruption of attentional mechanisms and information processing speed, in children, the deficits are not generalized. Simple motor speed is relatively intact, but visuomotor processing is more impaired (27). Specific memory deficits, verbal as well as visual memory, are also seen after pediatric TBI (28).

The prominence of visuospatial and motor deficits in the long-term follow-up of pediatric brain injury is consistent with the cortical space model. That language is relatively spared in children with severe diffuse brain injuries, as well as focal left hemisphere lesions, probably speaks to the vigor with which language develops in early life. A 7-year-old child has, for all practical purposes, the linguistic ability of a mature adult. Vocabulary and syntactic complexity continue to advance as the child matures, but the essential components of language function have achieved maturity by the age of 7. Motor development, conversely, especially the fine motor coordination and visuospatial abilities that are required for activities such as music and sports, heart surgery and needlepoint, do not fully mature until years into adult life. In children, the relatively underdeveloped visuospatial compartment seems to be vulnerable to the aggressive development of the language function.

The concept of equipotentiality does not imply that there is no functional specialization in the young brain. Interhemispheric transfer of function occurs in young children and is best illustrated by language sparing. Careful evaluation of children with TBIs has demonstrated at least some impairment of language-based abilities, especially when the injuries involve the left hemisphere, and this suggests a degree of early specialization even in the brains of very young children (29,30).

The neurobehavioral sequelae of pediatric, in contrast to adult, TBI, are not recognizably different from what used to be called "functional disorders," that is, psychiatric conditions occurring in the general pediatric population. The only typically "organic" patterns detected in the British studies were "disinhibited patterns of behavior," comparable with one form of the frontal lobe syndrome seen in adults (25).

The attribution of psychiatric disorders to pediatric TBI is compromised by the well-known fact that children with behavioral and/or emotional problems are more likely to experience a TBI. In one study, as many as 19% of the children who sustained severe TBI had premorbid attention deficit/hyperactivity disorder (ADHD) (31). Nevertheless, the occurrence of novel psychiatric disorders after pediatric TBI, and persisting for 2 years, may be as high as 69%, depending on the severity of the injury (32).

ADHD symptoms, as one might expect, are the most common pediatric outcome after TBI; emotional instability, characterized by irritability, mood swings, and explosive outbursts, are another. Depression is not uncommon (33). There is nothing unique about the brain-injured child in the manifestation of these common childhood problems.

BRAIN PLASTICITY

Is it really better to have your brain lesion early (34)?

The question is not just whether it is better or worse to have your brain lesion early (25). If nature has contrived to expose the term fetus and the young child to extraordinary dangers, it only makes sense that she would endow it with natural protections. I have already alluded to some of the mechanical and metabolic advantages enjoyed by the fetus, and these continue to maintain protection during the first few years of life. It has also been a general belief that protection against the effects of injury is a property of the brain itself—that the young brain is plastic, that it can recover from a traumatic event with minimal sequelae. The general question of brain plasticity, which is discussed throughout this book, has been a central focus of the study of perinatal and pediatric brain injuries. That is where the most research, and the most definitive research, has been done and where the complexity of the problem can be best appreciated.

The early ablation studies by Margaret Kenard (35) gave rise to the general conclusion that brain lesions early in life led to lesser deficits than similar lesions occurring in maturity. She found that although unilateral injury to the motor cortex in adult monkeys generally resulted in severe hemiplegia, comparable lesions in infancy resulted in less severe deficits. As it happens, the same is true in humans.

The psycholinguist Lenneberg (36) is also remembered for having advanced the case for brain plasticity. Even later in childhood, as he pointed out, focal damage to the left hemisphere rarely, if ever, results in aphasia, and recovery of normal language is the rule. It was supposed that children in the first decade of life recovered completely from a lesion to the language-dominant hemisphere, presumably because the cortical substrates of language are capable of redistribution or vicariation (37). Vicariation is another expression of the principle of equipotentiality.

At the same time, however, David Hebb (38) was advancing the opposite position, arguing that early brain damage limits intellectual capacity (intelligence A) and thus restrains the formation of new "cognitive products" (intelligence B) over the growth span. His position was supported by a frequently cited study by Myer and Byers (39), who described the sequelae of measles encephalitis in children. In this classic study, adverse long-term consequences were more apparent in children who had had encephalitis at an earlier age. In addition, the cognitive effects of encephalitis on IQ became more evident as the children grew older. The authors argued that "the younger ones had to attempt the acquisition of the more elementary adaptations with defective tools" (pp. 552–553).

Two generations ago, most writers were emphasizing the plasticity of the young brain; a few were emphasizing its vulnerability. It was the former position that captured the imagination of people in positions of influence and was very much in accord with the spirit of the time. Over the ensuing years, and as discussed in the next section, a great deal of effort was spent addressing the promise implicit in the concept of brain plasticity. In recent years, conversely, more has been written in support of early vulnerability. Recent surveys of research on the developmental consequences of early brain insults, however, have failed to provide unequivocal support for either the plasticity or the vulnerability hypothesis (40). There is support for, and limitations to, both positions.

Plasticity and vulnerability are conceptual positions; in some instances, they have been rhetorical, even ideologic positions. They are not physiologic absolutes. The brain is plastic and can recover from insults; it is also vulnerable, although the manifestations of its vulnerability may not be immediately apparent. Plasticity characterizes the brains of newborns and children in the first decade of life. It characterizes the adult brain and even the aged brain, as long as it remains healthy. What matters is not the conceptual position, plasticity versus vulnerability, but the specific influences that operate within and without the injured brain.

Developmental Influences on Recovery from Brain Injury

There was a tendency for cognitive test scores, and especially for measures of scholastic attainment, to show greater impairment in children younger than 5 years of age at the time of injury (25).

The Kenard principle holds that the younger the age at which brain damage of any cause occurred, the better the outcome (35). New evidence, however, suggests that age-related brain plasticity may be more complex (25,40–42). In some circumstances, children younger than 6 years of age have less favorable outcomes than older children. After TBI, most studies indicate that recovery is less complete in children injured at age 6 years of age or younger than in older children and adolescents. Infants are more likely than older children to show serious intellectual impairment after meningoencephalitis or therapeutic radiation of the brain. It may be that unilateral cortical injury produces more extensive language impairment in older patients compared with young children, but most follow-up studies of children with focal lesions demonstrate adverse effects on later development when more sophisticated measures of linguistic function are used. It is also well known that children are more prone to posttraumatic epilepsy than adults. Even mild head injuries in children younger than 6 years of age can affect the child's ability to acquire new skills (25,40–42).

The consequences of pediatric brain injury may even be more severe in some circumstances than the consequences of similar injuries sustained later in life. They can be different in degree and in kind. Brain injury in early childhood is more likely to lead to general intellectual impairment and to poor scholastic performance, and not as much to highly specific neuropsychological deficits. With respect to specific abilities, perceptual motor and spatial skills, verbal and written abilities, and attention are particularly susceptible to early insult (25,40).

As a rule, immature organs are more susceptible to injury than mature organs, and organs tend to be most vulnerable during periods of rapid growth. In the case of the brain, this is the prenatal period and the first 2 years of life. From the cognitive perspective, young children possess fewer consolidated abilities. The younger the child, the fewer are his or her mature cognitive abilities. Future acquisition of cognitive abilities can be compromised by injury. Brain injuries can lead to greater impairments in children, simply because they have more new learning to undertake and less accumulated knowledge and fewer established skills on which to rely (18,25).

The pliancy of the child's skull is protective against particular kinds of injury, like the forces generated during parturition, but in response to other kinds of trauma, it is more prone to generate shear forces and thus damage the brain. The age at which a brain injury is sustained is not unimportant in terms of plasticity and outcome. Age, however, is only one element among many that influences plasticity and outcome.

Biologic Mechanisms of Brain Plasticity

When one looks carefully at the specific mechanisms that mediate plasticity in response to injury, one discovers that the same principle holds: they are equally capable of promoting recovery or pathologic outcomes.

One such element is programmed cell death or apoptosis. The embryonic brain gives rise to many more nerve cells than will ultimately be needed by the mature brain. Neurons that fail to establish a suitable target and to accumulate some minimal amount of trophic factor or synaptic sites undergo devolution and death. Neuronal branching, which is quite prolific during early development, is pruned by a process known as axonal retraction. Neither of these events resembles necrosis, an excited state that is accompanied by toxic levels of amino acids, ion fluxes, free-radical generation, and proinflammatory secretions. Rather, apoptosis is a silent process and entirely harmless to surrounding tissues. Neurons or neuronal processes that have failed to establish meaningful connections simply fade away, which is just as well because it is such a widespread phenomenon. It has been estimated that close to one-half of all neurons die off during the process of establishing connectivity in early development.

The superimposition of perinatal injury on this massive process of neuronal sculpting has mixed effects. For example, diffuse asphyxial injury results in infarcted and spared areas of cells within a brain region. The spared areas should therefore have proportionately lower rates of normal cell degeneration because there is less competition for target space and trophic factors. In the very young brain, many neurons that would die off naturally in the normal course of events are able to establish connectivity and survive because the cells they are competing with have been destroyed by hypoxic injury. Thus, the redundancy of the young brain, simply in the numbers of neurons trying to establish functional relationships, provides an avenue for the recovery of function not available in the adult brain.

In contrast, circumscribed injury within a particular region permits neurons on the margins of the injured area to survive, neurons that would normally degenerate. In such cases, neonatal connections are preserved. That may not necessarily be a good thing because the surviving neurons are equally prone to establish inappropriate or dysfunctional connections. If a perinatal brain injury leads to stabilization of immature patterns of synaptic connectivity, the result is that functions are spared that ought to be lost. A similar lesion occurring in an older child or an adult would have no such effect. Inappropriate immature connectivity is likely to be disruptive in the long run and can compromise the development of undamaged capacities (43).

Finally, brain injury, perinatal and otherwise, ischemic or traumatic, can actually increase apoptosis.

Because programmed cell death is an active process, requiring an intact cellular matrix to begin with, it does not occur within an ischemic focus or the actively traumatized brain region. However, in cells surviving in the penumbra of the injury focus, one finds proteins being expressed that mark the inception of the apoptotic process. This occurs after contusive, excitotoxic, or ischemic injury and contributes to the secondary injury process that continues for some time after acute injury. It has also been targeted, as previously mentioned, as a potential target for therapeutic intervention with antiapoptotic drugs (44–46).

Virtually all the cellular mechanisms thought to underlie brain plasticity may also promote vulnerability. Sprouting, for example, is the growth of new axonal sprouts from the cell body of one cell to another. It occurs in the CNS in response to injury, but it too might generate inappropriate connections that are functionally embarrassing. The same is true for events such as denervation supersensitivity, the accommodation of a synaptic bed to diminished availability of its usual ligand, and neurononeogenesis, the birth of new nerve cells. The same is also true for unmasking, the awakening of quiescent neuronal connections that are inhibited in the normal state but disinhibited after injury (47).

Psychosocial Effects in Pediatric Brain Injury

The results of the Collaborative Perinatal Project tended to minimize the deleterious effects of perinatal asphyxia (HII) associated with prematurity (11). They also highlighted the importance of psychosocial variables on the development of the child. Thus, one of the most ambitious undertakings ever devised for the study of perinatal brain injury fell fully in line with the thinking of that era: that the child's brain was plastic and that environmental manipulation could be counted on to ameliorate the negative effects of perinatal and psychosocial adversity.

The conclusions of the British studies, however, were different (25). They concluded that cognitive outcome after childhood brain injury was determined almost entirely by the severity of the injury. Measures of severity included PTA, duration of unconsciousness, treatment for cerebral edema, posttraumatic seizures, and abnormalities on the neurologic examination. "No association was found between non-neurological features and any of the cognitive sequelae" (25). In these studies, the psychiatric sequelae of perinatal and childhood brain injury were clearly associated with psychosocial adversity but not the cognitive sequelae.

The conclusions of the Collaborative Perinatal Project had a greater impact at the time because its results fueled an area of interest that was already developing in the United States: studies of psychoeducational interventions to reduce the occurrence of cognitive disability in children who were at risk for MR. This brings us to a subject that is some distance from the specific problem of pediatric brain injury, but not too far. The underlying principles are entirely germane.

Most mentally retarded children are only mildly or moderately retarded. The cause of mild-moderate MR is mainly familial. It is related to familial genetics (as opposed to spontaneous, nonheritable genetic causes of MR, such as Down's syndrome) or to psychosocial variables such as poverty, poor prenatal and obstetric care, inappropriate parenting, and lack of stimulation. Forty years ago, it was the prevailing belief that the latter were more important. Therefore, it was proposed that if one could correct the intervening psychosocial variables, then one might prevent the development of mild MR, or stated more directly, that early intensive psychosocial intervention could raise a child's IQ.

We look back on the attitudes of 40 years ago as hopelessly optimistic and perhaps naïve, but at the time they were entirely defensible. The times were ripe for studies of special treatments to ameliorate the condition of the developing brain. The zeitgeist was favorable, and there were even scientific studies in laboratory animals to support the approach.

Rosenzweig, an American psychologist, is most closely associated with a series of experiments on the effects of environment on brain growth and development. His animal studies won wide attention because they clearly proved that "brain changes in response to experience" (48). This was the classic experiment. Rat litter mates were randomly assigned to one of three environmental conditions: a standard laboratory colony cage, an "enriched" environment (a cage with a lot of rats, plenty of room, and a lot of things to play with and explore), or an "impoverished" environment (a single rat in a small cage). After several months of living like this, the rats were killed, and their brains examined.

The typical results in this experimental paradigm were that rats from the enriched environment had heavier brains, thicker cerebral cortex, and enhanced activity of particular enzymes. In other words, brain changes in response to experience. This was the first demonstration of an observable brain effect related to experiential variables (at least since 1780). The scientific world was skeptical at first and then duly impressed. The experiment was repeated in other laboratories, and the findings were replicated and extended, including the observation that synaptic density was increased in the enriched-environment rats (48).

As a matter of fact, this new and exciting discovery was no more than a replication of the work of an Italian anatomist, Michele Gaetano Malacarne, in the late eighteenth century, who also had demonstrated that experience produced observable changes in brain structure. He performed the same experiment that Rosenzweig had done but in sibling pairs of dogs, parrots, finches, and blackbirds. One animal of each pair received special training and the other none at all. When he examined their brains, the trained animals were found to have more convolutions in their cerebellar cortex. These extraordinary results won little attention at the time and were soon forgotten (48). If they were remembered at all, it was in the same vein as one of Herodotus' old stories.

Herodotus told the story of an Egyptian pharaoh, Psammetichus, who subjected two children to isolation at birth to settle an argument about which language—Egyptian or Phrygian (Phrygia was a kingdom in Asia Minor)—was the more ancient. The boys were raised by caretakers who were mute; for their entire lives, they were never exposed to spoken language. After a number of years, finally, one of the boys spontaneously uttered the word *becos*, which turned out to be the Phrygian word for bread. This settled the argument, at least as far as Psammetichus was concerned.

It is difficult to evaluate Malacarne's experiments because the raw data are no longer available, but looking back at the experiments of Rosenzweig and others, I suggest that what a psychologist considers an enriched environment is simply the kind of world that the rat in nature is used to. The standard laboratory colony cage, not to mention the impoverished environment, represents to the average rat an extraordinary state of psychosocial deprivation. The experiments did not really prove that enrichment promotes brain development but rather that the lack of appropriate stimulation retards brain development. (By the same token, I doubt that the children imprisoned by Psammetichus said any recognizable word at all; humans raised in states of extreme deprivation tend to be mute, and if they remain in such conditions for several years, they lose the capacity ever to develop language.)

Rosenzweig cautioned against applying his surmises to the human condition, but the temptation was too much to resist. The zeitgeist of the postwar years was deeply opposed to any suggestion of biologic determinism and entirely supportive of the idea that cultural experience was the dominant force in human psychology. Even the great Russian neuropsychologist Luria had begun his career as a developmental psychologist, studying the thinking of preliterate societies in Uzbekistan: "We were able to establish that basic changes in the organization of thinking can occur in a relatively short time when there are sufficiently sharp changes in socio-historical circumstances, such as those that occurred after the 1917 Revolution" (49).

The prevailing belief of the time was influenced by the Kenard principle (35) that the brain was plastic and capable of surmounting an untoward beginning, be it perinatal trauma or psychosocial deprivation. All that was needed was an intervention properly engineered and applied with diligence. This was the philosophical background that led to the longitudinal studies of at risk children who were given early training in specially designed enriched educational environments. It was proposed that children at risk of suffering cognitive impairment could attain normal levels of intelligence if they were educated in an enriched atmosphere.

Several national projects were begun on this question; one of the most important was in Chapel Hill, NC (the Abecedarian Project). In the Chapel Hill project and in various centers around the country, the experimental design was straight out of Malacarne. Subjects would be selected on the basis of demographic and clinical variables that put them at high risk of developmental delay. They were given enriched day care, with high staff-to-child ratios, parent training and support, good nutrition, and free health care. Control children from similar circumstances were given health care and nutrition, but no special psychological interventions. The children were followed from infancy to high school. Subject attrition thereafter has been a problem for most such projects around the country, but not for the Carolina project. (Of all the 50 states, people born in North Carolina are the most likely to stay there.)

The results of these extraordinary experiments were exactly as Malacarne, Rosenzweig, or Luria might have predicted, at least for a while. As they grew up, the disadvantaged children in enriched day care scored much higher on IQ tests and on tests of academic achievement than the controls did. Environmental stimulation reversed the untoward effects of an adverse beginning. The brain was plastic, after all.

Unhappily, whenever one addresses the question of brain plasticity in babies and children, one meets with problems that are unfriendly to the idea or at least that limit its boundaries. After a few years, the effect of the special interventions began to diminish. By the end of the first decade, the children in the treatment group had declined significantly in their performance on intellectual tests. Their IQ scores began to correlate with those of their (similarly disadvantaged) parents. When they were tested recently, in their 20s, their scores had fallen to the low average range. They were still scoring approximately three IQ points higher than the untreated controls (50,51), a small difference that was attributed by critics to no more than training for the tests.

The results of the Abecedarian Project, however, were not entirely unfriendly to the plasticity hypothesis. As we shall see later on with respect to childhood lead exposure, a small difference in IQ scores may be meaningless to individuals but quite important for groups. Even though the at-risk children who enjoyed early intervention scored lower on cognitive testing than middle-class children in the community, they had fewer social and behavioral problems than the untreated controls and were much less likely to fail at school than at-risk children who had no such advantage. They were more likely to go to college and more likely to finish college (50,51). Therefore, the special interventions were useful, at least to a degree, not so much in the direction of cognitive enhancement, but rather in the direction of improved psychosocial adjustment. This, in fact, is precisely the result one would predict on the basis of the British studies. The British studies, as discussed previously, had demonstrated that psychiatric sequelae after pediatric TBI, but not cognitive deficits, were significantly more likely to occur in the presence of marked psychosocial adversity, such as marital discord, paternal criminality, or maternal psychiatric disorder (25,28).

The longitudinal studies were not oriented to the specific problem of pediatric brain injury. However, the studies do speak to the issue of brain plasticity that is so central to the issue. They are raised, like the story of Psammetichus, for the reader's diversion, and also because they underscore the limitations of brain plasticity, even in an experimental paradigm that is specially constructed to make the most of it. They also complement the results of pediatric brain injury studies: when severity of injury is controlled, no less than 25% of the variance in outcome is accounted for by measures of the child's family environment.

Improving the psychosocial and educational environment of the child is clearly one way to improve the outcome of cerebral insult. The experiments of Rosenzweig and others suggest that they do so by fostering brain growth and the richness of synaptic connectivity. The longitudinal studies of children obviously did not look at cerebral convolutions or synaptic density. The IQ score is only an indirect measure, at best, of the biologic brain matrix. The fact that psychosocial performance clearly improved, while cognitive function did not improve very much at all, suggests that behavioral compensation is the mechanism that accounts for brain plasticity in this paradigm (47).

A new dimension of the concept of plasticity is the potential for biologic treatments that may be developed to promote recovery from brain injury. There are potential new drugs that might affect apoptosis, stimulate trophic factors, or promote neurononeogenesis. When such treatments are available, it will be interesting to see whether young patients with brain injury respond better than older patients.

Brain plasticity is not a special attribute that is unique to the brains of young children, nor is it an overriding principle that invariably mitigates the effects of injury. Plasticity is a metaconcept that speaks to many different biologic and psychosocial processes. The concept of plasticity is less interesting than its dimensions.

EFFECTS OF DRUGS AND TOXINS ON THE DEVELOPING BRAIN

If we direct our attention to more specific kinds of brain insult, can we amplify our understanding beyond the continuum of casualty model? Let us turn, then, to a series of specific insults and examine the question: if gross injuries cause diffuse damage, do more specific injuries lead to more circumscribed deficits? To that end, we examine behavioral neurotoxicity associated with a number of centrally acting drugs, including illicit drugs, toxic substances, and viral infections with limited tropism. Our investigation is limited by the formidable methodologic difficulties that inhere to this kind of research, but some general, if tentative, conclusions are possible.

The stages of brain development in early life are extraordinarily prolific but highly dependent on the timing of events within a delicately balanced chemical milieu. The proliferation of neurons, neuronal migration, the establishment of functional connectivity, programmed cell death, myelination, synaptogenesis are all processes that are vulnerable to disruption by untoward chemical influences. Exogenous substances such as drugs, or toxins are capable of disrupting the process, sometimes directly by exerting a direct toxic effect and sometimes indirectly by impeding the supply of blood, oxygen, or nutrients to the embryonic brain. Drugs that are not particularly harmful to the mother may have exaggerated effects on the fetus, which has only a limited capacity to detoxify and excrete foreign substances.

It is not easy to evaluate the negative cognitive or behavioral effects of drugs, or even of overt toxins such as lead, on the developing brain. Unless the drug also causes overt dysmorphic features or congenital anomalies, physicians are slow to suspect toxic effects on the CNS. Even if a drug is associated with neonatal withdrawal symptoms, as heroin is, or restlessness and dysphoria, as cocaine is, that does not mean that permanent CNS impairment will necessarily ensue. Clinical manifestations of CNS fetotoxicity may not be apparent until years have passed, when learning disabilities or behavioral problems develop in later childhood, when behavioral and emotional problems arise during adolescence, or when psychiatric disorders appear in adult life. Even then, it is hard to disentangle the effects of drug-induced fetotoxicity from the effects of a suboptimal family environment or from a suboptimal genetic endowment.

TERATOGENIC DRUG EFFECTS: MEDICAL DRUGS

Psychotropic Drugs

In 1978, the prevailing view in psychiatry was that *"these drugs pose relatively little hazard for the fetus and newborn. Permanent or long-lasting adverse effects occur no more frequently among births to women treated with psychotropics that they do among women treated with nonpsychotropic drugs or no drugs" (52).*

That was enlightened opinion at that time. It is still the prevailing view, although circumstances have changed. There are many new psychotropic drugs, of course, and many more people are taking them. Women of childbearing age are taking psychotropics for relatively new indications, such as premenstrual syndrome, social anxiety, ADHD, and chronic dysthymia. Some of the new psychotropic drugs are also AEDs, a class that has always been associated with fetal teratogenicity. Attitudes against drug consumption during pregnancy have hardened considerably, even against "soft" drugs like caffeine, tobacco, and alcohol. In 1978, there were no "wrongful life" lawsuits against physicians to compensate parents for the birth of defective offspring.

What is the same, in 2001 as in 1978, is that there is not a strong base of systematic research on which to base a prediction that a given drug is perfectly safe to take during pregnancy and that it will have no effect on the development of the exposed child. As a matter of fact, only two foreign substances, ethanol and lead, have been given the kind of systematic, epidemiologic attention that one would like to give to any drug that a pregnant woman might take.

Three primary effects are associated with medication use during pregnancy: teratogenicity, perinatal syndromes or neonatal toxicity, and postnatal behavioral or developmental sequelae. Exposure to psychotropic drugs during pregnancy may increase the relative risk for some specific congenital abnormalities, but the rate of occurrence of these abnormalities even with an increased risk remains low. The available data indicate that first-trimester exposure to low-potency phenothiazines, lithium, certain anticonvulsants, and benzodiazepines, but not antidepressants or psychostimulants, may increase the relative risk for congenital abnormalities (53).

Antidepressants

The tricyclic antidepressants are not associated with fetal abnormalities, and the results of large-scale studies are in agreement. The new antidepressants appear to be equally safe. Animal studies of fluoxetine (FXT), paroxetine, and sertraline in very large doses have failed to show an increased risk of fetal dysmorphology or other perinatal complications. In a prospective, multicenter study conducted at nine teratology information centers in the United States, with a total of 267 women exposed to FXT, paroxetine, or sertraline, there was no evidence of increased risk of congenital malformations or perinatal complications (54).

In 1996, Chambers (191) reported a prospective study of 228 women who were pregnant while taking FXT. FXT exposure was not associated with fetal loss or major malformations, but exposed infants had more minor physical anomalies than controls. Exposure to FXT during the third trimester was associated with prematurity, admission to special-care nurseries, poor neonatal adaptation, and jitteriness. The results of this study were questioned, however, because of confounding elements associated with the control group; five other cohort studies were cited, comprising 450 pregnancies, with no untoward outcome on perinatal status or subsequent development related to FXT (55). A study of 55 children whose mothers had been treated with FXT during pregnancy, compared with controls, failed to find differences in mood, temperament, IQ, language, or behavior. The children were 16 to 86 months old when they were evaluated (56).

Neonatal withdrawal syndrome has been reported for FXT (57), sertraline (58), and paroxetine (59), characterized by tremors, tachypnea, and increased tone. Sustained jitteriness in one infant lasted for a month and then subsided. There were, apparently, no long-term sequelae.

Psychostimulants

Like the neuroleptics, stimulants are known to effect neurochemical changes in the brains of rat fetuses, and cognitive and behavioral abnormalities have been cited during early development (60). These animal findings are probably relevant to the fetotoxic effects of cocaine and methamphetamine taken in high doses by drug abusers. They are probably not germane to the low doses of stimulants women might take for ADHD or antidepressant augmentation (61).

Antipsychotic Drugs

It is possible that low-potency phenothiazines are associated with congenital anomalies (62), although the data from large-scale studies is conflicting. No such association has been suggested for high-potency neuroleptic drugs, and there are few data, one way or the other, for the atypical antipsychotics. Transient extrapyramidal symptoms (rigidity, restlessness, and tremor) have been noted in babies born to neuroleptic-treated mothers, but they are transient and disappear within a few weeks (53,63).

The neuroleptics are the most overtly neurotoxic of all the psychotropic drugs, and even low doses can cause side effects such as dystonia, akathisia, bradykinesia, and the tardive syndromes. They act on the dopamine system, which is highly vulnerable to the effects of exogenous toxins. If any class of psychotropic drug were to have a teratogenic effect, one would predict that the neuroleptics would (60). They have been given to millions of women, however, since 1954 and for psychiatric conditions that do not ordinarily permit "drug holidays" of 9 months' duration. In the old days, they were even used as antiemetics for pregnant women. If they were teratogenic, we would probably know by now.

Anxiolytics

Early studies indicated relatively high rates of congenital anomalies in association with maternal use of meprobamate and chlordiazepoxide, especially oral clefts. In 1989, Swedish investigators reported dysmorphic features, growth aberrations, and CNS anomalies similar to FAS (64). The Collaborative Perinatal Project examined the issue, however, and found no physical or developmental effects in the offspring of mothers who took anxiolytic drugs, and the association with oral clefts has also been questioned (1,65). Benzodiazepine withdrawal syndromes have been described in newborns (63). Behavioral and cognitive abnormalities have been described in rats exposed *in utero* to diazepam (66,67).

Lithium

Of all the traditional psychiatric drugs, lithium is most strongly associated with congenital anomalies, especially malformations of the heart and great vessels (Ebstein's anomaly). The association is not inevitable, and healthy babies have been born to mothers taking lithium, but it is sufficiently strong to contraindicate the drug during pregnancy. In 1978, the Registry of Lithium Babies reported 25 of 217 babies born to mothers on lithium were malformed (68). Later studies suggested that lithium teratogenesis may not be nearly as common as was once thought (69,70).

Thus far, the five classes of traditional psychotropic drugs have been considered. The antidepressants and psychostimulants are clearly safe and the antipsychotics and benzodiazepines are probably safe as well. They are safe, despite the facts that these drugs all cross the placental barrier and that the fetus is relatively incapable of metabolizing the drugs effectively, and transient neonatal drug effects are often observed. It has been necessary to examine congenital anomalies in general as a surrogate marker for CNS embryopathy because very few studies have actually examined long-term behavioral or developmental effects. This is hardly a secure footing on which to base any conclusive remarks. It does appear, however, that the action of these drugs, in altering neurotransmitter actions and receptor dynamics, does not exercise a readily observable effect on brain development.

The case of lithium is another matter entirely. It is unequivocally associated with congenital anomalies, although it is arguable how frequently they occur. Simply because lithium causes cardiac or limb anomalies, though, does not mean that it also affects brain development. In terms of fetotoxicity, lithium is comparable to the anticonvulsants, carbamazepine and valproate. They are similar to lithium in their psychiatric effects, and they are also prone to cause congenital anomalies.

In the next section, we shall consider the possible mechanisms of their embryopathic effects.

Antiepileptic Drugs

An accurate appraisal of the teratogenic risk of the AEDs has been complicated by the fact that epilepsy itself in either parent is related to an increased risk of having a malformed child (65). That said, one must acknowledge that all the AEDs have been associated with congenital anomalies, independent of maternal (or paternal) epilepsy, that animal models and *in vitro* studies have confirmed their potential for fetotoxicity, and that credible mechanisms have been proposed to explain the association (71–73).

The irony is that at different times, virtually every AED has been considered more (or less) teratogenic. Twenty years ago, phenobarbital was said to be the AED of choice for pregnant women. We have since learned that early barbiturate exposure in animals reduces brain weight, with corresponding changes in brain biochemistry and neuromorphology; and that babies exposed to phenobarbital *in utero* tend to have smaller heads (74,75). Phenobarbital and hydantoin are associated with cardiac, urogenital, and orofacial malformations in infants. A fetal hydantoin syndrome was described in 1976 by Hanson et al. (76), characterized by craniofacial anomalies, digital hypoplasia, growth deficiency, and MR. When similar anomalies were also described in infants exposed to trimethadione, primidone, and carbamazepine, the term fetal anticonvulsant syndrome was coined (77,78).

Many neurologists believe that carbamazepine is the least teratogenic of the anticonvulsant drugs, but it too has been associated with major malformations, including neural tube defects (79,80). The similarities of the anomalies caused by hydantoin and carbamazepine has fueled speculation that it is the epoxide metabolite (a breakdown intermediate formed by both drugs) that is responsible for the teratogenic effect (79). If that is the case, then oxcarbazepine should be less teratogenic than carbamazepine (81).

Valproate is clearly the most teratogenic of the major anticonvulsant drugs. It produces a varied pattern of major malformations, neural tube defects, and cardiovascular, urogenital, craniofacial, and skeletal anomalies (e.g., limb reduction defects) (82,83). It has been classed as a human teratogen since 1983, and well before then it was known to have adverse effects on brain growth in animals (84,85).

Whatever the relative merits or demerits of individual anticonvulsants in terms of teratogenesis, the consensus is that polytherapy raises the likelihood of congenital malformations. It is also accepted that anticonvulsant fetotoxicity is not limited to overt organ maldevelopment or, behaviorally, to a neonatal withdrawal syndrome. AEDs have a negative effect on cognitive development when the children are tested at age 6 (72,86) or in adolescence (87). MR and autism have been described in fetal anticonvulsant syndrome.

It is possible to overstate the embryopathic effects of AEDs. Most women on AEDs during pregnancy deliver normal babies, and, even with valproate, the rate of spina bifida is no more than 2% above the population baseline. Indeed, influential neurologists have gone so far as to claim that "since no agreement has been reached regarding which AED is the most teratogenic, the present consensus opinion is that the AED that stops seizures in a given patient should be used" (77).

It is also possible to overstate the potential fetotoxicity of the various psychotropic drugs; compared with the AEDs, they are remarkably safe. The exception is lithium. Even in the case of lithium, however, nothing as dramatic as fetal anticonvulsant syndrome has been described, and long-term follow-up of "lithium babies" has never uncovered developmental or neurobehavioral deficits.

There are numerous theories to explain why the anticonvulsants are teratogenic. We have already mentioned the epoxide metabolite of phenytoin and carbamazepine. Another possibility is the anticonvulsant effect on trace minerals and folic acid. Reduced levels of folic acid occur in patients on anticonvulsant drugs, in pregnant women, and especially in women with epilepsy who are pregnant. Because neural closure defects are associated with low folate levels, it is presumed that this is a mediating factor in the increased occurrence of spina bifida, anencephaly, and encephalocele in babies who were exposed to AEDs (88,89).

Anticonvulsant drugs, especially valproate, tend to accumulate in fetal tissues. If they block certain forms of electrical activity in the developing neuron during cell migration, axonal sprouting, and synaptogenesis, they may compromise neuronal survival. In neuronal cell cultures, all the AEDs are known to interfere with cell growth and the formation of dendritic spines, and all of them promote cell loss *in vitro*. Valproate has been shown to decrease protein and DNA content in the embryo, to impede mitosis, cell motility, and the metabolism of lipids, and to interfere with glutathione and thus increase oxidative stress in the developing brain. AEDs interfere with microtubule assembly and the organization of the cytoskeleton. Hypoxia and genomic imprinting have also been suggested as possible mechanisms (90–97).

These are, of course, all mechanisms that have been worked out *in vitro*, so their clinical salience is still an open question. No such effects have been described for any of the psychoactive drugs. The effect of lithium has been related to inositol depletion; many developmental neurotoxicants do seem to have an effect on protein phosphorylation, which is discussed in Chapters 20 and 21, when lithium, carbamazepine, and valproate in their roles as psychotropic agents are considered (98,99). Of all the psychotropic drugs, lithium is most closely identified with second messenger effects that influence the intracellular milieu, gene expression, and protein synthesis. Carbamazepine and valproate exert similar effects on what is called signal transduction; valproate and lithium seem to have a great deal in common in this regard.

If the traditional psychotropic drugs are comparatively free of fetotoxic effects, the opposite is the case for nonmedical psychotropics, which is discussed in the next section.

TERATOGENIC DRUG EFFECTS: NONMEDICAL DRUGS

In our society there are three, possibly four, mainstream drugs—psychoactive drugs that are widely used, freely available without a prescription, and generally considered safe, if not by the U.S. Food and Drug Administration, at least by users. They are caffeine, nicotine, and alcohol; the fourth, an emerging mainstream drug, is cannabis. Of the four, only alcohol is overtly teratogenic. The use of nicotine and (of course) cannabis is strongly discouraged in pregnant women. Caffeinated beverages can be consumed, not with impunity, but rather, in moderation.

In 1980, the U.S. Food and Drug Administration actually removed caffeine from its list of compounds generally regarded as safe, citing animal evidence that caffeine caused birth defects, fetal death, and reduced birth weight (100). In fact, the dose of caffeine necessary to cause anomalies in fetal mice or rats is enormous; if extrapolated to a 50-kg woman, it is the equivalent of 100 double lattes per day (101). There is modest evidence that it has a small effect on birth weight, and it may potentiate the teratogenic effects of smoking, alcohol, or other drugs, but, by itself, caffeine is not a human teratogen (102,103).

With regard to smoking, as late as 1998, no fewer than 25% pregnant women smoked, despite the fact that smoking tends to reduce fertility (104). Infants born to women who smoke during pregnancy weigh an average of 200 g less than those born to nonsmokers, and the incidence of low birth weight babies is doubled. The effect is dose dependent and independent of other factors known to influence birth weight (105,106). Carbon monoxide is a constituent of cigarette smoke, and carboxyhemoglobin is increased in both maternal and fetal blood, with a reduction in oxygen binding capacity and chronic fetal hypoxia. Nicotine can adversely affect uterine and placental blood flow by causing vasoconstriction. Nicotine levels are higher in the fetal circulation by approximately 15%; there are hundreds of different chemical substances in tobacco smoke, and although we know very little about their toxicity, most of them find their way into the fetal circulation as well (104,107).

Nicotine itself is a neuroteratogen, as evidenced by the effect of the transdermal patch, without the confounds of other constituents of tobacco smoke or of episodic hypoxic-ischemic insult. Nicotine effects neuronal proliferation, differentiation, and synaptogenesis. In animal studies, it affects the development of the cholinergic and catecholaminergic systems. Abnormalities of cortical and hippocampal morphology have been described (108–110). Long-term cognitive effects are seen in exposed rats (111,112).

Are there similar effects in humans? The children of smokers do seem to have lower scores on spelling and reading tests and more problems with hyperactivity and short attention span compared with the children of nonsmokers (113). There is also a higher incidence of childhood behavioral disorders and drug dependence during adolescence (114,115). Deficits in stature, cognitive ability, temperament, and behavior are consistently reported in the children of smoking parents, which may be related to intrauterine exposure, psychosocial and genetic influences, and perhaps exposure to passive smoke (116–118).

Fetal Alcohol Syndrome

Behold, thou shalt conceive, and bear a son; and now drink no wine or strong drink... (Judges, 13:7)

Foolish and drunken and harebrained women most often bring forth children like unto themselves, morose and languid. (Aristotle)

What must become of the infant who is conceived in gin? with the poisonous distillations of which it is nourished both in the womb and in the breast. (Henry Fielding)

FAS refers to a constellation of physical, behavioral, and cognitive abnormalities. It is characterized by dysmorphic facial features, growth retardation, and MR. In the developed countries, it is the number one cause of preventable birth defects; the incidence rate in the United States is 5.2 per 10,000 livebirths. It accounts for as many as 5% of all congenital anomalies (119).

Since biblical times, people have suspected that drinking alcohol had teratogenic effects on the fetus, but it was not until the publications of Lemoine and Lemoine (120) and Jones et al. (121) that a distinct dysmorphic condition associated with MR was definitively recognized (122). The facial features are characteristic, most notably short palpebral fissures (blepharophimosis), short upturned nose, maxillary hypoplasia, hypoplastic philtrum, and thinned upper vermillion. Growth retardation is moderate (less than the third percentile for height and weight), and microcephaly is usually the first indication of CNS dysfunction (123).

The diagnostic criteria for FAS are given in Table 2.1. Clinicians have also used the term fetal alcohol effects to describe children with a variety of problems, including growth deficiency, behavioral mannerisms, and developmental delays, but who lack the

TABLE 2.1. *Diagnostic criteria for fetal alcohol syndrome*

A. Confirmed, excessive maternal exposure; either substantial, regular intake or heavy episodic drinking. Evidence includes frequent episodes of intoxication, tolerance or withdrawal, social or legal problems related to drinking, physically hazardous behavior while drinking, and alcohol-related medical problems.
B. Characteristic facial anomalies: blepharophimosis (short palpebral fissures), flattened midface, thin vermillion, absent philtrum.
C. Low birth weight and/or growth retardation.
D. Central nervous system neurodevelopmental abnormalities such as decreased cranial size at birth and/or structural brain abnormalities (e.g., microcephaly, partial or complete agenesis of the corpus callosum, cerebellar hypoplasia).
E. Neurologic hard or soft signs: impaired fine motor skills, neurosensory hearing loss, poor tandem gait, poor eye-hand coordination.
F. Behavior or cognitive abnormalities such as learning difficulties, deficits in school performance, poor impulse control, problems in social perception, deficits in higher level receptive and expressive language, poor capacity for abstraction, specific deficits in mathematical skills, or problems in memory, attention, or judgment.
G. Birth defects associated with alcohol exposure include
   1. Cardiac
      a. Atrial septal defects
      b. Tetralogy of Fallot
      c. Aberrant great vessels
      d. Ventricular septal defects
   2. Skeletal
      a. Hypoplastic nails
      b. Clinodactyly
      c. Shortened fifth digits
      d. Radiolunar synostosis
      e. Flexion contractures
      f. Camptodactyly
      g. Pectus excavatum and carinatum
      i. Klippel-Feil syndrome
      j. Hemivertebrae
      k. Scoliosis
   3. Renal
      a. Aplastic, dyplastic, hypoplastic kidneys
      b. Horseshoe kidneys
      c. Ureteral duplications
      d. Hydronephrosis
   4. Ocular
      a. Strabismus
      b. Refractive problems secondary to small globes
      c. Retinal vascular anomalies
   5. Auditory
      a. Conductive hearing loss
      b. Neurosensory hearing loss

full complement of FAS criteria. It has been necessary to describe an intermediate condition because from the beginning, it was apparent that each individual anomaly can vary in severity and any subcombination of anomalies could occur (122).

There is a spectrum of ethanol teratogenesis, just as there is a spectrum of maternal behavior with respect to alcohol consumption. The earliest studies related FAS to daily, heavy use— the equivalent of six hard liquor drinks a day. Subsequent studies established that even moderate drinking—one or two drinks per day—could have a deleterious effect on the fetus and that there was a dose-response curve relating maternal alcohol intake to outcome of pregnancy. Clinical studies have been consistent with animal studies, especially with respect to neurodevelopmental outcomes, which are related in linear fashion down to the lowest nonzero levels of exposure, without a threshold. The risk of a low birth weight baby is doubled if the mother drinks one or two drinks a day, and an increased risk of spontaneous abortion occurs in women who drink two drinks twice per week (76,122, 124–126).

Alcohol readily crosses the placental barrier, and in humans, fetal blood ethanol levels rapidly approximate those in maternal blood. The fetus lacks alcohol dehydrogenase, so the ethanol has to be cleared by maternal metabolism. It also tends to accumulate in the amniotic fluid. Alcohol is particularly toxic during the first trimester of fetal life, during the stages of neuronal proliferation and migration. As a result, significant structural alterations of the CNS are observed in children and in experimental animals exposed to alcohol *in utero*. Brain weight is reduced, and multiple heterotopic cell clusters are found, especially on the brain surface. Microcephaly, heterotopias, and cerebellar dysplasia are among the most common neuropathologic findings. Others include hydrocephaly, neural tube defects, agenesis of the corpus callosum, polymicrogyria, and abnormalities of the basal ganglia (122,127–129).

Precisely how ethanol acts as a teratogen is not clearly understood. Sixty years ago, alcohol researchers recognized that there was a higher rate of fetal casualty in alcoholic mothers, but they attributed it to poor nutrition and a chaotic home life. Alcohol abuse is often associated with nutritional deficiencies. It is possible that there is a nutritional component to FAS, but it is not because alcoholic mothers eat poorly. Animal studies effectively quashed that idea. If nutrition plays any role at all role, it may be because alcohol impedes the placental transfer of nutrients (130).

Fetal hypoxia may play a role in FAS because ethanol can cause constriction of the umbilical arteries and veins. Alcohol effects prostaglandin metabolism, which can influence cell division, hormone secretion, and neurotransmitter systems, e.g., dopamine, serotonin, γ-aminobutyric acid, glutamate, acetylcholine, and endorphins. It is also an oxidative stressor, inhibiting mitochondrial respiratory chain components and thus generating reactive oxidative species; the fetus is comparatively unprotected by endogenous antioxidants (130,131).

The fact that the ethanol effect is strongest when migratory events are prominent in the early stages of pregnancy implies a negative influence on pathway guidance and the establishment of an appropriate connectivity pattern. Ethanol triggers widespread apoptotic degeneration among neurons in the developing rat forebrain. This effect occurs during the stage of synaptogenesis, which in humans extends from the third trimester to several years after birth. During this period, even transient ethanol exposure can delete millions of neurons from the developing brain (127,132).

Many children with FAS are mentally retarded, usually in the mild-to-moderate range, and the severity of the dysmorphic features is related to the degree of MR. Specific neurocognitive deficits are seen in attention, memory, visuospatial skills, problem solving, cognitive flexibility, and planning. Naturally, the children do poorly at school, and there is a high rate of learning disabilities, including nonverbal. The typical behavioral outcome is ADHD, but the children are also prone to eating and sleeping problems and head and body rocking stereotypies. Their problems tend to persist into adult life. The fact that children with FAS are small creates psychological problems in school, but, as a rule, children with FAS are not prone to extremes of emotional dysregulation. Autism has been related to FAS (76,123,133–137).

Many children with FAS come from pathologic families and grow up in chaotic and nonsupportive environments. Nevertheless, even when psychosocial variables are controlled, longitudinal studies indicate persistent cognitive and neurobehavioral problems that are related to degree of dysmorphology and therefore to the severity of ethanol exposure.

Cocaine

Cocaine-using women have higher rates of spontaneous abortion and premature birth. Low birth weight, low Apgar scores, perinatal asphyxia, intracranial hemorrhage, and withdrawal syndrome are all associated with cocaine exposure (138,139). Cocaine-exposed babies have smaller heads and smaller brains.

Cocaine-exposed infants tested at 43 weeks post-conception are more jittery and inattentive and have more sensory, movement, and tone abnormalities compared with nonexposed infants. Hypertonic tetraparesis has been described in as many as two-thirds of infants with prenatal cocaine exposure (140,141). They have significant depression of interactive behavior and poor organizational response to environmental stimuli. Their neonatal status is even impaired compared with babies exposed to alcohol, tobacco, or cannabis, although the effect is aggravated by concurrent exposure. As can best be determined, the cocaine effect is dose dependent. (138,142,143).

The recent crack cocaine epidemic gave rise to media reports of "crack babies," a blighted generation who are incapable of forming social attachments, making eye contact, or integrating into families or society. In fact, there is a spectrum of developmental outcomes associated with prenatal cocaine; not every child has developmental problems, and a positive family environment has been shown to attenuate many of the cognitive and behavioral problems. Cocaine-exposed children are prone to attentional problems and hyperactivity and to conduct problems, as well as cognitive delays, even when they are raised in optimal home environments. Many of them are diagnosed with ADHD; interestingly, they tend to respond less favorably to psychostimulant treatment (140,144–147) because of the supposed mechanism of cocaine fetotoxicity.

Most of the usual neurotoxic mechanisms have been supported in preclinical studies of cocaine-exposed fetuses: maternal vasoconstriction, hypoxia-ischemia, oxidative stress, increased cell death, ion channel effects, and diminished response to trophic factors. What may be unique about prenatal cocaine exposure is its effect on the development of monoaminergic neurons. Cocaine is selectively neurotoxic, especially to dopamine and serotonin neurons, and the effects, at least in laboratory animals, are long-lasting (148–150). Stimulants are indirect monoamine agonists and require an intact presynaptic neuron to be effective.

Similar, selective neurotoxicity has been described with prenatal exposure to methamphetamine, although there is not much clinical literature (151). The ill-fated appetite suppressant fenfluramine was also linked to serotonin neurotoxicity in developing rats and monkeys (152,153).

Cannabis and Heroin

Worldwide cannabis is the most commonly used illicit substance and, after alcohol and tobacco, the most commonly used drug during pregnancy. Early studies suggested an effect on intrauterine growth and length of gestation, but the more recent data are equivocal or negative (154–157). Cannabis-exposed neonates are jittery, tremulous, and given to startles and altered responsiveness (158,159). At 4 to 6 years of age, they are said to have problems with verbal ability, attention, and memory and later on problems with psychological tests that require impulse control and visual analysis/hypothesis testing (160,161).

Infants born to heroin-addicted mothers have a high incidence of intrauterine growth retardation and neonatal abstinence syndrome. As neonates they tend to be less alert, are less likely to attend or react to stimuli, and are tremulous and irritable. Attachment behavior, sleeping, and feeding are compromised in infancy. At 3 to 6 years of age, they are rated as less well adjusted socially and perform less well on perceptual-motor tests (162,163).

Chronic Hypoxia

Hypoxic brain injury is one of the proposed mechanisms for drug-induced fetotoxicity. The earlier discussions of hypoxic-ischemic and diffuse anoxic injuries dealt with the consequences of transient but severe depressions of the oxygen supply to brain. Chronic hypoxia is a different case altogether: the oxygen supply is diminished over a long period of time.

Chronic hypoxia in adults is usually associated with chronic obstructive pulmonary disease. Mild hypoxic injuries can occur during cardiac surgery or even after traveling to high altitudes. In children, chronic hypoxia may be associated with anemia or with cyanotic congenital heart defects.

Children with chronic hypoxia related to congenital heart defects have lower IQ scores, poor perceptual-motor skills, poor gross motor coordination, and slower reaction times compared with noncyanotic children. Sustained attention and freedom from distractibility are adversely affected, but the children are usually underactive, not hyperactive (164). In children with iron-deficiency anemia, mild deficits are reported in performance IQ, fine and gross motor development, perceptual speed, and quantitative reasoning (165). This pattern is suggestive of subcortical injury.

Hypoxia may be one of the mechanisms by which fetotoxic drugs cause damage, but there is not much similarity between the observed effects of hypoxic injury and the patterns of deficit observed after prenatal drug exposure. Chronic hypoxia may be a contributing factor to brain injury caused by drugs, but it is probably not the major event.

Brain Damage from Antenatal Drug Exposure: Summary

The impact of antenatal drug exposure is measured at term by physical problems: early parturition, obstetric complications, low birth weight, congenital anomalies, dysmorphic features, neonatal withdrawal, and sensorimotor abnormalities. As a rule, drugs that elicit such abnormalities also interfere with brain growth and development, and to the degree to which they are manifest is the degree to which the developing brain is likely to be injured. Brain damage is rarely evidenced by overt neurologic findings on examination or by neonatal seizures but rather by the newborn's pattern of responsiveness and his or her behavior during the neonatal period. The severity of cognitive and behavioral difficulties in later childhood is predicted by the severity of the initial presentation. Children whose neonatal status appears quite normal may develop mild-to-moderate impairments that are apparent only in later childhood.

The range of cognitive impairment resulting from prenatal drug exposure is wide, ranging from a moderate degree of mental handicap to mild learning disabilities. The range of behavioral outcomes includes disorders of conduct, an ADHD-like syndrome, and disorders of attachment and affective regulation. Generally, the effects of prenatal drug exposure, when they do occur, are diverse as well as general. They are not associated with specific neurocognitive or neurobehavioral abnormalities.

The psychotropic drugs are remarkably free of teratogenic or fetotoxic effects, even though neonatal symptoms are occasionally encountered. The exception is lithium, which has a good deal in common with the anticonvulsant drugs, especially in terms of ionic conductance, second messenger, and genomic effects (Chapters 20 and 21). The various nonmedical psychotropics are fetotoxic, some more than others, and their effects are compounded by coconsumption of multiple drugs.

LEAD

Lead encephalopathy occurs in adults in the context of industrial exposure. For children, there are many sources. Most cases of lead poisoning are in pica-prone toddlers living in homes built before the 1940s, when lead was commonly used for interior paint. In 1892, cases of lead poisoning were reported from Australia in 10 children who had ingested leaded paint flakes (166). Lead may be absorbed from water in places where the mineral content of the water is low, and lead pipes are still in use. (Hence, "plumber," from the Latin word *plumbum*, for lead. Plumbism is lead poisoning.) When gasoline was leaded, organic or tetraethyl lead was ingested through roadside dust contaminated with automobile emissions or habitual gasoline sniffing. Prenatal lead exposure occurs when mothers accumulate a lead burden from lead pipes or industrial dust. After it is absorbed, it is stored in bone, where it is tightly bound and nontoxic, and in liver, kidney, erythrocytes, and soft tissues, from where it is freely exchangeable and does much harm. Lead intoxication leads to an acute encephalopathy with cerebral edema, neuronal degeneration, and proliferation of the vascular endothelium, and then to obliteration of small-caliber vessels. Peripherally, there is degeneration of the myelin sheath and axis cylinders (167). Lead is very slowly excreted, so even very small amounts of ingested lead tend to accumulate.

It has been know since Roman times that lead is neurotoxic, and the acute effects of lead poisoning have been described by Western physicians for hundreds of years. That subclinical lead intoxication has encephalopathic effects in childhood has only been known since 1943, when Byers and Lord reported that chronic lead exposure, at levels that were not high enough to cause acute encephalopathy, led to the subsequent development of academic problems, sensorimotor deficits and behavior problems, including "violent, aggressive behavioral difficulties, such as attacking teachers with knives and scissors."

In the 1960s, concerns over the risk of subclinical lead intoxication led to screening programs in several American cities, and the discovery that many asymptomatic children in inner-city slums had evidence of excessive lead absorption. Several studies were undertaken to examine the effect of lead load on developmental achievement. The initial results were mixed but suggestive of a mild global effect, expressed in terms of IQ reduction of three or four points, in children exposed chronically to a lead burden of more than 60 μg/dL. Since then, the intellectual and behavioral effects of low-level lead exposure have been well established, albeit not without controversy. The effects are small, indeed; no specific pattern of neuropsychological deficit (or of congenital anomalies) has been established, but the finding of an IQ decrement has held up (169–171). The neurocognitive effects of childhood lead exposure are persistent, even 20 years later (172,173). As the evidence has mounted, the consensus on what level of lead burden is toxic has changed; the neurotoxic threshold is now 10 µg/dL.

The neurotoxic effects of lead differ in expression and sensitivity between young children and adults. The latter express inorganic lead toxicity as a peripheral neuropathy (e.g., wrist drop). Children, however, are more likely to develop an overt encephalopathy; their vulnerability to lead is explained by the immaturity of the blood-brain barrier. Adult exposure, however, is not without danger. Organic lead poisoning in adults may be manifest as a change in mood or affect or overt psychosis. Occupational studies have also demonstrated subtle neurocognitive deficits in adults, even with low-level exposure, that are persistent even after chelation therapy and that may even lead to progressive long-term decline (174–176).

Lead is a chemical stressor to the CNS, and there is no threshold below which it remains without effect (177). The developing hippocampus is uniquely sensitive to the neurotoxic effects of lead, and impairment of synaptogenesis, myelination, and dendritic arborization can have significant effects on intellectual development (178).

Lead: A Digression

There are three additional points to make with respect to lead intoxication. They are only peripherally related to the thrust of this chapter, but appropriate to set before the reader in any event.

First, environmental lead is an anthropogenic neurotoxin, perhaps the most common, but clearly the most historical. Lead production began approximately 6,000 years ago and flourished during classical times. Elemental lead is found in proximity to silver and is a product of silver mining. It is easy to work and was widely used for eating utensils and water pipes. At the height of the Roman Empire, lead production reached 80,000 metric tons per year, a level of production that was not exceeded until modern times. Smelter emissions are believed to have resulted in significant local and even regional pollution throughout Europe, and lead poisoning has been cited as one of the causes of the fall of the Roman Empire in the West (179). Lead levels in bone are approximately 100 times higher today than they were 5,000 years ago (180).

Second, consider the demographic and sociologic consequences of widespread, subclinical lead intoxication. We know that low levels of lead exposure in young children leads to a small decrement in IQ scores but only a small decrement (171). A four-point difference in IQ means very little if one is comparing two individuals. In very large groups, however, a mean IQ score that is four points lower is very important. It means that in the afflicted group, a much larger number of individuals score in the below-average range and a much smaller number score in the above-average range. The implications for the population are apparent: a larger number of people functioning at the marginal levels of society and a much smaller number who can function in positions of leadership and responsibility. A small degree of brain damage may be something an individual can learn to cope with. A small degree of brain damage to an entire population may have an incalculable toll.

In children, lead is associated with learning disabilities and school failure, but it is also associated with hyperactive, delinquent, and aggressive behavior. Within a circumscribed population of lead-exposed children, therefore, not only is there a substantial reduction in academic ability but a corresponding increase in maladaptive and criminal behavior. The impact is only aggravated by the fact that the lead exposure, in modern times, is much more likely to occur in minority populations, living in urban ghettoes, with low income, poor nutrition, and other risk factors, all of which compound, directly or indirectly, the effect of lead (168). Therefore, it is no surprise that long-term trends in exposure to paint lead and gasoline lead, going back to 1900, are strongly correlated with trends in violent crime and unwed pregnancy (181).

Finally, there are the postdevelopmental effects of early neurotoxicity. It is possible, even likely, that most people exposed to high levels of environmental lead as young children will have compensated for the neurotoxic insult. What will happen to those people as they age and as their nervous systems lose plasticity and functional reserve? Is it possible that the residual damage associated with early lead intoxication will be unmasked? In the industrial world, there is a large cohort of people who as children were exposed to levels of lead that would now be considered neurotoxic. They carry with them a persistent lead burden, stored silently in their bodies, mainly in the mineral compartment. Efflux of lead from bone stores has been observed in aging people. What will be the consequence to the aging brain of this reexposure added to the subclinical damage that occurred in early childhood (182)? Is it possible that early exposure to environmental lead will accelerate an age-related decline in function (21)?

VIRAL INFECTIONS

Children are particularly vulnerable to severe and diffuse cognitive impairment after viral infections of the CNS. The pattern was first appreciated in studies of survivors of epidemic encephalitis (von Economo's disease or encephalitis lethargica) after World War I. Afflicted adults tended to develop parkinsonism, children developed personality and behavioral disturbances (minimal brain damage, hyperkinesis), and infants were left with global intellectual deficits. As a rule, generalized dementia did not develop when the mature brain was infected.

Herpes simplex virus (HSV) causes an acute necrotizing encephalitis that selectively effects the temporal and orbitofrontal lobes. Although there are many viral causes of acute encephalitis in childhood, HSV encephalitis (HSVe) is particularly grave, with the risk of death or severe disability more than double that associated with other causative agents. Young children are particularly vulnerable. The risk of death or severe disability in infants is five times that of children who contract the virus after 1 year of age (183). Is that because the infant's brain is more vulnerable to viral insult or because the infant is relatively immunodeficient? It is probably the latter (184). It appears that HSV can persist in the CNS, even after a course of antiviral treatment, and that periodic activation of the latent virus may lead to continued or intermittent neural damage (185,186).

Viral infections are difficult to study with respect to one of our central issues (plasticity versus vulnerability) because the effects of acute infection can be compounded by the effects of persistent infection and/or the effects of immune-mediated response to the virus, which may by itself lead to disseminated demyelination. Such may be the case in subacute sclerosing panencephalitis, a rare but particularly destructive process that is related, directly or indirectly, to CNS infiltration by the measles virus. The white matter lesions that are typical of subacute sclerosing panencephalitis are identical to those of progressive rubella encephalitis, subacute acquired immunodeficiency syndrome encephalomyelitis, and other postviral conditions (187).

Congenital rubella infection is associated with a devastating constellation of deficits including hearing loss, cataracts, motor impairment, heart defects, microcephaly, cognitive impairment, and behavioral disturbances. Multiple handicaps occur in approximately 50% of rubella children with normal intelligence and in virtually all who are mentally retarded. The severity of handicap is related to the duration of intrauterine exposure, that is, how early or late during the course of pregnancy that the mother is exposed to infection (188,189). Severe neuropsychiatric conditions, including autism and schizophreniform psychosis, may be seen (190).

HSVe has a distinctive pathology, with localization of inflammation and necrosis to the mediotemporal and orbitofrontal lobes; it is the only virus that characteristically presents with signs and symptoms suggesting temporal lobe localization: hemiparesis with greater involvement of the face and arm, aphasia, superior quadrant visual field defects, paresthesias, and psychiatric symptoms such as terror, hallucinations, and bizarre behavior (191). The structures damaged by HSV are indeed part of an anatomic and functional unit—the limbic system; the limbic system is selectively vulnerable for anatomic and chemical reasons (192).

HSVe is a grave condition, and the outcome is more often than not death or severe disability. The outcome is less favorable in children than in adults, and children are more likely to experience diffuse cognitive impairment. In adults, focal deficits are the rule, but focal deficits are not uncommon in children, for example, aphasia, memory impairment, and Klüver-Bucy syndrome (193–197).

POSTIMMUNIZATION ENCEPHALOPATHY

The 1964 rubella epidemic in the United States left 30,000 children with congenital deformities. The goal of rubella vaccination (available since 1969) has been to immunize all preschool children, with the goal of eradicating rubella. A secondary goal was to vaccinate susceptible women of childbearing age, but it was discovered that the vaccine virus could cross the placental barrier and infect the fetus. The risk of fetal abnormalities was small, but nonzero, and therefore vaccination for pregnant women was discouraged (198).

The idea that vaccination [for measles, mumps, rubella, diphtheria, pertussis, tetanus (DPT), polio, and hepatitis B] might have adverse neurologic consequences has aroused a great deal of concern, especially among parents' groups and medicolegal circles. Public health advocates point to the extraordinary benefits of vaccination programs, not only against the diseases themselves but also against encephalitis, which, in children, can be a complication of most common childhood infections (199). Appeals to the public health, however, are little solace to parents of the rare child who develops an encephalopathic event temporally related to an immunization.

Questions have been raised about the safety of vaccines against DPT in young children (200). In some children, there may be seizures, hypotonic-hyporesponsive episodes, persistent crying, high fevers, and encephalopathy within days of immunization. Vaccine-related encephalopathy is also claimed to be associated with persistent developmental delays, many of them quite severe. The public reaction has been entirely predictable. There has been litigation against physicians and vaccine manufacturers. It is said to have impeded the success of national immunization programs and even led to small epidemics of diseases like pertussis in the most highly developed countries (201,202).

Reassurances issued by august bodies, like the Institute of Medicine, have done little to quench public concerns raised by small, vocal, and sometimes strident groups. The range of excess risk of acute encephalopathy after DPT immunization is said to be approximately 10 cases per million immunizations, a very small number from the perspective of the public health. The evidence, however, is insufficient to support either the presence or absence of a causal relationship between DPT vaccination and permanent neurologic damage (203).

Not long ago, an investigative group in Great Britain postulated that measles immunization might cause autism. The observation that the incidence of autism seemed to increase since measles immunization was introduced also fueled concerns of advocacy groups. Since autoimmunity has been implicated in the cause of autism, and brain autoantibodies have been detected in the sera of autistic children, there seemed to be a scientific basis for the association (204,205). In fact, the incidence of autism has not been increasing, although the diagnosis is probably made more frequently now than it used to be, and a recent epidemiologic study from California demonstrated convincingly that no association existed between autism and measles vaccination (206).

Nevertheless, encephalopathic reactions have been credibly reported after immunization for measles and DPT (202,207). Some toxoids are known to be associated with neurologic syndromes such as brachial neuritis and Guillain-Barré syndrome, and most (if not all) vaccines can cause severe anaphylactic reactions (208). It is also possible for encephalopathy to follow immunizations that are administered to adults, such as hepatitis, influenza, or yellow fever vaccines (209–211).

The putative risk of postimmunization encephalopathy is hardly sufficient to warrant a change in national policies toward the vaccination of children or adults. The anecdotal literature is troubling, but the epidemiologic studies are reassuring. It is not unlikely that a busy neuropsychiatric practice will on occasion treat a young patient whose developmental disability is attributed to a postimmunization catastrophe or an adult patient whose neuralgias and neuropsychological deficits are temporally related to vaccination. Sometimes the referral may be about a medicolegal question and sometimes about the application of an innovative treatment of dubious merit. Unfortunately, unless one has the capacity to measure antibrain autoantibodies, the clinical workup is not likely to be decisive. One is left with the possibility of association, and the necessity of developing a systematic differential diagnosis. As will be seen when the case of fluoxetine and suicide is discussed, a rare side effect is difficult to disprove even with the largest numbers. When dealing with only one case, establishing causation is a formidable problem.

PEDIATRIC BRAIN INJURY: PRINCIPLES AND CONCLUSIONS

Are there conclusions to be drawn about brain injury in early life? There is one perhaps: that children are neither different from adults nor are they the same. In considering the impact of brain injury, there are differences and similarities. The elements they have in common can be stated in terms of general principles, but the differences are best considered in terms of specific factors.

Therefore, the continuum of casualty is a venerable principle in developmental medicine, but it also holds true for brain injuries at any age; the severity of the cerebral insult is always related to the severity of outcome. There are threshold effects for children, as discussed, referring to mild insults that have no enduring sequelae. These are exemplified in hypoxic injury, in which the neonate has a certain degree of protection. There are also exponential effects, in which we see how each additional increment of risk magnifies the severity of outcome, exemplified by studies of very low birth weight babies. The negative effect of nonbiologic risk factors, especially familial and psychosocial, also has an exponential effect on the severity of outcome. This principle is expressed in virtually every domain considered in this chapter but is most prominent in studies of lead intoxication and fetotoxic drug effects. All these principles are relevant to the outcome of adult brain injury as well.

The mechanisms of brain injury, the mechanics, the cell physiology, and the biochemistry share a number of similarities, but major points of divergence have also been emphasized. The mechanical, anatomic, and metabolic properties of the child's skull and brain confer relative advantages and disadvantages. The mechanisms of brain plasticity are also similar and different. The young brain is not perfectly equipotential but is more so, certainly, than the adult brain. Apoptosis, axonal sprouting, and behavioral compensation are equally relevant to the study of adult and pediatric brain injury, but in different ways.

In terms of outcome, relative to focal injuries, nonspecificity is the rule for pediatric injuries, at least for very young children, but it is not an inviolate rule. Cerebral palsy, MR, epilepsy, ADHD, and nonverbal learning disabilities are the most important sequelae of pediatric brain injury, but subtle deficits in memory and language development adumbrate the typical effects of brain injury in adult life.

In terms of treatment, the fields of pediatric and adult brain injury have been historically divergent. In fact, the principles of treatment are remarkably similar, even if different vocabularies are used; differences lie only in the specifics.

REFERENCES

1. Hartz S, Heinonen OP, Shapiro S, et al. Antenatal exposure to meprobamate and chlordiazepoxide in relation to malformations, mental development, and childhood mortality. *N Engl J Med* 1975;292:726–728.
2. Robinson RO. Equal recovery in child and adult brain? *Dev Med Child Neurol* 1981;23:379–383.
3. Simon NP. Long-term neurodevelopmental outcome of asphyxiated newborns. *Clin Perinatol* 1999;26:767–778.
4. Cowan F. Outcome after intrapartum asphyxia in term infants. *Semin Neonatol* 2000;5:127–140.
5. Spreen O, Tupper D, Risser A, et al. *Human developmental neuropsychology*. New York: Oxford, 1984.
6. Gadian D, Aicardi J, Watkins K, et al. Developmental amnesia with early hypoxic-ischaemic injury. *Brain* 2000;123:499–507.
7. Volpe JJ. Intraventricular hemorrhage in the premature infant—current concepts. Part I. *Ann Neurol* 1989;25:3–11.
8. Volpe JJ. Intraventricular hemorrhage in the premature infant—current concepts. Part II. *Ann Neurol* 1989;25:109–116.
9. Volpe JJ. Intraventricular hemorrhage and brain injury in the premature infant; diagnosis, Prognosis, and prevention. *Clin Perinatol* 1989;16:387–411.
10. Scarr S. Effects of birth weight on later intelligence. *Soc Biol* 1969;16:249–256.
11. Niswander K, Gordon M. *The women and their pregnancies: the Collaborative Perinatal Study of the NINCDS*. Philadelphia: WB Saunders, 1972.
12. Pasman J, Rotteveel J, Maassen B. Neurodevelopmental profile in low-risk preterm infants at 5 years of age. *Eur J Pediatr Neurol* 1998;2:7–17.
13. Hack M, Taylor H, Klein N, et al. School-age outcomes in children with birth weights under 750 g. *N Engl J Med* 1994;331:753–759.
14. Silverstein FS, Barks JD, Hagan P, et al. Cytokines and perinatal brain injury. *Neurochem Int* 1997;30:375–383.
15. Robertson NJ, Edwards AD. Recent advances in developing neuroprotective strategies for perinatal asphyxia. *Curr Opin Pediatr* 1998;10:575–580.
16. Shapiro K. Head injury in children. In: Becker DP, Povlishock JT, eds. *Central nervous system. Trauma status report: 1985*, 1985:243–253.
17. Michaud L, Duhaime A, Batshaw M. Traumatic brain injury in children. *Child Dev Disabil* 1993;40:553–565.
18. Fenwick T, Anderson V. Impairments of attention following childhood traumatic brain injury. Neuropsychol Dev Cogn Sect C Child Neuropsychol 1999;5:213–223.
19. Benoit R, Watts D, Dwyer K, et al. Windows 99: a source of suburban pediatric trauma. *J Trauma* 2000;49:477–481.
20. Macgregor D. Injuries associated with falls from beds. *Inj Prev* 2000;6:291–292.
21. Holland A, Liang R, Singh S, et al. Driveway motor vehicle injuries in children. *Med J Aust* 2000;173:192–195.
22. DiScala C, Barthel M, Sege R. Outcomes from television sets toppling onto toddlers. *Arch Pediatr Adol Med* 2001;155:145–148.
23. Mulford J. Coconut palm-related injuries in the Pacific Islands. *Australian and New Zealand Journal of Surgery*. 2001;71:32–34.
24. Rosenthal B, Bergman I. Intracranial injury after moderate head trauma in children. *J Pediatr* 1989;115:346–350.
25. Rutter M. Developmental neuropsychiatry: concepts, issues, and prospects. *J Clin Neuropsychol* 1982;4:91–115.
26. Schatz J, Craft S, Koby M, et al. Associative learning in children with perinatal brain injury. *J Int Neuropsychol Soc* 1997;3:521–527.
27. Catroppa C, Anderson V, Stargatt R. A prospective analysis of the recovery of attention following pediatric head injury. *J Int Neuropsychol Soc* 1999;5:48–57.
28. Max JE, Roberts MA, Koele SL, et al. Cognitive outcome in children and adolescents following severe traumatic brain injury: influence of psychosocial, psychiatric, and injury-related variables. *J Int Neuropsychol Soc* 1999;5:58–68.
29. Dall'Oglio A, Bates E, Volterra V, et al. Early cognition, communication and language in children with focal brain injury. *Dev Med Child Neurol* 1994;36:1076–1098.
30. Brookshire B, Chapman S, Song J, et al. Cognitive and linguistic correlates of children's discourse after closed head injury: a three-year follow-up. *J Int Neuropsychol Soc* 2000;6:741–751.
31. Gerring J, Brady K, Chen A. Premorbid prevalence of ADHD and development of secondary ADHD after closed head injury. *J Am Acad Child Psychiatry* 1998;37:647–654.
32. Bloom D, Levin H, Ewing-Cobbs L, et al. Lifetime and novel psychiatric disorders after pediatric traumatic brain injury. *J Am Acad Child Psychiatry* 2001;40:572–579.

33. O'Brien G, Cheesebrough B. Traumatic brain damage. In: Gillberg C, O'Brien G, eds. *Developmental disability and behaviour*. London: MacKeith Press, 2000: 64–76.
34. Schneider GE. Is it really better to have your brain lesion early? A revision of the "Kennard principle." *Neuropsychologia* 1979;17:557–583.
35. Kenard M. Reorganization of motor function in the cerebral cortex of monkeys deprived of motor and premotor areas in infancy. *J Neurophysiol* 1938;1:477–496.
36. Lenneberg E. *Biological foundations of language*. New York: Wiley, 1967.
37. Levere ND, Gray-Silva S, Levere TE. Infant brain recovery: the benefit of relocation and the cost of crowding. In: Finger S, Levere TE, Almli CR, et al., eds. *Brain injury and recovery*. New York: Plenum, 1988: 133–150.
38. Hebb DO. Cerebral organization and consciousness. *Res Publ Assoc Res Nerv Mental Dis* 1967;45:1–7.
39. Myer E, Byers R. Measles encephalitis. *Am J Dis Child* 1998;84:853–879.
40. Taylor HG, Alden J. Age-related differences in outcomes following childhood brain insults: an introduction and overview. *J Int Neuropsychol Soc* 1997;3: 555–567.
41. Young B, Rapp RP, Norton JA, et al. Failure of prophylactically administered phenytoin to prevent posttraumatic seizures in children. *Childs Brain* 1983;10: 185–192.
42. Gronwall D, Wrightson P, McGinn V. Effect of mild head injury during the preschool years. *J Int Neuropsychol Soc* 1997;3:592–597.
43. Janowsky J, Finlay B. The outcome of perinatal brain damage: the role of normal neuron loss and axon retraction. *Dev Med Child Neurol* 1986;28:375–389.
44. Bar P. Apoptosis—the cell's silent exit. *Life Sci* 1996; 59:369–378.
45. Huang P, Esquenazi S, Le Roux P. Cerebral cortical neuron apoptosis after mild excitotoxic injury in vitro: different roles of mesencephalic and cortical astrocytes. *Neurosurgery* 1999;45:1413–1422.
46. Ng I, Yeo T, Tang W, et al. Apoptosis occurs after cerebral contusions in humans. *Neurosurgery* 2000;46: 949–956.
47. Bach-y-Rita P. A Conceptual approach to neural recovery. In: Bach-y-Rita P, ed. *Comprehensive neurologic rehabilitation, volume 2: traumatic brain injury*. New York: Demos Publications, 1989:81–85.
48. Rosenzweig MR, Bennett EL, Colombo PJ, et al. Short-term, intermediate-term, and long-term memories. *Behav Brain Res* 1993;57:193–198.
49. Luria AR. The making of mind: a personal account of Soviet psychology. Cambridge, MA: Harvard University Press, 1979.
50. Campbell F, Ramey C. Cognitive and school outcomes for high-risk African-American students at middle adolescence: positive effects of early intervention. *Am Educ Res J* 1995;32:743–772.
51. Swartz K, Liu F, Sewell D, et al. Interleukin-6 promotes post-traumatic healing in the central nervous system. *Brain Res* 2001;896:86–95.
52. Gerbino L, Oleshansky M, Gershon SI. Clinical use and mode of action of lithium. In: Lipton MA, Dimascio A, Killiam KF, eds. *Psychopharmacology: a generation of progress*. New York: Raven Press, 1978:1261–1275.
53. Altshuler LL, Cohen L, Szuba MP. Pharmacologic management of psychiatric illness during pregnancy: dilemmas and guidelines. *Am J Psychiatry* 1996;153: 592–606.
54. Kulin NA, Pastuszak A, Sage SR. Pregnancy outcome following maternal use of selective serotonin reuptake inhibitors. *JAMA* 1998;279:609–610.
55. Robert E. Treating depression in pregnancy. *N Engl J Med* 1996;335:1056–1058.
56. Nulman I, Rovet J, Stewart DE. Neurodevelopment of children exposed in utero to antidepressant drugs. *N Engl J Med* 1997;336:258–262.
57. Spencer M. Fluoxetine hydrochloride dependence in a neonate. *Pediatrics* 1993;92:721–722.
58. Kent L, Laidlaw J. Suspected congenital sertraline dependence [Letter]. *Br J Psychiatry* 1995;167:412–413.
59. Dahl M. Paroxetine withdrawal syndrome in a neonate [Letter]. *Br J Psychiatry* 1997;171:391–392.
60. Breese GR, Mueller RA, Lipton MA. Developmental neuropsychopharmacology. In: Lipton MA, Damasio A, Killam KF, eds. *Psychopharmacology: A Generation of Progress*. New York: Raven Press, 1978: 609–620.
61. Tachibana T. Behavioral teratogenic effect of methylmercury and amphetamine: meta-analysis and power analysis of data from the Collaborative Behavioral Teratology Study of National Center for Toxicological Research. *Teratology* 1989;40:93–100.
62. Rumeau-Rouquette C, Goujard J, Huel G. Possible teratogenic effect of phenothiazines in human beings. *Teratology* 1977;15:57–64.
63. Bernstein JG. *Handbook of drug therapy in psychiatry*, 3rd ed. St. Louis: Mosby, 1995.
64. Laegreld L, Olegard R, Walstrom J, et al. Teratogenic effects of benzodiazepine use during pregnancy. *J Pediatr* 1989;114:126–131.
65. Shapiro S, Hartz SC, Siskind V, et al. Anticonvulsants and parental epilepsy in the development of birth defects. *Lancet* 1976:272–275.
66. Kellogg C, Tervo D, Ison J, et al. Prenatal exposure to diazepam alters behavioral development in rats. *Science* 1980;207:205–207.
67. Gruen RJ. Perinatal diazepam exposure: alterations in exploratory behavior and mesolimbic dopamine turnover. *Pharmacol Biochem Behav* 1990;36:169–175.
68. Calabrese JR, Gulledge AD. Psychotropics during pregnancy and lactation: a review. *Psychosomatics* 1985;26:413–426.
69. Zalzstein E, Koren G, Einarson T, et al. A case-control study on the association between first trimester exposure to lithium and Ebstein's anomaly. *Am J Cardiol* 1990;65: 817–818.
70. Cohen LS, Friedman JM, Jefferson JW, et al. A reevaluation of risk of in utero exposure to lithium. *JAMA* 1994;271:146–150.
71. Hecht JT, Annegers JF. Familial aggregation of epilepsy and clefting disorders: a review of the literature. *Epilepsia* 1990;31:574–577.
72. Steinhausen H-C, Losche G, Koch S, et al. The psychological development of children of epileptic parents. I. Study design and comparative findings. *Acta Paediatr* 1994;83:955–960.
73. Waters CH, Belai Y, Gott PS, et al. Outcomes of pregnancy associated with antiepileptic drugs. *Arch Neurol* 1994;51:250–253.

74. Fishman RH, Yanai J. Long-lasting effects of early barbiturates on central nervous system and behavior. *Neurosci Biobehav Rev* 1983;7:19–28.
75. Gaily EK, Granstrom M, Hiilesmaa VK, et al. Head circumference in children of epileptic mothers: contributions of drug exposure and genetic background. *Epilepsy Res* 1990;5:217–222.
76. Hanson J, Streissguth A, Smith D. The effects of moderate alcohol consumption during pregnancy on fetal growth and morphogenesis. *J Pediatrics* 1978;92: 457–460.
77. Delgado-Escueta AV, Janz D. Consensus guidelines: preconception counseling, management, and care of the pregnant woman with epilepsy. *Neurology* 1992; 42:149–160.
78. Moore S, Turnpenny P, Quinn A, et al. A clinical study of 57 children with fetal anticonvulsant syndromes. *J Med Genet* 2000;37:489–497.
79. Jones KL, Lacro RV, Johnson KA, et al. Pattern of malformations in the children of women treated with carbamazepine during pregnancy. *N Engl J Med* 1989; 320:1661–1666.
80. Rosa FW. Spina bifida in infants of women treated with carbamazepine during pregnancy. *N Engl J Med* 1991;324:674–677.
81. Bennett GD, Amore BM, Finnell RH, et al. Teratogenicity of carbamazepine-10, 11-epoxide and oxcarbazepine in the SWV mouse. *J Pharmacol Exp Ther* 1996;279:1237–1242.
82. Kaneko S, Battino D, Andermann E. Congenital malformations due to antiepileptic drugs. *Epilepsy Res* 1999;33:145–158.
83. Arpino C, Brescianini S, Robert E, et al. Teratogenic effects of antiepileptic drugs: use of an international database on malformations and drug exposure. *Epilepsia* 2000;41:1436–1443.
84. Diaz J, Shields WD. Effects of dipropylacetate on brain development. *Ann Neurol* 1981;10:465–468.
85. Oakeshott P, Hunt GM. Valproate and spina bifida. *BMJ* 1989;298:1300–1301.
86. Losche G, Steinhausen H-C, Koch S, et al. The psychological development of children of epileptic parents. II. The differential impact of intrauterine exposure to anticonvulsant drugs and further influential factors. *Acta Paediatr* 1994;83:961–966.
87. Koch S, Titze K, Zimmerman RB, et al. Long-term neuropsychological consequences of maternal epilepsy and anticonvulsant treatment during pregnancy for school-age children and adolescents. *Epilepsia* 1999;40:1237–1243.
88. Dansky LV, Andermann E, Rosenblatt D, et al. Anticonvulsants, folate levels, and pregnancy outcome: a prospective study. *Ann Neurol* 1987;21:176–182.
89. Bower C. Epilepsy in pregnancy: neural tube defects and folate. *Med J Aust* 1994;160:56–57.
90. Estus S, Blumer JL. Role of microtubule assembly in phenytoin teratogenic action in the sea urchin (*Arbacia punctulata*) embryo. *Mol Pharmacol* 1989;36: 708–715.
91. Ransom BR, Elmore JG. Effects of antiepileptic drugs on the developing central nervous system. *Adv Neurol* 1991;55:225–237.
92. Cotariu D, Zaidman JL. Minireview: developmental toxicity of valproic acid. *Life Sci* 1991;48:1341–1350.
93. Kaneko S, Otani K, Kondo T, et al. Malformation in infants of mothers with epilepsy receiving antiepileptic drugs. *Neurology* 1992;42:68–74.
94. Azarbayjani F, Danielsson BR. Pharmacologically induced embryonic dysrhythmia and episodes of hypoxia followed by reoxygenation: a common teratogenic mechanism for antiepileptic drugs? *Teratology* 1998;57:117–126.
95. Walmod PS, Foley A, Berezin A, et al. Cell motility is inhibited by the antiepileptic compound, valproic acid and its teratogenic analogues. *Cell Motil Cytoskel* 1998;40:220–237.
96. Walmod PS, Skladchikova G, Kawa A, et al. Antiepileptic teratogen valproic acid (VPA) modulates organisation and dynamics of the actin cytoskeleton. *Cell Motil Cytoskel* 1999;42:241–255.
97. Beck SL. Does genomic imprinting contribute to valproic acid teratogenicity. *Reprod Toxicol* 2001;15: 43–48.
98. Hausman RE, Bonincontro A, Cametti C, et al. Rescue of the Li+-induced delay of embryonic myogenesis in vitro by added inositol. *Biochim Biophys Acta* 1989; 1013:92–96.
99. Di Luca M, Caputi A, Cattabeni F. Synaptic protein phosphorylation changes in animals exposed to neurotoxicants during development. *Neurotoxicology* 1994; 15:525–532.
100. Mills JL, Holmes LB, Aarons J, et al. Moderate caffeine use and the risk of spontaneous abortion and intrauterine growth retardation. *JAMA* 1993;269: 593–597.
101. Nehlig A, Debry G. Potential teratogenic and neurodevelopmental consequences of coffee and caffeine exposure: a review on human and animal data. *Neurotoxicol Teratol* 1994;16:531–543.
102. Santos IS, Victora CG, Huttly S, et al. Caffeine intake and low birth weight: a population-based case-control study. *Am J Epidemiol* 1998;147:620–627.
103. Eskenazi B, Stapleton AL, Kharrazi M, et al. Associations between maternal decaffeinated and caffeinated coffee consumption and fetal growth and gestational duration. *Epidemiology* 1999;10:242–249.
104. Economides D, Braithwaite J. Smoking, pregnancy and the fetus. *J R Soc Health* 1994;114:198–201.
105. Fielding JE. Smoking: health effects and control (first of two parts). *N Engl J Med* 1985;313:491–498.
106. Ellard GA, Johnstone FD, Prescott RJ, et al. Smoking during pregnancy: the dose dependence of birthweight deficits. *Br J Obstet Gynecol* 1996;103:806–813.
107. Lambers DS, Clark KE. The maternal and fetal physiologic effects of nicotine. *Semin Perinatol* 1996;20: 115–126.
108. Slotkin TA. Fetal nicotine or cocaine exposure: which one is worse? *J Pharmacol Exp Ther* 1998;285: 931–945.
109. Oliff HS, Gallardo KA. The effect of nicotine on developing brain catecholamine systems. *Frontiers Biosci* 1999;4:883–897.
110. Slawecki CJ, Thomas JD, Riley EP, et al. Neonatal nicotine exposure alters hippocampal EEG and event-related potentials (ERPs) in rats. *Pharmacol Biochem Behav* 2000;65:711–718.
111. Levin ED, Briggs SJ, Christopher NC, et al. Prenatal nicotine exposure and cognitive performance in rats. *Neurotoxicol Teratol* 1993;15:251–260.
112. Cutler AR, Wilkerson AE, Gingras JL, et al. Prenatal

cocaine and/or nicotine exposure in rats: preliminary findings on long-term cognitive outcome and genital development at birth. *Neurotoxicol Teratol* 1996;18: 635–643.

113. Naeye RL, Peters EC. Mental development of children whose mothers smoked during pregnancy. *J Am Coll Obstet Gynecol* 1984;64:601–607.
114. Weissman MM, Warner V, Wickramaratne PJ, et al. Maternal smoking during pregnancy and psychopathology in offspring followed to adulthood. *J Am Acad Child Psychiatry* 1999;38:892–899.
115. Kandel DB, Udry JR. Prenatal effects of maternal smoking on daughter's smoking: nicotine or testosterone exposure? *Am J Public Health* 1999;89: 1377–1383.
116. Rush D, Callahan K. Exposure to passive cigarette smoking and child development. A critical review. *Ann N Y Acad Sci* 1989;562:74–100.
117. Bauman K, Koch G, Fisher L. Family cigarette smoking and test performance by adolescents. *Health Psychol* 1989;8:97–105.
118. Bauman K, Flewelling R, LaPrelle J. Parental cigarette smoking and cognitive performance of children. *Health Psychol* 1991;10:282–288.
119. American Academy of Pediatrics. Committee on Substance Abuse and Committee on Children With Disabilities. Fetal alcohol syndrome and alcohol-related neurodevelopmental disorders. *Pediatrics* 2000;106: 358–361.
120. Lemoine P, Lemoine P. Outcome of children of alcoholic mothers (study of 105 cases followed to adult age) and various prophylactic findings. *Ann Pediatr (Paris)* 1992;39:226–235.
121. Jones K, Smith D, Ulleland C, et al. Pattern of malformation in offspring of chronic alcoholic mothers. *Lancet* 1973;1267–1271.
122. Clarren S, Smith D. The fetal alcohol syndrome. *N Engl J Med* 1978;298:1063–1067.
123. Streissguth A, Aase J, Clarren S, et al. Fetal alcohol syndrome in adolescents and adults. *JAMA* 1991; 265:1961–1967.
124. Mills J, Graubard B, Harley E, et al. Maternal alcohol consumption and birth weight: How much drinking during pregnancy is safe? *JAMA* 1984;252:1875–1879.
125. Jacobson J, Jacobson S. Drinking moderately and pregnancy. Effects on child development. *Alcohol Res Health* 1999;23:25–30.
126. Sampson P, Streissguth A, Bookstein F, et al. On categorizations in analyses of alcohol teratogenesis. *Environ Health Perspect* 2000;108:421–428.
127. Dow K, Riopelle R. Neurotoxicity of ethanol during prenatal development. *Clin Neuropharmacol* 1987;10: 330–341.
128. Roebuck T, Mattson S, Riley E. A review of the neuroanatomical findings in children with fetal alcohol syndrome or prenatal exposure to alcohol. *Alcohol Clin Exp Res* 1998;22:339–344.
129. Riikonen R, Salonen I, Partanen K, et al. Brain perfusion SPECT and MRI in fetal alcohol syndrome. *Dev Med Child Neurol* 1999;41:652–659.
130. Hoyseth K, Jones P. Minireview: ethanol induced teratogenesis: characterization, mechanisms, and diagnostic approaches. *Life Sci* 1989;44:643–649.
131. Heaton M, Mitchell J, Paiva M. Amelioration of ethanol-induced neurotoxicity in the neonatal rat central nervous system by antioxidant therapy 48. *Alcohol Clin Exp Res* 2000;24:512–518.
132. Ikonomidou C, Bittigau P, Ishimaru M, et al. Ethanol-induced apoptotic neurodegeneration and fetal alcohol syndrome. *Science* 2000;287:1056–1060.
133. Steinhausen H, Nestler V, Spohr H. Development and psychopathology of children with the fetal alcohol syndrome. *Dev Behav Pediatr* 1982;3:49–54.
134. Streissguth A, Bookstein F, Sampson P, et al. Neurobehavioral effects of prenatal alcohol: part III. PLS analyses of neuropsychologic tests. *Neurotoxicol Teratol* 1989;11:493–507.
135. Steinhausen H, Willms J, Spohr H. Long-term psychopathological and cognitive outcome of children with fetal alcohol syndrome. *J Am Acad Child Psychiatry* 1993;32:990–994.
136. Harris S, MacKay L, Osborn J. Autistic behaviors in offspring of mothers abusing alcohol and other drugs: a series of case reports. *Alcohol Clin Exp Res* 1995; 19:660–665.
137. Olson H, Feldman J, Streissguth A, et al. Neuropsychological deficits in adolescents with fetal alcohol syndrome: clinical findings. *Alcohol Clin Exp Res* 1998;22:1998–2012.
138. Chasnoff I, Burns W, Schnoll S, et al. Cocaine use in pregnancy. *N Engl J Med* 1985;313:666–669.
139. Roland E, Volpe J. Effect of maternal cocaine use on the fetus and newborn: review of the literature. *Pediatr Neurosci* 1989;15:88–94.
140. Kosofsky B. Cocaine-induced alterations in neuro-development. *Semin Speech Lang* 1998;19:109–121.
141. Singer L, Arendt R, Minnes S, et al. Neurobehavioral outcomes of cocaine-exposed infants. *Neurotoxicol Teratol* 2000;22:653–666.
142. Martin J, Barr H, Martin D, et al. Neonatal neurobehavioral outcome following prenatal exposure to cocaine. *Neurotoxicol Teratol* 1996;18:617–625.
143. Eyler F, Behnke M, Conlon M, et al. Birth outcome from a prospective, matched study of prenatal crack/cocaine use: I. Interactive and dose effects on health and growth. *Pediatrics* 1998;101:229–237.
144. Chasnoff I, Anson A, Hatcher R, et al. Prenatal exposure to cocaine and other drugs. Outcome at four to six years. *Ann N Y Acad Sci* 1998;846:314–328.
145. Koren G, Nulman I, Rovet J, et al. Long-term neurodevelopmental risks in children exposed in utero to cocaine. The Toronto Adoption Study. *Ann N Y Acad Sci* 1998;846:306–313.
146. Johnson J, Leff M. Children of substance abusers: overview of research findings. *Pediatrics* 1999;103: 1085–1099.
147. Delaney-Black V, Covington C, Templin T, et al. Teacher-assessed behavior of children prenatally exposed to cocaine. *Pediatrics* 2000;106:782–791.
148. Henderson M, McMillen B. Effects of prenatal exposure to cocaine or related drugs on rat developmental and neurological indices. *Brain Res Bull* 1990;24: 207–212.
149. Byrnes J, Pritchard G, Koff J, et al. Prenatal cocaine exposure: decreased sensitization to cocaine and decreased striatal dopamine transporter binding in offspring. *Neuropharmacology* 1993;32:721–723.
150. Olsen G. Potential mechanisms of cocaine-induced developmental neurotoxicity: a minireview. *Neurotoxicology* 1995;16:159–167.

151. Weissman A, Caldecott-Hazard S. In utero methamphetamine effects: I. Behavior and monoamine uptake sites in adult offspring. *Synapse* 1993;13:241–250.
152. Schuster C, Lewis M, Seiden L. Fenfluramine: neurotoxicity. *Psychopharmacol Bull* 1986;11:148–149.
153. Molliver D, Molliver M. Anatomic evidence for a neurotoxic effect of (+/–)-fenfluramine upon serotonergic projections in the rat. *Brain Res* 1990;511:165–168.
154. Day N, Richardson G. Prenatal marijuana use: epidemiology, methodologic issues, and infant outcome. *Clin Perinatol* 1991;18:77–91.
155. English D, Hulse G, Milne E, et al. Maternal cannabis use and birth weight: a meta-analysis. *Addiction* 1997; 92:1553–1560.
156. Balle J, Olofsson M, Hilden J. [Cannabis and pregnancy]. *Ugeskr Laeger* 1999;161:5024–5028.
157. Fried P, Watkinson B, Gray R. Growth from birth to early adolescence in offspring prenatally exposed to cigarettes and marijuana. *Neurotoxicol Teratol* 1999; 21:513–525.
158. Fried P. Marihuana use by pregnant women and effects on offspring: an update. *Neurobehav Toxicol Teratol* 1982;4:451–454.
159. Parker S, Zuckerman B, Bauchner H, et al. Jitteriness in full-term neonates: prevalence and correlates. *Pediatrics* 1990;85:17–23.
160. Fried P. Prenatal exposure to marihuana and tobacco during infancy, early and middle childhood: effects and an attempt at synthesis. *Arch Toxicol Suppl* 1995; 17:233–260.
161. Fried P, Watkinson B, Gray R. Differential effects on cognitive functioning in 9- to 12-year olds prenatally exposed to cigarettes and marihuana. *Neurotoxicol Teratol* 1998;20:293–306.
162. Wilson G, McCreary R, Kean J, et al. The development of preschool children of heroin-addicted mothers: a controlled study. *Pediatrics* 1979;63:135–141.
163. Householder J, Hatcher R, Burns W, et al. Infants born to narcotic-addicted mothers. *Psychol Bull* 1982;92: 453–468.
164. O'Dougherty M, Wright F, Loewenson R, et al. Cerebral dysfunction after chronic hypoxia in children. *Neurology* 1985;35:42–46.
165. Lozoff B, Jimenez E, Wolf A. Long-term developmental outcome of infants with iron deficiency. *N Engl J Med* 1991;325:687–694.
166. Smith M. Intellectual and behavioural consequences of low level lead exposure: a review of recent studies. *Clin Endocrinol Metab* 1985;14:657–680.
167. Menkes JH. *Textbook of child neurology*, 2nd ed. Philadelphia: Lea & Febiger, 1980.
168. Needleman HL, Riess JA, Tobin MJ, et al. Bone lead levels and delinquent behavior. *JAMA* 1996;275: 363–369.
169. Needleman HL, Rabinowitz M, Leviton A, et al. The relationship between prenatal exposure to lead and congenital anomalies. *JAMA* 1984;251:2956–2959.
170. Faust D, Brown J. Moderately elevated blood lead levels: effects on neuropsychologic functioning in children. *Pediatrics* 1987;80:623–629.
171. Needleman HL, Gatsonis CA. Low-level lead exposure and the IQ of children. *JAMA* 1990;263:673–678.
172. Needleman HL, Gatsonis CA. Low-level lead exposure and the IQ of children: a meta-analysis of modern studies. *JAMA* 1990;263:673–678.
173. Stokes L, Letz R, Gerr F, et al. Neurotoxicity in young adults 20 years after childhood exposure to lead: the Bunker Hill experience. *Occup Environ Med* 1998;55: 507–516.
174. Lucchini R, Albini E, Cortesi I, et al. Assessment of neurobehavioral performance as a function of current and cumulative occupational lead exposure. *Neurotoxicology* 2000;21:805–811.
175. Meyer-Baron M, Seeber A. A meta-analysis for neurobehavioural results due to occupational lead exposure with blood lead concentrations <70 microg/100ml. *Arch Toxicol* 2000;73:510–518.
176. Westbrook G. Seizures and epilepsy. In: Kandel E, Schwartz J, Jessell T, eds. *Principles of neural science*, 4th ed. New York: McGraw-Hill, 2000:910–935.
177. Finkelstein Y, Markowitz ME, Rosen JF. Low-level lead-induced neurotoxicity in children: an update on central nervous system effects. *Brain Res Rev* 1998; 27:168–176.
178. Verity MA. Comparative observations on inorganic and organic lead neurotoxicity. *Environ Health Perspect* 1990;89:43–48.
179. Hong W, Candelone J-P, Patterson CC, et al. Greenland ice evidence of hemispheric lead pollution two millennia ago by Greek and Roman civilizations. *Science* 1994;265:1841–1843.
180. Ericson JE, Shirahata HMS, Patterson CC. Skeletal concentrations of lead in ancient Peruvians. *N Engl J Med* 1979;300:946–951.
181. Nevin R. How lead exposure relates to temporal change in IQ, violent crime, and unwed pregnancy. *Environ Res* 2000;83:1–22.
182. Silbergeld EK. Mechanisms of lead neurotoxicity, or looking beyond the lamppost. *FASEB J* 1992;6: 3201–3206.
183. Rautonen J, Koskiniemi M, Vaheri A. Prognostic factors in childhood acute encephalitis. *Pediatr Infect Dis J* 1991;10:441–446.
184. Kohl S. A hypothesis on the pathophysiology of neonatal herpes simplex virus encephalitis: clinical recurrence after asymptomatic primary infection. *Pediatr Infect Dis J* 1990;9:307–308.
185. Gutman LT, Wilfert CM, Eppes S. *Herpes simplex* virus encephalitis in children: analysis of cerebrospinal fluid and progressive neurodevelopmental deterioration. *J Infect Dis* 1986;154:415–421.
186. Kimura H, Kosaburo A, Kuzushima K, et al. Relapse of *Herpes simplex* encephalitis in children. *Pediatrics* 1992;89:891–894.
187. Poser CM. Notes on the pathogenesis of subacute sclerosing panencephalitis. *J Neurol Sci* 1990;95:219–224.
188. Ziring PR. Psychiatric sequelae of the 1964–65 rubella epidemic. *Psychiatr Ann* 1978;8:57–69.
189. Desmond MM, Wilson GS, Vorderman AL, et al. The health and educational status of adolescents with congenital rubella syndrome. *Dev Med Child Neurol* 1985;27:721–729.
190. Chappell PB, Riddle MA, Scahill L, et al. Guanfacine treatment of comorbid attention-deficit hyperactivity disorder and Tourette's syndrome: preliminary clinical experience. *J Am Acad Child Adolesc Psychiatry* 1995; 34:1140–1146.
191. Chambers CD, Johnson KA, Dick LM. Birth outcomes in women taking fluoxetine. *N Engl J Med* 1996;335: 1010–1015.

192. Damasio AR, VanHoesen GW. The limbic system and the localisation of *Herpes simplex* encephalitis. *J Neurol Neurosurg Psychiatry* 1985;48:297–301.
193. Van Hout A, Lyon G. Wernicke's aphasia in a 10-year-old boy. *Brain Lang* 1986;29:268–285.
194. Pietrini V, Nertempi P, Vaglia A, et al. Recovery from herpes simplex encephalitis: selective impairment of specific semantic categories with neuroradiological correlation. *J Neurol Neurosurg Psychiatry* 1988;51: 1284–1293.
195. Pradham S, Singh MN, Pandey N. Kluver Bucy syndrome in young children. *Clin Neurol Neurosurg* 1998;100:254–258.
196. Utley TF, Ogden JA, Gibb A, et al. The long-term neuropsychological outcome of herpes simplex encephalitis in a series of unselected survivors. *Neuropsychiatry Neuropsychol Behav Neurol* 1997;10:180–189.
197. Fujii T, Yamadori A, Endo K, et al. Disproportionate retrograde amnesia in a patient with herpes simplex encephalitis. *Cortex* 1999;35:599–614.
198. Preblud SR, Stetler HC, Frank JA Jr, et al. Fetal risk associated with rubella vaccine. *JAMA* 1981;246: 1413–1424.
199. Koskiniemi M, Vaheri A. Effect of measles, mumps, rubella vaccination on pattern of encephalitis in children. *Lancet* 1989;31–34.
200. Mancini J, Chabrol B, Moulene E, et al. Relapsing acute encephalopathy: a complication of diptheria-tetanus-poliomyelitis immunization in a young boy. *Eur J Pediatr* 1996;155:136–138.
201. MMWR.Update: vaccine side effects, adverse reactions, contraindications, and precautions. Recommendations of the Advisory Committee on Immunization Practices. *MMWR Morb Mortal Wkly Rep* 1996;45:1–35.
202. Weibel RE, Caserta V, Benor DE, et al. Acute encephalopathy followed by permanent brain injury or death associated with further attenuated measles vaccines: a review of claims submitted to the National Vaccine Injury Compensation Program. *Pediatrics* 1998;101:383–387.
203. Cowan LD, Griffin MR, Howson CP, et al. Acute encephalopathy and chronic neurological damage after pertussis vaccine. *Vaccine* 1993;11:1371–1379.
204. Singh VK, Lin SX, Yang VC. Serological association of measles virus and human herpesvirus-6 with brain autoantibodies in autism. *Clin Immunol Immunopathol* 1998;1:105–108.
205. Connolly AM, Chez MG, Pestronk A, et al. Serum autoantibodies to brain in Landau-Kleffner variant, autism, and other neurologic disorders. *J Pediatr* 1999; 134:607–613.
206. Dales L, Hammer SJ, Smith NJ. Time trends in autism and in MMR immunization coverage in California. *JAMA* 2001;285:1183–1185.
207. Gale JL, Thapa PB, Wassilak SG, et al. Risk of serious acute neurological illness after immunization with diphtheria-tetanus-pertussis vaccine. A population-based case-control study. *JAMA* 1994;271: 37–41.
208. Stratton KR, Howe CJ, Johnston RB Jr. Adverse events associated with childhood vaccines other than pertussis and rubella. *JAMA* 1994;271:1602–1605.
209. Khan A, Mirolo MH, Claypoole K, et al. Low-dose thyrotropin-releasing hormone effects in cognitively impaired alcoholics. *Alcohol Clin Exp Res* 1993;17: 791–796.
210. Castresana-Isla CJ, Herrera-Martinez G, Vega-Molina J. Erythema nodosum and Takayasu's arteritis after immunization with plasma derived hepatitis B vaccine. *J Rheumatol* 1993;20:1417–1418.
211. Hayase Y, Tobita K. Influenza virus and neurological disease. *Psychiatry Clin Neurosci* 1997;51:181–184.

3

Mental Retardation

Of all Persons who are Objects of our Charity, none move my Compassion, like those whom it has pleas'd God to leave in a full state of Health and Strength, but depriv'd of Reason to act for themselves. And it is, in my opinion, one of the greatest Scandals upon the Understanding of others, to mock at those who want it. Upon this account I think the Hospital we call Bedlam, to be a Noble Foundation; a visible Instance of the sense our Ancestors had of the greatest Unhappiness which can befal Human Kind: Since as the Soul in Man distinguishes him from a Brute. So where the Soul is dead (for so it is to acting) no Brute so much a Beast as a Man. But since never to have it, and to have lost it, are synonymous in the Effect, I wonder how it came to pass, that in the Settlement of that Hospital, they made no provision for Persons born without the use of their Reason, such as we call Fools, or more properly, Naturals. We use such in England with the last Contempt, which I think is a strange Error, since tho' they are useless to the Commonwealth, they are only so by God's direct Providence, and no previous Fault. I think 'twould very well become this Wise Age to take care of such: And perhaps they are a particular Rent-Charge on the Great Family of Mankind, left by the Maker of us all; like a Younger Brother, who tho' the Estate be given from him, yet his Father expected the Heir should take some care of him.

If I were to be ask'd, Who ought in particular to be charg'd with this Work? I would answer in general, Those who have a Portion of Understanding extraordinary: Not that I would lay a Tax upon any man's Brains, or discourage Wit, by appointing Wise Men to maintain Fools: But some Tribute is due to God's Goodness for bestowing Extraordinary Gifts; and who can it better be paid to, than such as suffer for want of the same Bounty? (Daniel Defoe, 1697)

SUMMARY

Human beings have been caring for their disabled since prehistoric times. The fossil record indicates that people with what must have been severe brain injuries were able to survive and to live for many years in the most primitive societies, even in the time of the Neanderthals. Caring for the helpless is not an invention of the modern sensibility. It was fundamental to the spirit of cooperation and trust that guided the evolution of intelligent primates.

Not every human society in historical times espoused this virtue with equal assiduity. The Greeks and Romans, for example, whom we admire for their many accomplishments, practiced infanticide without compunction. In the West, it was not until the ascendancy of the Judeo-Christians that the unique value of each individual was firmly established, irrespective of his or her ability to contribute to the material well-being of society. The people of the Book, however, have not always lived up to their beliefs. Their attitudes toward the mentally retarded have not always been charitable, and their behavior was only slowly elevated to a level concordant with their professed faith.

Since the Middle Ages, the medical approach to mental retardation has been occupied mainly with issues of classification and etiologic factors. It is only in the past two centuries, and especially over the past 50 years, that real and enduring progress has been made in the service of education and treatment for the retarded. The extraordinary material prosperity of the postwar democracies has permitted the diversion of more than the usual pittance on behalf of the most severely disabled, but not much more than a pittance, and even this required vigorous interventions by organizations of parents and friends of the retarded.

The modern science of mental retardation has moved well beyond the sterile exercise of classification. The study of the causes of mental retardation has occupied the most fertile minds in genetics, biochemistry, and developmental neurobiology. Many of their discoveries have had a bearing on our understanding of the genetic and neural bases of behavior, as seen in Chapters 11–13.

MENTAL RETARDATION

With respect to classification, the ability to acquire effective language that distinguishes mildly mentally retarded people from the severely retarded is demonstrated. The presentation of neuropsychiatric conditions is very different in these two groups.

Twenty years ago, I was a young and aspiring academic and was given an assignment to escort the Grand Rounds speaker to dinner. I invited a couple of young, aspiring colleagues who promised to be good company. At the time, I was deeply involved in a research project that had to do with some of the neuropsychiatric problems of mentally retarded people. Tardive dyskinesia was one, and self-injury was another. Not necessarily dinner conversation, but then there were plenty of other things to talk about, mainly what our eminent speaker was up to.

It was pleasant enough for a while, but then one of the guests turned belligerent. A glass of wine can do that to some people. "Why," she said, condescendingly, "are you spending your career working with mentally retarded people? What can a psychiatrist possibly hope to accomplish with them that might do any good? After all, whatever you do, they're still going to be retarded."

I have never been particularly quick in verbal repartee and only remember stammering something defensive, or unbelieving, or both. It was an awkward moment, but the out-of-town guest rose to the occasion and changed the subject. The evening was redeemed, as best one might hope, given my poor choice for company. There are some people whom you just cannot invite to nice places.

This pithy vignette came to mind as I tried to present an introduction to the topic of mental retardation for psychiatrists. One usually begins a monograph like this with a series of definitions, a section on epidemiology and pathophysiology, and a few choice introductory remarks that segue into the main course. Another way to begin is to use a historical perspective, but it occurred to me that any serious discussion of severely disabled people should begin from a different direction, that is, to examine the problem of caring for the most severely disabled people. It has always been a low priority in the history of medicine in particular and in the history of human societies in general. It has usually been something that we have left to the saintly because the worldly rest of us have had more important things to do.

Now, I am no saint, but Defoe's suggestion, that some "tribute is due to God's Goodness for bestowing Extraordinary Gifts," has always struck a resonant cord. I might have recalled his words on that particular evening, but I suppose it was so deeply ingrained in my being as a physician that it was beyond articulation. Not that I have many extraordinary gifts to boast of, or any, for that matter, but compared with my little brother, who is profoundly retarded, I am a veritable polymath. Thus, the why of my gifts and his deprivation has been with me since earliest childhood. The imbalance of it was something that no little boy could understand. I still cannot. But Daniel Defoe urged us to pay some tribute, and I have tried.

So many of the people I know who work in child neurology, psychology, or special education have been influenced by the early experience of a handicapped sibling. Psychiatrists understand that; so many of us have entered the field because of an afflicted relative. We do ourselves a disservice when we attribute that to a neurotic impulse. I think that we have been influenced by a much more straightforward motivation. The near experience of extreme deprivation leads us to appreciate that a sound mind and a sound intellect are not, by any means, our birthright. They are, from one perspective, gifts; from another, the lucky roll of the dice. In either event, we have done nothing to earn them. The best we can do is to appreciate our good fortune and have the grace to pay some back. That is why many, if not most of us, have become psychiatrists, and why some of us actually like to work with severely disabled people.

It is a perfectly natural thing. A casual reading of history might incline the reader to think that caring for the severely disabled is something that does not come naturally to human societies, but, in fact, it is always something people have tried to do. We have just never done it very well, at least, until recently.

By the same token, it is a mistake to aver that the natural human reaction to severe disability is antipathetic. People who work with handicapped learn what the handicapped know too well, that the world is full of slights and barriers, cruel remarks and thoughtless people. Would that they were ill-intended; it would be that much easier to shame the world to do better. The severely handicapped are not despised; they just have the ill luck to be at the bottom of almost everyone's priority list. They have been the perennial victims of thoughtlessness rather than evil intention, of the moral poverty of society rather than its depravity. Daniel Defoe was only asking a rhetorical question when he wondered "how it came to pass...they made no Provision for Persons born without the use of their Reason." That the Hospital at Bedlam did as much as it did for the mentally ill, that society might develop even one humane institution, is a credit to our capacity for moral improvement. That it did not do more should not be the occasion for recrimination. It was a sign that society was trying to shed its ignorance; it was still an ignorant society. It was a sign that society had wealth to spend on something worthwhile; it was still a poor and struggling society. It is easy to be moralistic about past failings. In fact, it is more interesting, and more important, to reflect on why such an advance in our social conscience went so far, but no further.

If one were to study the history of mental retardation, the question that my erstwhile dinner guest raised recurs as an enduring theme. There are so many competing priorities for our charitable endeavors, how can we afford to elevate the interests of a class of people whose lives seem destined to be nothing if not brutish and short? The pursuit of scientific inquiry is so exquisite and so likely of success in so many dimensions, why should we channel its resources on behalf of those who are bereft of reason and destined to remain so? The best resources of medical science have been devoted to preventing mental handicap, not to treating the condition.

We cannot afford to dismiss such questions. They have to be met with respectful argument. It is necessary to address any niggardly view of the resources of the human heart, the timid belief that we can do so much and no more; that the resources of society are so limited that they can only be lavished on children who are likely to grow up; and the baleful view that medical science exists only for the sake of reward and that there is no tribute owed by those who are so well endowed. The proper study of humankind is, in large part, the study of that which lies beneath our reason. We are fortunate to live in an era that is coming to realize that the right measure of a society is how it measures the lives of its least members. We are richer and we are less ignorant and we are doing a better job of paying the tribute that we owe.

A PERSPECTIVE FROM PALEOBIOLOGY

Inasmuch as you have done it unto one of the least of these my brethren, ye have done it unto me. (Matthew, 25:40)

Human societies may be judged on their merits or their failings, just as people are. They are judged by history, usually on the basis of their external achievements. That, of course, is natural and understandable, but it is one of the fallacies of history and one reason why we pay history so little heed. It is a sterile and empty endeavor, as if we were to judge the value of an individual person simply in terms of what he or she had accomplished in material terms. The success of a human society is measured only to a small degree by its acquisitions, its artfulness, or the cleverness of its invention. The trust and kindness that join its members are the foundation of human society. It is the matrix for social organization, and without it there is no art, invention, or acquisition. The best way to judge whether a society of people is successful is the degree to which it nurtures and protects.

This is not simply a confessional point of view. Trust, protection, and nurturance are the psychological roots that gave rise to our existence as a species. They are our evolutionary foundation. Let us take a small digression on that point.

One of the signal problems in paleoanthropology has been to explain how large-brained homo sapiens evolved from the arboreal and ape-brained australopithecine, a particularly successful species that existed in Africa, largely unchanged, for a million and a half years. Then, approximately two million years ago, the first hominids appeared. They were large brained and fully bipedal, with the beginnings of a complex social structure and the capacity to fabricate tools.

The evolution of large brains and of human intelligence only happened because the first hominid were able to cooperate in the care of infants that were born less mature and more helpless than those of any other primate. A large-brained infant challenged the capacity of the primate birthing process—the "obstetric dilemma." The pelvis of a bipedal primate only allows the passage of a very small cranium. If that head is to contain a large brain, the infant must necessarily be born prematurely. Compared with other primates, the human newborn is 12 weeks premature. Even as the child's brain grows at an extraordinary rate in the first 12 months of life, his body is helpless, and the mother who takes care of him is equally helpless.

It was a signal, arguably miraculous, transformation that induced our African Eve to take that risk, and an equally unlikely event that led the males of her band to abide her experiment, indeed, to encourage her. She was larger, relative to the male of the species, than primate females had ever been. So presumably, she was better equipped to endure the risk of carrying a helpless infant; better equipped, one supposes, to assert maternal protectiveness as a social value for the band. Over a relatively short period of time, in evolutionary terms, but over many generations nevertheless, the hominid female grew progressively in size. Her offspring were born with larger brains but bodies that were woefully immature. The men in her tribe developed the capacity to cooperate to provide for the women and infants. It is hardly a mystery why, in the origins of our kind, trust, kindness, and cooperation anteceded the birth of intelligence, and, in fact, brought it to life (1).

Trust, kindness, and cooperation are such elemental components of all human societies that we tend to take them for granted, even to the point of forgetting how elemental they are. Therefore, in the study of history, we concentrate on pyramids and other such monuments even as we know that

> *Nothing beside remains. Round the decay*
> *Of that colossal wreck, boundless and bare*
> *The lone and level sands stretch far away.*
> *(Shelley)*

It is appropriate to reiterate this paleobiologic variant of the creation myth in a monograph devoted to the problem of mental handicap. Even today, it is necessary to defend the importance of these, the least of my brethren. Not that anyone would seriously argue that the value of severely disabled people was, in fact, metal of smaller worth. Rather, we have to remind ourselves every day that the allure of acquisition, art, and invention can grow into infatuation, that the exercise of intelligence itself can be intoxicating. Healers, in particular, can be so subsumed by their art that they spend their time working wonders. There is nothing wonderful about treating patients who never seem to get better. It is not that they are less valuable as people, just that they are a lower priority as patients.

No one will argue that a disabled child is less worthwhile than a healthy child. We must remind ourselves that they are beings of equal worth. It is easy to suggest that that comes naturally. The birth of a child with severe disabilities does indeed tax our capacity for good feeling and optimism. In the starkest terms, the birth of such a child violates the hope that attends new issue. It is the occasion, even among people of good will, for disappointment, grief, and anger. It does not come naturally to accept such an event as a signal of providential blessing. We look forward to the birth of a child for its promise of a limitless, perfect future. The birth of a disabled child dashes that promise from the very beginning. It conveys nothing more than the requirement to exercise continual, and unrequited, nurturance, protection, and charity. Most parents of handicapped children ultimately accept that gift with resignation, if not with grace. They are like the man whom Abraham Lincoln told about in one of his stories. For some transgression, he was tarred and feathered and ridden out of town on a rail. When they asked him how he felt about it, he said, "If it weren't for the honor, I'd rather have taken the train."

Psychiatrists are quite accustomed to dealing with our least brethren. They know all about how difficult it is to nurture without much hope, to protect the dangerous and unsavory, and to be charitable with little expectation of return. They certainly have enough patients whose mental problems have left them beyond the pale of normal social intercourse. Psychiatry has always been an activist field, devoted to treatment above all, and always optimistic that the treatments it had to offer were going to be successful—for better or worse, from the moral treatment of the nineteenth century to "direct analysis" and frontal lobotomies for schizophrenics, even before the era of psychotropic drugs. Treatment was what psychiatrists liked to do.

It is possible that the activist bent of our field has left us aground in dealing with the problems of the mentally handicapped. There never seemed to be anything that one could do. That, of course, was never really true, and it certainly is not true today. Modern psychiatry is one of the most important medical specialties for mentally handicapped individuals and for patients with brain injury in general. In turn, the study of neuropsychiatric problems in the handicapped is one of the most fertile areas for new development in neuropsychiatry. Psychiatry for the mentally handicapped is different, of course, but for that very reason, it is well worth studying.

HISTORY OF MENTAL RETARDATION

The evolution of *Homo sapiens* was associated with fundamental changes in the social organization that had characterized earlier primate societies. It comprised four essential elements: the adoption of a terrestrial rather than an arboreal habitat, thus increasing the vulnerability of the hominid band to predators; a prolonged period of infantile helplessness, which required a degree of parental investment in their offspring that is unique among mammals; an increase in the size of females relative to males, which was necessary to increase the strength and competence of the band and, presumably increased the relative weight of "maternal" psychology; and an increase in cooperation between male and female and between male and male. The care of infants and children in a new and hostile environment was the function of a new psychology characterized by trust and cooperation, kindness, and charity.

There is some evidence from the prehistoric remains of early humans and even Neanderthals that disabled individuals were cared for, participated in, and were valued by their small bands of fellows. Skeletal remains indicate that people with severe brain injuries were able to survive and recover and to live for years even in the most hostile environments, for example, in Ice Age Europe, where the Neanderthals lived, and in the high Andes. Even disabilities that were clearly congenital in nature could be tolerated—remarkable when one considers the low margin of surplus resources possessed by prehistoric bands. One must suppose that the division of labor left at least some duties available, even for disabled people. Alternatively, they may have been held in esteem as divine intermediaries of some sort.

It is important to emphasize that charity toward the handicapped is not exclusively a function of wealth or advanced civilization. Infanticide and exposure were of course prevalent in the ancient world. They remained so, even through the Roman era. The early Egyptians and Sumerians were known to be protective of children in general, but there is no indication of laws or admonitions to protect the disabled. Nevertheless, there are sufficient data to indicate at least a measure of kindness toward the disabled, even in the prehistoric world. The Hebrew Bible is nowhere explicit on the matter of mental handicap, but there are clear directives in the Torah to protect the poor and the helpless.

In the Western civilization, the renunciation of infanticide and the admonition to care for the disabled are inextricably linked to the triumph of Judaic and Christian values. Pagan emperors like Augustus, Vespasian, Trajan, and Nerva had tried to discourage infanticide, to encourage family care, and to open hospitals and homes for the disabled, but cruelty and indifference to human life were the prevailing attitudes of the Roman Empire. One may say that the triumph of Christianity was responsible for changing that attitude. It is equally likely that the revulsion of people, especially women, by the misanthropic attitudes of late antiquity led them to appreciate the moral teachings, first of the Jews, who were more populous and more influential in the Empire than most historians credit, and then, later, of the Christians. (The Late Roman Empire was violently misogynistic; selective female infanticide was widely practiced.) The quotation of Matthew that begins the previous section carries the weight of law in the Christian tradition; it is one of the best-remembered and often-cited verses from the New Testament, and it always has been. In the Roman world, it was truly revolutionary.

Of course, the subsequent history of care for the mentally disabled in the western countries has not always done credit to their biblical ideals. The extraordinary hardship of peasant life in Europe, the prevalence of wars, plague, and famine, and the evils of superstition always conspired against the disabled and the disadvantaged. The Church, however, always discouraged infanticide, and the first asylum for abandoned infants was founded in Milan in 787 AD. Foundling homes and orphanages were usually associated with monasteries or convents. The fundamental change brought forth by the Judeo-Christian ethic and its unique contribution was the assertion of the moral worth of every individual and the responsibility of the individual to cultivate virtue in the everyday world.

But the light did not always shine brightly. There was a time when enlightened Christians would say:

> *Changelings were merely a mass of flesh, a massa carnis, with no soul...the devil sits in such changelings where their soul should have been. (Martin Luther)*

But the light was never extinguished. In 1376, they were confined to a tower in the city wall of Hamburg called the "idiot's cage," but in 1497, the city councilors of Frankfurt-am-Main provided guardians for mentally handicapped people and even provided stipends for their families to keep them. As society was pacified and grew in wealth and as the wisdom and sensitivity of the people increased, it was only a matter of time before the benefits were felt by individuals with disabilities. However, it took a long time, and much longer in some places than in others. In the Middle Ages in Cairo, there was a hospital for the mentally ill and retarded that was idyllic even by modern standards, but that was unique in the Muslim world. In Christendom, the mentally ill and idiots were all too often confined to dungeons or dark cellars (2).

Very little was written about the mentally handicapped by the physicians and sages of the ancient world, the Middle Ages, and the Renaissance. There is ample dealing with lunatics, apoplectics, and epileptics in literature and medical treatises, but very little over "fools," "idiots," or "naturals" as they were called. [They were called "naturals" because they were by nature (i.e., congenitally) deficient in intelligence. Shakespeare uses the word.] Hippocrates was aware of microcephaly and craniosynostosis, Avicenna described a "watery swelling of the head," and Paracelsus observed that cretinism was associated with mental retardation. Paracelsus also distinguished between the mentally ill and the mentally retarded and recognized the variability that existed in both conditions.

The medical approach to mental handicap, however, has usually been no more than descriptive, concerned with classification and terminology, and pathologic, concerned with etiologies and associated conditions like epilepsy. Medical reformers, however, especially in the eighteenth and nineteenth centuries, also spoke to improvements in living conditions and for humane care and developed the concepts of moral treatment, occupational therapy, and special education. Advances in the education of the mentally handicapped have largely been the precinct of educators and psychologists during our century, but the origin of special education is mainly the invention of an extraordinary French physician, Itard, who worked personally with Victor, the so-called "wild boy of Aveyron." It is ironic that Itard ultimately felt that his efforts with the feral child had been futile because his treatment fell far short of cure. In fact, he laid down the framework that special education uses to this day. (Itard also gave us the first published descriptions of the syndrome of Gilles de la Tourette, although he never called it that. Autism and Tourette's syndrome both deserve to be called Itard's syndrome. Seguin was the student of Itard, and Maria Montessori was the student of Seguin.) Physicians always seem to have been pessimistic about the possibility of actually treating mentally handicapped people.

The contributions of physicians like Itard, Esquirol, Seguin, and Down are well appreciated by even the most superficial histories of psychiatry. During the eighteenth century, the understanding and care of mentally handicapped individuals gradually acquired the form that it is still in use today: categorization by degree of handicap, description of pathologic conditions that cause mental retardation, and distinction between genetic and environmental causes of the disorder. As society became increasingly prosperous and urbanized, hospitals and residential schools for the retarded were opened everywhere in Europe and the Americas. Physicians and educators began to take a special interest in mental handicap.

The cultivation of humane treatment for the mentally ill and the mentally retarded has been the concern of physicians for 200 years, but for much of that time, and in most of the world, the admonitions of reformers have had as little impact as the Holy Writ. The eleemosynary instincts behind the creation of residential schools for the retarded during the nineteenth century was everywhere overwhelmed by the magnitude of the population in need and the constraints of the public purse. The "training schools," like the state hospitals, were subject to the same problems that existed during the Middle Ages, when almshouses and asylums were afflicted by "indifferent attendants and no resident doctors" (2). The extraordinary expansion of wealth and culture during the nineteenth and twentieth centuries certainly improved the quality of care for the handicapped, but only in fits and starts. The contribution of the Church had also been favorable, in general, but Christian societies in the Middle Ages and Renaissance were given to occasional and entirely disgraceful lapses. The modern era was no different. The thrust of improvement was palpable, but then there was the hideous experience in Germany, where mentally retarded people were actually exterminated, or, more recently, the horrendous circumstances of orphans and handicapped children in Communist Romania.

It is too easy for us to decry, from our armchairs, the horrific experience of Nazi Germany or the excesses of the Inquisition and the Reformation. I am all too aware that inhumanity and atrocity are much closer to us all than that. In my lifetime and on these enlightened shores, I have seen conditions in "schools" for the retarded that were no less than barbarous. There is no need to go into the details. What is clear and apparent is that cruelty to the disabled has only very rarely been the result of articulated argument and systematic evil doing, as was the case in Nazi Germany. More often, it is because our good intentions and charitable instincts became overwhelmed by the sheer magnitude of the task at hand, and by our enduring willingness to be distracted from the pressing needs of wretched humankind.

THE MODERN ERA

The second half of the past century saw a transformation of the attitudes of people around the world toward the helpless and disabled. It is as if the extraordinary evils that that century endured were a crucible for forging a new moral point of view. It is ironic that a world order as secular and areligious as ours has generated sensitivity to "the least of my brethren" that is no less than a fulfillment of the Judeo-Christian ideal. If the Lord were to visit the Earth tomorrow, He would probably be more impressed that we take good care of handicapped children and less concerned by the fact that more people wash their cars on the weekend than go to worship.

Caring for the young is, of course, a biologic imperative that is pervasive in the animal kingdom. Prolonged caring for immature, helpless infants is virtually unique to hominid, and caring for the mildly disabled seems to have come naturally, even in prehistoric societies. Taking good care of the severely disabled is a thoroughly modern invention, having begun in the West in the nineteenth century and finally achieving a degree of universal acceptance only in the richest countries of the world over the past few decades.

To what can we ascribe this sanguine change? Clearly, the most important element is the fabulous prosperity of late twentieth-century societies. Unfortunately, our wealth has had to multiply many times over, before the small pittance assigned for the mentally disabled could be increased at all, and no one can argue that the balance is quite right yet. The second element has been the growth of a universal culture, characterized by education, communication, and dissemination of information. People are simply more aware of what is going on in the world and are more involved in striving to improve society. The third element has been the growth of democracy. Modern democratic societies tend to be attentive to the strongly felt opinions of small minorities. In our society, the parents of mentally retarded children have finally won the opportunity to affect public policy in beneficent ways.

The fourth reason is the most important. The profoundly handicapped are with us now, and they stay with us. They survive difficult births and are able to endure the risks of severe prematurity; respiratory infections can be treated and aspiration can be prevented. Even children who are nonambulatory can be cared for in attentive and stimulating environments and can survive for years. Overall, good medical care has reduced the number of children who are born mentally handicapped or who come to be that way from disease, but it has also assured that more children with profound handicaps will survive. Only a few years ago, it was reported that severely retarded, nonambulatory children in California were likely to survive only a matter of months (3). Now, with technology, resources, and special training for staff, even the most impaired individuals may live a long life. Indeed, the fastest growing problem in the field of mental retardation is the care of elderly patients.

The transformation that has occurred in our lifetime with regard to the severely handicapped has been almost entirely the result of political activity undertaken by their families. The most effective steps taken by the national government on behalf of the retarded were, indeed, initiated by President Kennedy, who had a handicapped sister. Kennedy's initiatives, however, began a full generation after the parents of mentally handicapped children in the United States had organized to form a group called the Association for Retarded Children and had developed educational programs in their communities on their own initiative. [Now, it is the Association for Retarded Citizens (ARC).] Parents were frustrated by the failure of local governmental entities, mainly school boards, to provide educational opportunities for their children. They were equally dismayed by the recommendations of physicians to consign retarded children to large, aggregate state-run facilities, where the living conditions were abysmal and the possibility for improvement was nil. They argued that no child was "ineducable."

The ARC deserves all the credit, as the first grassroots organization to mobilize political support for a disadvantaged group. It continues to exercise extraordinary influence, not only in the halls of government, but, on a day-to-day level, in generating opportunities for retarded citizens in communities. It remains the prototype for all the "special interest" lobbies that have developed since then. It began its work in the 1940s—hardly a decade that was supportive of that sort of thing.

It is appropriate to reflect on the success of the ARC movement, especially in contrast to some of the other social and political trends that have tried to have an impact on the lives of handicapped people but have not been nearly as successful. It allows us to consider what it is that comprises successful advocacy in contrast to some of the fallacies that always seem to intrude on the advocacy movement.

First, there is the contrast between the practical approach and the ideologic approach. The primary activities of the ARC have been in the community, but not in the ideologic community that has guided some of the worst aspects of the deinstitutionalization movement. The parents of retarded children have always been interested, first and foremost, in the development of community infrastructure: classrooms, workshops, respite services, group homes, small residential facilities, and local advocacy groups that include parents, physicians, educators, and other friends of the retarded. Within every community, therefore, there has developed a network of services for retarded people and an active group of local advocates. The closure of large residential institutions has never been a primary goal, but rather the goal was development of community services. The mental retardation "movement" has concentrated on infrastructure, not ideologic crusades. The availability of an effective network of services, however, has meant that deinstitutionalization of retarded people has been, by and large, a resounding success.

In contrast, the deinstitutionalization of the chronically mentally ill has been a recurring embarrassment. The original wave of deinstitutionalization for the chronically mentally ill in state hospitals during the 1950s and 1960s was driven by the success of drug treatment and was successful for the most part. During the 1970s and 1980s, the patients who remained hospitalized were largely people with complex and intractable conditions who had responded only partially to the new medications and who had little in the way of a psychosocial support network. During this blighted era, the main driving force behind psychiatric deinstitutionalization was an ideologic point of view that living in the community was preferable to hospital-based treatment under virtually any circumstances. The community-based infrastructure that was supposed to receive these difficult patients, however, was not in place, and the "experiment" was, for the most part, an egregious failure.

The second contrast is the reliance on local activism, which has always characterized the mental retardation movement, as opposed to reliance on government action, which has been the bane of the chronically mentally ill. Bureaucrats and legislators will always do only so much and no more. Relying on state-funded mental health centers or regional mental health authorities to meet the needs of the deinstitutionalized mentally ill was a good bureaucratic plan, but in the absence of the full range of services that severely disturbed individuals need and a broad community-based network of advocates and volunteers, it could never suffice. In fact, the care of mentally ill people in the community remained inadequate until the past few years when voluntary associations like National Alliance for the Mentally Ill and the Mental Health Association began to follow the lead of the ARC and actually work toward the development of such a network.

The third contrast has been the reliance on citizen leadership, which has characterized the mental retardation movement, as opposed to professional leadership, which has characterized the mental health movement. Psychiatrists, social workers, and lawyers are not as well placed to generate a network of community resources compared with the mass of ordinary people. A corollary is reliance on services as opposed to treatments. The mental retardation movement has concentrated on the development of resources, such as classrooms and workshops; the mental illness movement has, too often, concentrated on drugs. Speaking as a psychopharmacologist, psychiatric drugs are all right, as far as they go, but they don't go very far if there is nothing else working on the patient's behalf. It should be services first, then treatments.

A fourth contrast has been realism as opposed to faddism. The parents of autistic and learning disabled children, in particular, have been vulnerable to faddish treatments that promise dramatic results, even cures. In Chapter 14, some of the dubious treatments that have been proposed, with numbing regularity, for autistic children are discussed. Not much harm has been done by prescribing megavitamins, fenfluramine, secretin, eye exercises, auditory training, or any of the countless "cures" proposed by mountebanks, but it does take focus away from the main task. In contrast, the parents of mentally retarded children have been, in the main, a realistic lot.

Not that the field of mental retardation has been entirely free of ideologues, mountebanks, fads, bureaucratic clumsiness, or overvaluation of the promises of new technology. No human endeavor is. Mental retardation, after all, is where "politically correct" language had its origins. Retarded people have been subjected to "patterning" exercises, sheep-embryo injections, megavitamin therapy, "gentle teaching," "inclusion," and, most recently, "client-centered" programming. When Title XIX reviewers visit a mental retardation facility, the staff has to hide the stuffed animals because they are not "age appropriate." Changing psychotropic drugs, for example, from a neuroleptic to an atypical antipsychotic or from one selective serotonin reuptake inhibitor to another, requires the approval of a treatment "team" and review by a "human rights committee." I have seen small residential facilities closed down because they were located in idyllic rural settings and thus remote from the "community." At the same time, group homes are opened in the community, in inner-city neighborhoods where none of us would feel safe to walk the streets. Every field is prone to silly mistakes, and mental retardation is no exception.

Silliness is intrinsic to human nature. It is frustrating when it comes from well-meaning and well-educated adults who should know better. The strength of the mental retardation movement has been its ability to transcend these occasional lapses. As long as there are classrooms, well-trained teachers, workshops and employment opportunities, group homes and residential treatment centers, and support for families and local citizens' groups for advocacy and protection, mentally retarded people thrive. New fads just make their lives a little more interesting.

One signal problem that has developed as a byproduct of deinstitutionalizing the mentally retarded has concerned the provision of specialty services, especially in psychiatry. Not that all of the large aggregate facilities were superior in that regard, but many were; when there were lapses, they would soon be apparent to regulators and other visitors from the outside. But in the community, retarded people with psychiatric problems find it hard to obtain psychiatric services at all. Only a few mental health centers employ psychiatrists who know how to deal with the behavioral and emotional problems of retarded people. Medicaid and Medicare do not reimburse private psychiatrists very well, even when they are willing to look after these multiply handicapped individuals. Complicated pharmacologic regimes are often left to family practitioners who have little experience or training. As a result, the use of behavior-control medications among the retarded seems to be back on the upswing. Mentally retarded people with severe behavior problems are likely to be reinstitutionalized, and the state facilities, downsized as they are, are increasingly likely to concentrate large numbers of severely disturbed individuals. They are, in effect, becoming psychiatric hospitals for retarded people, which takes us back to the lesson of Bedlam.

Try as we may to do good things, there is always more that has to be done. As we solve one problem, new problems arise. When we improve medical care for severely handicapped infants, they survive and require even more care over a lifetime. As the life expectancy of handicapped people improves, the problem of geriatric care arises. When retarded people move into the community, the problem of access to specialized professional services becomes acute. If they live in the country, they may be too isolated. If they live in the city, they may be victimized. It never ends. There is no shortage of work to do, and this brings us back to the Book.

The ancients, who practiced infanticide, and the Nazis, who practiced genocide, looked on the retarded as liabilities. The Book, conversely, teaches that they are just special people. It tells us that the extension of caring and love toward "the least of my brethren" is one of the few ways that we might reflect the extraordinary generosity Providence has extended to the rest of us. It is not really "tribute" that is due, as Daniel DeFoe suggested, but the opportunity to exercise the spark of charity that is the source of our very nature.

MENTAL RETARDATION: DEFINITION AND STRUCTURE

Mental retardation has the dubious honor of having been the starting point of politically correct language. The terms that were used in the Middle Ages—idiots, fools, dunces, simpletons, naturals—and even the pseudoscientific terms that were coined during the past century—imbeciles, cretins, morons, mongoloids—have long since lost whatever descriptive value they once had and are now considered to be impossibly derogatory. In fact, they are, but that is not because of anything intrinsic in the old terminology. It appears to be an ongoing process. Even the current terminology is falling into disfavor, and schoolchildren use the adjective "retarded" as a pejorative for their unpopular classmates. In fact, it is usually preferred to say, "persons with mental retardation" in some quarters, whereas the English usage ("mental handicap") is growing in currency in the United States even as it is abandoned in the United Kingdom in favor of "learning disabled." This grasping at euphemisms (e.g., special children) is certainly well intentioned and is well received by the parents and teachers of handicapped children, who count a great deal more than you and I do. It is a sad fact, though, that whatever euphemism is coined, and even with the best intentions, its usage will soon degenerate and become the vehicle for derogation. That is simply because people overvalue "smartness," which we equate with all the virtues and shrink from its opposite. It is hard to believe that politically correct language will ever correct that flaw in human nature, but at least it puts a moving target to people with scurrilous tongues.

I use the terms mental retardation and mental handicap interchangeably and try to avoid euphemisms. Amentia is a term coined by Esquirol. I suppose that if we use the term dementia, we can use amentia, but hardly anyone does.

Amentia, or mental retardation, is defined by three elements: (i) intellectual deficiency measured on standard tests with scores that fall more than two standard deviations below the population mean (i.e., IQ less than 70), (ii) deficiency in social adaptation measured in the same way, and (iii) congenital onset. Other definitions have been proposed, but none that is better or more practical to use.

It is sometimes forgotten that the diagnosis of mental retardation is not made simply based on classroom performance or scores on an IQ test. It is possible to say that so-and-so has an IQ score that "falls in the mentally retarded range," but even that is gratuitous and potentially misleading. No one who works with learning disabled children is likely to say such a thing, for the obvious reason. Conversely, there are actually circumstances in which it is advantageous to be labeled "retarded." For example, in forensic settings, it is often convenient to forget the requirement for congenital onset and deficits in social adaptation. A prisoner is said to be mentally retarded and thus entitled to special consideration, simply based on a full-scale IQ in the high 60s. When journalists cluck about a "retarded man who was executed in Arkansas" or some other benighted Southern state, their sensitivity may be laudable, but they are almost invariably using inappropriate terminology.

Chronically mentally ill patients may be deemed by the courts to be inappropriately placed in a psychiatric hospital because they are mentally retarded. Chronic mental illness is sometimes associated with a decline in intellectual performance to be sure, but an IQ in the 60s does not make the diagnosis. Nevertheless, there has been a broad movement of such people from state hospitals to mental retardation facilities in the past several years, usually on the basis of a judicial decree.

Nevertheless, the IQ score is a major element in making the diagnosis, and, in fact, the epidemiology of mental retardation does reflect the normal curve for the distribution of IQ scores, but not perfectly. Three percent is the area under the normal curve two standard deviations down, but only approximately 1% to 2% of the population is diagnosed with mental retardation. Low IQ does not equal mental retardation, nor does it guarantee that social adaptation will be impaired, but it does correlate with both; therefore, for the population, the normal curve of IQ distribution predicts the occurrence of mental handicap. When dealing with individuals, however, it is inappropriate to make the diagnosis of mental retardation simply based on IQ.

IQ scores, however, may be used as a kind of clinical shorthand, and psychologists who are perfectly savvy about its limitations as a diagnostic instrument are usually quite comfortable in defining four levels of mental retardation according to the IQ score:

55 to 69: mild mental retardation
40 to 54: moderate mental retardation
25 to 39: severe mental retardation
Less than 24: profound mental retardation

In fact, the clinically useful classification defines two broad groups of mentally retarded people, and if there is an IQ cutoff, it is around 50 (4). The mild to moderately retarded represent most people with mental handicap. They are not, as a rule, particularly dysmorphic; they usually possess language, are usually capable of independent or semi-independent living, and include virtually all the people whose handicap is believed to be familial. Children from lower socioeconomic classes are overrepresented. Parents who are mildly retarded may have mildly retarded children but not severely retarded children. In the ancient world and in primitive societies, they would find a protected niche in village society.

Only a small proportion of the retarded fall into the severe to profoundly retarded range, in the tail of the normal curve, and more than four or five standard deviations below the population mean. People who are severely retarded are more likely to possess dysmorphic features; they do not have language, they live dependent lives, and the cause of their handicap is genetic (but not familial) or encephalopathic. They may be born to parents from any socioeconomic class and are much more likely to have significant sensory or motor handicaps and epilepsy. In primitive societies, such individuals usually do not survive.

Primitive people living in Nepal a generation ago divided the mentally handicapped into two groups: *laato* (dumb) and *adha-laato* (half-dumb). The distinction is based on whether the individual has useful language (*adha-laato*) or no language at all (*laato*). Verbal skill is found to be the defining characteristic in other primitive societies (5). In fact, it is, even to us, the central distinguishing element that that separates the mildly retarded from the severely retarded.

In fact, the normal curve does not accurately predict the number of people who are severely or profoundly retarded (IQ less than 40). There is an excess of people who fall into those unfortunate categories, the so-called pathologic bump, compared with what one might expect simply from the structure of the normal distribution of intelligence. There is a simple explanation. The normal curve represents the distribution of genetically permissible IQ scores. The human genome is permissive of a range of IQ scores between approximately 40 and 160. To generate a lower score, either the genome has to be defective (e.g., a chromosomal abnormality) or some pathologic event has to have damaged the developing brain.

As we shall see, there are considerable differences in the way neuropsychiatric issues are played out in these vastly different populations. Psychiatric conditions such as schizophrenia are very common among the mildly retarded but rare or nonexistent in the severely retarded. Behavior problems like stereotypy, self-injury, pica, and rumination are much more common in the severely retarded and seldom occur at all in the mildly retarded. Pathobehavioral conditions such as the fragile X syndrome are more likely to cause mild or moderate mental retardation, whereas others, such as the Cornelia de Lange syndrome, are more likely to cause a severe degree of mental handicap. Drug treatment for the mild to moderately retarded for the most part follows usual psychiatric practice; even psychostimulants may be prescribed successfully. Drug treatment for the severely retarded is rather different from conventional psychopharmacology, and stimulants, for example, are hardly ever effective. Seizure disorders are much more common in the severely retarded. They are probably more vulnerable to the severe side effects of neuroleptic drugs, such as tardive dyskinesia and tardive akathisia.

NEUROPSYCHIATRIC APPROACH TO MENTAL HANDICAP

There is no single way to approach the neuropsychiatric problems of mentally handicapped people. They have to be dealt with from different perspectives. The traditional psychiatric disorders occur more frequently in mentally retarded people than in the general population, although diagnosis is not always straightforward, and atypical conditions are commonly encountered. The mental retardation syndromes, what we refer to as pathobehavioral syndromes and what are elsewhere referred to as behavioral phenotypes, are often associated with specific, sometimes grotesque disorders of mood and behavior, and thus should be considered in their own right. Some of the problems retarded people have deserve to be considered as pure behaviors, divorced from any diagnostic category. This tripartite division is not definitive, and the three areas, psychiatric problems, pathobehavioral syndromes, and pure behaviors, are by no means mutually exclusive. But it is a convenient way to conceptualize the area for the purpose of a monograph, even if the differentiation is sometimes fuzzy.

It is impossible to consider the psychiatric problems of retarded people without recognizing the problem of epilepsy, which is so common and intrudes so often on the patient's mental state. Treatment issues in the management of epilepsy are extremely important to the mental health of retarded people.

REFERENCES

1. Stanley S. *Children of the ice age*. New York: Freeman, 1998.
2. Scheerenberger R. *A history of mental retardation*. Baltimore: Paul H. Brookes, 1983.
3. Eyman R, Grossman H, Chaney R, et al. The life expectancy of profoundly handicapped people with mental retardation. *N Engl J Med* 1990;323:584–589.
4. Pulsifer MB. The neuropsychology of mental retardation. *J Int Neuropsychol Soc* 1996;2:159–176.
5. Peters L. Concepts of mental deficiency among the Tamang of Nepal. *Am J Ment Deficiency* 1980;84:352–356.

4

Mechanisms of Brain Injury

SUMMARY

The primary mechanisms of brain injury (BI) are events such as cerebral contusion, hemorrhage, and diffuse axonal injury. They are sudden and direct, and their impact is immediate, but they also give rise to secondary events that are much more complex and evolve over time. These include disruption of the blood-brain barrier (BBB), derangement of neurotransmitter systems, excitotoxic cell damage, oxidative stress, and inflammatory reactions. The secondary mechanisms of BI are exaggerations of normal homeostatic mechanisms, normal reactions to an extraordinary event that overshoot their mark and cause additional tissue damage that sometimes exceeds the primary injury. The acute treatment of patients with BI is mainly to attenuate the impact of these secondary mechanisms. This has been the focus of a good deal of pharmacologic experimentation.

The mechanisms of brain recovery from injury include many of the same mechanisms described in Chapter 2 with respect to brain plasticity. During this prolonged phase, which can go on for years, normal physiologic mechanisms can be distorted by processes such as long-term depression, diaschisis, and kindling. These, in turn, can lead to delayed pathologic outcomes.

The neural events that lead to mental retardation (MR) are more diverse. They are less given to understanding as normal homeostatic mechanisms that have gone awry. Nevertheless, there are areas of commonality between BI and MR. This is exemplified in the study of dementia, which is a common outcome after severe traumatic BI (TBI) and in the severely retarded, and which is virtually universal in Down's syndrome (DS).

MR is defined, at least in part as a deficit in general intelligence, and severe BI results in general intellectual deficits. Biologic studies of intelligence indicate that it is a function of the quick, reliable, and efficient operation of neural syncytia. The neuropathology of MR is replete with circumstances that compromise the bioenergetics of neurons and their ability to establish quick, reliable, and efficient connectivity. These circumstances are described in general terms here and are brought up again when the specific MR syndromes are discussed.

MECHANISMS OF BRAIN INJURY

TBI leads to a number of neuropathologic events: epidural, subdural, subarachnoid, and intraparenchymal hemorrhages; multiple small petechial hemorrhages; cortical contusion; and diffuse axonal injury. The primary damage is caused by immediate mechanical disruption of neural pathways and vasculature. Secondary damage is caused by cellular, metabolic, and chemical events that evolve in the minutes, hours, and days after the injury.

Other forms of BI must also be considered in terms of the primary event that disrupts the activity of cerebral tissue, the supply of oxygen, or the integrity of the vasculature and also in terms of secondary events that develop over time in the damaged brain. It is often the case that more extensive and permanent damage is done by the secondary mechanisms. It is also the case that BIs of diverse types induce common pathways of chemical and histopathologic changes in cerebral tissue. The elucidation of these mechanisms in recent years has led to experiments with potential therapeutic interventions designed to mitigate the impact of cerebral insult by limiting the damage that is done by secondary mechanisms.

THE BLOOD-BRAIN BARRIER

The permeability of the BBB is a function of the cerebral capillary endothelium; it is accomplished by tight junctions between adjacent endothelial cells and a relative paucity of transport vesicles in the endothelium of capillaries, arterioles, and veins. It has long been appreciated that TBI, in animal models and in clinical studies, alters the permeability of the BBB. Cerebral edema and increased intracranial pressure are the inevitable result. In severe injuries, hemorrhage and frank vascular disruption contribute to barrier breakdown. In mild to moderate injuries, changes in endothelial integrity are induced by more subtle mechanisms. Perturbations in the BBB are reflected by abnormal permeability to protein and other components of plasma, which may contribute to the further evolution of cerebral damage. Alterations in the BBB may also impair transport into brain of important nutrients (1–3).

Breakdown of the BBB is also seen in acute hypertension and hypoxic injury. Hypoxia may also aggravate the effects of TBI in this regard; it is estimated that 30% to 50% of patients with TBI in a coma are hypoxic when they arrive at the emergency department (3,4).

DIFFUSE AXONAL INJURY

Direct trauma causes cerebral contusions and lacerations, typically in the frontal and temporal poles and on the inferior surface of the frontal and temporal lobes, where brain tissue comes in contact with bony protuberances at the base of the skull. As long as the lesions are not catastrophic, the fact that they are focal permits patients to make smooth and sometimes uneventful recoveries, even from severe contusions or lacerations. Healed contusions have been noted as incidental findings in no fewer than 2.5% of autopsies in a general hospital (5). Most of the time, however, recovery is compromised by the co-occurrence of diffuse axonal injury in the cerebral white matter, corpus callosum, cerebellum, and brainstem.

TBI in general, and closed head injuries (CHI) in particular, are known to produce diffuse, microscopic damage to the brain, especially to the subcortical white matter (6). Diffuse axonal injury is the characteristic pathology of CHI, especially in association with motor vehicle accidents, where there is abrupt acceleration and deceleration of the neuraxis. Cortical impact injury is transmitted, with particular vehemence, to axial structures, generating shear forces that cause scattered, multifocal subcortical and brainstem axonal damage (i.e., diffuse axonal injury) (6,7). Axonal damage throughout the neuraxis has been recognized as a consistent feature of severe, moderate, and even mild CHI, with the overall number of damaged neurons increasing with the severity of the respective injury (8). The shear and tensile forces associated with CHI physically tear neurons, causing them to retract and to expel a ball of axoplasm, resulting in the formation of a reactive axonal swelling commonly called a retraction ball (5).

It is possible for brain trauma to occur in acceleration-deceleration injuries (i.e., whiplash) in which the head itself never strikes a rigid surface (9). In primates, experimental whiplash has been shown to cause both surface and intracerebral petechial hemorrhages (10). The whiplash mechanism (inertial impulse loading) may be especially damaging to the limbic and frontotemporal cortices, zones of maximal centripetal, structural, and tissue-density susceptibility (11).

In moderate and severe TBI, it is possible to demonstrate pathologic effects of brain contusion on computed tomography or magnetic resonance imaging, and postmortem studies have demonstrated evidence of diffuse axonal injury. In mild traumatic brain injuries (MBIs), the demonstration of pathologic changes is not as easy. Therefore, the pathophysiology of MBI is based on animal models, for example, the angular acceleration model (12) and the fluid-percussion model (8). Because animal models of severe brain trauma demonstrate neuropathologic and neurochemical changes that are similar to those observed in severely injured humans (12,13), it is reasonable to assume that MBI in experimental animals is a valid model for what happens in patients with MBI. This is disquieting because it implies that any injury, even the most minor, causes some immediate and irrevocable axonal damage (8).

Cerebral contusion is not likely to be a component of the pathology of MBI, but in other respects, the only difference between MBI and severe TBI is the degree of diffuse and multifocal damage. Like severe TBI, the pathology of MBI involves diffuse axonal injury (5,8,14). MBI has also been shown to elicit axon terminal and preterminal degeneration within the brainstem (12). There are isolated descriptions of axonal damage in humans who have sustained MBI (15). Oppenheimer (16) described myelin destruction and axonal retraction balls in five patients with MBIs who died from other causes within days of their accidents.

There are three characteristics of axonal injury after TBI: the injury is both selective and diffuse, and the course of recovery is variable:

1. Selective injury: Large-caliber, long-tract decussating axons are preferentially vulnerable to injury through stretching or compression, the result of shear or rotational forces. However, an axon may be injured in direct proximity to other axons, neural elements, glia, and microvessels that are undamaged (8).
2. Diffuse injury: Multifocal axonal damage will not induce the dramatic changes that ordinarily occur when an entire tract in severed. Rather, the individual axons that are injured may be diffusely scattered throughout the afferent and efferent tracts of the brainstem. Thus, clinical effects are not confined to any particular functional system.
3. Variable outcome: The fate of axons damaged after TBI is variable. Over time, a damaged neuron may induce secondary effects on brain parenchyma that are immediate or delayed. Follow-up in animal models of TBI indicates that although some axonal swellings persist unchanged and some axons die back, still others manage to recover. Some of the damaged neurons exist in a relatively preserved brain microenvironment. As a result, they appear to be capable of mounting a sustained regenerative response. These features of the traumatically injured axon may contribute to an adaptive form of recovery (8).

Some subcortical neurons are damaged while others are not, damage is scattered among ascending and descending neuronal tracts and some damaged neurons die while others do not. What this suggests is that a quantitative or a parametric element is appropriate to the appreciation of TBI. In a parametric model, the severity of damage from TBI is proportional to the relative numbers of dead and damaged neurons, their relative functional importance, and their capacity for self-repair. The functional impact of diffuse axonal injury is also determined by the health of redundant systems, that is, their ability to compensate for tissue that is lost. The availability of compensatory systems is referred to throughout this book as cerebral reserve.

DERANGEMENT OF NEUROTRANSMITTERS

TBI activates the sympathoadrenomedullary axis, leading to a series of systemic derangements, such as increased intracranial pressure, sustained hypertension, cardiac arrhythmias, and pulmonary complications. Acute surges in epinephrine, norepinephrine (NE), dopamine (DA), and serotonin (5HT) have been noted in experimental animals and in human patients; the severity of the increase is in proportion to the severity of the injury (17,18). There is also an increase in the functional activity of opioid and cholinergic systems. Derangement of the BBB can also lead to inflow of blood-borne neurotransmitters into the brain (19). These dramatic changes in the neurochemical milieu may persist for days after acute injury and aggravate the effects of the primary injury by maintaining edema and causing vasospasm, decreased cerebral blood flow, and decreased oxygenation (20).

Hypoxic-ischemic BIs can also provoke a similar neurochemical response. In laboratory animals, drugs that attenuate the activity of these various neurotransmitters enhance recovery of function.

The acute surge of central nervous system (CNS) neurotransmitters after injury abates with time and then returns to baseline (21). The chronic postinjury state, however, is characterized by a relative decline in neurotransmitter metabolism, especially DA and NE (22,23). After CHI, for example, the axonal tracts that are most likely to be disrupted are monoaminergic projections from the brainstem to cortical and subcortical structures. Most of the monoaminergic neurons are located in the lower brainstem and project rostrally. They comprise an expansive chemical network, part of the reticular formation, organized in tightly clustered groups with extensive homotypic interconnections and long projections to interacting target areas (24). Their location, size, and pattern of connection render them especially vulnerable to the kind of injury that occurs in CHI. Experimental studies in laboratory animals and clinical experiments have been consistent in demonstrating persistent changes after CHI in the levels of various neurotransmitters, including acetylcholine and the catecholamines (19,25,26).

Because the monoamine neurotransmitters play a neuromodulatory rather than an executive role and because they exercise a facilitating effect on various CNS functions, damage to some of the neurons in several of the ascending monoamine pathways can have diffuse effects across the broad band of cerebral function. The diffuse effects of injury to monoamine systems should include alterations in arousal, attention, and information processing, mediated in large part by dopaminergic and noradrenergic neurons (27), and alterations in mood, appetite, sleep, sexual function, pain perception, circadian rhythms, motor activity, memory, anxiety, and aggression, mediated by serotonergic neurons (28).

If attenuating the effects of neurotransmitter release is a goal of early treatment for the chronic patient, enhancing the activity of various neurotransmitters, such as DA and NE, appears to promote recovery of function (29,30).

Because the neuromodulatory neurotransmitters are functionally interrelated (31), a derangement in one system is sometimes felt "downstream" in another system, for example, by influencing neuronal firing rates or the sensitivity of receptors. Such an effect may require weeks or months to evolve. The process is similar to what happens in mood disorders in which catecholamine receptors are down-regulated in response to prolonged states of stress-induced hypercortisolemia (32). Alterations in cholinergic neurotransmission can also produce a state of depression by perturbing the function of other neurotransmitters, namely, the monoamines (31).

In TBI, focal or diffuse injuries cause delayed changes in downstream systems, an event that is known as diaschisis. Diaschisis is functional shock or deactivation of intact brain regions remote from, but connected to, the area of primary injury (33). Although the idea was at one time controversial, it is now supported by demonstrations of altered regional blood flow and cerebral metabolism in remote sites with single photon emission computed tomography or positron emission tomography (34–37). For example, unilateral cortical injury evokes a widespread depression of cortical metabolism in the ipsilateral hemisphere and other sites. There is substantial evidence that perturbations of NE metabolism may be the mediating event in diaschisis (38,39). There is also evidence of diaschisis (or a similar pathologic process) in experimental models of concussion in the cat in which acetylcholine appears to be the mediating neurohumor (40).

EXCITOTOXICITY

When cerebral neurons are deprived of oxygen, the ischemic cell is soon depleted of adenosine 5′-triphosphate. When this happens, pumping mechanisms are hampered, sodium ions accumulate in the cell, and the neuron undergoes depolarization. As a result, excessive amounts of neuroactive substances accumulate in the extracellular space of the ischemic field (41). Chief among them are excitatory amino acid (EAA) neurotransmitters such as glutamate and aspartate. This massive and untoward concentration of EAA is elicited not only by hypoxia and ischemia but also by traumatic injury, hypoglycemia, stroke, and neurotoxic drug effects. When glutamate accumulates in the cellular interstitium, it acts persistently on receptors. This is referred to as paroxysmal receptor occupation or receptor abuse or excitotoxicity (42).

Glutamate is the principle excitatory neurotransmitter in the brain and is responsible for functions like cognition, memory, movement, sensation, and neuronal plasticity. Glutamate is present in approximately 30% of all synapses; in fact, most neurons in the CNS have receptors for one or another of the EAAs (43). The EAAs are the engines of excitatory neurotransmission; yet excessive activation of EAA receptors causes neuronal injury or death. When the natural balance of EAA neurotransmission is disturbed, a cascade of destructive events ensues. Excitotoxicity is not only central to the pathology of acute events such as stroke and TBI but also to chronic neurodegenerative conditions such as Alzheimer's disease (AD), Parkinson's disease, and even normal aging. The excitotoxin theory of cell death has aroused intense interest, particularly because it opens the possibility of therapeutic application for EAA antagonist drugs (44).

To balance EAA neurotransmission and prevent neurotoxicity, a delicate control system is required. There is only a small gradient between physiologic levels of glutamate and levels that may be toxic. The intracellular concentration of glutamate in brain tissue is approximately 10 μm/L. The normal extracellular concentration of glutamate is 0.6 mmol/L, and excitotoxic damage to neurons occurs when the extracellular concentration reaches 2 to 5 mmol/L. Thus, the brain has evolved with an extraordinary vulnerability to its own excitatory neurotransmitters and an exquisite system to control the concentration and compartmentalization of extracellular glutamate (45). Any condition that reduces the bioenergetics of the neuron can compromise the exquisite control mechanisms that hold the glutamate receptor in check, thereby allowing even physiologic concentrations of glutamate to induce an excitotoxic reaction (43).

In experimental studies of TBI, there is marked elevation of extracellular glutamate and aspartate adjacent to the trauma site, an increase that is proportional to the severity of injury and to the reduction in the cellular bioenergetic state (46). Cerebrospinal fluid levels of glutamate are elevated for days after severe TBI in humans (47). Thus, the idea has developed that glutamatergic excitotoxicity is central to the pathophysiology of TBI, as it is after stroke. Treatment with *N*-methyl-D-aspartate (NMDA) antagonists has been found to limit the resultant neurologic dysfunction (46), although there is a therapeutic window of only a few hours after injury (or stroke) during which the treatment may be effective.

It is not entirely clear how excessive excitation of NMDA receptors by abnormally high levels of glutamate leads to neuronal damage and death, but two mechanisms have been suggested: (i) increased membrane permeability to sodium and chloride, which leads to acute neuronal swelling, and (ii) increased calcium influx, which leads to delayed damage (18). Ethanol tends to aggravate glutamate excitotoxicity, which may account for the relative severity of TBI sequelae in patients who were intoxicated at the time of injury (48). In neurodegenerative conditions such as Parkinson's disease, Alzheimer's disease, and Huntington's disease, as well as in normal aging, excitotoxic damage may be the consequence of a pathologic chain of events that includes the generation of free radicals (43).

CHANGES IN ION CONCENTRATIONS, THE ARACHIDONIC ACID CASCADE, AND OXYGEN FREE RADICALS

The release of EAA neurotransmitters after BI leads to postinsult hyperexcitability. The EAAs open the calcium channels, and there is excessive intracellular accumulation of calcium (calcium overload). This unregulated increase in calcium leads to the activation of intracellular enzymes and the consumption of cellular adenosine 5′-triphosphate. Thus, neurons begin to catabolize themselves to maintain activity and in so doing are damaged to a degree that does not permit survival (49,50). Intracellular calcium triggers a number of metabolic events, including the generation of free radicals and the further release of EAAs into the interstitial space. The process, then, becomes self-sustaining, with characteristics of a feed-forward mechanism.

Calcium activates enzymes that liberate fatty acids from the cell membrane. It initiates the arachidonic cascade, leading to the production of prostaglandins, leukotrienes, thromboxanes, and oxygen free radicals (41,51).

The central role played by calcium in the propagation of untoward events explains the interest in calcium-channel blockade as an acute treatment after stroke and BI. The cerebroprotective effects of nimodipine and other L-channel antagonists have been well documented (18).

The magnesium ion has an important regulatory role with respect to calcium transport and accumulation and has been termed the physiologic antagonist of calcium. Magnesium concentrations tend to be depressed at the site of BI, the degree of depression correlating with the severity of the injury. Low levels of magnesium aggravate the effects of EAA toxicity, and administering magnesium salts has been found to attenuate tissue damage after experimental BI (18).

Under circumstances of stress, such as hypoxia-ischemia, the production of free-radical species in the mitochondria increases. The brain is particularly vulnerable to free-radical neurotoxicity because it is rich in cholesterol and polyunsaturated fatty acids, which are attacked by free radicals and easily broken down (lipid peroxidation). Among the free fatty acids that are generated is arachidonic acid, thus initiating a chain of events that only serves to increase oxidative stress on damaged tissue. The destructive effects of oxygen free radicals are catalyzed by the availability of free reactive iron (from extravasated blood); at the same time, and for unknown reasons, endogenous antioxidant concentrations are reduced (18,41).

INFLAMMATION OF THE BRAIN

The great Dostoyevsky was always one for characters with "brain fever" or an "inflamed brain." He may have been referring at times to encephalitis, but in the main, he was using the terms as we would use the word "feverish" to describe someone given to intense and inappropriate emotional reactions. One is taught in medical school that the brain is an "immunologically privileged site" and that events that normally characterize the inflammatory response do not transpire there.

It is true that the tight endothelium-capillary junctions that comprise the BBB are largely impervious to leukocytes, circulating antibodies, and the proinflammatory peptides known as cytokines. It is also true that the BBB is damaged during and immediately after brain trauma, that circulating elements foreign to the brain under normal circumstances can be detected, and that harm can attend such events. Neural tissue is itself capable of expressing the cytokine tumor necrosis factor, which results in leukocyte accumulation, adherence, and migration from capillaries into the brain (52). It is also true that the end products of the arachidonic cascade include proinflammatory elements. In the same vein, cyclooxygenase inhibitors such as indomethacin and ibuprofen prevent the conversion of arachidonic acid into proinflammatory prostaglandins, thromboxanes, and leukotrienes and in laboratory animals have reversed at least some of the deficits caused by percussive or ischemic BI (41).

We all know that the classical inflammatory response (tumor, rubor, calor, dolor) may sometimes be intense and inappropriate, and much of the damage done to tissues that are traumatized or infected is the result of the body's own excessive inflammatory response. So it is with the brain. Although inflammation is only one component of brain reaction to insults, every component yet identified tends to overshoot the mark. To adjust to trauma and to restore balance to a deranged system, mechanisms are set in motion that are self-sustaining and mutually reinforcing. An excess of zeal, as it were, only serves to cause more harm.

It is natural for the body to respond to stress, like BI, by activating the sympathoadrenomedullary axis, but the ensuing surge of circulating catecholamines is dangerous in its own right. It is natural for the damaged brain to shut down remote systems, if only to conserve energy. Metabolic depression in the face of a cerebral insult is an adaptive response; the neonatal brain is protected from hypoxia by its own limited metabolic requirements. Persistent depression (so-called diaschisis), however, may also be the occasion for prolonged disability after stroke or BI.

Intracellular calcium overload has a number of deleterious effects, but sublethal concentrations stimulate protein synthesis and generate neuroprotective factors. Free radicals are nasty things to have about, but they are the normal product of anaerobic metabolism in mitochondria deprived of oxygen. Anaerobic glycolysis leads to increased levels of lactate, and lactic acidosis is correlated with the severity of BI; conversely, lactic acid can protect cells by blocking calcium influx and preventing acetylcholine release (41,53). BI tends to reduce cerebral blood flow, but ultimately the injured area will be reperfused. Reperfusion, however, is associated with a dramatic increase in nitric oxide, which only increases oxidative stress in the injured tissue (54).

The pathology of BI and stroke, therefore, includes the primary event and then a cascade of secondary events in which normal homeostatic mechanisms react in predictable ways but overshoot the mark. These secondary events are sometimes as damaging as the initial trauma. Because they are predictable, they convey the potential for therapeutic intervention.

MECHANISMS OF NEURAL RECOVERY

The secondary pathologic events that evolve after contusive or ischemic BI are often described as cascades, with one untoward element generating another. They are more accurately described as feed-forward mechanisms or vicious circles. From any perspective, the injured cell is observed to respond in a manner quite in keeping with its normal physiologic capacity to preserve homeostasis. Rather than return the injured tissue to a state of balance, however, what begins as normal reactions only serves to aggravate the pathologic imbalance.

The initial contusive or ischemic event causes an immediate response in brain tissue. The cascade or vicious circle of secondary events described constitutes the stage of early response. Ultimately, these responses run their course, and what follows is a series of late responses that lead to healing and then, ultimately, to recovery.

The secondary events that constitute early response carry with them the elements of recovery. Macrophages migrate into the injured area from the peripheral circulation and are also generated from glial elements within the brain. Early on, they may contribute to neural damage by evoking an inflammatory response, but later they will be necessary to remove cell fragments and noxious substances from the site of injury. Early on, reperfusion of the injury site does more harm than good; later, an adequate supply of oxygen and nutrients contributes to healing. Ultimately, the fires of oxidative stress are quenched. Protein synthesis is restored, and neuroprotective and neurotrophic factors are generated. Endothelial cells proliferate and, after several days, the BBB reconstitutes itself. New capillaries are formed. Glial cells proliferate and migrate. Astrocytes produce nerve growth factor and other neurotrophic substances. Spreading metabolic depression reduces the brain's requirement for sustenance. The cascade of secondary events has run its course, and the injured brain musters its resources for the arduous business of repair and recovery.

Two repair processes have been mentioned: the clearance of posttraumatic debris by macrophages and the repair of partially damaged axons. Axonal repair is only occasionally successful, and the circumstances that promote repair are not readily amenable to therapeutic manipulation. In CHI, in which axonal damage is diffuse, the damaged neuron is able to survive as long as the surrounding microenvironment is intact (8). Conversely, axons that have been transected are incapable of regrowth, but not because they are unable to elongate; when the circumstances are right, axons can grow over comparatively long distances. After BI (or spinal cord injury), however, they find it impossible to do so. It is not entirely clear why that is so; neuronal cell bodies and dendrites are capable of remodeling in adult tissue after BI but not the axons (55).

Recovery of function seems to be accomplished by two physiologic responses: compensatory neural sprouting to restore lost synapses and biochemical adaptations to modify the effectiveness of existing synapses. Collateral sprouting has been known to occur in the peripheral nerves for more than 100 years and in the CNS for almost 50 years. When neurons die, vacancies appear where their dendritic arbors used to reside. Axons from nearby neurons sprout and form synapses to fill the empty spaces; dendrites sprout to receive them. Axonal sprouting reinnervates denervated zones only if their terminal field overlaps that of the damaged afferent; thus, they strengthen or rearrange previously existing connections. In the adult organism, sprouting does not create new pathways. The classic example is sprouting from surviving motoneurons to denervated muscle fibers in polio victims (56,57).

Synaptic reorganization occurs when synapses from secondary connections are strengthened. The connections between neurons have different strengths: primary, secondary, tertiary afferents, as it were. If the primary efferent is destroyed, secondary neurons acquire greater control over the target neuron. For example, many visual cortical cells also have auditory and somatosensory inputs, although the nonvisual inputs are weaker and have longer latencies. In a blind person, the visual cortex is metabolically active, presumably the result of increased activity from the nonvisual inputs. This is synaptic reorganization, by force of silent synapses or unmasking (57,58).

In a similar vein, secondary pathways may be unmasked during the course of recovery. The CNS has many redundant pathways; a secondary pathway may acquire increased importance when the primary pathway is destroyed (58).

When the innervation of a cell is reduced, its receptors are up-regulated or become supersensitive to the stimulation that remains. Receptor sensitization is another way for neurons to compensate for the loss of inputs. It appears that they may also develop receptors on extrasynaptic sites that are sensitive to neuroactive substances in the interstitial fluid, so-called diffusion neurotransmission (57).

What is clear is that the recovering brain is spending down its capital in the service of recovery. Redundant pathways, once employed in the service of a damaged system, cannot be reassigned as easily a second time. Collateral sprouting, too, has its costs, as the surviving neurons must be subject to more in the way of metabolic stress. Surviving motoneurons in poliomyelitis, for example, are given to collateral sprouting. They ultimately fail, exhausted, as it were, by the increased metabolic load they have to carry. This is the genesis of the post-polio syndrome.

The clinical concept of cerebral reserve is adumbrated by the limited resources that the brain has to rely on to compensate for injury. When considering pharmacologic approaches to the patient with BI, it is important to remember that we are dealing with a system that is already stressed.

All these dynamic changes in the neuropil are stimulated by the expression of immediate-acting genes and the production of nerve growth–promoting proteins and cytokines. They can be impeded by the administration of particular drugs, such as some anticonvulsants, and enhanced by others, such as amphetamine (AMP) (59,60). The thrust of pharmacologic research has been to find drugs that control the early-response events that aggravate the effects of BI and drugs that enhance the dynamics of sprouting and receptor reorganization.

Metabolic Depression and Long-Term Potentiation

Cerebral insult also leads to a state of functional depression in areas remote from the lesion (diaschisis). This state may resolve spontaneously or may persist for months at least (61). Resolution of remote functional depression is another aspect of the recovery process that is amenable to pharmacologic intervention.

Von Monakow coined the term diaschisis in 1914, postulating that BI and stroke can decrease regional blood flow and cerebral metabolism in distant areas of the brain. Diaschisis is a temporary functional deactivation of intact brain regions (33). It has been suggested that perturbations of NE activity may be a central event in the development of diaschisis (38). It can be blocked or reversed by intraventricular infusion of NE and by noradrenergic drugs such as AMP (62). Cortical injury in laboratory animals evokes widespread depression of cortical metabolism in various regions including the ipsilateral cortex and cerebellum. This metabolic depression is attenuated by AMP and exaggerated by lesions to the locus ceruleus (39,62).

Resolution of diaschisis is associated with functional improvement. Postlesion treatment with AMP enhanced motor recovery in cats with unilateral or bilateral frontal cortex ablation (38). Enduring recovery of function has also been demonstrated in cats subjected to cortical ablations treated with AMP, when drug treatment is combined with visual training (63). In rats, cortical ablation causes a motor deficit that is apparent when the animal has to traverse a narrow elevated beam. A single dose of AMP administered 24 hours after cortical ablation accelerates the rate of cortical recovery as long as the drug is coupled with beam-walking experience (64,65).

The pharmacologic mechanism of AMP-facilitated recovery is in all probability mediated by CNS noradrenergic neurons. Coadministration of haloperidol in the beam-walking paradigm blocks the AMP response; haloperidol blocks DA and NE but not 5HT (64). Intraventricular or cerebellar infusions of NE mimic the AMP effect, whereas infusions of DA do not. Antagonists or depleters of NE slow beam-walking recovery. The effect of methylphenidate is less robust than that of AMP. Taken together, these findings suggest that stimulant-induced recovery is mediated by central NE (66).

The element that is common to both the clinical and preclinical studies of AMP-induced recovery is the requirement for cotraining. That is, when drug treatment is combined with experience (training, therapy), a positive effect is seen but not with the drug alone. If resolution of metabolic depression is a form of brain plasticity, then it seems to require an optimal catecholamine environment; conversely, the catecholaminergic stimulants work best in the context of an optimal experiential environment (67). This suggests that the drug serves as a facilitator of the learning experience, and that experience augments the effects of the stimulant drug.

Long-term potentiation (LTP) is another mechanism of brain plasticity that is influenced by the catecholaminergic environment of the developing or the injured brain. LTP is a mechanism for memory formation—in the broadest sense of the term, memory (68). Although the mechanisms responsible for the development and persistence of LTP are unknown, consideration is usually given to changes in synaptic strength, neosynaptogenesis, and use-dependent sprouting.

Changes in synaptic strength are believed to be the basis for learning and memory; neocortical neurons, for example, can display sustained increase in synaptic efficacy after conditioning stimulation (69). In LTP, a brief tetanic stimulus to specific neural pathways produces an increase in synaptic responses that can last for days or weeks. The development of LTP is triggered by brief physiologic events, appears to be strengthened by repetition, and can persist indefinitely (70). In this sense, it is similar to learning and memory.

It is also similar to kindling. Kindling is also a process in which repeated, periodic administration of an initially subconvulsant electrical stimulus results in progressive intensification of seizure activity, culminating in a generalized clonic motor seizure (71). Both kindling and LTP are believed to model CNS plasticity. Both are induced by the localized application of brief, high-frequency trains of electrical pulses through implanted electrodes, and both result in a lasting increase in sensitivity to a constant stimulus (72). Similar mechanisms that modulate plasticity through use-dependent sprouting and neosynaptogenesis are proposed to play a role in kindling-induced pathologic states such as epilepsy (73) and the affective disorders (74).

Kindling is pharmacologically distinct from LTP, however. For example, depletion of central NE or destruction of noradrenergic fibers by 6-hydroxydopamine results in a dramatic acceleration in the rate of kindling with electrical stimulation of limbic or cortical sites. Depletion of NE does not affect established seizures, suggesting that the suppressive action of NE is limited to seizure development per se. Depletion of DA appears to have no effect on kindling (75), and with 5HT, the effect of depletion is ambiguous (76). In almost all the studies reported to date, treatments that interfere with NE transmission produce no effect of hippocampal LTP or reduce it, and treatments that enhance NE transmission produce no effect or facilitate it. Thus, if NE plays a role in LTP, it is a facilitatory one, in contrast to the inhibitory role it plays in kindling.

If drugs such as AMP facilitate cortical recovery by enhancing the learning process, it is likely that LTP is at least one of the pertinent mechanisms. If an optimal noradrenergic environment is necessary for the development of LTP in the service of recovery, a suboptimal NE environment may enhance the development of kindling, a potentially destructive variant of LTP.

In considering the problem of brain plasticity after injury, one is concerned with a dynamic process of reorganization of cell-to-cell communication. Axons and dendrites are capable of collateral sprouting, new receptors are generated at the synapse and extrasynaptically, and the strength of neuronal communication is enhanced by environmental stimulation. Even neurononeogenesis, occurring as it does only in privileged sites in the hippocampus and the olfactory system, is responsive to the organism's state of activation and level of activity. The processes of recovery are especially intense during the first days and weeks after injury and during the first year, but they also continue throughout life, as long as the brain remains healthy and free from ongoing noxious influence (77).

Cerebral insult is associated with a surge of neurotransmitter activity, followed by a relative depression, especially of NE. The widespread metabolic depression that persists after BI seems to be largely a function of an enduring hyponoradrenergic state. It is a condition that may self-correct ultimately, or it may be corrected by the judicious prescription of low doses of noradrenergic drugs, such as the psychostimulants, desipramine, and atomoxetine. Other drugs and dietary supplements may possibly enhance cerebral recovery. Their potential neuroprotective and neurotrophic properties are discussed in Chapters 18, 19, and 25.

BRAIN MECHANISMS OF MENTAL RETARDATION

General and Specific Deficits

It is difficult to discuss the encephalopathic mechanisms in conditions as broad and diverse as MR and acquired BI. In the previous section, we dealt with one member of the BI family, namely, TBI. Some of the components of TBI neuropathology are unique, while others are common to all cerebral insults, including stroke and hypoxic injury. Now, as we address the mechanisms of MR, we shall discover that some mechanisms are unique to particular MR syndromes, while other mechanisms are general and common to most forms of MR. Indeed, some mechanisms are shared by the acquired cerebral insults as well.

An appropriate starting point is just where we left off, as the brain is attempting to recover from a traumatic event and restore what it can of normal function. Surviving neurons reestablish function by growing new processes, reforming synaptic connectivity, normalizing their metabolic state, and reforming memory traces. Their goal is to reestablish an efficient and well-organized neural syncytium. The degree to which the brain is successful in accomplishing this end is the foundation for functional recovery. The degree to which it fails is the basis for functional deficit.

The functional deficits that follow acquired BI are either specific or general. The former is a specific lesion that compromises localized functions such as language and motor control. The latter is represented by diffuse damage that compromises generalized functions such as attention, memory, inhibition, processing speed, and intelligence.

Diffuse cerebral damage has four enduring pathologic consequences: neuronal loss, the loss of neuritic processes, synapses, and appropriate interneuronal communication; the development of aberrant connectivity or abnormal electrical activity; and functional metabolic depression at sites remote from the primary lesions.

The first three, and possibly the fourth, are also diffuse effects of MR. Loss of neural elements is not as germane as is failure to develop, but neuronal loss does occur in MR, for example in patients with Down's Syndrome, even in early childhood (78).

The generalized pathology attendant on BI and MR compromises the integrity of neural organization and the efficiency of neuronal communication. The most important general deficit in both events is measured by intelligence, a cognitive function considered a fundamental attribute of brain. In fact, intelligence is a meta-function, the summation of a number of more fundamental mental processes.

The Neural Basis of Intelligence

It is appropriate to turn our attention to the problem of intelligence because that, after all, is the defining element of MR. The very definition of MR carries the conviction that what one is dealing with is a general, not a specific, deficit. It is true that some MR syndromes are associated with specific neuropsychological deficits, but this chapter is devoted to general mechanisms, not exceptional cases, and the problem of low intelligence, a general deficit by any account, is where we should take up the neuropathology of MR.

A good psychological definition of intelligence is that it is the ability to deal with complex cognitive tasks. Its functional components include working memory and attention, coordination of goal-directed cognitive processes, and inhibition of goal-irrelevant processes. Classical psychometric theory posits the existence of *g*, a statistical expression of "pure fluid intelligence" that IQ tests approximate but never fully capture. Theoretically, at least, *g* should have a biologic correlate, but, if it exists, it has always been difficult to come by.

The psychologist Karl Lashley proposed that the biologic basis of intelligence resided in the mass action of functioning cortical tissue and that the loss of intelligence, for example, after BI, was a function of decreased efficiency in cortical operations (79). Several observations in recent years have tended to support Lashley's definition of intelligence as a manifestation of brain efficiency.

For example, there is a commonly observed correlation between reaction time (RT) and intelligence, a correlation that only grows stronger when the complexity of the RT task is increased (80). In experiments using both visual and auditory stimuli, the RT of low-intelligence subjects increases as more stimuli are added. In contrast, the RT of subjects with a high IQ decreases with more complex stimuli. They respond to the stimuli more quickly and more consistently.

Inspection time is a psychophysical measure like RT that requires more than simply an immediate response. In inspection time research, people with higher levels of intelligence are able to make more accurate judgments when stimuli are visible for very brief periods (81). Largely on the basis of RT and inspection time experiments, one general theory of intelligence holds that individual differences in information processing speed functionally determine individual differences in general intellectual ability (82,83).

Intelligence, however, is not simply a function of the speed of mental operations. This is clearly evidenced in evoked potential studies, in which response latencies are only weakly correlated with the subjects' IQ. What characterizes the evoked potentials of more intelligent subjects is diminished intrastimulus variability, that is, a more reliable waveform from one trial to another. This occurs, even though subjects with a high IQ generate more complex waveforms in response to the stimulus, and they fire more neurons in responding to it. They bring more resources to bear on the task, and they do so with a high degree of electrophysiologic reliability (81).

Another pertinent observation, in positron emission tomography studies of mentally retarded and normally intelligent people is that brain glucose metabolism in response to a cognitive task is inversely correlated with the subject's level of intelligence. In other words, the brains of more intelligent people work less hard to deal with the cognitive task than the brains of less intelligent people (84).

The neural operations of an intelligent brain, therefore, are "lashleyan," indeed, and characterized by efficient operation. The intelligent brain reacts quickly and consistently, mobilizes a greater mass of neuronal tissue, and, at the same time, utilizes less energy. On an ultrastructural level, one assumes that these attributes of intelligence are represented in superior neuronal connectivity and bioenergetics.

Hebb's rule defines learning in terms of synaptic plasticity. Hebb proposed that learning and memory are comprised of modifications in synaptic strength among neurons that are simultaneously active (85). In modern terms, the hebbian model is expressed in studies of LTP and long-term depression, which are experience-engendered changes in synaptic efficiency. Recently, proteins have been described that facilitate LTP and long-term depression within the synapse. Genetic modifications or chemical interventions that block proteins like Src and PSD-95 interfere with LTP and long-term depression and thus impair learning (86,87). Learning, of course, is not synonymous with intelligence, but theories of the latter have also been advanced in terms synaptic efficiency: "intelligence...is the summation of all of the factors which can affect the synaptic recognition process" (88).

The general intellectual impairment that accompanies severe BI and MR is associated with marked changes in the neuropil, reduced neuronal numbers or dysfunctional neuronal arrangements, and derangements of the neuritic elements that mediate neural connectivity. The connectivity of neural assemblies is thus compromised. As a result, in both conditions, information processing speed is markedly reduced (89,90).

The energy characteristics of the individual neuron are also impaired in MR by mitochondrial abnormalities, abnormal cellular inclusions, microtubules that are ill-formed or defective, and neuritic processes that are tortuous and poorly directed. After severe BI, a decreased number of neurons is forced to subserve the usual functions. They continue to function and compensate for the lost neurons, but only by taking on an unusual metabolic load.

When the bioenergetics of the neuron is thus compromised, the efficiency of signal transduction and genomic transcription in response to stimulation is also compromised. As a result, adaptation is impaired. One manifestation of impaired adaptation is electrophysiologic habituation to stimulus trains, which is attenuated or absent in studies of mentally retarded people (81).

A generalized reduction in the efficiency of central processing accounts for diminished intelligence in BI and MR. It is the consequence of impairments in neuronal connectivity and cellular bioenergetics.

Mental Retardation: Etiopathogenesis

There are more than 350 documented etiologies of MR. Virtually every aspect of brain development and maturation and virtually every cellular and biochemical element have been implicated in one or another. It is difficult to address the issue without being encyclopedic, and general rules are hard to extract from a wealth of technical and rapidly evolving information. Contradictions and paradoxes abound. Microcephaly is characteristic of many MR syndromes, and large heads are statistically correlated with intelligence, but large heads are also characteristic of people with fragile X syndrome and autism. Reduced neuronal numbers characterize some MR syndromes; in others, cortical neurons survive in increased numbers compared with normal brains and are more tightly packed. Abnormalities in neuritic development, of dendritic spines, and of synapses, are the most commonly observed neuropathologic findings in the brains of mentally retarded people, but such abnormalities are neither universal nor widely correlated with the degree of intellectual impairment. Even with all the advances of molecular medicine, almost half of the cases of MR are etiologically undiagnosable.

The old rule was that mild MR was sociofamilial in nature and that severe MR was biologic in nature, but increased familiarity with the various genetic syndromes that cause MR indicates a wide range of intellectual outcomes. The fragile X syndrome, for example, the second most common genetic cause of MR, is usually associated with only mild or moderate intellectual deficits. People with DS and de Lange syndrome can have IQ scores in the normal range.

Etiopathogenetic events that cause MR are typically associated with general deficits, namely, reduced intelligence. This should not obscure the importance of specific deficits in MR.

BI *in utero*, during childbirth, and in early childhood, as we have seen, is more likely to cause general deficits, especially in intellectual ability, and not specific neuropsychological deficits. This is the consequence of the diffuse nature of the traumatic event and of the reorganization of cerebral functions in the service of brain plasticity. Early BIs also have specific effects because some brain regions are more vulnerable than others, and cerebral reorganization attempts to protect certain functions at the expense of others.

When MR is the result of a genetic mistake—mutation, translocation, microdeletion, repeat amplification, or aneuploidy—the clinical outcome is usually thought of in terms of a general intellectual deficit. The genetic MR syndromes, however, are also associated with specific neuropsychological and neurobehavioral outcomes. Patients with DS, for example, are known to have memory and language deficits that are in excess of what would be predicted based on their mental age. Patients with Williams syndrome are fluent in language, even beyond their mental age, but deficient in visuospatial abilities. Patients with fragile X syndrome are poor in language pragmatics but high in vocabulary (79).

It is possible to trace in some cases of genetically determined MR the path that runs from the gene to the protein to the neural structure that is affected. What emerges from this extraordinary exercise in molecular biology is no less than a new window to the brain. It is comparable in importance, and in interest, to the early studies in experimental neuropsychology, when specific psychological functions were first attributed to specific lesions.

Genes that have generalized effects in the CNS are well known. In fragile X syndrome, the *FMR-1* gene is inactivated and the encoded protein is not produced. FMR protein plays a role in the development of dendrites, which are thin, tortuous, and underdeveloped in affected individuals (91). In phenylketonuria, a mutation in a gene on chromosome 12 that encodes phenylalanine hydroxylase leads to accumulation of phenylalanine in the blood, which has diffuse toxic effects on brain development (92). In DS, several genes identified on chromosome 21 are associated with general effects on brain development, such as *DYRK*, a gene that controls cell growth and development, whereas others nearby, such as the *APP* gene and superoxide dismutase-1, probably play a role in neuronal degeneration and the onset of dementia (93,94).

In other conditions, information is accruing about genes that have more specific effects on brain development and on specific areas of CNS function. The impairment of visuospatial performance in Williams syndrome is specifically associated with the *Lim-kinase1* gene on 7q11.23 (95). In Angelman syndrome, the gene for one of the γ-aminobutyric acid receptors is deleted, which may explain the particular kind of epilepsy that occurs in that condition. In Rett's syndrome, a mutation at MECP2 disrupts the normal sequence of CNS maturation and causes intellectual regression in late childhood (96).

Genetic abnormalities in the MR syndromes have general and specific effects. They can operate independently or in concert with other genetic deficits or environmental events. They can influence neuronal development at any stage of fetal development, in early childhood, or in later life.

Increasingly, the diagnosis of MR syndromes is made based on DNA analysis. This permits a degree of accuracy in diagnosis that was never possible when diagnosis was based on phenotypic characteristics. It also increases the number of people who are identified with the syndromes, many of whom do not have pronounced dysmorphic features, for example, or even intellectual impairment in the MR range. People are identified with relatively mild specific learning disabilities or psychiatric disorders that would never have been associated with a MR syndrome in the past.

Neuropathology of Mental Retardation

Gross anatomic abnormalities are not necessarily characteristic of MR, even severe MR. In 10% to 20% of severely retarded people, careful autopsy studies reveal a brain that appears perfectly normal.

As a rule, gross anatomic abnormalities and conventional microscopic examinations have little bearing on the severity of MR. The brain can be somewhat small or large. There can be gray matter heterotopias in the subcortical white matter. The cortex can demonstrate an unusually regular columnar arrangement, or neurons in the cortex may be more tightly packed than usual, but these changes rarely correlate with the severity of intellectual deficit (97). What, then, is the neural basis of MR?

Rather than searching for the pathology of MR in the gross structural abnormalities, investigators have found it more fruitful to examine the nature of dendritic and synaptic organization, especially in the cerebral cortex. In microscopic studies, using special techniques, striking abnormalities are demonstrated in the fine structure of the cerebral cortex, including terminal axons, dendrites, and synapses. Abnormalities of dendritic morphology have been documented in DS, with truncation of dendrites, simplification of dendritic arborization, malformed dendritic spines, and cytoskeletal abnormalities. Children with various forms of MR also show defects in the number, length, and spatial arrangement of dendrites and synapses (97–99).

Axonal and dendritic growth in the developing brain is particularly active during the last trimester of gestation and the first months of the postnatal period. The proper growth and development of axons, dendrites, and synapses, especially in the preterm infant, are vulnerable to toxic, metabolic, and nutritional disturbances. Postnatal hypothyroidism, for example, is associated with decreased dendritic and synaptic development, and postnatal axonal growth is stunted in postnatal malnutrition. Neonatal anoxia and postnatal ionizing radiation are associated with decreased development of the neuropil (100). In Rett's syndrome, in which there is increased neuronal packing, branching from pyramidal cells and dendritic arborization are markedly reduced (78).

In fragile X syndrome, there are abnormal dendritic spine patterns, with very thin, long tortuous spines and marked reductions in synaptic density (101). Genes associated with X-linked MR are involved in signal transduction mediated by rho proteins, which regulate the rearrangement of the actin cytoskeleton and thus neuronal motility and morphogenesis. Mutations in proteins involved in rho-dependent signaling compromise the formation of normal neuronal networks (102).

The most obvious mechanism by which dendritic pathology could lead to neurologic impairment is a decrease in the cortical synaptic surface, although the results of studies of synaptic density in mentally retarded individuals have been inconclusive thus far (78).

The pathology of MR is associated, therefore, with abnormalities of neuritic structure that reflect abnormal metabolic processes and compromise intraneuronal transport. Abnormal synaptic and dendritic organization is incompatible with efficient connectivity and interneuronal communication.

Gross abnormalities in the brains of mentally retarded people are associated with events that compromise neuronal proliferation and differentiation, which begins in the fifth week of gestation and continues through the fifth month. At this stage of development, the fetal brain is vulnerable to the effects of irradiation, intrauterine infections (especially rubella), maternal phenylketonuria, maternal alcoholism, and anticonvulsant drugs. These conditions are often associated with microcephaly (99).

Neurons are generated within the ventricular zone and then migrate radially toward the surface of the cerebral hemispheres, guided by climbing glial fibers and forming the cortex in an "inside-out" pattern. Neuronal migration occurs in two waves during the first gestational trimester. Disorders of neuronal migration primarily affect the development of the cerebral cortex; lissencephaly (smooth brain, i.e., the absence of gyri) is the best-known example. Cerebral heterotopias are collections of disorganized gray matter in inappropriate places, the result of aberrant migratory patterns. More than 25 MR syndromes of neuronal migration have been described, most resulting from incomplete neuronal migration to the cortex during the third and fourth months of gestation. Most are genetic conditions, including X-linked MR, but neuronal migration may also be impaired by viral infections, irradiation, retinoic acid, methylmercury, and alcohol (103,104).

MENTAL RETARDATION, BRAIN INJURY, AND DEMENTIA

There are five risk factors for the development of AD: aging, a family history of AD, the ApoE4 allele, DS, and severe BI. The high rate of dementia in MR and BI is an opportunity to examine the neuropathologic mechanisms that are common to both conditions and how they diverge.

Down's Syndrome

The association between AD and DS is so striking that the latter condition has been a virtual laboratory for the study of the former. Neuropathologic lesions characteristic of AD are found in the brains of all patients with DS past the age of 40, although they may not show behavioral or cognitive signs of decline until much later (105,106). A prospective study of dementia in institutionalized mentally retarded people with DS diagnosed clinically reported the prevalence to be 8% at 35 to 49 years, 55% at 50 to 59 years, and 75% at 60 years or older (107). In a population-based study of patients with DS 50 to 60 years of age, 24% had definite dementia and 24% had possible dementia (108).

The connection between DS and dementia was first reported in 1876: "in not a few instances, however, death was attributed to nothing more than general decay—sort of precipitated senility" (109). Because the association is so venerable, virtually every theory of dementia has been applied to explain it, and, as it happens, virtually every current theory of AD is relevant to the issue.

DS is a syndrome of premature aging; the average life span of patients with DS is just more than 40 years (110). People with DS look older than their chronologic age, with gray, thinning hair and dry, wrinkled skin. They develop cataracts, valvular pathology, and immunologic changes characteristic of elderly patients.

It has been proposed that the premature aging of patients with DS is the result of free-radical damage. The gene for the antioxidant enzyme superoxide dismutase-1, a key enzyme in free radical metabolism, is located on chromosome 21. The activity of this enzyme is elevated by approximately 50% in a variety of cells in patients with DS (111). Increased superoxide dismutase activity can generate free-radical stress through overproduction of hydrogen peroxide (93). Thus, DS neurons exhibit a three- to fourfold increase in intracellular reactive oxygen species and elevated levels of lipid peroxidation. Degeneration of DS neurons in culture is prevented by free-radical scavengers (112). The erythrocytes of adults with DS have an unbalanced antioxidant system, which may be indicative of the vulnerability of DS individuals to antioxidative stress (113). The observed changes in the cellular localization of superoxide dismutases in the neocortex and hippocampus in cases of DS and AD support a role for oxidative injury in neuronal degeneration and senile plaque formation (114).

Free-radical damage, therefore, has been presented as a key element in the etiopathogenesis of DS (115), as well as for the phenomena of premature aging (116) and dementia (117,118). Free-radical formation is also a component of secondary damage after TBI and ischemic BI.

The *APOE* Gene

A mutation in the amyloid precursor gene on chromosome 21, an unidentified gene on chromosome 14, and loci on other chromosomes are linked to the rare form of familial AD with onset before the age of 60, but the *APOE4* gene is associated with the more common late-onset disease form (119). In a multicenter study of 2,188 patients, 65% of those with pathologically confirmed AD had at least one ApoE4 allele (120).

Variants of the *APOE* gene seem to account for most cases of late-onset AD. The gene is located on chromosome 19 and has three major alleles: ε2, ε3, and ε4. Most of us have the ε3. The ε2 allele is protective, decreasing the risk of AD and delaying its onset, but the ε4 allele (ApoE4) is harmful, increasing risk and hastening onset. People with the ε4/ε4 genotype are especially vulnerable to AD (121).

The protein that is encoded by *APOE4*, apolipoprotein E isoform 4, is immunoreactive in the plaques that are characteristic of AD, with a greater avidity for β-amyloid (compared with the ApoE3 isoform). The ApoE4 isoform promotes a nonsoluble structure for amyloid protein. It also binds to neurofibrillary tangles where the major protein is tau, not amyloid (122–124). The *APOE4* gene is also associated with lower levels of endogenous antioxidants and increased oxidative stress (125).

Lipoproteins are molecules that are designed to complex with lipids to solubilize and recycle them. Apolipoprotein E plays a central role in plasma lipoprotein metabolism and in lipid transport within tissues. It is involved in brain development and repair.

It is central to this transport system and provides injured cells cholesterol and phospholipids for the maintenance and repair of membranes, the growth of neurites, dendritic remodeling and synaptogenesis (126).

The accumulation of β-amyloid in brain is more extensive in patients with the ApoE4 allele, even if they do not have AD (123). Elderly patients, for example, who are at risk of vascular dementia are more likely to experience cognitive decline if they carry the *APOE4* gene (127). Studies have indicated that the ApoE4 allele is a poor outcome factor for patients with head trauma, brain hemorrhage, and ischemia (128,129).

The characteristics of the ApoE alleles are reflected as well in the development of dementia in people with DS. ApoE2 appears to confer a degree of protection from symptomatic dementia, and ApoE4 increases the risk (130–132).

β-Amyloid and Tau

Severe TBI is associated with diffuse deposits of β-amyloid protein (BAP) in the brain. Even more widespread is immunoreactivity to the amyloid precursor protein (APP), especially in dystrophic neurites and neurons and in areas of axonal injury (133).

Amyloid plaques, the essential criterion for the pathologic diagnosis of AD, are extracellular deposits of a number of different proteins. The most important is BAP, a peptide formed by the cleavage of APP. APP itself is a transmembrane glycoprotein, synthesized in the brain and localized in synaptic endings (134).

Potentially amyloidogenic peptides are produced and secreted by most cells during normal metabolism and are present in soluble form in biologic fluids. BAP, however, is not normally generated, and production in the aging brain or in the brain of a person with AD requires an alteration in the normal processing of APP. The alternative proteolytic pathways responsible for the generation of BAP generate insoluble, β-pleated sheets that are deposited in plaques. This process appears, to a slight extent, during normal aging but it is markedly increased in AD (134,135). The ApoE4 allele promotes the formation of insoluble BAP.

The gene for APP is on chromosome 21; as a result, people with trisomy 21 (i.e., DS) overexpress the *APP* gene severalfold throughout their lives (136). By the age of 40, virtually all of them have developed the typical neuropathologic lesions of AD.

It was natural for scientists to consider BAP to be central to the cause of AD by virtue of its abnormal generation, its concentration in the hippocampus, amygdala, and cortical association areas, and the association of mutations in its precursor protein gene with some cases of early-onset AD. There is evidence that BAP is directly neurotoxic and that it increases cytosolic calcium, enhances neuronal vulnerability to excitotoxic neurotransmitters, and generates oxygen free radicals (137).

Conversely, not everyone agrees that BAP is the central mediating event in the genesis of AD, and there is even evidence to suggest that amyloid may have a protective effect on neurons, perhaps by preventing the excess accumulation of calcium. In the aging brain and in DS, there is not a clear association between the concentration of amyloid plaques and cognitive impairment. In fact, the signs and symptoms of AD correlate best with areas of high tangle formation (138).

There is still an active debate about whether the dementia of AD is primarily the result of extracellular BAP deposition, with subsequent formation of neurofibrillary tangles leading to neuronal death or whether the process is initiated by neurofibrillary damage, leading to the build up of extracellular amyloid. Neurofibrillary tangles are one of a number of cytoskeletal abnormalities characteristic of AD. They contain paired helical fragments that are formed primarily from abnormal aggregations of tau proteins. Tau proteins are associated with the microtubules that determine the shape of cells and the neuritic transport of cellular nutrients (including APP). Normal tau has only two or three phosphate groups per molecule. ApoE4 is associated with the hyperphosphorylation of tau (five to nine phosphate groups per molecule) and with the extra phosphates tau is no longer able to bind to tubulin, which makes microtubules (138).

The level of normal tau protein is markedly reduced in the brains of demented patients with DS (110). Paired helical fragments and neurofibrillary tangles also contain nontau materials, such as ubiquitin, which has been identified in the brains of boxers, including a number with dementia pugilistica (DP) (139).

It has been proposed that the deposition of BAP initiates a cascade of inflammatory events, but both senile plaques and neurofibrillary tangles represent in all probability a considerable inflammatory burden to the afflicted brain. They are found to contain a host of inflammatory proteins, including activated complement, complement inhibitors, inflammatory cytokines, acute phase reactants, lipoproteins, proteases, and trophic factors. As we have discussed, this inflammatory response may be more than just an epiphenomenon directed at detritus accumulating in the lesions and may also be a self-sustaining, autodestructive force that attacks bystander neurons in such a way that more lesions are produced (140,141). Here, also, ApoE may play a role, by modulating the inflammatory response (142).

An excessive inflammatory reaction typically contributes to the process of degeneration in any tissue in which it occurs. The clinical course of AD, beginning with the slow accumulation of plaques and tangles, a gradual loss of higher level cognitive abilities, and then a rapid clinical deterioration over a rather short period, suggests that the final stages are mediated by a vigorously self-sustaining, destructive reaction that may well be inflammatory in nature. It also provides, however, an avenue for potential treatment.

Dementia and Brain Trauma

Severe head trauma is almost always listed as one of the risk factors for the development of AD, and there is a great deal of evidence to support the association, but there are also conflicting data. That is surprising; the association is not only intuitive, it is venerable.

In 1928, an American pathologist, Martland, described the punchdrunk syndrome:

> *There may develop a peculiar tilting of the head, a marked dragging of one or both legs, a staggering, propulsive gait with the facial characteristics of the parkinsonian syndrome, or a backward swaying of the body, tremors, vertigo, or deafness. Finally, marked mental deterioration may set in necessitating commitment to an asylum (143).*

The English neuropathologist Corsellis published a classic article on DP in 1989, describing the "inexplicable alteration" in the neurons of former boxers, that is, neurofibrillary tangles without senile plaques. It was not inexplicable at all; when his specimens were reexamined using different staining techniques, large numbers of neuritic plaques were found. Subsequent studies have also indicated acetylcholine deficiency and tau immunoreactivity in DP. The pathology of DP is not much different from AD after all (144,145).

DP is a special case of posttraumatic dementia and the result of repetitive subconcussive blows over a span of time. A single concussion is not likely to exert any such effect, but severe TBI is.

The odds ratio, that is, the degree to which TBI will increase one's risk of developing a dementing condition, has ranged in different studies from 2.4 to 13.75 (146–151). Patients with TBI who go on to develop dementia are more likely to have had a severe injury, more than one head injury, a concurrent illness such as alcoholism, or small-vessel disease (152). Patients who have had severe BIs develop AD at an earlier age than patients with AD without a history of head trauma (153). Older patients with TBI are also more likely to develop cognitive decline after major head trauma (154). The absence of an association between mild head trauma and AD has been affirmed in studies in Olmstead County, MN (155,156) and from Europe (157–159).

Boxers (and other athletes prone to repetitive head trauma) have more severe deficits if they carry the ApoE4 allele (160,161). Posttraumatic dementia is more likely to develop in patients who possess the ApoE4 allele (80,151), and functional recovery after severe TBI is less successful (128).

Summary: Dementia, Down's Syndrome, and TBI

The connection between DS and AD derives from chromosome 21, where the APP originates, and superoxide dismutase and other pathogenic substances. The connection, therefore, is specific. Some of the elements that define that specific association are also reflected in the development of AD after severe TBI: amyloid, tau, ubiquitin, free-radical damage, even, as we have seen, ApoE4. There is also a nonspecific association between MR in general and AD. Simply put, mentally retarded people are more prone to dementia than the population at large. Based on a large sample of mentally retarded people, none of whom had DS, autopsy studies reveal a neuropathologic diagnosis of AD in 10% of those who died before the age of 50 years, 55% in those between 50 and 65, 70% in those between 66 and 75, and in 87% in those older than 75 (162,163). These numbers are extraordinary when compared with the normal population.

The explanation for this broader, nonspecific association between MR and AD is straightforward and intuitive. It relies on the well-established finding that people with more education are less likely to develop AD and that people with lower intellectual achievement are more likely to develop AD.

> *Scholars grow wiser as they age, but the noneducated become foolish. (The Babylonian Talmud)*

The origin of this striking observation, Talmudic scholars aside, was an epidemiologic study of dementia in Shanghai, and since then, it has been confirmed in studies in France, Italy, Sweden, Finland, Israel, and New York City. Illiterate or poorly educated subjects are two or three times more likely to develop AD than highly educated subjects. Higher occupational attainment has a similar, sanguine effect. It is not a function of relative facility with psychological testing, nor is it mediated by lifestyle differences or the availability of medical care. Fine-grained analysis, examining subjects whose intelligence had been tested for military service, indicates that both education and occupation are surrogate measures of intelligence, and it is the latter that is central to the protective effect (164–167).

Educational level is inversely correlated with the risk of AD, even in poorly educated, rural people (168). In DS, individuals with higher cognitive levels are less likely to develop symptomatic dementia (169).

The usual explanation is that education and its correlate intelligence reflect greater cerebral reserve, perhaps referring to synaptic density. This is consistent with evidence that the biologic basis for cognitive decline in AD is the loss of synapses. In fact, studies have shown that elderly patients with advanced neuropathologic findings of AD may be clinically nondemented as long as they have sufficient concentrations of intact neurons and that the variance in dementia severity, measured on psychological tests, is accounted for almost entirely by measures of synaptic density (86% to 92% of the variance) (165).

"Cerebral reserve" sounds like one of those imposingly transcendent but impossibly vague concepts that scholars call forth to explain phenomena for which they have no better explanation—like "mental energy" or the *élan vital* . Like intelligence itself, though, it appears to be rooted in the speed and efficiency of cerebral operations. It can be understood, in light of this discussion, in terms of synaptic organization and the efficiency of neuronal communication. It will be met with again, as we discuss some of the clinical consequences of TBI. It is a form of capital that is spent down every time the brain is injured. It is an asset that mentally retarded people never really manage to accumulate. Their poverty in this regard renders them vulnerable to dementia and to a number of other problems that are the subjects of later chapters.

REFERENCES

1. Cortez SC, McIntosh TK, Noble LJ. Experimental fluid percussion brain injury: vascular disruption and neuronal and glial alterations. *Brain Res* 1989;482: 271–282.
2. Jiang JY, Lyeth BG, Kapasi MZ, et al. Moderate hypothermia reduces blood-brain barrier disruption following traumatic brain injury in the rat. *Acta Neuropathol* 1992;84:495–500.
3. Tanno H, Nockels RP, Pitts LH, et al. Breakdown of the blood-brain barrier after fluid percussion brain injury in the rat: part 2: effect of hypoxia on permeability to plasma proteins. *J Neurotrauma* 1992;9: 335–347.
4. Mayhan WG. Disruption of the blood-brain barrier in open and closed cranial window preparations in rats. *Stroke* 1991;22:1059–1063.
5. Gennarelli TA, Thibault LE, Adams JH, et al. Diffuse axonal injury and traumatic coma in the primate. *Ann Neurol* 1982;12:564–575.
6. Bourke RS. *Head injury*. Bethesda, MD: NINCDS, 1988.
7. Blumbergs PC, Jones NR, North JB. Diffuse axonal injury in head trauma. *J Neurol Neurosurg Psychiatry* 1989;52:838–841.
8. Povlishock JT, Coburn TH. Morphopathological change associated with mild head injury. In: Levin HS, Eisenberg HM, Benton AL, eds. *Mild head injury*. New York: Oxford University Press, 1989:37–53.
9. Yarnell PR, Rossie GV. Minor whiplash head injury with major debilitation. *Brain Inj* 1988;2:255–258.
10. Ommaya AK, Faas F, Yarnell P. Whiplash injury and brain damage. *JAMA* 1968;204:285–289.
11. Ommaya AK, Gennarelli TA. A cerebral concussion and traumatic unconsciousness: correlation of experimental and clinical observations on blunt head injuries. *Brain* 1974;97:633–654.
12. Jane JA, Steward O, Gennarelli TA. Axonal degeneration induced by experimental non-invasive minor head injury. *J Neurosurg* 1985;62:96–100.
13. Clifton GL, McCormick WF, Grossman RG. Neuropathology of early and late deaths after head injury. *Neurosurgery* 1981;8:309–314.
14. Levin HS, Eisenberg HM, Benton AL. *Mild head injury*. New York: Oxford University Press, 1989.
15. Peerless SJ, Rewcastle NW. Shear injuries of the brain. *CMAJ* 1967;96:577–582.
16. Oppenheimer DR. Microscopic lesions in the brain following head injury. *J Neurol Neurosurg Psychiatry* 1968;31:299–306.
17. Bareggi SR, Porta M, Selenati A, et al. Homovanillic acid and 5-hydroxyindole-acetic acid in the CSF of patients after a severe head injury. I. Lumbar CSF concentration in chronic brain post-traumatic syndromes. *Eur Neurol* 1975;13:528–544.
18. McIntosh TK. Neurochemical sequelae of traumatic brain injury: therapeutic implications. *Cerebrovasc Brain Metab Rev* 1994;6:109–162.
19. Hayes RL, Lyeth BG, Jenkins LW. Neurochemical mechanisms of mild and moderate head injury: implications for treatment. In: Levin HS, Eisenberg HM, Benton AL, eds. *Mild head injury*. New York: Oxford University Press, 1989:54–79.
20. Armstead WM, Kurth CD. The role of opioids in newborn pig fluid percussion brain injury. *Brain Res* 1994; 660:19–26.
21. Markianos M, Seretis A, Kotsou A, et al. CSF neurotransmitter metabolites in comatose head injury patients during changes in their clinical state. *Acta Neurochir* 1996;138:57–59.

22. Goldstein L. Pharmacological approach to functional reorganization: the role of norepinephrine. *Rev Neurol* 1999;155:731–736.
23. Donnemiller E, Brenneis C, Wissel J, et al. Impaired dopaminergic neurotransmission in patients with traumatic brain injury: a SPECT study using 123I-beta-CIT a 123I-IBZM. *Eur J Nucl Med* 2000;27: 1410–1414.
24. Azmitia E. The CNS serotonergic system: progression toward a collaborative organization. In: Meltzer HY, ed. *Psychopharmacology: the third generation of progress*. New York: Raven Press, 1987:61–74.
25. Rosner MJ, Newsome HH, Becker DP. Mechanical brain injury: the sympathoadrenal response. *J Neurosurg* 1984;61:76–86.
26. Silver JM, Yodofsky SC, Hales RE. Depression in traumatic brain injury. *Neuropsychiatry Neuropsychol Behav Neurol* 1991;4:12–23.
27. Carlsson GS. Long-term effects of head injuries sustained during life in three male populations. *J Neurosurg* 1987;67:197–205.
28. Meltzer HY, Lowy MT. The serotonin hypothesis of depression. In: Meltzer HY, ed. *Psychopharmacology: the third generation of progress*. New York: Raven Press, 1987:513–526.
29. Boyeson MG, Harmon RL. Effects of trazodone and desipramine on motor recovery in brain-injured rats. *Am J Phys Med Rehabil* 1993;72:286–293.
30. Goldstein LB. Effects of amphetamines and small related molecules on recovery after stroke in animals and man. *Neuropharmacology* 2000;39:852–859.
31. Bartus RT, Dean RL, Flicker C. Cholinergic psychopharmacology: an integration of human and animal research on memory. In: Meltzer HY, ed. *Psychopharmacology: the third generation of progress*. New York: Raven Press, 1987:219–232.
32. Stokes PE, Sikes CR. Hypothalamic-pituitary-adrenal axis in affective disorders. In: Meltzer HY, ed. *Psychopharmacology: the third generation of progress*. New York: Raven Press, 1987:589–608.
33. Feeney DM, Baron JC. Diaschisis. *Stroke* 1986;17: 817–830.
34. Dobkin JA, Levine RL, Lagreze HL, et al. Evidence for transhemispheric diaschisis in unilateral stroke. *Arch Neurol* 1989;46:1333–1336.
35. Deuel RK. The functional anatomy of manual motor behavior after unilateral frontal lobe lesions. *Brain Res* 1992;580:249–254.
36. Baron JC, Levasseur M, Mazoyer B, et al. Thalamocortical diaschisis: positron emission tomography in humans. *J Neurol Neurosurg Psychiatry* 1992;55: 935–942.
37. Fulham MJ, Brooks RA, Hallett M, et al. Cerebellar diaschisis revisited: pontine hypometabolism and dentate sparing. *Neurology* 1992;42:2267–2273.
38. Feeney DM, Sutton RL. Catecholamines and recovery of function after brain damage. In: Stein DG, Sabel BA, eds. *Pharmacological approaches to the treatment of brain and spinal cord injuries*. New York: Plenum, 1988:121–142.
39. Feeney DM, Sutton RL, Boyeson MG, et al. The locus coeruleus and cerebral metabolism: Recovery of function after cortical injury. *Physiol Psychol* 1985;13: 197–203.
40. Hayes RL, Pechura CM, Katayama Y, et al. Activation of pontine cholinergic sites implicated in unconsciousness following cerebral concussion in the cat. *Science* 1984;223:301–303.
41. Novack TA, Dillon MC, Jackson WT. Neurochemical mechanisms in brain injury and treatment: a review. *J Clin Exp Neuropsychol* 1996;18:685–706.
42. Manev H, Costa E, Wroblewski JT, et al. Abusive stimulation of excitatory amino acid receptors: a strategy to limit neurotoxicity. *FASEB J* 1990;4:2789–2797.
43. Olney JW. Excitatory transmitter neurotoxicity. *Neurobiol Aging* 1994;15:259–260.
44. Chapman AG, Durmuller N, Lees GJ, et al. Excitotoxicity of NMDA and kainic acid is modulated by nigrostriatal dopaminergic fibres. *Neurosci Lett* 1989; 107:256–260.
45. Lipton SA, Rosenberg PA. Excitatory amino acids as a final common pathway for neurologic disorders. *N Engl J Med* 1994;330:613–622.
46. Faden AI, Demeduik P, Panter SS, et al. The role of excitatory amino acids and NMDA receptors in traumatic brain injury. *Science* 1989;244:798–800.
47. Baker AJ, Moulton R, MacMillian V, et al. Excitatory amino acids in cerebrospinal fluid following traumatic brain injury in humans. *J Neurosurg* 1993;79: 369–372.
48. Iorio KR, Tabakoff B, Hoffman PL. Glutamate-induced neurotoxicity is increased in cerebellar granule cells exposed chronically to ethanol. *Eur J Pharmacol* 1993;248:209–212.
49. Abe K, Aoki M, Kawagoe J, et al. Ischemic delayed neuronal death: a mitochondrial hypothesis. *Stroke* 1995;26:1478–1489.
50. Viola J, Ditzler T, Batzer W, et al. Pharmacological management of post-traumatic stress disorder: clinical summary of a five-year retrospective study, 1990-1995. *Mil Med* 1997;162:616–619.
51. Wauquier A, Edmonds HL Jr, Clincke GHC. Cerebral resuscitation: pathophysiology and therapy. *Neurosci Biobehav Rev* 1987;11:287–306.
52. Feuerstein GZ, Liu T, Barone FC. Cytokines, inflammation, and brain injury: role of tumor necrosis factor-alpha. *Cerebrovasc Brain Metab Rev* 1994;6:341–360.
53. Hovda DA, Becker DP, Katayama Y. Secondary injury and acidosis. *J Neurotrauma* 1992;9:S47–S60.
54. Mesenge C, Verrecchia C, Allix M, et al. Reduction of the neurological deficit in mice with traumatic brain injury by nitric oxide synthase inhibitors. *J Neurotrauma* 1996;13:209–214.
55. Landis D. The early reactions of non-neuronal cells to brain injury. *Annu Rev Neurosci* 1994;17:133–151.
56. LeVere T. Neural system imbalances and the consequence of large brain injuries. *Brain Inj Recov* 1988; 15–28.
57. Bach-y-Rita P. Recovery from brain damage. *J Neurorehabil* 1993;6:191–199.
58. Stroemer R, Kent T, Hulsebosch C. Neocortical neural sprouting, synaptogenesis, and behavioral recovery after neocortical infarction in rats. *Stroke* 1995;26: 2135–2144.
59. Almli C, Levy T, Han B, et al. BDNF protects against spatial memory deficits following neonatal hypoxia-ischemia. *Exp Neurol* 2000;166:99–114.
60. Swartz K, Liu F, Sewell D, et al. Interleukin-6 promotes post-traumatic healing in the central nervous system. *Brain Res* 2001;896:86–95.

61. Passineau M, Zhao W, Busto R, et al. Chronic metabolic sequelae of traumatic brain injury: prolonged suppression of somatosensory activation. *Am J Heart Circ Physiol* 2000;279:924–931.
62. Dail WG, Feeney DM, Murray HM, et al. Responses to cortical injury: II. Widespread depression of the activity of an enzyme in cortex remote from the focal injury. *Brain Res* 1981;211:79–89.
63. Hovda DA, Feeney DM. Amphetamine with experience promotes recovery of locomotor function after unilateral frontal cortex injury in the cat. *Brain Res* 1984;298:358–361.
64. Feeney DM, Gonzalez A, Law WA. Amphetamine, haloperidol and experience interact to affect rate of recovery after motor cortex surgery. *Science* 1982;217: 855–857.
65. Goldstein LB, Davis JM. Influence of lesion size and location on amphetamine-facilitated recovery of beam-walking in rats. *Behav Neurosci* 1990;104: 320–327.
66. McGilchrist I, Goldstein LH, Jadresic D, et al. Thalamo-frontal psychosis. *Br J Psychiatry* 1993;163: 113–115.
67. Exner M, Clark D. Subtle variations in living conditions influence behavioral response to d-amphetamine. *Neuroreport* 1993;4:1059–1062.
68. Brinton RE. Neuromodulation: associative & nonlinear adaptation. *Brain Res Bull* 1990;24:651–658.
69. Sutor B, Hablitz JJ. Long-term potentiation in frontal cortex: role of NMDA-modulated polysynaptic excitatory pathways. *Neurosci Lett* 1989;97:111–117.
70. Lynch G, Baudry M. The biochemistry of memory: a new and specific hypothesis. *Science* 1984;224: 1057–1063.
71. McNamara JO, Eubanks JH, McPherson JK, et al. Abstract: chromosomal localization of human glutamate receptor genes. *J Neurosci* 1992;12:2555–2562.
72. Cain D. Long-term potentiation and kindling: how similar are the mechanisms? *Trends Neurosci* 1989;12: 6–10.
73. Ben-Ari Y, Represa A. Brief seizure episodes induce long-term potentiation and mossy fibre sprouting in the hippocampus. *Trends Neurosci* 1990;13:312–317.
74. Post RM, Uhde TW, Putnam FW, et al. Kindling and carbamazepine in affective illness. *J Nerv Mental Dis* 1982;170:717–729.
75. Lewis J, Westerberg V, Corcoran M. Monoaminergic correlates of kindling. *Brain Res* 1987;403:205–212.
76. Wada Y, Nakamura M, Hasegawa H, Yamaguchi N. Intra-hippocampal injection of 8-hydroxy-2-(di-n-propylamino)tetralin (8-OH-DPAT) inhibits partial and generalized seizures induced by kindling stimulation in cats. *Neurosci Lett* 1993;159:179–182.
77. Kempermann G, van Praag H, Gage F. Activity-dependent regulation of neuronal plasticity and self repair. *Prog Brain Res* 2000;127:35–48.
78. Kaufmann W, Moser H. Dendritic anomalies in disorders associated with mental retardation. *Cereb Cortex* 2000;10:981–991.
79. Pennington BF, Bennetto L. Toward a neuropsychology of mental retardation. In: Burack JA, Hodapp RM, Zigler E, eds. *Handbook of mental retardation and development*. Cambridge: Cambridge University Press, 1998:80–114.
80. O'Meara E, Kukull W, Sheppard L, et al. Head injury and risk of Alzheimer's disease by apolipoprotein genotype. *Am J Epidemiol* 1997;146:373–384.
81. Deary I, Caryl P. Neuroscience and human intelligence differences. *Trends Neurosci* 1997;20:365–371.
82. Rabbitt P, Goward L. Age, information processing speed, and intelligence. *Quant J Exp Psychol* 1994; 47A:741–760.
83. Anderson M. Annotation: conceptions of intelligence. *J Child Psychol Psychiatry* 2001;42:287–298.
84. Buchsbaum MS, Haier RJ, Sostek AJ, et al. Attention dysfunction and psychopathology in college men. *Arch Gen Psychiatry* 1985;42:354–360.
85. Tang Y, Shimizu E, Dube G, et al. Genetic enhancement of learning and memory in mice. *Nature* 1999; 401:63–69.
86. Lu Y, Roder J, Davidow J, et al. Src activation in the induction of long-term potentiation in CA1 hippocampal neurons. *Science* 1993;279:1363–1367.
87. Migaud M, Charlesworth P, Dempster M, et al. Enhanced long-term potentiation and impaired learning in mice with mutant postsynaptic density-95 protein. *Nature* 1998;396:433–439.
88. Eysenck HJ. The nature of intelligence. In: Friedman MP, Das JP, O'Connor N, eds. *Intelligence and learning*. New York: Plenum, 1979:67–86.
89. Tromp E, Mulder T. Slowness of information processing after traumatic head injury. *J Clin Exp Neuropsychol* 1991;13:821–830.
90. Kail R. General slowing of information-processing by persons with mental retardation. *Am J Ment Retard* 1992;97:333–341.
91. Feng Y, Gutekunst C, Eberhart D, et al. Fragile X mental retardation protein: nucleocytoplasmic shuttling and association with somatodendritic ribosomes. *J Neurosci* 1997;17:1539–1547.
92. Simonoff E, Bolton P, Rutter M. Genetic perspectives on mental retardation. In: Burack JA, Hodapp RM, Zigler E, eds. *Handbook of mental retardation and development*. Cambridge: Cambridge University Press, 1998:41–79.
93. Antila E, Westermarck T. On the etiopathogenesis and therapy of Down syndrome. *Int J Dev Biol* 1989;33: 183–188.
94. Becker W, Joost H. Structural and functional characteristics of Dyrk, a novel subfamily of protein kinases with dual specificity. *Prog Nucl Acid Res Mol Biol* 1999;62:1–17.
95. Frangiskakis J, Ewart A, Morris C, et al. LIM-kinase1 hemizygosity implicated in impaired visuospatial constructive cognition. *Cell* 1996;86:59–69.
96. Amir R, Van der Veyver I, Wan M, et al. Rett syndrome is caused by mutations in X-linked MECP2, encoding methyl-CpG-binding protein 2. *Nat Genet* 1999;23: 185–188.
97. Huttenlocher P. Dendritic and synaptic pathology in mental retardation. *Pediatr Neurol* 1991;7:79–85.
98. Huttenlocher P. Synaptic and dendritic development and mental defect. *Brain Mech Ment Retard* 1975;123–140.
99. Pomeroy S, Kim J. Biology and pathobiology of neuronal development. *Ment Retard Dev Disabil Res Rev* 2000;6:41–46.
100. Benitez-Bribiesca L, De la Rosa-Alvarez I, Mansilla-Olivares A. Dendritic spine pathology in infants with severe protein-calorie malnutrition. *Pediatrics* 1999; 104:e21.

101. Wisniewski K, Segan S, Miezejeski C, et al. The Fra(X) syndrome: neurological, electrophysiological, and neuropathological abnormalities. *Am J Med Genet* 1991;38:476–480.
102. Ramakers G. Rho proteins and the cellular mechanisms of mental retardation. *Am J Med Genet* 2000; 94:367–371.
103. Dobyns W, Truwit C. Lissencephaly and other malformations of cortical development: 1995 update. *Neuropediatrics* 1995;26:132–147.
104. Dobyns W, Andermann E, Andermann F, et al. X-linked malformations of neuronal migration. *Neurology* 1996;47:331–339.
105. Lott IT. Down's syndrome, aging, and Alzheimer's disease: a clinical review. *Ann N Y Acad Sci* 1982;396: 15–27.
106. Thase ME, Tigner R, Smeltzer DJ, et al. Age-related neuropsychological deficits in Down's syndrome. *Biol Psychiatry* 1984;19:571–585.
107. Lai F, Williams RS. A prospective study of Alzheimer disease in Down syndrome. *Arch Neurol* 1989;46: 849–853.
108. Johannsen P, Christensen JEJ, Mai J. The prevalence of dementia in Down syndrome. *Dementia* 1996;7: 221–225.
109. Fraser J, Mitchell A. Kalmuc idiocy: report of a case with autopsy with notes on 62 cases. *J Ment Sci* 1876; 22:161:169–179.
110. Holland A, Oliver C. Down's syndrome and the links with Alzheimer's disease. *J Neurol Neurosurg Psychiatry* 1995;59:111–114.
111. Brugge KL, Nichols S, Delis D, et al. The role of alterations in free radical metabolism in mediating cognitive impairments in Down's syndrome. *EXS* 1992; 62:190–198.
112. Busciglio J, Yankner BA. Apoptosis and increased generation of reactive oxygen species in Down's syndrome neurons in vitro. *Nature* 1995;378:776–779.
113. Gerli G, Zenoni L, Locatelli GF, et al. Erythrocyte antioxidant system in Down syndrome. *Am J Med Genet* 1990;7:272–273.
114. Furuta A, Price DL, Pardo CA, et al. Localization of superoxide dismutases in Alzheimer's disease and Down's syndrome neocortex and hippocampus. *Am J Pathol* 1995;146:357–367.
115. Fujii J, Suzuki K, Taniguchi N. Physiological significance of superoxide dismutase isozymes. *Nippon Rinsho* 1995;53:1227–1231.
116. Bras A, Monteiro C, Rueff J. Oxidative stress in trisomy 21. A possible role in cataractogenesis. *Ophthalmic Paediatr* 1989;10:271–277.
117. Volicer L, Crino PB. Involvement of free radicals in dementia of the Alzheimer type: a hypothesis. *Neurobiol Aging* 1990;11:567–571.
118. Friedlich AL, Butcher LL. Involvement of free oxygen radicals in beta-amyloidosis: an hypothesis. *Neurobiol Aging* 1994;15:443–455.
119. Small G, Mazziotta J, Collins M, et al. Apolipoprotein E type 4 allele and cerebral glucose metabolism in relatives at risk for familial Alzheimer disease. *JAMA* 1995;273:942–947.
120. Mayeux R, Saunders A, Shea S, et al. Utility of the apolipoprotein E genotype in the diagnosis of Alzheimer's disease. *N Engl J Med* 1998;338: 506–511.
121. Reiman E, Caselli R, Yun L, et al. Preclinical evidence of Alzheimer's disease in persons homozygous for the e4 allele for apolipoprotein E. *N Engl J Med* 1996; 334:752–758.
122. Corder E, Saunders A, Strittmatter W, et al. Gene dose of apolipoprotein E type 4 allele and the risk of Alzheimer's disease in late onset families. *Science* 1993;261:921–923.
123. Polvikoski T, Sulkava R, Haltia M, et al. Apolipoprotein E, dementia, and cortical deposition of B-amyloid protein. *N Engl J Med* 1995;333:1242–1247.
124. Genis L, Chen Y, Shohami E, et al. Tau hyperphosphorylation in apolipoprotein E-deficient and control mice after closed head injury. *J Neurosci Res* 2000;60: 559–564.
125. Ramassamy C, Averill D, Beffert U, et al. Oxidative insults are associated with apolipoprotein E genotype in Alzheimer's disease brain. *Neurobiol Dis* 2000;7:23–37.
126. Graham D, Horsburgh K, Nicoll J, et al. Apolipoprotein E and the response of the brain to injury. *Acta Neurochir Suppl* 1999;73:89–92.
127. Haan M, Shemanski L, Jagust W, et al. The role of apoe e4 in modulating effects of other risk factors for cognitive decline in elderly persons. *JAMA* 1999;282: 40–46.
128. Lichtman S, Seliger G, Tycko B, et al. Apolipoprotein E and functional recovery from brain injury following postacute rehabilitation. *Neurology* 2000;55: 1536–1539.
129. McCarron M, Muir K, Nicoll J, et al. Prospective study of apolipoprotein E genotype and functional outcome following ischemic stroke. *Arch Neurol* 2000;57: 1480–1484.
130. Lai F, Kammann E, Rebeck G, et al. APOE genotype and gender effects on Alzheimer disease in 10 adults with Down syndrome. *Neurology* 1999;53:331–336.
131. Rubinsztein D, Hon J, Stevens F, et al. Apo E genotypes and risk of dementia in Down syndrome. *Am J Med Genet* 1999;88:344–347.
132. Deb S, Braganza J, Norton N, et al. APOE epsilon 4 influences the manifestation of Alzheimer's disease in adults with Down's syndrome. *Br J Psychiatry* 2000; 176:468–472.
133. Dale G, Leigh P, Luthert P, et al. Neurofibrillary tangles in dementia pugilistica are ubiquitinated. *J Neurol Neurosurg Psychiatry* 1991;54:116–118.
134. Yankner B, Mesulam M-M. B-Amyloid and the pathogenesis of Alzheimer's disease. *N Engl J Med* 1991; 325:1849–1857.
135. Nieto-Sampedro M, Mora F. Active microglia, sick astroglia and Alzheimer type dementias. *Neuroreport* 1994;5:375–380.
136. Neve R, McPhie D, Chen Y. Alzheimer disease: a dysfunction of the amyloid precursor protein (1). *Brain Res* 2000;886:54–66.
137. Richardson J, Zhou Y, Kumar U. Free radicals in the neurotoxic actions of B-amyloid. *Ann N Y Acad Sci* 1996;777:362–367.
138. Blass J. Pathophysiology of the Alzheimer's syndrome. *Neurology* 1993;43:25–38.
139. Kavaliers M, Ossenkopp K, Tysdale D. Evidence for the involvement of protein kinase C in the modulation of morphine-induced 'analgesia' and the inhibitory effects of exposure to 60-Hz magnetic fields in th snail, Cep. *Brain Res* 1991;554:65–71.

140. McGeer PL, McGeer EG. The inflammatory response system of brain: implications for therapy of Alzheimer and other neurodegenerative diseases. *Brain Res Rev* 1995;21:195–218.
141. Eikelenboom P, Rozemuller A, Hoozemans J, et al. Neuroinflammation and Alzheimer disease: clinical and therapeutic implications. *Alzheimer Dis Assoc Disord* 2000;14:54–61.
142. Lynch J, Morgan D, Mance J, et al. Apolipoprotein E modulates glial activation and the endogeno central nervous system inflammatory response. *J Neuroimmunol* 2001;114:107–113.
143. Corsellis A. Boxing and the brain. *BMJ* 1989;298:105–109.
144. D'Amico MFMS, Roberts DL, Robinson DS, et al. Placebo-controlled dose-ranging trial designs in phase II development of nefazodone. *Psychopharmacol Bull* 1990;26:147–149.
145. Jordan B. Chronic traumatic brain injury associated with boxing. *Semin Neurol* 2000;20:179–185.
146. Heyman A, Wilkinson WE, Stafford JA, et al. Alzheimer's disease: a study of epidemiologic aspects. *Ann Neurol* 1984;15:335–341.
147. French LR, Schuman LM, Mortimer JA, et al. A case-control study of dementia of the Alzheimer type. *Am J Epidemiol* 1985;121:414–421.
148. Henderson AS. The epidemiology of Alzheimer's disease. *Br Med Bull* 1986;42:3–10.
149. Shalat SL, Seltzer B, Pidcock C, et al. Risk factors for Alzheimer's disease: a case-control study. *Neurology* 1987;37:1630–1633.
150. Schofield P, Tang M, Marder K, et al. Alzheimer's disease after remote head injury: an incidence study. *J Neurol Neurosurg Psychiatry* 1997;62:119–124.
151. Guo Z, Cupples L, Kurz A, et al. Head injury and the risk of AD in the MIRAGE study. *Neurology* 2000;54:1316–1323.
152. Violon A, Demol J. Psychological sequelae after head trauma in adults. *Acta Neurochir* 1987;85:96–102.
153. Gedye A, Beattie B, Tuokko H, et al. Severe head injury hastens age of onset of Alzheimer's disease. *J Am Geriatr Soc* 1989;37:970–973.
154. Luukinen H, Viramo P, Koski K, et al. Head injuries and cognitive decline among older adults: a population-based study. *Neurology* 1999;52:557–562.
155. Kokmen E, Beard M, Offord KP, et al. Prevalence of medically diagnosed dementia in a defined United States population: Rochester, Minnesota, January 1, 1975. *Neurology* 1989;39:773–776.
156. Williams D, Annegars J, Kokmen E, et al. Brain injury and neurologic sequelae: a cohort study of dementia, parkinsonism, and amyotrophic lateral sclerosis. *Neurology* 1991;41:1554—1557.
157. Andersen K, Launer LJ, Ott A, et al. Do nonsteroidal anti-inflammatory drugs decrease the risk for Alzheimer's disease? *Neurology* 1995;45:8:1441–1445.
158. Launer L, Andersen K, Dewey M, et al. Rates and risk factors for dementia and Alzheimer's disease: results from EURODEM pooled analyses. EURODEM Inside Research Group and Work Groups. European studies of dementia. *Neurology* 1999;52:78–84.
159. Mehta K, Ott A, Kalmijn S, et al. Head trauma and risk of dementia and Alzheimer's disease: T Rotterdam Study. *Neurology* 1999;53:1959–1962.
160. Jordan B, Relkin N, Ravdin L, et al. Apolipoprotein E e4 associated with chronic traumatic brain injury in boxing. *JAMA* 1997;278:136–140.
161. Kutner K, Erlanger D, Tsai J, et al. Lower cognitive performance of older football players possess apolipoprotein E epsilon4. *Neurosurgery* 2000;47:651–657.
162. Popovitch E, Wisniewski H, Barcikowska M, et al. Alzheimer neuropathology in non-Down's syndrome mentally retarded adults. *Acta Neuropathol* 1990;80:362–367.
163. Silverman W, Popovitch E, Schupf N, et al. Alzheimer neuropathology in mentally retarded adults: statistical independence of regional amyloid plaque and neurofibrillary tangle densities. *Acta Neuropathol* 1993;85:260–266.
164. Fratiglioni L, Grut M, Forsell Y, et al. Prevalence of Alzheimer's disease and other dementias in an elderly urban population: relationship with age, sex, and education. *Neurology* 1991;41:1886–1892.
165. Katzman R. Education and the prevalence of dementia and Alzheimer's disease. *Neurology* 1993;43:13–20.
166. Stern Y, Guland B, Tatemichi T, et al. Influence of education and occupation on the incidence of Alzheimer's disease. *JAMA* 1994;271:1004–1010.
167. Plassman B, Welsh K, Helms M, et al. Intelligence and education as predictors of cognitive state in late life: a 50-year follow-up. *Neurology* 1995;45:1446–1450.
168. Prencipe M, Casini A, Ferretti C, et al. Prevalence of dementia in an elderly rural population: effects of age, sex, and education. *J Neurol Neurosurg Psychiatry* 1996;60:628–633.
169. Temple V, Jozsvai E, Konstantareas M, et al. Alzheimer dementia in Down's syndrome: the relevance of cognitive ability. *J Intellect Disabil Res* 2001;45:47–55.

5

Evaluation of the Neuropsychiatric Patient

SUMMARY

The four approaches to evaluation discussed are paradigmatic; that is, they introduce principles of diagnosis and differential diagnosis that are appropriate to many different types of neuropsychiatric patients. The TBI evaluation is appropriate for adult patients with a number of different neuropsychiatric conditions, including stroke and dementia, and it also raises issues that are pertinent to forensic evaluations. The ADHD evaluation is good for pediatric patients with BI in general, and elements of the evaluation are also appropriate for high-level adult patients who present with mild cognitive complaints. The autism evaluation addresses the differential diagnosis of severe developmental delay. The mental retardation (MR) evaluation covers important ground that is hardly ever addressed in the literature: the problem of long-term care for the patient with cognitive impairment, chronic mental illness, and the need for a lifetime of supervised care.

Patients who are treated with psychotropic drugs require a special kind of evaluation and regular monitoring. The way that this is done varies from one drug to another, and I try to cover the field.

All these matters serve to illuminate a vexing question: what exactly is a neuropsychiatrist? My position is practical and straightforward. A neuropsychiatrist is properly trained and equipped to carry out all these evaluations with efficiency, speed, and reliability. He or she ought to set up his or her clinic in a particular way, as I describe, and choose their confederates wisely.

THE TRAUMATIC BRAIN INJURY PATIENT

The History

The most important purpose of the clinical history is to understand the nature and severity of the traumatic event: exactly what kind of injury it was, the biomechanical forces that were generated, and the relative likelihood of BI. Unless one has at least some idea of the nature and severity of the traumatic event, it is impossible to make diagnostic attributions. If the injury occurred in a motor vehicle accident, this information may be obtained directly by studying the accident report to determine the relative velocities of the vehicles and the vectors of force. In other kinds of injury, there are salient details to uncover, for example, the duration and depth of hypoxia, blood levels of carboxyhemoglobin, and the amperage of an electrical discharge. Once the medical record attributes a patient's symptoms to BI, successive physicians tend to maintain the attribution, however unlikely it may be. A critical reexamination of the primary sources is always in order.

This information is not always available or is of dubious accuracy, in which case, one proceeds to the second step. That step is to examine the patient's acute response to injury: whether he or she experienced loss of consciousness and, if so, for how long; the depth of coma, defined by the Glasgow Coma

Scale; the occurrence and duration of posttraumatic amnesia or posttraumatic confusion; and the temporal course of acute recovery.

Computed tomography (CT) scans are usually done in the emergency department if the physician is at all suspicious of brain trauma. If the patient is admitted to the hospital, reviewing the medical record is essential. The neurosurgical record is important as are the records from rehabilitation. If a patient taking a particular drug presents, it is important to know exactly why the drug was prescribed. Never assume that the neurosurgeon's choice of phenytoin, metoclopramide, amitriptyline, or haloperidol was ill considered. It is necessary to know whether the patient had seizures after the trauma, and, if so, what kind of seizures they were and whether there are any important risk factors for posttraumatic epilepsy. Immediate posttraumatic seizures or psychosis are not necessarily indicators of a poor prognosis, but one looks the fool for changing the patient's medications in ignorance of same, and it may not be good for the patient.

Understanding the evolution of neurobehavioral sequelae after TBI requires familiarity with the specific BI syndromes and how they relate to the particular kinds of cerebral insult. Patients who have had mild BIs, for example, should never present with seizures, psychosis, or severe intellectual decline; if they do, the problem is more than simply mild BI, or less, as the case may be. Patients with hypoxic or electrical injuries, conversely, frequently present with hysterical symptoms that may obscure the underlying neuropathology.

The patient is not always capable of reporting all his or her symptoms and deficits directly; they may have to be drawn out by concise and pertinent questioning. Questionnaires and rating scales are available to complement the clinical history, such as the Neurobehavioral Rating Scale, the Memory Questionnaire, and the Head Injury Questionnaire (see Appendix). Symptoms of anxiety and depression, quite common in patients with TBI, can be measured on self-report measures such as the Beck scales. Such measures provide a great deal of information; even when the patient over- or understates symptoms, it is interesting.

It is also necessary to get information about the patient from family members, from people who knew the patient before the injury and sometimes from school transcripts, standardized academic tests (such as the CAT or the SAT), employment records, or previous medical records. Anosognosia (failure to appreciate the severity of one's deficits) and amnesia are BI sequelae that necessarily compromise the patient's accuracy as a historian. Current disability should not be attributed to a specific traumatic event unless one is quite sure that there was no preexisting morbid condition. Conversely, the existence of a premorbid condition does not, of itself, obviate the impact of a TBI; it may rather be a question of aggravation. BIs have the unnerving propensity to accentuate whatever negative traits the patient may have had before the injury.

The initial history should include the basics: medical history, family history (especially for psychiatric, neurologic, and developmental disorders), and medication history. The patient's premorbid characteristics should be discussed at length: personality traits, school and work history, family relations, sexuality, attitudes, psychological difficulties, high-risk behaviors, and substance abuse. The social history ought to be biographic: what the patient has done since high school, where he or she have lived and worked, and what he or she has done with his or her life.

It is often helpful to review medical records in the patient's presence. If a doctor along the way thought that the patient was exaggerating or malingering, that should be discussed openly with the patient. ("Look here. Doctor So-and-so wrote that 'The patient's memory problems were clearly exaggerated.' Why do think she said that?")

It is important to examine the patient's memory of events immediately before and after an alleged BI. It is always remarkable, but not uncommon, to meet a patient who claims to have experienced a disabling TBI but who can remember quite clearly and in striking detail all the details before and after the accident. It is possible to have sustained a penetrating BI or an electrical injury without amnesia but not a concussion or a closed head injury (CHI)]. Remember this: retrograde amnesia never occurs in patients who do not also have disabling anterograde amnesia. Patients who have had a severe concussion may experience a few hours of retrograde amnesia but they do not forget their birthday, when they graduated from high school, or their children's names.

Sometimes, the patient's biggest problems have to do with bitterness against the insurance company or against his or her former employer. Sometimes this is justified. Conversely, pseudo-patients who allege severe cognitive impairment and score in the demented range on neuropsychological tests are able to argue their case against the "company" fluently, with lucidity and in great detail. Most pseudo-patients are more concerned about the economic aspects of their claims than the diagnosis and treatment of their alleged neurologic impairments.

The patient should be asked to describe his or her current level of deficit on questionnaires completed before the evaluation, and the discussion of current difficulties can be based on these responses. There is then more time to expand on areas of difficulty, their development over the course of time after the injury, and their response to treatment interventions. It is essential to understand how a problem area is actually an impediment to normal function. How does the patient spend his or her day? Does he or she drive, shop, cook, clean house, and tend the garden or spend the day on the couch watching television?

The Examination

The history should be taken before, during, and after the physical examination. Patients tend to relax after the examination is over. Sometimes they are more willing to share intimacies after the laying on of hand in a physical examination.

The neuropsychiatric examination begins with a regular physical and then a complete neurologic examination. One looks for dysmorphic features that may speak to a preexisting developmental problem and to signs of alcoholism or drug abuse. The neurologic examination is directed especially at the motor system: strength and tone, gait, tandem gait, cerebellar testing (finger to nose, heel to shin), an expanded Romberg (feet together, eyes closed, arms outstretched, palms up), fine motor coordination (finger to nose, finger-thumb opposition), and motor sequencing [fist-ring, Luria three-step task, Mandrake (see below)]. One looks for subtle asymmetries in tone, strength, and deep tendon reflexes. One looks for tremor, dyskinesia, mannerisms, or stereotypies. One tests for cogwheeling and glabellar tap and looks for other signs of parkinsonism.

Testing for visual field and other sensory deficits may be the opportunity to discover nonphysiologic signs (e.g., tunnel vision, monocular diplopia.) The funduscopic examination may reveal arteriolar narrowing, a sign of premorbid white matter disease that is almost always a poor prognosis indicator.

The Mandrake test, properly executed, is a sensitive sign of prefrontal injury. The patient is asked to imitate the examiner, who gestures hypnotically, as Mandrake the Magician used to do. The patient is asked to overcome his or her inhibition at such a silly task and to perform smoothly and gracefully. After a while, the examiner thrusts his or her arms with fingers extended on one side, and a closed fist on the other, and alternate left to right, fingers and fist, and the patient is expected to spontaneously follow the examiner's lead without a prompt. Then, one may change the pattern of fist-fingers, left-right-right-left-right-right, and then change sets again, with increasing frequency and increasing difficulty to the pattern. This is a test of a variety of prefrontal functions including motor coordination and imitation, cognitive flexibility, preservation, frustration tolerance, and compliance. It is what Luria would call a kinetic melody task.

Testing for olfaction is a useful measure for frontal lobe injury. The small terminals of the first cranial nerve poke through the cribriform plate into the nasopharynx and are shorn when the brain is thrown forward and back during a CHI. Patients always enjoy the game of having to identify a number of familiar scents. Do it, however, with a control because even the most pungent scents lose their volatility over time. A good control is the patient's spouse, who, by this time, is probably eager for a bit of attention. The last scent to give the patient should be irritative, such as the scent of Listerine. A patient who is malingering anosmia will fail to respond to an irritative stimulus, which is detected by the fifth not the first cranial nerve. It is said that persistent anosmia is a bad prognosis indicator for CHI patients (1). (The Cross-Cultural Smell Identification Test is a standardized, self-administered test of olfaction.)

One checks for frontal release signs, such as the grasp reflex, Hoffmann's sign, the palmomental reflex, and the suck, snout, rooting, and corneomandibular ("bulldog") reflexes. The palmomental reflex is the most sensitive to frontal injury. It should be quantitated: left and right, mild, moderate, extreme, and one to six in succession, to test for extinction. The palmomental reflex, however, is a relatively nonspecific finding, and false positives are common.

The Mental State Examinations

There are two MSEs. One is psychiatric, concerned mainly with the patient's behavior, mood, affect, personality, manner of relating, concerns, and motivations, as well as the signs and symptoms of the traditional psychiatric disorders. The psychiatric MSE entails a very gross appraisal of the patient's cognitive ability. The neuropsychiatric MSE, conversely, involves a more systematic assessment of the patient's cognitive status.

The psychiatric MSE can usually be done during the course of taking a history and performing a physical examination. It does not take much time for an experienced clinician to write down the abbreviations listed in Table 5.1. For medicolegal purposes, it is probably better to write down one's observations in abbreviated terms. If any of these superficial observations are suspicious, the area of concern may be pursued at greater length after the physical examination is done.

The formal or neuropsychiatric MSE is a more elaborate undertaking, and the method advanced by Strub and Black (2), for example, may easily take an hour. For this reason, the entire examination is rarely done; rather, the examination is targeted to specific areas of concern. After all, if the patient's cognitive status is really at issue, one should probably recommend a full neuropsychological battery.

Structured MSEs, such as the Mini-Mental State Examination (3) or the Neurobehavioral Cognitive Evaluation (4) are quick and comprehensive. The former is better for patients with severe cognitive disabilities and the latter for patients with moderate disabilities. They are not particularly sensitive and are not diagnostic measures but are excellent for screening or serial assessment.

The bedside MSE is rather like the Mini-Mental State Examination: orientation to time and place, memory for four words at 5 and 10 minutes, verbal and/or semantic fluency, who is the president, name some recent presidents, serial sevens or threes, simple computations, draw a clock (house, cube), name this (a watch, a band, a crystal) and that (a pen, a tip, a clip), or do two things at once (answer a question during the Romberg test without breaking the pose or during tandem walk without losing one's balance).

There a few paper-and-pencil tests that are quick and easy to administer in the office setting, for example, the Controlled Oral Word Association Test (FAS, Verbal Fluency) (5), the Rey Auditory Verbal Learning Test, and the Rey Malingering Test (6). There are also several tests that can be administered on a computer: the Computerized Assessment of Response Bias, a test of factitious responding (i.e., malingering); a forced choice test such as the Portland Digit Recognition Test (7); Categories (8); and several good tests of attention, such as the Tests of Variables of Attention and the Neurobehavioral Evaluation System (9).

The office or bedside MSE, even when augmented by additional tests of frontal and temporal lobe function, fails to test for reaction-time and processing-speed impairments, two keys areas of CHI-induced impairment. Personal computer–based assessment systems show promise in addressing this deficit in assessment (9). An advantage of a computerized, office-based cognitive assessment is that it can be administered serially to measure recovery after TBI and to measure the effects of drug administration. However, the computerized battery is no substitute for an experienced neuropsychologist. It is an assessment tool, not a diagnostic instrument.

Neuropsychological Testing

A complete neuropsychological battery by a neuropsychologist who has experience with patients with TBI is probably the most sensitive diagnostic instrument, but it is arduous and expensive. There are several different approaches to the problem of neuropsychological assessment, and many good neuropsychologists have adopted an eclectic style that includes individual tests from several different batteries. The original role of formal neuropsychological testing was used to localize brain lesions; this obviously has been supplanted by modern neuroimaging. Now its purpose is to delineate specific and sometimes subtle areas of functional weakness, to help in planning specific treatment strate-

TABLE 5.1. *An abbreviated mental state examination*

NAD	No acute distress
NADF	No asymmetries or dysmorphic features
ASA	Appears stated age
WDANG	Well-dressed and neatly groomed
ANSOI	Alert, not sedated or irritable
ASFLAO	Affect stable, fluent, lucid, and oriented
NADADP	Not anxious, depressed, agitated, disorganized, or paranoid
NODOS	Not overtly depressed or suicidal
PWRCC	Pleasant, well related, cheerful, and cooperative
NOCMOAD	No overt conversational memory or attention deficit
NOHAOD	Not overtly hyperactive or distractible
NAMODAK	No abnormal movements or dyskinesia or akathisia
ACAHC	Appropriately concerned about his/her condition
NOEMOE	No overt evidence of malingering or exaggeration

gies, and to assess a patient's course and response to treatment.

Neuropsychological testing is essential and invaluable for the evaluation of patients with TBI, especially patients with moderate or severe BIs. The contributions of neuropsychologists to the study of TBI and the development of rehabilitative treatments have been signal. The neuropsychological literature is central to the understanding of BI. This said, it is necessary to at least mention the limitations of neuropsychological testing:

- Full batteries are arduous and expensive and therefore may not be appropriate for serial evaluation.
- Neuropsychological tests may determine where the areas of deficit reside but not what caused them or even whether the cause was organic or psychiatric in nature.
- Conventional neuropsychological tests may not be sensitive to minor deficits in reaction time and information-processing speed that characterize mild BIs.
- Not everyone who performs a neuropsychological examination is appropriately credentialed or skilled in the evaluation of TBI.
- Not every cognitive deficit necessarily requires a course of "cognitive remediation," especially early in the course of recovery when restoration of neurocognitive functions may occur spontaneously.

Neuropsychological testing is evaluative, not diagnostic. The diagnosis of BI, even subtle BI, rests on a thorough assessment of information from many different sources and should never rely simply on the results of a psychological test.

The complete neuropsychological battery is not a first-line diagnostic instrument, especially for people who have had mild TBI. Like any complex and expensive diagnostic test, it should not be considered a routine measure. Rather, it should be reserved for special cases, when the referring physician has a specific question to address.

Finally, the results of the neuropsychological battery, like the results of magnetic resonance imaging (MRI), generate not a single diagnosis but a differential diagnosis with which the results are consistent.

The Special Case of the Minnesota Multiphasic Personality Inventory

One particular test that has attained iconic status in the neuropsychological evaluation is the Minnesota Multiphasic Personality Inventory (MMPI). In fact, it is probably the only psychological test that referring agents (e.g., case managers) specifically request when they send the patient for an evaluation.

The MMPI does indeed enjoy a venerable status. It was originally developed in the 1930s and 1940s as a screening instrument for psychopathology (10). Proponents of the MMPI and its later revision, the MMPI-2, have even asserted "with confidence that no psychological test rests on stronger scientific foundations than the MMPI and its updated version, the MMPI-2."

For these reasons, it is necessary to address critically the utility of the MMPI in the evaluation of patients who have had BI. This question goes beyond mere quibbling because important decisions that can influence the patient's career, for example, return to work in a sensitive position, are made in part based on the results of a MMPI.

Lezak (11) summarized the pitfalls in the use of the MMPI in patients with various conditions affecting the central nervous system. For example, the original MMPI clinical scales were developed based on patients whose psychiatric diagnoses were current in the 1930s. Some of these categories, such as hysteria, psychasthenia, and psychopathic deviate, are no longer current and indeed are questionable by today's standards. Many of the patients whose 1930s-era diagnoses comprised the various normative groups of the MMPI would probably be diagnosed quite differently today. The revised version of the test, the MMPI-2, was restandardized in an attempt to correct the weaknesses of the original MMPI. However, items have remained in the scales in which they were originally placed when the original MMPI was first developed, thus the scales are essentially the same.

There are some general patterns that characterize the MMPI profile of patients who have neurologic disorders, but the MMPI profiles of patients with BI are in part an artifact of the test items and scale composition. Many of the neurologic symptom items are reflected in the schizophrenia scale. Many patients with TBI have elevations on three scales in particular: hypochondriasis, depression, and hysteria. Consequently, nonpsychiatric patients with central nervous system disease are found to have an elevated "neurotic triad" and higher than average schizophrenia scores. Elevations on these same scales have also been reported for workers who have been exposed to neurotoxic substances (12).

The problem, then, is that when BI patients take the MMPI, they are likely to show rather high levels of psychopathology. To put it another way, the physical, neurobehavioral, and neurocognitive symptoms of TBI will register on the MMPI as if they were symptoms of a psychiatric disorder. Clearly, one must exercise caution in the interpretation of these profiles.

Gass and Russell (13) recently offered empirical support for the application of an MMPI-2 correction factor in a clinical sample of nonlitigating individuals who had sustained recent and mild head trauma. Their results indicated that, unlike subjects in psychiatric sample, the MMPI-2 items that best distinguished the subjects with closed head trauma from normals had neurologic symptom content. Of the 15 items originally proposed, 10 were included in the 14-item correction (13). Thirteen of the 14 correction items effectively distinguished the cross-validation sample of subjects with CHI from normals. That is reassuring but beside the point.

The essential question is whether the MMPI or the MMPI-2 can yield information about a person with a TBI that cannot be obtained more efficiently by other means; whether it will distinguish between problems that derive from BI and problems that stem from a premorbid psychiatric condition or whether the test will detect malingerers, exaggerators, or people who are pathologically defensive about their problems. It may help the clinician to do all those things sometimes at least, but it is never a particularly efficient test. For individuals who have had moderate or severe BIs, the MMPI-2 is often difficult to complete. After all, it is very long: 567 items. Patients with significant motor, vision, or attentional problems often have difficulty completing it.

There are other measures to use, such as the Symptom Checklist-90-Revised (14), and rating scales such as the Beck Anxiety Inventory (15), the Beck Depression Inventory (16), the Leyton OCD (obsessive-cumpulsive disorder) inventory, and the ADHD Checklist, which are shorter and easier to complete and provide valid and reliable diagnostic information. The Personality Assessment Inventory is a shorter version of the MMPI that gives results in terms of *DSM-IV* categories.

In difficult diagnostic or forensic cases, one is still expected to do a MMPI, and it is still a useful and informative test. It is, however, only one test of several that might be given, and its results should never be permitted to stand on their own. There is more to a psychiatric or a neuropsychological evaluation than the MMPI.

Neurodiagnostic Testing

The delineation of a lesion with a standard neurologic examination or with direct imaging techniques such as CT scanning and MRI is a straightforward and simple way to establish an organic basis for the complaints of a patient with CHI. Nevertheless, there are many patients whose symptoms are severe and debilitating, but whose examination and scans are normal or equivocal. It is increasingly appreciated that functional imaging methods such as positron emission tomography, single photon emission computed tomography, and computerized brain mapping can define areas of abnormality not seen in anatomic studies. Further development of functional imaging techniques will eventually resolve a number of common diagnostic problems. Until these techniques are better validated, however, the physician has to rely on the clinical history, the MSE, and neuropsychological testing to infer the locus and extent of BI, particularly in cases of mild CHI.

The role of neurodiagnostic testing is sometimes misunderstood. It is not meant to be diagnostic but only to supplement clinical judgment. The CT scan is useful for demonstrating fractures, bone fragments, hemorrhage, missile particles, intracranial fluid collections, hydrocephalus, and other clinical features that are important for the acute management of head trauma. It is a fast test, too, so it is especially useful in the acute care setting. MRI takes a long time and requires the patient to lie still in a claustrophobic tube as the machine clinks and whirrs; it is not appropriate to the acute care setting and is not tolerable to the acutely agitated patient who is hard to sedate. Conversely, it is capable of demonstrating subtle lesions, especially in the white matter, that do not show up on CT, and this is where the neuropathic correlates of TBI are often to be found. MRI, therefore, is the test of choice for the stable patient with TBI for whom the aim is to define the location and extent of the lesion or to acquire a baseline for future comparison (e.g., against the development of hydrocephalus or cortical atrophy long after the injury). Archival MRI is essential for the patient with severe TBI, for comparative purposes if complications develop later.

Electroencephalography (EEG) may show diffuse slowing (acutely) that is compatible with CHI but not very specific, focal slowing that localizes a lesion, or paroxysmal discharge that is compatible with (but not diagnostic of) epilepsy. Sleep deprivation may enhance the value of EEG by evoking an epileptiform focus, but nasopharyngeal leads do not necessarily generate additional knowledge.

Computerized EEG is sometimes used to assess TBI patients, often in patients who have had mild injuries. In some communities, a small cottage industry has arisen around this test; in the spirit of charity, I do not descry how the tests are sometimes marketed, for example, to personal injury attorneys. Their clinical utility has yet to be fully developed.

Diagnosis and Medicolegal Considerations

The diagnosis of clinically significant TBI is not based on any one of the elements described. It is based on a consistent clinical picture drawn from all the sources, with the necessary skepticism concerning the importance of a single, isolated finding. The clinical utility, for example, of frontal release signs is limited in an elderly patient; neurologic "soft" signs such as dysdiadochokinesia are of limited utility in young patients or patients with developmental disabilities. MRI abnormalities may be ambiguous. Even the description of the patient's current problems may be confused or contradictory because people may minimize or exaggerate a symptom or may make attributions about a problem that colors its actual relationship to a traumatic event. The MMPI may indicate hypochondriasis, but the patient with chronic pain and disability often exaggerates his or her symptoms, especially if physicians are skeptical or unsympathetic.

In general, the clinical evaluation of mild TBI does not require expensive neurodiagnostic procedures or comprehensive neuropsychological testing. However, if the issue is litigation, one may be urged to spare no expense to identify an objective neuropathic finding. Unhappily, the findings that emerge from MRI or single photon emission computed tomography or from the neuropsychological battery in such cases are often nonspecific and less than objective. As the professional is pulled into the adversarial process, there are inevitable pressures to put spin on equivocal findings to benefit the plaintiff or the defense.

If the purpose is disability determination, the process may be equally daunting because there are no objective criteria to measure the degree to which mild symptoms such as fatigue, hypacusis, and motor incoordination affect the performance of a construction worker or the degree to which frontal lobe symptoms such as disorganization, inattention, difficulty planning, and indecision compromise the function of an executive or a professional. The assessment of disability after TBI is best made over time with serial assessment by the treating physician. The patient's difficulties should be assessed in terms of real-world performance at home, in school, at work, or at play. Disability cannot be established by neuropsychological tests alone. The validity of tests in predicting social and occupational performance has not been very well established. Consulting professionals should give due weight to the observations of the people who live and work with the patient. The sequelae of frontal lobe lesions, in particular, may be more evident in real life than in the artificial setting of the doctor's office.

EVALUATION OF THE PATIENT WITH ATTENTION DEFICIT/HYPERACTIVITY DISORDER

ADHD is not one of the conditions dealt with in this monograph, but the evaluation of the patient with ADHD is discussed. The reader is doubtless familiar with the enormous weight of recent writing on the subject, and no further explication is needed here. The reason why the evaluation is germane, however, is this: the assessment of ADHD is well established, especially in pediatric neuropsychiatry; the problems of patients with ADHD are similar to those of patients with TBI, especially patients with mild or moderate BI; one evaluates psychostimulant drug effects in patients with BI just as one does in patients with ADHD.

The essential ingredients of the neuropsychiatric evaluation for ADHD in children and adults are similar to what has already been described. The clinical history is guided by two important considerations. Obviously, it aims to delineate symptoms and the degree to which they are disabling, but the cognitive symptoms of ADHD, like the symptoms of mild BI, are relatively nonspecific and can arise as a result of stress, fatigue, ill health, medications, substance abuse, mood disorder, or anxiety.

The mere subjective experience of inattention, lack of focus, and distractibility is not diagnostic of ADHD; rather, it is the appropriate occasion for a differential diagnosis. A chronic history of impulsive, injudicious behavior is typical of ADHD, but in attention deficit disorder without hyperactivity, the diagnosis is based on cognitive disability alone, and the differential diagnosis of mild cognitive impairment is formidable, indeed. Table 5.2 lists the most common psychiatric diagnoses in adults who have presented to our Neuropsychiatry Clinic reporting ADHD or mild cognitive impairment. All these di-

TABLE 5.2. *Psychiatric conditions presenting as attention deficit/hyperactivity disorder*

Anxiety disorders, including panic
Depression
Bipolar affective disorder
Obsessive-compulsive disorder
Alcoholism, substance abuse

agnoses are also pertinent to the evaluation of the patient with MBI.

Rating scales can be used to evaluate ADHD in children and adults. There is even a standardized instrument, the Wender Utah Rating Scale, that captures childhood symptoms of ADHD in patients who present as adults. (The Wender scale can also be used to assess premorbid characteristics in patients with BI.) Rating scales are good for delineating symptoms and their perceived severity. They are also an efficient means for screening patients for symptoms of other conditions that may be comorbid with ADHD or that may have ADHD-like symptoms.

The psychiatric examination itself is not likely to reveal signs of ADHD because the patients are usually able to maintain their attention perfectly well in novel situations and one-on-one examinations. For the same reason, psychological testing may not indicate inattention or distractibility. Patients with ADHD, both children and adults, can do well enough in short bursts. It is the rare patient with ADHD who is overtly disorganized or disinhibited or who cannot persevere even in complex tests of balance or coordination; usually, they are very young children.

The evaluation thus far may be supportive of the diagnosis of ADHD, but two additional steps are recommended to confirm one's impression. We have come to rely on the computerized tests that have been developed for ADHD that measure sustained vigilance attention over time in a dull, boring task. The Continuous Performance Test is the paradigm, and several variants are commercially available, including the TOVA and the NES. They have been standardized, are expensive to administer, and take no more than 30 minutes.

The second step is the test dose. One can actually observe the cognitive effects of a short-acting stimulant drug within an hour. The patient is given a small dose of methylphenidate or dextroamphetamine, and then he or she is sent off to lunch. An hour later, the patient returns, and retakes the computerized test. The short onset of psychostimulant drugs allows one to assess, at least on a preliminary basis, the patient's subjective response to a single dose, acute side effects, and performance on tests of attention, reaction time, and information-processing speed. A positive response in this setting does not necessarily predict that stimulant treatment will be useful in the long term, but it is encouraging. Conversely, if the patient does worse after the test dose or experiences a dysphoric response to the stimulant, one might rethink the differential diagnosis and consider another form of treatment.

This test-dose method is appropriate for neuropsychiatric patients in general who have problems with attention, organization, memory, or information-processing speed. It is quick and inexpensive and yields an enormous amount of information. Indeed, we are inclined to propose this method as a standard of good medical care.

Patients who have sustained mild or moderate BI, especially children, develop a typical ADHD pattern of behavior. There is no established way to differentiate between acquired ADHD and the congenital form beyond the history of posttraumatic change; even this may not be helpful because premorbid ADHD occurs in approximately 5% of children in North America, and children with ADHD are more likely to experience injuries. Children with posttraumatic ADHD are more emotionally labile, but this is hardly sufficient to base a causal attribution.

EVALUATION OF THE AUTISTIC CHILD

Like the TBI and ADHD evaluations, this, too, is paradigmatic. It is the way one approaches children with severe developmental disabilities in general.

When a child with developmental delays (DDs) is referred to a psychiatrist, the question is usually about behavior and how to manage it and whether drug treatment is appropriate. Before one gets into that, however, it is necessary to address a more fundamental issue: the diagnostic basis of the child's developmental handicap. To the neuropsychiatrist, MR and autism are not sufficient diagnoses. Moderate MR secondary to prematurity and perinatal asphyxia is an acceptable diagnosis. Autism and mild MR secondary to Down's syndrome is acceptable. Even if the diagnosis is severe to profound MR of unknown origin, the physician is acknowledging that the issue of cause has at least been addressed.

It is always helpful if the child has already been seen by a developmental pediatrician, a pediatric neurologist, or a medical geneticist, but it is also necessary to establish whether that consultation was comprehensive. It is never a good idea to assume that it was. It may be up to the neuropsychiatrist to readdress the issue of cause. One does well to review the records of previous evaluations rather than rely on second-hand information.

Only a small minority of children with DDs receives an etiologic diagnosis when they are evaluated in the community. In one survey of mentally retarded 10-year-old children, only 22% were so diagnosed. Conversely, when they were evaluated by a pediatric neurologist attuned to the issue and a standard protocol was used, the proportion of children with an etiologic diagnosis increased to 63%. In one-half of the cases, the diagnosis was made based on the laboratory tests alone. Etiologic diagnosis modified the physician's appraisal of recurrence risk in 25% of the cases and influenced medical management in 10% (17).

The family history is very important. Most of the genetic causes of MR and autism are nonfamilial, but some are heritable. In fragile X syndrome, family members on the maternal side may have had affective or anxiety disorders or learning disabilities but not frank MR. Language-based learning disabilities, developmental language disorders, and abnormalities in social communication are frequently found in the families of autistic children.

One inquires about the pregnancy and delivery, the child's neonatal status, early childhood diseases, and early developmental milestones. Reduced optimality in the pre-, peri-, and neonatal periods is typical in autism, perhaps more than in other developmental disorders. Suboptimality includes bleeding during pregnancy, high maternal age, pre- and postterm birth, clinical dysmaturity, and hyperbilirubinemia.

When did people first suspect that the child might be developmentally delayed? In some autistic children, there is a peculiar pattern of normal early development, even the acquisition of some language, followed by a developmental regression. This pattern is not uncommon but has never been explained well. The regression is sometimes attributed to external factors, such as vaccination, or to the introduction of gluten in the child's diet; it is also characteristic of the Landau-Kleffner syndrome (see Chapter 14).

The diagnosis of epilepsy is extremely important in the treatment and the prognosis of children with autism and other developmental conditions. It is said that one-third of all autistic children develop seizures, most commonly during infancy or after puberty. Sometimes a child is referred for problems of inattention, hyperactivity, mood swings, aggression, or self-injurious behavior, and the cause is an undiagnosed or undertreated seizure disorder. It is not necessary to perform routine EEGs in children referred for a DD evaluation, but one should have a low threshold for ordering a study in children whose behavior problems are severe or unusual or paroxysmal in nature.

EEG abnormalities, even epileptiform spikes, are rather common in normal children and do not by themselves represent sufficient evidence for the diagnosis of epilepsy or for anticonvulsant treatment. When they occur in children with DDs with severe behavior or emotional problems, however, they may suggest the diagnosis of "subclinical epilepsy" or may predict a favorable behavioral response to an anticonvulsant drug.

Primary sensory abnormalities occur quite frequently in this population (20% to 50%) (17). Therefore, visual and auditory screening are essential components of the initial assessment.

The physical examination is very important. Growth retardation is essential to the diagnosis of conditions such as the fetal alcohol syndrome and de Lange syndrome. Autistic children tend to have large heads (but not macrocephaly or megalencephaly as such), and a large head is not by itself and indication for a CT scan or a MRI. Minor physical anomalies, similar to the anomalies that typify Down's syndrome, are frequent findings in children with DDs in general (Table 5.3); they are usually nonspecific and do not necessarily convey diagnostic information. Physical anomalies may, however, suggest a particular syndrome, and because the various syndromes are discussed here, their dysmorphic characteristics are mentioned.

Hepatosplenomegaly, cloudy cornea, and a cherry-red macula are suggestive of lysosomal storage diseases. Inborn errors of metabolism are associated with ataxia, unusual hair, and unusual odors.

Careful attention must be paid to the examination of the skin because tuberous sclerosis is one of the more common definable causes of autism, and it has important genetic, prognostic, and therapeutic ramifications. Depigmented macules are usually the first sign of the disorder and are often visualized only with the use of an ultraviolet Wood's light.

The standard neurologic examination is usually normal or nonspecific. Poor fine and gross motor coordination and nonspecific gait abnormalities are often noted. One is particularly interested in motor

TABLE 5.3. *Minor physical anomalies*

Fine electric hair
Multiple hair whorls
Low-set ears
Soft, floppy ears
Hypertelorism
Epicanthal folds
High arched palate
Furrowed tongue
Curved fifth finger
Single transverse palmar crease
Large gap between first and second toes
Third toe longer than second

asymmetries that may suggest cerebral palsy, although prematurity and perinatal asphyxia are more frequently associated with MR without autism.

Neurologic soft signs are abnormal findings that do not necessarily suggest any underlying neurologic or developmental abnormality. Their very character is indefinite, and their meaning is uncertain. In the examination of the child, they may simply represent isolated developmental dysmaturities; in the adult with mild BI, they may simply be dysmaturities that have persisted, or drug effects, or they may suggest an underlying but nonspecific brain dysfunction. The classic soft signs are isolated hyperreflexia, minimal intention tremor, mild choreoathetosis, finger agnosia, dysdiadochokinesis, astereognosis, motor impersistence, imbalance on tandem gait or single-leg standing, spooning or pronation on arm extension, mirror movements, agraphesthesia, right-left disorientation, and persistent infantile reflexes.

Hearing impairment should be excluded by formal audiologic examination or, if necessary, by brainstem evoked response. Sensorineural hearing loss is one of the consequences of perinatal asphyxia as is strabismus, and careful evaluation of extraocular movements is always necessary.

Brain imaging is rarely productive. Many different structural abnormalities have been described in autistic people, including increased brain volume, increased ventricular volume, increased white matter volume, cerebellar hypoplasia, parietal lobe hypoplasia, and abnormalities in the corpus callosum, hippocampus, and amygdala. When imaging is used as a routine screening tool, however, there is a low incidence of focal abnormalities; from the clinical perspective, abnormalities, when they occur might just as well be coincidental.

Examination of the cerebrospinal fluid is not usually part of the routine neurologic evaluation unless progressive encephalitis is suspected. Herpes simplex virus is a particularly noxious pathogen that may persist in the central nervous system even after a course of antiviral therapy and thus may cause significant damage.

Chromosomal studies, or karyotyping, should be considered if the child has multiple anomalies, especially of the face, ears, and distal extremities, or if the child is born small for gestational age. Other indications for karyotyping include a maternal history of repeated miscarriages, dermatoglyphic abnormalities, short stature, voracious appetite, simian crease, unusual facies, or a suspected genetic syndrome. Chromosomal anomalies as an etiologic diagnosis have been documented in 6% of children with subtle dysmorphic features and developmental delay (17).

It is no longer appropriate to use karyotyping (in a folate-deficient medium) to detect fragile X syndrome because the DNA probe is less expensive and more accurate. Fragile X syndrome is associated with physical anomalies, but they are not pathognomonic, and it is arguable that testing for this syndrome, the second most common genetic cause of MR and a frequent cause of autism, should be done in every male patient with DDs. There is no question it should be done for every male patient with a maternal family history of DDs.

Several chemical abnormalities have been reported in the autism literature, but there is no clinical justification for routine serotonin or endorphin level testing. The rationale for a complete blood count and a chemistry screening panel is no different from that for any other patient who may require drug treatment, namely, to establish a baseline against which future abnormalities may be measured. Of the inborn errors of metabolism, phenylketonuria is the most likely to be associated with autism. Of course, all the developed countries screen newborns for phenylketonuria, but most developed countries also have large immigrant communities; one cannot assume that screening was done if the child was born in an underdeveloped country. Congenital hypothyroidism is another condition that has been virtually eliminated in the developed world but that may still occur in poor countries.

The organic amino acidopathies, such as histidinemia and hyperlysinemia, are associated with DDs and autism. Serum and/or urinary screening is part of the evaluation, even if the yield is low. One may also screen for disorders of purine and pyrimidine metabolism. Metabolic screening is not necessarily routine, but the implications of diagnosing a metabolic disorder are such that it ought to be undertaken in the following circumstances: parental consanguinity, previously affected siblings, prominent feeding difficulties, multiple organ involvement, or developmental regression. Tests may include capillary blood gas, serum lactate/amino acids/ammonia/very long chain fatty acids as well as urinary amino acids (17).

The Diagnosis of Autism

Does it really matter whether a retarded child is autistic, mildly autistic, or not autistic at all? Indeed, from the perspective of the diagnostic workup, what is appropriate for the autistic child is equally appropriate for the nonautistic child with DDs. Conditions such as celiac disease may be common in autistic people, but it also common in other disorders, such as Down's syndrome. Epilepsy is a frequent occurrence in autistic children and in retarded children in general.

The diagnosis of autism is very important for education, behavior management, and treatment planning. It is important for family support and parent training. It is extremely important for understanding the symptoms of high-level autistic adults, so-called Asberger's syndrome; far too many such patients are misdiagnosed with other psychiatric labels. From the perspective of drug treatment, however, we have never discovered an effective approach that is not equally effective for mentally retarded people who were not autistic.

Early diagnosis of autism may be crucial, not because it will generate early intervention strategies, although that is not unimportant, but because Landau-Kleffner syndrome, a degenerative condition that may well be treatable, may be at issue.

EVALUATION OF THE MENTALLY RETARDED ADULT

The neuropsychiatrist does not have many opportunities to deal with the problems of the chronically mentally ill. The exceptions are mentally handicapped people and patients with TBI with severe disorders of behavior or emotional response. As we shall discuss, these two classes of patients pose some of the most challenging psychiatric problems. In terms of chronicity, poor response to psychotropic treatment, and the requirement for intensive management, they are not dissimilar to patients with chronic mental illness.

One thing that they all have in common is the difficulty of generating an accurate history. The adult patient who presents with a long history of challenging behaviors has often been seen by many different physicians and psychologists, with a number of inpatient stays, a litany of different medications, and innumerable workups of varying quality and salience. It is ironic that the more medical treatment such a patient has had along the way, the harder it is to reconstruct exactly what was done, when, and what was the result. The medical record that accompanies the patient to his or her initial evaluation can be at once massive and irrelevant. It is usually comprised of reams of consent forms, order sheets, and daily notes by health care technicians. Discharge summaries, specialist consultations, psychological evaluations, and neurodiagnostic test reports have usually been assiduously expunged from the record. With luck, one can find a list of previous medications; however, information on doses, side effects, and treatment responses is seldom there. It is an impenetrable morass—a mass of information in the service of ignorance.

Assume, however, that one is finally able to reconstruct a meaningful history of the patient's condition and course of treatment, that one has gathered the essential information, beginning with the pediatric workup described in the previous section, and capturing the evolution of the patient's psychiatric problem over the years, the circumstances that led to hospitalization and the success of residential placements, the drugs that were administered, and the results of treatment. One is secure that etiologic factors have been established, there are archival MRI results in the record, and the question of seizures, past or present, has been appropriately addressed. One knows all there is to know about catastrophic side effects, such as tardive dyskinesia (TD), neuroleptic malignant syndrome, and drug-induced leukopenia.

Finally, one is confident that the patient is residing in an appropriate setting, that caretakers are well trained and sensitive to his or her daily needs, and that ongoing medical care is in place. The patient is in a day program that is interesting and rewarding. Family disharmony, so devastating to the mentally handicapped child or adolescent, is no longer at issue.

A cynic can say that if one needs all this in place before evaluating the patient, the consultation will never take place. That is all too true, but the perfect should never be the enemy of the good, and one can make do with a fair approximation of what is prescribed above. Whenever a physician receives a chronic patient into his or her care, it is necessary to accommodate some uncertainty in the patient's history. It is hoped that it was not a catastrophic drug reaction or a particularly violent outburst whenever the antipsychotic dose was lowered even a little.

The physical examination is oriented to dysmorphic features, as always, to potentially painful physical conditions, such as arthritis, contractures, and skeletal deformities, and to systems that may be affected by chronic drug treatment (see below). It should also be an opportunity to review the patient's general medical state. Painful conditions, such as headache, menstrual cramps, and musculoskeletal and neuropathic pain are at least as common in the severely handicapped as they are in the general population, probably more so, and are woefully underdiagnosed and undertreated. Signs of self-injury should be documented, and signs of abuse should be investigated. We recommend a careful examination for abnormal involuntary movements. An appropriate examination form, the Tardive Dyskinesia and Tardive Akathisia, is found in Appendix 6.

The psychiatric examination of a nonverbal individual is based largely on the patient's appearance and affective state, his or her pattern of reactivity and relatedness, and level of activity. Positive psychiatric symptoms are readily elicited: hypervigilance, fearfulness, agitation, screaming, perseverative vocalizations, obstinacy and oppositional behavior, stereotypies, self-injurious behavior, hyperactivity, and disorganization.

Periodic psychological evaluations are appropriate, but little is gained by administering a complete neuropsychological battery. I strongly recommend testing adaptive behavior levels on an annual or biannual basis. Decline in adaptive function is a better way to detect early dementia, better certainly than a CT scan. ApoE genotyping is not a bad thing to have in the chart.

The chronic patient is probably going to remain on psychotropic medication for an indefinite length of time. There will be changes in dose along the way, new drugs may be introduced, and old ones lowered or withdrawn. How, then, does one monitor the patient's response over time?

The standard of care in the past has been direct behavioral observation, with accurate "counts" of behavioral mishaps, such as angry outbursts, aggressive behavior, or head-banging. There are two problems with this old standard: first, it is hard to generate reliable data in a residential setting that does not have expert psychological consultation available and second, the data are limited and may not capture important aspects of the patient's psychiatric condition, such as mood, sleep patterns, disorganization, or paranoia.

Rating scales are quick and easy to use, generate information across the spectrum of mood, performance, and behavior, and can be available from collateral sources. Two examples of rating scales, contained in the Appendix, are the Self-injurious Behavior Questionnaire for retarded people and the Neurobehavioral Rating Scale for patients with BI. Weekly ratings, by two or more caretakers (e.g., at home and at the workshop) are extremely useful to review when making decisions about drug treatment.

EXAMINING THE PATIENT ON PSYCHOACTIVE MEDICATION

Prudent pharmacotherapy requires a baseline examination and then serial examinations to monitor the patient for therapeutic response and anticipated side effects. Every candidate for pharmacotherapy requires a comprehensive physical and neurologic examination by the physician who prescribes the drug. It is, in my opinion, irresponsible to rely on the examination of another physician. It is even less responsible to prescribe without an examination at all. The fact that psychiatrists routinely administer psychoactive medications without performing even a screening physical examination is indefensible. One can only compare it with the situation in some underdeveloped countries where pharmacists dispense what are prescription drugs in the developed world simply based on the patient's reported symptoms.

In addition to the physical examination, every candidate for pharmacotherapy should have a baseline complete blood cell count and an automated lab panel with a thyroid profile. The general physical and laboratory studies should be repeated yearly or every other year. Blood pressure, pulse, and weight should be measured at every clinic visit, and height (in young patients) at 3-month intervals.

These are essential practices, defined by generations of medical custom, to ensure the good health of the patient at the beginning of treatment and his or her continued good health as pharmacologic treatment is administered. I feel no compunction to justify this recommendation beyond noting the high frequency of medical illnesses that are concurrent or causative in psychiatric patients (18), and reminding the reader of the amazing and unpredictable side effects of seemingly benign drugs, such as the occurrence of eosinophilia-myalgia in association with L-tryptophan (19), granulopenia with felbamate, or the recent disaster of fen-phen.

The routine of regular physical examination should not obscure the rationale for a specific examination and specific blood tests for patients who have specific problems or who are taking specific medications. Each drug and each disorder come with its obligate inquiries and warnings and its obligate laboratory and examination procedures.

Patients treated with stimulants and stabilized on an optimal dose should be monitored at 3- to 4-month intervals, with particular attention to pulse and blood pressure, rate of growth, mood (sedation, dysphoria, irritability), abnormal movements, tics or dyskinesias, and sleep and eating patterns. Headache (including classic migraine), abdominal pain, and dysphoria are probably the most frequent side effects of stimulant drugs. Tachycardia, atrial fibrillation, and hypertension are rare stimulant effects, but they may occur in adults. Although paradoxical excitement may occur with stimulants, it is more common to find depression. In a patient with head injury or a hyperactive child on stimulants, the greater risk is for depression, either as a consequence of drug treatment or after the drug is discontinued.

A stimulant-treated child with tics should be carefully evaluated, and the necessity of drug treatment should be reassessed. Stimulants do not cause irreversible tics, but that is no reason to continue treatment in the face of an annoying side effect. Tics can be reduced if the dose is lowered or if an alternative drug can be found. Adding hydroxytryptophan can eliminate stimulant-induced tics. Hydroxytryptophan supplementation also reduces the occurrence of rebound symptoms after the effects of a stimulant have worn off and may reduce the "on-off" phenomenon that often occurs with methylphenidate.

Stimulant dependence has proven to be such an uncommon occurrence in the patients at the Neuropsychiatry Clinic that no special warning is required. (Stimulant abuse is another problem altogether, especially in adolescent patients.) It is important to warn the patient of the risk of drug-induced depression or migraine.

The other dopamine agonists have a side-effect profile that is similar to that of stimulants, and monitoring is similar. Amantadine may cause pedal edema, for some reason, and a blotchy skin rash called livedo reticularis. Amantadine can also lower the blood levels of some anticonvulsant drugs. Patients should be warned of the risks of paradoxical excitement and seizures, especially if alcohol is consumed.

Monitoring tricyclic antidepressant therapy is similar to monitoring therapy with stimulants, although special attention should be given to the danger of antidepressant overdose, especially for patients who are potentially suicidal (e.g., patients with severe BI) and patients who have young children at home. Baseline cardiograms are not useful, as a rule, and do not guarantee the safety of subsequent treatment. The occurrence of arrhythmias, especially conduction defects, is the major concern with tricyclics. Sinus tachycardia is the most common cardiovascular effect of tricyclic antidepressants in children; resting heart rate elevation above 120 requires drug discontinuation or dose reduction.

The major warning that is required for the tricyclics is that of cardiac arrhythmia and accidental overdose. Weight gain may also be a problem on the tricyclics, and patients should be warned and monitored accordingly.

Tricyclics are not prescribed very often for psychiatric indications in the United States, largely because of the problems that arise with the high doses that are usually necessary. Low doses of amitriptyline or doxepin, prescribed for pain or sleep problems in neurologic patients are largely free of untoward effects.

Virtually all the typical stimulant side effects can occur with tricyclic antidepressants: tics, headaches (including migraine), dysphoria, and irritability. The clinical utility of determining antidepressant blood levels has not been convincingly demonstrated, except in special circumstances: in the geriatric population, in antidepressant nonresponders, in people with preexisting cardiovascular disease, and in people who are cotreated with certain selective serotonin reuptake inhibitors (SSRIs).

The new antidepressants are easier to monitor than the tricyclics because they are less prone to cardiovascular side effects and there is little if any danger of a fatal overdose. For trazodone, the warning should be about priapism; at every visit, one should inquire after the occurrence of unusual penile tumescence. The low dose of trazodone used for sleep problems does not cause priapism, but it may if you do not warn the patient. For maprotiline and bupropion, the warning should be about seizures, but maprotiline is hardly used any more, and bupropion is not notably epileptogenic.

The SSRIs hardly require medical monitoring because most of their side effects are appetitive, cognitive, or neurobehavioral. There have been problems with inappropriate medical workups for patients on SSRIs who are actually having drug side effects, such as sleep studies for hypersomnolence and the misdiagnosis of narcolepsy. It is not necessary to monitor vitamin C levels in patients on fluoxetine, but if they develop ecchymoses or other signs of capillary fragility, it is a good idea to prescribe supplemental C.

Long-term treatment with SSRIs or other new antidepressants sometimes gives rise to complaints of inattention, memory impairment, and anergia. It is not a bad idea to have a baseline NES (or similar neurocognitive profile) for patients who are likely to require long-term antidepressant therapy.

Patients on SSRIs (especially paroxetine), venlafaxine, amitriptyline, and gabapentin must be warned about withdrawal syndromes.

The examination of the patient on dopamine agonists or antidepressants must include inquiries about depression and irritability as well as observations of the patient's affect and mood. One examines the heart and appraises the patient for dyskinesia, increased muscle tone, and changes in fine motor coordination. One can measure verbal memory, attention, and fluency with simple paper-and-pencil tasks or with a computerized neuropsychological battery. No special laboratory measures are needed beyond the routine described.

In contrast to psychiatry's attitude toward most of the psychotropic drugs, careful physical evaluation of the lithium-treated patient has always been *de rigueur.* The baseline examination requires renal and thyroid studies, and these should be done subsequently at yearly intervals. Lithium blood levels require frequent monitoring, for example, at 6- or 12-month intervals.

The patient on lithium should be examined at 3-month intervals for signs of excessive sedation, motor incoordination, tremor, dyskinesia, increased tone, thyromegaly, edema, and acne vulgaris. Lithium-induced tremor may be a necessary evil, but the occurrence of motor incoordination, dyskinesia, or dystonia on lithium is a serious event. Patients on lithium should be warned that abrupt discontinuation may cause a withdrawal-induced psychosis (20,21).

Neuroleptic treatment is relatively contraindicated in encephalopathic patients in general. One reason is the high frequency of serious untoward effects. Careful monitoring, therefore, at 3-month intervals at least is required. Acute extrapyramidal reactions such as dystonia are easy to detect, but subtle extrapyramidal reactions such as akathisia may be hard to diagnose and may be misinterpreted as failure to respond. Akathisia should be suspected in any patient who is dysphoric or hyperactive on neuroleptic treatment. Coryza, urinary incontinence, and weight gain are side effects of thioridazine.

The problem of QT interval (QTc) prolongation (more than 450 milliseconds) has received a good deal of recent attention in connection with some of the older neuroleptics thioridazine, mesoridazine, and pimozide, as well as some of the atypical antipsychotic drugs including ziprasidone and risperidone. Age and underlying cardiac pathology contribute to the problem, which can result in the potentially fatal ventricular arrhythmia, and *torsade de pointes* (French, "twisting of the points"). Cotreatment with another drug that may also prolong the QTc (e.g., tricyclic antidepressant, sotalol, macrolides) or inhibit the metabolism of the antipsychotic may have a disastrous effect (22,23). Does this mean that serial electrocardiographic monitoring is necessary for patients at risk? It is better to select an alternative drug.

TD is not uncommon in neuroleptic-treated patients, and although most such occurrences appear to be short-lived, severe and persistent cases have been observed even in children (24). TD is usually characterized by choreoathetoid movements, but tics, dystonia, and akathisia may also occur. The major problem with TD monitoring is that maintenance neuroleptic treatment tends to mask early signs of the disorder. Therefore dose reduction or neuroleptic treatment also tends to mask early signs of the disorder. A standard examination for TD, the Abnormal Involuntary Movement Scale (AIMS), has been developed. (I prefer the TDAK, a scale developed by my colleagues and I, which includes the AIMS, but also conveys additional information of particular relevance to the neuropsychiatric patient; see the Appendix.) The AIMS examination can be reliably administered to most patients, even the severely handicapped, who have a high incidence of abnormal movements and stereotypies. Patients on neuroleptics should have an AIMS at 3-month intervals and should also be examined for sedation and dysphoria, abnormalities of muscle tone, and weight gain.

The neuroleptic malignant syndrome requires a special warning that may frighten patients even more than the standard TD warning. Inquiries about rigidity and hyperthermia should be made at every visit and should be accompanied by an admonition to avoid strenuous exertion and dehydration.

Although cholestatic jaundice and granulocytopenia are neuroleptic side effects, periodic laboratory tests beyond those just listed are not necessarily protective. Neuroleptic blood levels have no established clinical salience (25).

The atypical antipsychotics require the same kind of monitoring, except for clozapine, which is in a class by itself. The risk of extrapyramidal symptoms and of TD is less with the serotonin-dopamine antagonists, but unusual movement disorders may occur.

The major problem with the atypical antipsychotic drugs is weight gain, even to the point of inducing diabetes and hyperlipidemia. Patients need to be warned of this and monitored accordingly.

Carbamazepine (CBZ) is prescribed for the treatment of psychiatric patients, young and old, with increasing frequency. Monitoring CBZ requires examination for ataxia and nystagmus, sedation, dysphoria, nervousness or irritability, increased occurrence of seizures (especially absences), skin rash, easy bruising, or frequent infection. CBZ blood levels should be checked at 6-month intervals, along with a complete blood count and liver function tests. The tests should be done more frequently when treatment begins. Irritability or lethargy in a patient on CBZ may be a sign of hyponatremia.

One might mention the hematopoietic effects of CBZ when discussing the drug, but the warning does not have to be draconian. It is not at all clear that CBZ is more likely than valproate, for example, or the neuroleptic drugs, to cause agranulocytosis or thrombocytopenia.

The monitoring procedure for valproate is similar to that for CBZ, although checking serum ammonia levels may also be necessary to detect subtle changes in hepatic function. The warning about hepatic failure should never be omitted, especially in young patients and patients on concurrent drugs.

When a patient is stable on lithium, CBZ, or valproate, blood levels should be checked yearly.

Patients who may become pregnant should be warned about valproate, lithium, and even CBZ. If a patient is likely to become pregnant, an alternative drug should be used.

The new antiepileptic drugs lamotrigine and gabapentin are used a great deal by psychiatrists. Lamotrigine is associated with a serious skin reaction. What is required is not only a warning, but also a careful description of exactly what to do in the event of a skin eruption of any sort; namely, to stop the drug immediately and come right to the office. The toxicity of gabapentin and tiagabine is almost entirely neurobehavioral and easily managed, requiring no special precautions. Topiramate is safe and well tolerated but can cause severe depression, even years after it is introduced. A careful warning is necessary. None of the new antiepileptic drugs requires blood level monitoring, although there should be a baseline level in the chart.

The behavioral toxicity that frequently accompanies treatment with sedating anticonvulsants (phenytoin and the barbiturates) is not usually manifest during a neuropsychiatric examination, but a psychiatrist who consults on a patient treated with archaic anticonvulsants should consider recommending alternative anticonvulsant therapy before embarking on a course of psychiatric treatment.

Patients who are treated with propranolol or other beta-blockers require careful cardiovascular monitoring because bradycardia and hypotension are not uncommon side effects. The same is true for clonidine and the calcium-channel blockers. Beta-blockers are contraindicated in patients with asthma and some patients with diabetes. Patients who are smokers require a chest examination at every visit. One may want to keep track of serum triglycerides and cholesterol in patients on beta-blockers.

The general physical examination is supplemented by special measures aimed at detecting specific drug side effects. Balance and fine motor coordination are easily checked in a routine physical examination. Verbal memory, verbal and semantic fluency, and visual-perceptual processing are easily tested with a few simple neuropsychological tests. The entire procedure may require only 5 or 10 minutes. It is not inappropriate to do serial computerized neuropsychological testing in patients who will be on psychotropics for a long time (especially when they will be taking mood stabilizers or antipsychotics). At some point, that is likely to be the standard of care.

During this brief examination, the physician may make the most of the important interpersonal assessments that are part of the MSE. There is the opportunity for causal banter and for serious questions about sexuality, depression, or thoughts of suicide. Patients are far more comfortable discussing such issues with someone who behaves in a familiar, doctorly manner, competently goes about the job of a physical assessment, and will extend him- or herself in a bit of small talk. The physical examination is probably the best opening to a psychiatric interview. The intimacy that comes of physical contact can extend to a patient's inner side as well.

The physical examination is a bit of ritual but is an essential part of the doctor-patient relationship. It is not an empty ritual. It is no less than the occasion for the physician to remember: "I am giving this patient a drug. What should I be looking for? What harm may it be doing? What have I forgotten to look for? To worry about?" It is a ritual of touch, and an opportunity for self-examination that leads to the next questions: "What have I forgotten to ask? What have I forgotten to say?"

A ritual is not a substitute for thinking. It is a chance for thoughts to wander, to think again about the differential diagnosis, to observe the patient again from a slightly different angle, and to reflect on the principles that make psychopharmacology successful.

WHAT (IF ANYTHING) IS NEUROPSYCHIATRY?

Physicians more learned than I have tried to address this question, but it is really not very difficult. Historically, neuropsychiatry had economic ramifications. In the old days, neurologists found it hard to make a living in an office-based practice. So they hung out the neuropsychiatry shingle and made a living consulting with psychiatric patients.

Today, the neuro- prefix may or may not be economically advantageous; perhaps it is just a matter of prestige or perhaps self-inflation. Its popularity is attested by the proliferation of brain-care specialists who have affixed neuro- to their professional titles. We already have neuropsychologists and neuropsychiatrists and will soon have neurosocial workers, neurochiropractors, and neuromedical ethicists. "Whether this will be the sign of inflation that debases the currency or simply the adjustment required by a vigorous, expanding economy is still an open question. It depends, I suppose, on whether there is an increase in productivity..." (26). (I once saw an ad for a "neuroattorney.")

Increasingly, a neuropsychiatrist is someone who has taken independent training in neurology and psychiatry. That is a rather expensive way to get there in my opinion. It may not help to train in both specialties if psychiatry residents learn little in the way of neuropsychiatry and neurology residents learn little of behavioral neurology, and if both learn to relinquish cognitive evaluation to neuropsychologists. Unless men and women thus trained can win a post at an academic medical center, they are likely to spend their career practicing one specialty or the other. Office practice and the referral patterns that sustain it are not especially accommodating to this new-old hybrid.

To practice a subspecialty such as neuropsychiatry outside an academic center, one has to work hard to cultivate a referral train of neuropsychiatric patients. One also has to work hard to develop procedures for evaluation and treatment that represent added value for the patients and the professionals who refer them. I define neuropsychiatry as a subspecialty interest that resides fairly and squarely within the mainstream of psychiatry; it is further defined in terms of the patients one sees and the procedures one cultivates.

The patients whose medical problems are the subject of this book are bona fide neuropsychiatric patients. Others not dealt with here are also neuropsychiatric patients: patients with dementia, for example, and other neurodegenerative diseases; patients with chronic pain syndromes or perhaps even chronic fatigue; patients with ADHD or specific learning disabilities; patients with minor cognitive impairments such as so-called "benign senescence"; patients with certain types of movement disorders, such as TD and akathisia, Tourette's syndrome, and restless legs syndrome, and others.

The procedures that are the subject of this book are also the essentials of neuropsychiatric practice. The evaluation process goes beyond the conventional psychiatric and neurologic examination and necessarily includes neurocognitive assessment, dysmorphology, and genetic and biochemical analysis. The treatments addressed are special forms of counseling, drug treatment, and other somatic treatments that are oriented to the special requirements of the neuropsychiatric patient.

The rationale for office-based neuropsychiatry is not, as implied, the accretion of credentials but an improvement in day-to-day productivity. By this I mean that the practice is economically advantageous to the practitioner and medically advantageous to the patient. These twin criteria are not necessarily orthogonal, although in actual practice, they may be. I do not believe that a productive neuropsychiatric practice is represented by a machine in the back room, especially one of dubious merit, such as a brain-mapping device or a low-resolution single photon emission computed tomography scanner. I do not believe that it is routine referral for exorbitantly expensive tests. It is not the redefinition of run-of-the-mill anxiety and depression patients or people with ADHD, conjuring up pseudoneurologic explanations (such as "temporal lobe stuff") for their psychiatric symptoms.

Productivity is ultimately achieved by more accurate diagnosis and more efficient treatment. The design of one's practice can be amended to accommodate these goals. To this end, I recommend a hybrid model.

At present, there are two models for the outpatient practice of psychiatry. The advanced model is the psychopharmacology clinic or the clinical trials unit, where patients are seen in a setting that is wholly medical and for short periods of time. Drug prescription and brief counseling are the only treatments offered. (If the clinic is in the business of doing drug trials for pharmaceutical companies, even brief counseling may be a protocol violation.) The traditional model is the psychiatrist's office, which is still, for all practical purposes, a psychotherapist's suite. It is distinctly nonmedical. Drug treatment is undertaken as if it were an adjunct to various kinds of psychotherapy.

Both settings have their advantages. The first is well equipped to deal with all manner of medical issues, patients are often seen by more than one physician, and rating scales and other objective evaluation instruments are relied on, if somewhat obsessively. The second is more agreeable to visit, the practitioners are more open to wider issues in the patients' lives, and nonmedical therapists are used quite efficiently. Neither setting is ideal because each lacks the amenities provided by the other. In my opinion, the ideal neuropsychiatry clinic is a mix of the two.

The neuropsychiatry clinic is a medical clinic, equipped like a neurologist's office with examining rooms and all the necessary accoutrements but also with ample room for soft chairs, room for a relative to be present, and room for several people to talk together. Room, and at least some time, should be set aside for counseling or even psychotherapy. Smaller rooms are used for cognitive testing, especially computerized testing. There should be a place to take vital signs, a doctor's scale and a stadiometer, a laboratory for blood work, and an electrocardiography machine. Auxiliary staff includes physician's assistants, nurses, and neuropsychologists, but it is a distinct advantage to have therapists on board, too. Rating scales and computerized testing batteries are used freely because they generate a great deal of useful information and do not cost much. Neurodiagnostic tests are prescribed for the appropriate medical indications and not routinely.

Patients are seen for brief checks, for longer counseling visits, or for evaluations that may take several hours or a couple of days. Patients in crisis are seen frequently; routine follow-up is done quarterly or semiannually. If a patient is worked up by more than one professional, for example, a nurse and a physician, follow-up may be done by either of them, depending on the complexity of the problem and the patient's preference. With voice mail, e-mail, and pagers, and more than one professional familiar with the patient, communication between visits should be highly reliable, and simple medication changes can be made by phone.

The neuropsychiatry clinic is also defined by the patients who are treated there. Here, the clientele of a community-based office is usually different from that of a hospital practice. The majority of patients are the ones discussed in this monograph: patients with BI and with stroke, mentally retarded and autistic patients, ADHD and learning disabled people, and people with benign senescence and dementia. All these patients need three things: a good evaluation with a differential diagnosis; advice, counseling, and family support; and competent drug treatment.

An economically viable neuropsychiatry practice usually entails consultation arrangements with rehabilitation centers, residential treatment centers, nursing homes, and group homes in addition to the usual hospital affiliations.

If one is not sure that there are enough such patients to support all this overhead, be assured. A well-equipped neuropsychiatry clinic is increasingly popular among patients with traditional psychiatric diagnoses, many of whom prefer to see nonmedical therapists but who also prefer to deal with drug treatment in a more conventionally medical environment. They find it convenient to be seen in a setting where vital signs are taken by an office assistant, where blood samples can be drawn, and where cognitive testing may be done, if needed. They like the convenience of talking to a nurse or a physician's assistant who knows them when the psychiatrist is tied up. They appreciate a place where medical issues, such as headache or chronic pain, can also be dealt with.

A medical clinic is a familiar place for patients seeking an evaluation. The old psychiatric habit of 45-minute sessions is not well suited for the initial evaluation of a patient with a complex neuropsychiatric disorder; the new habit of 15-minute medication checks is not well suited for anything. An initial evaluation with rating scales and neurocognitive testing should take as long as 3 hours or more. Some evaluations require the better part of a day. At the end of such an evaluation, the patient is confident that his or her problem has been examined carefully and is grateful that treatment recommendations are being made on the basis of thorough understanding.

The degree to which managed care reimbursement will support such activities is problematic, to say the least. That is where efficiency is crucial, and the use of paraprofessionals, rating scales, and automated testing comes into play. A well-organized evaluation lasting 3 or 4 hours may be designed to take no more than 60 minutes of the physician's time. The well-trained and competent staffing that allows such an operation is also expensive, and not even the most efficient neuropsychiatrist can conduct a thorough evaluation for what most managed care companies allow for a psychiatric first visit. I offer no easy solution to this problem; the best advice is to keep track of your patient mix. Unfortunately, medical practice still relies on the economic principles set down by Robin Hood.

REFERENCES

1. Varney NR, Menefee L. Psychosocial and executive deficits following closed head injury: implications for orbital frontal cortex. *J Head Trauma Rehabil* 1993;8: 32–44.
2. Strub RL, Black FW. *The mental status examination in neurology*, 2nd ed. Philadelphia: FA Davis, 1985.
3. Folstein MF, Folstein SE, McHugh PR. Mini mental state—a practical method of grading the cognitive state of patients for the clinician. *J Psychiatr Res* 1975;12: 189–198.

4. Schwamm L, VanDyke C, Kiernan R. The neurobehavioral cognitive status examination. *Ann Intern Med* 1998;107:491.
5. Benton A, Hamsher K, Varney N, et al. *Contributions to neuropsychological assessment*. New York: Oxford University Press, 1983.
6. Rey A. *L'examen clinique en psychologie*. Paris: Presses Universitaires de France, 1964.
7. Binder L, Willis S. Assessment of motivation after financially compensable minor head trauma. *Psychol Assess* 1991;3:175–181.
8. Halstead WC. *Brain and intelligence: a quantitative study of the frontal lobes*. Chicago: University of Chicago Press, 1947.
9. Baker EL, Letz R, Fidler AT. A computer-administered neurobehavioral evaluation system for occupational and environmental epidemiology. *J Occup Med* 1985;27: 206–212.
10. Ben-Porath YS, Graham JR. Scientific basis of forensic applications of the MMPI-2. In: Ben-Porath YS, Graham JR, Hall GCN, et al., eds. *Foresnsic applications of the MMPI-2*. Thousand Oaks, CA: Sage Publications, 1995:1–17.
11. Lezak M. Recovery of memory and learning functions following traumatic brain injury. *Cortex* 1979;15: 63–72.
12. Lezak MD. *Neuropsychological assessment*, 2nd ed. New York: Oxford University Press, 1983.
13. Gass CS, Russell EW. MMPI profiles of closed head trauma patients: impact of neurologic complaints. *J Clin Psychol* 1991;47:253–260.
14. Derogatis LR. *Symptom Checklist-90-R*. Minneapolis: National Computer Systems, 1996.
15. Beck A. *Beck Anxiety Inventory*. San Antonio, TX: The Psychological Corporation, 1999.
16. Beck A. *Beck Depression Inventory*. San Antonio, TX: The Psychological Corporation, 1999.
17. Shevell M. The evaluation of the child with a global developmental delay. *Semin Pediatr Neurol* 1998;5:21–26.
18. Lorrin M, Koran M. Medical evaluation of psychiatric patients: 1. Results in a state mental health system. *Arch Gen Psychiatry* 1989;46:733–740.
19. Centers for Disease Control and Prevention/Morbidity and Mortality Weekly Reports. Eosinophilia-myalgia syndrome—New Mexico. *MMWR Morb Mortal Wkly Rep* 1989;38:765–767.
20. King JR, Hullin RP. Withdrawal symptoms from lithium: four case reports and a questionnaire study. *Br J Psychiatry* 1983;143:30–35.
21. Mander AJ. Is there a lithium withdrawal syndrome? *Br J Psychiatry* 1986;149:498–501.
22. Buckley N, Sanders P. Cardiovascular adverse effects of antipsychotic drugs. *Drug Saf* 2000;23:215–228.
23. Gury C, Canceil O, Iaria P. [Antipsychotic drugs and cardiovascular safety: current studies of prolonged QT interval and risk of ventricular arrhythmia]. *Encephale* 2000;26:62–72.
24. Gualtieri CT, Barnhill LJ, McGimsey J, et al. Tardive dyskinesia and other drug-induced movement disorders in children. *J Am Acad Child Psychiatry* 1980;19:491–510.
25. Gualtieri CT, Hicks RE, Patrick K, et al. Clinical correlates of methylphenidate blood levels. *Ther Drug Monit* 1984;6:379–392.
26. Gualtieri CT. The functional neuroanatomy of psychiatric treatments. *Psychiatr Clin North Am* 1991;14: 113–124.

6

Transient Sequelae of Traumatic Brain Injury

SUMMARY

The neurobehavioral consequences of brain injury are either transient, static, or delayed. Transient sequelae arise within hours or days of the injury; they can be very short-lived or can persist for months. That they are only transient does not diminish their importance, that is, the degree to which they are disabling and the anguish that they cause to patients and families. Transient problems can be quite severe. They pose some interesting diagnostic and therapeutic dilemmas.

The postconcussion syndrome is the most familiar example of a transient neurobehavioral sequela; posttraumatic headache is another. These problems are most commonly associated with mild brain injuries. It is ironic that the most severe posttraumatic headaches occur after relatively mild injuries.

The consequences of mild brain injury are usually transient. Persistent problems, when they occur, are invariably mild and hardly ever disabling. Because mild brain injuries are so numerous, it is inevitable that a physician will encounter patients whose clinical course defies the usual expectations. How does one contend with patients who complain of severe and enduring problems after a relatively minor blow to the head? A way to approach them is given here in some detail.

Severe brain injuries can also be the occasion of transient conditions. Severe agitation, aggression, and self-injurious behavior can occur as the patient with traumatic brain injury (TBI) emerges from coma. There are several behavioral and pharmacologic approaches to this dangerous condition. The *N*-methyl-D-aspartate antagonist amantadine is particularly useful.

Seizures and psychotic states that arise in the first few days after TBI require careful attention but do not necessarily predict the development of posttraumatic epilepsy or persistent posttraumatic psychosis. The latter are usually delayed in onset.

TRANSIENT SEQUELAE

Brain injury is considered to be permanent, but nothing is further from the truth. Some degree of functional recovery characterizes the course of virtually every survivor of traumatic brain injury (TBI). Often the sequelae of TBI are entirely transient, lasting only a few days, weeks, or months, followed by complete (or near-complete) remission. The best example, of course, is the postconcussion syndrome (PCS) that follows mild brain injury (MBI). The most severe example is agitation during coma recovery. Immediate posttraumatic seizures and immediate posttraumatic psychosis have nowhere near the prognostic gravity of epilepsy or psychosis with delayed onset.

MILD BRAIN INJURY

By convention, a TBI is considered mild if the following criteria are met (1):

- Brief loss of consciousness (LOC) of less than 20 minutes
- A short period of posttraumatic amnesia (PTA) (less than 24 hours)
- Initial score on the Glasgow Coma Scale no less than 13
- The neurologic examination is nonfocal
- Traditional neurodiagnostic tests [e.g., electroencephalography (EEG), computed tomography (CT), magnetic resonance imaging (MRI), skull films] are normal

A recent modification of the diagnostic criteria for mild TBI expanded the definition (2):

- LOC of less than 30 minutes and a Glasgow Coma Scale score of 13 to 15 after this period of LOC
- Any loss of memory of events immediately before or after the accident, with a period of PTA of less than 24 hours
- Any alteration in mental state at the time of the accident (e.g., feeling dazed, disoriented, or confused)
- Focal neurologic deficits that may or may not be transient

Yet another system for grading concussion (3):

- Grade I concussion: confusion without amnesia
- Grade II concussion: amnesia without LOC
- Grade III concussion: LOC of up to six hours

And another, again (4)

- Grade I: no LOC, transient mental state changes < 15 min duration
- Grade II: no LOC, transient mental state changes > 15 min duration
- Grade III : LOC, which may be brief (seconds) or prolonged (minutes)

For all practical purposes, the terms concussion and MBI are equivalent. Every concussion is a MBI, not every MBI is a concussion; concussion is, by definition, traumatic. As far as grading is concerned, it is useful for some specific applications, like the acute management of sports injuries (4). For clinical communications, it is better to be specific, e.g., concussion with no LOC but 2 hours of posttraumatic confusion. Different physicians use different grading systems.

Epidemiology

Of the 2,000,000 TBIs that occur in the United States each year (5), almost 90% are classified as mild (6). It is likely that the true incidence of MBI is higher because 20% to 40% of patients with MBI never seek medical attention (7). In one survey, no fewer than 24% of male and 16% of female college students reported a previous head injury with LOC (8).

Motor vehicle accidents, falls, and assaults account for most MBIs, but a considerable number occurs during sporting activities. It is interesting to note that the rate of concussion in soccer is as high or higher than it is in the more violent sports, football, ice hockey, and lacrosse (4,9).

The morbidity associated with MBI is not inconsiderable. It accounts for no less than three-fourths of all hospital admissions for TBI (10). Because MBIs are so numerous, they represent in aggregate a considerable proportion of complications, poor outcome, and prolonged hospital stay.

Signs and Symptoms of Mild Brain Injury

MBI is associated with two problems: an acute encephalopathy that lasts no more than a few days and PCS, which may last for weeks or months. The acute symptoms of MBI are nausea, vomiting, blurred vision, and somnolence. These are almost invariably short-lived (11) and require no special treatment. Persistence of acute encephalopathic symptoms beyond a few days is not consistent with MBI.

The symptoms of PCS are headache, fatigue, insomnia, irritability, emotional lability, anxiety, depression, hyposexuality, photosensitivity, hypacusis, dizziness, inattention, memory deficits, and alcohol intolerance. They generally arise within hours, days, or even weeks after MBI. The delayed onset of PCS does not imply a "neurotic" as opposed to an "organic" cause (12).

The neuropsychological deficits that follow MBI are well known and have been reviewed on several occasions. There is clear evidence that cognitive deficits arise within the first few days after MBI, especially in attention, memory, reaction time, and the efficiency of cognitive processing (12–18). Patients may describe problems like stuttering, difficulty in word retrieval, letter reversals, difficulties in reading, spelling, or math, especially when they are tired, but discrete cortical deficits (e.g., aphasia, agnosia, apraxia) are incompatible with MBI.

Diagnosis of Mild Brain Injury

The conventional definition of MBI comprises three essential points:

- A traumatic event of sufficient intensity to cause concussion

- A change in the mental state of the patient (LOC, PTA, confusion, lethargy) that is only transient
- No evidence of focal brain damage, hemorrhage, or skull fracture on examination or in diagnostic testing

All three points are essential to the diagnosis. A trivial blow, such as that sustained in a rear-end collision at 5 to 10 mph, is well below the threshold necessary to induce concussion. This has been established in biomechanical studies of experimental animals, including primates (19,20). Without a credible blow, a change in the patient's mental state is unlikely to be encephalopathic in nature.

A brain injury may occur in patients who do not lose consciousness. This may occur, for example, with a penetrating brain injury such as a gunshot wound (21) but not as a rule in CHI. It is hard to maintain that a patient was concussed if there was not even a hint of PTA, confusion, or disorientation. If the patient's memory of the event is reliable and detailed, the likelihood of concussion is slim indeed.

Conversely, a brief period of LOC or PTA does not mean that the brain injury was only mild. It is known that patients who have had only a brief change in the mental state may have serious pathology, such as a skull fracture, intracranial hematoma, or cerebral contusion (16). In one series, no fewer than 7.6% of patients with TBI with LOC of less than 10 minutes were found to have abnormalities on CT examination, usually small lesions in the tip or base of the frontal and temporal lobes adjacent to the skull (22). In a study of 658 patients with TBI whose Glasgow Coma Scale scores were 13 or higher, no fewer than 20% were found to have abnormalities on the CT scan (46 had skull fractures, 28 had hemorrhage or hematoma, 33 had contusions, 36 had diffuse brain swelling) (23). Had it been feasible in either of these surveys to do magnetic resonance imaging (MRI) rather than CT scans, the numbers would be even more dramatic. MRI is capable of demonstrating multiple small areas of increased T2 signal in subcortical or brainstem white matter; CT scans rarely show these white matter abnormalities (24). Finally, in a study of hospitalized patients with TBI, those admitted as mild cases constituted no fewer than 72% of the depressed skull fractures; 43% of the patients were severely disabled on discharge, and 48% of the patients stayed in hospital for more than 1 week (25).

From a sharp blow to the head and a subsequent period of amnesia, one infers that concussion has occurred. If there are focal findings on the neurologic examination and abnormalities on the CT or MRI, the TBI is defined as moderate or severe.

When the patient with MBI is evaluated using conventional techniques, it is not uncommon to detect abnormalities such as motor coordination and balance problems, pathologic reflexes, EEG dysrhythmias, and minute lucencies on the MRI, but these are nonspecific findings and seldom, if ever, diagnostic. The mental state examination and the Minnesota Multiphasic Personality Inventory often indicate somatic preoccupation, anxiety, and depression. Such findings are significant for the diagnosis of psychiatric disorders but hardly represent deviant findings in a patient with acknowledged PCS. Medical tests for attention and memory (e.g., digit span, serial 7s, the four-word test, the Mini-Mental State Examination) are not particularly sensitive for the MBI patient.

Evoked potentials, computerized EEG (e.g., brain electrical activity mapping), single photon emission computed tomography, and positron emission tomography scanning have been put forth as sophisticated and sensitive measures of cerebral dysfunction that may be otherwise inaccessible to conventional measurement. Preliminary research indicates that such tests are more sensitive in the sense that they demonstrate abnormal features in patients with TBI whose examination is otherwise normal and that they indicate abnormal function beyond the areas shown to be damaged on CT or MRI (26–31). The specificity of abnormal findings, however, may be open to question in individual cases. The utility of such measures has not been tested in rigorous fashion for groups of patients with MBI compared with suitable controls (32). Functional neurodiagnostics are expensive and impressive, but they may not necessarily increase the level of diagnostic certainty in cases that are ambiguous for other reasons. A diagnostic test that merely adds to a mountain of ambiguous data is not much of a test.

Conventional neuropsychological batteries are expensive but seem to be the appropriate thing to do for a patient with neurocognitive problems. On the other hand, the focal cortical deficits that are the specific target of a neuropsychological battery are not at issue in the case of MBI. In fact, focal neuropsychological findings (e.g., aphasia, agnosia, apraxia) or a drop in the IQ score from premorbid estimates are incompatible with the diagnosis of MBI.

More to the point are paper-and-pencil tests of memory [e.g., auditory memory tests such as the Rey (33) or the Buschke (34)] or of sustained attention [e.g., the Paced Auditory Serial Addition Test (35)]. There are also brief computerized batteries that emphasize tests of attention, memory, reaction time, and processing time. They are quick, inexpensive, and reliable (36) and may be administered serially. One may argue that the best way to diagnose MBI is to document mild deficits in attention, memory, and reaction time that improve as the symptoms of PCS diminish.

Differential Diagnosis of Postconcussion Syndrome

The differential diagnosis of PCS includes a number of medical, neurologic, and psychiatric disorders that can cause symptoms such as headache, fatigue, depression, and memory lapses. In fact, the symptoms of PCS, although typical, are relatively nonspecific and may overlap with a number of other clinical entities that may be temporally (if not causally) related to a traumatic injury. For example, soft-tissue injuries of the neck and back may also cause headache, irritability, and insomnia. The stress of pain and disability may cause depression, anergia, inattention, and memory impairment.

Posttraumatic stress disorder (PTSD) represents an intense, pathologic response to an extreme event. Obviously, patients may develop PTSD after a life-threatening accident. There is substantial overlap between the symptoms of PTSD and PCS: insomnia, depression, difficulty concentrating, attentional lapses, irritability, emotional lability, and so on. However, the cardinal symptoms of PTSD (intrusive memories, emotional blunting) are not encountered in the PCS. If a patient with PCS experiences avoidance behavior, it is usually brief and entirely understandable, for example, feeling uncomfortable about highway driving or not wanting to work again on high scaffolding. It is neither pathologic nor persistent. However, to reexperience the traumatic event in nightmares or flashbacks requires an event that has been encoded in long-term memory. Because true MBI is almost invariably accompanied by amnesia for the event (brief retrograde, a longer period of anterograde), PTSD and PCS are considered by some to be incompatible diagnoses. Many psychiatrists believe, however, that the two conditions may sometimes coexist, that despite a brief interval of amnesia, enough is retained in the way of toxic memory of pre- and postaccident events to cause PTSD. In my opinion, both views are correct: the first is generally true and the latter occurs sometimes but not often.

Dissociative reactions (e.g., hysterical conversion reactions, fugue states, retrograde amnesia) are known to arise after a traumatic event. It has even been suggested that the unique neuropathology of TBI may cause hysteria or somatoform disorder by damaging diencephalic structures that mediate cortical gating, loss of hedonic responsiveness, and will (37). That is an interesting but speculative view. An alternative construction is offered in the discussion below.

The terms compensation neurosis (38) and accident neurosis (39) refer to a posttraumatic syndrome (e.g., PCS, cervical whiplash, low back pain) that is maintained in the face of litigation in the hopes of winning a favorable award. Prevailing wisdom places it somewhere to the left of hysteria because it does not serve the resolution of "unconscious conflict" but clearly to the right of malingering because it does not represent a conscious effort to deceive. This too is the focus of later discussion.

Complications of Postconcussion Syndrome

In patients with persistent symptoms of PCS, the main complication seems to be major depression. Long-term studies of patients with persistent PCS agree that emotional symptoms tend to grow more prominent relative to the physical and cognitive symptoms (40–44).

Although depression (feeling sad, unhappy, dysphoric, or irritable) is a cardinal symptom of the PCS, few patients actually meet the criteria for major depression. Patients with PCS freely admit to feeling depressed but usually designate their emotional condition to a secondary status. It is, they say, a reaction to pain, disability, uncertainty, and behavioral changes that they do not understand. This is not denial. As the months pass, the same patient will readily concur with the primacy of his or her emotional symptoms as the physical symptoms have subsided, but depression, discouragement, and chronic stress have only increased. Affective disorders, especially depression, are probably the most common psychiatric sequelae of TBI in general (32), but posttraumatic depression is usually a delayed consequence of MBI (45).

The occurrence of major depression can contaminate one's interpretation of neuropsychological deficits after MBI. Patients with major depression, for example, are known to exhibit deficits in attention and vigilance, abstraction, fluency, memory, visuospatial, and motor skills (46). Depressives are likelier to have deficits in visuospatial, motor, and memory skills than in verbal skills. However, verbal tasks that require sustained attention may also be impaired in depression (46). It is not always possible, therefore, to make a clear diagnostic distinction between depression and PCS simply based on neuropsychological test results.

The distinction may be made on clinical grounds over time by a clinician who knows the patient well. Because the performance of a depressed patient on neuropsychological tests is largely a function of poor motivation, personal distress, and distraction, his or her performance may be expected to improve with personal encouragement to increase the level of motivation. It is certainly expected to improve with the application of successful therapy (47).

Posttraumatic headache is usually described as mixed, with elements of muscle contraction headache and vascular headache. It is controversial whether TBI can actually cause migraine in an individual who is not predisposed, but it is clear that migraine will develop after TBI in some patients, especially children (48). Posttraumatic narcolepsy may occur in patients with TBI but only, it seems, in patients with a genetic predisposition (49).

Posttraumatic seizures do not occur after MBI. Patients with PCS may describe spells or brief periods of affective alteration, weakness, dystonia, inattention, or confusion (50). Such intermittent interruptions of behavior are known to occur in a number of neuropathic states, for example, stroke (51), demyelinating disease (52), and aging (53). They are not ictal in nature. The EEG is normal, they remit spontaneously, and treatment with antiepileptic drugs is not appropriate. [The discussion of postconcussional disorder in the *DSM-IV* refers to "posttraumatic onset of seizures," influenced, no doubt by Brown et al. (54), who were, in turn, influenced by Verduyn et al. (50). In fact, seizures do not arise from concussion, and they are not symptomatic of the postconcussive state.]

Pathology of Mild Brain Injury

CHI is known to produce diffuse, microscopic damage to the brain, especially to the subcortical white matter (55). Cortical impact injury is transmitted, with particular vehemence, to axial structures, generating shear forces that cause scattered, multifocal subcortical and brainstem axonal damage (diffuse axonal injury) (55,56). Axonal damage throughout the neuraxis has been recognized as a consistent feature of severe, moderate, and even mild CHI, with the overall number of damaged neurons increasing with the severity of the respective injury (57). The shear and tensile forces associated with CHI physically tear neurons, causing them to retract and to expel a ball of axoplasm, resulting in the formation of a reactive axonal swelling commonly called a retraction ball (58).

It is possible for brain trauma to occur in acceleration-deceleration injuries (i.e., whiplash), in which the head itself never strikes a rigid surface (59). In primates, experimental whiplash has been shown to cause both surface and intracerebral petechial hemorrhages (60,61). The whiplash mechanism (inertial impulse loading) may be especially damaging to the limbic and frontotemporal cortices, zones of maximal centripetal, structural, and tissue-density susceptibility (61).

In moderate and severe CHI, it is possible to demonstrate pathologic effects of brain contusion on CT or MRI, and postmortem studies have demonstrated evidence of diffuse axonal injury. In MBI, obviously, the demonstration of pathologic changes is not as easy. Therefore, the pathophysiology of MBI is based on animal models, for example, the angular acceleration model (62) and the fluid-percussion model (63). Because animal models of severe brain trauma demonstrate neuropathologic and neurochemical changes that are similar to those observed in severely injured humans (62,64), it is reasonable to assume that MBI in experimental animals is a valid model for what happens in patients with MBI. This is disquieting because it implies that any injury, even the most minor, causes some immediate and irrevocable axonal damage (57).

Cerebral contusion is not likely to be a component of the pathology of MBI, but in other respects, the only difference between MBI and severe CHI is the degree of diffuse and multifocal damage. Like severe CHI, the pathology of MBI involves diffuse axonal injury (57,58,65). MBI has also been shown to elicit axon terminal and preterminal degeneration within the brainstem (62). There are isolated descriptions of axonal damage in humans who have sustained MBI (66). Oppenheimer (67) described myelin destruction and axonal retraction bulbs in five patients with minor brain injuries who died from other causes within days of their accidents.

There are three important features of axonal injury after MBI: the injury is both selective and diffuse, and the course of recovery is variable:

- *Selective injury*: Large-caliber, long-tract decussating axons are preferentially vulnerable to injury through stretching or compression, the result of shear or rotational forces. However, an axon may be injured in direct proximity to other axons, neural elements, glia, and microvessels that are undamaged (57).
- *Diffuse injury*: This kind of focal damage will not induce the dramatic changes that ordinarily occur when an entire tract is severed. Rather, the individual axons that are injured are diffusely scattered

throughout the afferent and efferent tracts of the brainstem. The clinical effects of MBI are not confined to any particular functional system.

- *Variable outcome*: The fate of axons damaged after MBI is variable. Over time, a damaged neuron may induce secondary effects on brain parenchyma that are immediate or delayed. Follow-up in animal models of MBI indicate that although some axonal swellings persisted unchanged and some axons die back, still others seem to mount a regenerative effort. Some of the damaged neurons exist in a relatively preserved brain microenvironment. As a result, they appear to be capable of mounting a sustained regenerative response. These features of the traumatically injured axon may be expected to lead to an adaptive form of recovery (57).

The pathologic anatomy of CHI is accompanied by derangements in neurotransmission that mediate some of the symptoms of PCS. Experimental studies in laboratory animals and clinical experiments have been consistent in demonstrating persistent changes after CHI in the levels of various neurotransmitters (68–70). The diffuse effects of injury to monoamine systems include alterations in arousal, attention, and information processing, mediated in large part by dopaminergic and noradrenergic neurons (71), and alterations in mood, appetite, sleep, sexual function, pain perception, circadian rhythms, motor activity, memory, anxiety, and aggression, mediated by serotonergic neurons (72).

Outcome

The course and outcome of MBI have been well defined by a series of studies of relatively large patient groups. There is a degree of variability in the observed results, of course, owing to differences in experimental method, in the clinical populations from which the samples were derived, screening for premorbid characteristics, and so on. The research was done, after all, in several countries by clinicians from different backgrounds and over a span of 50 years. The results are, in fact, strengthened by the diversity of approach. They can be summarized in the most general terms.

Mild Brain Injury Has a Good Prognosis

Most patients with MBI improve and are able to return to school or work within days or weeks of their injury (12,35). At the very least, two-thirds of patients with MBI are able to return to their jobs within 3 months (12,35). Most patients are asymptomatic after 6 months (73).

Mild Brain Injury Symptoms May Be Persistent

Even among patients who improve and return to school or work, posttraumatic symptoms may continue for several weeks or months. Persistent symptoms are described as somatic (headache, dizziness, tinnitus, diplopia), neurobehavioral/vegetative (irritability, fatigue, weakness, anxiety, depression), or neurocognitive (memory, attention, information-processing speed). The latter are of particular interest because they can be measured on objective tests and compared with normative values. In the Virginia studies, neuropsychological impairments were demonstrated at 3 months after MBI (74). In the collaborative multicenter study reported by Levine et al. (75), neurocognitive deficits were present in patients with MBI at 1 month after discharge from hospital; by 3 months, most patients had improved and their neuropsychological performance was comparable with that of controls. However, for some of the patients a residue of isolated neurocognitive defects persisted for a longer period.

Postconcussion Syndrome Improves with the Passage of Time

As time passes, the proportion of patients who describe persistent symptoms declines. In the Virginia study of 587 MBI cases, the incidence of posttraumatic symptoms declined from 65% to 67% at discharge, to 38% to 63% at 3 months, to 23% to 44% at 6 months, to 23% to 44% at 9 months, and to 13% to 40% at 12 months (76). In the Belfast studies, 51% of the cases were symptomatic after 6 weeks (77) and 15% were symptomatic after 1 year (78). Denker (79) reported a rate of 33% at 1 year and 15% at 3 years.

Some People May Never Get Better

The gradual decline of the population with PCS does not appear to achieve a zero asymptote. Although the quality of the long-term data is not nearly so strong, there are respectable descriptions of persistent symptoms after 3 years (80) or longer [14 years, Merskey and Woodforde (40); 16 years, Amphoux et al. (81)].

Healthy Individuals Have a Very Good Prognosis.

When studies are done of highly selected groups of healthy individuals, the outcome is uniformly good. For example, in Cook's (82) study of 303 rugby players who had sustained MBIs followed by a short period of impaired consciousness, posttraumatic headache lasted less than 48 hours in three-fourths of the sample, and only 17% missed any work at all. That may be because sporting injuries are less traumatic than motor vehicle accidents. However, in a study of 20 patients who were hospitalized briefly for MBI and who were carefully screened for premorbid conditions such as alcoholism, previous head injury, and psychiatric disorders, Dikmen et al. (14) reported only mild neurocognitive deficits (memory, attention) persisting after 1 month, with complete resolution after 12 months.

Persistent Symptoms Are Usually Subjective in Nature

In the study by Dikmen et al. (14), many of the patients with MBI continued to complain of persistent symptoms after a year (e.g., headache, fatigue), but the sample of patients with MBI did not differ in their complaints from a matched group of normal controls. This finding highlights a failing in the literature with respect to persistent postconcussion symptoms. It is clear that authors have described patients with subjective complaints that are consistent with persistent PCS. The complaints, however, are rarely if ever supported by objective findings, for example, deficits in neuropsychological tests, or comparisons to matched controls.

There is near unanimity in the literature to the effect that persistent symptoms of PCS, lasting 12 months or longer, are heavily weighted toward the somatic (e.g., headache, dizziness, chronic pain) and the neurobehavioral/vegetative (e.g., depression, anxiety, fatigue) (40,43,83). The observations of clinicians are supported by a cluster analysis of postconcussion symptoms in 155 patients in a multicenter study reported by Levine et al. (75). PCS, therefore, begins as an encephalopathy and evolves in a small number of patients as a functional problem of chronic pain or depression.

Factors That Predict Outcome.

It is interesting to consider the variables that are predictive of outcome from MBI. Recovery is known to be slower in patients who have had a previous concussion (84). The older patient is at greater risk for prolonged disability (13,78,85,86); patients more than 40 years old are twice as likely to have persistent symptoms than patients under the age of 30 (79). Persistent symptoms are more frequent in women than in men (11).

Persistent disability is more common in patients from low socioeconomic classes compared with the managerial classes (12); this is often attributed to differences in motivation or to the fact that managers have more flexibility in arranging their work when they do not feel well. One should not, however, overlook the fact that social class is, in modern society, highly correlated with IQ. In studies of TBI, high IQ is one of the strongest predictors of a good outcome (87).

In addition to IQ, pretraumatic personality characteristics are known to be predictive of outcome of MBI (88). It is known that a tendency to psychological difficulties premorbidly may contribute to lingering disability in soldiers sustaining head injuries in wartime (89), just as it does to the development of severe PTSD. Unemployment after MBI was found to be more common in patients who had significant life stress before injury (12). Patients with MBI with preexisting emotional problems were more likely to complain of persistent neurocognitive symptoms as well as neurobehavioral-emotional symptoms than patients with no such premorbid history (44).

One class of patients who sometimes experience prolonged and debilitating symptoms after a MBI are highly intelligent, high achievers (or overachievers) with a premorbid obsessive-compulsive personality.

Effects of Litigation

It is possible that litigation, the adversarial process, and compensation seeking may influence the course of recovery from MBI, but the effect is not nearly as strong as some authors, such as Miller (39), have represented. Patients who are involved in litigation may take more time off work than those without claims (90) and are likelier to have persistent symptoms (11), and their symptoms are more likely to be subjective in nature (91,92). Individuals who attribute their injury to the fault of an employer or to some large, impersonal organization are twice as likely to report persistent symptoms than individuals who only blame themselves or attribute their injury to an act of God (11).

Conversely, the PCS symptoms of litigation patients are the same as the symptoms of nonlitigation patients, and persistent symptoms have been described in patients for whom compensation was not at issue (12,81). It is well known that patients with PCS usually return to work, even in the face of outstanding claims or continued symptoms (12,13,86,93). Complete remission of PCS is not uncommon in litigation patients, even before their claims are settled (11), and prolonged PCS is not necessarily resolved by settlement of a claim (40,79,94,95).

In response to Miller's (39) cynical prediction that patients with accident neurosis never respond to treatments until their claims are resolved, Kelly (96) argued that withholding treatment from litigation patients may only aggravate their posttraumatic symptoms. The fact is that most people do not exaggerate symptoms or concoct disabilities to win undeserved compensation, but that does not mean that no one ever does or even that it should be surprising when someone does.

Catastrophic Outcomes

The literature contains no credible descriptions of patients with MBI who have developed seizures or psychosis, whose IQ has declined, or who have suffered catastrophic disability as a result of a MBI, without some significant premorbid condition or some alternative etiologic factor that is at least as credible as the link to MBI.

THE CONCEPT OF CEREBRAL RESERVE

In view of the previous section, the famous quote from Symonds (97) that "the effects of concussion are never completely reversible" may seem off base. It is not. In his response to Miller, who was in his day a famous skeptic, Symonds marshaled data from neuropathologic studies and from clinical observations to make this point:

> *In (concussion) there may be rapid and complete recovery of cerebral function; but this does not necessarily exclude the possibility that a small number of neurons may have perished—a number so small as to be negligible at the time, but leaving the brain more susceptible as a whole to the effects of further damage of the same kind (97, p 5).*

The concept of cerebral reserve may be vague and abstract, but its clinical manifestations are apparent in a host of familiar conditions: for example, the development of parkinsonism in postencephalitic patients; the abrupt decompensation of an elderly patient who is removed from familiar surroundings; the loss of ambulation in middle age in mentally retarded people who had cerebral palsy as youngsters; and even, on a spinal level, the postpolio syndrome. Its foundation is the redundancy of neurons in the central nervous system. Recovery is possible if redundant tissue can take up the slack, but the capacity of the organism to recover from future stressors will necessarily be diminished.

The effects of two or more severe brain injuries are known to be cumulative, even in the face of good recovery (71). The same is true of MBI. In boxers, the effects of repeated concussions are cumulative, and beyond a certain number of concussions, the effects are likely to be irreversible (98). In boxers, multiple subconcussive blows to the head were thought to be a plausible etiologic factor for abnormal neurologic findings, including abnormal examinations, abnormal EEGs, and abnormal CT scans (99). There is a direct relationship, in fact, between the development of cerebral atrophy and the number of matches a boxer has had (99).

When the test scores of patients with MBI who have experienced a second or third injury are compared with those who have never had an MBI before, the former are more severely affected and take longer to recover (84). Patients with MBI who have made a recovery that is seemingly complete may be shown to have deficits on neuropsychological testing under conditions of hypoxia (100).

It is disturbing, therefore, to consider that the effects of even a single MBI may have far-reaching effects, even in the face of a complete clinical recovery. Apparently, the brain is able to compensate for the deficits created by multifocal lesions and diffuse axonal injury, but with each succeeding injury, the cerebral reserve—the ability to compensate for lost neurons—is diminished.

Many of the predictive outcome elements discussed in the preceding section are consistent with the theory of cerebral reserve. The recovery of children from TBI in general and from MBI in particular is more robust than that of adults, and the recovery of elderly patients is almost invariably compromised. IQ and social class (which is highly correlated with IQ) also predict good recovery; patients who are better endowed with intelligence and/or socio-econommic advantage are more likely to make a better recovery. Patients with a low IQ are also more likely to experience clinically significant damage from a mild neurotoxic insult (101). Patients with premorbid psychiatric conditions, especially alcoholic patients, are at particular risk for neurobehavioral sequelae from TBI in general (10,87) and MBI in particular (102), and their clinical course is more complicated.

MBI: Summary

Symptoms of PCS may be severe and debilitating, but severe symptoms are transient, except in the unusually fragile patient. PCS symptoms may persist for months or years, but persistent symptoms are mild and rarely debilitating. Severe, persistent symptoms are incompatible with MBI, which means that something else is going on.

PCS is a well-defined syndrome that arises from MBI, with clear and irrefutable neuropathologic correlates. In most patients, full recovery is likely because redundancy of neurons is characteristic of the central nervous system, especially in young people. Recovery is possible because in the healthy brain, there is a certain capacity for neuronal self-repair. Remote functional changes, such as diaschisis, seem to be reversible with the appropriate pharmacologic intervention or just with the passage of time. PCS may be persistent, for months or even years, but the weight of evidence indicates that persistent symptoms are relatively mild and should not lead to permanent disability.

The problem of MBI is the catastrophic case: the patient with persistent symptoms and severe disability. In evaluating such a patient, it is necessary to consider four explanations:

- There was, in fact, a brain injury, but it was not a mild one. A contusion or hematoma was present early on, but the opportunity for diagnosis was missed, and any footprints that are left are obscure and hard to interpret, or the patient's premorbid state was precarious because of age, a bleeding diathesis, small-vessel disease, and so on.
- There was MBI, and then PCS. Then, the patient developed major depression. Depression was not recognized, probably because somatic and neurocognitive deficits were the focus of treatment. The patient has not had the benefit of appropriate treatment for posttraumatic depression.
- There was MBI or a traumatic event of some sort that may or may not have caused MBI. The patient, however, had a premorbid psychiatric condition, such as paranoia, antisocial personality, borderline personality, or substance abuse. The patient developed a fixation on the accident as the source of his or her problems, a preoccupation that is reinforced by the attention of professionals who were not aware of his or her premorbid condition.
- There was MBI or a traumatic event that may or may not have involved MBI. The patient has subsequently developed a functional disorder, i.e., somatoform disorder, somatoform pain disorder, compensation neurosis, or malingering.

None of these alternative explanations should be a serious problem to an experienced physician who takes the time to understand the patient and is capable of exercising critical judgment in the service of a differential diagnosis.

A Minor Injury with a Major Impact

We know that what seems at first to be MBI may contain elements of major pathology. Even if an early CT scan was never done, however, and the results of a late MRI are nonspecific, there will usually be some credible indicator that the initial injury was, in fact, a severe one. The clinical course will show improvement of at least some symptoms; not all symptoms will persist. If new symptoms arise, they will be the expected ones, such as depression or migraine, not unusual or catastrophic ones, such as paresis, psychosis, or seizures. Neuropsychological deficits will be consistent with the hypothesized lesion and will show improvement or stasis, not deterioration, from test to test. A biomechanical analysis of the accident will document G forces sufficient to cause moderate or severe brain injury.

A careful history may indicate vulnerability to major injury even from a minor blow, for example, a previous TBI, a bleeding diathesis, white matter disease, or risk factors for small-vessel disease such as hyperlipidemia or smoking.

Symptomatic treatments will have a measure of success. Posttraumatic depression will clear with nonsedating antidepressants, attentional problems will improve with stimulants, and headache will improve with the usual treatments. The residue of persistent pathology will be of the kind that is normally resistant to treatment, such as memory deficits.

One cannot place too much credence in the manner of a patient's self-presentation. A tendency to overstate problems or to exaggerate one's distress may simply be a cultural heritage or a personal quirk. Referral by an attorney should not, of itself, discredit the patient or diminish his or her problems. A preoccupation with financial issues or the unfairness of the adversarial system should not be held against a patient. The system is not always fair, and it is almost always annoying. A tendency to doctor-shop may simply be the appropriate adaptation to an unsympathetic medical community. The habit of relying on analgesic or sedating drugs may not be indicative of a purely functional disorder.

There may be inconsistencies in the clinical record, but they are usually understandable. A&O in the emergency department record sometimes means that the patient was alive and his or her eyes were open; it does not always reflect a real test of the mental state. The patient did not complain of postconcussion symptoms when he or she saw a neurosurgeon 3 days after the accident, probably because the interview was only 5 minutes long. The diagnosis of TBI was not made until 6 months had passed because no one had even entertained the possibility. Inconsistencies and ambiguities invariably arise in the evaluation and treatment of patients. One or two minor inconsistencies are not important if the overall picture is consistent with moderate or severe brain injury.

A disabling outcome may be the result of moderate or severe brain injury when the initial presentation was no more than a concussion. It is not a common event, but it does happen. Before one actually concludes that was the case, however, it is also necessary to exclude the alternatives that follow.

Posttraumatic Depression

Persistent PCS may lead to major depression. The neuropathology of MBI, perturbations of neuromodulatory neurotransmitters and diaschisis, provides a theoretical underpinning for this common phenomenon. It is possible that some of the severe, persistent problems that stem from MBI may be depressive conditions that were not treated adequately. In fact, surveys have demonstrated that, even among psychiatrists, the treatment of depressed patients is often suboptimal (103).

There are no controlled studies of treatment of posttraumatic depression or anxiety, and I do not recommend that high priority be given for such research. The usual treatments are generally successful. Treatment-refractory depression has never been described in association with MBI. Over a long career treating patients with TBI, I have yet to encounter depression after MBI that was not amenable to conventional treatments.

A Premorbid Psychiatric Condition

Given the high rates of (i) MBI and (ii) psychiatric disorders, it is inevitable that many patients who present with (i) will have also had (ii). In fact, epidemiologic studies show that TBI patients have a higher rate of premorbid psychopathology, especially conditions associated with alcohol or drug abuse, impulsive behavior, and poor judgment, compared with the baseline population rate.

In such cases, it is possible that the pain and stress associated with MBI may cause the psychiatric patient to decompensate. It is also possible that the neuropathic and neurochemical changes that attend MBI may aggravate the premorbid psychiatric condition or make it more difficult to treat.

The psychiatric patient's premorbid coping style may be characterized by these "defense mechanisms": projection, denial, distortion, externalization, hypochondriasis, somatization, or dissociation. If so, posttraumatic symptoms that are entirely subjective in nature may be more likely the manifestation of their premorbid condition. A pre-existing psychiatric condition can turn a mild traumatic event into a new focus for the patient's psychopathology.

The Persistent Problem Is Not What It Appears to Be

When symptoms are far in excess of what one is capable of explaining in terms of pathophysiologic mechanisms or when they fly in face of same, it is necessary to consider one of these alternatives: somatoform disorder (hysteria), somatoform pain disorder, compensation neurosis, and malingering.

Malingering and Compensation Neurosis

Are these not really the same thing or is it possible to make a differentiation based on inferences, e.g., about the patient's level of awareness or his or her underlying motivational set. In Miller's words:

> *Whether exaggeration and simulation are "conscious" or "unconscious," their only purpose is to make the observer believe that the disability is greater than it really is. To compensate a man financially because he is stated to be deceiving himself as well as trying to deceive others is strange equity and stranger logic (39, p. 993).*

Miller's trenchant prose is hardly equal to the real problem. After all, malingering is not of a kind with pathologic somatization. In our culture, it is a brazenly antisocial act. It is an assault on the integrity of the physician-patient relationship and on the sincere concern of civilized society to redress wrongs and to protect the sick and the injured. By all accounts, it is an extremely rare event in the diagnosis and treatment of MBI.

> *Compensation neurosis is not the equivalent of malingering. In the former instance, the injury is real. The sequelae of the injury are exaggerated and kept alive because the patient is convinced that some person, institution or agency is responsible for his suffering...(he) becomes involved in a stubborn, unyielding struggle against those he blames.... It seems as if the patient somehow senses that he must persist in and nurture his illness and sufferings, which serve as his main argument in blaming those who are to compensate him. He is, therefore, unwilling to relinquish his illness until his claims are recognized (38).*

The psychological mechanism is neither obscure nor oblique. It is simple and straightforward: You did this to me and you owe me for it. I am not the same person I was. The patient is not trying to deceive anybody; he or she is seeking simple justice, and is only taking the compensation system at its word. If there is a fault to this behavior, it is only, perhaps, an inflated notion of the importance of his or her suffering and entitlement to reward.

Or else the patient is being a good negotiator. It is a peculiar irony to our system of justice that lawyers and insurance companies are permitted to undervalue a patient's claims without loss of face, but a patient who overvalues his or her damages loses credibility. I suppose it is because we expect lawyers and insurance companies to be dishonest and patients to be stoical.

The two circumstances are further differentiated by the proper role of the treating physician. In cases of suspected malingering, the role of the physician is to be a good detective. In cases of compensation neurosis, the proper role is to be a fair mediator. It is not strange logic to propose a medical contribution on behalf of this kind of equity.

Somatoform Disorders

The reader may be forgiven for thinking that the issue has been settled, that hysteria is not an organic affliction at all, but rather a psychological disturbance. Centuries of medical opinion, culminating in Charcot's demonstrations of the neurology of hysteria, were quietly put to rest by his loyal student, Babinski, who attributed it all to suggestion.

However, the frequent occurrence of somatoform disorders after TBI in general and MBI in particular has given rise to new speculations that they may well have a biologic basis. Eames (37), for example, found that 54 of 167 patients with TBI referred to a neurobehavioral unit had three or more primary symptoms of hysteria and raised "the possibility that some aspect of physical damage to the brain (was) responsible" (p. 1051). Yarnell and Rossie (59) described major debilitation in 27 patients after cervical whiplash injuries, none of whom experienced LOC, PTA, or "significant other-system injuries." The sequelae included many of the usual postconcussion symptoms and also "hypochondriacal ruminations, depersonalization, phobias...(and even) paranoid psychosis." They attributed these problems to "inertial impulse loading...(producing) injury to the limbic and frontotemporal cortices." In the summary discussion of Trimble and Cummings (104) of hysteria and neurosis after TBI, they agree that the same symptoms can be both "psychologically induced and organically induced" but that behavioral changes after concussion are probably related to "small structural lesions in the midbrain and diencephalon...(with) similar subtle changes in the limbic system."

It is possible that the somatoform disorders represent the end point of a neuropsychopathologic process set in motion by axonal injury, neurochemical changes, and then diaschitic changes in remote systems or possibly the result of petechial hemorrhages in the limbic system or in the frontal and temporal lobes. The stress of such a cascade of events may be exerted against a *locus minoris resistentiae*, a specific area of psychological weakness (105). If this combination of neuropathic and psychological stressors exceeded a certain threshold and if the process were excited by external events that undermined the patient's self-confidence and will to recover, a hysterical condition would presumably emerge.

It is always interesting to entertain a hypothetical mechanism of how a minor neuropathic event can turn into a major psychiatric disability. As a hypothesis, however, it must stand in line with some others. As a mechanism, I think that it is impossibly vague.

A logical problem arises when one posits such far-reaching consequences of a relatively minor neuronal event. If one concedes the importance of one minor element, what is the logical basis for discounting the potential impact of other minor elements, for example, the desire for economic security, the urge to set aside the burdens of self-reliance, the tendency that all people have sometimes to make irrational attributions, the desire for retribution, and finally the impact of suggestion, especially in the face of the extravagant treatments some patients with PCS may receive? When should a physician select the neurologic (or pseudo-neurologic) explanation in preference to these other explanations? How is it possible to raise any to the level of an etiologic factor?

It is well known that hysterical patients have a high rate of comorbidity, especially disorders of the central nervous system (106). It is probably true that "neurotic symptoms are apt to emerge...whenever the resources of the personality have suffered through injury to the brain" (107). It is a fallacy, however, to presume that because A (brain injury) may sometimes cause B (hysteria), then if B exists, A is necessarily the cause.

If an ordinary person is hurt, especially by concussion, he or she will naturally be in a vulnerable state. If the patient is dealt with unkindly by doctors, the boss, or an insurance company, he or she may succumb to dismay and a crisis of self-confidence. The resolution of such a crisis may take some peculiar turns. If the patient is dealt with gently, given some relief and appropriate encouragement, events will likely turn out well. If, however, the preoccupation of doctors is with extravagant diagnostics, therapeutic expeditions of dubious merit, and endless talk about damage to the brain, is it surprising that some people may take up the role of Charcot's ladies?

In 1975, Kelly (96) demonstrated that disability after MBI could be the result of therapeutic nihilism and believed that the posttraumatic syndrome was an iatrogenic disease. The point of Miller's (39) arguments was not that the injuries were concocted but that they were exaggerated by a system that rewarded disability rather than encouraging recovery. It is ironic that a generation later, the system has changed little, whereas a philosophy of therapeutic excess may well be creating a new kind of iatrogenic disease.

Levels of Certainty

Sometimes physicians are asked whether a patient's enduring disabilities were, in fact, caused by MBI. Because the theater for such inquiry is usually forensic, an opinion is required at the level of reasonable medical certainty or probability, which means, more likely than not, 51% certainty.

Physicians, relieved of the strictures of scientific certainty, may underestimate the intellectual rigor of reasonable medical certainty. The physician is well aware of the known neuropathic consequences of MBI. He or she may look on the MBI as the "straw that broke the camel's back," believing that a minor event may indeed set in motion an inexorable chain of destructive circumstances. The patient is perceived as an individual whose previous adjustment was tenuous and who has little reserve to compensate for the physical, social, and economic consequences of a minor injury. Swayed, doubtless on an unconscious level, by the knowledge that an unsettled account is more likely to be resolved by an outcome favorable to the patient and with a "shrug of the medical shoulders," the physician's reasoning achieves the cherished goal of 51%.

"More likely than not," however, is a standard that means no less than this: the direct neuropathic effects of the MBI were so formidable and so persistent that they exceed in likely impact the sum of all other possible causes of the patient's current condition. That standard may indeed be met in many cases of transient, severe PCS or mild, persistent PCS. It is less likely to be met in cases of severe, persistent PCS.

There is a level of certainty for scientific publication ($p < 0.05$) and a level of certainty for medicolegal endeavors ("more likely than not"). However, medical treatment, on the day-to-day level, often proceeds on the basis of inescapable uncertainty.

Treatment of Postconcussion Syndrome

There are two essential treatments for PCS: psychological and pharmacologic. The most important element of psychological treatment is counseling about the normal course of recovery. Patients need to be educated about the problems they are having and how they stem naturally and physiologically from the injury they have sustained. They have to know what to expect and the meaning of what they are experiencing. They need guidance in how to cope with their physical and psychological symptoms, their neuropsychological deficits, and their altered temperament, level of energy, and sexuality. They need counseling about their jobs, family relations, and legal proceedings. They need an advocate, a guiding hand, and a source of reassurance. Their somatic complaints require respectful attention. Referral to other specialists and recourse to neurodiagnostics should be intelligent and prudent. Patients deserve to be kept out of the hands of quacks. They need to be protected from physicians whose point of view is so thoroughly objective that they believe no problem exists unless it is demonstrated on a scan of some sort. They need to be protected as well from physicians and psychologists who believe that every patient with PCS needs a single photon emission computed tomography scan and a brain map, a full neuropsychological battery, cognitive remediation, and language and occupational therapy.

When a patient is told that he or she has a brain injury, there is the inevitable conclusion that the situation is irremediable. The patient should be told, and told with conviction, that nothing is further from the truth. The brain is more capable of healing than any other organ system, and healing is a natural process fostered by a positive attitude and a rapid return to one's normal occupations. The patient should also be told that healing can be delayed by impatience, frustration, rage, and self-pity.

Pharmacologic treatment should not be used because drugs have an uncertain effect in patients with head injury, and their side effects may actually retard the course of recovery. There are, however, occasions when prudent pharmacotherapy can accomplish a great deal. For problems with sleep, the serotonergic antidepressant trazodone is the preferred drug. Amitriptyline is another choice, but it is an anticholinergic drug (108). The benzodiazepines are not usually necessary and have their disadvantages to be sure, but sometimes they may be useful. Diazepam may be good if the patient cannot sleep because of muscle spasm pain. If the severe insomnia of PCS can be controlled, much of the daytime anguish and irritability may disappear as well.

For problems with low energy, mild depression, abulia, inattention, and poor memory, the psychostimulants such as methylphenidate are preferred. For emotional lability, irritability, and depression, a serotonergic antidepressant or bupropion is recommended. For problems of anxiety, restlessness, akathisia, and somatic preoccupation, the drug of choice may be buspirone.

POSTTRAUMATIC STRESS DISORDER

PTSD is not necessarily a transient disorder but is included in this chapter because it is transient at least half the time and because it is necessary to distinguish between PTSD, which is a psychopathologic state that occurs in only a fraction of trauma patients, from "adjustment reactions" or acute stress disorder (ASD), which is virtually universal after trauma or any unpleasant experience.

It is said that 40% of the American population has experienced a severely traumatic event and that PTSD develops in one-fourth of the trauma-exposed population. The prevalence of PTSD, therefore, should be high. Lifetime prevalence rates in community samples range from 1% to 9% (the latter is almost certainly an overestimate). In approximately one-half of the cases, symptoms persist for many years.

PTSD may be malingered, especially in cases in which compensation is at issue. True victims of PTSD tend to downplay symptoms, whereas malingerers tend to exaggerate them. Patients with PTSD do not like to talk about the traumatic event, and malingerers relish the telling. The nightmares of PTSD are not usually replays of the incident but rather derivatives—dreams of helplessness or disembodied terror. Malingerers describe accurate replays in their dreams. Malingerers may also recount atypical symptoms, deny little-known symptoms of PTSD, and reflect at length over the injustices of the compensation system. Guilt is the prevailing emotion in PTSD. In malingering and compensation neurosis, it is anger (109).

PTSD is a pathologic condition that develops in some people who have experienced an extreme life-threatening event. It is distinguished from ASD, a much more common reaction to a traumatic event. The symptoms of ASD are similar to those of PTSD, but the condition is, by definition, time limited. PTSD is a long-term condition, and its psychological components exercise a destructive, almost cancerous growth over time. ASD is really just a severe variant of the normal human reaction to trauma. PTSD is one of the most debilitating of all the psychiatric disorders.

Obviously, patients may develop ASD or PTSD after a life-threatening accident. When such an accident may have caused concussion, it may be difficult to know whether the patient is experiencing an acute stress reaction or PCS. There is, after all, a great deal of overlap between the symptoms of ASD and PCS: insomnia, depression, difficulty concentrating, attentional lapses, irritability, emotional lability, and so on. One may simply finesse the problem by giving the patient a tentative diagnosis of posttraumatic syndrome, a term that could refer to ASD or PCS. Both conditions are likely to clear in short order; symptomatic treatment is similar for both conditions.

The full panoply of PTSD symptoms is not usually encountered in the patient with PCS. If a patient with PCS experiences avoidance behavior, for example, it is usually brief and understandable, for example, feeling uncomfortable about highway driving or not wanting to work on high scaffolding. This kind of reaction is neither pathologic nor persistent. It is simply be a mild manifestation of ASD.

The symptoms of true PTSD are quite different from those of PCS. The persistence of intrusive thoughts and images in PTSD (nightmares, flashbacks, intrusive memories) sets up a chronically disordered pattern of arousal in which the patient reacts to a host of reminders with a physiologic intensity appropriate to the original trauma. At the same time, there is a loss of appropriate reactivity to stimuli and situations that normally elicit an arousal response: interpersonal relationships, personal ambition, and hopes for the future. Although the patient with PTSD can be hyperaroused by trivial events, he or she may be "emotionally numb" to important aspects of everyday life. This is sometimes referred to as a loss of stimulus discrimination (110).

The pathogenesis of PTSD requires the persistence of a memory that behaves in a pathologic way, but an intrusive memory has to have been encoded. Because CHIs are always accompanied by amnesia of the event (brief retrograde, a longer period of anterograde amnesia), PTSD and CHI are considered by some to be incompatible or "mutually exclusive" diagnoses (111). The patient with PTSD is expected to retain a "highly charged" memory of the traumatic event, whereas the patient with CHI should have none at all. In a study of 47 patients who had experienced moderate brain injury, none met the all the criteria for the diagnosis of PTSD. A few of the patients had avoidance or arousal symptoms, a "form of PTSD without the reexperiencing symptoms" (112).

Many physicians and psychologists who treat patients with CHI, however, believe that the two conditions may sometimes coexist and that PTSD may sometimes be a sequela of CHI or even of concussion. Although Sbordone and Liter (111) were not able to identify any cases of PTSD in their sample of patients with MBI, in another survey, Bryant and Harvey (113) diagnosed ASD (or "subsyndromal ASD") in almost 20% of a sample of 79 patients who had sustained MBI in motor vehicle accidents. In another survey of 100 adults with TBI, PTSD was one of the most common psychiatric diagnoses (114). In a study of children with TBI, two of 46 developed PTSD, and no less than 68% had at least one symptom of ASD at 3 months post-TBI (115). They also concluded that ASD and PTSD were, in fact, common sequelae of TBI, at least in children. There are several other reports of PTSD in patients with TBI (116–119)

Some of these authors have made efforts to explain how a pathologic engram might be laid down even in the face of organic amnesia. If the interval of amnesia is brief, for example, enough may be retained in the way of toxic memory of pre- and postaccident events to cause PTSD (120). "Islands" of memory may be preserved within a period of PTA (118). It is possible that the traumatic event may be comprised of secondary circumstances, such as the ambulance trip to the emergency department, the air-evacuation, or the experience of being bloody and alone and confused and afraid in an emergency department. In other words, if the amnestic experience is less than total, enough may be retained to cause ASD or PTSD.

That explanation may be sufficient for cases of mild concussion, in which PTA may indeed be "patchy" or short-lived. It is hardly sufficient to explain the occurrence of PTSD in patients who have had severe brain injuries, in whom it is difficult to maintain that the amnesia is less than total. The pathophysiologic mechanism that causes PTSD to develop in patients with TBI is probably more complex and much more interesting. It may have to do with something known as "unconscious memory."

"Intraoperative awareness" is a significant problem in anesthesiology. Patients who have been under general anesthesia may recall sounds or voices, visual perceptions, anxiety and fear, and even pain (121–124). It is not clear whether this is a common (123) or rare problem (122,124), but it does occur and may lead to the subsequent development of "traumatic neurosis" (125). If patients under general anesthesia are read a word list and then given a forced-choice task to assess recognition memory, they demonstrate memory for the material that was presented (126). Patients are capable of processing information that they receive intraoperatively, even though they are entirely unconscious throughout.

In an interesting paper that is hardly ever referenced in this regard, Tosch (127) described patients' recollections of posttraumatic coma. These were patients with Glasgow Coma Scores less than 8 for at least 6 hours. Eight of 15 were able to relate having experienced sensory experiences, a sense of imprisonment, or death-like experiences.

The mnemonic process is not entirely cortical, and the extraordinary phenomenon of unconscious memory suggests that subcortical structures may generate lasting memory traces even in the absence of cortical participation. If PTSD can, in fact, develop in patients after general anesthesia or in patients who have had CHI, then one may surmise that subcortical memory is sufficient to set in motion the events that ultimately lead to PTSD. One may suppose that PTSD represents a flooding of the subcortical substrate for memory by an extraordinary life-threatening event.

Hippocampal atrophy is the one neuropathologic finding that has been identified in association with PTSD (110). It is usually explained as a secondary phenomenon, the consequence of persistently elevated levels of cortisol in the patient with PTSD. Whether primary or secondary, PTSD may well be a subcortical disorder: the evidence includes prominent autonomic and neuroendocrine abnormalities, fundamental derangement of the arousal system, neurovegetative symptoms, and loss of stimulus discrimination.

PTSD and TBI are not mutually exclusive. The fact that PTSD does happen in patients who have had a TBI may, in fact, reveal something about the pathophysiology of the condition.

POSTTRAUMATIC HEADACHE

Headache is the most common problem after mild head injury. It is central to the diagnosis of PCS, but it is a less common problem in patients who have had severe TBI. This paradox has led many neurologists to discount the importance of posttraumatic headache.

Muscle contraction headaches, sometimes associated with occipital neuralgia, account for perhaps 85% of all posttraumatic headaches (128). The typical posttraumatic headache is described as a dull ache or less frequently as a throbbing sensation. It may be focal or diffuse, unilateral or bilateral. It is not typically paroxysmal, although it is not uncommon to find a patient who complains of a constant, dull headache on which are superimposed intermittent, paroxysmal attacks. The cephalgias may be described as stabbing, bursting, or hammering, or there may simply be a sense of fullness, dizziness, or fuzziness in the head (120). There may be elements suggestive of migraine, such as nausea and vomiting or the need to rest quietly in a dark room.

Headache is one of the most persistent symptoms after MBI, and it can be one of the most difficult symptoms to treat. Two elements make posttraumatic headache a therapeutic challenge: outstanding compensation issues and medication rebound. Ergotamine, sumatriptan, narcotics, and even mild analgesics may aggravate tension headache and migraine if they are taken daily. Several studies have reported substantial improvement in the severity and frequency of headache when daily analgesics are stopped. Unfortunately, not many patients have read those studies.

Sudden withdrawal from a selective serotonin reuptake inhibitor antidepressant may precipitate headache and even migraine, even if headache was not a prior symptom.

It is said that true migraine is uncommon after TBI (120). That is probably an overstatement. "Footballer's migraine" is well described in athletes after mild head trauma, such as "heading" a ball in soccer (129). Posttraumatic migraine may be more commonly encountered in children than adults (130). It has also been suggested that transient global amnesia or delayed mental state changes in patients with MBI might represent a variant of traumatic migraine (131,132). Posttraumatic migraine in patients with MBI or whiplash injuries may be chronic, but response to typical treatments, such as propanolol and amitriptyline, has been described as gratifying even in patients whose compensation claims had not been settled (133).

Although muscle contraction headaches and migraine variants account for most posttraumatic headaches, virtually every form of headache has been described after TBI (128) (Table 6.1)

We do not really understand the mechanism of posttraumatic headaches. They may be related to scars or small neuromas in the scalp, to meningeal adhesions, scars, or cysts, or to neurochemical events in the innervation of the cerebral vasculature. They may be related to cervical whiplash injuries, i.e., headaches of musculoskeletal or tension type with neck pain and vertigo.

TABLE 6.1. *Posttraumatic headaches*

Muscle contraction headaches
Occipital neuralgia
Migraine
Cervical injury
Temporomandibular joint injury
Infraorbital neuralgia
Supraorbital neuralgia
Cluster headache
Dysesthesia around scalp lacerations
Basilar artery migraine
Orgasmic cephalgia
Dysautonomic cephalgia

Posttraumatic headaches do not necessarily arise immediately after the injury. In fact, the onset of generalized headache is usually some time after the injury (120).

Treatment of posttraumatic headache is the same as treatment of headache in general. It is appropriate to consider the same range of treatments that are effective for patients whose headache is not traumatic in origin. Drugs with negative cognitive effects, such as amitriptyline, and drugs that may cause depression, such as the beta-blockers, should be used with care. Fortunately, there are rarely problems associated with the short-term use of these drugs. If headache is not relieved by ibuprofen or similar nonsteroidal anti-inflammatory drugs or by acetaminophen, one may consider a serotonergic antidepressant such as fluoxetine. Posttraumatic headaches with migrainoid features may require a beta-blocker, a calcium-channel blocker, or a triptan. Tension headaches may require a muscle relaxant, especially diazepam. Nonpharmacologic treatments such as biofeedback, relaxation training. and cranial electrostimulation are occasionally helpful.

Although the pharmacologic and behavioral treatments for posttraumatic headache are less than ideal, they can still be reassuring to the patient. Posttraumatic headache may be persistent, but it usually subsides with the passage of time, and the patient may be thus reassured. Often one will observe alleviation of posttraumatic headache when other neurobehavioral sequelae of CHI, such as anxiety, fatigue, depression, and social isolation, are successfully handled.

Basilar Artery Migraine

Basilar migraine (basilar artery migraine) is a commonly misdiagnosed disorder, an intense vascular headache preceded by aura or prodromata to indicate dysfunction in the brainstem, cerebellum, and occipital cortex (134), the areas supplied by the basilar artery and its branches. The accompanying symptoms may include visual impairment (transient amaurosis, reduction in vision, diplopia), vertigo, ataxia, paraesthesias, weakness, and dysarthria (135). There may be transient LOC, and EEG abnormalities are not uncommon. The latter may be persistent, even between headaches; therefore, basilar artery migraine may be misdiagnosed as epilepsy (136). The fact that both basilar artery migraine and complex partial epilepsy may respond to the anticonvulsant carbamazepine may complicate the diagnosis, although it is customary to treat basilar migraine with a beta-blocker or a calcium-channel blocker rather than carbamazepine. Because the symptoms of basilar migraine are so dramatic and peculiar, hysteria or malingering may be suspected.

Basilar artery migraine occurs most commonly in adolescent girls (135). It may arise after concussion or uncomplicated whiplash (137).

DIZZINESS AND VERTIGO

Dizziness is a common complaint after MBI, occurring in 53% of patients within 1 week of the injury and persisting in 18% after 2 years. Dizziness, vertigo, tinnitus, and hearing loss may be caused by labyrinthine concussion, temporal bone fracture, perilymph fistula, or disruption of the ossicular chain (128).

Dizziness, vertigo, and tinnitus can cause significant disability. Sometimes patients with these problems get depressed and are referred to psychiatrists. There is not much one can do for the secondary depression, if the primary problem is severe and disabling. Antidepressants, antihistamines, sedatives, muscle relaxants, and analgetics can all make dizziness or vertigo worse.

STUTTERING

Stuttering is a form of dysfluent speech characterized by prolongations, hesitational blocks, and involuntary repetitions. Common or developmental stuttering begins in childhood or adolescence and has a prevalence of approximately 4% in children and 1% in the adult population (138,139). Acquired stuttering differs from the developmental form clinically: speech blocks are not confined to word initial sounds or syllables alone; it is not associated with secondary symptoms such as anxiety, tension, articulatory struggles, facial grimaces, and contortions. Acquired rhythm disturbances are usually transient (140).

Acquired or neurogenic stuttering from stroke, trauma, and degenerative or metabolic brain damage, is not common. It is often, but not always, associated with aphasia. It has been reported after left, right, and bilateral cortical injury. Subcortical pathology, unilateral and bilateral, has been reported. Acquired lesions in adults have rekindled childhood stuttering but have also cured stuttering (139). It is rare for acquired stuttering to persist unless both hemispheres or the corpus callosum are damaged (141).

There are no reports in the medical literature that document an association between persistent stuttering and MBI. Stuttering rarely occurs after concussion, but it is always mild and transient. Persistent stuttering in a patient with MBI is a sign of hysteria or malingering.

The speech-motor system is tied into the limbic system. For this reason, speech output, like other finely controlled motor outputs, is affect sensitive. The term "scared speechless" reflects this phenomenon (142). Stammering refers to speech hesitancy induced by anxiety, stress, or fatigue. Stuttering is not a symptom of anxiety disorder or PTSD. It may, however, be a clue to malingering.

In 1991, Brady (138) reviewed the psychopharmacology of stuttering. The literature is comprised largely of case reports. Controlled studies were done, but the results usually did not confirm the optimistic reports of success from case studies. The exception is haloperidol, which is effective for many of the elements of common stuttering. Not surprisingly, patient acceptance is low. Sedatives are not effective, but there is reason to believe that psychostimulants and calcium-channel blockers (e.g., verapamil) may occasionally be helpful. The serotonergic antidepressants have not been tested. There are no drug studies of acquired stuttering (138).

TRANSIENT SEQUELAE OF SEVERE BRAIN INJURIES

Agitation After Coma Recovery

As the patient with TBI emerges from a coma, there is often a period of extreme behavioral instability, with confusion, disorientation, agitation, or aggression. The symptoms arise in the context of low arousal, punctuated by episodes of hypervigilance, with intense reactivity to environmental stimuli. Distractibility is high, and the patient is extremely resistant to anything that requires sustained attention. The patient is usually amnestic. Stereotyped motor behaviors are not uncommon, including elements of Klüver-Bucy syndrome (143). Emotional lability is the rule. There may be intense reactions to people and to therapeutic interventions, with hostility, assaultiveness, and violent epithets. If the patient is ambulatory, he or she may wander, with no regard to personal safety or to the norms of decency. The behavior is disorganized, and the most common element of affective expression is agitation (69).

This condition hardly merits the word normal, but it is an expected phase of the recovery process. Because it is such a common event in any hospital unit that cares for patients recovering from coma, one should expect a degree of sophistication in behavior management among staff. A heavy therapeutic hand, e.g., physical restraints or neuroleptic drugs, should hardly ever be necessary in a specialized TBI unit. The patient is best treated with environmental or behavioral intervention rather than controlled or suppressed with sedating drugs or restraints. Principles of specialized treatment include maintaining a small, familiar staff, limiting stimulation, restricting therapy time to what the patient can tolerate, and waiting for the condition to pass. If the patient is upset about some particular thing, just walk away for a while. Because he or she is amnestic as well as stimulus bound, he or she will settle down quickly, and you can come back in a minute or two.

It is remarkable what simple environmental measures will do to alleviate the problems of the agitated patient recovering from coma: keeping the patient with one familiar nurse, adjusting the level of light and ambient noise, redirecting the patient to a safer environment, and putting Velcro tape on the doorknobs to discourage attempts to escape. It is only in the most severe and prolonged cases of postcoma agitation that pharmacologic intervention is necessary. When agitation occurs in the neurosurgical intensive care unit, with a patient pulling tubes and resisting treatments that are life sustaining, it may be necessary to intervene sooner with an effective drug. In the rehabilitation unit, however, there has to be at least some tolerance for difficult behaviors and some capacity to adjust the physical environment and level of staffing.

The evaluation of the patient recovering from coma who is agitated or hypoaroused requires first a medical workup to exclude metabolic or infectious disorders and neurologic evaluation for seizures, hydrocephalus, or intracranial hemorrhage. The alcoholic patient may require thiamine injection. The psychological evaluation should address environmental measures that can increase agitation, especially overstimulation or confusion arising from isolation and unfamiliarity.

The conventional psychiatric differential that would include schizophreniform psychosis, organic affective disorder, and intermittent explosive disorder is not usually helpful, and one's choice of medication is usually guided more by trial and error than by psychiatric diagnosis. There is the clinical inclination to treat temporal lobe patients with carbamazepine, whether they are psychotic, affective, or explosive. Diagnosis by location of the injury is of limited value; coma and the agitation that occurs during coma recovery are almost invariably associated with brainstem injury. Conversely, the brain map may be a guide to pharmacotherapy, and because coma and postcoma are states of axial compromise, monoamine agonists may represent rational pharmacotherapy. The location of cortical injury may also explain why a patient is disturbed by a particular circumstance, however, and a proper environmental program should be developed. The patient with an occipital lesion may not respond to a program that requires processing visual information. A patient with extensive temporal lobe injuries may have Klüver-Bucy syndrome symptoms that are disturbing to staff and to family, who must be counseled to tolerate these problems to a degree, to redirect activities when possible, and to abide patiently their passage. It is said that carbamazepine is effective in Klüver-Bucy syndrome; that may be an overstatement, but it is reasonable to try it and other drugs, guided by trial and error.

The first principle of pharmacotherapy during the coma-recovery stage is to avoid drugs that may impede the recovery process or impair the patient's limited ability to process information and to respond effectively. The second principle, or, rather, a corollary of the first, is to minimize the prescription of neuroleptic drugs. Although neuroleptic drugs are probably the most commonly prescribed agents for patients with postcoma agitation, the only unequivocal indication for this class of drugs is central hyperthermia. (In fact, central hyperthermia may be distinguished from septic pyrexia by the patient's response to neuroleptic drugs.)

Drug treatment should be guided by a presumption that the state of agitation represents a general failure of arousal and mental processing. Therefore, drugs that sedate a patient or reduce clarity of thought are relatively contraindicated. These include the sedating anticonvulsants, antispasticity drugs, benzodiazepines, and neuroleptics. Metoclopramide, a dopamine blocker that is used to enhance gastrointestinal motility, should be avoided. In fact, many cases of postcoma agitation can be resolved by withdrawing the patient from potentially sedating drugs such as haloperidol, phenytoin, metoclopramide, amitriptyline, and carbamazepine.

If the problem of postcoma agitation is severe and prolonged and if the problem cannot be mitigated by behavior management or withdrawing unnecessary medications, pharmacologic intervention may be necessary. The neuropsychiatrist has a number of alternatives from which to choose: the psychotropic anticonvulsants (oxcarbazepine and valproate), lithium, beta-blockers—all of them have been successful in some cases (144). None has achieved primacy, however, because patient response is unpredictable, and it may not be possible to explore each of the possible alternatives. There has been recent research, however, to support an additional alternative: the dopamine agonists, especially amantadine. The rate of success for amantadine in one case series was greater than 50% (145).

In the rehabilitation centers where I have worked, the drug of choice for postcoma agitation is amantadine (145). My colleagues and I originally explained the rationale for amantadine therapy as if it were a mixed dopamine agonist (146). The idea was to compensate for damage to monoaminergic neurons that were subcortical or axial in origin and that project to striatal, limbic, and frontal cortex. The monoamine neurotransmitters have been figured in the neuropharmacology of CHI and the maintenance of appropriate levels of arousal (147,148). Because agitation during coma recovery is supposed to be an arousal disorder, monoamine therapy was said to be rational (146).

As discussed in Chapter 18, the therapeutic action of amantadine is probably not explicable in terms of its direct effect on dopamine but rather on the excitatory amino acid neurotransmitter *N*-methyl-D-aspartate. That did nothing for the "rational pharmacotherapy" idea, although it did explain why the actions of amantadine were different from those of the other monoaminergic drugs. The change in our understanding of the drug mechanism, however, did not diminish the therapeutic utility of the agent.

One may expect success with amantadine in more than half of the patients recovering from coma treated with the drug; it is not sedating and, at moderate doses, may actually raise the seizure threshold and promote arousal, attention, and motor performance. The side-effect profile is favorable, especially when it is compared with the usual alternatives, and the major problems are paradoxical excitement, which is a rare event, and seizures, which are extremely rare in doses of 300 mg per day or less.

Acute agitation in patients with TBI in general hospital intensive care unit settings often requires urgent treatment to prevent injury. In this situation, serial trials of dopamine agonists and other nonsedating drugs may not be feasible. In such cases, neuroleptics and benzodiazepines are the main options and are used as in the treatment of any agitated delirium. However, because neuroleptics and benzodiazepines have negative effects on cognition and motor ability, they are not appropriate for long-term treatment. Further, there is one preclinical study that suggests that neuroleptics can retard the course of recovery from brain injury (149). Therefore, strong consideration should be given to tapering and discontinuing neuroleptics or benzodiazepines when the crisis is over and to exploring the nonsedating alternatives if agitation recurs and interferes with rehabilitation.

Peduncular Hallucinosis

The delayed psychoses that follow TBI stand in contrast to transient psychoses that occur much earlier, during the state of delirium that sometimes accompanies coma recovery, and the psychotic states that are associated with static lesions. Peduncular hallucinosis is an example of the latter in patients with lesions in the cerebral peduncles, thalamus, or substantia nigra. It is characterized by visual images of people, animals, plants, and scenes that are often vividly colored (150). The images are transient and usually nonthreatening, without the disorganization and agitation that characterizes a true psychosis.

Lhermitte hypothesized that damage to midbrain or thalamic tissues allows dream states to enter wakeful consciousness, the phenomenon of dream release, similar to what happens in narcolepsy (151).

Antipsychotic treatment is not always necessary in such cases. The condition is self-limiting, although the patients usually have severe and persistent cognitive deficits.

Immediate Posttraumatic Seizures

These occur most commonly in the first 24 hours after injury and are usually generalized tonic-clonic seizures. There is a 25% chance that patients with immediate posttraumatic seizures will develop posttraumatic epilepsy. That means that there is a 75% chance that they will not. If the patient did not have other risk factors for posttraumatic epilepsy, such as dural penetration or intracerebral hemorrhage, and if his or her EEG is nonepileptiform, then it may be possible to discontinue anticonvulsants after 6 months or even sooner. In such cases, it is seldom necessary to continue treatment past 1 year.

Posttraumatic Chorea

Patients with severe brain injury may have severe choreiform, ballistic or athetoid movements, or akathisia, especially during the unstable phase of coma recovery. Agitation often accompanies these movements. The clinical appearance is striking, not dissimilar to patients with Huntington's disease. Low doses of a potent neuroleptic such as haloperidol are usually effective, one of the few circumstances in which neuroleptics are indicated during TBI recovery (152).

Autonomic Instability

The other unequivocal indication for neuroleptics during the early postinjury phase is for autonomic storm, the dramatic fluctuations of body temperature that occur in some coma patients. Low doses of chlorpromazine (e.g., 25 to 50 mg) are sometimes effective (153).

REFERENCES

1. Evans R. The postconcussion syndrome and the sequelae of mild head injury. *Neurol Clin* 1992;10: 815–843.
2. Esselman PC, Uomoto JM. Classification of the spectrum of mild brain injury. *Brain Inj* 1995;9:417–424.
3. Ommaya AK. Biomechanics of head injury: experimental aspects. In: Nahum AM, Melvin J, eds. *The biomechanics of trauma*. Norwalk, CT: Appleton-Century-Crofts, 1985:245–269.
4. Kelly JP, Rosenberg JH. The development of guidelines for the management of concussion in sports. *J Head Trauma Rehabil* 1998;13:53–65.
5. Goldstein M. Traumatic brain injury: a silent epidemic. *Ann Neurol* 1990;27:327.
6. Miller JD. Head injury. *J Neurol Neurosurg Psychiatry* 1993;56:440–447.
7. Frankowski RF, Annegers JF, Whitman S. The descriptive epidemiology of head trauma in the United States. In: Becker DP, Povlishock JT, eds. *CNS trauma status report*. Bethesda, MD: NINCDS, NIH,1985:33–43.
8. Crovitz HF, Horn RW, Daniel WF. Inter-relationships among retrograde amnesia, post-traumatic amnesia and time since injury: a retrospective study. *Cortex* 1983;19:407–412.
9. Baroff GS. Is heading a soccer ball injurious to brain function? *J Head Trauma Rehabil* 1998;13:45–52.
10. Kraus JF, Black MA, Hessol N, et al. The incidence of acute brain injury and serious impairment in a defined population. *Am J Epidemiol* 1984;119:186–201.
11. Rutherford WH. Postconcussion symptoms: relationship to acute neurological indices, individual differences and circumstances of injury. In: Levin HS, Eisenberg HM, Benton AL, eds. *Mild head injury*. New York: Oxford University Press, 1989:217–228.
12. Rimel RA, Giordani B, Barth JT, et al. Disability caused by minor head injury. *Neurosurgery* 1981;9: 221–228.
13. Binder LM. Persisting symptoms after mild head injury: a review of the postconcussive syndrome. *J Clin Exp Neuropsychol* 1986;8:323–346.
14. Dikmen S, Temkin N, McLean A, et al. Memory and head injury severity. *J Neurol Neurosurg Psychiatry* 1987;50:1613–1618.
15. Jakobsen J, Baadsgaard SE, Thomsen S, et al. Prediction of post-concussional sequelae by reaction-time test. *Acta Neurol Scand* 1987;75:341–345.
16. Hayes RL, Lyeth BG, Jenkins LW. Neurochemical mechanisms of mild and moderate head injury: implications for treatment. In: Levin HS, Eisenberg HM, Benton AL, eds. *Mild head injury*. New York: Oxford University Press, 1989:54–79.
17. Gronwall D. Cumulative and persisting effects of concussion on attention and cognition. In: Levin HS, Eisenberg HM, Benton AL, eds. *Mild head injury*. New York: Oxford University Press, 1989:153–162.
18. Ruff RM, Levin HS, Mattis S, et al. Recovery of memory after mild head injury: a three-center study. In: Levin HS, Eisenberg HM, Benton AL, eds. *Mild head injury*. New York: Oxford University Press, 1989:176–188.
19. Ommaya AK, Yarnell P. Subdural haematoma after whiplash injury. *Lancet* 1969;2:237–239.
20. Ommaya AK, Hirsch AE. Tolerances for cerebral concussion from head impact and whiplash in primates. *J Biomechanics* 1971;4:13–21.
21. Teuber H-L. Neglected aspects of the post-traumatic syndrome. In: Walker AE, Caveness WF, Critchley M, eds. *The late effects of head injury*. Springfield, IL: Charles C. Thomas, 1969:13–34.
22. Sekino H, Nakamura N, Yuki K, et al. Brain lesions detected by CT scans in cases of minor head injuries. *Neurol Med Chir (Tokyo)* 1981;21:677–683.
23. Stein SC, Spettell C, Young G, et al. Limitations of neurological assessment in mild head injury. *Brain Inj* 1993;7:425–430.
24. Levin HS, Amparo E, Eisenberg HM, et al. Magnetic resonance imaging and computerized tomography in relation to the neurobehavioral sequelae of mild and moderate head injury. *J Neurosurg* 1987;66:706–713.
25. Jennett B. Some international comparisons. In: Levin HS, Eisenberg HM, Benton AL, eds. *Mild head injury*. New York: Oxford University Press, 1989:23–36.
26. Rao N, Turski P, Polcyn RE, et al. 18F Positron emission computed tomography in closed head injury. *Arch Phys Med Rehabil* 1984;65:780–785.
27. Langfitt TW, Obrist WD, Alavi A, et al. Computerized tomography, magnetic resonance imaging, and positron emission tomography in the study of brain trauma. *J Neurosurg* 1986;64:760–767.
28. Gray BG, Ichise M, Chung D, et al. Technetium-99m-HMPAO SPECT in the evaluation of patients with a remote history of traumatic brain injury: a comparison with X-ray computed tomography. *J Nucl Med* 1992; 33:52–58.
29. Oder W, Goldenberg G, Spatt J, et al. Behavioural and psychosocial sequelae of severe closed head injury and regional cerebral blood flow. *J Neurol Neurosurg Psychiatry* 1992;55:475–480.

30. Newton MR, Greenwood RJ, Britton KE, et al. A study comparing SPECT with CT and MRI after closed head injury. *J Neurol Neurosurg Psychiatry* 1992;55:92–94.
31. Segalowitz SJ, Unsal A, Dywan J. CNV evidence for the distinctiveness of frontal and posterior neural processes in a traumatic brain-injured population. *J Clin Exp Neuropsychol* 1992;14:545–565.
32. Gualtieri CT. Pharmacological interventions for cognitive and behavioral impairments. In: Finlayson MAJ, Garner S, eds. *Brain injury rehabilitation: clinical considerations*, 1st ed. Baltimore: Williams & Wilkins, 1993:264–278.
33. Lezak MD. *Neuropsychological assessment*, 2nd ed. New York: Oxford University Press, 1983.
34. Buschke H, Fuld PA. Evaluating storage, retention and retrieval in disordered memory and learning. *Neurology* 1974;14:1019–1025.
35. Gronwall D, Wrightson P. Delayed recovery of intellectual function after minor head injury. *Lancet* 1974; 2:605–609.
36. Arcia E, Gualtieri CT. Association between patient report of symptoms after mild head injury and neurobehavioural performance. *Brain Inj* 1993;7:481–489.
37. Eames P. Hysteria following brain injury. *J Neurol Neurosurg Psychiatry* 1992;55:1046–1053.
38. Noy P. New views of the psychotherapy of compensation neurosis: a clinical study. In: Arieti S, ed. *New dimensions in psychiatry: a world view*. New York: John Wiley & Sons, 1975:162–168.
39. Miller H. Accident neurosis. *BMJ* 1961;1:919–925.
40. Merskey H, Woodforde JM. Psychiatric sequelae of minor head injury. *Brain* 1972;95:521–528.
41. Dikmen S, Reitan RM. Emotional sequelae of head injury. *Ann Neurol* 1977;2:492–494.
42. Bornstein RA, Miller HB, Van Schoor JT. Neuropsychological deficit and emotional disturbance in head-injured patients. *J Neurosurg* 1989;70:509–513.
43. Alexander MP. Neuropsychiatric correlates of persistent postconcussive syndrome. *J Head Trauma Rehabil* 1992;7:60–69.
44. Bohnen N, Twijnstra A, Jolles J. Post-traumatic and emotional symptoms in different subgroups of patients with mild head injury. *Brain Inj* 1992;6:481–487.
45. Gualtieri CT, Cox DR. The delayed neurobehavioral sequelae of traumatic brain injury. *Brain Inj* 1991;5: 219–232.
46. Cassens G, Wolfe L, Zola M. The neuropsychology of depression. *J Neuropsychiatry* 1990;2:202–213.
47. Sternberg DE, Jarvik ME. Memory functions in depression. *Arch Gen Psychiatry* 1976;33:219–224.
48. Horn LJ. Post-concussive headache. In: Horn LJ, Zasler ND, eds. *Rehabilitation of post-concussive disorders*. Philadelphia: Hanley & Belfus, 1992:69–78.
49. Good JL, Barry E, Fishman PS. Posttraumatic narcolepsy: the complete syndrome with tissue typing. *J Neurosurg* 1989;71:765–767.
50. Verduyn WH, Hilt J, Roberts MA, et al. Multiple partial seizure-like symptoms following 'minor' closed head injury. *Brain Inj* 1992;6:245–260.
51. Fisher CM. Intermittent interruption of behavior. *Trans Am Neurol Assoc* 1968;93:209–210.
52. Sethi KD, Hess DC, Huffnagle VH, et al. Acetazolamide treatment of paroxysmal dystonia in central demyelinating disease. *Neurology* 1992;42:919–921.
53. Haimovic IC, Bereford R. Transient unresponsiveness in the elderly. *Arch Neurol* 1992;49:35–37.
54. Brown SJ, Fann JR, Grant I. Postconcussional disorder: time to acknowledge a common source of neurobehavioral morbidity. *J Neuropsychiatry Clin Neurosci* 1998;6:15–22.
55. Bourke RS. *Head injury*. Bethesda, MD: NINCDS, 1988.
56. Blumbergs PC, Jones NR, North JB. Diffuse axonal injury in head trauma. *J Neurol Neurosurg Psychiatry* 1989;52:838–841.
57. Povlishock JT, Coburn TH. Morphopathological change associated with mild head injury. In: Levin HS, Eisenberg HM, Benton AL, eds. *Mild head injury*. New York: Oxford University Press, 1989: 37–53.
58. Gennarelli TA, Thibault LE, Adams JH, et al. Diffuse axonal injury and traumatic coma in the primate. *Ann Neurol* 1982;12:564–575.
59. Yarnell PR, Rossie GV. Minor whiplash head injury with major debilitation. *Brain Inj* 1988;2:255–258.
60. Ommaya AK, Faas F, Yarnell P. Whiplash injury and brain damage. *JAMA* 1968;204:285–289.
61. Ommaya AK, Gennarelli TA. A cerebral concussion and traumatic unconsciousness: correlation of experimental and clinical observations on blunt head injuries. *Brain* 1974;97:633–654.
62. Jane JA, Steward O, Gennarelli TA. Axonal degeneration induced by experimental non-invasive minor head injury. *J Neurosurg* 1985;62:96–100.
63. Jiang JY, Lyeth BG, Kapasi MZ, et al. Moderate hypothermia reduces blood-brain barrier disruption following traumatic brain injury in the rat. *Acta Neuropathol* 1992;84:495–500.
64. Clifton GL, McCormick WF, Grossman RG. Neuropathology of early and late deaths after head injury. *Neurosurgery* 1981;8:309–314.
65. Eisenberg HM, Levin HS. Computed tomography and magnetic resonance imaging in mild to moderate head injury. In: Levin HS, Eisenberg HM, Benton AL, eds. *Mild head injury*. New York: Oxford University Press, 1989:133–141.
66. Peerless SJ, Rewcastle NW. Shear injuries of the brain. *CMAJ* 1967;96:577–582.
67. Oppenheimer DR. Microscopic lesions in the brain following head injury. *J Neurol Neurosurg Psychiatry* 1968;31:299–306.
68. Rosner MJ, Newsome HH, Becker DP. Mechanical brain injury: the sympathoadrenal response. *J Neurosurg* 1984;61:76–86.
69. Gualtieri CT. *Neuropsychiatry and behavioral pharmacology*. Berlin: Springer-Verlag, 1990.
70. Silver J, Shin C, McNamara J. Antiepileptogenic effects of conventional anticonvulsants in the kindling model of epilepsy. *Ann Neurol* 1991;29:356–363.
71. Carlsson GS. Long-term effects of head injuries sustained during life in three male populations. *J Neurosurg* 1987;67:197–205.
72. Meltzer HY, Lowy MT. The serotonin hypothesis of depression. In: Meltzer HY, ed. *Psychopharmacology: the third generation of progress*. New York: Raven Press, 1987:513–526.
73. Grant I, Alves W. Psychiatric and psychosocial disturbances in head injury. In: Levin HS, Grafman J, Eisenberg HM, eds. *Neurobehavioral recovery from head*

injury, 1st ed. New York: Oxford University Press, 1987:232–261.

74. Barth JT, Macciochi SN, Giordani B, et al. Neuropsychological sequelae of minor head injury. *Neurosurgery* 1983;13:529–533.
75. Levine MJ, Gueramy M, Friedrich D. Psychophysiological responses to closed head injury. *Brain Inj* 1987; 1:171–181.
76. Alves W, Macciocchi SN, Barth JT. Postconcussive symptoms after mild head injury. *J Head Trauma Rehabil* 1993;8:48–59.
77. Rutherford WH, Merrett JD, McDonald JR. Sequelae of concussion caused by minor head injuries. *Lancet* 1977;1:1–4.
78. Rutherford WH, Merrett JD, McDonald JR. Symptoms at one year following concussion from minor head injuries. *Injury* 1979;10:225–230.
79. Denker PG. The postconcussion syndrome: prognosis and evaluation of the organic factors. *N Y S Med J* 1944;44:379–384.
80. Fee CRA, Rutherford WH. A study of the effect of legal settlement on postconcussion symptoms. *Arch Emerg Med* 1988;5:12–17.
81. Amphoux M, Gagey P-M, Le Flem A, et al. The development of the postconcussion syndrome. *Rev Med Travail* 1977;5:53–75.
82. Cook JB. Effects of minor head injuries sustained in sports and the postconcussional syndrome. In: Walker AE, Caveness WF, Critchley M, eds. *The late effects of head injury*. Springfield, IL: Charles C. Thomas, 1969: 408–413.
83. Lahz S, Bryant RA. Incidence of chronic pain following traumatic brain injury. *Arch Phys Med Rehabil* 1996;77:889–891.
84. Gronwall D, Wrightson P. Cumulative effect of concussion. *Lancet* 1975;2:995–997.
85. Russell WR. *The traumatic amnesias*. New York: Oxford University Press, 1971.
86. Wrightson P, Gronwall D. Time off work and symptoms after minor head injury. *Injury* 1981;12:445–454.
87. Gianotta SL, Weiner JM, Karnaze D. Prognosis and outcome in severe head injury. In: Cooper PR, ed. *Head injury*, 2nd ed. Baltimore: Williams & Wilkins, 1987:464–487.
88. Mach A, Horn LJ. Functional prognosis in traumatic brain injury. In: Horn LJ, Cope DN, eds. *Traumatic brain injury*. Philadelphia: Hanley & Belfus, 1989: 13–26.
89. Symonds CP, Russell WR. Accidental head injuries: prognosis in service patients. *Lancet* 1943;1:7–10.
90. Cook JB. The post-concussional syndrome and factors influencing recovery after minor head injury admitted to hospital. *Scand J Rehabil Med* 1972;4:27–30.
91. McKinlay WW, Brooks DV, Bond MR. Post-concussional symptoms, financial compensation and outcome of severe blunt head injury. *J Neurol Neurosurg Psychiatry* 1983;46:1084–1091.
92. Kozol HL. Pretraumatic personality and the psychiatric sequelae of head injury. *Arch Neurol Psychiatry* 1946;56:245–275.
93. Oddy M, Humphrey M, Uttley D. Subjective impairment and social recovery after closed head injury. *J Neurol Neurosurg Psychiatry* 1978;41:611–616.
94. Jacobson SA. Mechanism of the sequelae of minor craniocervical trauma. In: Walker AE, Caveness WF, Critchley M, eds. *The late effects of head injury*. Springfield, IL: Charles C. Thomas, 1969:35–45.
95. Steadman JH, Graham JG. Head injuries: an analysis and follow-up study. *Proc R Soc Med* 1970;63:23–28.
96. Kelly R. The post-traumatic syndrome: an iatrogenic disease. *Forensic Sci* 1975;6:17–24.
97. Symonds C. Concussion and its sequelae. *Lancet* 1962;1:1–5.
98. Kaste M, Vikki J, Sainio K, et al. Is chronic brain damage in boxing a thing of the past? *Lancet* 1982;2: 1186–1188.
99. Casson IR, Sham R, Campbell EA, et al. Neurological and CT evaluation of knocked-out boxers. *J Neurol Neurosurg Psychiatry* 1982;45:170–174.
100. Ewing R, McCarthy D, Gronwall D, et al. Persisting effects of concussion shown by impaired performance at altitude. *J Clin Neuropsychol* 1981;2:147–155.
101. Bolla KI, Briefel G, Spector D, et al. Neurocognitive effects of aluminum. *Arch Neurol* 1992;49:1021–1026.
102. Kraus JF, Nourjah P. The epidemiology of mild head injury. In: Levin HS, Eisenberg HM, Benton AL, eds. *Mild head injury*. New York: Oxford University Press, 1989:8–22.
103. Keller MB, Lavori PW, Klerman GL, et al. Low levels and lack of predictors of somatotherapy and psychotherapy received by depressed patients. *Arch Gen Psychiatry* 1986;43:458–467.
104. Trimble MR, Cummings JL. Neuropsychiatric disturbances following brainstem lesions. *Br J Psychiatry* 1981;138:56–59.
105. Dreifuss FE. Cognitive function—victim of disease or hostage to treatment? *Epilepsia* 1992;S1:S7–S12.
106. Whitlock FA. *The aetiology of hysteria. Acta Psychiatr Scand* 1967;43:144–162.
107. Stengel E. Borderlands of neurology and psychiatry. *Recent Prog Psychiatry* 1949;11:1.
108. Mattila MJ, Liljequist R, Seppala T. Effects of amitriptyline and mianserin on psychomotor skills and memory in man. *Br J Clin Pharmacol* 1978;5:53S–55S.
109. Simon RI. *Posttraumatic stress disorder in litigation*. Washington, DC: American Psychiatric Press, 1995.
110. van der Kolk B. *The psychobiology of posttraumatic stress disorder. J Clin Psychiatry* 1997;58[Suppl 9]: 16–24.
111. Sbordone RJ, Liter JC. Mild traumatic brain injury does not produce post-traumatic stress disorder. *Brain Inj* 1995;9:405–412.
112. Warden DL, Labbate LA, Salazar AM, et al. Post-traumatic stress disorder in patients with traumatic brain injury and amnesia for the event? *J Neuropsychiatry Clin Neurosci* 1997;9:18–22.
113. Bryant RA, Harvey AG. Relationship between acute stress disorder and posttraumatic stress disorder following mild traumatic brain injury. *Am J Psychiatry* 1998;155:625–629.
114. Hibbard MR, Uysal S, Kepler K, et al. Axis I psychopathology in individuals with traumatic brain injury. *J Head Trauma Rehabil* 1998;13:24–39.
115. Max JE, Roberts MA, Koele SL, et al. Cognitive outcome in children and adolescents following severe traumatic brain injury: influence of psychosocial, psychiatric, and injury-related variables. *J Int Neuropsychol Soc* 1999;5:58–68.
116. McMillan TM. Post-traumatic stress disorder and severe head injury. *Br J Psychiatry* 1991;159:431–433.

117. McMillan TM. Post-traumatic stress disorder following minor and severe closed head injury: 10 single cases. *Brain Inj* 1996;10:749–758.
118. King NS. Post-traumatic stress disorder and head injury as a dual diagnosis: "islands" of memory as a mechanism. *J Neurol Neurosurg Psychiatry* 1997;62: 82–84.
119. Trudeau DL, Andersen J, Hansen LM, et al. Findings of mild traumatic brain injury in combat veterans with PTSD and a history of blast concussion. *J Neuropsychiatry Clin Neurosci* 1998;10:308–313.
120. Sandyk R, Tsagas N, Anninos PA. Magnetic fields mimic the behavioral effects of REM sleep deprivation in humans. *Int J Neurosci* 1992;65:61–68.
121. Bailey AR, Jones JG. Patients' memories of events during general anaesthesia. *Anaesthesia* 1997;52:460–476.
122. Nordstrom O, Engstrom AM, Persson S, et al. Incidence of awareness in total i.v. anaesthesia based on propofol, alfentanil and neuromuscular blockade. *Acta Anaesthesiol Scand* 1997;41:978–984.
123. Schwender D, Kunze-Kronawitter H, Dietich P, et al. Conscious awareness during general anesthesia: patients' perceptions, emotions, cognition and reactions. *Br J Anaesthesiol* 1998;80:133–139.
124. Ranta SO, Laurila R, Saario J, et al. Awareness with recall during general anesthesia: incidence and risk factors. *Anesthesiol Analg* 1998;86:1084–1089.
125. Smith TL, Zapala D. The evolution of the auditory midlatency response in evaluating unconscious memory formation during general anesthesia. *Clin Res Nurses Assoc* 1998;9:44–49.
126. Bonebakker AE, Bonke B, Klein J, et al. Information processing during general anesthesia: evidence for unconscious memory. *Mem Cognit* 1996;24:766–776.
127. Tosch P. Patients' recollections of their posttraumatic coma. *J Neurosci Nurs* 1988;20:223–228.
128. Evans R. The postconcussion syndrome and the sequelae of mild head injury. *Neurol Clin* 1992;10: 815–843.
129. Matthews WB. Footballer's migraine. *BMJ* 1972;2: 326–327.
130. Heyck H. *Der Kopfschmerz*, 4th ed. Stuttgart: Georg Thieme Verlag, 1975.
131. Guthkeich ANMC. Benign post-traumatic encephalopathy in young people and its relation to migraine. *Neurosurgery* 1977;1:101–106.
132. Haas DC, Ross GS. Transient global amnesia triggered by mild head trauma. *Brain* 1986;109:251–257.
133. Weiss HD, Stern BJ, Goldberg J. Post-traumatic migraine: chronic migraine precipitated by minor head or neck trauma. *Headache* 1991;31:451–456.
134. Bickerstaff ER. Basilar artery migraine. *Lancet* 1962; 1:15–17.
135. Sturzenegger MH, Meienberg O. Basilar artery migraine: a follow-up study of 82 cases. *Headache* 1985; 25:408–415.
136. Jacome DE. EEG features in basilar artery migraine. *Headache* 1987;27:80–83.
137. Jacome DE. Basilar artery migraine after uncomplicated whiplash injuries. *Headache* 1986;26:515–516.
138. Brady JP. The pharmacology of stuttering: a critical review. *Am J Psychiatry* 1991;148:1309–1316.
139. Nass R, Schreter B, Heier L. Acquired stuttering after a second stroke in a two-year-old. *Dev Med Child Neurol* 1994;36:70–83.
140. Bhatnagar SC, Andy OJ. Alleviation of acquired stuttering with human centremedian thalamic stimulation. *J Neurol Neurosurg Psychiatry* 1989;52:1182–1184.
141. Rosenfield DBM. Stuttering. In: Scheinberg PM, ed. *Neurology and Neurosurgery*, 5th ed. Princeton, NJ: Continuing Professional Education Center, 1985:2–8.
142. Rosenfield DB. Spasmodic dysphonia. *Adv Neurol* 1988;50:537–545.
143. Gerstenbrand F, Aichner PF, Saltuari L. Kluver-Bucy syndrome in man: experiences with postraumatic cases. *Neurosci Biobehav Rev* 1983;7:413–417.
144. Gualtieri CT. Pharmacotherapy and the neurobehavioral sequelae of closed head injury. *Brain Inj* 1988; 2:101–129.
145. Gualtieri CT, Chandler M, Coons T, et al. Amantadine: a new clinical profile for traumatic brain injury. *Clin Neuropharmacol* 1989;12:258–270.
146. Chandler MC, Barnhill JB, Gualtieri CT. Amantadine for the agitated head-injury patient. *Brain Inj* 1988;2: 309–311.
147. van Woerkom TCAM, Teelken AW, Minderhoud JM. Difference in neurotransmitter metabolism in frontotemporal-lobe contusion and diffuse cerebral contusion. *Lancet* 1977;1:812–813.
148. Vecht CJ, van Woerkom TCAM, Teelken AW, et al. Homovanillic acid and 5-hydroxyindoleacetic acid cerebrospinal fluid levels. *Arch Neurol* 1975;32:792–797.
149. Feeney DM, Gonzalez A, Law WA. Amphetamine, haloperidol and experience interact to affect rate of recovery after motor cortex surgery. *Science* 1982;217: 855–857.
150. Nicolai A, Lazzarino LG. Peduncular hallucinosis as the first manifestation of multiple sclerosis. *Eur Neurol* 1995;35:241–242.
151. Matthews MK, Alter M, Sirken DH. Recognition of peduncular hallucinosis prompted by magnetic resonance images. *Neuropsychiatry Neuropsychol Behav Neurol* 1995;8:64–69.
152. Silver BV, Yablon SA. Akathisia resulting from traumatic brain injury. *Brain Inj* 1996;10:609–614.
153. Childers MK, Rupright J, Smith DW. Post-traumatic hyperthermia in acute brain injury rehabilitation. *Brain Inj* 1994;8:335–343.

7

The Static Neurobehavioral Syndromes

SUMMARY

The long-term behavioral and cognitive deficits of patients with brain injury are understood in terms of the nature of the injury, the brain regions that were damaged, and their known function. The enduring consequences of brain injury are either general or specific.

General deficits are typically associated with closed head injury (CHI), hypoxic-ischemic injury, and electrocution, in which tissue destruction is diffuse and involves the cortex, subcortical white matter, and brainstem. Diffuse axonal injury causes general deficits in arousal, attention, and information-processing speed. This, in turn, influences behavior and cognitive operations in a general way. The general capacity of the organism to compensate and to adapt to injury is compromised.

In contrast, penetrating brain injuries are usually associated with focal lesions, especially to the frontal and temporal lobes. Focal cortical injuries tend to have a better prognosis than diffuse injuries.

Focal cortical injuries, especially in the frontal lobes, were interesting to the early students of neuropsychology because they were associated with specific rather than general patterns of cognitive and behavioral impairment. Extensive damage to the convexity of the frontal lobes is associated with specific deficits in motivation, planning, and perseverance; damage to the orbitomedial surface is associated with deficits in affective regulation and self-control. This approach to lesion analysis has been quite fruitful and is discussed in some detail.

Regions of the cerebral cortex, however, are not so much the seat of the higher cortical functions as they are participants in complex functional systems. Neuropsychological constructs, such as the executive functions of the frontal lobes, are actually descriptions of complex functional systems that also involve subcortical structures, the cerebellum, and the brainstem. The enduring consequences of a cortical lesion are not simply the result of subtracting an essential function from the patient's behavioral repertoire. They are also the result of secondary changes in remote structures that participate in the functional system that was damaged.

Lesions in the frontal and temporal lobes, basal ganglia, and thalamus, therefore, have both general and specific characteristics. Their specific attributes entail different approaches, for example, pharmacologically.

Over the long term, however, the personality of the patient with brain injury is affected, not only by the specific nature of the primary lesion but by general effects that influence compensation and adaptation to injury. The evolution of psychopathology in patients with brain injury is not only a function of the specific lesion but also the summation of numerous dimensional inputs, including events and circumstances in the patient's wider ecology.

STATIC SYNDROMES

The pathology of moderate to severe brain injuries has an irreversible component that can be either focal or diffuse. Focal brain injuries are associated with specific deficits, depending on the specific area that is damaged. Diffuse brain injury is associated with general impairments such as mental and physical slowness, inattention and poor memory, anergia, and low arousal. Loss of intellect is more likely to be the result of diffuse injury.

Penetrating brain injuries are most commonly associated with focal damage to the frontal lobes, and closed head injuries are most likely to cause focal contusions or hemorrhages in the frontal and temporal lobes. These areas are vulnerable to TBI by virtue of their anterior position and exposure to the cribriform plate, a bony structure against which brain tissue may be shorn during a traumatic episode. In closed head injury, the pathology is also diffuse, with damage to the brainstem and subcortical white matter in addition to areas of focal pathology. Hypoxic-ischemic, toxic, and infectious injuries are usually, but not always, associated with diffuse damage.

The neurobehavioral syndromes associated with focal injury, especially to the frontal and temporal lobes, have been of great interest historically and have given rise to an extensive literature. Several syndromes have been described in patients with focal lesions and reproduced in laboratory animals. Lesion analysis has a venerable history in experimental neuropsychology and, before dynamic imaging, was the only basis for understanding cortical localization. In clinical practice, however, most brain-injured patients have elements of both focal and diffuse injury.

In conventional parlance, lesions are referred to as static, if they are attributable to a discrete event, and nonprogressive. That a lesion is static, however, does not imply that its effects are immutable. A static lesion may be irritative, for example, epileptogenic or prone to "kindle" seizures locally or in a remote locus. Perhaps there is also a form of neurobehavioral kindling. A static lesion may also induce a state of remote functional depression, a process known as diaschisis (1). A static lesion may thus induce a chain of secondary pathologic events. Secondary changes, however, are not only mediated by active biologic processes. The mere fact of disability has far-reaching personal consequences. The particular disabilities that patients with BI have, especially their emotional and interpersonal difficulties, can be more damaging in the long run than the original injury was. They can lead to new complications: isolation from family and friends, alienation from treatment, or injudicious or even self-destructive behavior. If one understands the evolution of such secondary events, biologic and psychosocial, one might be able to change their course. Thus, it is possible to attenuate or reverse the functional consequences of a static lesion.

THE FRONTAL LOBE SYNDROMES

Neuropsychology has advanced beyond the *"curious situation...(when) some authors looked upon the frontal lobes as one of the more important sections of the human brain, as the 'organ of civilization'* (2) *or as the 'seat of abstract intelligence'* (3), *whereas others were inclined to deny it any special function in human mental activity"* (4).

The frontal lobes are a vast expanse of brain tissue that occupies no less than a third of the cerebral hemispheres. Although they possess natural boundaries (the central sulcus, the corpus callosum, and the sylvian fissure), no single organizing principle can be attributed to them. They subsume a wide range of disparate functions: motor control (the motor strip and the premotor strip), expressive language (Broca's area), regulation (the orbitofrontal surface), and executive behavior (the convexity). By the same token, the deficits attributable to frontal lobe lesions are quite diverse. So it is presumptuous to talk about a unitary "frontal lobe syndrome."

Of course, it is done all the time. In fact, clinicians refer to two frontal lobe syndromes, at least in terms of neurobehavioral consequences. One is related to lesions in the convexity, and the other is related to lesions in the orbitomedial surface. Convexity lesions are associated with deficit or negative symptoms and orbitofrontal lesions with positive or expressive symptoms: abulia on the one hand, disinhibition on the other. It is clinical shorthand, and it is efficient, if shallow. Abbreviated terminology does little justice to the complexity of patients with frontal lobe lesions. Discrete lesions are sometimes encountered, but pure types are rare.

The Primate Frontal Cortex

The distribution and relative redundancy of functions in different brain regions are such that similar, although not precisely equal, syndromes can result from damage at different neural sites. Complex psychological activities cannot be viewed as the result of the operation of a single area or even a single functional region. They are, rather, the consequence of concerted activity in networks made up of multiple regions (5). In the words of Luria: "The higher mental functions may be disturbed by a lesion of one of the many links of the functional system; nevertheless, they will be disturbed differently by lesions of different levels" (4). The issue, therefore, is not what the frontal lobes do or what specific functions find their seat in the frontal lobes. It is more useful to deem frontal lobe structures as participants in the physiology of complex, integrated systems that also include the brainstem, subcortical nuclei, cerebellum, and other cortical areas. By virtue of their efflorescence over millions of years of primate evolution, they have amplified those functions to an extraordinary degree. When we consider the psychologic functions of the frontal lobes, we are, once again, using clinical shorthand to describe their role as the head ganglion in several networks of functional connectivity.

As neuropsychiatrists use the term, "frontal lobe syndrome" hardly ever refers to deficits arising from lesions in the precentral-premotor areas. Damage to this component of the frontal lobes results in weakness, alteration of muscle tone, release of grasp reflexes, incontinence, akinesia, mutism, aprosody, apraxia, and some of the motor components in unilateral neglect and Broca's aphasia (6). The changes in personality, behavioral aberrations, and cognitive deficits that contribute to the concept of a frontal lobe syndrome are associated with damage to the prefrontal cortex (the convexity) and the limbic cortex (the orbitomedial surface) of the frontal lobes. Even when usage is thus limited, however, it is neither precise nor satisfactory. The term refers to an amorphous, varied group of deficits that result from various etiologic factors in different anatomic subunits. Frontal lesions vary in laterality and size and in their impact on connecting systems. Their functional impact is influenced by the rate at which they develop and the timing of their occurrence at different points in the life cycle (7). They may be irritative or silent.

We confine our interest to the specific cognitive and behavioral affiliates of lesions in the heteromodal or dorsolateral cortex (the convexity) and in the paralimbic or orbitomedial area of the frontal lobes (6). Lesions in these regions exercise profound effects on one's style of thought and temperament, on one's patterns of responding to internal stimuli and of interacting with external events; in fact, on some of the fundamental elements of personality. Rather than proposing a frontal personality type, however, it is better to ponder the specific functional deficits that are associated with prefrontal lesions. If we consider the list of specific deficits and aberrations, the reader may recognize many of the pathologic components that are assembled, in varying patterns, to create the clinically recognized personality disorders.

THE COGNITIVE IMPACT OF FRONTAL LOBE LESIONS

The cognitive functions that are most closely identified with the frontal lobes are conceptual ability, executive ability, attention and arousal, perseverance, awareness, and empathy.

Conceptual Ability

Conceptual thinking comprises the ability to draw abstractions from perceptual experience and to manipulate abstract ideas in an organized and effective way. The frontal lobes are central to conceptual thought, although brain lesions in other sites are also known to induce conceptual dysfunctions. If a patient has difficulty with similarities or interpreting proverbs during the examination, for example, one may suspect an organic brain disorder but not necessarily frontal lobe damage. Nevertheless, frontal lobe lesions are sufficient to induce conceptual dysfunction and "concrete thinking" is a typical sign of frontal lobe injury.

Conceptual ability can be measured quite nicely during the clinical examination. One may test the patient's ability to draw abstract similarities or differences between words or analogies, and one may do the same with figures, mazes, mathematical problems, or proverbs. The Halstead Categories Test (2) measures one's ability to abstract a simple concept from a series of stimulus figures, the correct concept growing more obscure as the test proceeds, requiring a trial-and-error approach that may be extremely frustrating to vulnerable patients.

Deficits in conceptual thinking are encountered in many different kinds of patients, not only patients with brain injury with frontal lobe lesions. Children do not have much in the way of conceptual thinking, adolescents show it in only spurts, and schizophrenics, like demented people, have lost it. It is not well developed in patients of low intelligence. Patients with attention deficit/hyperactivity disorder (ADHD) are capable of thinking conceptually, but it does not seem to "tag" their limbic system. That means that the patient has the capacity for abstract thought, for example, following the rules, but sufficient emotional impact to motivate behavior is not generated. They have the right ideas, but they do not necessarily put them to good use.

Cognitive Flexibility

Cognitive flexibility refers to the ability to shift sets, i.e., to move from one operating principle to another as circumstances require. The classic test of cognitive flexibility is the Wisconsin Card Sort (8). Cards are presented to the subject, and sorted according to the shape, color, or number of figures on the cards. As the test proceeds, the examiner changes the sorting rules, and the patient has to infer the new rule by trial and error. The patient with frontal lobe injury has difficulty with changing rules and tends to perseverate, even in the face of negative feedback from the examiner.

Dual-task tests that require the patient to respond to different stimuli with different response patterns are also extremely difficult for patients with frontal lobe lesions because they cannot shift from one response set to another. If a computer administers the test, it may be possible to record the patient's response time on a dual-task test; a slower response time indicates mild difficulty with shifting sets that may indicate a mild frontal lobe injury.

Cognitive flexibility and the ability to shift sets are central to one's ability to function effectively, especially in social interactions when one sometimes has to relate to different people on different levels in close proximity if not at the same time. It is key to effective performance in managerial occupations and in science, in which paradigms change constantly. Artistic achievement may also be conceived as the ability to shift effortlessly between sets or paradigms or even to maintain antithetical sets simultaneously in the service of creating a unique synthesis. Conceptual ability and flexibility are two functions that have suggested that the frontal lobes are the seat of higher intelligence. A failure therein contributes to the perceived "shallowness" of the patient with frontal lobe injury.

Perseveration, the tendency to maintain a cognitive set that is inappropriate to the situation, is a symptom of frontal lobe injury, but so is the inability to maintain a set when it is necessary to do so in the face of distracting or competing stimuli. This conceptual disability may be elicited by the Stroop Test (9).

Executive Functions

The executive functions of the prefrontal cortex refer to the capacity for autonomous behavior beyond the structure of external guidance. In clinical terms, this refers to initiative, motivation, spontaneity, planning, judgment, insight, goal-directed behavior, the ability to operate in favor of a remote or an abstract reward, the capacity for self-monitoring, and the flexibility required for self-correction. The executive functions are activity-related behaviors that are necessary for appropriate, socially responsible, and self-serving adult conduct. In the clinical literature concerned with deficits in executive behavior, lesions of the frontal lobes are most commonly implicated, although other cortical and subcortical structures may also be involved (10).

The central element in this concept is autonomy, i.e., the capacity to formulate goals, make plans for their execution, carry them out in an effective way, change course or improvise in the face of obstacles or failure, and do so successfully in the absence of external direction or structure. The capacity of the individual to generate goals and to achieve them is something that we consider an essential aspect of a mature and effective personality. It is not a social convention or an artifact of culture. It is "hard-wired" in the construction of the prefrontal cortex and its connections.

Patients with frontal lobe lesions retain the individual functional subunits necessary to achieve a given end. They are incapable, however, of developing a conceptual framework for complex, goal-directed behavior and for assembling the functional subunits in an effective way without external guidance. With structure and appropriate feedback from the outside, they do well. As soon as structure is removed, they lapse into inactivity or pursue idle, self-defeating impulses. Patients with frontal lobe lesions also have the unnerving habit of justifying their failure with rationalizations or expressions of external blame. When their external feedback system fails, they are incapable of self-monitoring. They may recite with perfect recall the words of advice that they were given to deal with an untoward circumstance, but they are unable to use verbal mediation to direct their behavior (4).

Because patients with frontal lobe lesions have significant deficits in sustained attention, they are easily distracted by irrelevant stimuli or by an immediate stimulus from the more important requirements of a remote goal. Behavior is, therefore, said to be stimulus bound rather than goal bound. Bakchine et al. (11) refer to an environmental dependency syndrome in patients with frontal lobe lesions—the excessive control of behavior by external stimuli at the expense of behavioral autonomy.

Extreme deficits in executive behavior may be observed in the clinical setting. The patient may respond appropriately to questions, for example, but offers no spontaneous questions or remarks; he or she may move perfectly well on command but has few, if any, spontaneous gestures or expressions. A deficit in spontaneity may be obscured in a patient who is also depressed, as patients with frontal lobe lesions often are. Clinical observations by an experienced examiner, however, can usually distinguish lack of spontaneity from psychomotor retardation. The patient with frontal lobe lesions responds appropriately when he or she is led to do so, but the depressed patient will require much more encouragement, and expressions of sadness, hostility, or disinterest usually accompany his or her response.

Deficits in initiative and motivation are not always apparent in the clinical setting, and the patient with frontal lobe lesions hardly ever complains about it. The information sometimes must be gleaned from family members.

Confabulation in the face of examination in an area of weakness is easy for the examiner to detect. It is harder to realize that the arguments and rationalizations of patients with frontal lobe lesions are cut from the same cloth. Patients with frontal lobe lesions may be argumentative, even to the point of legalisms, when confronted over an area of difficulty, for example, an impulsive act, an ill-considered spree, or a lapse in safety awareness. When they are denied the gratification of an immediate impulse, they behave like surly teenagers, churning the argument over small and irrelevant details. The problem is a paradigm conflict. The doctor is speaking from the vantage point of an abstract or remote goal: safety, maturity, and socially responsible behavior. Abstractions like that are meaningless to the patient with frontal lobe lesions who is driven, like an adolescent, by the compelling demand of immediate gratification.

The inability to self-monitor and respond flexibly in the face of a minor failure or obstacle is often the occasion for self-serving recriminations. The failure to execute a plan or the failure of a plan that was defective from the beginning may occasion the same response. The patient with frontal lobe lesions, singularly lacking in insight and the capacity for detached perspective, tends to fix blame on some trivial element or, more commonly, a lapse on the part of someone else. The psychiatrist recognizes the defense of externalization, but the underlying deficit is an executive and conceptual failure. It is not confabulation, but the germ of it is there. The laws of reasoned discourse are set aside in the service of the self-image of an ineffectual individual.

When Lhermitte introduced the idea of an environmental dependency syndrome in frontal lobe injuries, he described the patient who saw a tongue depressor and proceeded to give the professor a medical checkup. Psychiatrists are not likely to have a similar experience unless they see many young, hyperactive children who are patients with frontal lobe deficits of a different stripe. To the patient Lhermitte described, the mere sight of an object elicited the compulsion to use it. The tongue depressor was a cue that evoked a stereotyped response appropriate to the setting but not to the context (6). The behavior is socially inappropriate because it is stimulus bound rather than goal directed. Just as perseveration is the converse of cognitive flexibility, stereotyped, stimulus-bound responses are the converse of autonomous executive ability.

Attention and Arousal

Arousal is the ability of the organism to be awakened, maintain wakefulness, and follow stimuli or respond to commands. The frontal lobes participate in the functions of arousal and attention as the rostral pole of a brainstem–frontal lobe axis that includes the thalamus and the ascending reticular activating system. The brainstem–frontal lobe system provides tonic levels of arousal and alertness through the reticular apparatus, phasic levels of alertness through the diffuse thalamic projection system, and selected and directed attention through the frontal-thalamic gating system (7).

The state of akinetic mutism is a dramatic demonstration of failure in the frontal lobe–brainstem axis that mediates arousal. It is a condition of silent, inert-appearing immobility in which sleep-wake cycles exist, but externally obtainable evidence for mental activity remains almost entirely absent and spontaneous motor activity is lacking (12). The patient lies inert and speechless. Akinetic mutism is associated with lesions that interfere with reticulocortical or limbic-cortical integration, e.g., large lesions in the postero-medial-inferior frontal lobes or small lesions in the paramedian reticular formation.

Disorders of the frontal lobe may lead to deficits in arousal, e.g., akinetic mutism, clouding of consciousness with diminished alertness, hypersomnolence, easy fatigue, or to deficits in attention, e.g., short attention span, decreased concentration, distractibility. The clinical signs are readily observable, and the patients frequently complain of the symptoms. Patients with frontal lobe lesions are inattentive and easily distracted by extraneous stimuli. Similar problems are observed in children with developmental disorders of attention. Indeed, frontal lobe dysfunction has been demonstrated in patients with ADHD (13–16). The cause of developmental attentional disorders is sometimes related to neuropathic events, but, more commonly, it has a familial basis. Presumably, it represents a lag in the development of a frontal lobe attentional system. Psychostimulants are equally effective for attentional problems in patients with frontal lobe lesions (17) and in patients with ADHD. Dopaminergic drugs have been successful in rousing patients from states of akinetic mutism.

Just as the patient with frontal lobe lesions has difficulty in maintaining a cognitive set, he or she also has difficulty in sustaining attention to an important but dull and necessary task. By the same token, the routine chores of day-to-day schoolwork are impossible for the child with ADHD. Conversely, like the child with ADHD, the patient with frontal lobe lesions is capable of intense concentration on matters that are novel, stimulating, or intensely gratifying. The appropriate concept with which to understand this is limbic tagging. Because several areas of the prefrontal cortex project to the limbic system via the cingulate and from there to the hippocampus, input from the frontal lobe may be protected from abnormally rapid decay by the necessary limbic reinforcement. The preservation of a prefrontal activity, such as concentration or maintaining a set, may be blunted if there is not a high level of limbic activation to begin with.

Digression: The Delayed-Response Paradigm

A fundamental demonstration of the role of the prefrontal cortex in developing and maintaining an appropriate cognitive set is the delayed-response paradigm (18). The experiment requires a monkey with bilateral frontal lobe resections who is trained to find a piece of food hidden beneath one of two cups. If the monkey is allowed to respond immediately, he usually gets it right, but there is a sharp decrement in performance if a time delay (a few seconds) is interposed before the monkey can respond. The discovery of impaired performance in delayed response and a related experiment, delayed alternation, was a landmark in neuropsychology because it was the first robust experimental demonstration of a double-dissociable frontal lobe function. The fact that the preclinical experiment was irreproducible in humans did not diminish its importance to experimental neuropsychologists who had a long and frustrating search for an explanation of the underlying deficit (19). Because failure in the delayed-response test could not be attributed simply to impairments in memory, attention, or visual discrimination, for example, the real nature of the deficit remained a riddle for many years.

The delayed-response experiment is presented because the solution to the riddle shows how the conceptual functions of the frontal lobe actually find their origin in the premotor functions of the frontal lobe. By focusing on the motor functions, Teuber (20) proposed that frontal lobe structures were responsible for corollary discharge, i.e., discharge from motor to sensory systems, to prepare the sensory system for an anticipated movement. The motor system exerts a preparatory action on the sensory system to announce the intention of an incoming movement, to correct for displacement of perception, and to assure smooth perceptual continuity once movement is carried out (5). Thus, during a voluntary shift of gaze, the environment stands still because a corollary discharge from the oculomotor to the visual mechanism prepares the latter for the change in relative position that will result from ocular motion (21). A grasp elicits a contact sensation that is anticipated because it matches the anticipation of contact, and this in turn serves as a brake to the grasping movement (20). The coordination of motor and sensory systems to guide successful, goal-directed behavior requires the development and maintenance of what is called a kinesthetic set, in other words, a sensorimotor concept.

In the delayed-response paradigm, the monkey locates the cue (the food under a cup) and selects an appropriate motor response. This is understood to involve "programming the self-regulation of future actions" by forming a "kinesthetic guidance system" (19). To preserve this cognitive set in the face of temporal delay, the monkey's attention to cue location and the formation of internalized stimulus-response associations must be resistant to distracting internal and external stimuli. It must also be free from the effects of proactive interference from previous trials. A new response set (or kinesthetic guidance system) must be developed that is appropriate to the trial at hand and that is liberated from well-established but inappropriate response sets.

Although the delayed-response deficit is not directly reproducible in humans, the function of frontal lobe structures in developing kinesthetic guidance systems in a simple sensorimotor task is not irrelevant to clinical studies. Self-regulated behavior in humans also requires the development of guidance systems and programs that are appropriate to a chosen goal, flexible in the face of obstacles, protected from extraneous or internal distracters, and liberated from the proactive interference of previously learned programs. This chain may be interrupted in the patient with frontal lobe lesions by deficits in initiative, cognitive flexibility, distractibility, and perseveration. The fact that the delayed-response paradigm is demonstrated in subprimate monkeys suggests that the formation of a kinesthetic set, or a sensorimotor concept, is an early evolutionary step toward the conceptual and executive ability of the frontal lobes in Homo sapiens.

Self-Awareness and Empathy

In 1908, Flechsig suggested that the fundamental role of the prefrontal cortex was self-awareness or consciousness of the self (7). Lesions of the parietal lobes are also known to disorder the "consciousness of person" (22), but it is clear that unconcern, unawareness of deficit, and indifference are features that typify patients with frontal lobe lesions. Insight, a fundamental concept in psychiatric assessment and treatment, is one of the cardinal functions of the frontal lobes.

The clinical manifestations of this frontal lobe deficit are dramatic. Anosognosia, for example, is the incapacity to appreciate the nature or the degree of one's impairment. It is a formidable clinical problem in patients with right frontal lesions. Unilateral inattention or neglect is even more striking because the patient is unable to register information from a sensory hemifield, even to the point of denying one-half of his or her own body. Reduplicative paramnesia is associated with severe bifrontal pathology. The patient remains convinced that a familiar place or person has been duplicated. The reduplication of persons is referred to as Capgras' syndrome in the psychiatric literature. Cotard's syndrome involves the denial of one's own existence and that of the external world; a key feature is the delusion that one is dead (23).

A patient with chronic pain who has been treated with a stereotactic lesion in the frontal lobe continues to be aware of his or her pain but no longer experiences the unpleasant sensation of painfulness. In fact, one purpose of prefrontal lobotomy was to reduce the characteristics of self-concern: brooding, self-preoccupation, and self-consciousness (7).

Safety awareness is a practical term that one is compelled to apply to the management of patients with frontal lobe lesions who are capable of wandering onto a thoroughfare crowded with traffic, inattentive to danger, or who insist on a restoration of their privilege to drive an automobile, cook, or go out partying on a Saturday night. When indifference to one's personal safety is coupled with impulsive behavior and poor judgment, the results are potentially dangerous, and management issues become paramount.

Frontal lobe apathy, or lack of concern, comprises limited awareness with none of the appropriate limbic "tagging." The patient with frontal lobe lesions may be aware of his or her deficiencies but is indifferent to their impact. Awareness of the right and wrong of a situation does not necessarily guide his or her behavior. Awareness of a tendency to make errors, for example, in a psychological test, does not lead to self-correction. Error evaluation, in other words, does not translate into error utilization.

The awareness of the dimension of time (time perception) may also be impaired in patients with frontal lobe lesions who tend to respond only to concrete, present contingencies with no regard to the future or the consequences that it may bring. [Impairment in time perception is seen most commonly in patients with ADHD and in people drinking alcohol (why one loses track of time at a cocktail party).]

During complex behaviors, especially in social situations, self-monitoring and self-correction require ongoing awareness of one's position with respect to one's circumstances. Effective performance in such circumstances also requires awareness of the position of other people and their own agendas—the ability to project the effect that one's own actions may have on the thoughts or feelings of another at the present time or far in the future. The patient with frontal lobe lesions with Capgras' syndrome cannot even concede the identity of a person with whom he or she is familiar or even intimate (a rare disorder). More common is the shallow egotism of the patient with frontal lobe lesions who is insensitive to the thoughts and feelings of his or her fellows. Empathy in social intercourse is based on the maintenance of an abstract but compelling concept of individuality and mutuality. The patient with severe frontal lobe injury cannot even raise the concept. The less severely afflicted patient can afford the concept as long as it is gratifying or at least inexpensive.

Clinical interventions are compromised by patients' inability to self-monitor, their failure to appreciate the seriousness of their circumstances, and their failure to sustain a sense of self that is concordant with the perceptions of other people. Patients with frontal lobe lesions with anosognosia represent only the most extreme examples. The most frequent example is the adolescent patient who finds it painful to reflect on the nature of his or her problematic behavior. An adolescent's conceptual sense of self is so tenuous and ill-formed that the attentions of a helping adult are perceived as invasions or assaults. (As we shall see, the adolescent is a "frontal lobe patient" of slightly different stripe.)

The self-deception of alcoholics is a form of anosognosia that can be a function of the neurotoxic effects of alcohol on frontal structures. Addicts to cocaine or cannabis have a similar problem. The integrity of one's self-concept can be overwhelmed by a strong appetitive urge, even a destructive one. Patients with mania or hypomania are also prone to denial. Manic depression is not a frontal lobe disorder, but, as in appetitive disorders, deep limbic hyperactivity can overwhelm the capacity of frontal systems to self-monitor.

BEHAVIORAL CHARACTERISTICS OF FRONTAL LOBE LESIONS

Many of the behavioral attributes of the patient with frontal lobe lesions are, in large part, a function of specific cognitive deficits. Goldstein (24) referred to this as "the personality change owing to impairment of abstract attitude." Other behavioral attributes of the patient with frontal lobe lesions can be formulated in terms of impairment of the regulatory apparatus.

Concrete Behavior

The patient with frontal lobe lesions has a deficit in conceptual thinking. His or her actions are guided by a concrete interpretation of events and circumstances. This, in turn, gives rise to behaviors that seem shallow, misguided, peculiar, or even bizarre. The performance of familiar tasks is unimpaired, and under ordinary circumstances, the patient appears quite normal, but the patient finds it taxing to modify his or her behavior to meet an unfamiliar demand and is easily overwhelmed by the novel circumstances. Thus distracted, the patient is unable to abstract a familiar essence from the new situation.

It is a capacity for abstracting the essence of a novel situation that allows one to behave appropriately when dealing with situations that are superficially different but conceptually quite similar. Goldstein (24) described the case of a skilled mechanic who was able to do his familiar work satisfactorily and was still considered an excellent worker. Nevertheless, a new, complicated piece of machinery would give him a great deal of trouble. He continued to be adept at the execution of familiar behavioral sets but was incapable of manipulating them in novel ways or modifying them to meet a new challenge. When confronted with such a challenge, he was prone to what Goldstein called a "catastrophic reaction" of confusion and anxiety.

In social situations, the actions of other people may be interpreted in the shallowest terms. If a friend bestows his or her attention on a third person, the act may be interpreted as a personal slight or an act of betrayal. The patient is unable to understand the event in terms of his friend's point of view because that would require what Piaget called a formal operation, that is, an act of conceptual abstraction. The patient with frontal lobe injury, performing at the level of "concrete operations," interprets the event from a limited perspective. In psychiatric terms, this behavior may be said to be highly personalized, idiosyncratic, or perhaps even paranoid.

Executive behaviors such as planning and executing complex goal-directed behaviors and anticipating problems are areas of deficit for the patient with frontal lobe lesions that arise out of his or her relative conceptual failure. The patient is incapable of maintaining a steady course toward the attainment of a remote goal. Even though he or she is able to articulate the appropriate goal, he or she cannot use verbal mediation to prevent distraction or deflect a momentary impulse.

Perseveration and Stereotyped Behavior

Cognitive inflexibility is a term that describes the patient's weakness at manipulating conceptual sets to solve new problems. The behavioral manifestations of this cognitive deficit are perseveration or stereotyped behavior and lack of initiative.

Perseveration is an extreme example of the stereotyped behavior of the patient with frontal lobe injury who is only comfortable with familiar routines. Perseveration is the abnormal repetition of a specific behavior, and the term is usually applied to behavioral fragments that have no utility whatever, such as turning a faucet on and off or repeating a phrase over and over. Stereotypy refers to similar behavior but at a much lower level, such as hand flapping in an autistic child or repetitive finger movements in a patient with Pick's disease. The stereotyped behavior of a patient with frontal lobe lesions, however, usually transpires at a much higher level, for example, the patient who met every person on the ward with the same cheerful smile and friendly hello but who was unable to follow any of these encounters with a meaningful conversation. Such behavior is sometimes referred to as "shallow."

The "chesterfieldian" manners of a patient with frontal lobe lesions are also a form of stereotyped interaction, guided by an exquisite attentiveness to the superficialities of social intercourse. The patient's manners, however, are hardly a reflection of an empathic nature. The patient is incapable of the formal operations necessary for mutuality. Such manners are, in fact, the mask of empathy, and behind the mask, one frequently meets an individual who is at best indifferent and at worst predatory and remorseless. The charming con man is the prototype.

Initiative, Motivation, and Perseverance

If patients with frontal lobe injury are ill equipped to deal with novel circumstances, it is easy to understand why they seem perfectly content to persist in behaviors that are routine and familiar. Naturally, initiative will be a problem, and they will hardly be motivated to seek out novel situations. Deficits in initiative and motivation are common complaints by family members of patients with frontal lobe lesions, although the patients are unlikely to complain. They may sit at home doing nothing, never speaking spontaneously, not asking for anything, and not seeming to desire anything.

The extreme clinical example is abulia, literally, the absence of appetite. It is a syndrome associated with lesions of the lateral convexity of the frontal lobes. The patient is apathetic in the face of normal human desires. Not only does the patient lack the drive necessary to satisfy them, but also he or she lacks the desire. (To be differentiated from anhedonia. If you ask the patient with frontal lobe injury, "Would you like to go to a restaurant to eat?", he or she would respond politely that he or she would. If you asked if he or she had enjoyed him/herself, he or she would respond sincerely, yes, indeed. But that would never demonstrate the initiative to request another such outing, nor would it occur to him or her to do so.)

Even if patients with frontal lobe lesions are able to generate an action program, they are incapable of bestowing it with the necessary "limbic drive" to overcome inertia. The patients may even verbalize a plan, if pressed to do so, but cannot recruit the energy to initiate action. Complaints of low energy and easy fatigue are not uncommon in patients with frontal lobe lesions. Even if they can initiate a plan, they find it difficult to sustain, and if there are obstacles, they find it difficult to persevere.

Perseverance deficits are easy to demonstrate in the examining room by asking the patient to perform a complex motor task and in computerized tests, such as the Continuous Performance Task.

Effective goal-directed behavior, especially in complex situations, requires not only the ability to maintain a plan—an abstract guidance set—but also the energy to see it through. It is the role of frontal lobe projections to subcortical areas to recruit the tonic stimulation that is necessary to sustain motivation in the service of a conceptual set. If the conceptual set is extremely weak, but tonic stimulation is strong, the patient demonstrates perseveration or stereotypy. If the set is well developed, but there is a failure in recruitment, the patient grows fatigued or discouraged. If both components are weak, the patient will be abulic.

The developmental disorder ADHD is an appropriate model for understanding the problems of a patient with frontal lobe lesions. Distractibility and impulsivity represent failures in maintaining an appropriate cognitive or behavioral set. That may be postulated as a primary frontal lobe dysfunction. Patients with ADHD, however, are also referred to specialists because of lack of motivation and initiative in school, especially when they are adolescents. By then, they have acquired some degree of frontal lobe control of their overt behaviors, but their capacity for developing a sustained effort remains impaired. Limbic drive may be given to phasic eruptions of anger or frustration but not to tonic stimulation in the service of sustained achievement. It is interesting that drugs such as methylphenidate and amantadine can strengthen both components, decreasing impulsiveness and distractibility and sustaining levels of motivation and initiative, and the drugs appear to be as successful in patients with frontal lobe lesions as they are in children with ADHD.

Behavioral inertia in the patient with frontal lobe lesions, like the underachieving adolescent, may respond to stimulant or dopaminergic drugs or to external structure, or it may not. Physicians, like parents, may discover that their encouragement or blandishments are met with a degree of stubbornness or obstinacy that is positively mule-like. The issues that provoke such a reaction are predictable: in a patient who has limited insight into the nature of his or her limitations, it will be over a privilege denied, such as a driver's license, or it will be over the need to cooperate with some form of treatment. In a patient whose horizons have been limited from lack of initiative or venturing forth, it will be over a proposed change of routine.

Disorders of Mood

The frontal lobes are not the nexus of the emotions but rather their governing body. The fact that affective and emotional disorders are the most dramatic signs of frontal lobe disease is, indeed, a consequence of its regulatory activity. Frontal lobe structures mediate the cognition necessary to modulate lower forms of response. Frontal lobe disease downgrades the quality of gate mechanisms and allows less elaborate responses to complex environmental situations to take place (5).

The limbic system, for example, influences the frontal lobes and modulates externally directed higher forms of drives. In turn, the prefrontal cortex influences internally directed limbic drive states. Lesions of the frontal lobes, therefore, produce dissociation between these systems: there is less neocortical influence on the limbic system and the hypothalamus, which monitor the internal milieu and induce drive states. There is also less limbic influence on neocortical function, for example, externally directed activity aimed at preservation of the self or the species (25).

The clinical manifestation of reduced frontal lobe influence over subcortical drive states is commonly referred to as disinhibition. The orbitofrontal cortex has extensive connections to the septal area and the amygdala. Lesions in the orbitofrontal cortex produce disinhibition of these areas. Patients with orbitofrontal lesions not uncommonly demonstrate inappropriate irritability, anger, or rage (25). Instinctual functions such as eating may be released if the normal inhibitory influences on the hypothalamus and the hunger drive are no longer kept in check. Thus, overeating is a common observation in primates with lesions of the orbitofrontal cortex. The sexual drive may also be disinhibited by prefrontal lesions, leading to overt eroticism or hypersexuality. The disinhibition of instinctual drives seems to be fostered by a concomitant loosening of conventional moral restraints (26). However, there is no indication that disinhibited behavior is pleasurable.

Euphoria is a striking feature of patients with orbitofrontal lesions, rarely appearing as a pure feeling of elation but occurring in sporadic or recurrent fashion and resembling the affect of the hypomanic state, with its nervous, irritable, and sometimes paranoid quality. It is usually accompanied by a kind of compulsive, shallow, and childish humor that has been called puerilism, moria, or *witzelsucht* (26). The patient with orbitofrontal damage may be hyperkinetic, as if driven by ceaseless energy and impulsivity, and require little sleep. The patient has no brake to control excitability.

In contrast, the emotional consequence of damage to the dorsolateral aspect of the frontal lobes is referred to as blunting. This area has input into the cingulate gyrus and the reticular activating system. Patients with lesions of the convexity often have a deficit in phasic arousal: although they can develop the correct cognitive state in response to external stimuli, they fail to be aroused. When they encounter an event that ordinarily should evoke an emotional response, they appear unemotional or apathetic (25). The apathetic syndrome in patients with extensive lesions of the prefrontal convexity is characterized by low awareness, lack of initiative, hypokinesia, and decreased spontaneity. In the affective sphere, its hallmark is the generalized blunting of affects and emotional responses (26). The patient is often unkempt and indifferent to the slovenly appearance of his or her person or quarters.

The apathy of patients with frontal lobe injury has been referred to as pseudodepression (27), but the patients rarely show the self-concern and preoccupation that depressed patients do.

The patient with frontal lobe lesions also shows a restricted response to pain. On the other hand, he or she is not necessarily tame or docile. Moods are changeable, and apathy or indifference may alternate with sudden outbursts of irritability and aggression. The emotional and moral lapses are not so much vicious as inappropriate, inconsiderate, and self-defeating.

Regulation

If there is one principle around which the cognitive and behavioral components of the frontal lobe unite, it is the "psychoregulation" of Bekhterev (28) or the concept of behavioral regulation of Luria (29). It regulates the arousal mechanism, the coupling of sensory information to autonomic activity, and the integration of complex, goal-directed behavior.

The nonspecific activating system of the brainstem is closely bound to the cerebral cortex, especially the cortex of the limbic region and medial parts of the frontal lobes, and descending impulses from the frontal lobes regulate the activating system by modifying the state of cortical activity (29). The reticulothalamocortical system regulates the activity of brainstem and midline subcortical structures having to do with activation, arousal, alerting, and attention.

The orbital surface of the frontal lobes is the most rostral sympathetic ganglion that inhibits both somatomotor and visceromotor activities and couples these core systems with areas directly or indirectly involved in processing sensory information. The role of the frontal cortex is necessary for psychological factors to influence these core systems, whereby basic homeostatic systems may be influenced by external events (30,31).

The actions of regulation and modification are in the service of stability of behavior and mood and the successful execution of complex behaviors. Maintaining a constant cortical tone is essential for the regulation of goal-directed behavior. When the cortex is in an inhibitory phasic state, when the individual is asleep or half-awake, organized thought is impossible, and selective connections are supplanted by nonselective associations that have no purposeful character, e.g., the peculiar logic of dreaming (29).

Derangements in the regulation of states of neural activity arising from lesions of the frontal cortex must inevitably lead to marked disturbance of complex forms of behavior. The frontal lobes control the active state of the cortex, which is necessary for the accomplishment of complex tasks. Lesions in the orbitofrontal cortex compromise the ability to maintain a protracted state of cortical tone necessary for the task at hand. The behavioral set is diminished by the failure to regulate the necessary balance between selective (relevant) associations and diffuse (irrelevant) associations. Attention is scattered and intention is lost.

Problem-solving behavior is impaired because the patient never begins with a preliminary analysis of the conditions of the task. To do so requires a stable network of selective associations. Instead, the patient with frontal lobe lesions embarks on a solution with characteristic impulsiveness. Behaviors that are elective and purposive are replaced by emerging fragments of inert stereotypes. Impulsive responding, therefore, emerges as a stereotyped solution.

It has been proposed that the unique contribution of the dorsolateral surface of the frontal lobes is to serve as a "buffer register" to bring about and to maintain relative facilitation in those neuronal elements that are appropriate to a complex schema that is in the process of execution, regardless of minor interruptions, to "preserve an anticipated future," the yet-to-be-activated plan (31). What Goldstein referred to as the capacity for abstraction has been termed a "working memory" by Pribram and Luria (32), in which various action plans could be stored while awaiting execution. This is why the consequence of a frontal lobe lesion is almost invariably a disturbance of the independent choice of programs of action, the inability to readjust action programs to the changing requirements of the external situation, or to modify internal drive states to adjust to changing situations (29).

Fuster (26) emphasized the critical role of the prefrontal cortex in the temporal organization of behavior, involving provisional memory, anticipatory set, and control of interference. The prefrontal cortex is not essential for the execution of any motor act per se, for example, but for the orderly and purposive execution of novel and complex behavioral structures of which motor acts, along with perceptual and mnemonic acts, are a part. The prefrontal cortex confers to movement the spontaneity, intentionality, and active quality that characterize all the essential components of purposive behavior (26).

THE FRONTAL LOBE CONTRIBUTION TO PSYCHOPATHOLOGY

The regulatory and integrative functions of the frontal cortex are of intense importance to understanding pathologic behavior, not only in patients with frontal lesions, but also in patients with psychiatric disorders, as illustrated in the foregoing discussion. The elements of frontal lobe disease are no less than the clinical manifestations of the common psychiatric disorders. No psychiatrist is a stranger to clinical signs and symptoms such as concrete thinking, cognitive inflexibility, poor judgment, impulsiveness, inattention, irritability. Dysregulation and disintegration are at the heart of psychopathology. Dynamic brain imaging studies demonstrate abnormalities in frontal lobe metabolism—"hypofrontality"—in most of the common psychiatric disorders: schizophrenia (33), obsessive-compulsive disorder (34), ADHD (16), and depression (35).

There have always been limits, however, to a localizationist approach to the psychiatric disorders. Psychopathology cannot be localized to specific cortical lesions in the frontal lobes or elsewhere. By the same token, although patients with lesions may resemble psychiatric patients or may develop psychiatric disorders as a complication of their injury, it is usually a mistake to apply conventional psychiatric terminology to a patient with a frontal lobe injury and equally so to apply a lesional diagnosis to a psychiatric patient. A clinician might be inclined to diagnose depression in a patient with a convexity lesion or sociopathic personality disorder in a patient with an orbitomedial lesion. Clinicians may argue that ADHD is a frontal lobe disorder. There are germs of truth to all these, but they are imperfect models for two reasons: they overrepresent the cogency of lesion analysis and understate the multiple dimensions that contribute to psychopathology. Neuropsychology and psychiatry are complementary disciplines, but they are not concurrent.

The paradigms of lesion analysis and experimental neuropsychology are familiar to clinicians and have been addressed cursorily in the previous sections, but their contribution to psychopathology is as obscure as it is, in some quarters, overstated. Lesion analysis addresses the localization of cortical functions. Psychiatrists are equally concerned with the patient's underlying impairment, or at least they ought to be, but they are also concerned with processes that govern compensation or decompensation in the face of an underlying impairment. Psychopathology, as the psychiatrist views it, is the outcome of an underlying weakness, a genotype or a biotype that has interacted over the years with the unique events of the patient's personal history (see Chapter 26).

A cortical lesion can cause functional impairment, which does not necessarily indicate that the function is localized to the structure in question or that it is the seat of the function. Rather, it indicates that the damaged structure is a participant in a dynamic functional system, a structural network that is internally redundant and reduplicative and is also capable of recruiting other structural networks in a systematic way. The treatment of patients with brain injuries is aimed at strengthening other elements in a redundant functional system and undoing the pathologic processes that inhibit their powers of compensation.

Experimental studies of the cognitive and behavioral concomitants of frontal lobe lesions indicate a large number of functional networks that are vulnerable to impairment. Neuropsychologists take those impairments as predictive of behavioral and cognitive types. Patients with convexity lesions are expected to have one type of behavior, and patients with orbitofrontal lesions another type.

In the system that psychiatrists use, the representative types are identified *a priori*. Then, in a process that is like reverse engineering, they try to determine which functional networks are impaired. The two disciplines approach the problem from different perspectives. They have identified their conceptual approaches with their starting points: the neuropsychologist with the lesion, the psychiatrist with the patient's clinical state. Neither is a better starting point, and neither, as a conceptual position, is sufficient. A truly synthetic view would be to address the intervening events that govern the evolution of a cortical impairment to a psychopathologic condition.

Convexity Lesions

Lesions of the frontal convexity typically are associated with abulia, lack of motivation and initiative, anergia, failure to plan, and inability to execute complex behavioral programs, such as getting up in the morning, getting dressed, having breakfast, and going to work. This clinical presentation may be misinterpreted as anergic depression or an inadequate or avoidant personality.

Patients with convexity lesions have been described as pseudodepressed (27) because of their apathy, lack of drive, inability to plan ahead, total unconcern, and the appearance of decreased mentation. Clearly, they are not patients with major depression, chronic dysthymia, or bipolar disorder. Patients with frontal lobe lesions are not, as a rule, anhedonic, pessimistic, suicidal, or preoccupied with a state of inner suffering. There is also evidence that they should be treated with dopamine agonists such as bromocriptine (36) and amantadine (37) or the psychostimulants (17) rather than the conventional antidepressants.

Something that a psychiatrist may refer to as denial or lack of insight is the phenomenon of anosognosia, usually associated with lesions of the right frontal lobe or right parietal lobe (38). Anosognosia is the inability to appreciate the nature of one's impairment or even that one is impaired. The typical presentation is an unconcerned patient with an intensely concerned family.

The companion symptoms are really quite extraordinary: the patients may deny their disability (anosognosia), may be compliant to a fault, or, alternatively, may be as stubborn as mules. These patients are not flexible as people or as thinkers and prefer to deal with simple, agreeable issues. They have difficulty when the rules are changed, when there is the requirement for readjustment to a new set of demands. They tend to get stuck in a rut—a personal or cognitive rut. In extreme cases, this may be so dramatic that they perseverate or engage in stereotyped behavior. They tend to be socially inappropriate but in an innocent kind of way, like a bumpkin. These patients are not very good in complex or ambiguous situations, prefer structure and predictability in their environment, are not good planners, and have real difficulty with complex tasks. They are easily distracted, can be absentminded, and can stare off for long periods without a thought in their head.

One of my patients had bifrontal lesions of the convexity. He took the earnings from his settlement and built a small grocery at a country crossroads. There was no business. He stayed there. The milk in his cooler was out of date, the cans of food were old and dusty, and the few customers who lived nearby—hardly anyone lived nearby—stopped coming. He did not leave the place until his money ran out and he had used up all his credit. Then he moved back to town. The store was a total write-off.

Another patient had bilateral lesions in the frontal pole when he got tossed around in a cement mixer. He was prone to spells; he would sit and stare into space, immobile, attentive to nothing in his environment, and responsive to no stimulus except physical touch. He was not in nonconvulsive status; he had severe attentional lapses, which responded favorably to dopamine agonist treatment.

Some patients with frontal lobe injury are said to be abulic, from the Greek for without appetite. Such patients are not especially motivated to do anything, simply for lack of will, and spend their days quietly, doing as little as they possibly can. It is not that they are uninterested or disinterested; it is the capacity for interest at all that is missing. They may also have parkinsonian signs: mask-like faces, cogwheeling, and positive glabellar tap. They also respond favorably to the antiparkinsonian drug amantadine (37).

One patient with bilateral lesions of the convexity was really quite polite and responsive during the examination and during the interview would respond appropriately, although passively and without much expressiveness. When she was sitting in the waiting room, however, she would just sit immobile and stare into space. She would never read or fidget or talk to the receptionist. She lived by herself. At home, she would just sit, sometimes watching television, sometimes not. She hardly had the initiative to feed herself. She made instant coffee, but that was about all. As time went on, she just seemed to waste away.

The ardent clinician may believe that a simple series of interventions may correct the problem. He or she is eager to steer aright such a simple, aimless soul: structure, guidance, counseling; amantadine or a psychostimulant; or moving away from a dead-end situation. These are the usual clinical recommendations. It is instructive how the patient will resist the physician's best advice. Good therapeutic intentions run headlong against the stubbornness of the patient with frontal lobe lesions.

Orbitofrontal Lesions

Lesions of the orbitomedial surface of the frontal lobes typically are associated with inattention and distractibility, excitability, impulsiveness, disinhibition, and socially inappropriate behavior. Psychiatrists might interpret this syndrome as sociopathic behavior or as ADHD.

The disinhibited patient may be an innocent, not unlike a hyperactive child, with *witzelsucht*, the compulsion to joke, excitability, short attention span, impulsiveness, restlessness, and emotional lability. He or she may be sexually disinhibited, with either promiscuous behavior or lewd talking or both. Impulsive behavior and extremes of temperament may take a destructive turn, with substance abuse, reckless driving, or scrapes with the law. As a rule, such patients do not seem to be as violent as patients with temporal lobe injuries, but they are extremely susceptible to the effects of alcohol and other depressants (like the benzodiazepines); they may be prone to what is called pathologic intoxication, and under such circumstances they can be assaultive. The patient with orbitofrontal injury has lost his or her capacity for self-control or, more commonly, is capable of losing it very easily in unstructured settings or when stressed or under the influence of an intoxicant.

I had the privilege during my youth to serve as a general physician in a couple of rough, rural Southern communities. There I grew familiar with the Saturday night denizen of the emergency room: the young man whose idea of a good time was a few beers at a roadhouse and then a good fight. It was not until many years later that the behavioral neurology of the American redneck became apparent. Combine the impulsive, aggressive behavior of the patient with frontal lobe lesions with an elevated pain threshold (also the consequence of an orbitofrontal lesion), the disinhibiting influence of even a small amount of alcohol, and the inability to learn enduring lessons from unpleasant experience, and you have the regulars of a country emergency room.

Conversely, under structured circumstances, the patient with orbitofrontal lesions does quite well. When scrutiny is intense or when the situation is structured or novel, he or she may be polite and compliant—"chesterfieldian" in manners and consideration for others. Let the structure lapse, however, and Lord Chesterfield will retire, and the devil will rise again. (Psychiatrists who work with prisoners are all too familiar with this paradox.)

The orbitofrontal surface is the rostral projection of the ascending reticular activating system, a latticework of neurons that arises in the brainstem and projects monoaminergic neurotransmitters to the diencephalon, limbic cortex, and frontal lobe. The function of this network is regulation: at the brainstem level, it is regulation of arousal; in the diencephalon, of appetitive behaviors; and in the limbic and frontal cortex, of higher level behavior and emotional expression. The frontal patient with a lesion in this region has a limited capacity to regulate and control behavior in response to feedback from the environment; he or she has difficulty conforming to societal norms or social cues, cannot control overreactions to novel or to stressful circumstances, and is likelier to respond to stress by acting out some untoward motor program than by internalizing his or her reactions and getting anxious, worried, or insecure. In fact, such people have a limited capacity for experiencing such emotions at all. Psychosurgical procedures are still done to ablate this pathway, in fact, in patients with severe, disabling anxiety who do not respond to conventional treatments. Surgical procedures in this area may also be brought to bear to control some intense pain syndromes.

Psychiatrists occasionally talk about "pure" sociopaths, people who are capable of the most egregious transgressions but who are wholly incapable of experiencing remorse for their actions, even when confronted. Some of these people are similar to patients with frontal lobe lesions of the orbital surface. It is a kind of disconnection syndrome. Impulsive behavior is released from inhibitory cortical regulation, and the capacity to integrate behavior in line with established social norms has been removed. There is no capacity to self-reflect or to view oneself in an alternative framework, for example, as others do. There is limited capacity for self-correction, most notably when the consequences of misbehavior are painful. There is a tendency to repeat the transgression whenever the opportunity presents itself, and there is agnosia for the deficit.

Processes of Transformation

The types represented by injuries to the convexity or orbitomedial surface of the frontal lobes are clinical "familiars" to a neuropsychiatric practice. They also bear a resemblance to a couple of psychiatric conditions. Convexity patients are pseudodepressed. Patients with orbitofrontal injury are "pseudosociopathic," but between the neuropsychological impairment and the psychiatric disability are several intervening variables, biologic and psychological processes that govern the transformation from functional impairment to behavioral disability.

Those intervening variables are the functional adjustments that the system undertakes when one of its essential parts is disabled. In children, the process is in large part governed by the plasticity of the developing brain. One such mechanism is compensation and reassignment of function, sometimes referred to as vicariation (39). Serving to augment the strength of this biologic response, the world of the child mounts an active investment in protection, guidance, and education.

In elderly people who have had strokes or brain injuries, compensatory adjustments are less active, and the course of age-related deterioration is accelerated. The resulting state of chronic undercompensation and functional loss is matched socially by a less vigorous investment in rehabilitation.

The adjustment to disability may be a pathologic state of secondary imbalance, such as a depressed focus (e.g., diaschisis) that will aggravate functional impairment or an irritative focus that can kindle epilepsy or psychosis (40). If the secondary imbalance is corrected, spontaneously or pharmacologically, impairment is reduced. If it is not corrected, impairment grows out of proportion even to the primary disability. If the consequence is a severe behavioral disturbance, there will be an inexorable deterioration in the patient's social links and a progressive, downward spiral.

Psychopathology is not caused by a cortical lesion or neuropsychological disability, any more than a psychiatric disorder can be localized to a cortical lesion. The disability represents a "setting event" or a nidus around which psychopathology may develop. The processes that govern the transformation may be intrinsic to the patient's age or premorbid condition, may represent a cascade of secondary biologic events, or may be a function of the social response to the patient's difficulties.

Sociopathic Personality

The patient with an orbitomedial lesion is sometimes described as pseudopsychopathic (27), by virtue of impulsive, self-serving behavior, disinhibition, irritability, aggression, and a distinct lack of empathy or concern for moral standards. Such patients, however, are not really sociopaths; they are not vicious or predatory and lack the ability to premeditate. Frontal lobe pathology may be a necessary participant in the genesis of the antisocial personality, but it is not sufficient.

The orbitomedial surface of the frontal lobes participates in a functional system that regulates the impact of reinforcement, especially negative reinforcement, on the development of complex patterns of behavior. Hare (41) and others have found reduced autonomic activity in sociopathic individuals and have suggested that certain features of psychopathic behavior may be related to hypoarousal induced by prefrontal dysfunction. It appears that high autonomic activity is associated with anxiety. Because the sociopath has reduced anxiety and fear, his or her behavior is not modified by punishment (42). Similarly, an orbitomedial lesion diminishes the apperception of pain, and it is well established that sociopaths are less prone than normals to learn new behaviors in response to painful stimuli (43). In monkeys with prefrontal resections, reinforcement, whether reward, punishment, or error, is processed sluggishly. The feedback to actions from their outcomes is impaired, and reinforcers become relatively ineffective (44).

It is not appropriate to refer to a patient with an orbitomedial lesion of the frontal lobe as a sociopath nor is it appropriate to refer to a sociopath as a patient with a frontal lobe lesion. It is appropriate to say that both entail disabilities in a functional system that is responsible for the integration and assimilation of the effects of reinforcement.

The patient with a frontal lobe lesion acquired during adult life has a static disorder that will impair his or her capacity for experiential learning and compel at least some degree of external supervision, but the lesion is not likely to be circumscribed. Other functional systems that require the participation of the frontal lobe are also likely to be damaged. The patient with frontal lobe lesions may be less dangerous than the sociopath because he or she lacks a strong sense of personal identity or will, initiative and energy level are low, and there is no ability to make or carry out a plan.

If the sociopath has a similar deficit in experiential learning, it is congenital, not acquired, dynamic, not static, and circumscribed, with no deficit of will, initiative, energy, or planning. If this formidable arrangement is coupled with an abusive childhood, an indifferent education, and the company of like-minded individuals, the outcome will not be sanguine. It is easy to appreciate how the attachments to family and society that are weakened by a frontal lobe injury are never even laid down in the developing sociopath.

What the psychology of the frontal lobes tells us, then, is that a neocortical system exists to guide the development of social integration through reinforcement, empathy, and attachment. If the system is damaged in later life, the individual may nevertheless be sustained by the linkages he or she has previously acquired. If the system has never developed at all, the necessary links are never made. Treatment of the patient with frontal lobe injury involves strengthening and sustaining linkages that have already been laid down. Treatment of the sociopath is obviously a more formidable chore.

There are other elements of frontal lobe function, such as the capacity for empathy, that are also disabled in the sociopathic individual and the patient with TBI. The principle is the same. If a patient sustains a traumatic injury to the orbitomedial surface of the frontal lobes during early adult life, he or she acquires the necessary substrate for some dangerous pathologic transformations. It is as if the genotype has been changed, although obviously nothing is different about the patient's DNA. Rather, one should say the patient's biotype has been altered, but a biotype, like a genotype, may or may not find expression in the patient's phenotype.

With respect to personal characteristics, personality traits, and indeed many forms of psychopathology, the phenotype is evoked from the genotype by influences external to the individual. The phenotype of height is evoked by optimal nutrition. The phenotype of intelligence is evoked by optimal stimulation. The same is true for the genotype for sociopathic behavior. In studies of children of criminal parents who were adopted away, for example, the expression of their potentially criminal genotype is influenced to a significant degree by the characteristics of their adoptive parents. The child is more likely to develop a criminal phenotype if his or her adoptive family is given to criminal behavior and less likely to do so if they are not. Elements in the child's environment evoke the genotype.

The patient with orbitofrontal lobe injury may have a sociopathic biotype, but the circumstances of his or her subsequent life will determine whether that biotype is ever expressed phenotypically. Treatment is aimed at suppressing the biotype. There are two treatments that work: psychostimulant drugs, presumably because they alter the patient's response to environmental rewards and punishments, and structure because it limits the patient's freedom to follow his or her untoward impulses into a destructive cycle. Structure locks the patient into relationships with other people in which mutuality is necessary. It forces him or her to experience the negative consequences of punishment.

There are also elements that can increase the likelihood than the biotype will be evoked: a premorbid proclivity toward risk-taking or antisocial behavior, a family that is tolerant of sociopathic role models, the use of alcohol or other drugs, lack of structure and guidance. The relationship then between frontal lobe lesions and sociopathic behavior requires an evolution of the condition, in concert with other events, internal and external.

Attention Deficit/Hyperactivity Disorder

The frontal lobe basis for ADHD has been established by clinical studies that have demonstrated striking similarities between patients with ADHD and patients with frontal lobe injury (14), by positron emission tomography studies that demonstrate frontal hypometabolism in patients with ADHD with correction of the deficit by psychostimulant drugs (45), and by pharmacologic studies that demonstrate similar therapeutic responses to the psychostimulants in patients with ADHD and in patients with frontal lobe injury (17). Children who sustain TBI to the frontal lobe develop a clinical syndrome that is identical to ADHD. This fact led to the original name of the syndrome: minimal brain damage. The functional systems that are disabled in ADHD and are inherent in the frontal lobes are the frontothalamoreticular arousal system that mediates tonic attention, the orbitomedial structures that recruit limbic input, subserving initiative and motivation, a complementary system that regulates and controls internal drive states, and a superordinate system that mediates goal-directed behavior by protecting the autonomy of executive functions.

The genesis of ADHD is usually not traumatic or acquired. The syndrome is familial, probably polygenetic (46). It is best understood as a dysmaturational disorder, a failure of attentional and self-regulatory mechanisms to develop at a normative rate. The threshold for phenotypic expression is mutative, relative to the social and educational demands that are placed on children and adolescents at a point in time. Therefore, it is hardly surprising that the past decade has seen a virtual explosion in the diagnosis and treatment of ADHD, especially in the United States. Our preoccupation with efficiency and productivity has led to an explosion in the adult diagnosis of ADHD as well.

Because clinical studies of ADHD date back more than 40 years, there has been ample opportunity to follow the children into adult life. The information from longitudinal studies is a telling commentary on the longitudinal course of a form of frontal lobe dysfunction. In essence, we have the opportunity to learn from a natural experiment, not from a small number of patients with lesions but from a vast number of patients with ADHD.

Like most of the important discoveries in medicine, the result of longitudinal studies of children with ADHD may be summarized in very clear, simple terms (47). A large number of children, perhaps one-third, actually becomes asymptomatic during adolescence. This represents in all probability the maturation of frontal lobe systems that were slow in developing but not necessarily defective. Another large number of children, perhaps one-third, remains symptomatic; with continued mild cognitive difficulties and some mild instability of behavioral control and emotional expression. They are not psychopathologic patients. They are diagnosed with adult ADHD and respond perfectly well to the psychostimulants (13).

The last one-third has a poorer outcome: the continuance of ADHD symptoms combined with a predisposition to psychopathology in general. The only specific conditions that occur in significant numbers, however, are the antisocial personality disorder and alcohol and substance abuse. This finding is consistent with the observation that the families of children with ADHD contain histrionic, sociopathic, and alcoholic individuals (46). (The fact that histrionic personality disorder does not occur in the ADHD follow-up studies is probably because of the preponderance of male subjects.)

The dramatic personality disorders, which include the antisocial and histrionic types, are characterized by dysregulation of the stress response, emotional instability, including dysphoria, anxiety, anger, impulsive and maladaptive behavior, and, as a result, disordered interpersonal relationships. These are all elements discussed in relation to frontal lobe disease. In fact, neuropsychological deficits that are characteristic of frontal lobe dysfunction have been reliably demonstrated in the dramatic personality disorders (48), but they are not simply a more complicated iteration of the frontal lobe syndrome that is ADHD. There is clearly something else at issue. It is proposed that a deficit in the functional system regulating experiential learning, the integration and assimilation of reinforcement, is central to the maladaptive behaviors of the personality disorders.

If we examine the predictors of adult psychopathology in the child with ADHD, it is not the severity of the initial symptoms but rather the occurrence of comorbid symptoms. For example, childhood aggression and familial antisocial behavior are the main predictors of adult sociopathy in children with ADHD (47). What leads to adult psychopathology are not the deficits in attention, motivation, behavioral inhibition, and executive function that characterize ADHD. It is the interaction with other predispositions, the involvement of multiple systems that creates the untoward result. To phrase this idea in terms of the functional systems of the frontal lobes: the pathophysiology of ADHD involves the systems listed above: attention-arousal, limbic recruitment in the service of motivation, inhibition of drive states, and superordinate, goal-directed behavior. The comorbidity of the personality disorders may be superimposed if the system that regulates the assimilation of reinforcement is also deranged.

The psychopathologic outcome of frontal lobe lesions is different, then, from the neurobehavioral sequelae. The latter are relatively circumscribed and more closely related to the known functions of the lesioned area. They may even be studied in primates. The transformation of a neurobehavioral proclivity, a biotype as it were, into a psychopathologic state involves the interaction of a large number of intervening variables, many of which are inherent to the patient, his or her premorbid weaknesses and proclivities, and many of which are external and thus are open to therapeutic manipulation.

Psychopathology may well be derived from a neurobehavioral lesion, but it also entails additional dimensions of the patient's internal life and environment. The development of psychopathology is an evolutionary process, not the inevitable outcome of a single lesion.

THE TEMPORAL LOBE SYNDROMES

The clinical elements associated with temporal lobe injury (or disease) are more variable and more diverse even than the frontal lobe syndromes. For that reason, we have been mercifully spared overarching theories of temporal lobe function. Different regions of the temporal lobes are responsible for specific functions: receptive language, memory, and emotional expression. When clinicians refer to the temporal lobe syndromes, they are usually talking about disorders of receptive language, some of the amnestic syndromes, and a number of emotional or functional psychiatric disorders.

If the temporal lobes are at all comparable with the frontal lobes, it is because of their associative function with respect to the high-level integration of sensory input. If there is a theoretical structure to be gleaned from the multiple functions of the temporal lobes, it is as an integrator of sensory input (including language), a comparator of new inputs to stored data, as a marker of the salience of new data (limbic tagging), and an activator of appropriate response modes. The behavioral pathology of temporal lobe disease is expressed, therefore, in terms of the faulty integration of sensory data that may be manifest as psychotic symptoms, faulty comparisons with information stored (and time coded) in memory that may be manifest as misperceptions or aberrant sensations (e.g., *déja vu*), and faults in salience marking and activation that are manifest as affective symptoms (e.g., anxiety, depression, mania, explosiveness).

The concept of a temporal lobe personality is ambiguous if not controversial. If there are two frontal lobe personalities, there are several residing in the temporal lobes. The best known is the interictal personality, said to be associated with temporal lobe epilepsy, and is dealt with extensively in the psychiatric literature (49); the same attributes may also be seen with temporal lobe lesions that do not give rise to overt seizures (50). Somatic preoccupations, even to frank hypochondriasis, may also be symptoms of temporal lobe disease (10). Then there are anxious, depressive, and explosive personalities.

Psychiatrists, like all people, tend to refer to personality types when some particular trait or constellation of traits is so predominant that other elements of the person are obscured. It is usually a form of shorthand, an abbreviated way of describing people, and an economical way of letting other clinicians know what they may expect from a patient. It is not particularly useful for understanding people, let alone how their brains work. One does better to consider the traits and elements of which they are composed.

Memory

Bilateral temporal lobe injuries around the anterior horn of the hippocampus are invariably associated with severe impairments of memory. Thus, in discussions of temporal lobe amnesia, it is customary to refer to the experiences of H.M., whose medial temporal lobes were excised in 1953 by Penfield to alleviate a particularly severe seizure disorder. H.M.'s seizures did, in fact, improve, but the patient has had a profound anterograde amnesia ever since. H.M. is able to recall events from his preoperative days but nothing since. It is said that every time he is told of the death of his beloved father, he grieves as if the information were new.

Although H.M. lost utterly the ability to acquire certain kinds of information, his capacity to learn has not been entirely lost. He cannot remember events from an hour ago, but he retains the ability to acquire new visuospatial skills. His memory impairment, the result of bilateral medial temporal lobe lesions, is limited to what neuropsychologists call explicit or declarative memory, the ability to recollect new events in one's life or new events in the world. What was left intact is implicit or procedural memory.

When clinicians speak of amnesia, they are usually referring to explicit memory, i.e., recall or recognition. Like H.M., patients with Alzheimer's disease are impaired in their ability to store and consciously recall words, facts (semantic memory), and life events (episodic memory). Their ability to learn procedural skills, like motor acts or puzzle solving, usually is left unimpaired. Patients with Parkinson's disease, conversely, have deficits in procedural memory, while explicit memory is spared. There is dissociation between the different forms of memory that reflects the functions of their anatomic substrates. This has been well established in clinical studies and has been replicated in primates and lower mammals. Explicit memory is a reflection of the work of the medial temporal lobes, thalami, septum, and other structures. Procedural or implicit memory is based in the neostriatum, emotional conditioning is based in the amygdala and neocortex, classic conditioning of the skeletal musculature in the cerebellum, and perceptual priming in the posterior neocortex (51,52).

The functional and neuroanatomic distinction among different forms of memory and learning has implications for diagnosis and treatment. The amnesia of TBI usually refers to explicit memory and is measured by tests of recall and recognition. The temporal lobes, of course, are especially vulnerable to closed head injury, and the amnesia of TBI is usually "patchy," meaning that some memories are successfully encoded and others are not. It is rarely "dense," like the amnesia of H.M., especially in patients with closed head injuries because their pathology is diffuse. Because surgeons seldom do bilateral medial lobe extirpations, the only dense amnesias that one encounters in clinical practice occur in demented patients with severe cortical pathology, in a few patients after encephalitis, and in patients with brain injury with diffuse cognitive impairment of the severest kind.

It is much more difficult to test the memory of a developmentally handicapped individual who has limited powers of speech and understanding, but memory impairment related to particular areas of cerebral damage is not uncommon. The unique pathology of the autistic person, for example, may be attributed to deficits in explicit memory and emotional conditioning. Both are suggestive of medial temporal lobe pathology. Because autistic people are not thought to have basal ganglia pathology, it is not surprising that their education almost invariably emphasizes procedural or habitual learning. That approach is not only anatomically correct but ontogenetically correct as well. Explicit memory has a clear maturational course, as one would expect in a function that is cortical in origin, whereas procedural learning, hard-wired in subcortical structures, shows no such maturational course (53).

Although educational approaches emphasizing the acquisition of motor skills and habitual associations are the hallmark of treatment for retarded people in general, and autistics in particular, the treatment of memory deficits in patients with TBI has tended to emphasize cognitive remediation techniques. The rationale is to strengthen what is left of the declarative memory system and to give the patient behavioral strategies to compensate for it. The approach is successful only to the degree that remnants of the system exist to be revived.

Drug Effects on Memory

Remnants of an injured memory system may be revived, at least to a degree, by pharmacologic interventions. The psychopharmacology of memory, however, is not especially well advanced. Because it is as economical to measure declarative memory as it is complicated to measure implicit memory or emotional conditioning, little is known about the relative effects of the various drugs on the different forms of learning and memory. It is ironic that we know more about drugs that impair memory than we do about the memory enhancers.

If little is known about drug effects on the different forms of memory, even less is understood about drug effects on the specific biologic processes that underlie the formation of memory, for example, on long-term potentiation. On a molecular level, the encoding of a memory trace—the engram, as Lashley called it—relies on a series of events. The process begins with the binding of neurotransmitters to receptor molecules, release of second messengers, activation of protein kinases and early intermediate genes, protein synthesis, and ultimately leads to the creation of a hebbian web of synaptic connections wherein presumably resides the engram (54). The hippocampus, where the process begins, is also one of two areas in the adult brain that is routinely given to neuroneogenesis.

It is possible that the effects of the benzodiazepines on memory have been studied more than the effects of any other class of drugs because they are prescribed so frequently and their negative effects on the memory process are so important. The benzodiazepines augment the actions of γ-aminobutyric acid (GABA), the major inhibitory neurotransmitter of brain. The benzodiazepine receptor forms a macromolecular complex with the $GABA_A$ receptor and the chloride ionophore. As it happens, the highest densities of the $GABA_A$-benzodiazepine receptor complex are located in structures that are most involved in the formation of the memory trace (e.g., thalamus, hippocampus, septum). This pattern of localization is consistent with the benzodiazepine effect on explicit (as opposed to procedural) memory (55).

The negative memory effects of the neuroleptic drugs are tricky to measure because one has to control for the confound of neuroleptic-induced motor impairment in normal subjects and the improvement in attention, organization, and cooperation that occurs in psychotic patients after they are treated with neuroleptics. One would predict a negative effect on procedural learning from the dopamine antagonists similar to what is experienced by patients with Parkinson's disease.

In contrast to the benzodiazepines, amphetamine exercises a positive effect on learning and memory (14). The amphetamine effect is more consistently demonstrated in studies of laboratory animals in paradigms that measure procedural learning, but they are also observed in humans in semantic memory tests. The actions of psychostimulants are mediated in all likelihood by the monoamine neurotransmitters. Insofar as they are dopamine agonists, their effect on procedural memory should be the opposite of that of the neuroleptics.

After TBI, temporal lobe amnesia is usually complicated by a component of inattention, which is frontal or axial rather than temporal. This has an important bearing of the psychopharmacology of memory in patients with brain injury. When psychostimulants are effective for the patient with amnesia, it may simply be an attentional effect that strengthens the encoding process. The stimulants, however, are also known to affect the consolidation of long-term memory in animals as well as in humans, a direct effect on explicit memory (56).

The acetylcholinesterase inhibitors, such as galanthamine, tetrahydroaminoacridine, and donepezil, are known to improve explicit memory in patients with brain injury or dementia. There is substantive evidence that the cholinergic system is the primary neuromediator of memory (e.g., administration of scopolamine produces memory impairment in healthy individuals, an effect that is attenuated by physostigmine). Patients with Alzheimer's disease have significant neuronal atrophy in areas of the basal forebrain (the septal nuclei, nuclei of the diagonal band of Broca, and nucleus basalis of Meynert) that contribute extensive cholinergic innervation to medical temporal lobe structures such as the hippocampus and amygdala (57).

The effects of antidepressants and mood stabilizers on signal transduction pathways and hippocampal plasticity are interesting and potentially important, but as yet unproven, at least as far as memory is concerned. This important topic is discussed in Chapters 19 and 20. It is arguable that the natural course of the major affective disorders is complicated by a degree of cognitive decay and that effective treatment averts this consequence. In certain circumstances, however, antidepressants and mood stabilizers may have a negative effect on memory.

Affective Instability

Emotional instability is a central element of some temporal lobe syndromes. Patients with temporal lobe injuries are prone to the full range of anxiety disorders: extreme emotionalism or pseudobulbar affect to explosive rage attacks to affective and schizophreniform psychoses (58–61).

When early neurosurgeons operated to alleviate intractable temporal lobe epilepsy, they sometimes went as far back as the anterior hippocampus; had they gone further, they would have reproduced the experiment of Klüver and Bucy (62). Monkeys with bilateral temporal lobectomies involving the amygdala appear to be incapable of mounting an emotional response to any circumstance, and their day is passed in bland endeavors, especially stereotyped activity such as mouthing and self-stimulation. Klüver-Bucy syndrome is occasionally seen in patients with severe TBI during the coma-recovery period. Partial Klüver-Bucy syndrome, a grossly incapacitating condition with symptoms that resemble those of autism, may persist in some patients.

Rather than emotional indifference or "psychic blindness," the patient with temporal lobe injury is usually given to excess of emotional expression, for example, uncontrollable rage attacks, sudden unprovoked episodes of crying or laughing (emotional incontinence), or sudden changes in mood (emotional lability). The psychiatrists sometimes use the term intermittent explosive disorder, and neurologists prefer the term "episodic dyscontrol." After aphasia, it is probably the most common behavioral manifestation of temporal lobe injury and certainly the most dramatic, with significant forensic and interpersonal aspects. The animal model for episodic dyscontrol is a lesion in the septum or amygdala: two deep temporal nuclei that are usually included as part of the limbic brain.

The traditional treatment for episodic dyscontrol is carbamazepine, and alternatives are valproic acid, lithium, lamotrigine, beta-blockers, and, more recently, the serotonergic antidepressants. Buspirone is an occasional augmenter. It is not a difficult disorder to treat as long as the patient is compliant with treatment.

Patients with lesions of the orbital surface of the frontal lobe may also be prone to episodes of violent rage, and the distinction between patients with frontal and temporal lobe damage may not always be made based on the topography of the behavior. Rather, the correlates of the behavior and the results of neurodiagnostic and neuropsychological testing are required to localize the source. However, closed head injury is usually associated with damage to both areas of brain.

Major affective disorders frequently arise in patients with temporal lobe injury, although there is disagreement whether they are more likely to occur in right (59) or left (63) temporal lobe lesions. In fact, it is likely that the anterior region of both hemispheres plays a role in the expression of affective symptoms (64). The affective disorders that occur after TBI may be either unipolar or bipolar and are virtually indistinguishable from the functional affective disorders that psychiatrists contend with all the time. In fact, affective disorders arising from temporal lobe lesions are probably the only neurobehavioral consequence of TBI that is indistinguishable from the conventional psychiatric condition.

The treatment of affective disorders after TBI is usually the same as one would prescribe for a conventional psychiatric disorder, and antidepressants and mood stabilizers are usually effective. One may be more inclined to consider a dopamine agonist or stimulant to treat anergic depression; virtually all the tricyclics may have negative effects on motor performance (17), and some of the anticholinergic antidepressants may impair memory performance (65). Bupropion would be an ideal antidepressant for patients with TBI were it not for its ability to lower the seizure threshold; that side effect, however, may well be overstated because most antidepressants have the same effect. The serotonergic antidepressants are, as a consequence, enjoying primacy among psychiatrists who treat patients with TBI.

Lithium is a drug that may impair motor performance, and it is said to slow the speed of mental processing (66,67). Carbamazepine, valproate, lamotrigine, or gabapentin may be a better choice for the patient with TBI who is bipolar.

Anxiety and Panic

Positron emission tomography scans of patients with panic disorder have shown areas of hypermetabolism in the temporal poles during a panic attack (68). This does not prove, of course, that the temporal lobes are the locus of anxiety or panic, but the fact that anterior temporal lesions are sometimes associated with anxiety and panic strengthens the case.

There is an anecdotal footnote to the association of $GABA_A$ receptor density in the temporal lobes to the presumably unrelated problems of amnesia and anxiety: H.M. was thought to have a number of attributes associated with temporal lobe pathology, such as hyposexuality. At times, he was also said to describe "feelings of apprehension to which it is difficult for others to assign a cause" (69). Anxiety, like amnesia, is a sign of temporal lobe disease. The GABA-mimetic benzodiazepines are, in a sense, temporal lobe drugs. They may depress the expression of anxiety but at the expense sometimes of depressing the formation of explicit memory.

Psychosis

Flor-Henry (59) is identified with the attribution of schizophreniform psychosis to left temporal lobe injury. This observation, however, has been superseded by subsequent descriptions of the psychosis of temporal lobe epilepsy; although the association between a left temporal focus and schizophrenia may well be correct, at least statistically; a unilateral temporal lesion will likely kindle a mirror focus long before psychotic symptoms develop. The psychosis of temporal lobe epilepsy, furthermore, is not identical to typical schizophrenia; negative symptoms are less likely to occur—a relative sparing of the ego, and the patient will usually show additional features suggestive of the interictal personality of temporal lobe epilepsy. The delusions and hallucinations, for example, are more commonly religious in nature, and the patient may be prone to typical rage outbursts and violent behavior. The treatment of the psychosis of temporal lobe epilepsy is primarily with an anticonvulsant such as carbamazepine or valproic acid, and only secondarily with low doses of a high-potency neuroleptic, such as fluphenazine or pimozide, which will not lower the seizure threshold as much as the other neuroleptics. It is not uncommon for psychotic patients with temporal lobe injury to develop depressive symptoms, which, in turn, require specific antidepressant therapy. These depressive episodes are not always prevented by treatment with thymoleptic drugs.

Sexuality

Hyposexuality is a typical temporal lobe symptom. I have seen several patients with TBI with mixed temporal and frontal lobe syndromes with disinhibition and sexually explicit language combined with hyposexuality and absolute disinterest in acting on the consequences of their leering insinuations.

I was once called to consult on behalf of a middle-aged man who had sustained severe temporal and frontal lobe damage in a motor vehicle crash. He had been a Nashville policeman who was in pursuit of a criminal when his squad car was struck broadside by a city garbage truck. The city of Nashville was committed to this man's rehabilitation, and no expense was spared to find the best services money could buy.

He had a preoccupation with sex and talked about nothing else. He wandered off at every opportunity toward downtown where he intended to find a woman of the night on Music City Row. Finally, desperate to suppress this preoccupation and willing to go any length to gain his cooperation with rehabilitation, the staff at the home where he was living resolved to satisfy his desires. They even found one of his old girlfriends who was willing to make the ultimate sacrifice on behalf of his recovery.

Their assignation was uneventful. Our patient was polite and solicitous but as disinterested in the act as he had been preoccupied with its pursuit. However, this epiphany had no lasting effect on his rambling and preoccupations, just on our notion how to treat it. He responded to a slight increase in his dose of carbamazepine.

The sexual dysfunction associated with selective serotonin reuptake inhibitors is either a loss of erectile competence, which is responsive to sildenafil, or loss of libido, which is not. The sexual dysfunction of temporal lobe patients reveals that disorders of libido itself may be sub-divided into two components. Patients on selective serotonin reuptake inhibitors can experience an absolute loss of interest in sexuality. Patients with temporal lobe lesions and some patients with frontal lobe damage can retain a preoccupation with sex but lose all interest in the actual sexual act.

The Interictal Personality

The interictal personality of patients with temporal lobe epilepsy, and the development of posttraumatic temporal lobe psychosis are dealt with at length in Chapters 8 and 17. It is appropriate to emphasize at this juncture, however, that epilepsy is not the primary mediating event in the development of personality traits or symptoms that have been traditionally described in association with temporal lobe epilepsy.

Aphasia

The treatment of aphasia is rarely discussed in terms of drug effects. The recent literature alludes to occasional success with bromocriptine or other dopamine agonists in patients who have posttraumatic aphasia after severe injuries, a subject that is reviewed in Chapter 18. Attention is also given to the apparent success of amphetamine at enhancing motor recovery, including speech, after stroke (70).

It was reported that propanolol improved communication in a small group of stroke patients (71), which is interesting because psychiatrists often use propanolol for the emotional volatility and behavioral instability that sometimes accompanies Broca's aphasia. It is one of the few conditions that, in my experience, responds favorably to beta-blockers.

Impairment of communication characterizes chronic schizophrenia, a negative symptom of the disease, and autism, in which it is a primary symptom. In both cases, it is said that communication is enhanced after treatment with *N*-methylglycine, an amino acid (72). Conversely, virtually any psychotropic drug or anticonvulsant may enhance communication in a patient whose clinical state is compromised by recurrent seizures or psychiatric illness. It cannot be said that there is a specific drug to enhance communication or restore language to the aphasic patient. One is probably dealing with nonspecific effects that are secondary to improvement in the patient's general state.

THE BASAL GANGLIA

If the basal ganglia are taken to include the thalamus and other nearby structures, they represent a little brain that does almost everything the cortex does, although with less elaboration or proficiency. There are animals that manage with no more than a striate cortex. Even the rat has only a thin layer of cortical mantle overlying its basal ganglia. It is arguable that children are striatal organisms; the executive functions that they have are mediated by their basal ganglia (see below).

Therefore, we never speak of a striatal syndrome to capture the signs and deficits of a striatal lesion. Rather, we have a long list of deficits and signs that are hard to assemble into syndromic terms because they never co-occur and are hard to attribute to the basal ganglia because they are not unique to the basal ganglia.

Traumatic hemorrhage of the basal ganglia is observed in approximately 3% of severe CHIs. It can occur in isolation or in association with other more common consequences of brain trauma, such as diffuse axonal injury, cortical contusion, or subdural or epidural hematoma. It can happen after moderate traumatic injuries with brief loss of consciousness or after severe injuries with prolonged coma. In the former instance, patient outcome may be quite good, with few lasting sequelae. The clinical manifestations include motor deficits contralateral to the lesion; muteness, hypophonia, aphasia, and apraxia with left-sided lesions; and left neglect, visuospatial impairment, flat affect, anosognosia, and motor impersistence with right-sided lesions. Inattention and mental slowing are common findings (73).

Injury to the structures of the basal ganglia occurs more commonly as the result of toxic exposure (e.g., carbon monoxide), electrocution, or cerebral anoxia. Although intelligence is often intact, neuropsychological deficits are seen in attention, memory (especially procedural memory), processing speed, perseveration, and mental flexibility. Spontaneous activity is restricted but improves greatly when stimulated by the examiner. Perseverance is diminished in the face of a difficult task. Neurologic signs are not prominent, although some patients may have tics or parkinsonian findings. Affect is severely constricted, and depression is not uncommon. Obsessions, compulsions, tourettisms, and motor stereotypies occur in many patients (74).

Bilateral calcification of the basal ganglia may be familial or related to other causes including birth trauma, carbon monoxide or lead intoxication, radiation, long-term anticonvulsant therapy, and infectious and inflammatory diseases. Sometimes it is a serendipitous finding on the computed tomography scan, with little in the way of pathologic correlates. When it is the manifestation of a hereditary condition, neuropsychiatric disorders such as dementia, epilepsy, and extrapyramidal symptoms often coexist, but it is less clear that calcifications that are occasional findings have any special neuropsychiatric significance beyond the effects of the primary condition that caused them (75).

The cognitive deficits associated with basal ganglia calcifications are those of subcortical dementia: executive dysfunction, slowed information processing, motor programming, memory, and visuospatial skills. The pattern of neuropsychological deficit has a frontal lobe quality that is explained by the disruption of prefrontal-subcortical loops that characterizes virtually all the striatal conditions. Affective disorders and obsessive-compulsive disorders are the psychiatric conditions most often spoken of in connection with basal ganglia calcification, although other conditions, such as paranoia, have been noted (76,77).

Caudate infarcts also have typical but far-ranging clinical manifestations: contralateral weakness that is usually mild or transient, occasional hyperreflexia and dysarthria, and most notably cognitive and behavioral abnormalities. The most frequent behavioral abnormality is abulia (decreased spontaneity, motor and cognitive slowing, and impersistence). Hyperactivity, restlessness, agitation, disinhibition, euphoria, and confusion occur almost as frequently, sometimes alternating with abulia. There may be psychiatric symptoms, such as depression, anxiety, paranoia, hallucinations, and manic depression. Deficits in executive function, memory, and attention are very common. Contralateral neglect occurs with right-sided infarcts (78,79).

All the clinical findings associated with damage to the basal ganglia are contained quite naturally in the clinical pathology of Parkinson's disease and Huntington's chorea, the prototypic striatal diseases. The pathologic conditions of the striate cortex virtually contain the cannon of psychopathology. Yet schizophrenia, anxiety, and manic-depression are not considered striatal diseases. When we think of psychiatric disorders that originate in the basal ganglia, we think of obsessions, compulsions, tics, and stereotypies and the disorders that they delimit.

Obsessions, compulsions, tics, and stereotypies represent the inappropriate expression of cognitive or motor programs that are intrinsic to the basal ganglia and that are normally inhibited or appropriately directed by cortical inputs. Lesions of the basal ganglia interfere with highly stereotyped and species-specific integrated displays or fixed-action patterns. The striatum also seems to be involved in the execution of overlearned automatic behaviors. The motor patterns and automatic behaviors expressed in psychiatric conditions such as Tourette's syndrome, obsessive-compulsive disorder, and autism also occur with lesions of the basal ganglia and suggest that striatal pathology is central to the manifestations of those conditions (80). The drugs that are used to treat Tourette's syndrome, obsessive-compulsive disorder, and autism (dopaminergics, antidopaminergics, serotonergics, *N*-methyl-D-aspartate antagonists) are appropriate to use for Parkinson's disease, Huntington's chorea, and all the conditions associated with injury or degeneration of the basal ganglia.

The anatomy, chemistry, and connectivity of the basal ganglia are well preserved in all amniotes (birds, reptiles, mammals). In all amniotes, these factors play a key role in the control of movement (specifically, promoting desired movement and suppressing unwanted movement) (81). There also exists a level of phylogenetic development in which the striatum is the highest formation of the brain. Such species are able to display variable behavior possessing a variety of capacities and functions. The behavior of a totally decorticated animal with the striatum preserved is much better organized than that of a thalamic preparation and in simple situations is almost indistinguishable from that of normal animals. Respective cortical and striatal regions are discovered to subserve the same function, although not necessarily with the same proficiency (82). The striatum also seems to be involved in the sparing of cortical function so that those behavioral deficits resulting from cortical damage are not demonstrable in the adult if the damage is incurred in infancy. It may be assumed that in the young animal, the striatum has functions that it loses as the cortex develops (83).

The simple motor and behavioral programs that are elicited in Tourette's syndrome and obsessive-compulsive disorder are elements contained in the phylogenetically ancient basal ganglia, as are the fragmentary motor programs that characterize chorea. They are released in response to certain pathologies and suppressed by others. The defects in procedural memory that result from striatal lesions or disease represent an inability to develop new motor programs, a deficit in habitual learning, but the fact that the neurocognitive and motor deficits associated with basal ganglia lesions usually subside with time reflects the redundancy of striatal systems with the higher cortices and the organism's capacity to shift functions from the striatum to the cortex in response to injury, just as it does during the course of development.

The Child as a Striatal Organism

The fully developed but prepubertal child, age 10 or 11 years, is one of the supreme creations of nature, and a walking example of the extraordinary capacities of the corpus striatum. He or she has developed a full range of adaptive behaviors and is fully capable of independent action, even in complicated, modern societies. He or she has mastered the skills of reading and calculation—arts that it has taken the species a thousand centuries to develop—and can use those skills to master new, more complicated endeavors. He or she understands social relationships and builds his or her own social structures, which are sometimes extraordinarily subtle and complex, and does it all with good cheer, deference to his or her elders, and a moral sense that is sometimes painful to the adults they live with. Moralistic may be an appropriate word for it.

Then, it all goes to hell. My patients and friends usually attribute the change to "hormones."

In fact, the prepubertal child is largely operating on the basis of striatal functions. The striatum is capable of subserving a wide range of sophisticated behaviors that are largely procedural, what one might call social learning. Like the lower mammals and birds, the child is able to perform adequately in a social environment, to master its rules, and to use them in creative ways. He or she has the opportunity for extensive elaboration. The transition, however, is not entirely seamless, and there is ample opportunity for instability and misdirection. Thus, the docile and moralistic child becomes a surly and provocative adolescent.

In the experiments alluded to previously, like the delayed-response paradigm, an immature primate can learn to master the task, using, it is presumed, only its striatum to learn it. If it is then subjected to frontal lobe ablations, it retains its mastery of the task. If the frontal lesion is applied, however, after it has passed puberty, it loses its mastery. After puberty, the substrate for performing the task has been transferred, as it were, to the frontal lobes. If the frontal cortex never develops because of a lesion, the skill resides in the striatum where it originated. An adult primate with a frontal lobe lesion can never learn to master the task, even though its striatum is intact and fully functional. As the primate matures, the frontal lobe takes over certain functions that were originally the domain of the basal ganglia.

Thus, it is with children and adolescents. In the interest of acquiring the expanded capacities of the mature human being, they are subjected to a redistribution of function from the corpus striatum to the frontal lobes. In the long run, this works to the better. In the short run, important social functions are being transferred from a competent striatum to an immature frontal cortex. The transition is sometimes unstable.

THE THALAMUS

Lesions of the thalamus are associated with dementia, amnesia, or aphasia. Thalamic lesions may cause behavioral disorders, including psychosis, mania, depression, and a variant of the frontal lobe syndrome. So-called central pain syndromes do not always involve the thalamic nuclei but often do. Thalamic injury is usually a consequence of stroke or tumors or chronic alcohol toxicity and it is uncommon for a circumscribed injury to the thalamus to occur after TBI. Thalamic hemorrhage after TBI is not a rare event either.

Even a small thalamic lesion may affect the function of remote cortical, subcortical, or cerebellar regions, with which the thalamus has extensive connections. It is the most important subcortical relay center for exteroceptive and proprioceptive stimuli and plays a fundamental role in the integration and coordination of information going to the cerebral cortex. It is also an essential part of the ascending reticular activating system and the limbic system; it has important connections to the basal ganglia and receives input from the cerebellum. Therefore, it is not surprising that metabolic depression is observed in diverse regions of brain (by positron emission tomography) after small thalamic lesions. The distribution of the metabolic depression is determined by the location of the thalamic lesion (84). The frontal lobe syndrome that sometimes accompanies a thalamic lesion is probably a manifestation of diaschisis.

Dejerine and Roussy first described thalamic syndrome in 1906, and it is sometimes referred to as Dejerine's syndrome. Thalamic pain syndrome is another term by which it is known, but it is not invariably associated with an identifiable lesion of the thalamus (85). It arises after a variable length of time has elapsed after an insult to the thalamus, and as sensation begins to recover, the patient develops pain and hyperpathia on the side contralateral to the lesion. In patients with TBI, the problem is often bilateral. The pain is spontaneous or else provoked by external stimuli that one would ordinarily not consider noxious. It is usually constant but may be paroxysmal. The quality is often described as an unfamiliar disagreeable sensation, like paresthesia, formication, gnawing, crushing, burning, or freezing (86).

Patients with TBI with elements of thalamic syndrome are almost never able to actually describe their experience of pain and dysesthesia because there are usually cognitive and linguistic deficits as well. Like Klüver-Bucy syndrome after TBI, it is most commonly observed during the coma-recovery phase, when the patient is confused and disoriented as well as dysesthetic. This may complicate the problem of diagnosis. A typical manifestation after TBI is a patient at Rancho level 3 or 4 who reacts intensely and in the most negative way to any new stimulus: a noise, the physical touch of attendants or therapists, or the mere approach of another individual. The patient may scream, utter obscenities, or lash out physically. The provocative stimulus may be the approach of any new person, although the patient can sometimes tolerate the proximity of a familiar attendant.

The appropriate treatment for such a problem when it occurs in a coma-recovery patient is simple. Minimize stimulation, rely on familiar faces and familiar stimuli, and introduce new things slowly and gradually. Wait for the problem to pass, as it usually does.

The treatment of central pain syndromes in general, or of thalamic syndrome in particular, usually involves an antidepressant or anticonvulsant drug. The rationale for the use of analgesic anticonvulsants such as carbamazepine, phenytoin, and valproate is entirely empirical, but it may speak to the irritative nature of the mechanism of central pain. The new antiepileptic drug gabapentin is winning strong support among practitioners who treat patients with chronic pain syndromes, although very high doses are sometimes needed.

The alternative mechanism is related to disinhibition because it has been established that serotonergic projections from the dorsal raphe to the intralaminar nucleus of the thalamus are responsible for the inhibition of nociceptive neurotransmission (87), which may explain the utility of serotonergic antidepressants such as amitriptyline for dysesthesia. In a recent study, in fact, amitriptyline was found to be more effective than carbamazepine for the control of post-stroke pain (85). It appears that the other serotonergic antidepressants are as effective as amitriptyline, at least in some patients (88).

There is a small class of patients who exhibits a total lack of spontaneous activity at rest and extremely intense symptoms only under stimulation. One such patient, described by Bakchine et al. (89), was described as hypersyntonic, referring to an exacerbated, immediate apprehension of the external world, with immediate reaction associated with difficulty in apprehending the relative salience of stimuli. This may also be described as hypervigilance with intense hyperreactivity. One such patient had manic symptoms under stimulation, with bilateral orbitofrontal lesions and right temporoparietal injury (89). Another patient, with similar symptoms, had a circumscribed right thalamic infarct (90). Disinhibition, loss of selectivity, irritability, and lack of initiative and perseveration, ordinarily thought to be signs of frontal lobe injury, are not unknown in association with thalamic lesions as a consequence of disruption of frontal lobe projections, especially from the dorsomedian nucleus (90). Bakchine et al. (89) described successful treatment with clonidine. I have used the combination of beta-blockers and clonidine. Amantadine is another alternative.

Affective disturbance is not uncommon after thalamic infarction and usually takes the form of apathy, lack of initiative, and irritability. In some patients, this state may alternate with periods of agitation, psychosis, or overt mania, and secondary mania has been described after several different kinds of thalamic lesions (91,92). The dorsomedial nucleus of the thalamus is a relay between the frontal and temporal cortices and the subcortical structures of the limbic system, especially the hypothalamus. It is possible, however, that the relay also regulates the effectiveness or gain of its neuronal connections, a role that may be mediated by the voltage-sensitive conductance of the *N*-methyl-D-aspartate receptor (93). An irritative lesion in the thalamus, therefore, might amplify the gain of cortical or sensory input to limbic structures; thus, the hyperreactivity of mania or explosive behavior.

In at least two cases studies, secondary mania caused by a thalamic lesion alternated with periods of hypersomnolence (91,94). The thalamus does play a central role in the regulation of the sleep-wake cycle. A lesion of the thalamus will rob the hypothalamus and brainstem structures of inhibitory cortical control and thus derange the endocrine and autonomic homeostasis that derives from a normal circadian rhythm. Thalamic degeneration has been observed in cases of fatal familial insomnia (95). Dysregulation of the sleep-wake cycle is, of course, characteristic of manic depression as well as Klein-Levin syndrome.

The thalamic gating system enables conscious, directed behavior. It appears to be under the influence of ascending reticular projections and descending impulses from the frontal cortex. Thus, afferent and efferent impulses can be integrated, interpreted, and used to control sensory pathways. Pathology in this system results in disorders of more complex behaviors, such as planning, selection of behavior, and monitoring of performance (7).

REFERENCES

1. von Monakow C. "Diaschisis," localization in the cerebrum and functional impairment by cortical loci (1914). In: Pribram KH, ed. *Brain and behavior, volume I*. Baltimore: Penguin, 1969:27–36.
2. Halstead WC. *Brain and intelligence: a quantitative study of the frontal lobes*. Chicago: University of Chicago Press, 1947.
3. Goldstein K. The significance of the frontal lobes for mental performances. *J Neurol Psychopathol* 1936;17:27.
4. Luria AR. *Higher cortical functions in man*, 2nd ed. New York: Basic Books, 1977.
5. Damasio A. The frontal lobes. In: Heilman K, Valenstein E, eds. *Clinical neuropsychology*. New York: Oxford University Press, 1979:360–412.
6. Mesulam MM. Frontal cortex and behavior. *Ann Neurol* 1986;19:320–325.
7. Stuss DT, Benson DF. *The frontal lobes*. New York: Raven Press, 1986.
8. Berg EA. A simple objective test for measuring flexibility in thinking. *J Gen Psychol* 1948;39:15–22.
9. Stroop JR. Studies of interference in serial verbal reactions. *J Exp Psychol* 1935;18:643–662.
10. Lezak MD. *Neuropsychological assessment*, 2nd ed. New York: Oxford University Press, 1983.
11. Bakchine S, Chain F, Lhermitte F. Syndrome de Kluver-Bucy humain complet apres une encephalite a herpes simplex type 2. *Rev Neurol* 1986;142:126–132.
12. Plum F, Posner JB. *The diagnosis of stupor and coma*, 3rd ed. Philadelphia: FA Davis, 1980.
13. Gualtieri CT, Hicks RE. The neuropharmacology of methylphenidate and a neural substrate of childhood hyperactivity. *Psychiatr Clin North Am* 1985;8:875–892.
14. Evans RW, Amara I, Gualtieri CT. Methylphenidate and memory: dissociated effects in hyperactive children. *Psychopharmacology* 1986;90:211–216.
15. Zametkin AJ, Nordahl TE, Gross M. Cerebral glucose metabolism in adults with hyperactivity of childhood onset. *N Engl J Med* 1990;323:1361–1366.
16. Ernst M, Zametkin A, Matochik J, et al. Presynaptic dopaminergic deficits in Lesch-Nyhan disease. *N Engl J Med* 1996;334:1568–1572.
17. Gualtieri CT, Evans RW. Stimulant treatment for the neurobehavioral sequelae of traumatic brain injury. *Brain Inj* 1988;2:273–290.
18. Jacobsen CF. Studies of cerebral function in primates: I. The functions of the frontal association areas in monkeys. *Comprehens Psychol Monogr* 1936;13:3–60.
19. Stamm JS. The riddle of the monkey's delayed-response deficit has been solved. In: Perecman E, ed. *The frontal lobes revisited*. Hillsdale: Lawrence Erlbaum, 1987.
20. Teuber HL. The riddle of frontal lobe function in man. In: Warren JM, Akert K, eds. *The frontal granular cortex and behavior*. New York: McGraw-Hill, 1964:410–444.
21. Sperry RW. Neural basis of the spontaneous optokinetic response produced by visual inversion. *J Comp Physiol Psychol* 1950;43:417–429.
22. Denny-Brown D. The frontal lobes and their function. In: Freiling A, ed. *Modern trends in neurology*. London: Butterworth, 1951:13–89.
23. Young AW, Robertson IH, Hellawell DJ, et al. Cotard delusion after brain injury. *Psychol Med* 1992;22: 799–804.
24. Goldstein K. The mental changes due to frontal lobe damage. *J Psychol* 1944;17:187–208.
25. Heilman K, Valenstein E. *Clinical neuropsychology*. New York: Oxford University Press, 1979.
26. Fuster JM. *The prefrontal cortex*, 2nd ed. New York: Raven Press, 1989.
27. Blumer D, Benson DF. Personality changes with frontal and temporal lobe lesions. In: Benson DF, Blumer D, eds. *Psychiatric aspects of neurologic disease*. New York: Grune & Stratton, 1975:151–169.
28. Bekhterev VM. *Fundamentals of brain function*. St. Petersburg: The St. Petersburg Psychoneurological Research Institute, 1907.
29. Luria AR. The frontal lobes and the regulation of behavior. In: Pribram KH, Luria AR, eds. *Psychophysiology of the frontal lobes*. New York: Academic Press, 1973:3–28.
30. Sauerland EJ, Clemente CD. The role of the brain stem in orbital cortex induced inhibition of somatic reflexes. In: Pribram KH, Luria AR, eds. *Psychophysiology of the frontal lobes*. New York: Academic Press, 1973.
31. Grueninger W, Grueninger J. The primate frontal cortex and allassostasis. In: Pribram KH, Luria AR, eds. *Psychophysiology of the frontal lobes*. New York: Academic Press, 1973:253–292.
32. Pribram KH, Luria AR. *Psychophysiology of the frontal lobes*. New York: Academic Press, 1973.
33. Andreasen N, Nasrallah HA, Dunn V, et al. Structural abnormalities in the frontal system in schizophrenia. *Arch Gen Psychiatry* 1986;43:136–144.
34. Machlin SR, Harris GH, Pearlson GD, et al. Elevated medial-frontal cerebral blood flow in obsessive-compulsive patients: a SPECT study. *Am J Psychiatry* 1991; 148:1240–1242.
35. Coffey CE, Wilkinson WE, Weiner RD, et al. Quantitative cerebral anatomy in depression. *Arch Gen Psychiatry* 1993;50:7–16.
36. Ross ED, Stewart RM. Akinetic mutism from hypothalamic damage: successful treatment with dopamine agonists. *Neurology* 1981;31:1435–1439.
37. Gualtieri CT, Chandler M, Coons T, et al. Amantadine: a new clinical profile for traumatic brain injury. *Clin Neuropharmacol* 1989;12:258–270.
38. Prigatano GP, Schacter DL. *Awareness of deficit after brain injury*. New York: Oxford University Press, 1991.
39. LeVere ND, Gray-Silva S, Levere TE. Infant brain recovery: the benefit of relocation and the cost of crowding. In: Finger S, Levere TE, Almli CR, et al., eds. *Brain injury and recovery*. New York: Plenum, 1988: 133–150.
40. Stevens JR, Livermore A. Kindling of the mesolimbic dopamine system: animal model of psychosis. *Neurology* 1978;28:36–46.

41. Hare RD, Quinn MJ. Psychopathy and autonomic conditioning. *J Abnormal Psychol* 1971;77:223–235.
42. Denckla MB, Heilman KM. The syndrome of hyperactivity. In: Heilman KM, Valenstein E, eds. *Clinical neuropsychology*. New York: Oxford University Press, 1979:574–597.
43. Lykken DT. A study of anxiety in the sociopathic personality. *J Abnorm Social Psychol* 1957;55:6–10.
44. Pribram KH. The primate frontal cortex—executive of the brain. In: Pribram KH, Luria AR, eds. *Psychophysiology of the frontal lobes*. New York: Academic Press, 1973:293–314.
45. Giannini AJ, Houser WL, Louiselle RH, et al. Antimanic effects of verapamil. *Am J Psychiatry* 1984;141: 1602–1603.
46. Morrison JR, Stewart MA. Bilateral inheritance as evidence for polygenicity in the hyperactive child syndrome. *J Nerv Ment Dis* 1974;158:226–228.
47. Weiss G, Hechtman LT. Hyperactive children grown up. New York: Guilford, 1986.
48. Burgess JW. Neurocognitive impairment in dramatic personalities: histrionic, borderline, and antisocial disorders. *Psychiatry Res* 1992;42:283–290.
49. Bear DM, Fedio P. Quantitative analysis of interictal behavior in temporal lobe epilepsy. *Arch Neurol* 1977;34: 454–467.
50. Barnhill LJ, Gualtieri CT. Late-onset psychosis after closed head injury. *Neuropsychiatry Neuropsychol Behav Neurol* 1989;2:211–218.
51. Knowlton BJ, Mangels JA, Squire LR. A neostriatal habit learning system in humans. *Science* 1996;273: 1399–1400.
52. Robbins TW. Refining the taxonomy of memory. *Science*, 1996;273:1353–1354.
53. Homberg V, Bickmann U, Muller K. Ontogeny is different for explicit and implicit memory in humans. *Neurosci Lett* 1993;150:187–190.
54. Rosenzweig MR, Bennett EL, Colombo PJ, et al. Short-term, intermediate-term, and long-term memories. *Behav Brain Res* 1993;57:193–198.
55. Ghoneim MM, Mewaldt SP. Benzodiazepines and human memory: a review. *Anesthesiology* 1990;72:926–938.
56. Evans RW, Gualtieri CT, Patterson DR. Treatment of chronic closed head injury with psychostimulant drugs: a controlled case study and an appropriate evaluation procedure. *J Nerv Ment Dis* 1987;175:106–110.
57. Morris MK, Bowers D, Chatterjee A, et al. Amnesia following a discrete basal forebrain lesion. *Brain* 1992; 115:1827–1847.
58. Delgado-Escueta AV, Mattson RH, King L. The nature of aggression during epileptic seizures. *N Engl J Med* 1981;305:711–716.
59. Flor-Henry P. On certain aspects of the localization of the cerebral systems regulating and determining emotions. *Biol Psychiatry* 1979;14:677–698.
60. Mellow AM, Sunderland T, Cohen RM, et al. Acute effects of high-dose thyrotropin releasing hormone infusions in Alzheimer's disease *Psychopharmacology (Berl)* 1989;98:403–407.
61. Krauthammer C, Klerman GL. Secondary mania: manic syndromes associated with antecedent physical illness or drugs. *Arch Gen Psychiatry* 1978;35: 1333–1338.
62. Kluver H, Bucy PC. "Psychic blindness" and other symptoms following temporal lobectomy in rhesus monkey. *Am J Physiol* 1937;119:352–353.
63. Robinson RG, Starr LB, Kubos KL, et al. A two-year longitudinal study of post-stroke mood disorders: findings during the initial evaluation. *Stroke* 1983;14:736–741.
64. Ross ED, Rush AJ. Diagnosis and neuroanatomical correlates of depression in brain- damaged patients. *Arch Gen Psychiatry* 1981;38:1344–1354.
65. Mattila MJ, Liljequist R, Seppala T. Effects of amitriptyline and mianserin on psychomotor skills and memory in man. *Br J Clin Pharmacol* 1978;5:53S–55S.
66. Judd LL, Hubbard B, Janowsky DS, et al. The effect of lithium carbonate on the cognitive functions of normal subjects. *Arch Gen Psychiatry* 1977;34:335–357.
67. Kusumo KS, Vaughn M. Effect of lithium salts on memory. *Br J Psychiatry* 1977;131:453–457.
68. Reiman E. The application of positron emission tomography to the study of normal and pathologic emotions. *J Child Psychol Psychiatry* 1997;58:4–12.
69. Milner B, Corkin S, Teuber H-L. Further analysis of the hippocampal amnesic syndrome: 14-year follow-up study of H.M. *Neuropsychologia* 1968;6:215–234.
70. Small SLM. Pharmacotherapy of aphasia: a critical review. *Stroke* 1994;25:1282–1289.
71. Porch B, Wyckes J, Feeney DM. Haloperidol, thiazides and some antihypertensives slow recovery from aphasia. Proceedings of the Annual Meeting of the Society for Neuroscience, 1985;52.
72. Leiderman E, Zylberman I, Zukin S, et al. Preliminary investigation of high-dose oral glycine on serum levels and negative symptoms in schizophrenia: an open-label trial. *Biol Psychiatry* 1996;39:213–215.
73. Katz DI, Alexander MP, Seliger GM, et al. Traumatic basal ganglia hemorrhage: clinicopathologic features and outcome. *Neurology* 1989;39:897–904.
74. Laplane D, Levasseur M, Pillon B, et al. Obsessive-compulsive and other behavioural changes with bilateral basal ganglia lesions. *Brain* 1989;112:699–725.
75. Forstl H, Krumm B, Eden S, et al. Neurological disorders in 166 patients with basal ganglia calcification: a statistical evaluation. *J Neurol* 1992;239:36–38.
76. Trautner RJ, Cummings JL, Read SL, et al. Idiopathic basal ganglia calcification and organic mood disorder. *Am J Psychiatry* 1988;145:350–353.
77. Lopez-Villegas DM, Kulisevsky JM, Dues JP, et al. Neuropsychological alterations in patients with computed tomography-detected basal ganglia calcification. *Arch Neurol* 1996;53:251–256.
78. Mendez MF, Adams NLPD, Lewandowski KS. Neurobehavioral changes associated with caudate lesions. *Neurology* 1989;39:349–354.
79. Caplan LR, Schmahmann JD, Kase CS, et al. Caudate infarcts. *Arch Neurol* 1990;47:133–143.
80. Saint-Cyr JA, Taylor AE, Nicholson K. Behavior and the basal ganglia. *Behav Neurol Mov Disord* 1995;65:1–28.
81. Medina L, Reiner A. Neurotransmitter organization and connectivity of the basal ganglia in vertebrates: implications for the evolution of basal ganglia. *Brain Behav Evol* 1995;46:235–258.
82. Divac I. Functions of the caudate nucleus. *Acta Biol Exp* 1968;2:107–120.
83. Buchwald NA, Hull CD, Levine MS, et al. The basal ganglia and the regulation of response and cognitive sets. In: Brazier MAB, ed. *Growth and development of the brain*. New York: Raven Press, 1975:171–189.
84. Szelies B, Herholz K, Pawlik G, et al. Widespread functional effects of discrete thalamic infarction. *Arch Neurol* 1991;48:178–182.

85. Leijon G, Boivie J. Central post-stroke pain—a controlled trial of amitriptyline and carbamazepine. *Pain* 1989;36:27–36.
86. Levin AB, Ramirez LF, Katz J. The use of stereotactic chemical hypophysectomy in the treatment of thalamic pain syndrome. *J Neurosurg* 1983;59:1002–1006.
87. Westlund KN, Sorkin LS, Ferrington DG, et al. Serotoninergic and noradrenergic projections to the ventral posterolateral nucleus of the monkey thalamus. *J Comp Neurol* 1990;295:197–207.
88. Nuzzo JL, Warfield CA. Thalamic pain syndrome. *Hosp Pract* 1985;32:32c–32j.
89. Bakchine S, Lacomblez L, Benoit N, et al. Manic-like state after bilateral orbitofrontal and right temporoparietal injury: efficacy of clonidine. *Neurology* 1989;39: 777–781.
90. Bougousslavsky J, Ferrazzini M, Regli F, et al. Manic delirium and frontal-like syndrome with paramedian infarction of the right thalamus. *J Neurol Neurosurg Psychiatry* 1988;51:116–119.
91. McGilchrist I, Goldstein LH, Jadresic D, et al. Thalamo-frontal psychosis. *Br J Psychiatry* 1993;163: 113–115.
92. Kulisevsky J, Berthier ML, Pujol J. Hemiballismus and secondary mania following a right thalamic infarction. *Neurology* 1993;43:1422–1424.
93. Koch C. The action of the corticofugal pathway on sensory thalamic nuclei: a hypothesis. *Neuroscience* 1987; 23:399–406.
94. Bogousslavsky JM, Martin RM, Regli FM, et al. Persistent worsening of stroke sequelae after delayed seizures. *Arch Neurol* 1992;49:385–388.
95. Lugaresi E. The thalamus and insomnia. *Neurology* 1992;42:28–33.

8

Delayed Neurobehavioral Sequelae of Brain Injury

SUMMARY

The clinical consequences of brain injury are general or specific, transient or persistent, immediate or delayed. The delayed neurobehavioral sequelae arise months or years after the event. A few examples are described here.

Posttraumatic migraine, chronic pain, and fatigue are associated with relatively mild brain injuries. The nature of the connection is obscure; that there even is a causal connection has been a matter for debate. There is no consensus on the pathophysiologic mechanism, and it is possible that events external to brain trauma, such as cervical whiplash or "spinal shock" are at play. Attributions to patients' premorbid personality traits or psychiatric disorders have not been wholly convincing. What is clear is that physicians will attend many such patients, and treatment can be as frustrating to them as it is to the patients.

Posttraumatic depression, conversely, is a regular consequence of brain injuries, both mild and severe, and there is no controversy surrounding the association. Prolonged postconcussion syndrome (PCS) almost invariably leads to depression. It is simple depression that responds to the usual antidepressant drugs. Sometimes, however, psychostimulants work better. The rate of depression after severe brain injury is also very high, equal to or greater than the rate of poststroke depression. Complicated affective conditions, including explosive disorder and bipolar disorder, occur as well; they are rarely, if ever, found after mild brain injury. Treatment also is complicated, and the usual psychiatric approaches are not always successful.

Affective instability is the most common psychiatric complication of brain injury, mental retardation, stroke, and the neurodegenerative disorders. One presumes that is the consequence of a persistent derangement in the governing neurotransmitters, i.e., a persistently suboptimal monoamine environment.

Posttraumatic epilepsy and posttraumatic psychosis tend to arise 2 to 5 years after severe brain injury. The former is predictable, based on the nature of the injury, and responds well to antiepileptic drugs. The latter is unpredictable, responds poorly to drug treatment, and can take a catastrophic course. Severe brain injury is an important risk factor for dementia of the Alzheimer type.

DELAYED SEQUELAE

Some of the sequelae of brain injury evolve over time. The evolution of neurobehavioral sequelae may be the consequence of a particular kind of traumatic event such as electrocution and radiation necrosis, the result of a pathophysiologic process such as kindling or long-term depression, or psychological factors such as discouragement and chronic frustration. Delayed sequelae may be, therefore, a biologic mandate, a pathologic turn, or an artifact of circumstance. The delayed neurobehavioral sequelae of traumatic brain injury (TBI) are as debilitating as any direct consequence of the injury, but they are not present, even in nascent form, during the acute recovery process. They arise after a year or after several years.

The delayed sequelae addressed are:

- Two delayed effects that follow concussion: chronic fatigue and chronic pain,
- Affective disorders, especially depression,
- Delayed posttraumatic amnesia,
- Posttraumatic narcolepsy,
- Posttraumatic movement disorders,
- Posttraumatic epilepsy,
- Posttraumatic psychosis, and
- Dementia, which is a long-term problem.

It appears that TBI increases the risk over basal rates for the general population to this degree: for depression, by a factor of 5 or 10; for seizures, by 2 to 5; for psychotic disorders, by the same factor; and for dementia, by 4 or 5. Severe TBIs or injuries with special characteristics increase the risk of delayed sequelae even more.

Other problems arise in patients with TBI with the passage of time, but the ones listed here are the major clinical problems. Posttraumatic headache, in contrast, usually begins within the first few days or weeks after TBI, and although the nature of headache evolves over time and may even turn into a long-term problem, it is not usually delayed in onset. Sexual dysfunction or anosmia may not appear for many months or even years after an injury, but that is more a question of detection; the problem was always there, but no one thought to inquire about it, and the patient did not think to relate it to the injury. Cognitive disability may not be evident until after the patient has returned to work or to school. Cognitive deficits, especially in highly placed people, may not be recognized for a very long time. Personality changes are detected almost immediately by family members who assume that they are transient and will pass with time. Only after months go by do they complain about it to a physician; the patients themselves seldom realize that their personalities have changed.

Late pathologic transformation after a serious insult to the central nervous system is remarkably common. In many of the other encephalopathic conditions considered in this book, such as epilepsy, stroke, and mental retardation, the evolution of delayed sequelae follows a predictable course. Several neurologic conditions are also prone to late transformation: the weakness, fatigue, and pain of postpoliomyelitis syndrome (1); postencephalitic Parkinson's disease (PD); early dementia in people who are mentally retarded by virtue of viral encephalitis (2); Alzheimer's disease (AD) in patients with Down's syndrome; tardive dyskinesia; epilepsy in autism; brain atrophy after leukotomy (3); the psychosis of temporal lobe epilepsy; the intellectual decline of epileptic patients; and the delayed neurotoxicity produced by methylmercury (4). Even major psychiatric disorders such as schizophrenia and manic-depression are associated with delayed changes that follow a regular pattern and are not dissimilar to those described in TBI.

It is unlikely that a single mechanism can be held to account for such a long and diverse list. Even the mechanisms that we think we understand are vague or speculative. Nevertheless, thinking about mechanisms of delayed neurotoxicity is important for guiding treatment. Effective treatment is not only about suppressing untoward symptoms but also promoting recovery and preventing delayed neurotoxicity.

DELAYED SYMPTOMS OF THE POSTCONCUSSION SYNDROME

Most of the time, symptoms of PCS develop soon after the injury, within hours or days. In some patients, however, PCS symptoms such as headache, memory loss, inattention, and hyposexuality may not be apparent until several days or weeks have passed. In one well-known study, patients who had sustained mild brain injuries actually complained of more postconcussion symptoms at 3 months than they did immediately after the accident (5). Delayed symptoms are commonly interpreted in terms of psychogenic etiologic factors or worse; depression, hysteria, and malingering do indeed account for most cases.

Postconcussion symptoms almost invariably resolve within weeks or months of the injury. In Chapter 6, some problems attendant on the diagnosis of severe, persistent symptoms after mild brain injury were discussed. The development of depression in postconcussives, especially after 6 to 12 months, was also mentioned. Two additional problems may arise after mild brain injury: chronic fatigue and chronic pain.

Chronic fatigue and chronic pain are important conditions in their own right. They are also formidable diagnostic confounders. Patients with fatigue and/or pain often complain of cognitive impairment, and when they are given neuropsychological tests, they do poorly. All too often the inexperienced examiner attributes cognitive impairment to the mild brain injury that the patient may have sustained some months or years before. That is almost always a misattribution.

Chronic Pain

Three kinds of persistent pain are associated with mild brain injury: posttraumatic headache, fibromyalgia, and chronic pain from a concurrent injury (e.g., neck pain, back pain).

Posttraumatic headache (see Chapter 6) is usually a transient event and not usually delayed in onset. The dull, continuous headache described by patients with PCS is often associated with neck injury and muscle spasm in the neck and upper back. It has the characteristics of tension headache and is treated accordingly. It usually remits over a course of days, weeks, or months. Sometimes, however, this typical posttraumatic headache evolves and grows increasingly migrainoid. Auras are rare in posttraumatic migraine, but the headaches are described as "throbbing," and there are all the typical migrainoid correlates such as nausea and vomiting, photo/sonosensitivity, and exercise intolerance. Drug-rebound headache can also present this way.

Neck or back pain, for example, after whiplash injury, is also a transient problem, and the onset is usually within a day or so after the event. The patient's experience of the pain, reaction to it, and means of coping are, of course, influenced by his or her personality and psychological state at the time. The evolution of posttraumatic back pain into a more chronic, debilitating condition is an unusual event, but it sometimes happens and may or may not be a function of the patient's personality or psychological state.

Sometimes mild traumatic events, such as concussion with cervical whiplash, can evolve into a peculiar condition known as fibromyalgia (also known as fibrositis or myofascial pain). Fibromyalgia is a chronic pain syndrome associated with diffuse musculoskeletal pain. It is accepted as a rheumatologic condition, but neither the pain nor the pathology is articular. As a matter of fact, there is no overt pathology in the fibromyalgia syndrome. Nothing consistent has ever shown up in electrodiagnostic studies, muscle biopsies, or laboratory tests. Neither the etiology nor the pathophysiology of the disorder is understood. For these and other reasons, the diagnosis has been controversial (6).

Fibromyalgia is 10 times more common in women than in men. The cause is unknown, but there seems to be a relationship to trauma, surgery, medical illness, or chronic physical stress at work. The symptoms are sometimes quite intense and disabling: diffuse aching muscle pain, morning stiffness, poor sleep, chronic fatigue, intolerance to weather changes or cold weather, or emotional distress. Anxiety and depression are common correlates. When patients with fibromyalgia are asked about their quality of life, they rate themselves lower than patients who have rheumatoid arthritis, chronic obstructive pulmonary disease, or insulin-dependent diabetes mellitus (7,8).

The characteristic signs of fibromyalgia are trigger points or tender points, areas on the body, especially the upper back, that elicit exquisite pain on deep palpation. More formal evaluation of patients with fibromyalgia, however, for example with dolorimetry, has called into question the discriminative validity of trigger points. Patients with fibromyalgia are more pain sensitive to controls, at their trigger points, and elsewhere (9).

Critics of the condition usually attribute patients' complaints to an underlying psychiatric condition, e.g., somatoform pain disorder or hypochondriasis. The fact that many patients with fibromyalgia are on long-term disability as a result of their condition has fueled both sides of the controversy. There is a high incidence of major affective disorder in patients with fibromyalgia, but aggressive antidepressant treatment rarely alleviates the condition (10). In fact, the psychological profile of patients with fibromyalgia is no different from that of patients with rheumatoid arthritis or other chronic pain conditions of known organic etiology (11,12). I can shed no new light on the "validity" of the disorder, but in my experience, patients with fibromyalgia do not resemble any class of psychiatric patients.

Chronic Fatigue Syndrome

Fibromyalgia is often comorbid with chronic fatigue, and patients with chronic fatigue syndrome frequently complain of diffuse aching pain, poor sleep, and morning stiffness. Both conditions are characterized by an extreme degree of exercise intolerance and a high rate of depressive symptoms. They are both related to trauma or surgery. It has been suggested that fibromyalgia and chronic fatigue are related disorders, conditions that exist on a spectrum, as Tourette's syndrome and obsessive-compulsive disorder do.

Neurasthenia was described in 1869 by George Beard, an American neurologist, and popularized by no less a luminary than Silas Weir Mitchell. "Nervous prostration" and "nervous exhaustion" were nineteenth-century synonyms. Beard's first patient was a young man, a physician, who complained that he was "living on a plane lower than normal" (13). This is an accurate description of what the patient with chronic fatigue experiences, although it hardly captures their degree of disability and unhappiness. It is glib to state that chronic fatigue is just "a culturally sanctioned form of illness behavior" or that the diagnosis will "meet the same fate as neurasthenia" (14), but it is inevitable that some physicians will feel that way. Chronic fatigue syndrome, like fibromyalgia, has been grouped by the skeptics with multiple chemical sensitivity syndrome, alien abduction, systemic yeast infection, and hypersensitivity to electricity.

I have seen too many patients with chronic fatigue and/or fibromyalgia to share this trenchant view. I have also seen too many patients with hysteria, compensation neurosis, malingering, and atypical depression to believe that all or even most patients with fatigue or fibrositis inevitably fit into one or another of those categories. They are potentially disabling physical conditions that deserve to be dealt with on their own terms.

However, one would be more secure in a discussion of chronic fatigue syndrome if one knew exactly what those terms should be; for example, if some objective measure were brought forth in terms of etiopathogenesis or if there were some indication that the condition was responsive to treatment. Its relation to head trauma is nonspecific and unpredictable; like fibrositis, it is more likely to be seen in patients who sustained mild injuries and is hardly ever encountered in patients who have had severe TBI. It is not an uncommon outcome of severe viral illness, but a specific association, for example, with Epstein-Barr virus, has been excluded. It is possible that viral infection might initiate a sequence of abnormal immune reactions or generate excessive amounts of interferon. Obscure retroviruses have been implicated (but not replicated). Chronic fatigue has also been related to neurally mediated hypotension and thus treated with fludrocortisone with some success (15), but not in controlled studies (16).

Patients with chronic fatigue do not respond to aggressive antidepressant therapy. More troubling, they do not respond very well to stimulants, amantadine, or dopamine agonists, the usual treatment for neuropsychiatric patients who are anergic, hypoaroused, or hypersomnolent. Chronic fatigue is different somehow. It may not be a central nervous system disease at all.

Chronic fatigue syndrome and fibromyalgia may be poles on a spectrum or unrelated but occasionally comorbid conditions. They may be central, peripheral, or systemic, and some people still maintain that they are imaginary. Be that as it may, they are occasionally manifested in patients who have had a mild brain injury. Sometimes, the evaluation of such patients is in the context of a forensic undertaking. When that is the case, one must remember that cognitive deficits are inevitably a component of physical conditions characterized by pain and/or fatigue. Measures of attention, memory, reaction time, and information-processing speed are the cognitive areas most frequently affected (17,18).

AFFECTIVE DISORDERS

The prevalence and incidence of affective disorders in general are influenced by the diagnostic criteria that are being used at the time and by the ascertainment criteria and the sampling method of the particular survey. There is no statistic that is universal for any of the affective disorders as there is for schizophrenia, which occurs at the same rate across national boundaries and continents and appears to have occurred at the same rate over the years. The prevalence of the various affective disorders is usually found to vary with gender, race, and culture, and there has even been commentary to the effect that the prevalence of affective disorders, especially depression, is increasing in modern times. One reads that 13% or 20% of the general population in this country will have at least one clinically significant depressive episode at some time in their lives (19). The number is much smaller, however, if one refers to the most severe forms of affective illness, such as bipolar disorder, affective psychosis, or melancholia (1.9% to 3.5%) (19).

Mood disorders are clearly associated with significant morbidity and are a major public health problem around the world. They also carry significant mortality. The lifetime risk of suicide may be as high as 15% for patients with a major affective disorder (20). Depression and related affective disorders also contribute to mortality from other causes such as accidents and natural diseases. The standardized mortality ratio is increased in people with depression, and for such patients it is 1.5, a 50% increase over the mortality rate of the general population; 2.1 for men, 1.2 for women (21).

The most definitive statement concerning the epidemiology of affective disorder is based on the National Institute of Mental Health Epidemiologic Catchment Area Program in which 18,571 people were interviewed in five U.S. cities: New Haven, CT; Baltimore, MD; St. Louis, MO; Durham, NC; and Los Angeles, CA. The prevalence of affective disorders was determined within a specific time frame: more than 1 month, 6 months, and lifetime. The three categories were manic depression (bipolar disorder), major depressive disorder, and dysthymic disorder (depressive neurosis). The prevalence rates for the total U.S. sample were determined (22) (Table 8.1).

One may therefore assume, for the sake of argument, a lifetime prevalence rate for a major depressive disorder at approximately 6% for the general population and approximately 3% for dysthymic disorder. It is clear, then, that major insults to the central nervous system, such as TBI or stroke, carry a significant increase in the probability of occurrence.

For example, McKinlay et al. (23) reported that more than half their patients with TBI complained of depressive symptoms at 3, 6, and 12 months after the injury. Levine et al. (24) reported that the prevalence

TABLE 8.1. *Prevalence of affective disorders in the United States*

	1 mo (%)	3 mo (%)	Lifetime (%)
Bipolar disorder	0.4	0.5	0.8
Major depression	2.2	3.0	5.8
Dysthymia	3.3	3.3	3.3

of depressive symptoms in a three-center study of patients who had sustained mild head injury was 34% to 39%, but the rate must be higher for patients who have sustained a moderate or a severe head injury because it is known that the severity of the injury is directly related to the severity and prevalence of the residual affective disorder (25). The suicide rate for wartime victims of TBI has been reported at 14% over 18 years (26), a statistic that is equal to the suicide rate of patients with major depression. The frequency of bipolar disorder, conversely, may not be increased by TBI (5). Even if one were to grant the weakness of these surveys from an epidemiologic and a diagnostic perspective, one concedes an increase in the liability to affective disease in patients with TBI by a factor of 5 or 10.

Mood disorder after TBI is roughly comparable with other encephalopathic conditions. Patients who have sustained a cerebrovascular accident may be at greater risk of developing affective symptoms than patients with TBI. In one survey, 60% of patients who had a stroke had clinically significant depression compared with only 20% of the patients with TBI (27). In another study, 50% of patients who had a cerebrovascular accident developed clinically significant depressive symptoms and 25% developed major depression (28). Perhaps age plays a role; patients with TBI, as a rule, are younger than patients who had a stroke and are less likely to have concomitant disease or take multiple medications.

Poststroke depression is sometimes a persistent problem, and it may be difficult to treat. The duration of poststroke depression is at least 7 to 8 months, on the average, and there is an increase in the prevalence of depression even in the second year after cerebrovascular accident (29). The same is true of other neurologic conditions. The combination of depression and neurologic disease in general has been described as a particularly lethal combination. In one study, 83 patients with a neurological disease and depression were compared to 44 patients with a neurologic disease without depression and with 43 depressives who had no neurologic disease. The patients with a neurologic disease and depression were less likely to respond to antidepressant treatments than the depressed patients without neurologic disease and did less well than the patients with pure neurologic disease in terms of their medical outcome (30).

Mood disorders are highly prevalent in neurologic conditions in general. James Parkinson himself (31) noted depression in conjunction with PD. Brown and Wilson (31a) reported a 52% rate of clinically significant depression in patients with PD. Mayeux et al. (31) reported a depression rate of 47% in PD; 31% of the depression was mild, 13% moderate, and 4% severe.

It has also been noted that depression is more likely in patients with PD who have severe intellectual impairment, suggesting a connection between the dementia of PD and the affective symptoms (31,32). On the other hand, intellectual impairment is not necessary for the development of depression, and the latter can certainly develop even when there are no signs of cognitive deterioration (33). Patients with severe PD are more likely to be depressed than patients with mild or moderate manifestations of the syndrome (34), a pattern that also holds for TBI and stroke.

The prevalence of affective disorders is also high (42%) in patients with multiple sclerosis (35). One concludes, therefore, that depression after TBI follows the established pattern of other severe central nervous system disorders. The prevalence rate is increased dramatically; the condition is long-standing and difficult to treat, and its presence confers a negative influence on the course of the neurologic condition.

There have been attempts to relate the occurrence of affective symptoms after brain trauma with a specific lesion site, although the results of such attempts have not been conclusive. There is a long-standing belief that symptoms of depression, dysphoria, anxiety, and sadness relate to functional alterations in the frontotemporal regions of the right hemisphere (36), and this has been attributed to the functional organization of the right hemisphere for the "modulation of affective components of language and behavior" (37). The studies of Robinson and co-workers (38) did not agree with this formulation, and they actually alluded to a left hemisphere predominance in terms of poststroke depression. They also suggested that poststroke depression may be related to lesion proximity to the frontal poles bilaterally (27). Starkstein et al. (39) found that patients with poststroke depression were more likely to have evidence of subcortical atrophy. Cummings and Mendez (40) asserted that the focal lesions most commonly associated with secondary mania are diencephalic, whereas others asserted that damage to orbitofrontal structures in the right hemisphere is associated with secondary mania (41).

The cerebral localization of poststroke depression seems to have eluded the experts. In TBI, especially closed head injury (CHI), the cerebral damage is more diffuse than in stroke and less likely to be lateralized. One presumes that depression after TBI is a consequence of damage to anterofrontal and temporal lobe structures or to the ascending monoamine pathways or both. At this point, one cannot be more specific.

It is not possible to identify a particular group of patients with TBI or stroke who are more likely to develop mood disorders, which is why the failure of the anatomic model is so disappointing. One may assume, however, that the problem of posttraumatic depression will be more serious in women compared with men, in older patients, in patients who must take medications that are potential depressants, and in patients with preexisting mood disorders or family histories of mood disorders. One might also expect to see more serious problems with depression in patients with more severe injuries, in patients whose residual handicaps are more severe, in patients with subcortical and cortical damage, and in patients whose psychosocial support systems are less effective.

One cannot say that there is a peak period during which affective disorders are most likely to develop and after which the risk necessarily subsides. Based on clinical observations and surveys, the prevalence of affective disorders is very common in the first 2 years after TBI, just as it is after stroke. The studies of Vauhkonen (26) and Robinson et al. (29) suggest that the risk is carried for a long time after the insult.

The pathophysiologic basis for the delayed onset of behavioral sequelae, especially affective disorders, may reside in the theory of diaschisis or late functional depression. Diaschisis is roughly comparable with denervation atrophy. When the activity of a particular brain structure is impaired, the activity of other structures to which it is functionally linked may also be compromised. The phenomenon of late functional depression is consistent with descriptions of deficits in monoamine metabolism after TBI. Altered levels of catecholamines, for example, may result from damage to catecholaminergic neurons, with a shift from neurotransmitter production to protein synthesis for repair (42,43). The gradual evolution of functional depression occurs over a span of weeks after TBI.

Functional depression of monoamine systems may account for reduced arousal, inattention, difficulty concentrating, memory lapses, fatigue, anergia, comprehension difficulties, lack of flexibility, extreme sensitivity to environmental stressors such as bright light and loud noises, and irritability. It may also lead to the development of major depression. It is interesting that recovery from brain injury in experimental paradigms is enhanced by treatment with psychostimulants and antidepressants. This has been attributed to the correction of late functional depression.

Treatment

Mood disorders associated with stroke and other neurologic diseases tend to be prolonged and difficult to treat (29). Posttraumatic depression, however, may have a better prognosis. There are no controlled studies, but psychiatrists who specialize in the treatment of patients with TBI tend to be confident about the likelihood of a favorable response to conventional antidepressants (44,45).

Posttraumatic depression is usually treated with an antidepressant. The new antidepressants are the first-line agents for all the obvious reasons. Patients with TBI may be vulnerable to akathisia with the selective serotonin reuptake inhibitors. Bupropion is an appropriate drug for patients with TBI despite the admonitions on the package insert. The tricyclic antidepressants may be problematic because of their sedating, orexigenic, and anticholinergic effects.

If a patient with TBI fails to respond to a reasonable trial of antidepressant therapy, it is appropriate to try a psychostimulant or dopamine agonist by itself or combined with the antidepressant. The deficits in monoaminergic neurotransmission that occur in brainstem nuclei after TBI are amenable to treatment with simple monoaminergic drugs such as the psychostimulants (46). The stimulants enhance recovery from experimentally induced brain injury (47), and double-blind studies have shown favorable effects of stimulants on depressive symptoms and cognitive function in patients with TBI (48). Drugs that enhance monoaminergic neurotransmission then, such as the psychostimulants and antidepressants, represent rational pharmacotherapy for posttraumatic depression (47,49).

Secondary Mania

This term refers to manic behavior occurring secondary to medical and/or pharmacologic antecedents (50). The diagnosis should be made, not based on the nonspecific symptoms such as hyperactivity, insomnia, and emotional instability, but only when patients have symptoms that are unequivocally manic, e.g., increased energy, euphoria, grandiosity, pressured speech, flight of ideas. It is not a common outcome of TBI and hardly appears at all in the follow-up studies. Among patients admitted to psychiatric care however, a small number of manic patients will be seen whose symptoms developed with a year or two of TBI. Most often, these are patients with diencephalic or orbitofrontal lesions (40,51). Many patients have a family or personal history of depression (but not of manic-depression) (52). Secondary mania is usually treated as one normally treats mania, although lithium may be less well tolerated than the usual alternatives. In my experience, mood-stabilizing drugs in general are less effective than atypical antipsychotics in cases of secondary mania.

DELAYED POSTTRAUMATIC AMNESIA

In 1964, Smith reported that a number of post-lobectomy patients had deteriorated on tests of complex mental functioning many years after surgery and after an initial postsurgical recovery (52a). In the early 1970s, secondary regression of intellectual performance, especially memory, was reported in patients who had severe TBIs, a clear decrement from their initial recovery (53,54), and in 1979, Lezak (55) affirmed the observation. The decline in cognitive function was not explicable in terms of any active neurologic or psychiatric condition and did not appear to presage the onset of AD.

It is not entirely clear why this should happen. Mortimer and Pirozzolo (56) suggested that dementia pugilistica is a model for delayed cognitive deterioration after TBI. Although AD has been observed in boxers, the course of punchdrunk syndrome or chronic posttraumatic encephalopathy is not usually a rapidly progressive dementia. It is a gradual deterioration that develops over the years after a number of subconcussive injuries but without a rapid, inexorable downhill course, and the process may arrest.

Secondary cognitive regression after TBI would appear to be then the result of a mildly dementing process. It is less florid than what happens in Alzheimer's or Pick's disease but probably contains elements of the pathophysiology of dementia. It is possible that the effects of remote functional depression (diaschisis) grow in severity, turn chronic and irreversible, but progress only to a point.

Head trauma is known to cause a transient derangement of the blood-brain barrier, allowing serum proteins to enter the brain parenchyma (57). If contact between leukocytes with specific brain antigens were to sensitize the immune system, brain-specific antibodies can develop. With further disruption of the blood-brain barrier from subsequent trauma or aging, there might be an increased secondary response with damage to neuronal elements. Disruption of the blood-brain barrier might open the brain to viruses or neurotoxins such as aluminum that may also have damaging effects (56).

All this is very theoretical, even speculative. Gradual deterioration of memory in particular or cognitive function in general, without dementia, is a rare consequence of severe brain injury. It may simply be the consequence of chronic depression, lack of stimulation, or concomitant medication. In cases of mild brain injury, it is not encountered except as a complication of depression or chronic pain or as a sign of malingering or conversion disorder.

SECONDARY NARCOLEPSY

Excessive daytime somnolence is not uncommon in patients with brain injury, but true posttraumatic narcolepsy is relatively rare (58). Reviews of narcolepsy seldom mention trauma as an etiologic consideration (59). There are a few reports of narcolepsy confirmed by sleep polysomnography secondary to brain tumors or multiple sclerosis involving the brainstem. When narcolepsy occurs in a patient with TBI, HLA antigens may be absent, affirming the traumatic cause (60), or present, suggesting an interaction between trauma and genetic proclivity (61). When it does occur, the onset may be weeks or months after injury.

MOVEMENT DISORDERS

Most cases of torticollis are idiopathic, and trauma is a rare cause. There have been case reports of secondary torticollis after trauma. Occasionally, the onset of torticollis may be years after a TBI. A similar latency is seen in patients with stroke or other structural lesions, which may evolve from hemiparesis to hemidystonia over the course of weeks, months, or years. (62). Posttraumatic tremor, choreoathetosis, tics, and parkinsonism usually have a delayed onset (63).

POSTTRAUMATIC EPILEPSY

Seizures that arise in the first 24 hours or in the first 7 days after TBI are the result of acute trauma. The fact that a patient has had one such seizure, or even several, does not mean that he or she has posttraumatic epilepsy. Electroencephalographic abnormalities in the first year after TBI are not necessarily predictive of posttraumatic epilepsy, although persistence of an epileptiform electroencephalogram may well be (64).

Patients who are recovering from TBI, even a mild injury, may have spells during the first year in which they may experience focal weakness, paroxysms of abnormal movement, sudden unusual sensations, or sudden behavioral lapses; these may be indistinguishable from focal or absence seizures. These spells do not necessarily recur nor necessarily develop into overt epilepsy.

The onset of true posttraumatic epilepsy may be in the first year, but it usually comes later. In the study by Salazar et al. (65), the onset of posttraumatic epilepsy in Korean War veterans who had sustained penetrating brain injuries was 57% in the first year, 18% after 5 years, and 7% after 10 years. Caveness et al. (66) reported that 50% to 80% of the cases of posttraumatic epilepsy after wartime brain injury arose during the first 2 years.

The incidence of epilepsy after penetrating head injuries is much higher than it is after CHIs. The overall prevalence of posttraumatic epilepsy in the study of penetrating head injuries by Salazar et al. (65) was 53%, whereas the prevalence of epilepsy after CHIs is 2% (67) to 5% (68). Severe CHIs may have a higher rate: 7.1% at 1 year and 11.5% after 5 years (67). McQueen et al. (69) reported the incidence of posttraumatic epilepsy after severe CHI to be 7% in the first year and 10% after 2 years. In children, the rates are higher: the incidence of epilepsy is 9.8% after severe TBI, and most patients have their first seizure in the first year (70).

By way of comparison, the frequency of epilepsy after stroke is 6.5% to 13% (71,72).

In terms of predictive factors, posttraumatic epilepsy after penetrating head injuries is related to the depth of dural penetration and to injury in the region of the central sulcus (66), to the presence of focal neurologic signs, especially hemiparesis and aphasia, and to the size of the lesion (65) but not to a family history of epilepsy or the patient's premorbid IQ (65). For CHI, the predictive factors are coma duration and duration of posttraumatic amnesia, evidence of focal cortical injury associated with a mass lesion or depressed skull fracture, the presence of focal neurologic signs, and seizures in the first week after injury (68). The occurrence of early fits raises the prevalence of posttraumatic epilepsy to approximately 25% (73). Patients with stroke who develop seizures are much more likely to have a cortical lesion; in one study, no fewer than 50% of patients with stroke with persisting paresis and a specific cortical lesion developed epilepsy (71).

An algorithm was developed to estimate the probability of posttraumatic epilepsy (74). The predictive elements and their relative weight are given in Table 8.2. Weiss et al. (75) developed an algorithm for predicting epilepsy after penetrating head injury.

Young children are more likely to develop posttraumatic epilepsy than children older than 2 years of age. In children, the latency to seizure onset is delayed compared with adults. For children 2 years or younger, the latency to onset is as long as 13 years; for children 3 to 14 years, it is 6 years; and for children older than 15 years, it is 3 years on average (76).

The follow-up studies of posttraumatic epilepsy suggest that one-half of the patients cease having seizures after 5 or 10 years (65,66). These are studies of penetrating head injuries, however, that generally show a good prognosis; there are no epidemiologic data on the outcome of posttraumatic epilepsy after CHI.

Other problems may arise, however, as a consequence of epilepsy. Complex-partial seizures are the most common form of epilepsy after brain trauma, and lesions of the temporal lobe or limbic cortex are frequently involved. The long-term psychiatric consequences of temporal lobe epilepsy have been covered extensively in the literature (77), but the most elegant epidemiologic study is that of Lindsay et al. (78), published over 2 years in Developmental Medicine and Child Neurology. In their 13-year follow-up of 100 children with temporal lobe epilepsy, five had died, 33 were living independently and were seizure free, 32 were more or less independent but not seizure free and on anticonvulsants, and 30 were completely dependent and severely handicapped. Only 15% were completely free of psychological problems. The most common psychiatric problems were attention deficit/hyperactivity, explosive rage attacks, and antisocial personality. No fewer than 10% developed an overt psychosis (79).

TABLE 8.2. *Prediction of posttraumatic epilepsy*

Centroparietal lesion	0.25
Dural penetration	0.20
Hemiparesis or aphasia	0.20
Hemorrhage	0.20
Early seizures	0.15
Temporal lesion	0.15
Depressed skull fracture	0.10
Persistent EEG abnormality	0.10
Prefrontal lesion	0.10
Occipital lesion	0.10
CNS infection	0.10
LOC, PTA >1 h	0.05
Linear skull fracture	0.05

EEG, electroencephalograph; CNS, central nervous system; LOC, loss of consciousness; PTA, posttraumatic amnesia.

People with posttraumatic epilepsy have shorter life expectancy than the general population or victims of TBI without epilepsy. The death rate (death from any cause) of men with posttraumatic epilepsy is higher at all ages but especially after age 45 (80). As these men age, they are prone to increasing disability from their original physical handicaps and are more prone to early dementia (80).

The final element of risk that is introduced by posttraumatic epilepsy are the neurotoxic effects of long-term anticonvulsant treatment, especially phenytoin, associated with encephalopathy, dementia, benign intracranial hypertension, and cerebellar atrophy (81–83), and barbiturates, associated with depression (84) and rheumatism (85). For women, there is the problem of teratogenesis, a dilemma that is posed by virtually all the anticonvulsants.

If one assumes, therefore, a basal rate for epilepsy in the general population of less than 1%, a moderate CHI may be conservatively estimated to increase the risk of epilepsy by a factor of 2 to 5. A severe head injury or stroke will increase the risk by a factor of 10; a severe stroke or a penetrating brain injury (PBI) will increase the risk by a factor of 50. If posttraumatic epilepsy develops, there is a 50% probability that the disorder will not remit. If the seizure disorder involves a temporal or limbic focus, there is a 33% risk that severe psychiatric sequelae will develop.

Anticonvulsant Prophylaxis

The relatively high rates of posttraumatic epilepsy among wartime victims who sustained penetrating head injuries and among patients who had neurosurgical procedures gave rise to the use of anticonvulsant prophylaxis, a practice that has lost its value in the current era of CHI. Although the prescribing habits of some practitioners appear to ignore the results of clinical studies, it does not appear that anticonvulsant prophylaxis will diminish the likelihood of posttraumatic epilepsy (65,69,70).

This prescribing practice may cause depression or neuropsychological deficits in convalescent patients with TBIs owing to the side effects of prophylactic anticonvulsants. When a patient with a TBI on a prophylactic antiepileptic drug presents with depression or cognitive impairment, it is usually a good idea to reconsider the utility of anticonvulsant treatment (86–88).

Anticonvulsant prophylaxis may not be altogether inappropriate in cases in which the patient's injury was characterized by events that render the likelihood of posttraumatic seizures very high. In the case of open or penetrating head injuries, when the dura is breached or when there is extensive intracerebral hemorrhage, it may not be unreasonable to continue treatment with moderate doses of a nonsedating anticonvulsant, especially if the patient has made an excellent recovery. The occurrence of a seizure can compromise the patient's return to work or his or her driving privilege. In such cases, the patient may be treated for a year or two, as if he or she has had a seizure. At the end of the treatment period, the anticonvulsant is withdrawn. Research does not indicate that an electrocephalogram predicts the success of anticonvulsant withdrawal, but one should think twice before withdrawing a patient who has an epileptiform electroencephalogram.

LATE-ONSET PSYCHOSIS

Psychosis is the most severe and devastating outcome of brain injury. It may not be as dehumanizing as dementia or as dangerous as epilepsy or depression, but there is nothing that is so destructive to the human personality or the relationships that one has with family and friends. There are drugs that can control at least some of the severe manifestations of a psychotic disorder, but they are not pleasant drugs to take, their side effects are cumulative, and they are seldom completely effective.

Psychosis immediately after TBI occurs during states of delirium, in which orientation and anterograde memory are also impaired (89). Such psychotic states are accompanied by hallucinations, poorly systematized delusions, agitation, combativeness, and marked fluctuations in the mental state. This form of psychosis occurs in patients in the early stages of recovery from coma and is not germane to the problem of late-onset psychosis. It usually clears as the patient's mental state improves.

After the coma-recovery stage but within the first few months of coma recovery, patients with a clear sensorium may develop psychosis. These psychotic symptoms are not as a rule related to acute perceptual and orientation deficits. Delusions, for example, have been reported in patients with lesions in the basal ganglia (90,91), thalamus (50,89), mesencephalon (92, 93), and various limbic structures (94). In these cases, the delusions involve referential thought, persecutory beliefs, fears of illness and death, and jealousy. The complexity and organization of these more systematized delusions are related to the level of general cognitive and intellectual functioning of the patient (90,92). Delusions of misidentification (Capgras' syndrome) are often seen.

The psychosis of the coma-recovery stage is associated with delirium, confusion, and cerebral disorganization. Postrecovery psychosis is attributed to the effects of specific cortical or subcortical lesions or diffuse cortical disease, as in dementia. For late-onset psychosis, however, it is likely that another process must be brought to bear.

Filley and Jarvis (95) described late-onset psychosis 3 years after CHI, a case of "delayed reduplicative paramnesia" related to right hemisphere and bifrontal pathology. Delayed psychoses after stroke in one patient and after CHI in another were described by Hayman and Abrams (96), although the intervals were contaminated by the seizures in the first case and by alcoholism in the second. Levine and Finkelstein (97) reported delayed psychotic reactions after right temporoparietal stroke or trauma in eight patients, seven of whom had seizures. Epilepsy, then, is a common feature but not a necessary ingredient in the development of delayed psychosis after cerebral insult.

Barnhill and Gualtieri (98) reported two cases of late-onset psychosis after CHI: one was a young woman whose condition developed abruptly after 3 years and the second was a young man whose condition developed abruptly after 4 years. Although in both cases, there were elements suggestive of the psychosis of temporal lobe epilepsy, in neither case was there clinical evidence of seizures. Both patients were severely aphasic, and it is likely that left temporal lobe damage was one element of the diffuse injuries that they had sustained. It is possible that they also sustained damage to deep temporal lobe structures and that the kindling phenomenon could explain the late development of psychosis (99). In both cases, at least a measure of relief came from treatment with carbamazepine.

In Thomsen's survey (100,101) of 40 patients in Denmark followed up 10 to 15 years after severe CHI, the incidence of posttraumatic psychosis was 20%. Six of the eight psychotic patients had a late-onset condition; none had a preexisting psychiatric condition and none had seizures.

Patients with late-onset posttraumatic psychosis are among the most challenging patients. Their disordered thinking is laced with hostility against caregivers or with invitations or accusations of a bizarre sexual nature. Such symptoms are especially repellent to the people who must be intimately involved with the patient for his or her day-to-day care.

Most studies of the neurobehavioral sequelae of TBI have come from wartime patients with penetrating central nervous system injuries. In the follow-up study of 3,552 Finnish war veterans with TBI, the prevalence of psychosis was 8.9% (102). In Lishman's review (103) of 670 patients with TBI 1 to 5 years after injury, significant psychiatric sequelae were described in 144 patients (21.5%). Risk factors for neurobehavioral symptoms related to localization and extent of the penetrating injury, the degree of subcortical involvement, duration of coma, and emergence of posttraumatic epilepsy. Pertinent neurologic findings included severe cognitive deficits, sensorimotor impairments, dysphasia, and visual field deficits to confrontation. In general, the severity of psychiatric disease correlated with the extent of the central nervous system lesion (24,103).

Although there have been no epidemiologic studies of sufficient strength to establish clear incidence and prevalence rates for delayed- or late-onset psychosis, it is reasonable to surmise a prevalence that is similar to that of posttraumatic epilepsy: 2% to 5% after moderate injuries and 10% or more after severe TBI.

The treatment of posttraumatic psychosis depends on the underlying pathology. If a delusional state occurs in the context of delirium, no pharmacologic treatment is necessary, and the patient may even improve when sedating drugs are withdrawn. Amantadine may be useful. Postrecovery psychosis may require low-dose antipsychotics. For late-onset psychosis, clinicians used to rely on the psychotropic anticonvulsants carbamazepine and valproate as maintenance drugs augmented by antipsychotic drugs during periods of extreme disorganization or disabling positive symptoms. Buspirone can augment the psychotropic effects of carbamazepine and valproate in patients with temporal lobe disease (104). Currently, atypical antipsychotic drugs are probably prescribed more than any other drugs.

DEMENTIA

There are four established risk factors for the development of senile dementia of the Alzheimer's type, none of which can be foreseen or prevented. They are a family aggregate of AD or Down's syndrome, the ApoE4 allele or a severe TBI sustained earlier in life (105). Other than that, there is only the incidence of dementia with every passing year beyond the age of 65, which has been estimated in the past to be approximately 1% (106). The prevalence of dementia in people older than the age of 65 is 3.5%, and the prevalence of AD in the same age cohort is 2% for men and 2.7% for women (107). More recent epidemiologic studies, however, suggest that the prevalence of AD is much higher: 3% in people aged 65 to 74; 19% in people aged 75 to 84, and no less than 47% in people 85 and older (108).

After a dementing condition such as AD is diagnosed, the outcome is first dependence and then death. Five years after AD is first diagnosed, 73% of patients are in nursing homes and 30% have died. After 7 years, 84% are in nursing homes and 44% have died (109).

As pointed out in Chapter 4, the degree to which TBI increases one's risk of developing a dementing condition ranges from 2.4 to 13.75 (106,110–114). Patients with TBI who go on to develop dementia are more likely to have had a severe injury, more than one head injury, or a concurrent illness such as alcoholism or small-vessel disease (115). Patients who have had severe brain injuries develop AD at an earlier age than AD patients without a history of head trauma (116). Older patients with TBI, for example, people who are older than 60 years, are also more likely to develop posttraumatic dementia. (117). Posttraumatic dementia is more likely to develop in patients who possess the ApoE4 allele (114,118,119).

One should place the morbidity ratio therefore at 4 or 5 for dementia after TBI. That is to say, a person who has sustained a severe brain injury is four or five times more likely to develop a dementing condition later in life, and the problem is likely to arise at an earlier age. If the prevalence of dementia in the population at large is 3.5%, then the prevalence of dementia in the brain-injured population should be 14% to 17.5%, which is less than the prevalence of dementia associated with PD (20% to 40%) (111,120) but comparable in order of magnitude.

REFERENCES

1. Cashman NR, Maselli R, Wollman RL, et al. Late denervation in patients with antecedent paralytic poliomyelitis. *N Engl J Med* 1987;317:7–12.
2. Townsend JJ, Baringer JR, Wolinsky JS, et al. Progressive rubella panencephalitis. *N Engl J Med* 1975;292:990.
3. Pakkenberg B. What happens in the leucotomised brain? A post-mortem study of brains from schizophrenic patients. *J Neurol Neurosurg Psychiatry* 1989;52:156–161.
4. Rice DC. Evidence for delayed neurotoxicity produced by methylmercury. *Neurotoxicology* 1996;17:583–596.
5. Grant I, Alves W. Psychiatric and psychosocial disturbances in head injury. In: Levin HS, Grafman J, Eisenberg HM, eds. *Neurobehavioral recovery from head injury*. New York: Oxford University Press, 1987:232–261.
6. Bohr T. Problems with myofascial pain syndrome and fibromyalgia syndrome. *Neurology*, 1996;46:593–597.
7. Wolfe F. Fibrositis, fibromyalgia, and musculoskeletal disease: the current status of the fibrositis syndrome. *Arch Phys Med Rehabil* 1988;69:527–531.
8. Bennett R. Disabling fibromyalgia: appearance versus reality. *J Rheumatol* 1993;20:1821–1824.
9. Cohen M, Quintner J. Fibromyalgia syndrome, a problem of tautology. *Lancet* 1993;342:906–909.
10. Hudson J, Pope H, Goldenberg D, et al. Comorbidity of fibromyalgia with medical and psychiatric disorders. *Am J Med* 1992;92:363–367.
11. Ahles T, Khan S, Yunus M, et al. Psychiatric status of patients with primary fibromyalgia, patients with rheumatoid arthritis, and subjects without pain: a blind comparison of DSM-III diagnoses. *Am J Psychiatry* 1991;148:1721–1726.
12. Birnie D, Knipping A, van Rijswijk M, et al. Psychological aspects of fibromyalgia compared with chronic and nonchronic pain. *J Rheumatol* 1991;18:1845–1848.
13. Martensen R. Was neurasthenia a 'legitimate morbid entity'? *JAMA* 1994;372:1243.
14. Abbey S, Garfinkel P. Neurasthenia and chronic fatigue syndrome: the role of culture in the making of a diagnosis. *Am J Psychiatry* 1991;148:1638–1646.
15. Bou-Holaigah I, Rowe P, Kan J, et al. The relationship between neurally mediated hypotension and the chronic fatigue syndrome. *JAMA* 1995;274:961–967.
16. Rowe P, Calkins H, DeBusk K, et al. Fludrocortisone acetate to treat neurally mediated hypotension in chronic fatigue syndrome. *JAMA* 2001;285:52–59.
17. Moss-Morris R, Petrie K, Large R, et al. Neuropsychological deficits in chronic fatigue syndrome: artifact or reality? *J Neurol Neurosurg Psychiatry* 1996;60:474–477.
18. Hart R, Martelli M, Zasler N. Chronic pain and neuropsychological functioning. *Neuropsychol Rev* 2000;10:131–149.
19. Blazer D, Swartz M, Woodbury M, et al. Depressive syndromes and depressive diagnoses in a community population. *Arch Gen Psychiatry* 1988;45:1078–1084.
20. Black DW, Winokur G, Nasrallah A. Suicide in subtypes of major affective disorder. *Arch Gen Psychiatry* 1987;44:878–880.
21. Murphy JM, Monson RR, Olivier DC, et al. Affective disorders and mortality. *Arch Gen Psychiatry* 1987;44:473–480.
22. Regier DA, Boyd JH, Burke JD, et al. One-month prevalence of mental disorders in the United States based on five epidemiologic catchment area sites. *Arch Gen Psychiatry* 1988;45:977–986.
23. McKinlay WW, Brooks DN, Martinage DP, et al. The short-term outcome of severe blunt head injury as reported by relatives of the injured person. *J Neurol Neurosurg Psychiatry* 1981;44:527–533.
24. Levine MJ, Gueramy M, Friedrich D. Psychophysiological responses to closed head injury. *Brain Inj* 1987;1:171–181.
25. Levin HS, Grossman RG. Behavioral sequelae of closed head injury: a quantitative study. *Arch Neurol* 1978;35:720–727.
26. Vauhkonen K. Suicide among the male disabled with war injuries to the brain. *Acta Psychiatr Neurol Scand* 1959;137[Suppl]:90–91.
27. Robinson RG, Szetela B. Mood change following left hemispheric brain injury. *N Ann Neurol* 1981;9:447–453.
28. Robinson RG, Starr LB, Price TR. A two year longitudinal study of mood disorders following stroke: prevalence and duration at six months follow-up. *Br J Psychiatry* 1984;144:256–262.
29. Robinson RG, Kubos KL, Starr LB, et al. Mood

changes in stroke patients: relationship to lesion location. *Compr Psychiatry* 1983;24:555–566.
30. Berrios GE, Samuel C. Affective disorder in the neurological patient. *J Nerv Ment Dis* 1987;175:173–176.
31. Mayeux R, Stern Y, Rosen J, et al. Depression, intellectual impairment and Parkinson disease. *Neurology* 1981;31:645–650.
31a. Brown GL, Wilson WP. Parkinsonism and depression. *Southern Med J* 1972;65:540–545.
32. Huber SJ, Paulson GW, Shuttleworth EC. Depression in Parkinson's disease. *Neuropsychiatry Neuropsychol Behav Neurol* 1988;1:47–51.
33. Taylor AE, Saint-Cyr JA, Lang AE, et al. Parkinson's disease and depression: a critical re-evaluation. *Brain* 1986;109:279–292.
34. Santamaria J, Tolosa E, Valles A. Parkinson's disease with depression: a possible subgroup of idiopathic parkinsonism. *Neurology* 1986;36:1130–1133.
35. Joffe RT, Lippert GP, Grey TA, et al. Mood disorder and multiple sclerosis. *Arch Neurol* 1987;44:376–378.
36. Flor-Henry P, Koles ZJ. EEG studies in depression, mania and normals: evidence for partial shifts of laterality in the affective psychoses. *Adv Biol Psychiatry* 1980;4:21–43.
37. Ross ED, Rush AJ. Diagnosis and neuroanatomical correlates of depression in brain- damaged patients. *Arch Gen Psychiatry* 1981;38:1344–1354.
38. Robinson RG, Starr LB, Kubos KL, et al. A two-year longitudinal study of post-stroke mood disorders: findings during the initial evaluation. *Stroke* 1983;14: 736–741.
39. Starkstein SE, Robinson RG, Price TR. Comparison of patients with and without poststroke major depression matched for size and location of lesion. *Arch Gen Psychiatry* 1988;45:247–252.
40. Cummings JL, Mendez MF. Secondary mania with focal cerebrovascular lesions. *Am J Psychiatry* 1984; 141:1084–1087.
41. Starkstein SE, Robinson RG, Berthier ML, et al. Differential mood changes following basal ganglia vs thalamic lesions. *Arch Neurol* 1988;45:725–730.
42. Feeney DM, Sutton RL, Boyeson MG, et al. The locus coeruleus and cerebral metabolism: Recovery of function after cortical injury. *Physiol Psychol* 1985; 13:197–203.
43. Feeney DM, Sutton RL. Catecholamines and recovery of function after brain damage. In: Stein DG, Sabel BA, eds. *Pharmacological approaches to the treatment of brain and spinal cord injuries*. New York: Plenum, 1988:121–142.
44. Cassidy SB, Gainey AJ, Butler MG. Occupational hydrocarbon exposure among father of Prader-Willi syndrome patients with and without deletions of 15q. *Am J Hum Genet* 1989;44:806–810.
45. Silver JM, Yodofsky SC, Hales RE. Depression in traumatic brain injury. *Neuropsychiatry Neuropsychol Behavioral Neurol* 1991;4:12–23.
46. Feeney DM, Baron JC. Diaschisis. *Stroke* 1986;17: 817–830.
47. Feeney DM, Gonzalez A, Law WA. Amphetamine, haloperidol and experience interact to affect rate of recovery after motor cortex surgery. *Science* 1982;217: 855–857.
48. Gualtieri CT, Evans RW. Stimulant treatment for the neurobehavioral sequelae of traumatic brain injury. *Brain Inj* 1988;2:273–290.
49. Clay TH, Gualtieri TC, Gullion C. Clinical and neuropsychological effects of the novel antidepressant, buproprion. *Psychopharmacol Bull* 1988;24:143–148.
50. Krauthammer C, Klerman GL. Secondary mania: manic syndromes associated with antecedent physical illness or drugs. *Arch Gen Psychiatry* 1978;35:1333–1338.
51. Starkstein SE, Boston JMA, Robinson RG. Mechanisms of mania after brain injury. *J Nerv Ment Dis* 1988;176:87–100.
52. Starkstein SE, Pearson GD, Boston JMA, et al. Mania after brain injury: a controlled study of causative factors. *Arch Neurol* 1987;44:1069–1073.
52a. Smith JL. Some neuro-ophthalmological aspects of head trauma. *Clin Neurosyrgery* 1964;12:181–192.
53. Naquet R, Baurand C, Benayoun R. Donnees EEG et psychologiques chez un groupe de traumatises craniens adultes. *Med Leg Dommage Corp* 1970;3:32–38.
54. Vigouroux RP, Baurand C, Naquet R. A series of patients with cranio-cerebral injuries studies neurologically, psychometrically, electroencephalographically and socially. In: *International symposium on head injuries*. Edinburgh: Churchill-Livingstone, 1971.
55. Lezak M. Recovery of memory and learning functions following traumatic brain injury. *Cortex* 1979;15:63–72.
56. Mortimer JA, Pirozzolo FJ. Remote effects of head trauma. *Dev Neuropsychol* 1985;3:215–229.
57. Rapoport SI. *Blood-brain barrier in physiology & medicine*. New York: Raven Press, 1976.
58. Guilleminault C, Faull KF, Miles L, et al. Posttraumatic excessive daytime sleepiness: a review of 20 patients. *Neurology* 1983;33:1584–1589.
59. Maccario M, Ruggles KH, Meriwether MW. Post-traumatic narcolepsy. *Mil Med* 1987;152:370–371.
60. Rivera VM, Meyer JS, Hata T, et al. Narcolepsy following hypoxic ischemia. *Ann Neurol* 1986;19:505–508.
61. Good JL, Barry E, Fishman PS. Posttraumatic narcolepsy: the complete syndrome with tissue typing. *J Neurosurg* 1989;71:765–767.
62. Isaac K, Cohen JA. Post-traumatic torticollis. *Neurology* 1989;39:1642–1643.
63. Katz DI, Alexander MP, Seliger GM, et al. Traumatic basal ganglia hemorrhage: clinicopathologic features and outcome. *Neurology* 1989;39:897–904.
64. Aicardi J. *Epilepsy in children*. New York: Raven Press, 1986.
65. Salazar AM, Jabbari B, Vance SC, et al. Epilepsy after penetrating head injury. I. Clinical correlates: a report of the Vietnam Head Injury Study. *Neurology* 1985;35: 1406–1414.
66. Caveness WF, Meirowsky AM, Rish BL. The nature of post-traumatic epilepsy. *J Neurosurg* 1979;50:545–553.
67. Annegers JF, Grabow JD, Groover RD, et al. Seizures after head trauma: a population study. *Neurology* 1980;30:683–689.
68. Jennett B. Posttraumatic epilepsy. *Adv Neurol* 1979; 22:137–147.
69. McQueen JK, Blackwood DHR, Harris P, et al. Low risk of late post-traumatic seizures following severe head injury: implications for clinical trials of prophylaxis. *J Neurol Neurosurg Psychiatry* 1983;46:899–904.
70. Young B, Rapp RP, Norton JA, et al. Failure of prophylactically administered phenytoin to prevent post-

traumatic seizures in children. *Childs Brain* 1983;10: 185–192.
71. Olsen TS, Hogenhaven H, Thage O. Epilepsy after stroke. *Neurology* 1987;37:1209–1211.
72. Faught E, Peters D, Bartolucci A, et al. Seizures after primary intracerebral hemorrhage. *Neurology* 1989; 39:1089–1093.
73. Jennett B, Teasdale G. *Management of head injuries*. Philadelphia: FA Davis, 1981.
74. Feeney DM, Walker AE. The prediction of posttraumatic epilepsy: a mathematical approach. *Arch Neurol* 1979;36:8–12.
75. Weiss GHP, Salazar AN, Vance SC, et al. Predicting posttraumatic epilepsy in penetrating head injury. *Arch Neurol* 1986;43:771–773.
76. Manaka S, Takahashi H, Sano K. The difference between children and adults in the onset of post-traumatic epilepsy. *Folia Psychiatr Neurol* 1981;35:301–304.
77. Bear DM, Fedio P. Quantitative analysis of interictal behavior in temporal lobe epilepsy. *Arch Neurol* 1977; 34:454–467.
78. Lindsay J, Ounsted C, Richards P. Long-term outcome in children with temporal lobe seizures. IV: genetic factors, febrile convulsions and the remission of symptoms. *Dev Med Child Neurol* 1980;22:429–439.
79. Lindsay J, Ounsted C, Richards P. Long-term outcome in children with temporal lobe seizures. III: psychiatric aspects in childhood & adult life. *Dev Med Child Neurol* 1979;21:630–636.
80. Walker AE, Blumer D. The fate of World War II veterans with posttraumatic seizures. *Arch Neurol* 1989;46: 23–26.
81. Masur H, Elger CE, Ludolph AC, et al. Cerebellar atrophy following acute intoxication with phenytoin. *Neurology* 1989;39:432–433.
82. Kalanie H, Niakan E, Harati Y, et al. Phenytoin-induced benign intracranial hypertension. *Neurology* 1986;36:443–444.
83. Reynolds EH. Chronic anti-epileptic toxicity: a review. *Epilepsia* 1975;16:319–352.
84. Rovet JF, Ehrlich RM. The effect of hypoglycemic seizures on cognitive function in children with diabetes: a 7 year prospective study. *J Pediatr* 1999;134: 503–506.
85. Taylor LP, Posner JB. Phenobarbital rheumatism in patients with brain tumor. *Ann Neurol* 1989;25:92–94.
86. Temkin NR, Dikmen SS, Wilensky AJ, et al. A randomized, double-blind study of phenytoin for the prevention of post-traumatic seizures. *N Engl J Med* 1990;323:497–502.
87. Hernandez TD, Naritoku DKM. Seizures, epilepsy and functional recovery after traumatic brain injury: a reappraisal. *Neurology* 1997;48:803–806.
88. Hernandez TD. Preventing post-traumatic epilepsy after brain injury: weighing the costs and benefits of anticonvulsant prophylaxis. *Trends Pharmacol Sci* 1997; 18:59–62.
89. Cummings JL. Organic delusions. *Br J Psychiatry* 1985;146:184–197.
90. Cummings JL, Gosenfeld LF, Houlihan JP, et al. Neuropsychiatric disturbances associated with idiopathic calcification of the basal ganglia. *Biol Psychiatry* 1983;18:591–599.
91. Bogerts B, Meertz E. Basal ganglia & limbic system pathology in schizophrenia. *Arch Gen Psychiatry* 1985;42:784–790.
92. Trimble MR, Cummings JL. Neuropsychiatric disturbances following brainstem lesions. *Br J Psychiatry* 1981;138:56–59.
93. Trzepacz PT, Murko AC, Gillespie MP. Progressive supranuclear palsy misdiagnosed as schizophrenia. *J Nerv Ment Dis* 1985;173:377–378.
94. Nasrallah HA, Fowler RC, Judd LL. Schizophrenic-like illness following head injury. *Psychosomatics* 1983;22:359–361.
95. Filley CM, Jarvis PE. Delayed reduplicative paramnesia. *Neurology* 1987;37:701–703.
96. Hayman MA, Abrams R. Capgras' syndrome and cerebral dysfunction. *Br J Psychiatry* 1977;130:68–71.
97. Levine DN, Finkelstein S. Delayed psychosis after right temporoparietal stroke or trauma: relation to epilepsy. *Neurology* 1982;32:267–272.
98. Barnhill LJ, Gualtieri CT. Late-onset psychosis after closed head injury. *Neuropsychiatry Neuropsychol Behav Neurol* 1989;2:211–218.
99. Furgerson SM, Rayport M. Psychoses in epilepsy. In: Blumer D, ed. *Psychiatric aspects of epilepsy*. Washington, DC: American Psychiatric Press, 1984:229–270.
100. Thomsen IV. Late psychosocial outcome in severe blunt head trauma. *Brain Inj* 1987;1:131–143.
101. Thomsen IV. Late outcome of very severe blunt head trauma: a 10–15 year second follow-up. *J Neurol Neurosurg Psychiatry* 1984;47:260–268.
102. Horvath K, Stefanatos G, Sokolski KN, et al. Improved social and language skills after secretin administration in patients with autistic spectrum disorders. *J Assoc Acad Minor Phys* 1998;9:9–15.
103. Lishman WA. Brain damage in relation to psychiatric disability after head injury. *Br J Psychiatry* 1968;114: 373–410.
104. Gualtieri CT. Psychopharmacology and the fragile X syndrome. In: Hagerman RJ, McKenzie P, eds. *1992 International Fragile X Conference Proceedings* . Dillon, CO: Spectra Publishing, 1992:167–178.
105. Amaducci L, Lippi A. Risk factors and genetic background for Alzheimer's disease. *Acta Neurol Scand* 1988;77:13 18.
106. Henderson AS. The epidemiology of Alzheimer's disease. *Br Med Bull* 1986;42:3–10.
107. Kokmen E, Beard M, Offord KP, et al. Prevalence of medically diagnosed dementia in a defined United States population: Rochester, Minnesota, January 1, 1975. *Neurology* 1989;39:773–776.
108. Evans DA, Funkenstein H, Albert MS, et al. Prevalence of Alzheimer's disease in a community population of older persons. *JAMA* 1989;262:2551–2556.
109. Berg L, Miller JP, Storandt M, et al. Mild senile dementia of the Alzheimer type: 2. Longitudinal assessment. *Ann Neurol* 1988;23:477–484.
110. Heyman A, Wilkinson WE, Stafford JA, et al. Alzheimer's disease: a study of epidemiologic aspects. *Ann Neurol* 1984;15:335–341.
111. French LR, Schuman LM, Mortimer JA, et al. A case-control study of dementia of the Alzheimer type. *Am J Epidemiol* 1985;121:414–421.
112. Shalat SL, Seltzer B, Pidcock C, et al. Risk factors for Alzheimer's disease: a case-control study. *Neurology* 1987;37:1630–1633.

113. Schofield P, Tang M, Marder K, et al. Alzheimer's disease after remote head injury: an incidence study. *J Neurol Neurosurg Psychiatry* 1997;62:119–124.
114. Guo Z, Cupples L, Kurz A, et al. Head injury and the risk of AD in the MIRAGE study. *Neurology* 2000; 54:1316–1323.
115. Violon A, Demol J. Psychological sequelae after head trauma in adults. *Acta Neurochir* 1987;85:96–102.
116. Gedye A, Beattie B, Tuokko H, et al. Severe head injury hastens age of onset of Alzheimer's disease. *J Am Geriatr Soc* 1989;37:970–973.
117. Luukinen H, Viramo P, Koski K, et al. Head injuries and cognitive decline among older adults: a population-based study. *Neurology* 1999;52:557–562.
118. O'Meara E, Kukull W, Sheppard L, et al. Head injury and risk of Alzheimer's disease by apolipoprotein genotype. *Am J Epidemiol* 1997;146:373–384.
119. Lichtman S, Seliger G, Tycko B, et al. Apolipoprotein E and functional recovery from brain injury following postacute rehabilitation. *Neurology* 2000;55:1536–1539.
120. Brown RG, Marsden CD. How common is dementia in Parkinson's disease? *Lancet* 1984;2:1262–1264.

9

Psychiatric Disorders in Mentally Retarded People

SUMMARY

Mentally retarded people are especially prone to emotional and behavioral problems. In mildly retarded people, they present more or less like typical psychiatric disorders. Diagnosis and treatment follow the usual guidelines. In the severely retarded, however, psychiatric diseases seldom present in typical form. Schizophrenia, for example, is quite common in the mildly retarded. In the severely retarded, it is very difficult to diagnose; some authorities contend that it is nonexistent. Were that the case, they would be the only human beings on the planet who were, as a group, protected from the condition.

Affective disorders are the most common neurobehavioral conditions in retarded people. Here, the pattern is similar to BI. In mildly retarded people, simple depression is the most common type, and treatment is usually quite straightforward. In the severely retarded, complex patterns of emotional instability are the rule, often accompanied by unusual behavioral manifestations. Treatment is more complicated.

Anxiety disorders and panic are extremely common in retarded people, especially in retarded people who are autistic. They tend to be underdiagnosed, however. Consequently, the anxiolytic drugs are underused. It is difficult to recognize a panic attack if its primary manifestation is aggression or self-injury.

Young women who are mildly or moderately retarded can develop an affective psychosis that may be precipitated by a sexual assault or that can present in the form of a paranoid belief that such an assault has occurred. It is difficult sometimes to discover the truth of the matter.

PSYCHIATRIC DISORDERS

When the neuropsychiatric disorders of patients with brain injury (BI) were discussed in Chapters 6, 7, and 8, three broad divisions were made: transient posttraumatic disorders, static conditions, and delayed neurobehavioral sequelae. It is a system that makes sense physiologically, is essential to the prognosis, and bears on treatment. Virtually all the psychiatric problems of patients with BI fall into one or another of these three broad categories.

The neuropsychiatric problems of mentally retarded people are not open to a neat scheme like that. The retarded are a much more diverse group than BI patients. The nature and origins of their neuropsychiatric problems must be considered in a different way. As it happens, it is again convenient to use three general divisions:

Mentally retarded people are prone to all the conventional psychiatric disorders such as depression and schizophrenia. They also are prone to behavioral disorders that are less complex than the psychiatric disorders and much less likely to manifest themselves in the nonretarded population. They are, however, no less troublesome to treat. The classic example is self-injurious behavior, but there are others, such as rumination and copraxia, that are less well known. Finally, the mentally retarded have neuropsychiatric problems that are specific to the cause of their condition. These problems are often unique and stereotyped, like Lesch-Nyhan and Prader-Willi syndromes, and are referred to here as pathobehavioral syndromes. Others use the term behavioral phenotypes.

These divisions are not necessarily physiologic or prognostic nor do they have a strong bearing on treatment. There is substantial overlap as well. Down's syndrome, for example, is a pathobehavioral disorder, by my reckoning, but a patient with Down's syndrome may be autistic or depressed—psychiatric diagnoses to be sure. He or she may also be self-injurious, a condition that the behaviorists have arrogated to their own sphere. One cannot pretend that this system is transcendent or without fault, but it is useful for the purpose of exposition.

Therefore, one uses different categories to understand the neurobehavioral problems of people with congenital brain insult and people with acquired BI, but there are areas of commonality as well. For example, both Down's syndrome and severe TBI are risk factors for the development of Alzheimer's disease. Self-injurious behavior is a problem for mentally retarded people and for patients with severe BI as well. Certain types of temporal lobe injury lead to Klüver-Bucy syndrome, a compelling model for autism. "Organic hyperphagia" in mental retardation (MR) and in BI have a great deal in common. Affective disorders, in all their varied manifestations, are the most important neuropsychiatric problems in both groups.

It is worthwhile to consider the neuropsychiatric problems of mentally retarded people juxtaposed with those of patients with BI because both demand a change in one's professional orientation. In both conditions, neuropsychiatrists have to remove themselves from the orthodox kraepelinian position that dominates modern psychiatry and occupy a more adaptationist stance. Psychiatrists identify this point of view with Adolf Meyer and neuropsychiatrists with Kurt Goldstein.

Neurobehavioral disorders after BI arise when the adaptive capacity of the organism is overwhelmed by the severity of injury, if the adaptive process itself goes awry, or if the process of recovery does not find sufficient support or is thwarted in some way. Treatment involves three corresponding steps: to support the process of recovery, to deal with the pathologic processes that lead to maladaption or deterioration, and to compensate for the limited adaptive capacity of the organism.

In the mentally retarded person, the development of adaptive systems occurs in the context of a system that has never been fully functional. Unlike acquired BI, there are no surviving systems on which to draw. The thrust of treatment, therefore, is to support the laborious development of a functional "infrastructure," and that often involves removing obstacles to development. Neurobehavioral problems arise if the limited adaptive capacity of the person is unable to cope with impulses, appetites, moods, or environmental events. They arise when elements of personality and temperament interact with functional limitations and an inhospitable environment. Tendencies to habitual responding, emotional instability, or impulsive behavior become exaggerated, especially if the patient's limitations are not expanded or if his or her environment remains inhospitable.

The pathologic processes that lead to maladaptive behaviors in patients with BI are conceptualized in terms of specific or diffuse lesions that impair functional systems. In the mentally retarded, the conceptual roots are diverse and offer no such unity. In some MR syndromes, genetics and biochemistry are the root cause, even to the point of allowing accurate syndromic reproduction in animal models. In others, maladaptive behaviors are nothing more than infantile behaviors that have never been supplanted by more effective behaviors but have become exaggerated and increasingly pathologic with time, in other words, a formal of developmental arrest. In any event, understanding and treating psychopathology are only possible if one appreciates the adaptive limitations of the patient, the available functional infrastructure, and the system of external compensations that can be brought to bear.

Finally, it is appropriate to iterate three terms that are essential both to habilitation (MR) and rehabilitation (BI): impairment, disability, and handicap. Impairment refers a specific pathologic event, e.g., retinitis pigmentosa. Disability refers to the physical incapacity that results, e.g., the patient with retinitis pigmentosa has reduced visual acuity or is totally blind. Handicap refers to the functional incapacity that may or may not be the result of the disability. A blind person is handicapped with respect to reading unless he or she is facile in braille, in which case they are not handicapped at all.

The impairments that patients with BI and patients with MR sustained are encephalopathies and more or less static. These necessarily result in some level of disability in terms of cognition, motor control, impulse control, and regulation of emotional expression. The degree to which the disabilities are handicapping is a function of compensatory systems that can be brought to bear. When the disabilities in question are neurobehavioral in nature, they are almost always significantly handicapping, far more so in my experience than cognitive or motor disabilities.

In Chapters 10 and 11, a few different approaches to the neurobehavioral aberrations of mentally retarded people are considered. We begin with the traditional psychiatric conditions, as they occur, albeit in atypical form. As a rule (and one that finds many exceptions), the conventional psychiatric disorders are most likely to be seen in people whose cognitive development is not so impaired to preclude language, that is, the mild to moderately mentally retarded. In the severe to profoundly retarded, the manifestations of psychiatric disease are obscure and undifferentiated. In all mentally retarded individuals, psychotic disorders are probably overdiagnosed, whereas the affective and anxiety disorders and chronic pain are probably underdiagnosed.

Chapter 10 addresses the particular behavior disorders of retarded people that do not fit into traditional categories. These disorders are defined in purely behavioral terms such as aggression, pica, self-injurious behavior, and stereotypy. They tend to occur in people who are severe or profoundly retarded who have not developed effective language. It is possible that they represent elemental forms of psychopathology. Like the animal behaviors that are studied in the neuropharmacology laboratory, they may be, to a degree at least, amenable to relatively simple neurochemical correlates. The evolutionists have a word, neoteny, to describe the selective preservation of infantile traits in certain individuals. The behavior disorders of the severely retarded are almost all problem behaviors of infants and very young children that are continued into adult life with unfortunate results.

In Chapter 11, the pathobehavioral syndromes are introduced. These are MR syndromes, genetic in origin and usually associated with dysmorphic features. They are associated with predictable constellations of pathologic behaviors (e.g., Lesch-Nyhan syndrome and self-injurious behavior) or with the development of a specific neuropsychiatric disorder (e.g., Down's syndrome, Alzheimer's disease). Another group of pathobehavioral syndromes associated with abnormalities of the X and Y chromosome is discussed in Chapter 13.

Chapters 15 and 16 on self-injurious behavior are a discussion on one particular behavioral disorder. Self-injurious behavior has a differential diagnosis that reiterates my approach to differential diagnosis in MR.

In the chapter on Autism (Chapter 14), we discuss the neurobehavioral problems of autistic people. Autistic people are a unique group, but most of their behavioral difficulties are met with mentally retarded people who are not autistic. Autism is not by any means a pathobehavioral syndrome. It is classified in the *Diagnostic and Statistical Manual of Mental Disorders* (DSM-IV) as a psychiatric disorder, but it is, in fact, a mongrel condition that borrows features from the static encephalopathies, developmental communication disorders, and anxiety disorders (especially obsessive-compulsive disorder).

The problem of epilepsy and its neurobehavioral and neurocognitive correlates is addressed in Chapter 17. The principles raised in that chapter are germane to the mentally retarded and to patients with BI.

It is not my intent to cultivate a new theory of how the abnormal behaviors of mentally retarded people should be classified. I only propose that several alternative models, or schemata, are necessary to embrace the full range of abnormal behaviors that occur in retarded individuals, just as several systems are necessary to embrace all the neurobehavioral disorders that occur in patients with BI. The overall prevalence of neurobehavioral disorders is between 30% and 40% in mentally retarded adults and between 40% and 60% in mentally retarded children (1). It would be surprising, indeed, if any one model could account for all of them.

AFFECTIVE DISORDERS

Epidemiology

For more than 60 years, writers have agreed that the full range of affective disorders occur in people who are mentally retarded (2). Their contributions are primarily in the form of individual case reports; survey data are less conclusive. In the Camberwell study, for example, when ICD-8 criteria were used, only 22 of 402 retarded people with psychiatric disorders had current or prior episodes of unipolar or bipolar depression (3). In the Nebraska study, using DSM-III criteria, the diagnosis of affective disorder was never made in 114 subjects referred for psychiatric consultation (4). The survey data are spurious, however, the consequence of inappropriate diagnostic methods. When Reiss (5) applied a broader diagnostic basis to a sample of 66 mentally retarded outpatients, he found that 13.6% of the patients were in fact depressed. It is a more credible number but still an underestimate. It is higher than survey results of the prevalence of depression in the general population (6) but lower than the number of depressives in any psychiatric clinic and much lower than the rates of depression after stroke or head injury. In my opinion, the prevalence of affective disorders is at least as high in mentally retarded people as it is in patients with stroke or TBI.

The epidemiologic studies do not demonstrate this, but that is a reflection on their methodologic weakness not on the truth of the matter. Consider this: compare depression with two clinical conditions that are extremely common in the general population but are rarely diagnosed in mentally retarded people: migraine and chronic pain. They, like depression, are conditions that rely strongly on patient self-report. The diagnosis of migraine or chronic pain in a patient of limited understanding and verbal ability is problematic. It must rely on the correct inference of a sensitive and perceptive examiner who in turn relies on the reports of caregivers. Migraines occur in approximately 15% of the general population, but in 30 years of practice, I have consulted only once on behalf of a retarded migraineur. Can anyone seriously maintain that the retarded are somehow protected from migraine or is it simply a diagnosis that is overlooked? The latter is more likely.

It is not unlikely that migraine and chronic pain underlie many of the behavioral disorders for which mentally retarded people are referred to psychiatrists. The same is true of depression. When a physician treats the maladaptive behaviors or challenging behaviors of a mentally retarded person with an antidepressant, a mood stabilizer, or an atypical antipsychotic drug, it is possible that he or she is inadvertently treating migraine, chronic pain, or depression, all of which happen to respond favorably to the same drugs.

Diagnosis

The perceived rate of affective disorders in mentally retarded people is a function of the criteria that are used to define affective disorder. Because mentally retarded people are less effective at relating their subjective state, the diagnosis relies almost entirely on the examiner's observations and the reports of caregivers. These, of course, are a function of their presuppositions and points of view. If the patient does not complain of being depressed, if the examiner is not looking for depression, and the caregiver does not even know what to look for, the diagnosis will never be made.

One may make the diagnosis of major affective disorder in a mildly retarded person or in a moderately retarded person who is suitably verbal by applying traditional DSM criteria. In the severely to profoundly retarded person, however, self-report of mood is not an appropriate criterion, and the diagnosis can only be inferred. It is risky to try to infer someone else's mood state from overt behaviors, but sometimes there is no alternative. Because the treatments of affective disorder are so effective, it is important that we have a low threshold for making the diagnosis.

The diagnosis of a major affective disorder may be made in mentally retarded people based on the following clinical elements (7):

1. A change is observed in the patient's emotional state, in a negative direction and from an established baseline.
2. This change persists for at least 2 months.
3. The emotional state of the depressed patient may be described consistently as sad, melancholic, or prone to tears or as irritable and prone to angry outbursts or tantrums.
4. Symptoms include emotional lability; anhedonia or lack of interest in things that were formerly agreeable; anxiety, fearfulness, panic, or agitation; somatic complaints, hypochondriasis, or somatic delusions; morbid thoughts, memories, or preoccupations; suicidal thoughts or gestures; self-injury.
5. The patient's emotional state may be inferred from behavioral changes such as social isolation, withdrawal, anergia, hypoactivity, psychomotor retardation, or agitation.
6. It may be inferred from the development of vegetative symptoms such as anorexia or hyperphagia, weight loss or gain, constipation, insomnia, or hypersomnolence.
7. It may be inferred based on developmental regression or a fall off in performance in school or in the workshop.
8. Manic behavior and hypomania are given to a similarly wide range of symptoms: emotional such as euphoria or agitation or irritability; behavioral such as distractibility, off-task, out-of-seat, hyperactivity, aggressiveness, destructiveness, and disorganization; vegetative such as insomnia, anorexia, and hyperphagia. One may observe a dramatic increase in whatever target behavior the patient was usually prone to. Social interactions and workshop performance may deteriorate.

The diagnosis of a depressive or a manic episode is easy when it hinges on a clearly observed change in the patient's mental state or when the changes follow a well-defined up-down pattern suggestive of cycling or rapid cycling. There are two problems, however. One is that some depressive episodes may have persisted for such a long time that no one will have remembered a discrete change; chronic depression (or dysthymia) may be a lifelong condition. Thus, evidence for a change in mental state is not always available to the consultant, and the diagnosis is therefore less secure.

The other problem is that of cyclical behavior. As you should remember from having read the Italian philosopher Vico, everything occurs in cycles. Every biologic system, the heavenly bodies, and perhaps all of creation is organized around the continual reoccurrence of cycles. Since Vico, no one seems to be more adept at detecting subtle but ineluctable cycles in human misbehavior than the psychiatrist with a low threshold for the diagnosis of bipolar disorder. There is, indeed, credible new evidence to the effect that bipolar disorder is underdiagnosed and that partial manifestations of the condition may present in atypical ways. Conversely, the mere suggestion of an on-off or up-down pattern to a patient's mood state is not sufficient for the diagnosis of bipolar disorder. It is all too easy to attribute a circular pattern to the day-to-day variability that characterizes the emotional state of the mentally retarded or patients with BI, but that is not necessarily rapid cycling bipolar disorder.

The affective disorders include a number of diagnoses, e.g., dysthymia, major depression, bipolar disorder, mixed anxiety and depression, rapid cycling bipolar disorder, cyclothymia. All these conditions occur in the retarded, but a substantial number of mentally retarded people are prone to affective conditions that are not quite as differentiated. Their problems are characterized by emotional instability, irritability, dysphoria, and occasional outbursts. The negative mood state is neither persistent nor pervasive, nor is it immediately obvious.

Emotional instability, dysphoria, and irritability are central to the diagnosis of organic mood disorders, organic affective disorders, and intermittent explosive disorders. These are the most common psychiatric symptoms that occur in mentally retarded people and in patients with stroke and traumatic brain injury (TBI).

Affective Disorders in Special Populations

In patients with head injury, MR, epilepsy, stroke, and other encephalopathic conditions, affective symptoms are quite common, often debilitating, and usually require pharmacologic management. Only occasionally do they meet diagnostic criteria for a discrete major affective episode. In these special populations, affective symptoms tend to be more variable, more changeable from day to day, and more given to sudden extremes of emotional expression. They are less prone to the pervasive cognitive dimension (pessimism, hopelessness, anhedonia) that affective disorders have in adults with normal cortical function.

The same is true for affective disorders that occur in children and the demented elderly. Indeed, the characteristic of affective disorders in special populations is the comparative rarity of discrete affective episodes in contrast to the extreme frequency of transient negative mood states and the comparative rarity of prolonged extremes of mood in contrast to the extreme frequency of emotional instability or lability.

Transient mood swings are typical of retarded people, and also people with TBI, stroke, and dementia. They are most often negative moods, including anger, screaming, crying, and aggressive behavior. In young and vigorous retarded people, for example, young men with fragile X syndrome, the displays can be rather athletic, for example, jumping up and down, running about (or away), breaking things, or else they can just be dysphoric, for example, irritable, grumpy, oppositional, growly, and churlish. Then the mood passes, and they are all right.

The most dramatic mood swings occur in patients with BI during the coma-recovery phase. These extraordinary outbursts of inchoate rage are usually elicited by some innocent intrusion or another, such as the ministrations of a nursing attendant, but nothing personal. To end the episode, leave the room. Return 30 seconds later, the patient is calm, and, being amnestic, has forgotten all about the episode.

Such an event gives a clue to the origins of emotional instability in the patient with an encephalopathic condition. What the patient is experiencing is mood, dissociated from thought, reflection, or motivation. In pure form, the phenomenon is manifest as emotional incontinence. Other terms for the problem are emotionalism, pseudobulbar affect, and pathologic laughing and crying. This peculiar condition, in which the patient responds with appropriate but excessive emotion to ordinary events, is met with in a number of conditions, including TBI, stroke, white matter disease, Alzheimer's disease, and, often, in mentally retarded people as well. Much to the patient's embarrassment, he or she will endure paroxysms of laughter or crying in response to the blandest event: a TV commercial or an oversized American flag flying over a car dealership. There is no specific anatomic basis for the phenomenon, but it is associated with diffuse cortical disease of various kinds. One presumes that cortical inhibition is removed from the expression of emotion generated in the brainstem.

The serotonergic antidepressants are particularly effective in controlling emotionalism. Indeed, on occasion patients who take selective serotonin reuptake inhibitors complain that the drugs dampen to an unacceptable degree their normal range of affective expression. Conversely, we have seen the occasional patient on a selective serotonin reuptake inhibitor who actually complains of emotionalism as a side effect of the drug.

Sometimes affective events in patients with TBI are described in terms of mania (8). There is a syndrome that occurs in patients with brainstem injuries, especially during the recovery phase of coma, that is associated with extreme hypervigilance, hyperactivity, and mood swings. It is not inappropriate to call such behavior manic, but it is a stretch to maintain that it is a variant of manic-depression. A similar behavioral syndrome is encountered in autistic people in whom an extreme form of hyperreactivity and agitated vigilance is sometimes described as panic (9). Because treatment with α_2 adrenergic agonists and beta-blockers is often effective for such patients and hypervigilance and hyperreactivity are also seen in cases of stimulant toxicity, it is not unreasonable to propose a noradrenergic mechanism that is attributable to brainstem injury. This is not an easy condition to treat pharmacologically, and sometimes only antipsychotic drugs are successful.

The psychiatric condition that clinicians refer to as chronic dysthymia or depressive personality includes a large group of people whose energy level is somewhat low, whose outlook is perennially dim, and whose capacity for pleasure is circumscribed, to say the least. When such a patient is encountered in a BI clinic, the appropriate diagnosis is abulia, and the syndrome is usually attributable to a frontal lobe lesion in the convexity. Some mentally retarded patients have a similar syndrome, associated with low energy, social withdrawal, anhedonia, and resistance to novelty or change. A similar form of anergic depression is frequently found in elderly patients. The syndrome may also have a more active dimension, with negativism, oppositional behavior, and resistance to change, especially in patients with frontal lobe injury and in children with affective disorders. Treatment is better with the so-called dopamine agonists such as the psychostimulants, amantadine, L-dopa, and bromocriptine.

There are rapid cyclers and emotionally unstable individuals who are given to extremes of emotional highs and lows and who may bounce frequently from one extreme to another. One may refer to such patients as atypical bipolars. This is different from the hypervigilance/hyperreactivity syndrome discussed because the emotional events may occur without even the most trivial offense. Many of these patients have temporal lobe disease, and treatment is probably more rational with a psychotropic anticonvulsant.

All the variants of emotional dysregulation that are engendered by TBI and stroke are also encountered in mentally retarded people. All the medications that are useful for affective disorders in patients with TBI and stroke are similarly effective in the mentally retarded.

ANXIETY DISORDERS

The anxiety disorders are closely related to the affective disorders:

1. There is overlap of symptoms; it is rare to find an anxious patient who has no symptoms of depression or a patient with panic disorder who is not anxious and depressed (10).
2. There is overlap among the treatments. Anxiety, panic, and depression are all treated, for better or worse, with antidepressants and benzodiazepines (11).
3. There is no neuropathic differentiation between anxiety and depression, i.e., a lesion, hemisphere, or disease, that is reliably associated with anxiety and not depression or the other way around.
4. The disorders do not breed true: within families, people may have slightly different manifestations of what may be thought of as a genetic proclivity to affective dysregulation: one member of the family may be depressive, another more anxiety prone, and a third given to panic attacks. A fourth might drink to excess, but that might be because he or she has to live with "one, two, and three."

This is no less true of mentally retarded people in whom anxiety and depression are often intermixed. There is very little difference in the principles of treatment. The antidepressants, especially the serotonergics, benzodiazepines, and the atypical anxiolytic buspirone, are all effective, although, as a rule, effective doses may be somewhat lower.

The manifestations of anxiety states, panic, and mixed anxiety depression are not much different in mentally retarded people, nor are they manifestly different in patients with BI, patients with stroke, the demented elderly, and children. It is probably true that severe anxiety, the type that leads to total emotional breakdown, is more common in encephalopathic cases. It is certainly true that encephalopathic patients with severe, disorganizing anxiety are often thought to be psychotic and are treated with antipsychotic drugs. The antipsychotic drugs are, after all, effective for severe anxiety. They are not, by any means, the treatment of choice. Indeed, the misdiagnosis of anxiety has always been one of the sources of inappropriate neuroleptic treatment in the mentally retarded.

Symptoms of anxiety and panic are not uncommon in developmentally handicapped people and are very common in autistic people. In some cases, they fit neatly into DSM categories and respond to the conventional treatments. In other cases, alternative constructions may be appropriate. Irrational fear and panic may be ictal or peri-ictal, related especially to lesions in the temporal lobe. What appears to be panic may be an expression of hypervigilance/hyperreactivity syndrome.

Mentally retarded people may be referred because of problems with angry outbursts or aggressive behavior. Some of these patients are, in fact, subject to anxiety and/or panic attacks. It may be difficult to know for sure. If the patient is also autistic, one might be more inclined to suspect an anxiety disorder. If the patient responds to a long-acting benzodiazepine or an anxiolytic anticonvulsant drug such as gabapentin or tiagabine, one may assume that anxiety was the correct diagnosis.

Anxiety is a universal human emotion. Everyone has experienced anxiety in circumstances of insecurity. Because a person who is cognitively impaired is less well equipped to master an unfamiliar or a threatening situation, feelings of insecurity and anxiety are more common, and coping strategies to mitigate anxiety are less successful. Because emotions tend to grow stronger as they are repeatedly experienced, anxiety disorders are necessarily more common and more disabling in the cognitively impaired.

Are the anxiety disorders more common in the mildly retarded compared with the severely retarded, as is the case with schizophrenia? Or, like depression, are they equally common at every level of mental handicap? There is not a vast body of evidence to rely on in addressing this question. At one time, I was convinced that the severely handicapped were less prone to anxiety disorders than people who are only mildly retarded. More recently, the impressive success of treatment with anxiolytic drugs, especially in the severely retarded, has given pause.

There are plenty of examples of a small degree of handicap proving to be more troublesome, in some dimensions at least, than a profound handicap. The psychiatric consequences of epilepsy, for example, are much more common in people who only have occasional seizures. Retarded people who have severe seizure disorders, seize every day, and have several seizures every day are extremely unlikely to have psychiatric disorders. Patients with mild BIs are much more likely to complain of headache than people who have had severe BIs. There are circumstances in which large cortical lesions have less impact over the long term than smaller lesions (12).

All that is true, but it begs the question. Anxiety and depression, it must be remembered, are closely related states. They are probably expressed with equal vigor across the spectrum of mental handicap.

SCHIZOPHRENIA

All the typical functional psychoses occur in mentally retarded people with a frequency that equals or exceeds the population at large: manic depression, affective psychosis, schizoaffective disorder, transient schizophreniform reactions, and schizophrenia. There are problems with accurate diagnosis, to be sure, just as there are among patients who are not retarded. There are physicians who make the diagnosis too frequently, and those who never make the diagnosis at all. In the past, psychoses were certainly overdiagnosed in the mentally retarded and overtreated as well. Now one encounters the opposite problem.

As recently as 1978, it was possible to make the diagnosis of psychosis in severely retarded people based on bizarre behavior (e.g., stereotypies) or psychotic withdrawal (e.g., poor eye contact) and to maintain that 23% of the severely retarded were in fact psychotic (13). This kind of thinking began with Kraepelin, who maintained than no fewer that 7% of all cases of dementia praecox arose based on "idiocy" and who coined the term *pfropfschizophrenia* for the combined disorder. In 1932, no less a luminary than Critchley maintained that stereotypies in mentally retarded patients with tuberous sclerosis were indicative of catatonia (14). It was clearly a turn away from the nineteenth-century tradition of drawing a line between "idiotism" and mental illness. During that enlightened century, psychiatric conditions were known to occur in the retarded, but "insanity" was thought to be rare in the severest forms of "amentia" (15).

Schizophrenia does occur in retarded people. The major prevalence studies done in the United Kingdom affirmed that it is indeed a problem in the mild to moderately retarded but that it cannot be diagnosed on clinical grounds in the more severe and profound ranges of retardation. Its prevalence among the former is approximately 3% (16). In general, there is nothing unique or esoteric in the symptomatology of schizophrenia in mentally retarded people (16).

Much of what was once thought to be schizophrenia is now known to be something else. Today, it is rare to hear autistics referred to as "psychotic children," and autism is no longer thought to be a form of childhood schizophrenia. We recognize, as Bleuler did, that the stereotypies of the severely mentally retarded are really quite different from the stereotypies of schizophrenic patients. When a schizophreniform psychosis arises in a retarded person as a discrete episode, it is usually diagnosed as an affective psychosis and treated accordingly. The prognosis is usually quite good. The psychosis of epilepsy, toxic psychoses from psychotropic and anticonvulsant drugs, and the peculiar mannerisms of Tourette's syndrome may all be mislabeled as schizophrenia.

It is arguable that the first rank symptoms are undetectable in the severely retarded because they are nonverbal but that a "schizophrenic core" may fester beneath the surface. Certainly, one may see severely retarded people who are unrelated and withdrawn, whose behavior is disorganized and even bizarre, who are paranoid sometimes, and who may even seem to hallucinate. It is not a common clinical event, but it occurs frequently enough. The differential diagnosis of such behavior includes a number of alternatives that are more convincing than the diagnosis of schizophrenia. It is rare, indeed, to be secure in the diagnosis of schizophrenia in a severely mentally retarded person.

Schizophreniform psychosis occurs in some MR syndromes more commonly than in others. The sex chromosome disorders (fragile X syndrome, Klinefelter's syndrome, XYY syndrome) are more prone to psychosis than most of the other pathobehavioral syndromes. They also happen to be syndromes, however, typified by only mild to moderate degrees of mental handicap.

Schizophrenia in its traditional kraepelinian form (dementia praecox) behaves like an adolescent-onset encephalopathy, with a deteriorating course that not infrequently leads to significant mental handicap. In fact, state facilities for the mentally retarded have more and more referrals from the downsizing state hospitals of chronic schizophrenics who are adjudicated "retarded" by virtue of an IQ score below 70. But that is another story.

The nineteenth-century distinction, therefore, between MR and insanity is thus upheld. Obviously, the two conditions are not incompatible, but their co-occurrence is now understood to be limited to mentally retarded people who possess language, i.e., the mild and moderately retarded.

In my opinion, the affective psychoses are much more prevalent than schizophrenia among the mentally retarded at every level of mental handicap. Instability of mood is one of the most common characteristics of retarded people who are psychotic. When they have disorganized or bizarre behavior, hallucinations, or paranoia, it is usually mood syntonic. The antidepressants, mood stabilizers, and high-potency benzodiazepines are much more likely to control symptoms over the long run than the antipsychotics care.

I am, of course, influenced by my experience with patients with TBI who are, like patients with stroke, extremely prone to severe affective illness, including the affective psychoses. We have already described the extremely high rate of affective disorders in patients with severe TBI (40% to 60%), and the relatively low rate of posttraumatic psychosis (2% to 5%). When the patient with TBI develops a schizophreniform psychosis, its clinical manifestations and appropriate treatments are closer to those of the psychoses of epilepsy than they are to those of schizophrenia. The classic presentation of paranoid schizophrenia, for example, is hardly ever found in patients with TBI or in the severely retarded for that matter.

From the perspective of treatment, the acute treatment of a psychotic disorder that derives from a neuropathic condition is not necessarily different from classic schizophrenia. Acute symptomatic treatment with antipsychotic drugs is usually the only successful approach. It is over the long-term, however, that the treatments diverge. Long-term antipsychotic therapy is not always necessary in patients with severe TBI or mentally retarded persons who have been psychotic. High-dose neuroleptic treatment is almost never required. The long-term mood stabilizers lithium, valproate, and carbamazepine are the primary long-term treatments. As the years go by, the relapses that occur will usually be affective in nature and will require augmentative antidepressant or benzodiazepine therapy.

In mentally retarded people, autistic people, patients with fragile X syndrome, patients with TBI, and the demented elderly, the treatment of psychosis is guided by what is necessary and what is possible. If treatment is possible with a drug that is more agreeable and less toxic than an antipsychotic drug, the patient is lucky and the physician is relieved. One should never shrink, however, from the judicious application of a neuroleptic if that is what the circumstances demand. People who care for the mentally retarded sometimes disapprove of antipsychotic drugs because of their blunting effects. The cognitive toxicity of a neuroleptic is never so destructive as a persistent psychosis can be.

There is a rough equivalence in the programmatic treatment of the psychotic disorders, whatever their origin or diagnostic affiliation. Structure, protection, and limited demands are the essence of long-term behavioral management. It is ironic that the chronic schizophrenics who succeed in transferring to an MR facility usually do quite well there, better than they used to do in the state hospitals, in fact. There is more structure, and the programs are habilitative. The environment is safer and more homelike, and the demands of social integration are more easily met.

Sexual Psychosis

Young mentally retarded people, especially females in late adolescence and their early 20s, are prone to an affective psychosis characterized by extreme anxiety, irrational fears, emotionalism (especially tearfulness), disorganization, loss of self-help skills, and complete dependence on a parental figure, most often the mother. The psychosis usually has an abrupt onset and is not preceded by premorbid symptoms or personality deficits. It is most common in patients who are mild to moderately retarded and is not associated with autism or epilepsy. Its initial symptoms are those of an anxiety disorder or of agitated depression, but then the patients grow increasingly disorganized and finally, psychotic. It may be precipitated by a sexual encounter or a sexual assault. Alternatively, accusations of sexual assault may be an early paranoid symptom. It is sometimes very difficult to determine the truth, and the accused is often another retarded individual at school, on the bus, or in the workshop. Sometimes, one suspects that the patient's sexual preoccupations are delusional or erotomanic. On the other hand, instances of sexual abuse against mentally retarded females are so common that one can never be sure.

Parents are understandably dismayed at the dramatic change that overtakes their child, the severe loss of adaptive skills, and the emotional regression. They are not reassured by the failure of early treatments with antidepressants or anxiolytics, and because the course of the disorder may carry on for months, they begin to fear that the changes may be permanent in nature. They are dismayed by the possibility of alleged sexual assault and tortured by the uncertainty of not knowing whether it happened. They develop a morbid but understandable fear that a chronic mental illness is developing. Because all this is occurring in a retarded child who has already negotiated the most difficult challenges of the school years and whose habilitation is almost complete, their dismay is understandable.

The patient will ultimately respond to low or moderate doses of an appropriate antipsychotic, but a full recovery will take months or longer. Fortunately, full recovery is the rule, and long-term treatment with antipsychotics is rarely, if ever, indicated. In fact, full recovery seldom occurs until the patient finds an agreeable mood stabilizer.

Varley (17), Collacott (18), Ghaziuddin and Tsai (19), Cooper and Collacott (20), and McGuire et al. (21) described psychotic conditions of this type. The descriptions are all fairly recent, probably a function of community placement, where mentally retarded girls live in less protected environments and are exposed to the pressures of sexuality in their day-to-day lives. It is not surprising that retarded people find this to be a dangerous period of transition.

REFERENCES

1. Dosen A. Diagnosis and treatment of psychiatric and behavioural disorders in mentally retarded individuals: the state of the art. *J Intellect Disabil Res* 1993;37:1–7.
2. Sovner R, Hurley A. The management of chronic behavior disorders in mentally retarded adults with lithium carbonate. *J Nerv Ment Dis* 1981;169:191–195.
3. Corbett JA. Psychiatric morbidity and mental retardation. In: James FE, Smith RP, eds. *Psychiatric illness & mental handicap*. London: Gaskell Press, 1979:11–25.
4. Eaton LF, Menolascino FJ. Psychiatric disorders in the mentally retarded: types, problems, and challenges. *Am J Psychiatry* 1982;139:1297–1303.
5. Reiss S. Psychopathology and mental retardation: survey of a developmental disabilities mental health program. *Ment Retard* 1982;20:128–132.
6. Blazer D, Swartz M, Woodbury M, et al. Depressive syndromes and depressive diagnoses in a community population. *Arch Gen Psychiatry* 1988;45:1078–1084.
7. Gualtieri CT. The differential diagnosis of self-injurious behavior in mentally retarded people. *Psychopharmacol Bull* 1989;25:358–363.
8. Bakchine S, Lacomblez L, Benoit N, et al. Manic-like state after bilateral orbitofrontal and right temporoparietal injury: efficacy of clonidine. *Neurology* 1989;39:777–781.
9. Grandin T, Scariano MM. *Emergence labelled autistic*. Novato, CA: Arena Press, 1986.
10. Kendler KS, Heath AC, Martin NG, et al. Symptoms of anxiety and symptoms of depression: same genes, different environments? *Arch Gen Psychiatry* 1987;44:451–460.
11. Rickels K, Schweitzer EE. Current pharmacotherapy of anxiety disorders. In: Meltzer HY, ed. *Psychopharmacology: the third generation of progress*, 3rd ed. New York: Raven Press, 1987:1193–1203.
12. Irle E. Lesion size and recovery of function: some new perspectives. *Brain Res Rev* 1987;12:307–320.
13. Haracopos D, Kelstrup A. Psychotic behavior in children under the institutions for the mentally retarded in Denmark. *J Autism Child Schizophr* 1978;8:1–12.
14. Reid AH. Psychoses in adult mental defectives: II. Schizophrenic and paranoid psychoses. *Br J Psychiatry* 1972;120:213–218.
15. Turner TH. Schizophrenia and mental handicap: an historical review, with implications for further research. *Psychol Med* 1989;19:301–314.
16. Reid AH. Schizophrenia in mental retardation: clinical features. *Res Dev Disabil* 1989;10:241–249.
17. Varley CK. Schizophreniform psychoses in mentally retarded adolescent girls following sexual assaults. *Am J Psychiatry* 1984;141:593–595.
18. Collacott RA. Erotomanic delusions in mentally handicapped patients: two case reports. *J Ment Defic Res* 1987;31:87–92.
19. Ghaziuddin M, Tsai L. Depression-dependent erotomanic delusions in a mentally handicapped woman. *Br J Psychiatry* 1991;158:127–129.
20. Cooper SA, Collacott RA. Pathological jealousy and mental handicap. *J Intellect Disabil Res* 1993;37:195–199.
21. McGuire BE, Akuffo E, Choon GL. Somatic sexual hallucinations and erotomanic delusions in a mentally handicapped woman. *J Intellect Disabil Res* 1994;38:79–83.

10
Disorders of Behavior

SUMMARY

Severely retarded people are prone to problems that are not listed in the psychiatric manuals. I refer to them here simply as behavioral disorders. Perhaps they are just symptoms of an underlying condition. Certainly, problems such as oppositional behavior and aggression can be symptoms of an underlying psychiatric disorder, a behavioral phenotype, seizures, or drug toxicity.

Conversely, repetitive behavioral problems and patterns of emotional reactivity in the severely retarded can be extremely primitive and undifferentiated. It is not always accurate to attribute them to an underlying pathologic process, beyond the limitations of severe intellectual deficit compounded by sensorimotor impairment, environmental deprivation, or both. The repetitive behaviors that retarded people manifest usually serve purposes that are no more complex than self-stimulation, self-calming, or pain control.

The regulation of behavior in severely retarded people is governed by subcortical mechanisms, perhaps in the striatum. There is little direct evidence for this idea, but it is consistent with the fact that similar behavior disorders can be elicited in lower organisms, under circumstances of stress, even in rodents, who do not have even have a cerebral cortex. In any event, subcortical behaviors are typified by a sluggish response to reinforcers. They are less goal directed and more driven by stereotypy, habit, or compulsion.

Undifferentiated patterns of emotional reactivity in severely retarded people include irritability, withdrawal, and affective lability. These could be attributed to underlying depression or anxiety, but it is more likely that they represent primitive patterns of affective expression.

The literature on self-injurious behavior usually presents it as a pure disorder of behavior, and that is true, at least to a degree. Self-injury is dealt with at some length in Chapters 15 and 16.

BEHAVIOR DISORDERS

In mentally retarded people, some problems are defined in terms of the particular behavior that is at issue, e.g., noncompliance, stereotypy, self-injurious behavior. They often occur in retarded people who have psychiatric diagnoses or pathobehavioral syndromes but also occur by themselves with no other diagnostic hallmark.

NONCOMPLIANCE

Child psychiatrists use the term oppositional. Clinicians who work with schizophrenics or patients with brain injury call it negativism. In mental retardation, this target behavior is usually referred to as noncompliance. The condition is found frequently in its different forms, but there is virtually no literature on it. Stubbornness and nay-saying are not events that excite scientific interest. They do excite literary interest, as in *Oblomov*, Bartleby the Scrivener, and *The Loneliness of the Long Distance Runner*.

Writers have interpreted noncompliance or oppositional behavior as a form of individual expression, albeit a negative one. Oblomov was a lazy aristocrat, a slob; the polite expression is *ennui du siecle*. The long distance runner, in Alan Sillitoe's story, was expressing the outrage of an oppressed class, if you will, or, alternatively, a sense of despair over his father's meaningless life and death. In both stories, and, of course, in Bartleby, the dramatic hinge is "no."

Writers understand negativism and oppositional behavior. In fact, they tend to live it. If you ever tried to convince an author to abandon his or her Underwood and buy a word processor, you have probably encountered a good case of oppositional behavior. Scientific writers have been reluctant to take the problem on; perhaps it is because of their own ineluctable positivism. Have you ever read a paper that ended with the words: "no more research is needed" or "this topic is simply too dull and unimportant to carry on"? Probably not. Anyway, literary allusions aside, it may be that no one writes about oppositional disorder because no one has found an interesting context in which to frame the problem. In fact, there is.

When I worked in a child psychiatry clinic, the question of oppositional behavior would occasionally come up. When I worked at facilities for mentally retarded people, there would be behavioral graphs to peruse that referred to episodes of noncompliant behavior. In either event, I shrugged my shoulders, made a recommendation, and then carried on to the next patient. It was not the red meat of neuropsychiatric practice. The prescription would be this: look for specific areas of cognitive weakness or emotional vulnerability that were the "setting event" for negativistic behavior and deal with them, structure the patient's experiences in a developmentally appropriate way, and handle transitions in a gentle and a creative way. That was all.

It was not until I began to work with patients with traumatic brain injuries that the problem of oppositional behavior got interesting because it finally began to make sense. In brain injury, oppositional behavior and noncompliance are the manifestations of frontal lobe injury, especially the right frontal lobe. Patients with lesions in this area can be very stubborn. Adult patients with lesions of the convexity can be as intractable and truculent as the most oppositional child. They are inflexible and usually have difficulty "changing sets."

The idea of cognitive flexibility refers to one's capacity to change behavioral or cognitive sets in response to changing circumstances. It is a term that arose in neuropsychology and is demonstrated in tests such as the Wisconsin Card Sort, the Categories Test, and in a number of Luria tasks. The extreme of cognitive inflexibility is perseveration, which is well demonstrated on these tests. In the Stroop Test, the patient with frontal lobe injury has great difficulty operating out of two simultaneous cognitive sets, suppressing one while the other is active.

The function of the frontal lobes is to execute complex programs of activity, form the orienting basis for action, and organize its strategy (1). Lesions of the frontal convexity lead to motor stereotypy and a derangement in complex forms of organized behavior against the background of intact consciousness. Patients with such lesions have an inertia to maintain the present set. They are inflexible in the face of changing external demands because they cannot dissociate their responses or pull their attention away from what is in their present field (2). They eschew novel circumstances because they have difficulty maintaining organization in the face of insufficient redundancy (3). Once they get going in a new set and when redundancy or at least familiarity is established, they continue in a perfectly suitable way. It is the transition that is hard for them.

Patients with frontal lobe injury, like primates with dorsolateral lesions, are sluggish in response to reinforcers. The feedback to actions from their outcomes is impaired, so reinforcers become relatively ineffective (3). Therefore, it is no easy matter to induce them to be more accommodating by rewarding or punishing selected behaviors.

The pathophysiology of noncompliance, therefore, has to do with the physiology of frontal lobe function in distributing attention and organized behavior in response to appropriate external requirements and in registering novelty so that habituation or assimilation can take place.

It should not be surprising when similar difficulties arise in a troubled child who, in the first decade of life, has little in the way of frontal lobe resources or in severely retarded people who have a diffuse encephalopathy and little in the way of cortical executive function at all. It is frequently encountered in adolescent patients. The executive powers of their frontal lobes are as yet underdeveloped, even as the executive powers of their basal ganglia have faded away.

Understanding the physiology should direct treatment. The principles of treatment for oppositional behavior, based on this understanding, are to look for specific areas of cognitive weakness or emotional trauma that would be a setting event for the negativistic behavior and to contend with them, to structure the patient's experiences in a developmentally appropriate way, and to handle transitions in a gentle and a creative way.

The psychopharmacology of oppositional behavior, noncompliance, and negativism is relatively straightforward. In patients with brain injury, we rely on the activating properties of the psychostimulants (and related drugs such as amantadine). In children who have oppositional-defiant disorder, the underlying pathology is usually attention deficit/hyperactivity disorder or affective disorder. Thus, one uses a stimulant or antidepressant. The negativism of schizophrenic patients may improve with one of the atypical antipsychotic drugs, especially clozapine. Stimulants, amantadine, and antidepressants may also mitigate the problem in schizophrenics.

In their pattern of drug response, retarded people resemble patients with brain injury and children with oppositional-defiant disorder. Noncompliance is dealt with, first behaviorally and then pharmacologically. Stimulants, amantadine, and various antidepressants are sometimes helpful.

STEREOTYPY

Stereotypies are repetitious, topographically invariant motor behaviors or action sequences in which reinforcement is noncontingent (4). They are a normal behavioral variant in infancy and early childhood (5) but are far more dramatic when they occur in retarded and autistic people and in the congenitally deaf and the blind ("blindisms"). Stereotypies occur in approximately two-thirds of these populations (6).

The most common stereotypies are whole-body movements or postures (rocking, twirling), other repetitive movements (head rolling, head banging), nonrepetitive movements (posturing, sucking), complex hand movements, manipulation of objects, and meaningless utterances (7). For the most part, the stimuli that initiate, guide, and reward stereotyped behavior have their origin within the organism performing the act (8). This feature renders stereotypies relatively resistant to behavioral treatment.

Stereotypies arise in two different contexts. They are more likely to occur in people with severe sensory impairments—the congenitally blind and deaf (9,10). They occur in circumstances of confinement (11), restriction (12), or sensory deprivation (13,14). This suggests a functional end in the service of self-stimulation. Zoo behavior or stereotypy in animals (especially foraging animals such as bears) occurs when they are confined, frustrated, or isolated. The motor patterns include scratching, hair pulling, masturbation, and endless pacing (15).

Stereotypies may also have a purpose in the service of tension reduction. They are likely to occur in response to intense environmental stimuli (16), frustration (17), or novel situations (12). The animal equivalent is displacement behavior or stereotyped motor acts (or fixed motor patterns) that are excessive and inappropriate. The particular behaviors, such as pecking, grooming, digging, or head turning, are typical within a species but vary greatly between species. They are invariably triggered by an emotionally laden situation, such as sexual or territorial conflicts, and it is believed that their purpose is to reduce tension associated with conflict (15).

Stereotyped motor activity has a well-known neuropharmacologic basis because it can be evoked quite reliably in laboratory rats by lesions or chemical agents that induce a state of hypersensitivity in the postsynaptic striatal dopamine receptor (18). Apomorphine-induced stereotypy after a 6-hydroxydopamine–induced lesion is a classic preparation. It is reversed by D_2 dopamine receptor antagonists such as haloperidol. In clinical circumstances, neuroleptics are very effective in reducing stereotypies. Dopamine agonists, like L-dopa and the psychostimulants, evoke stereotyped behavior, especially in high doses.

Noncompliance, rituals, preoccupation with sameness, tyrannical behavior, and stereotypies are all manifestations of frontal lobe dysfunction or, to be more precise, dysfunctions of a complex integrative system in which the frontal cortex participates to an important degree. They may be conceptualized as a failure of executive control of motor programs embedded in the basal ganglia. They are much more complex than the simple dyskinesias attributed to diseases of the basal ganglia, such as Huntington's chorea, but they respond, like chorea, to low doses of dopamine antagonists and are aggravated, like chorea, by low doses of dopamine agonists.

The pharmacologic treatment of stereotyped behavior should therefore be with neuroleptics to mitigate the influence of striatal hyperreactivity. That is hardly ever a good idea, however, because the treatment may be, in the long term, worse than the disease. The classic neuroleptics in the long run are also toxic to the dopamine receptor and actually produce severe dyskinesia. Some of the clinical manifestations of tardive dyskinesia, in fact, resemble stereotyped mannerisms. The atypical neuroleptics may be better, but they are not free from serious side effects either.

An alternative treatment strategy is to activate frontal modulation, as one does in the treatment of abulic states, with a stimulant or a dopamine agonist such as amantadine. However, it seems to be impossible to stimulate dopaminergic projections to frontal structures without also increasing dopaminergic neurotransmission to the striatum, and that, of course, is only going to make the stereotypies worse.

The pharmacologic strategies appear to be contradictory, although it should never be a surprise when opposite stimuli evoke the identical behavioral response. Stereotypies may be evoked by high doses of amphetamine (19) or can be suppressed by amphetamine (15). As we have also seen, stereotypies can be elicited clinically under circumstances of sensory deprivation or intense sensory activation.

There is a solution to this paradox in considering the mutual and interrelated roles of frontal cortex and corpus striatum in ritual and stereotyped behavior. Some light may be shed by considering the example of obsessive-compulsive disorder (OCD), and this may also be pertinent clinically. It is argued that the rituals and stereotyped behavior of autistic and retarded people are variants or prototypes of OCD. Certainly, the serotonergic treatments that are helpful for OCD are also good for treating the former conditions.

The similarity between rituals and stereotyped motor behaviors in developmentally handicapped people and people with OCD does not mean that the former is a brain-damage variant of OCD. That is a naive construction. A better way to frame the idea is to propose that the neural substrate for ritual behavior is the same in both disorders. The occurrence of stereotypies (zoo behavior and displacement behavior) in lower animals suggests that the neural substrate is subcortical. Thus, one's interest in the functional anatomy of stereotyped behavior, which begins with the consideration of the consequence of frontal lobe lesions, and extends caudally along frontal projections to the corpus striatum. This is a natural progression because the basal ganglia subserve what are usually considered to be frontal lobe functions in immature primates and in lower mammals, such as the rat, which hardly possesses a frontal cortex (20).

The basal ganglia probably participate in the ritual behavior of patients with OCD, and there is clinical evidence for lesions in the basal ganglia associated with OCD (21,22). One of the functions of the basal ganglia is presumably to release species-specific motor patterns (23). Its function is also to respond to levels of motivation, either to persist in motor patterns that are internally driven or to respond to external stimuli (24). It may be considered as a gate or a filter between the incentive system, which is input to the caudate, and the motor system, which is output (25). The incentives come from above; the appropriate response patterns are delivered to effector systems below.

The release of repetitive, meaningless stereotypes, for example, in OCD, are probably the result of something like an aberrant feedback loop around the frontal lobes, limbic cortex, basal ganglia, and thalamus (21,26,27). One may conceptualize the disorder as dissociation of the motivational from the motoric, with all the doubt, dismay, and confusion that will necessarily ensue. A reverberating circuit, if you will, and one that is badly out of balance.

The release of repetitive, meaningless stereotypes in developmentally handicapped individuals probably has a more diffuse origin, but it probably also involves a deficit in cortical modulation of striatal activity. It is not dissociation between the motivational and the motoric. It is a lapse in the capacity of frontal structures to respond to new external stimuli and to generate the motivation for adaptational motor patterns in the striatum. This is the model of a caged animal that is unable to forage and who finds nothing external that is sufficient to motivate a motor pattern. So it relies on repetitive, internal motor patterns. There is no incentive to do anything else.

This is the kind of stereotypy that occurs in severely handicapped people in circumstances of sensory deprivation. It is also the type of stereotypy that should be expected to respond favorably to a dopamine agonist (15,28) or to an antagonist (26), and it does.

For the second variant of clinical stereotypy, the mechanism is different, although the output is the same. The release of repetitive meaningless stereotypes in the face of intense novel stimuli occurs when frontal structures, inefficient in their response to novel external stimuli, are overwhelmed. New stimuli overflow the circuitry, paralyzing the system, as it were. This leaves the striatal generator once again at the mercy of a much lower, intrinsic order of motivation.

One usually will discover a degree of success against ritualized behavior in handicapped people by manipulating the serotonin system, as in OCD, but it does not always work. The effects of serotonergic drugs on movement disorders, another manifestation of striatal dysfunction, like tics and dyskinesias, are weak and unpredictable. They are better for stereotypies, tyrannical behavior, and preoccupation with sameness, but they are not invariably successful. The combination of a serotonergic with amantadine is sometimes necessary, and in severe cases, an atypical antipsychotic drug may be necessary.

RITUALS, PREOCCUPATION WITH SAMENESS, AND TYRANNICAL BEHAVIOR

The motor stereotypies that occur in patients with severe brain injuries, congenital or acquired, are also represented in more complex behavioral and emotional manifestations. Rituals are extremely complex, stereotyped behaviors that grow by accretion over the years. The bedtime rituals of autistic people are classic. If the same pattern of activity is not pursued in the same order and with the same emphasis night after night, sleep is impossible, and a horrible scene may take its place. One of my patients heard a doorbell ring during a nighttime ritual that lasted about an hour; thereafter, doorbell ringing at precisely that time had to be incorporated into the ritual.

The other symptom that is classic for autistic people is preoccupation with sameness: the same arrangement of furniture around the house, going to school by exactly the same route, the same teachers every day, the same, invariant task at work every day.

Tyrannical behavior refers to the development of stereotyped activities over the years, especially when a severely handicapped person lives at home. As parents grow elderly, they learn that the course of least resistance is to accommodate the rituals and sameness behavior of the handicapped child. Confronting the individual and failing to gratify his or her demands only lead to an outburst of rage. It is easier to give in, which only serves to expand the repertoire of stereotyped activity until the whole day is spent in gratifying ritual preoccupations. Extricating a family from this dead end can be a major operation.

PICA

Pica is the Latin word for magpie, a bird that was once believed to eat inedible things. That is also the definition of the behavioral syndrome, although it also pertains to scavenging for inedibles or mouthing them (29). Pica is a developmental variant in children with a normal IQ. It is seen in approximately half of all 1-year-old children and 10% of 4-year-old children (30,31). The most frequently ingested items are paper, clothing, dirt, matches, toilet items, plaster, writing materials, and tobacco.

Pica has been observed in 26% of a population of 991 institutionalized retarded people (32). The occurrence of pica was more common in younger patients and in patients who were more severely handicapped intellectually. Its co-occurrence with low levels of iron suggests a nutritional context and with low levels of zinc, which causes dysgeusia.

Zinc deficiency in children is associated with hypogeusia, dysgeusia, and pica (33). Supplemental zinc has been reported to eliminate pica in children (34) and in a mentally retarded adult (Lofts, unpublished data, 1986). In severe zinc deficiency, plasma levels are less than 6 µmol/L (normal range, 10 to 17) (33).

A small number of patients with habitual pica can develop serious medical consequences such as lead poisoning or intestinal obstruction. In such patients, treatment or prevention is a high priority. There is, however, no current psychopharmacologic treatment. The proper treatment strategy is to investigate the possibility of a nutritional deficiency, such as low zinc levels, or an addiction, such as tobacco, and then to determine whether pica is a function of boredom, frustration, unhappiness, idleness, or some other emotional state that might be corrected programmatically. The behavioral alternatives are contingent restraint (Singh and Dowson, unpublished data, 1980) and overcorrection (35). If pica is oriented to cigarette butts, one may consider the nicotine patch as a substitute.

The frequent occurrence of pica in infants and young children, in mentally retarded people, and especially in autistic children is a reflection of the hyperorality that characterizes Klüver-Bucy syndrome. In the autism literature, mouthing objects, touching, licking, or smelling them are referred to as near-receptor preference. The near receptors (smell, touch, taste) are distinguished from the far receptors (vision and hearing). Theoretically, autistic people prefer the stimulation of near receptors because they are phylogenetically older, subcortical, and less reliant on the efficient function of cortical association areas. Near-receptor preference is therefore a manifestation of a cortical lesion (e.g., Klüver-Bucy syndrome), cortical immaturity (infants), or cortical maldevelopment (retarded people).

COPROPRAXIA

This term refers to rectal digging, playing with feces, feces smearing, and coprophagia, repugnant behaviors that are rarely seen outside institutions (36). It is usually a function of idleness, rage, or severe disorganization. Psychiatrists are most likely to encounter the problem in psychotic patients and in the chronically mentally ill. Autistic children and patients with OCD may sometimes exhibit smearing. It also happens in jails and prisons.

In mentally retarded people, copropraxia was just one of the awful problems that used to happen in large public institutions, when people were neglected and appropriate programming was not available. Under such circumstances, severely regressed behavior was not infrequent, and psychiatric disorders were neither diagnosed nor treated.

Copropraxia sometimes occurs in a chain, from scavenging to pica to digging to smearing to coprophagia, although this pattern is by no means invariant. Rectal digging, for example, may be masturbatory, or it may be a response to parasites, pruritus ani, or hemorrhoids (37). The treatment is usually behavioral (38). When pharmacology is entertained, the differential diagnosis should include OCD, episodic rage, and psychosis.

RUMINATION

Rumination, or ruminative vomiting, consists of repeated vomiting, chewing, and reingestion of the vomitus. Rumination is not difficult to distinguish from vomiting as an acute response to illness or toxic ingestion or as a manifestation of altered taste sensitivity from burns, cancer, renal failure, zinc or lead toxicity, medication, or hypothalamic disease or as a symptom of anorexia or bulimia nervosa (39). In contrast, rumination is said to have a significant learned component that is maintained by sensory reinforcement. It is a complex, chronic problem that is highly resistant to therapeutic intervention. Like pica and copropraxia, it may occur in normal children as a developmental variant (40,41).

Rumination occurs in 5% to 10% of the institutionalized retarded population (42, Singh and Dowson, unpublished data, 1980), especially in the severe and profoundly retarded and in autistic individuals. The onset is usually after years of institutionalization, and because it is often accompanied by stereotypies, it appears to be a form of self-stimulation. It is only rarely associated with an anatomic or a physiologic abnormality (e.g., hiatal hernia). It is not life threatening, as a rule, but it may lead to weight loss, dehydration, respiratory infections, periodontitis, halitosis, and caries, as well as social isolation (39). The behavioral treatment is multiple small feedings to satiety, with active involvement in activities that are stimulating and diverting (43).

There is no established pharmacotherapy for rumination. It is possible that some of the pharmacologic investigations currently applied in the treatment of hyperphagia in Prader-Willi syndrome or in anorexia and bulimia nervosa may be applicable to some individuals with these disorders. A drug that speeds the gastric emptying time may be useful for rumination.

SEXUAL MISBEHAVIOR

There is an old text that advises students how to counsel parents of children newly diagnosed as mentally handicapped. It suggests assuring them that their child will never grow up to be an Edison or a Mozart, but then he will never be a Hitler or a Richard Speck either. Consolation, I suppose, for some, but then hardly anybody has a child who grows up to be an Edison, Mozart, Hitler, or Speck. In fact, it is false consolation. The burden of raising a handicapped child is not limited to the obvious disappointments: the loss of the promised child, the endless drudgery and hard work, and the petty humiliations that crop up in unexpected places. The overt injury is sometimes compounded by the development of behavioral aberrations that are gross and humiliating. Nothing is quite so difficult to contend with for most families as sexual misbehavior. Nothing is quite so destructive of the possibility of living in the community.

Paraphilias and sexual compulsions occur in mild and moderately retarded people just as they do in the population at large. The full range of difficult behaviors and every level of severity are represented. What is different, however, is the poor judgment and lack of discretion that characterizes mildly retarded people. Because they usually find themselves in supervised circumstances, their indiscretions are more likely to be detected. The prejudicial stereotype of retarded people as potentially dangerous may aggravate the community response to a relatively minor infraction, such as peeping or stealing shoes. Even as the large aggregate facilities for retarded people have succeeded in downsizing their populations, they have come to accrue an increasing number of mentally retarded sex offenders whose hope of community reintegration is necessarily diminished.

The psychiatric approach to compulsive sexual misbehavior, especially aggressive misbehavior, has not been wildly successful. Sexual offenders who are mentally retarded or brain injured are no more or less likely to attain a successful result. Individual programs, inpatient programs, and community programs have met with success, but they are usually a low priority for public funding. Even if the legislatures of our less progressive states might be induced to support such programs, there would be a shortage of skilled professionals to staff them.

Treatment often begins with a serotonergic antidepressant, as one might expect, and some anecdotal reports cite the usefulness of selective serotonin reuptake inhibitors for compulsive paraphilias. There are, however, no published controlled studies or clinical trials. Virtually every other class of psychotropic drug has been used at one time or another with varying degrees of success. The androgen antagonist cyproterone acetate is not available in the United States, but one wishes that it were (44,45). Intramuscular medroxyprogesterone (Depo-Provera) is used sometimes, but it would be helpful to have an alternative such as cyproterone (46).

HYPERACTIVITY

Hyperactivity is one of the most common behavior problems in mentally retarded people, especially children. It is discussed in Chapters 7, 13 and 14 as an attribute of patients with brain injury with frontal lobe lesions, during coma recovery, and as a characteristic of autistic children and children with fragile X syndrome.

Childhood hyperactivity is most commonly encountered in attention deficit/hyperactivity disorder. The diagnosis of attention dysfunction in retarded children, however, is almost always problematic, and therefore the diagnosis is rarely made, except perhaps in older children with borderline or mild mental handicap. Response to psychostimulant drugs in retarded children is not nearly as good as it is in hyperactive children of normal intelligence. They are sometimes effective for mildly retarded children, occasionally helpful for moderately retarded children, and seldom successful in the treatment of hyperactivity in the severely retarded. Amantadine, with or without a stimulant, is the drug of choice for hyperactivity in retarded children (28).

AGGRESSION

Aggression is a common and sometimes severe problem in mentally retarded individuals and patients with brain injury, but the stereotype of a violent, aggressive brain-damaged person is hardly valid. In neuropsychiatric patients, aggressive behavior, when it occurs, is usually mild and easily controllable.

Just as there are many theories of aggression, the problem has many forms when it occurs in neuropsychiatric patients.

Most aggressive behavior is "temperamental" or "instrumental." An autistic child who is hyperactive-disorganized with very active exploratory behavior and hypermetamorphosis will sometimes be aggressive if attempts are made to interrupt or redirect the behavior. Mentally retarded people respond the same way when they are engaged in self-stimulatory behavior or stereotyping. Interrupting an autistic ritual can be the occasion of an aggressive outburst. The aggression is usually mild and short-lived, such as hitting someone to warn him or her away, as it were, as a 2-year-old child might do. Patients with traumatic brain injury during the delirious stage of coma recovery are also aggressive in response to intrusion.

Practically anyone can be aggressive when he or she is in a bad mood, and no less is true of neuropsychiatric patients. Aggressive behavior can be a symptom of mood disorder in mental retardation and brain injury. It may also be the expression of a painful physical condition such as headache. Mild hypoglycemia, fatigue, and anxiety are overlooked causes of aggression.

Disorders such as autism, developmental communication disorders, and some frontal lobe syndromes are typified by a relative weakness in perceiving or interpreting social cues or in conforming to social expectations. If one is going to conform an energetic, assertive nature to social expectations, one needs the ability to read social cues and interpret them correctly, to appreciate and respect the feelings, opinions, and expectations of other people, or even on a more fundamental level to understand that such things exist. We know that some neuropsychiatric conditions are associated with an incapacity to establish empathic bonds with other people.

The capacity for social learning is deficient in some mentally retarded individuals and patients with brain injury. One needs the capacity to learn from past experience and to adapt one's behavior in light of it. Mentally retarded people who are prone to stereotyped and habitual behavior are singularly refractory to social learning. Patients with frontal lobe orbitomedial lesions develop habitual patterns of responding, including aggression, that persist in the face of the most utter social derogation and are unresponsive even to repeated correction.

Aggressive behavior may be more overtly pathologic. The typical example is the paroxysmal, explosively aggressive behavior that occurs in patients with deep temporal lobe lesions and some forms of epilepsy. Another is the volatile aggression of patients with fragile X syndrome. Explosive behavior in such instances is not necessarily preceded by a negative mood state and is usually unprovoked. It serves no clear instrumental function, except perhaps the exhaustion of a discharge.

Another example of aggressive behavior that is clearly pathologic is the compulsive aggression of Lesch-Nyhan syndrome and de Lange syndrome. In both instances, the aggression is usually mild, such as hitting or pinching, but it is repetitive, unprovoked, unpredictable. and senseless. Sometimes the caretakers of patients with de Lange syndrome get the idea that the children are teasing them or just being mischievous.

Autistic people can also develop unique or even bizarre patterns of compulsive aggression. Sometimes the aggression is rare but directed against only one individual under particular circumstances. It can be preplanned, accompanied by threats or warnings, and can be quite severe. This form of monomaniacal aggression is particularly difficult to deal with pharmacologically.

Self-injurious behavior in mentally retarded people is closely related to aggression. Most self-injurious patients are also prone to aggression. It is amazing to see a retarded person who tries to be aggressive with another person but is thwarted and then turns to beating himself.

Four Components of Aggressive Behavior

The four components of aggressive behavior are threshold, amplitude, duration, and the postdischarge state. These are clinical descriptors and have a small degree of diagnostic specificity, but only a small degree. The aggressive behavior of adults with fragile X syndrome is characterized by volatility, which indicates a low threshold. It tends to be high-amplitude behavior, with severe aggression and much yelling and carrying on. The duration of their aggressive outbursts is variable, and there is not usually postdischarge depression, withdrawal, or remorse. The compulsive aggression of people with Lesch-Nyhan syndrome and the provocative aggression of people with de Lange syndrome have an extremely low threshold. When these people are aggressive, it is usually unprovoked. It is low amplitude, that is, not very severe, and the duration is very short. Patients with Lesch-Nyhan syndrome have a postictal phase, i.e., postaggression sadness and remorse, but children with de Lange syndrome generally do not.

Explosive aggression in patients with temporal lobe lesions has a variable threshold, high amplitude, short duration, and a pronounced refractory phase. Patients with frontal lobe orbitomedial lesions have a low threshold to aggression and a variable amplitude, but control systems are weak and thus the duration may be prolonged. They do not usually have a refractory phase.

Treatment

The four components of aggression have some bearing on psychopharmacologic treatment. If drug treatment is effective, the threshold might be raised, the amplitude lowered, or the duration shortened. It is not clear that a specific drug is more or less likely to affect one phase over another, but research has not been done with this model in mind.

Conversely, a two-stage model of aggression lends itself to a philosophy of treatment. The treatment of temperamental aggression is simply this: teaching the patient to direct his or her energies in appropriate directions and rewarding him or her for doing so, teaching the patient to read external cues more accurately, and structuring the patient's environment to guarantee the success of the lessons that one has taught. The treatment of temperamental aggression, therefore, is largely behavioral, educational, and environmental. If psychopharmaceuticals are useful at all, they are drugs such as the stimulants, which tend to reduce impulsive behavior and increase reflective behavior. As in the treatment of attention deficit/hyperactivity disorder, stimulants are intended to increase cortical regulation of impulsive and excitable behavior. It is a good example of what is discussed in Chapter 26, the "dimensional" effect of psychoactive drugs.

The treatment of pathologic aggression, conversely, like the treatment of self-injurious behavior, which is discussed in Chapters 15 and 16, is aimed at the underlying pathologic process. It is not specific to aggression as such; it is specific to the underlying pathologic process. That is why it is probably an idle endeavor to try to develop a class of antiaggression drugs. Because aggression itself is not a unitary construct, it is unlikely that there could be a unitary treatment. In fact, the psychopharmacology of aggression is quite diverse.

The notable success of the psychotropic anticonvulsant carbamazepine is thought to have a "tropism" for temporal lobe structures such as the amygdala, which is an organ that is linked to a particular manifestation of intense aggressive behavior. Carbamazepine, however, is not effective for all cases of explosive aggression, although it is a very good drug. Valproate is an anticonvulsant with a preference for centrencephalic epilepsies, but it is sometimes effective when carbamazepine fails.

There is no unitary mechanism to account for the success of other antiaggressive agents such as lithium, beta-blockers, alpha agonists, and serotonergics for cases of pathologic aggression. Lithium probably acts as a serotonergic drug or as a drug that reduces abnormal neuronal excitability by virtue of its effect on second messenger systems. The beta-blockers and the α_2-adrenergic agonists probably reduce noradrenergic overdrive in response to stress. Buspirone is sometimes effective, alone or in combination. Caffeine, a drug that increases irritability, aggression, and self-injurious behavior, does so by antagonizing the inhibitory neurotransmitter adenosine, and carbamazepine, a useful drug for some cases of pathologic aggression, is an adenosine agonist.

It is ironic that the drugs most commonly prescribed for aggressive patients are in the long run probably the least effective. The antipsychotics are dramatically effective in reducing aggressive behavior in acute or emergency situations and are irreplaceable in the treatment of aggressive schizophrenic patients. Their long-term usefulness for the control of aggression in most retarded patients, however, is quite marginal. In fact, because they may cause a prolonged state of akathisia even after they are withdrawn, they may actually aggravate the problem in the long term. Conversely, the atypical antipsychotics, which also bind to the serotonin receptor, seem to be more specific and more effective for the long-term management of severely aggressive individuals.

REFERENCES

1. Luria AR. *Higher cortical functions in man*, 2nd ed. New York: Basic Books, 1977.
2. Lezak MD. *Neuropsychological assessment*, 2nd ed. New York: Oxford University Press, 1983.
3. Sauerland EJ, Clemente CD. The role of the brain stem in orbital cortex induced inhibition of somatic reflexes. In: Pribram KH, Luria AR, eds. *Psychophysiology of the frontal lobes*. New York: Academic Press, 1973:167–184.
4. Schroeder SR. Abnormal stereotyped behaviors. In: American Psychiatric Association, ed. *Treatments of psychiatric disorders*. Washington, DC: American Psychiatric Association, 1989:44–49.
5. Sallustro F, Atwell C. Body rocking, head banging and head rolling in normal children. *J Pediatr* 1978;93: 704–708.
6. O'Brien F. Treating self-stimulatory behavior. In: Matson JL, McCartney JR, eds. *Handbook of behavior modification with the mentally retarded*. New York: Plenum Press, 1981.
7. Berkson G. Abnormal stereotyped motor acts. In: Zubin J, Hunt HF, eds. *Comparative psychopathology*. New York: Grune & Stratton, 1967:76–94.
8. Berkson G. Repetitive stereotyped behaviors. *Am J Ment Defic* 1983;88:239–246.
9. Guess D, Rutherford G. Experimental attempts to reduce stereotyping among blind retardates. *Am J Ment Defic* 1967;71:984–986.
10. Kaufman ME, Levitt H. A study of three stereotyped behaviors in institutionalized mental defective. *Am J Ment Defic* 1965;69:467–473.
11. Warren SA, Burns NR. Crib confinement as a factor in repetitive and stereotyped behavior in retardates. *Ment Retard* 1970;8:25–28.
12. Berkson G, Mason WA, Saxon SV. Situation and stimulus effects on stereotyped behaviors of chimpanzees. *J Comp Physiol Psychol* 1963;56:786–792.
13. Higgenbottam JA, Chow B. Sound-induced drive, prior motion restraint and reduced sensory stimulation effects on rocking behavior in retarded persons. *Am J Ment Defic* 1975;80:231–233.
14. Tizard B. Observations of overactive imbecile children in controlled and uncontrolled environments. *Am J Ment Defic* 1968;72:548–553.
15. Insel TR. Obsessive-compulsive disorder: new models. *Psychopharmacol Bull* 1988;24:365–369.
16. Forehand R, Baumeister AA. Effect of frustration on stereotyped body rocking: follow-up. *Percept Motor Skills* 1970;31B:894.
17. Baumeister AA, Forehand R. Effects of extinction of an instrumental response on stereotyped body rocking in severe retardates. *Psychol Record* 1971;21:235–240.
18. Lewis MH, Baumeister AA. Stereotyped mannerisms in mentally retarded persons: animal models and theoretical analyses. In: Ellis NR, ed. *International review of research on mental retardation*, 2nd ed. New York: Academic Press, 1983.
19. Iversen S. Striatal function and stereotyped behaviour. In: Cools AR, Lohman AHM, van den Bercken JHL, eds. *Psychobiology of the striatum*. Amsterdam: Elsevier/North-Holland, 1977:99–118.
20. Divac I. Functions of the caudate nucleus. *Acta Biol Exp* 1968;2:107–120.
21. Rapoport JL, Wise SP. Obsessive-compulsive disorder: evidence for basal ganglia dysfunction. *Psychopharmacol Bull* 1988;24:380–384.
22. Weilburg JB, Mesulam MM, Weintraub S, et al. Focal striatal abnormalities in a patient with obsessive-compulsive disorder. *Arch Neurol* 1989;46:233–235.
23. Stahl SM. Basal ganglia neuropharmacology and obsessive-compulsive disorder: the obsessive-compulsive disorder hypothesis of basal ganglia dysfunction. *Psychopharmacol Bull* 1988;24:370–374.
24. Cools AR, van den Bercken JHL. Cerebral organization of behaviour and the neostriatal function. In: Cools AR, Lohman AHM, van den Bercken JHL, eds. *Psychobiology of the striatum*. Amsterdam: Elsevier/North-Holland, 1977:119–140.
25. Broekkamp CLE, van Dongen PAM, van Rossum JM. Neostriatal involvement in reinforcement and motivation. In: Cools AR, Lohman AHM, van den Berken JHL, eds. *Psychobiology of the striatum*. Amsterdam: Elsevier/North-Holland, 1977:61–72.
26. Stevens JR. Interictal clinical manifestations of complex partial seizures. *Adv Neurol* 1975;11:85–112.
27. Modell JG, Mountz JM, Curtis GC, et al. Neurophysiologic dysfunction in basal ganglia/limbic striatal and thalamocortical circuits as a pathogenetic mechanism of obsessive- compulsive disorder. *J Neuropsychiatry Clin Neurosci* 1989;1:27–36.
28. Chandler M, Barnhill LJ, Gualtieri CT. Amantadine: profile of use in the developmentally disabled. In: Ratey JJ, ed. *Mental retardation: developing pharmacotherapies*. Washington, DC: American Psychiatric Press, 1991:139–162.
29. Kruck S. Pica in the mentally retarded. In: American Psychiatric Association, ed. *Treatments of psychiatric disorders*. Washington, DC: American Psychiatric Association, 1989:51–53.
30. Barltrop D. The prevalence of pica. *Am J Dis Child* 1966;112:116–123.
31. Lourie RS, Layman EM, Millican FK. Why children eat things that are not food. *Children* 1963;10:143–146.
32. Danford DE, Huber AM. Pica among mentally retarded adults. *Am J Ment Defic* 1982;87:141–146.
33. Hambidge KM. Zinc deficiency in man: its origins and effects. *Philos Trans R Soc Lond B Biol Sci* 1981;294: 129–144.
34. Hambidge KM, Silverman A. Pica with rapid improvement after dietary zinc supplementation. *Arch Dis Child* 1973;48:567–568.
35. Mulick JA, Barbour R, Schroeder SR, et al. Overcorrection of pica in two profoundly retarded adults: analysis of setting effects, stimulus, and response generalization. *Appl Res Ment Retard* 1980;1:241–252.
36. Frieden BD. Clinical issues on the physical restraint experience with self-injurious children. *Res Retard* 1977; 4:1–6.
37. Schroeder SR. Rectal digging, feces smearing, and co-

prophagy. In: American Psychiatric Association, ed. *Treatments of psychiatric disorders*. Washington, DC: American Psychiatric Association, 1989:43–44.
38. Frieden BD, Johnson HK. Treatment of a retarded child's feces smearing and coprophagic behavior. *J Ment Defic Res* 1979;23:55–61.
39. Schroeder SR. Rumination. In: American Psychiatric Association, ed. *Treatments of psychiatric disorders*. Washington, DC: American Psychiatric Association, 1989:53–55.
40. Richmond J, Eddy E. Rumination: a psychosomatic syndrome. *Psychol Res Rep* 1957;8:1–11.
41. Kanner L. *Child psychiatry*. Springfield, IL: Charles C. Thomas, 1959.
42. Ross RT. Behavioral correlates of levels of intelligence. *Am J Ment Defic* 1972;76:545–549.
43. Mulick JA, Schroeder SR, Rojahn J. Chronic ruminative vomiting: a comparison of four treatment procedures. *J Autism Dev Dis* 1980;10B:203–213.
44. Bradford JM, Pawlak A. Double-blind placebo crossover study of cyproterone acetate in the treatment of the paraphilias. *Arch Sexual Behav* 1993;22:383–402.
45. Cooper AJ. Review of the role of two antilibidinal drugs in the treatment of sex offenders with mental retardation. *Ment Retard* 1995;33:42–48.
46. Emory LE, Cole CM, Meyer WJ III. Use of Depo-Provera to control sexual aggression in persons with traumatic brain injury. *J Head Trauma Rehabil* 1995;10:47–58.

11

The Pathobehavioral Syndromes

SUMMARY

The most extraordinary manifestations of human behavior are associated with the pathobehavioral mental retardation syndromes (Table 11.1). The pathobehavioral syndromes, or behavioral phenotypes as they are sometimes called, are genetic disorders associated with dysmorphic features and organ anomalies, developmental delays, and behavioral patterns that are absolutely stereotypical. In many of the syndromes, the actual gene mutation has been identified. In some cases, the protein expressed by the gene has been also been identified, and the way it influences neuronal development has been traced.

For example, in Down's syndrome (DS), the gene for the antioxidant enzyme, superoxide dismutase-1 causes oxidative stress, which leads to premature aging and Alzheimer's dementia. In Rett's syndrome, a mutation at MECP2 on the X chromosome disrupts the normal sequence or brain maturation; as a result, girls with Rett's syndrome (RS) undergo a profound developmental regression in late childhood. In phenylketonuria (PKU), a mutation in the gene that encodes phenylalanine hydroxylase results in elevated levels of phenylalanine, with a corresponding reduction in the levels of other amino acids. Amine neurotransmitter synthesis is therefore reduced, and brain development occurs in a persistently suboptimal monoamine environment.

Genetic analysis of the pathobehavioral syndromes is an important window to brain function and dysfunction, just as lesion analysis was a generation ago. People born with one or another of the pathobehavioral syndromes have amazing physical, behavioral, and neurocognitive similarities. Children with Williams syndrome (WS), for example, are sociable and have a particular manner of conversing with other people, but as they grow older, they become withdrawn and obsessive. Children with Angelman syndrome (AS) walk like marionettes and are prone to outbursts of laughter. Self-injurious behavior, occurring in unique and utterly stereotypical ways, is typical of Smith-Magenis syndrome and Smith-Lemli-Opitz syndrome (SLOS).

The characteristics of the pathobehavioral syndromes are found nowhere else in neuropsychiatry. In no other conditions is the chain from gene to protein to neuron to behavior so well defined or so bizarre.

PATHOBEHAVIORAL SYNDROMES

The eponymous mental retardation syndromes considered here are genetic in origin. Their genetic basis may have been identified (Lesch-Nyhan syndrome, fragile X syndrome) or not (de Lange syndrome). In all the syndromes just mentioned, there is a behavioral stereotype. In others, such as DS and the neurocutaneous syndromes, the behavioral manifestations are variable, but certain aspects of their psychiatric complications are unique and predictable.

There are no more abiding examples of genetic determinism than the pathobehavioral syndromes. Consider this: given a microdeletion on the q arm of chromosome 15, if the active segment was derived from the father, the individual is obese, volatile, and hyperphagic with small arms, feet, and genitals. If the active segment is maternal in origin, the resulting individual is lithe and well formed but walks like a marionette and laughs uncontrollably.

TABLE 11.1. *Pathobehavioral syndromes of mental retardation*

Angelman syndrome
- Chromosome 15 (15q11q13), maternal segment active
- "Puppet-like" gait, epilepsy, inappropriate laughter
- High frequency of autism

Brunner syndrome
- X chromosome
- Intermittent impulsive, aggressive behavior with sleep disturbance

de Lange syndrome
- Short stature, hirsutism, facial and skeletal abnormalities
- Gastroesophageal reflux, peripheral neuropathy
- Self-injurious behavior, aggression

Down's syndrome
- Chromosome 21
- Flat facies, slanted eyes, epicanthal folds, small ears, short fingers
- Premature aging, predisposition to Alzheimer's disease

Fragile X syndrome
- X chromosome (Xq27.3)
- Long face, prominent forehead, large ears, macro-orchidism
- Hyperactive, impulsive, temperamental children; mood swings, explosiveness, and aggression in adults

Klinefelter's syndrome
- 47,XXY
- Tall, hypogonadal males with gynecomastia and a eunuchoid habitus
- Speech and language disabilities, "asexual" delinquency

Landau-Kleffner syndrome
- Seizures, receptive aphasia, and developmental regression in early childhood
- Sometimes a cause of autism

Lesch-Nyhan syndrome
- X chromosome
- Dystonia, choreoathetosis, hyperuricemia
- Aggression and self-mutilation

Lowe's syndrome
- X chromosome (Xq25–26)
- Hypotonia, cataracts, renal tubular acidosis
- Hyperexcitable, hyperactive, tantrums, obsessive, compulsive, and stereotyped behaviors

Möbius syndrome
- Cranial nerve palsy, expressionless face
- Psychosocial adjustment problems, autism

Neurofibromatosis type 1 (von Reckinghausen disease)
- Café-au-lait spots, neurofibromas in nerves, meninges, and various organs
- Seizures, mental retardation, hyperactivity, and other behavioral problems

Phenylketonuria
- Chromosome 12
- Fair hair and skin
- Impulsive, irritable, immature, aggressive, poor interpersonal relations

Prader-Willi syndrome
- Chromosome 15 (15q11q13), paternal segment active

TABLE 11.1. *(continued)*

- Hypotonia; small genitals, hands, and feet
- Severe hyperphagia, obesity, compulsive and explosive behaviors

Rett's syndrome
- X chromosome (Xq28)
- Girls with abnormal gait and stereotyped hand-wringing
- Autism, severe cognitive deterioration in late childhood

Smith-Lemli-Opitz syndrome
- Microcephaly, multiple anomalies, cholesterol deficiency
- Irritability, sleep disturbance, self-injurious behavior, autism

Smith-Magenis syndrome
- Chromosome 17 (17p11.2)
- Broad, flat face; hoarse, deep voice; scoliosis; eye, ears, nose, and throat abnormalities
- Severe self-injurious behavior, mood instability, hyperactivity, disturbed sleep

Sturge-Weber syndrome
- Cutaneous hemangiomata of face and meninges, cortical atrophy
- Seizures, paresis

Tuberous sclerosis
- Adenoma sebaceum, cortical tubers
- Epilepsy, autism, attention problems, aggression, sleep disturbance

Turner's syndrome
- 45,X
- Short stature, nuchal webbing, broad chest, sexual immaturity
- VIQ > PIQ, visuospatial deficits, passive, meek, overly compliant

Williams syndrome
- Chromosome 7 (7q11.23)
- Cardiovascular anomalies, hypertension, hypercalcemia, "elfin facies"
- "Cocktail chatter," socially disinhibited, attention deficit/hyperactivity disorder; later, anxiety and social withdrawal

Velocardiofacial syndrome
- Chromosome 22 (22q11)
- Congenital heart disease, dysmorphic facies, palatal abnormalities
- Bland affect, poor social interactions, psychosis in adults, paranoid schizophrenia

XYY males
- Tall, long facies, prominent glabella, large teeth and ears
- Temper outbursts, aggression

VIQ, verbal IQ; PIQ, performance IQ.

St. Augustine, believing in a perfect and all-powerful God who loves humankind, was forced to concede that every person's fate must, of necessity, be preordained or predestined by Providence. But as a practical matter, he said, it is better to live as if one had free will. When we think about conditions such as Prader-

Willi syndrome and AS, we are confronted by no less than genomic predestination. They are contrived in such intricate detail by the subtraction or duplication of a few bases on a fraction of a chromosome. It lays to rest the conceit that we are masters of our fate.

Fortunately, we are not confronted with such stark examples very often. The pathobehavioral syndromes are common causes of mental handicap, but they do not comprise a very large segment of the general population. That they are prototypes for a genetic determinism that affects us all is questionable at best. The strongest links between genotype and behavioral phenotype are only clearly apparent in a few simple souls among us.

For the rest of us, the traverse from our chromosomes to our behavioral phenotype is much wider. It is separated by a broad expanse of accident, complexity, ambiguity, and concealment. As St. Augustine advised, we pretend that that is free will.

DOWN'S SYNDROME

DS (trisomy 21) is the prototypical mental retardation syndrome, with a phenotype that is familiar to people who know little of dysmorphology. It is named for the English physician John Langdon Down, who described the condition in 1866.

DS is the most common known genetic cause of mental retardation, closely followed by fragile X syndrome. The incidence of DS is one in 800 live births, and people with DS comprise approximately 16% of the mentally retarded population (1). If the incidence of DS births is declining, by virtue of prenatal screening, the prevalence of DS is increasing because of increased longevity.

Most cases of DS (95%) are caused by nondisjunction of chromosome 21. During meiosis, the chromosomes divide and separate (disjunction). If they fail to do so, and both remain in one of the daughter cells, that is called nondisjunction. The result is a state of aneuploidy, i.e., an abnormal number of chromosomes in both of the daughter cells. Nondisjunction of chromosome 21 is usually maternal in origin (95%) (2) and is strongly influenced by maternal age. At age 35, a woman has a one in 400 chance of conceiving a child with DS; at 40, one in 110; and at 45, one in 35 (National Down Syndrome Society). There is no current explanation for the age effect (3).

Approximately 3% to 4% of cases of DS are the result of robertsonian translocation, in which material from chromosome 21 is rearranged onto chromosome 14 and thus exists in triplicate, although the total number of chromosomes is normal. The remainder of DS cases is characterized by mosaicism, with an admixture of cells with a normal karyotype and cells with trisomy 21. As a rule, individuals with mosaic DS are less dysmorphic, have higher IQ scores, and are less likely to develop Alzheimer's disease (AD) (4).

One presumes that the mechanism by which the extra chromosome in DS produces an abnormal phenotype is the overexpression of genes located on a small portion of the chromosome on its long arm, known as the DS critical region (on 21q). There may be 20 to 50 genes in the DS critical region that contribute to the DS phenotype. In Chapter 4, we discussed how these extra genes lead to overproduction of amyloid precursor protein and superoxide dismutase-1 in DS. Other genes have also been identified, if tentatively, such as *DYRK*, a gene for the protein kinases that control cell growth and development, including neurogenesis (5,6).

Increased superoxide dismutase-1 activity may generate free-radical stress through overproduction of hydrogen peroxide (7). Free-radical damage, therefore, has been presented as a key element in the etiopathogenesis of DS (8) as well as in the phenomena of premature aging (9) and dementia (10). People with DS are prone to signs of early senescence such as thin hair, dry, wrinkled skin, and cataracts as well as neuropathic changes as early as the third decade (11). In fact, virtually all patients with DS develop neuropathic changes in brain tissue characteristic of AD by the age of 40, although they may not show behavioral or cognitive signs of decline until much later (12,13).

The neuropathology of DS is characterized by reduced numbers of cortical neurons, especially in the temporal lobe. There are also reductions in dendritic spines, reduced synaptic dimensions, and abnormalities in electric membrane properties. These are the types of changes one expects would compromise the strength and efficiency of mental operations (14).

It is hardly necessary to reiterate the characteristic dysmorphic features of DS or its association with disorders of the immune, endocrine, and cardiovascular systems. DS people are mentally retarded, of course, although not every person with DS is retarded, and many are only mildly or moderately retarded.

Physicians and psychologists who work with patients with DS, beginning with Langdon Down, have been inclined to characterize their personality traits, generally in positive terms. As people, DS patients tend to be sociable, positive in outlook, amiable, easily amused, affectionate, and sometimes obstinate.

Writers have also remarked on the social competence of individuals with DS and their relative freedom from the conduct problems that all too often afflict mentally handicapped individuals. Nevertheless, they are not immune to psychopathologic conditions

(15). People with DS are less likely to have problems such as hyperactivity, aggression, disruptive, destructive, or self-injurious behavior, personality disorders, or paranoia, compared with similarly retarded controls (16,17). But I have consulted on many cases of patients with DS who were hyperactive, aggressive, paranoid, or self-injurious, and similar cases have been described in the literature.

It has been suggested that mania is incompatible with DS (18), but there is a good deal of evidence to the contrary (17). Conversely, everyone agrees that depression is a common problem in individuals with DS. Some have argued that it occurs at a higher rate than in other retarded people; others disagree. Cases of autism have been described in people with DS, perhaps at a lower rate than in retarded controls, perhaps not.

What emerges from a somewhat confusing literature is that although individuals with DS are not absolutely protected against the development of psychiatric conditions, they may enjoy at least a relative degree of protection. With the possible exception of depression, however, they are not uniquely prone to any particular constellation of behavioral or emotional problems, in the way that individuals with fragile X syndrome are, for example.

The striking psychopathologic association, however, is with AD. Patients with DS are uniquely prone to AD. Indeed, as mentioned in Chapter 4, DS has been a natural laboratory for the study of AD. The prevalence of dementia in one prospective study of people with DS is 8% at 35 to 49 years, 55% at 50 to 59 years, and 75% at 60 and older. Seizures develop in 84% of the patients with DS with dementia, and 20% have parkinsonian features. Brain tissue loss as shown on computed tomography (CT) is most pronounced in the temporal lobes (19).

The diagnosis of dementia in patients with DS is made based on personality changes or developmental regression on standardized tests. The onset of dementia may be heralded by seizures, gait deterioration, sphincteric incontinence, frontal release signs, or personality change. Serial CT scans may establish the diagnosis (12). Conversely, the cause of dementia, even in a patient with DS, may be a reversible condition, such as hypothyroidism (20). Depression also may mimic the symptoms of dementia or presage its onset.

Preventive Treatment

When it comes to treating behavioral problems and psychiatric disorders in patients with DS, the appropriate behavioral and pharmacologic therapies are usually brought to bear. The literature does not suggest that special considerations be made because the patient has DS nor does my experience. The problem of dementia in DS, however, does raise a couple of special treatment issues. The first has to do symptomatic treatment and the second with prevention.

Physicians are, of course, concerned with psychopharmacology for the neurobehavioral symptoms of dementia: impulsive behavior, aggression, emotional instability, psychosis, sleep disturbance, screaming, and seizures. This happens to be one of the more frustrating areas of psychopharmacology. In contrast to most patients with brain injury and developmentally handicapped people, most of whom are young, the dementing patient is deteriorating. Symptomatic control, therefore, may be lost at any point in the face of a deteriorating brain.

Every psychiatrist knows that the benzodiazepines are relatively contraindicated in dementing patients, that the drugs of choice are usually the modern antidepressants, buspirone, and the mood stabilizers (21).Treatment with a low-dose antipsychotic drug is often necessary. It is less well appreciated that something may be gained early in the course of a dementing condition from a trial of stimulants or amantadine (22).

Cholinergic drugs, the acetylcholinesterase inhibitors, to be precise, are the best treatment for early dementia. They stem the downward course of the condition, at least for a year or so. Memory and the executive functions improve. The drugs sometimes ameliorate neurobehavioral symptoms of dementia. The effect is modest but appreciable nonetheless. The cholinesterase inhibitors are probably equally effective for dementia in patients with DS, in mentally retarded people in general, and in patients whose dementia is attributable to brain injury. The evidence base is narrow, but there is at least one report of clinical improvement in adults with DS treated with donepezil, with improvement in communication, expressive language, attention, and stability of mood (23); similar findings have appeared in the literature on traumatic brain injury (24,25).

This is hardly surprising because cholinergic dysfunction is characteristic of AD, whatever the patient's background. A more interesting question is when to begin treatment. Should patients with DS be treated with a cholinergic drug even before the symptoms of dementia are manifest? After all, the neuropathic changes of AD arise in DS long before any behavioral or cognitive symptoms of dementia are manifest. Is there any harm in beginning low-dose or intermittent treatment at age 40, when the amyloid plaques have begun to appear? Is any long-standing benefit likely to accrue? Will early presymptomatic treatment with a cholinergic drug delay the onset of dementia or will it diminish the utility of cholinergic treatment after the symptoms of dementia are manifest?

Questions like this are normally the impulse for multicenter, longitudinal studies, if the issue is a medical condition of national importance, but they have rarely generated attention or support when the patients at risk are retarded or when the issue is an "orphan" condition such as DS or traumatic brain injury. They do introduce the important issue of dementia prevention, however, and in that regard, we are fortunate to have a couple of better alternatives to the acetylcholinesterase inhibitors, compounds that are less expensive, less troublesome, and theoretically more interesting. Consider the antioxidants and the anti-inflammatory drugs.

It has been asserted that the premature aging of patients with DS is the result of free-radical damage and that oxygen-derived free radicals, such as the superoxide and hydroxyl species, may be responsible for the progressive neuronal degeneration in AD (26). There is also evidence for increased free-radical formation in DS. DS neurons exhibit a three- to fourfold increase in intracellular reactive oxygen species and elevated levels of lipid peroxidation that precede neuronal death. Degeneration of cultured DS neurons is prevented by free-radical scavengers (27). The erythrocytes of adults with DS have an unbalanced antioxidant system, which may be indicative of the vulnerability of individuals with DS to antioxidant stress (28). The observed changes in the cellular localization of superoxide dismutases in the neocortex and hippocampus in cases of DS and AD support a role for oxidative injury in neuronal degeneration and senile plaque formation (29). Indeed, oxidative damage to brain cells occurs in patients with DS well before the deposition of amyloid (30).

Oxidative stress may be central to the development of AD in DS or it may be epiphenomenal, but no one can assert that it is irrelevant. More important, it is something that can be addressed therapeutically. Antioxidant therapy is discussed at length in Chapter 25. There the potential neuroprotective effects of antioxidants that are readily available, inexpensive, and free of adverse effects are addressed. Evidence of efficacy is preliminary. Physicians who are familiar with the literature, however, have found it hard to resist recommending aggressive antioxidant therapy for children with DS as soon as they can tolerate the treatment (7).

Another interesting approach to dementia prevention involves acetylsalicylic acid and other nonsteroidal anti-inflammatory drugs, which may also inhibit the course of AD. This astounding suggestion arose from the observation that elderly patients taking aspirin or other anti-inflammatory drugs to treat arthritis were much less likely to develop AD. The idea that there is an inflammatory component to the pathophysiology of AD is also supported by the demonstration of acute phase reactants and other markers of immune reaction in the postmortem brains of patients with AD. This line of thinking led some to hypothesize that drugs limiting immunologic activity may reduce the risk of AD or slow its progression. Several controlled studies have in fact demonstrated that AD occurs at a lower rate in patients who have had long-term treatment with nonsteroidal anti-inflammatory drugs, for example, people with rheumatoid arthritis or osteoarthritis, and that a course of treatment with anti-inflammatory drugs may slow the progression of dementia in patients with AD. The issue is taken up in some detail in Chapter 25.

The question then is whether antioxidant supplements and low-dose acetylsalicylic acid should be recommended to the families of patients with DS or severe brain injury. There is not a definitive answer to that question. I am inclined, however, to respond with a qualified yes.

PHENYLKETONURIA

PKU is a genetic disorder, inherited as an autosomal recessive trait. It is an inborn error of metabolism that causes seizures, spastic paraparesis, and mental retardation but is treatable by environmental manipulation. The incidence is one in 10,000 in Northern Europeans but lower in other groups. Dietary restriction of phenylalanine-containing foods has been successful in reducing the occurrence of mental retardation as a consequence of PKU. Thus, admission of patients with PKU to mental retardation facilities has declined dramatically since the introduction 35 years ago of newborn screening and dietary treatment (31).

Classical PKU is caused by a mutation in a gene on the short arm of chromosome 12 that encodes phenylalanine hydroxylase. Either an absolute or partial relative deficiency in the enzyme phenylalanine hydroxylase leads to accumulation of phenylalanine in the blood or hyperphenylalaninemia (32). As a result, central nervous system levels of phenylalanine are elevated, with a corresponding decrease in other large neutral amino acids, especially methionine and tyrosine. Brain protein synthesis is therefore decreased, neurotransmitter synthesis is also decreased, and myelin turnover is increased. Concentrations of amine neurotransmitters, including dopamine, norepinephrine, serotonin, and epinephrine are reduced in plasma and the brain (33,34).

There are several PKU phenotypes, defined in terms of different components of the phenylalanine hydroxylating system, and at least one of the phenotypes is associated with a malignant neurologic course, even in the face of dietary restriction. In malignant PKU, caused by a deficiency in tetrahydrobiopterin, there is impairment of the tyrosine and tryptophan hydroxylases, and the condition is characterized by deficiency of catecholamines and serotonin in the central and peripheral nervous systems (35).

In untreated PKU, pathologic changes occur in brain structures that develop after birth. There are abnormalities in the myelination of subcortical white matter and spinal cord and in the growth of axons, dendrites, and synapses in the cerebral cortex. In a small number of patients, there is evidence for progressive white matter degeneration or leukodystrophy (36).

Severe mental retardation and other neurologic consequences of PKU are averted by early introduction of the low protein diet. Conversely, collaborative studies of treated children have revealed subtle neuropsychological impairments, which might be attributable to inadequate control of hyperphenylalaninemia or to premature resumption of a normal diet (37,38). Workers who have identified decrements in cognitive performance after diet termination have suggested that a chronic metabolic encephalopathy can arise, even in adults, possibly related to phenylalanine interference with neurotransmitter synthesis (39).

Children with PKU are believed to have a selective reduction of dopaminergic innervation to prefrontal cortex, perhaps because their ability to convert the amino acid phenylalanine to the dopamine precursor tyrosine is impaired. An optimal monoamine environment, as previously discussed, is critical for normal development of the cerebral cortex, and the neurotransmitter dopamine is essential to the development of the prefrontal cortex (40,41). Patients with PKU who are untreated are known to have selective impairment of the cognitive executive functions subserved by the dorsolateral prefrontal cortex (41), and similar findings have been reported even in treated children (38,42).

In PKU, there may also be alterations in serotonin metabolism by virtue of competition between phenylalanine and tryptophan for uptake into neurons (43). Even in treated PKU with good metabolic control, there may be a chronic inhibition of 5-hydroxytryptophyl synthesis (44). It may be an exaggeration to define PKU as a primary disorder of serotonin metabolism, but that is an important component of the neurochemistry of the disorder and certainly may have a bearing on the behavioral manifestations. Laboratory animals with PKU have been compared with low-serotonin preparations; they are anxious, "in a state of general preparedness" (45). Chronic dietary administration of phenylalanine to monkeys produces lethargy, irritability, and diminished reactivity in a normal environment but abnormally heightened levels of activity in response to novelty or to stress (45). Patients with PKU are not dissimilar and may be treated successfully with a selective serotonin reuptake inhibitor in low to moderate doses or with a serotonin precursor.

Behavioral and emotional disturbances and overt psychiatric disorders are known to be associated with PKU, even when the disorder is treated successfully and mental retardation does not occur (46). Children with PKU have been described as impulsive, irritable, immature, and aggressive, and studies have documented poor interpersonal relationships and mood and behavioral problems (47). The occurrence of behavioral problems is correlated with control of phenylalanine levels (48). The diverse and nonspecific nature of these difficulties speaks to the broad band of neurotransmitter abnormalities that have been associated with hyperphenylalaninemia.

There are several avenues of rational pharmacotherapy for neuropsychiatric problems in children and adults with PKU. The first step is to reinstitute a low phenylalanine diet (49,50). That is an unpalatable intervention, to be sure, and unfortunately the results are sometimes insufficient.

Excessive levels of phenylalanine inhibit the synthesis of carnitine and the polyunsaturated fatty acids arachidonic acid and docosahexanoic acid. Dietary supplementation with carnitine, omega-6, and omega-3 fatty acids should be contemplated as a second step in rational pharmacotherapy (51).

Psychotropic drugs that influence dopamine or serotonin metabolism are the third approach to treatment; the psychostimulants, amantadine, and serotonergic antidepressants are probably the most commonly used treatments for children and adults with PKU. The literature is scarce on the use of dietary precursors such as tyrosine and tryptophan or dopaminergic drugs such as amantadine or L-dopa, and my experience in this regard is limited. In the occasional case, however, supplementation may be appropriate.

The success of PKU screening and dietary treatment has resulted in a population of more or less normal adults who no longer require a restrictive diet and are able to tolerate persistent hyperphenylalaninemia without undue effects. The result can be catastrophic however, if the patient is a woman of childbearing age. Elevated maternal phenylalanine levels during pregnancy are teratogenic, and the offspring are subject to microcephaly, growth retardation, dysmorphic features, and congenital heart disease. If a mother with PKU is chronically depressed or impulsive with a low IQ, she is less likely to adhere to the restrictive diet that is necessary to assure a successful pregnancy (52).

RETT'S SYNDROME

RS occurs only in girls and is characterized by autistic behavior, dementia, apraxia of gait, loss of facial expression, and stereotyped hand wringing. Andreas Rett, a Viennese physician, first described the syndrome in 1966 (52a); the more influential paper was by Gillberg et al. in 1985 (53). Based on studies in Sweden and Scotland, the prevalence of RS has been estimated to be 1.0 to 1.2 per 15,000 girls (54).

The onset is toward the end of the first year of life or early in the second year, after a period of normal development. Then, there is a period of developmental stagnation or regression accompanied by loss of communication skills and purposeful use of the hands. Thereafter, it follows a progressive, deteriorating course with characteristic hand movements, gait disturbance, and slowing of the rate of head growth (55,56). The patient then stabilizes in a severely retarded state that can last for decades.

Children with RS are quite autistic. Features of the syndrome include loss of functional use of the upper extremities, jerky truncal ataxia, apraxia, acquired microcephaly, spastic paraparesis, vasomotor disturbances of the lower limbs, intermittent hyperventilation, bruxism, and seizures (53). Atypical variants, mildly retarded girls or women, are in the minority, but because of increasing identification, it is an expanding cohort (57). There are eight cases of male RS-like syndrome in the medical literature (58).

The syndrome was always thought to be genetically determined, but the mode of transmission was not convincingly compatible with any known pattern. The more or less exclusive affliction of females, correlated with findings from pedigree analysis, suggested a dominant mutation on the X chromosome that results in affected girls and nonviable male hemizygous concepti (53,59). In fact, RS is an X-linked disorder with a high rate of new mutations; only 0.5% of cases represent familial reoccurrences. The gene for RS is *MECP2* on the long arm of the X chromosome (Xq28). The gene product MecP2 is a protein critical for brain development; it controls the complex expression patterns of other genes through its interaction with methylated DNA. What is does apparently is control the biochemical switches that turn other genes on and off. A mutation at MECP2 disrupts the normal sequence of central nervous system maturation (60). *MECP2* mutations have been discovered in patients with several different clinical syndromes, ranging from mild learning disabilities in females to severe mental retardation, seizures, ataxia, and sometimes neonatal encephalopathy in males (61).

It is believed that RS comprises a fundamental failure in neuronal maturation and dendritic arborization, intracellular connectivity, and thus the integration of sensory, emotional, motoric, and autonomic function. It is not a degenerative process but rather a maturational or developmental arrest during a period of dynamic brain growth. The failure is selective rather than diffuse. Both basal forebrain afferents and monoaminergic systems have been implicated in the pathogenesis of the condition.

The disorder is associated with cortical atrophy, extrapyramidal dysfunction, diminished dopamine activity in the basal ganglia (62), and decreased cholinergic activity in the nucleus basalis of Meynert (63). Depigmentation in the substantia nigra has been described (59). There are reduced levels of metabolites of the biogenic amines norepinephrine, dopamine, and serotonin in cerebrospinal fluid, and elevated levels of biopterin (64). Cortical atrophy in RS is associated with a normal number of neurons in the gray matter but increased cell packing density. It is suggested that early deficits in dopaminergic and cholinergic neurons projecting to the cortex from the brainstem and basal forebrain can disrupt axodendritic development in the cerebral cortex (63,65).

Some of the clinical elements of RS have been compared with the effects in laboratory animals of exogenously administered opiate compounds. In rodents, exogenous opiates lead to a deceleration of brain growth and development, stereotypies (e.g., excessive grooming behavior), respiratory depression and apnea, myoclonic jerks and seizures, indifference to pain, nystagmus, decreased rapid eye movement sleep, and motor incoordination. The cerebrospinal fluid of patients with RS indicates a significant elevation of β-endorphin-like immunoreactivity, and improvement in sleep, apnea, and seizure control has been described in patients with RS treated with the opiate antagonist naltrexone (54).

RS has been particularly interesting to students of autism, not only because the girls are autistic but also because the pattern of developmental regression after a period of normal development is often seen in autistic children who do not have RS. The stereotyped handwringing movements of patients with RS are also familiar to parents of autistic children. It is likely that there are several degenerative diseases involving brainstem and subcortical tissues that cause variants of autism.

WILLIAMS SYNDROME

WS was first described in the 1960s by cardiologists who noted an association between supravalvular aortic stenosis in patients with cognitive impairment and characteristic facial features. It is a relatively rare disorder (one in 20,000) that in most cases is attributed to a microdeletion involving the elastin gene locus on chromosome 7 (7q11.23). The locus contains at least 17 genes, including several that are highly expressed in the brain (66) Most cases of WS appear to represent a *de novo* or spontaneous mutation, although there are a few reports of familial cases.

The characteristic facial features of patients with WS include supraorbital fullness with a broad forehead, short palpebral fissures, and a flat nasal bridge with a full tip and anteverted nostrils. There is a tendency toward ocular hypertelorism, and many patients may have strabismus or a stellate iris. There is malar hypoplasia with a definitely wide mouth and a full lower lip. It has been referred to as the elfin face syndrome.

Cardiovascular abnormalities are present in most patients with WS (>75%), although the spectrum and severity are highly variable. A relatively characteristic feature is supravalvular aortic stenosis. Peripheral pulmonic stenosis is frequently present in addition to supravalvular aortic stenosis. Less commonly associated findings include atrial septal defect, ventricular septal defect, abdominal coarctation, and renal artery stenosis. Systemic hypertension or some degree of elevation in blood pressure is usually present in patients with WS. Hypercalcemia is another common feature.

Patients with WS have a distinct neurodevelopmental profile including mild to moderate mental retardation with relative verbal strengths, marked motor and perceptual deficits, and an outgoing personality (67). Hyperactivity and short attention span are the most common behavioral features. The social demeanor of these patients is friendly, loquacious, and socially disinhibited, and their language is described as "cocktail chatter" (68). Other characteristics include sleep disturbance, hypacusis, and musical strengths.

The neuropsychological profile is striking, with fluency in language and facility in reading, in contrast to a substantial deficit in visuospatial performance. The patients are overly talkative and have no obvious problems with vocabulary or syntax, but they also tend to overuse clichès, and there tends to be a tangential quality to their language. They say much more than they mean, and their capacity to express is far in excess of what they are capable of processing. Impressed by their fluency, people may overestimate their intellectual abilities.

What all this represents is a developmental variant of fluent aphasia. It is characteristic of patients with WS, although it is by no means limited to that group. Cocktail chatter is also described in hydrocephalic children.

One is inclined to attribute the neuropsychological profile of WS to a relative strength in left hemisphere linguistic processing and a relative weakness in communicative pragmatics in the right hemisphere. Such a formulation would predict a relative weakness in other right hemisphere–mediated abilities such as visual-motor performance, which is, of course, exactly what is observed in these patients. The pragmatics of language are the rules that govern its appropriate use, depending on the situational context (69). It is also this component of language that is impaired in patients with right hemisphere lesions, but there is no evidence beyond the functional to support the idea of a hemispheric deficit in WS.

Although children with WS are usually friendly, sociable, affectionate, empathic, and attentive to social cues, there sometimes seems to be an undercurrent of anxiety related to social situations. As they grow up, they change and become less lively, active, quarrelsome, and overly friendly, better balanced, and more withdrawn. As adults, others may have behavioral and emotional difficulties, such as poor social relationships, preoccupations and obsessions, and high levels of anxiety, depression, and distractibility. As children, they are most often are diagnosed with attention deficit/hyperactivity disorder and treated with psychostimulants (and/or amantadine). In adult life, more aggressive forms of management may be required.

There have been cases of autism in WS, but as a rule autism is uncommon, and it has been argued that autism and WS are incompatible. Some children with WS do very well on facial recognition tasks, consistent with their quality of attentiveness to the emotional states of other people (70–73). In WS, there is a dissociation between language processing and pragmatics; in some autistic people, language processing and pragmatics are poor, but fluency is intact.

Senile plaques and neurofibrillary tangles were reported in the brain of a 35-year-old man with WS, an interesting but as yet isolated report. The condition is not notably associated with early cognitive decline (74).

LOWE'S SYNDROME

Lowe's syndrome (LS), or the oculocerebrorenal syndrome of Lowe, was first recognized in 1952. It is a rare condition that occurs in approximately one to 10 boys per million people, and there are estimated to be 200 to 2,000 cases in the United States. It is caused by an X-linked recessive gene, although female heterozygotes may have mild ocular or renal symptoms. The *OCLR1* gene is located in Xq25–26 (75). Neuroimaging studies indicate cystic lesions, gliosis, and demyelination (76,77).

The ocular symptoms are cataracts with or without glaucoma. Renal involvement is Fanconi's syndrome or renal tubular acidosis. The disorder is also characterized by generalized hypotonia and mental and growth retardation. Seizures occur in approximately one-half of the patients. Frontal bossing and a protuberant abdomen are sometimes prominent.

Children with LS tend to be moderately mentally retarded, but in one series, no fewer than 25% had normal IQ scores (78). They are not prone to specific neurocognitive weaknesses, but maladaptive behaviors are very common.

Behaviorally, the children are hyperexcitable, with a high-pitched scream and stereotyped arm movements. They are typically happy, loving, and sociable, but they are also given to behavioral problems. They may be stubborn, hyperactive, distractible, destructive, aggressive, or self-injurious. They are prone to minor snits and major temper tantrums and perseverative questions and unusual obsessions and compulsions. Their behavioral problems are said to peak at 8 to 13 years of age.

The specific behavioral problems described in more than 50% of children with LS are twirling, rubbing, shaking, or repetitively moving body parts or objects; strong attachment to or fascination with certain things or objects resulting in inappropriate behavior or conversation; talking and chattering excessively; incapacitating fear of neutral objects, noises, places, animals, and so on; yelling or screaming; hitting, biting, or scratching self or others; destroying personal or household objects; resisting requests or demands (79).

There is treatment preference for the serotonergic antidepressants, especially paroxetine, for some reason. It does work occasionally, although there is no reason to think it is better than the alternative selective serotonin reuptake inhibitors. Amantadine, buspirone, and low doses of risperidone may sometimes be effective.

ANGELMAN (HAPPY PUPPET) SYNDROME

Children with AS belong to the large group of mentally retarded children with epilepsy. It is named for Harry Angelman who described "puppet children" in 1965 (79a). In French, it is *marionette joyeuse* or *pantin hilare*, but "happy puppet" is perhaps too derisive for modern use, and the parents prefer the eponymous name.

Children with AS are distinguished by a peculiar facial appearance (protruding jaw and tongue, flattened occiput, and a smiling but otherwise expressionless face), ataxia and a special puppet-like gait (walking as though controlled by strings), seizures, and paroxysms of inappropriate laughter (80). A severely abnormal electroencephalogram, epilepsy, muteness, and delay in establishing upright walking are the rule. The unprovoked laughter often encountered in this syndrome may have led to the mistaken notion that they are happy, sociable people. In one survey of 98 children with mental retardation, there were four with AS, and all four were also autistic (81).

AS is associated with a partial deletion at location q11–13 on chromosome 15, which is also the genetic basis of Prader-Willi syndrome. In AS, the source of the microdeletion is maternal, and in Prader-Willi syndrome, it is paternal (81,82).

Most genes have two alleles, one on the maternal and one on the paternal chromosome. When a gene is "turned on," both alleles are transcribed equally, and functional protein is produced from both chromosomes. Most, but not all genes, behave in this manner. Some genes are "imprinted." That means that only one of the alleles is expressed when the gene is turned on, and the other is silent because it has been imprinted. Methylation of DNA is one mechanism by which imprinting occurs.

In AS, the relevant region on chromosome 15q is normally imprinted on the paternal chromosome and expressed on the maternally derived chromosome. Although the maternal copy is deleted, the paternal allele is unable to compensate because it remains imprinted. The opposite circumstance arises in the case of PWS. There are genetic variants of both conditions, of course, and the mechanisms at work are more complex, involving a number of different genes, but the essential principle holds. Which disorder arises in a given individual is determined by whether the deletion occurs on the maternal or paternal chromosome (83,84).

In both conditions, the deleted region includes many genes, and one in particular, called *UBE3A*, is of particular interest because a mutation at this site is sufficient to cause most of the symptoms of AS. *UBE3A* is expressed from both maternal and paternal alleles in all tissues except the central nervous system, where the paternal allele is normally imprinted, and only the maternal allele is expressed. The gene expresses an enzyme (ubiquitin ligase 3) that is necessary for normal protein turnover within cells. The failure to degrade proteins can lead to deleterious accumulation within cells (83).

The proximal long arm of chromosome 15 is where the gene for one of the γ-aminobutyric acid receptors is located, and that gene is in the region that is deleted in individuals with AS. In one autopsy study, there was reduced benzodiazepine binding in the brain. In another, there was reduced γ-aminobutyric acid concentration in the cortex. This may be responsible for the fact that patients with AS have a particular form of epilepsy. Dendritic hypoplasia has also been described (85,86).

The high rate of autism in children with AS is in contrast to Prader-Willi syndrome, in which autism is rare. Children with AS, however, also tend to be more severely cognitively impaired than children with Prader-Willi syndrome and are more likely to have severe seizures (81). Treatment primarily addresses their seizure disorders. One hopes that behavior and communication improve with optimal anticonvulsant therapy, and the availability of a wider range of new anticonvulsant drugs raises one's hopes further.

As patients with AS grow up, they continue to have epileptic seizures but are less prone to outbursts of laughter (87).

LANDAU-KLEFFNER SYNDROME

This rare form of acquired aphasia is mostly associated with very heterogeneous epileptic manifestations. Seventy percent of patients have clinical seizures (88). Between 4 and 7 years of age (usually), the children develop receptive aphasia. Hearing impairment is suspected, but there is none. Then spontaneous speech begins to change; the children speak in short sentences and show articulation problems. The period of language breakdown may be fast (1 day) or slow (several months), and the outcome often resembles global aphasia in adults (89).

Because autism sometimes begins as a regression in language during the second year, there has been interest in the association between Landau-Kleffner syndrome and autism. Without seizures or an electroencephalogram diagnostic of epilepsy, it is not possible to make the diagnosis of Landau-Kleffner syndrome. It may, however, be a cause of acquired autism (90). Landau-Kleffner syndrome is discussed at length in Chapter 17.

MÖBIUS SYNDROME

Möbius syndrome (MS) is a rare congenital condition of unknown cause that involves nuclear agenesis of the sixth and seventh nerves. Frequently, the lower cranial nerves (IX, X, and XII) are also involved. The most striking feature is an expressionless face because the facial musculature does not develop or is inactive. Feeding issues are paramount initially, but the expressionless face takes on greater importance as the children begin to interact at age 3 or 4 years. The psychosocial implications are enormous. The children are often rejected by their peers, with devastating consequences. Psychosocial adjustment is often disturbed (91).

Two cases have been described with deletions on chromosome 13 (91a), but the condition is more likely related to embryopathy, perhaps a transient ischemic-hypoxic insult or a vascular event that causes brainstem/cerebellar pathology (92,93).

Gillberg and Winnergard (94) described one mentally retarded autistic child with Möbius syndrome. Then they reported a series of 17 children with Möbius syndrome, eight of whom were mentally retarded, seven were autistic, and two behaviorally disturbed. Only six of the 17 were free of developmental or behavioral problems (95).

SMITH-MAGENIS SYNDROME

Smith-Magenis syndrome is probably underdiagnosed because of its mild clinical features. High-resolution chromosome analysis indicates an interstitial deletion of chromosome 17p11.2 (96). The clinical features include a broad, flat face, brachycephaly, broad nasal bridge, brachydactyly, and a hoarse, deep voice. Eye, ear, nose, and throat abnormalities, scoliosis, and ventriculomegaly occur in most cases. Most patients are moderately mentally retarded, and the IQ range in a series of 27 cases was 20 to 78 (97).

The neuropsychiatric disturbances may be especially troublesome. These are disturbed sleep, hyperactivity, self-injurious behavior, and instability of mood (98). Children with Smith-Magenis syndrome are given to a few behaviors that are very unusual, such as onychotillomania (pulling out fingernails or toenails), polyembolokoilamania (inserting foreign bodies into body orifices), and arm hugging/hand squeezing when excited. Self-injurious is nearly universal in Smith-Magenis syndrome, increases with age, and is directly correlated with intellectual function (99). (In Lesch-Nyhan and de Lange syndromes, self-injurious behavior is inversely correlated with intellectual level.)

Pharmacologic treatment is similar to that for fragile X syndrome. Stimulants are used for attention deficit/hyperactivity disorder symptoms, α_2 agonists, and possibly amantadine; the selective serotonin reuptake inhibitors and mood stabilizers for tantrums or aggressive behavior, and sometimes an atypical antipsychotic drug.

SMITH-LEMLI-OPITZ SYNDROME

SLOS is an autosomal recessive disorder characterized by multiple malformations (microcephaly, corpus callosum agenesis, male pseudohermaphroditism, finger anomalies), growth retardation, and mental retardation. The facial features are sometimes subtle and hard to recognize. The diagnosis is often missed, an error of no little import because SLOS is the result of an inborn error of metabolism and can be treated.

SLOS is a syndrome of not enough cholesterol. In SLOS, there is reduced activity of the enzyme 7-dehydrocholesterol-Δ^7-reductase (DHCR7) that converts 7-dehydrocholesterol to cholesterol. The gene for DHCR7 has been mapped to chromosome 11q12–13.

As a result of this enzyme deficiency, there is a generalized cholesterol deficiency and an accumulation of 7-dehydrocholesterol, which may be toxic, in body tissues. Cholesterol is a major constituent of cell membranes and myelin and is necessary for the synthesis of steroid hormones and bile acids. The severity of the syndrome is proportional to the extent of cholesterol deficiency. The diagnosis is made by demonstrating elevated levels of 7-dehydrocholesterol in plasma or amniotic fluid (100).

The behavioral phenotype of SLOS includes mental functioning from borderline to severe retardation, sensory hyperreactivity, irritability, language impairment, sleep-cycle disturbance, self-injurious behavior, and autism. In a recent study of 28 patients with SLOS, one-half exhibited a behavior called opisthokinesis (throwing themselves backward in a characteristic upper body movement). In a study of 13 children with SLOS, one-half were autistic (101).

SLOS is probably the only human condition that is appropriately treated by increasing dietary cholesterol. This may be done with powdered egg yolk. Treatment leads to increased plasma levels of cholesterol and ultimately reduced tissue levels of 7-dehydrocholesterol, which is probably a good thing (102). Treatment with dietary supplementation (including bile acids) is associated with improvement in growth, behavior, and general health. Older children and adults have shown improved intellectual function (103).

VELOCARDIOFACIAL SYNDROME

The velocardiofacial syndrome (VCFS) is caused by a deletion of band 11 on the long arm of chromosome 22. Phenotypically, individuals present with congenital heart disease, palatal abnormalities, facial dysmorphism, and developmental delay. The incidence is one in 4,000 livebirths. An autosomal dominant mode of inheritance is demonstrated in some families (104). The phenotypic expression of the VCFS abnormality is highly variable.

VCFS is associated with borderline or mild retardation and learning, language, or attention problems. As children, they have a bland affect, monotonous voice, and poor social interactions, with extremes of disinhibited or shy behavior. As adults, there is an high incidence of psychotic disorders (105).

Patients with VCFS have abnormalities in the white matter, cerebellum, septum pellucidum, and frontal and right temporal lobes (106).

VCFS was first described in 1968. As patients with the condition were followed into adult life, more than 10% were found to have developed chronic psychotic disorders, in particular, paranoid schizophrenia. In a recent survey of 50 adults with the syndrome, 24% met criteria for the diagnosis of schizophrenia, and 6% had major depression but without psychotic features (107). This extraordinary association has fueled interest in 22q11 as a candidate region to search for genes responsible for major psychiatric disorders.

Psychotic disorders in patients with VCFS may be particularly hard to treat, with poor response to conventional neuroleptic drugs or electroconvulsive therapy. Parkinsonism was described in a 30-year-old man with VCFS. The utility of clozapine has been mentioned in a couple of reports, but patients with VCFS are also prone to seizures (108,109).

THE NEUROCUTANEOUS SYNDROMES

The neurocutaneous syndromes or phakomatoses are genetic aberrations of cell differentiation characterized by the appearance of malformations and tumors of the skin, nervous system, and other organs. The syndromes are tuberous sclerosis, neurofibromatosis (1 and 2), Sturge-Weber syndrome, ataxia-telangiectasia, and von Hippel-Lindau syndrome. They have certain elements in common: a wide range of severity; a large number of subclinical patients who are only identified if a close relative is severely afflicted; a course that may be progressive and deteriorating, but that may arrest at any time; a tendency to malignant transformation; and in severe cases, mental retardation and neurobehavioral disorders. The seizures that occur in the neurocutaneous disorders may be of virtually any type; by the same token, the behavioral disorders are relatively nonspecific, although autism is well represented among patients with tuberous sclerosis.

Tuberous Sclerosis

Tuberous sclerosis is a disorder of cellular differentiation associated with multisystem hamartomatous changes and characterized by specific skin lesions, seizures, and developmental delay. It was first described by the German pathologist Friedrich von Recklinghausen in 1862, but von Recklinghausen's disease is the *other* neurocutaneous disorder. The external manifestations of tuberous sclerosis include the well-known adenoma sebaceum, hypomelanotic macules, shagreen patches, facial angiofibromas, and periungual fibromas. Ophthalmoscopic examination may reveal gray or yellow retinal plaques, and ultrasonographic examination of the kidneys and heart may also reveal hamartomas.

There are three kinds of abnormalities in the central nervous system of people with tuberous sclerosis: (i) cortical tubers, areas of disordered lamination with gliosis, most common in the cerebral convexities but also found in the brainstem, cerebellum, and spinal cord; (ii) white matter heterotopias consisting of disorganized, enlarged neurons, generally in the cerebral white matter and believed to represent migration arrest; and (iii) subependymal giant cell nodules along all the ventricular surfaces. Giant cell astrocytomas arise from these nodules (110).

The characteristic CT findings in tuberous sclerosis are multiple calcified nodules adjacent to the ventricular system, often associated with ventricular dilation, calcified lesions in the superficial brain parenchyma or cerebellum, and low-density lesions in the cerebral hemispheres. Magnetic resonance imaging (MRI) is better for imaging the cortical lesions, and there seems to be a quantitative relationship between the density of the cortical lesions on MRI (but not CT) and the degree of clinical impairment. However, MRI is less reliable at picking up the periventricular calcifications that are diagnostic of tuberous sclerosis, therefore, CT is a more specific neurodiagnostic tool. Cerebellar lesions have been documented by MRI in one-fourth of patients with tuberous sclerosis, but brainstem lesions are rare (111,112).

Tuberous sclerosis is an autosomal dominant disorder estimated to afflict one in 10,000 persons, but extreme variability in the clinical manifestations may make mild disorders difficult to detect. Family studies using the full range of diagnostic tools have determined that as many as 44% of cases are familial. The rest are presumably the result of spontaneous mutation (113).

Epilepsy, mental retardation, and behavioral disorders are closely interrelated in cases of tuberous sclerosis. That is to say, patients with severe mental retardation are the most likely to have seizures, patients without seizures are likely to be behaviorally and cognitively normal, and patients with the most severe seizure disorders are likely to have the most difficult behavioral problems. A substantial number of patients with tuberous sclerosis are also autistic or have autism-spectrum disorders such as Asberger's syndrome or pervasive developmental disorder. Hyperactivity, attention problems, aggressive behavior, and sleep disorders are frequently found (114).

Treatment follows the rule of the primacy of antiepileptic treatment. Behavioral improvement will, as a rule, follow seizure control, but an alternative antiepileptic drug might be selected for its psychotropic effects even if seizure control is optimal. If additional psychotropic drugs are used, attention must be paid to their effect on the seizure threshold. Of course, no treatment is particularly effective if the patient has a progressive condition.

Neurofibromatosis

The neurofibromatoses consist of two distinct disorders, the genes for which have been located on separate chromosomes. Neurofibromatosis 1 is also known as von Recklinghausen's disease/neurofibromatosis. It is characterized by multiple brown skin macules (café-au-lait spots), intertriginous freckling, iris hamartomas (Lisch nodules), and multiple skin neurofibromas. It may be associated with optic gliomas, spinal and peripheral nerve neurofibromas, macrocephaly, neurologic or cognitive impairment, or scoliosis and other bone abnormalities. It has an incidence of one in 3,000 in all ethnic and racial groups and is one of the most common autosomal dominant disorders of humans. Neurofibromatosis 2, bilateral acoustic neurofibromatosis, is considerably less frequent and is not, as a rule, associated with neuropsychiatric problems (115).

Although von Recklinghausen's disease is associated with intracranial neoplasia, and the *NF1* gene is a tumor-suppressor gene, the high proportion of cases with abnormal cranial MRI scans (74%) is probably related to abnormal but nonmalignant brain parenchyma, such as hamartomas, heterotopias, and dysplasias. They are found most frequently in the basal ganglia, cerebellum, optic tract, and brainstem. The presence of MRI abnormalities, however, does not correlate with clinical indices of neurocognitive deficit (116).

It is estimated that intellectual handicap in one form or another occurs in at least 40% of patients with neurofibromatosis, but frank mental retardation only occurs in 2% to 5% of patients. Seizures and behavior problems such as hyperactivity occur with similar frequency (117–119).

REFERENCES

1. Fryns JP, Kleczkowska A, Kubien E, et al. Cytogenetic findings in moderate and severe mental retardation. *Acta Paediatr Scand Suppl* 1984;313:3–23.
2. Antonarakis S. Parental origin of the extra chromosome in trisomy 21 as indicated by analysis of DNA polymorphisms. *N Engl J Med* 1991;324:872–876.
3. Petersen M, Mikkelsen M. Nondisjunction in trisomy 21: origin and mechanisms. *Cytogenet Cell Genet* 2000;91:199–203.
4. Fishler K, Koch R. Mental development in Down syndrome mosaicism. *Am J Ment Retard* 1991;96:345–351.
5. Becker W, Joost H. Structural and functional characteristics of Dyrk, a novel subfamily of protein kinases with dual specificity. *Prog Nucleic Acid Res Mol Biol* 1999;62:1–17.
6. Kentrup H, Joost H, Heimann G, et al. Minibrain/DYRK1A gene: candidate gene for mental retardation in Down's syndrome. *Klin Paediatr* 2000;212:60–63.
7. Antila E, Westermarck T. On the etiopathogenesis and therapy of Down syndrome. *Int J Dev Biol* 1989; 33:183–188.
8. Fujii J, Suzuki K, Taniguchi N. Physiological significance of superoxide dismutase isozymes. *Nippon Rinsho* 1995;53:1227–1231.
9. Bras A, Monteiro C, Rueff J. Oxidative stress in trisomy 21. A possible role in cataractogenesis. *Ophthalmic Paediatr* 1989;10:271–277.
10. Friedlich AL, Butcher LL. Involvement of free oxygen radicals in beta-amyloidosis: an hypothesis. *Neurobiol Aging* 1994;15:443–455.
11. Gualtieri CT. *Neuropsychiatry and behavioral pharmacology*. Berlin: Springer-Verlag, 1990.
12. Lott IT, Lai F. Dementia in Down's syndrome: observations from a neurology clinic. *Appl Res Ment Retard* 1982;3:233–239.
13. Thase ME, Tigner R, Smeltzer DJ, et al. Age-related neuropsychological deficits in Down's syndrome. *Biol Psychiatry* 1984;19:571–585.
14. Scott B, Becker L, Petit T. Neurobiology of Down's syndrome. *Prog Neurobiol* 1983;21:199–237.
15. Gath A, Gumley D. Behaviour problems in retarded children with special reference to Down's syndrome. *Br J Psychiatry* 1986;149:156–161.
16. Collacott R, Cooper S, McGrother C. Differential rates of psychiatric disorders in adults with Down's syn\drome compared with other mentally handicapped adults. *Br J Psychiatry* 1992;161:671–674.
17. Collacott RA. People with Down syndrome and mental health needs. In: Bouras N, ed. *Psychiatric and behavioral disorders in developmental disabilities and mental retardation*. Cambridge: Cambridge University Press, 1999:200–211.
18. Sovner R, Desnoyers Hurley A, Labrie R. Is mania incompatible with Down's syndrome? *Br J Psychiatry* 1985;146:319–320.
19. Lai F, Williams RS. A prospective study of Alzheimer disease in Down syndrome. *Arch Neurol* 1989;46: 849–853.
20. Thase ME. Reversible dementia in Down's syndrome. *J Ment Deficiency Res* 1982;26:111–113.
21. Reifler BV, Teri L, Raskind M, et al. Double-blind trial of imipramine in Alzheimer's disease patients with and without depression. *Am J Psychiatry* 1989;146:45–49.
22. Erkulwater S, Pillai R. Amantadine and the end-stage dementia of Alzheimer's type. *South Med J* 1989;82: 550–554.
23. Kishnani P, Sullivan J, Walter B, et al. Cholinergic therapy for Down's syndrome. *Lancet* 1999;353: 1064–1065.
24. Taverni J, Seliger G, Lichtman S. Donepezil medicated memory improvement in traumatic brain injury during post acute rehabilitation. *Brain Inj* 1998;12:77–80.
25. Whelan F, Walker M, Schultz S. Donepezil in the treatment of cognitive dysfunction associated with traumatic brain injury. *Ann Clin Psychiatry* 2000;12:131–135.
26. Volicer L, Crino PB. Involvement of free radicals in dementia of the Alzheimer type: a hypothesis. *Neurobiol Aging* 1990;11:567–571.
27. Busciglio J, Yankner BA. Apoptosis and increased generation of reactive oxygen species in Down's syndrome neurons in vitro. *Nature* 1995;378:776–779.
28. Gerli G, Zenoni L, Locatelli GF, et al. Erythrocyte antioxidant system in Down syndrome. *Am J Med Genet* 1990;7:272–273.
29. Furuta A, Price DL, Pardo CA, et al. Localization of superoxide dismutases in Alzheimer's disease and Down's syndrome neocortex and hippocampus. *Am J Pathol* 1995;146:357–367.
30. Nunomura A, Perry G, Pappolla M, et al. Neuronal oxidative stress precedes amyloid-beta deposition in Down syndrome. *J Neuropathol Exp Neurol* 2000;59: 1011–1017.
31. Scriver CR, Clow CL. Phenylketonuria: epitome of human biochemical genetics. *N Engl J Med* 1980;303: 1336–1342.
32. Simonoff E, Bolton P, Rutter M. Genetic perspectives on mental retardation. In: Burack JA, Hodapp RM, Zigler E, eds. *Handbook of mental retardation and development*. Cambridge: Cambridge University Press, 1998:41–79.
33. Lasala JM, Coscia CJ. Accumulation of a tetrahydroisoquinoline in phenylketonuria. *Science* 1979;203: 283–284.
34. Surtees R, Blau N. The neurochemistry of phenylketonuria. *Eur J Pediatr* 2000;159:109–113.
35. Kapatos G, Kaufman S. Peripherally administered reduced pterins do enter the brain. *Science* 1981;212: 955–956.
36. Huttenlocher P. The neuropathology of phenylketonuria: human and animal studies. *Eur J Pediatr* 2000;159:102–106.
37. Azen C, Koch R, Friedman E, et al. Summary of findings from the United States Collaborative Study of children treated for phenylketonuria. *Eur J Pediatr* 1996;155:29–32.
38. Arnold G, Kramer B, Kirby R, et al. Factors affecting cognitive, motor, behavioral and executive functioning in children with phenylketonuria. *Acta Paediatr* 1998;87:565–570.
39. Seashore MR, Friedman E, Novelly RA, et al. Loss of intellectual function in children with phenylketonuria after relaxation of dietary phenylalanine restriction. *Pediatrics* 1985;75:226–232.

40. Welsh MC. A prefrontal dysfunction model of early-treated phenylketonuria. *Eur J Pediatr* 1996;155: S87–S89.
41. Diamond A. Evidence for the importance of dopamine for prefrontal cortex functions early in life. *Philos Trans R Soc Lond B Biol Sci* 1996;351:1483–1493.
42. White D, Nortz M, Mandernach T, et al. Deficits in memory strategy use related to prefrontal dysfunction during early development: evidence from children with phenylketonuria. *Neuropsychology* 2001;15:221–229.
43. Wurtman RJ, Fernstrom JD. Control of brain neurotransmitters synthesis by precursor availability and nutritional state. *Biochem Pharmacol* 1976;25:1691–1696.
44. Giovannini M, Valsasina R, Longhi R, et al. Serotonin and noradrenaline concentrations and serotonin uptake in platelets from hyperphenylalaninaemic patients. *J Inherit Metab Disord* 1988;11:285–290.
45. Chamoye AS. Long-term learning deficits of mentally retarded monkeys. *Am J Ment Defic* 1984;88:352–368.
46. Graham PJ, Rutter ML. Organic brain dysfunction and child psychiatric disorder. *BMJ* 1968;3:695–700.
47. Realmuto GM, August GJ, Garfinkel BD. Clinical effect of buspirone in autistic children. *J Clin Psychopharmacol* 1989;9:122–124.
48. Smith I, Knowles J. Behaviour in early treated phenylketonuria: a systematic review. *Eur J Pediatr* 2000; 159:89–93.
49. Harvey E, Kirk S. The use of a low phenylalanine diet in response to the challenging behaviour of a man with untreated phenylketonuria and profound learning disabilities. *J Intellect Disabil Res* 1995;39:520–526.
50. Baumeister A, Baumeister A. Dietary treatment of destructive behavior associated with hyperphenylalanemia. *Clin Neuropharmacol* 1998;21:18–27.
51. Infante J, Huszagh V. Impaired arachidonic (20:4n-6) and docosahexaenoic (22:6n-3) acid synthesis by phenylalanine metabolites as etiological fact the neuropathology of phenylketonuria. *Mol Genet Metab* 2001;72:185–198.
52. Koch R, Friedman E, Azen C, et al. The International Collaborative Study of Maternal Phenylketonuria: status report 1998. *Eur J Pediatr* 2000;159:156–160.
52a. Rett A. On an until now unknown disease of a congenital metabolic disorder. *Krankenschwester* 1966;19:121–122.
53. Gillberg C, Wahlstrom J, Hagberg B. A "new" chromosome marker common to the Rett syndrome and infantile autism? The frequency of fragile sites at X P22 in 81 children with infantile autism, childhood psychosis and the Rett syndrome. *Brain Dev* 1985.
54. Brase DA, Myer EC, Dewey WL. Minireview: possible hyperendorphinergic pathophysiology of the Rett syndrome. *Life Sci* 1989;45:359–366.
55. Rett A. *Uber ein zerebral-atrophisches Syndrome bei Hyperammonamie*. Wein: Bruder Hollinek, 1966.
56. Hagber B, Aicardi J, Dias K, et al. A progressive syndrome of autism, dementia, ataxia, and loss of purposeful hand use in girls: Rett's syndrome: report of 35 cases. *Ann Neurol* 1983;14:471–479.
57. Hagberg G. Rett syndrome: clinical peculiarities and biological mysteries. *Acta Paediatr* 1995;84:971–976.
58. Christen HJ, Hanefeld F. Male Rett variant. *Neuropediatrics* 1995;26:81–82.
59. Hillig U. On the genetics of the Rett syndrome. *Brain Dev* 1985;7:368–371.
60. Amir R, Van der Veyver I, Wan M, et al. Rett syndrome is caused by mutations in X-linked MECP2, encoding methyl-CpG-binding protein 2. *Nat Genet* 1999;23: 185–188.
61. Shahbazian M, Zoghbi HY. Molecular genetics of Rett syndrome and clinical spectrum of MECP2 mutations. *Curr Opin Neurol* 2001;14:171–176.
62. Wenk GL. Alterations in dopaminergic function in Rett syndrome. *Neuropediatrics* 1995;26:123–125.
63. Johnston MV, Hohmann C, Blue ME. Neurobiology of Rett syndrome. *Neuropediatrics* 1995;26:119–122.
64. Zoghbi HY, Milstien S, Butler IJ, et al. Cerebrospinal fluid biogenic amines and biopterin in Rett syndrome. *Ann Neurol* 1989;25:56–60.
65. Dunn HG, MacLeod PM. Rett syndrome: review of biological abnormalities. *Can J Neurol Sci* 2001;28: 16–29.
66. Schultz R, Grelotti D, Pober B. Genetics of childhood disorders: XXVI. Williams syndrome and brain-behavior relationships. *J Am Acad Child Psychiatry* 2001;40:606–608.
67. Pagon RA, Bennett FC, LaVeck B, et al. Williams syndrome: features in late childhood and adolescence. *Pediatrics* 1987;80:85–91.
68. MacDonald GW, Roy DL. Williams syndrome: a neuropsychological profile. *J Clin Exp Neuropsychol* 1988; 10:125–131.
69. Blumstein SE. Neurolinguistic disorders: language-brain relationships. In: Filskov SB, Boll TJ, eds. *Handbook of clinical neuropsychology*. New York: John Wiley & Sons, 1981:227–256.
70. Reiss AL, Feinstein C, Rosenbaum KN. Autism associated with Williams syndrome. *J Pediatr* 1985;106: 247–249.
71. Gosch A, Pankau R. Personality characteristics and behaviour problems in individuals of different ages with Williams syndrome. *Dev Med Child Neurol* 1997;39: 527–533.
72. Davies M, Udwin O, Howlin P. Adults with Williams syndrome. Preliminary study of social, emotional and behavioural difficulties. *Br J Psychiatry* 1998;172: 273–276.
73. Mervis C, Klein-Tasman B. Williams syndrome: cognition, personality, and adaptive behavior. *Ment Retard Dev Disabil Res Rev* 2000;6:148–158.
74. Golden J, Nielsen G, Pober B, et al. The neuropathology of Williams syndrome. Report of a 35-year old man with presenile beta/A4 amyloid plaques and neurofibrillary tangles. *Arch Neurol* 1995;52:209–212.
75. Nussbaum R, Orrison B, Janne P, et al. Physical mapping and genomic structure of Lowe syndrome gene OCRL1. *Hum Genet* 1997;99:145–150.
76. Ono J, Harada K, Mano T, et al. MR findings and neurologic manifestation in Lowe oculocerebrorenal syndrome. *Pediatr Neurol* 1996;14:162–164.
77. Schneider J, Boltshauser E, Neuhaus T, et al. MRI and proton spectroscopy in Lowe syndrome. *Neuropediatrics* 2001;32:45–48.
78. Kenworthy L, Park T, Charnas L. Cognitive and behavioral profile of the oculocerebrorenal syndrome of Lowe. *Am J Med Genet* 1993;46:297–303.
79. Kenworthy L, Charnas L. Evidence for a discrete behavioral phenotype in the oculocerebrorenal syndrome of Lowe. *Am J Med Genet* 1995;59:283–290.
79a. Angelman H. "Puppet" children: a report on three cases. *Dev Med Child Neurol* 1965;7:681–688.
80. Elian M. Fourteen happy puppets. *Clin Pediatr* 1975;14:902–908.

81. Steffenburg S, Gillberg C, Steffenburg U. Psychiatric disorders in children and adolescents with mental retardation and active epilepsy. *Arch Neurol* 1996;53: 904–912.
82. Smeets DFCM, Hamel BCJM, Nelen MR, et al. Prader-Willi syndrome and Angelman syndrome in cousins from a family with a translocation between chromosomes 6 and 15. *N Engl J Med* 1998;326:807–811.
83. Lalande M, Minassian B, DeLorey T, et al. Parental imprinting and Angelman syndrome. *Adv Neurol* 1999; 79:421–429.
84. Lombroso P. Genetics of childhood disorders: XVI. Angelman syndrome: a failure to process. *J Am Acad Child Psychiatry* 2000;39:931–933.
85. Jay V, Becker L, Chan F, et al. Puppet-like syndrome of Angelman: a pathologic and neurochemical study. *Neurology* 1991;41:416–422.
86. Odano I, Anezaki T, Ohkobu M, et al. Decrease in benzodiazepine receptor binding in a patient with Angelman syndrome detected by iodine-123 iomazenil and single-photon emission tomography. *Eur J Nucl Med* 1996;23:598–604.
87. Laan LA, den Boer AT, Hennekam RC, et al. Angelman syndrome in adulthood. *Am J Med Genet* 1996; 66:356–360.
88. Mouridsen SE. The Landau-Kleffner syndrome: a review. *Eur Child Adolesc Psychiatry* 1995;4:223–228.
89. Broekkamp CLE, van Dongen PAM, van Rossum JM. Neostriatal involvement in reinforcement and motivation. In: Cools AR, Lohman AHM, van den Berken JHL, eds. *Psychobiology of the striatum*. Amsterdam: Elsevier/North-Holland Biomedical Press, 1977:61–72.
90. Roulet E, Deonna T, Gaillard F, et al. Acquired aphasia, dementia, and behavior disorder with epilepsy and continuous spike and waves during sleep in a child. *Epilepsia* 1991;32:495–503.
91. Braye R, Souchere B, Franc C, et al. Moebius syndrome: therapeutic proposals from 2 cases. *Rev Stomatol Chir Maxillofac* 1996;97:332–337.
91a. Slee JJ, Smart RD, Viljoen DL. Deletion of chromosome 13 in Möbius syndrome. *J Med Gen* 1991;28:413–414.
92. Lipson AH, Webster WS, Brown-Woodman PD, et al. Moebius syndrome: animal model-human correlations and evidence for a brainstem vascular etiology. *Teratology* 1989;40:339–350.
93. Harbord MG, Finn JP, Hall-Craggs MA, et al. Moebius' syndrome with unilateral cerebellar hypoplasia. *J Med Genet* 1989;26:579–582.
94. Gillberg C, Winnergard I. Childhood psychosis in a case of Moebius syndrome. *Neuropediatrics* 1984;15: 147–149.
95. Gillberg C, Steffenburg S. Autistic behaviour in Moebius syndrome. *Acta Paediatr Scand* 1989;78:314–316.
96. Lacombe D, Moncla A, Malzac P, et al. Smith-Magenis syndrome. *Arch Pediatr* 1997;4:438–442.
97. Greenberg F, Lewis R, Potocki L, et al. Multi-disciplinary clinical study of Smith-Magenis syndrome (deletion 17p11.2). *Am J Med Genet* 1996;62:247–254.
98. Fischer H, Oswald H, Duba H, et al. Constitutional interstitial deletion of 17(p11.2) (Smith-Magenis syndrome): a clinically recognizable microdeletion syndrome. Report of two cases and review of the literature. *Klin Padiatr* 1993;205:162–166.
99. Finucane B, Dirrigl K, Simon E. Characterization of self-injurious behaviors in children and adults with Smith-Magenis syndrome. *Am J Ment Retard* 2001; 106:52–58.
100. Malgorzata J, Gorski A. T cell adhesion to the extracellular matrix proteins as a determinant of pregnancy success or failure. *Immunol Lett* 1998;63:135–140.
101. Tierney E, Nwokoro N, Kelley R. Behavioral phenotype of RSH/Smith-Lemli-Opitz syndrome. *Ment Retard Dev Disabil Res Rev* 2000;6:131–134.
102. Linck L, Lin D, Flavell D, et al. Cholesterol supplementation with egg yolk increases plasma cholesterol and decreases plasma 7-dehydrocholesterol in Smith-Lemli-Opitz syndrome. *Am J Med Genet* 2000;93: 360–365.
103. Nowaczyk M, Whelan D, Heshka T, et al. Smith-Lemli-Opitz syndrome: a treatable inherited error of metabolism causing mental retardation. *CMAJ* 1999; 161:165–170.
104. Thomas J, Graham J Jr. Chromosomes 22q11 deletion syndrome: an update and review for the primary pediatrician. *Clin Pediatr* 1997;36:253–266.
105. Chow E, Bassett A, Weksberg R. Velo-cardio-facial syndrome and psychotic disorders: implications for psychiatric genetics. *Am J Med Genet* 1994;54:107–112.
106. Amelsvoort T, Daly E, Robertson D, et al. Structural brain abnormalities associated with deletion at chromosome 22q11: quantitative neuroimaging study of adults with velo-cardio-facial syndrome. *Br J Psychiatry* 2001;178:412–419.
107. Murphy K, Jones L, Owen M. High rates of schizophrenia in adults with velo-cardio-facial syndrome. *Arch Gen Psychiatry* 1999;56:940–945.
108. Krahn L, Maraganore D, Michels V. Childhood-onset schizophrenia associated with parkinsonism in a patient with a microdeletion of chromosome 22. *Mayo Clin Proc* 1998;73:956–959.
109. Gothelf D, Frisch A, Munitz H, et al. Clinical characteristics of schizophrenia associated with velo-cardio-facial syndrome. *Schizophr Res* 1999;35:105–112.
110. Dotan SA, Trobe JD, Gebarski SS. Visual loss in tuberous sclerosis. *Neurology* 1991;41:1915–1917.
111. Roach ES, Williams DP, Laster DW. Magnetic resonance imaging in tuberous sclerosis. *Arch Neurol* 1987;44:301–303.
112. Roach ES, Kerr J, Mendelsohn DMC, et al. Detection of tuberous sclerosis in parents by magnetic resonance imaging. *Neurology* 1991;41:262–265.
113. Cassidy SB, Pagon RA, Pepin MMS, et al. Family studies in tuberous sclerosis: evaluation of apparently unaffected parents. *JAMA* 1983;249:1302–1604.
114. Gillberg IC, Gillberg C, Ahlsen G. Autistic behaviour and attention deficits in tuberous sclerosis: a population-based study. *Dev Med Child Neurol* 1994;36:50–56.
115. Martuza RL, Eldridge R. Neurofibromatosis 2 (bilateral acoustic neurofibromatosis). *N Engl J Med* 1988; 318:684–688.
116. Duffner PK, Cohen ME, Seidel FG, et al. The significance of MRI abnormalities in children with neurofibromatosis. *Neurology* 1989;39:373–378.
117. Riccardi VMM. von Recklinghausen neurofibromatosis. *Neurofibromatosis* 1981;305:1617–1626.
118. Huson SM, Harper PS, Compston DAS. von Recklinghausen neurofibromatosis. *Brain* 1988;111:1355–1381.
119. Korf F, Carrazana E, Holmes GL. Patterns of seizures observed in association with neurofibromatosis. *Epilepsia* 1993;34:616–620.

12

Disorders of Eating, Drinking, and Sleeping

SUMMARY

Organic hyperphagia and organic bulimia are clumsy terms by today's standards, but they aptly describe a troublesome problem that can arise in a number of different neuropsychiatric conditions. Uncontrollable hyperphagia, whatever the cause, is an extremely difficult problem to treat pharmacologically or behaviorally. It usually requires a degree of control over the patient's access to food, which is extraordinarily restrictive in day-to-day life.

Prader-Willi syndrome (PWS) is a prototypical pathobehavioral disorder characterized by hyperphagia and morbid obesity, obsessions and compulsions, and affective instability. It is thought to be a hypothalamic disorder, at least in part. Hypothalamic lesions in patients with brain injury (BI) or in children after resection of a craniopharyngioma lead to similar patterns of hyperphagia and behavioral dysregulation.

The most common cause of organic hyperphagia, of course, is drug treatment, and the problem of drug-induced obesity, especially with the new antidepressant and antipsychotic drugs, is discussed here. Many psychiatric drugs can cause obesity, usually by virtue of carbohydrate craving and hyperphagia.

If life were fair, there would also be drugs that controlled hyperphagia and obesity—if only that was the case. Treatment of organic hyperphagia with stimulants, naltrexone, high-dose fluoxetine, topiramate, felbamate, and modafinil is discussed.

Kleine-Levin syndrome (KLS) is a neuropsychiatric disorder characterized by hypersomnia and hyperphagia and is related neither to BI nor mental retardation (MR). It may be related to abnormal activity of hypocretin, a hypothalamic neuropeptide that regulates food intake and the sleep-wake cycle. It is possible that hypocretin activity is also abnormal in PWS, narcolepsy, and other conditions typified by hyperphagia and/or hypersomnia.

High-quality, restorative sleep is the hallmark of well-balanced, rhythmic brain function, and disruptions of brain function almost always compromise the integrity of the sleep-wake cycle. Therefore, it is hardly surprising that mentally retarded and brain-injured people are prone to sleep disorders. Hypoarousal, hypersomnia, and posttraumatic narcolepsy are disorders of sleep excess. Intractable insomnia and sleep-phase reversal are the opposite.

EATING DISORDERS IN MENTAL RETARDATION AND BRAIN INJURY

Prader-Willi Syndrome

Prader, Labhart and Willi described PWS in 1956 as a syndrome of MR, short stature, obesity, hypogonadism, and muscular hypotonia. More than 700 cases have been reported; the estimated incidence is approximately five to 10 in 100,000 livebirths (1,2). It is one of the five most common syndromes seen in birth defects clinics, is only one-fifth to one-tenth as common as Down's syndrome (3), but is the most common dysmorphic form of obesity (1).

Children with PWS have typical facies: a narrow bifrontal diameter, almond-shaped eyes, and a triangular mouth, features that may be lost after they gain weight. They have small hands and feet and abnormal development of sexual characteristics. They have feeding problems in infancy and failure to thrive. Then, during the preschool years, there is a sudden increase in weight.

Although most people with PWS are mild to moderately mentally retarded, approximately 40% are not retarded at all. There is a decrement in cognitive development at approximately the same time that they begin to engage in hyperphagia. It has been suggested that children with PWS whose hyperphagia is controlled at an early age may continue to develop intellectually (4).

Although hyperphagia and food-seeking behavior are the most striking behavioral abnormalities of children with PWS, they are also prone to psychiatric problems that are not food related. Virtually all patients with PWS have obsessive thoughts about food but also have obsessive-compulsive behaviors such as hoarding, compulsive speech, rewriting, ordering, arranging, symmetry, exactness, and cleanliness. Other typical behavioral difficulties include stubbornness, temper tantrums, aggression, skin picking, sadness, and verbal perseveration. Autism and pervasive developmental disorder (PDD) have been described in association with PWS (5).

Genetics and Pathophysiology

Several specific chromosomal abnormalities were hypothesized to account for PWS until high-resolution cytogenetic studies revealed the cause to be a deletion on chromosome 15 (15q11q13) (6). The chromosomal deletion might be apparent cytogenetically or it might be a microdeletion detectable only by molecular genetic techniques.

Every chromosome pair is diploid, with one maternal and one paternal contribution. In PWS, the paternal contribution to chromosome 15 in the 15q11–13 region is missing, i.e., the deletion is of paternal origin. This particular region of chromosome 15 is made up of tandem inverted repeats, a structural feature that may predispose the DNA to structural instability and thus mutation (7). Speculations have been raised about paternal hydrocarbon exposure as a possible etiologic factor of PWS (8–10).

If it is the lack of some paternal gene in the 15q11–13 region that causes PWS, one likely candidate is *SNRPN*. *SNRPN* is an imprinted gene, i.e., a gene that is modified during development, in this case by methylation. *SNRPN* is methylated in the maternal allele and unmethylated and therefore expressed in the paternal allele. The gene encodes a protein that is expressed in most tissues but especially in the brain and in particular in the hypothalamus. Another candidate gene is *NDN*, which encodes a protein that regulates neuronal growth and is also expressed vigorously in the hypothalamus.

The cause and pathophysiology of PWS may be imperfectly understood, but virtually all the observed abnormalities point to a disturbance in the development and function of midline structures, including the thalamus and hypothalamus (11). Indeed, most of the clinical features of PWS may be attributed to hypothalamic dysfunction including hypersomnia, thermoregulatory disturbance, growth retardation, genital hypoplasia, hyperphagia, and obesity.

Autopsy findings in patients with PWS have been nonspecific (12–14), although subtle reductions in hypothalamic neurons responsible for the regulation of food intake have been described (15).

Hyperphagia in Prader-Willi Syndrome

Children with PWS begin to gain weight during the preschool years, after an infant period with failure to thrive; thereafter, there is a rapid increase to morbid obesity if eating is not controlled. In fact, hyperphagia is the most compelling behavioral symptom of PWS, and it may be severe, bizarre, and life threatening. Eating behaviors include an insatiable appetite, stealing, foraging, and gorging. People with PWS try to consume enormous amounts of food with no concern for taste or quality: garbage, dog food, frozen bread, and other unappetizing things. They may be devious to the level of minor genius in their attempts to get at food and may be aggressive or prone to tantrums when their attempts are thwarted. They are not bulimic because they do not eat in binges and there is no induced vomiting. It may be that people with PWS cannot vomit. Nor is what they do pica because they confine their intake to recognized if unappetizing foodstuffs.

The driving force behind the obesity of people with PWS is hyperphagia and increased caloric intake. Measures of fat mobilization are normal (16). Glucose tolerance is normal as is the growth hormone response to insulin-induced hypoglycemia (compared with obese controls). The thyrotropin-releasing hormone response to thyroid-stimulating hormone is elevated (17). Because hypogonadism is a defining characteristic of PWS, it is no surprise that the normal rise in follicle-stimulating hormone and luteinizing hormone in response to gonadotropin-releasing hormone is blunted or absent (17). The activity level of children with PWS is not invariably reduced (18). In the absence then of any peripheral mechanism or any clearly defined endocrinopathy aside from luteinizing hormone, one surmises that a hypothalamic mechanism is responsible for the hyperphagia and its attendant morbidity.

The treatment of hyperphagia in PWS requires a program of behavior management that is often no less than heroic. Control of caloric intake must begin when the child is quite young and must be done in cognizance of the fact that the caloric needs of children with PWS are lower than those of normal children. It requires major modifications in the home economy including absolute control of access to foodstuffs of any kind including pet food, leftovers, and garbage. School personnel, neighbors, relatives, and friends must be included in a compact of absolute restriction. It is easier said than done, and many children with PWS have to be managed, ultimately, in structured residential settings where the discipline of food management can be professionally guided.

Treatment with growth hormone increases muscle tone and enhances growth in children with PWS, increasing height, decreasing central obesity, and normalizing the body habitus (5). Androgens and human chorionic gonadotropin may correct genital abnormalities such as micropenis and cryptorchism.

Neuropharmacology

Because serotonergic neurons are known to modulate appetitive behavior, there has been interest in applying treatment with drugs that enhance serotonin neurotransmission to the treatment of eating disorders such as anorexia and bulimia nervosa (19,20). PWS is an extraordinary disorder of appetitive instability that may also be related to abnormal serotonin metabolism (21).

The neuropharmacology of eating behavior is complex, and all the monoamine neurotransmitters are implicated in some way, although which neurochemical effects are most salient to PWS remains to be seen. Through α-adrenergic receptors in the paraventricular nucleus of the hypothalamus, norepinephrine can be a powerful inducer of eating behavior in rats (22,23). Lesions of ascending dopaminergic pathways have been associated with aphagia in laboratory animals (24); dopamine agonists are known to produce anorexia (25), and dopamine antagonist drugs, such as the neuroleptics, are known to lead to obesity, especially in mentally retarded people. Manipulations that increase serotonin synthesis are known to reduce appetite (22), and the serotonergic antidepressant fluoxetine sometimes has impressive effects in reducing appetite and weight (26).

It has been natural, therefore, to explore the possibility that hyperphagia, self-injurious behavior, and emotional instability in PWS might respond to treatment with serotonergic drugs. The results of published accounts and clinical experience have been mixed, but the selective serotonin reuptake inhibitor (SSRI) fluoxetine is probably the most frequently prescribed psychotropic drug for children and adults with PWS.

Fluoxetine was reported useful for hyperphagia and self-injurious behavior in a 35-year-old woman with PWS and quite remarkably induced menstruation in two women with PWS who had been amenorrheic (27). SSRI antidepressants have also been suggested for the self-excoriating skin picking that is so common in PWS (28). Other behaviors characteristic of patients with PWS that may respond to serotonergic drugs are irritability, stubbornness, obsessions and compulsions, trichotillomania, arguing, and defiance. I had success with one mildly retarded man with PWS whose weight and hyperphagia had been stabilized behaviorally but who still was given to episodes of angry aggression and who improved behaviorally on L-tryptophan at 4 g daily. L-tryptophan in daily doses as high as 15 g, however, had no effect on eating behavior in a larger group of patients with PWS (17).

Serotonergics may or may not reduce the hyperphagia associated with PWS but are used more frequently than any other class of drugs for some of the temperamental and behavioral aspects of the disorder. The SSRIs are, as of this writing, the drugs of choice, although high doses are usually necessary, and unfortunately even normal doses may be poorly tolerated (5).

The effects of psychostimulants on hyperphagia in PWS and other conditions characterized by organic bulimia are unpredictable. Sometimes they work, at least for a while. They may work better with augmentation by amantadine. The ill-fated antiepileptic drug felbamate looked promising for a while; one really cannot use it for hyperphagia anymore except in the most dire cases. Topiramate may be a reasonable alternative and deserves consideration.

Patients with PWS with rage outbursts may require a mood-stabilizing drug (29). I had used carbamazepine (CBZ) in the past but now would use oxcarbazepine. Neuroleptics used to be prescribed often in PWS, and antipsychotic drugs are still required sometimes (30). One must be careful, however, with drugs such as the mood stabilizers and atypical antipsychotics, which tend to cause weight gain (31).

Organic Hyperphagia

PWS is a paradigm for the study of organic hyperphagia. For example, it bears an interesting resemblance to Frölich's syndrome or adiposogenital dystrophy, a syndrome of obesity and genital underdevelopment usually related to a tumor of the pituitary or the hypothalamus. It too may be associated with aggression, angry outbursts, and antisocial behavior.

Organic hyperphagia is usually (but not invariably) associated with hypothalamic lesions. Brain trauma can occasionally cause hyperphagia and intractable obesity, although the frequency is not known. It is only seen in severe BI and is usually accompanied by considerable cognitive, behavioral, and emotional impairment.

Patients with traumatic BI (TBI) who are hyperphagic tend to prefer palatable foodstuffs and are given to "pressured overeating." Like patients with PWS, they sometimes consume uneatables, such as garbage and pet food, but this is unusual and probably more common in young patients. In contrast, mentally retarded people with pica and patients with BI with Klüver-Bucy syndrome consume foodstuffs, eatable and uneatable, as well as inedible things, such as cigarette butts, stones, and string (32).

Hyperphagia occurs in a substantial proportion (10% to 25%) of elderly patients with dementia, especially during the middle stages of the condition. It is not a function of memory because they have not forgotten that they have eaten. It may be more common in wanderers who are compensating for increased caloric expenditure, but it is more often dissociated from caloric need and the patient's level of physical activity. It is said to be more common in severely demented people with frontal lobe involvement. Perhaps it is a form of "stimulus-bound" behavior (33–35).

Organic hyperphagia is sometime called hypothalamic obesity, although neither term is entirely satisfactory, considering the complexity of the sensory, cognitive, and motivational sources of feeding behavior, and the complexity of the neural systems that participate in it. There is a satiety center in the ventromedial hypothalamus and an appetite center in the ventrolateral hypothalamus. Lesions in the medial hypothalamus lead to overeating and severe obesity. Lesions in the lateral hypothalamus lead to severe neglect of eating (aphagia). Chemical stimulation of the respective centers can either stimulate or inhibit the function; the peptide CRF inhibits feeding when injected into the medial hypothalamus and neuropeptide Y stimulates feeding. [Only a very small minority of obese people has medial hypothalamic lesions. Of overriding importance in common obesity are genetic factors (e.g., the number or lipocytes that one inherits) and environmental/behavioral factors, especially a sedentary lifestyle in a food-laden society.]

There is actually an obesity gene (*ob*) that expresses a hormonal product, leptin, in lipocytes; this circulating hormone is part of a feedback system that signals the hypothalamus about the abundance of fat. Animals with mutations in the *ob* gene are obese but lose weight when they are given leptin, which leads to weight loss by suppressing the appetite and increasing the metabolic rate. Most obese people, however, are relatively insensitive to leptin (36).

The modulation of hunger and satiety, food-seeking behavior, body image, and the long-term regulation of adiposity and weight is a complicated process that is usually related to serotonin but is hardly explicable in terms of a single neurotransmitter system. Norepinephrine, for example, produces an appetite stimulant effect. One way that the tricyclic antidepressants stimulate food intake may be by activating the norepinephrine system in the paraventricular nucleus (37).

The endogenous opiate system is known to exercise a stimulatory effect on eating behavior in lower animals (38). Endogenous opiates (endorphins) and exogenous opiates (morphine) induce feeding when injected into the paraventricular nucleus, and opiate antagonists decrease feeding. This, of course, is the rationale for opiate antagonist treatment for eating disorders. Naloxone, an opiate antagonist, is known to suppress eating behavior induced in animals by stress or benzodiazepines (38,39). Naloxone has also been found to reduce daily caloric intake in obese subjects (40). The results of trials of opiate antagonists in patients with PWS and those with bulimia nervosa however have not been impressive (37,41). There are anecdotal reports of success with naltrexone for hyperphagia in patients with TBI, but no controlled trials.

Dopamine is the transmitter substance most closely involved with self-administration behaviors and reward. Dopaminergic neurons in the ventral tegmentum comprise a system that is stimulated by reinforcing events such as feeding. They project to the striatum, limbic system, and cortex, generating complex behaviors such as movement, emotional states, ideation, and planning. In animals, low doses of dopamine agonists stimulate feeding and high doses inhibit feeding.

Bulimia Nervosa

Bulimia (or bulimia nervosa) is an eating disorder characterized by massive binge eating followed by the induction of vomiting and excessive use of laxatives. It is closely related to anorexia nervosa; people with anorexia are frequently given to binge eating, and in both groups of patients, there are disturbances in attitudes toward weight and the perception of body shape.

The most effective pharmacologic approach to the psychiatric eating disorders to date has been antidepressant therapy, although the anticonvulsant topiramate has excited recent interest (42). The rationale for antidepressant therapy for eating disorders is the impressive comorbidity of eating and affective disorders and the observation that semistarvation in normal individuals can lead to depressive symptoms. The fact that many patients with eating disorders have obsessive-compulsive behaviors unrelated to food and that body dysmorphic disorder is closely related to obsessive-compulsive disorder has stimulated interest in the serotonergic antidepressants in particular.

Indeed, there is ample evidence for serotonin dysfunction in anorexia nervosa and serotonin hypofunction in bulimia. Serotonergic activity appears to be related to the development of satiety. Serotonin injected into the paraventricular nucleus suppresses deprivation-induced and norepinephrine-induced eating. The serotonergic antidepressants, especially fluoxetine, are probably used more frequently, and perhaps with more success, than any other class of medications for the treatment of patients with eating disorders. However, high doses of fluoxetine (e.g., 60 mg/d) are needed, and the normal antidepressant dose is not usually effective.

However, the success of antidepressant therapy has always been modest. Pharmacology to induce weight gain in patients with anorexia or to control excessive weight gain in those with bulimia has generally been disappointing, although treatment in the postacute phase to maintain emotional stability and optimal weight and prevent relapse has been more successful (43).

Drug-Induced Obesity

Most of the neuroactive drugs are associated, to some degree, with weight gain, sometimes to the point of frank obesity, and type II diabetes: virtually all the antidepressants, all the antipsychotic drugs (except molindone and ziprasidone), and all the mood stabilizers (except topiramate and lamotrigine).

Within categories, there is marked variation, although the statistical data do not always predict what will happen to individual patients. Among the antidepressants, for example, the tricyclics and the monoamine oxidase inhibitors are more troublesome than the new antidepressants. Amitriptyline is notorious for inducing carbohydrate craving and weight gain, desipramine much less so, and fluoxetine still less. (44). Among the newer antidepressants, mirtazapine is more likely than the others to cause weight gain, but much less than the tricyclic antidepressants, and bupropion and nefazodone are least likely, even when compared with the SSRIs (45).

Weight gain with the SSRIs is controversial. People recovering from depression should be expected to regain the weight they lost when they were depressed. In fact, when the SSRIs were first introduced, there were reports of clinically significant weight loss in elderly patients in nursing homes (46). However, over the long term, all the SSRIs can cause hyperphagia and weight gain, paroxetine perhaps more than the others. Perhaps sertraline is the least orexigenic SSRI, but it is fluoxetine that has received the most attention as a potential weight-loss drug and as a treatment for bulimia nervosa (47).

Among the antipsychotic drugs, weight gain is pronounced with clozapine, olanzapine, sulpiride, thioridazine, chlorpromazine, and somewhat less with quetiapine. Risperidone, sertindole, zometapine, and haloperidol are intermediate, and ziprasidone seems to induce only slight body weight changes (48,49).

The relative affinities of the atypical antipsychotic drugs for the histamine H_1 receptor appears to be the most robust correlate of the clinical findings (50). In sulpiride-induced obesity, there is no increase in circulating leptin or insulin (51). Atypical antipsychotic drugs that antagonize the 5-HT_{1A} receptor may decrease the responsiveness of pancreatic beta cells to blood sugar levels (52), which may explain the occurrence of type II diabetes with these agents.

The anticonvulsants (e.g., phenytoin, valproate, CBZ) and mood-stabilizing drugs (e.g., lithium) are notorious for inducing weight gain. Gabapentin, lamotrigine, and tiagabine are less likely to have an effect on weight (53–55). Topiramate does not cause weight gain and may be a good treatment for various conditions associated with hyperphagia.

There is no clear consensus on what it is about the various neuroactive drugs that leads to weight gain. It is unlikely that they all access a common mechanism.

Kleine-Levin Syndrome

KLS is a peculiar disorder that primarily affects adolescent males. First described by Kleine (56), the syndrome is characterized by alternating episodes of hypersomnia and hyperphagia. Critchley (57) included disturbance of mood and other appetitive functions as symptoms of KLS. The symptom list has grown with succeeding descriptions. The incidence of KLS is unknown, but it is not a common disease. It is given to a relapsing course and often remits entirely after a number of years with no clear residua (58,59).

Patients with KLS present with acute onset of stupor, relative ease of arousal, irritability on awakening, and hyperphagia. Hypersexuality has been described in several patients and seems to be associated with a generalized increase in appetitive behaviors. Subsequent descriptions by Lewis (60), Levin (61), and Daniels (62) corroborated a clinical picture of recurring hypersomnia (16 to 20 hours per day), awakening only for urination and defecation, excessive food intake, and mild confusion and mood disturbances ranging from euphoria to extreme irritability. These symptoms arise in marked contrast to the patient's premorbid state of health. Powers and Gunderman (63) added fire setting as an associated symptom in a single case study. Orlosky (64) added confusion, amnesia for the episode, (unspecified) movement disorder, delusional thinking, and auditory and visual hallucinations to the list of KLS symptoms.

Despite the dramatic presentation, few positive findings have been reported on neurologic examination. The symptoms associated with KLS are commonly seen in other neurologic diseases. Hypersomnia has been reported in connection with medial mesencephalic lesions (65), medial thalamic lesions (66), posterior hypothalamic lesions (67), and lesions that affect elements of the reticular activating system. Hyperphagia and mood instability have been reported in lesions of the hypothalamus (68), orbitofrontal cortex (69), and periventricular areas (70). No such findings, however, have been reported in KLS.

In KLS, positive neurologic findings are infrequent and are often confined to atypical cases. Popoviciu and Corfariu (71) reported a single case with modest enlargement of the third ventricle on pneumoencephalogram. In contrast, Ferguson (72), Goldberg (73), Thompson et al. (74), Merriman (75), Orlosky (64), and Mayer et al. (58) reported normal findings on computed tomography and magnetic resonance imaging. Kleine (56) and Daniels (62) reported that some patients with KLS had an influenza-like illness before the onset of the syndrome but no definitive signs of encephalitis. Critchley (57), Takrani and Cronin (76), Carpenter et al. (77), and Merriman (75) reported cases of KLS after viral encephalitis. Critchley (57) described two cases with upper respiratory illness and headache preceding the onset of KLS.

KLS was described in a 25-year-old man with encephalitis (75), a 9-year-old boy with PWS (78), two adolescent males with Asberger's syndrome (79), and three patients with "interepisodic brain dysfunction" (80).

Neuropathologic findings have included neuronal loss, glial proliferation, and perivascular changes in the hypothalamus, amygdala, and anteromedial temporal cortex (76), depigmentation of the locus ceruleus and substantia nigra (81), and microglial proliferation suggestive of localized encephalitis (82). Thalamic lesions have also been reported (77,83).

The results of neurophysiologic studies have been ambiguous. Merriman (75) described nonspecific slow-wave activity in one patient with documented encephalitis. Critchley (57) and Orlosky (64) reported acute-phase changes that included bursts of bilaterally synchronous 2- to 4-cycle per second activity, consistent with sleep. There was no reported epileptiform activity.

Green and Cracco (84), Garland et al. (85), Lavie et al. (86), Elian and Bornstein (87), and Thacore et al. (88) reported a different set of electroencephalographic irregularities. Lavie et al. (86) reported a male patient with KLS whose electroencephalogram was characterized by instability in the sleep architecture. Their second case was a female patient with sleep-onset rapid eye movement (REM) activity reminiscent of narcolepsy. Kupfer and Heninger (89) described a similar pattern of sleep-onset REM sleep during multistep sleep provocation, but Chesson et al. (90) found reduced REM sleep. Elian and Bornstein (87) reported paroxysmal episodes of high-voltage, 2.5- to 3.0-Hz activity during sleep episodes. The degree of electroencephalographic abnormality seems to be related to the duration of symptoms. Thacore et al. (88) reported similar bursts of delta activity but also noted bursts of 8- to 12-Hz activity alternating with slow-wave activity, activation of slow-wave activity with eye opening, and a reduction in sleep spindles. The latter finding has also been described in patients with thalamic lesions (65).

Conversely, Orlosky (64) noted that polysomnographic studies of 30 patients with KLS were consistently negative. Despite this negative result, he recommended sleep polysomnography for patients with KLS. Kupfer and Heninger (89) and Lavie et al. (86) supported this recommendation, especially in atypical cases, to rule out narcolepsy or sleep apnea. Sleep-onset REM activity is pathognomonic for narcolepsy but uncommon in typical cases of KLS.

Sleep apnea might be confused with KLS based on hypersomnia, but polysomnography should reveal episodes of apnea not present in KLS (91).

Physicians have long suspected an endocrine or neuroendocrine cause for the extraordinary symptoms of KLS, but the results of various tests of hypothalamic function have been disappointing (56,74, 92). It would be surprising, however, if there were not some connection between KLS and the recently discovered hypocretins (see below).

The existence of the syndrome is hardly in doubt, although few physicians have ever had the opportunity to attend a case. There is often an association with some encephalopathic event, but the association is nonspecific. Where, then, does KLS fit?

In 1990, a colleague and I described two typical cases of KLS in adolescent males (93). In one case, the prodromata included a brief period of hyperactivity, insomnia, and euphoric mood, and in the other, it was precipitated by a mild head injury and an episode of sexual assault. Both patients responded to lithium treatment and did well in follow-up for 2 years. The first patient had some initial symptoms suggestive of hypomania, but no family history of major affective disorder. The second patient had a strong family history of bipolar disorder, responsive to lithium, in two first-degree relatives, and a dexamethasone suppression test that was strongly positive during an acute episode.

Lithium has been recommended for KLS more frequently than any other drug (94–98). It is not unreasonable to suggest that KLS may be a peculiar variant of adolescent major affective disorder. Hypersomnia is known to be associated with the depressive phase of bipolar disorder (99), and episodic hyperphagia has also been described in major affective disorder (100). Other symptoms associated with KLS that are known to occur in bipolar patients are hypersexuality, irritability, withdrawal, and intermittent aggression (100–104).

Psychostimulants have been a traditional treatment for KLS (64); the rationale is that KLS is a disorder of arousal (104). Stimulant treatment, however, may not prevent recurrences of KLS (94,95,105), and it did not do so in either of our two cases. It is our opinion that lithium should be considered the treatment of choice for recurrent KLS. In patients with KLS who do not respond to lithium or cannot tolerate the drug, treatment with the usual alternative drugs for bipolar disorder (oxcarbazepine, valproic acid, lamotrigine, or topiramate) should be considered: (106–110). There has never been a controlled drug trial in KLS.

Of course, lithium response does nothing to finalize the diagnosis of major affective disorder. Lithium has been helpful in the management of self-injurious behavior (108,109), violent and aggressive behavior (108), and other nonspecific behavioral difficulties associated with BI and MR (111). By the same token, it is virtually impossible to establish a connection between two syndromes whose manifestations are entirely behavioral and whose underlying pathophysiology is unknown.

DRUG TREATMENT FOR ORGANIC HYPERPHAGIA

In the previous sections, the available treatments for organic hyperphagia were discussed. As we have seen, bulimia nervosa and KLS are special cases. They have no structural underpinnings and no regular association with an encephalopathic condition. The antidepressants and mood stabilizers, respectively, are the drugs of choice insofar as any drug might be helpful at all. Psychostimulants and naltrexone are sometimes effective. Topiramate is promising, but the data are preliminary.

Mood stabilizers are appropriate for patients with PWS and KLS, but are more effective in controlling the emotional instability that usually attends those peculiar syndromes. Patients who are treated with lithium or CBZ may be more agreeable and less volatile, but they may remain as hyperphagic and hypersomniac as ever. One hopes that topiramate will be better. When specific agents are developed to influence the hypocretin system, rational pharmacotherapy may finally be achieved.

High-dose fluoxetine is still the drug of choice for organic hyperphagia in patients with PWS and BI. Naltrexone sometimes works better when it is combined with high-dose fluoxetine. It may take months, however, before the beneficial effects of naltrexone are seen.

Felbamate is sorely missed. It was an excellent anorexigenic drug. Fenfluramine, however, is not missed at all.

SLEEP-RELATED PROBLEMS IN MENTAL RETARDATION AND BRAIN INJURY

The normal sleep-wake cycle is an active neurophysiologic process that originates in the brainstem, hypothalamus, and basal forebrain, with relay nuclei in the thalamus; the target organ is the cerebral cortex. Wakefulness is a functional component of the generalized arousal system maintained by tonic activity in the reticular activating system. Norepinephrine- and acetylcholine-containing neurons are active during wakefulness. Wakefulness is enhanced by neurons containing various peptides and histaminergic neurons; antipsychotic and antidepressant drugs that induce somnolence often exercise an antihistamine effect. Sleep is generated by the activity of neurons in the raphe nuclei of the brainstem, thalamus, hypothalamus, preoptic area, and basal forebrain. Serotonin, adenosine, γ-aminobutyric acid and a variety of peptides are active in promoting sleep. The serotonin precursor tryptophan is a mild soporific, and caffeine is an adenosine antagonist. A complex balance among anatomic regions and neuroactive substances maintains the integrity of the sleep-wake cycle. It is eminently vulnerable to disruptions of brain function, local and systemic in origin, and to lesions in the pertinent brain structures (112).

During gestation and through early childhood, sleep architecture evolves and matures. By the age of 2 years, children achieve a normal proportion of REM sleep but spend more sleep time in stages three and four than adults do, which may explain why they are more prone to parasomnias such as nightmares, night terrors, and somnambulism. A normal adult pattern is not achieved until the end of adolescence. Adults spend progressively less time in stage three and four sleep; past the age of 75, stage four sleep virtually disappears. The sleep of elderly people is also characterized by the number and duration of nocturnal arousals and by sleep that is increasingly light and more vulnerable to external or internal disruptions. Nonrestorative sleep and insomnia are common problems in elderly people. Their circadian cycle is shortened. Their sleep-wake cycle is less plastic, and therefore they are more vulnerable to time-zone changes (112,113).

The changes in sleep patterns that occur in normal elderly people are difficult to distinguish from the changes that occur with degeneration, but there are differences. Sleep disruption, in general, is more common in demented patients than in elderly controls; nocturnal confusion, agitation, combativeness, and wandering are characteristic of dementia but not normal aging. In patients with dementia, sleep/wake disruption is correlated with severity of cognitive impairment (114).

High-quality, restorative sleep is the hallmark of well-balanced, rhythmic brain function, and disruptions of brain function almost always compromise the integrity of the sleep-wake cycle (112). Therefore, it is natural to encounter sleep disorders in patients with BI or MR. Insomnia and hypersomnia are the most common clinical problems, but virtually every kind of sleep disorder may occur. Conceptually, one expects the sleep problems of retarded children to be the manifestation of an immature sleep pattern, and the sleep problems of retarded adults and most patients with BI to be similar to those encountered in normal aging, cerebrovascular disease, and dementia.

In any patient who presents with a sleep-related complaint, it is necessary to distinguish between primary and secondary sleep disorders and between sleep problems that are central in nature and those related to systemic dysfunction. The differential diagnosis of sleep-related problems includes pain, chronic or otherwise, headache, seizures, medication effects, systemic disease, and virtually all the psychiatric disorders. Before attributing a sleep problem to the nonspecific effect of encephalopathy, one should also consider specific conditions such as sleep apnea, restless legs syndrome, periodic leg movements of sleep, nocturnal myoclonus, isolated sleep paralysis, KLS, and PWS.

Sleep-Related Problems Attendant on Brain Injury

Sleep disturbance is very common after BI. Patients with TBI often complain of sleep-related problems, and they are not unlike the sleep problems of elderly patients. Early in the course of recovery from severe TBI, most patients complain of difficulty falling asleep and/or frequent awakenings during the night. Over the longer term, however, excessive daytime sleepiness is the most common problem (115).

Problems with sleep initiation and maintenance may be more common in patients who have had mild TBI. Postconcussion insomnia, however, tends to be transient and is commonly treated with low doses of trazodone or amitriptyline. Physical pain, such as headache and neck and back pain, tends to aggravate sleep problems in postconcussion syndrome and in other BI syndromes. Sleep problems in patients with BI are correlated with fatigue and cognitive deficits during the day (116,117).

Posttraumatic delayed sleep phase syndrome, in contrast to simple insomnia, is caused by a delay in the patient's normal sleep-wake pattern, a circadian setback but with preservation of normal sleep architecture. It is said to respond favorably to melatonin (118,119).

Parasomnias are not described in the TBI literature, although nocturnal bruxism has been (120).

The differential diagnosis of sleep disorders in patients with BI should always include posttraumatic stress disorder, a particularly troublesome condition that is usually associated with severe sleep disturbance and much more difficult to treat successfully.

Hypoarousal

Hypersomnia, or excessive sleep, is characteristic of diseases such as encephalitis lethargica and trypanosomiasis, traumatic or vascular lesions affecting the midbrain or the diencephalon. It is also characteristic of PWS and KLS.

Excessive daytime sleepiness, or somnolence, is a relatively nonspecific syndrome with a host of different causes including certain forms of depression, medication effects, systemic disease, chronic fatigue syndrome, sleep apnea, and neurologic diseases such as dementia and multiple sclerosis. It may be the consequence of insomnia with all its causes. In the postconcussion syndrome, diurnal somnolence is almost always associated with insomnia.

Hypersomnia and excessive daytime sleepiness are both encountered in patients with TBI. More commonly, however, people who have had severe BI, especially closed head injury, experience a state of chronic hypoarousal. This state is not characterized by sleeping or drowsiness but rather a chronic state of reduced activity and responsiveness that is hardly ever interrupted except perhaps by occasional outbursts of dysphoria or agitation. Not only is spontaneous behavior reduced, but reactive behavior as well. The patient is engaged only with difficulty and responds only to a minimal degree, even to the most vigorous forms of stimulation.

Drugs such as phenytoin, amitriptyline, metoclopramide, and haloperidol aggravate the condition of chronic posttraumatic hypoarousal; indeed, virtually any neuroactive drug can aggravate the problem. It tends to respond favorably to psychostimulant drugs, amantadine, and dopamine agonists. Sometimes, however, the cost of increased arousal is increased agitation. If that occurs, a second course of treatment, some months later, may have a more positive effect.

Posttraumatic Narcolepsy

Narcolepsy is a disorder characterized by REM sleep attacks, flaccid paralysis (cataplexy), and excessive daytime sleepiness. No specific morphologic abnormalities are found in the central nervous system of affected patients, and the condition is not related, even in a nonspecific way, with encephalopathy. Excessive daytime somnolence is not uncommon in patients with BI, for example, but true posttraumatic narcolepsy is relatively rare (121). Rather, narcolepsy has a strong familial basis, with a strong association with the HLA-DR and HLA-DQ antigens. Not everybody who is HLA-DR2 positive is narcoleptic, obviously, but most authors now concede that the presence of specific HLA antigens is necessary for the diagnosis (122). The HLA-DR2 antigen is found in 20% to 35% of the general population (123).

Studies of human narcoleptics and of animal models of the condition have concentrated on the function of the pertinent neurotransmitter systems. The feature of abnormal control of REM sleep in narcolepsy focused the attention of researchers on neural generators/modulators of REM sleep in the brainstem, especially their cholinergic neurons. REM sleep is the result of acetylcholine activity. In Alzheimer's disease, for example, cholinergic deficiency is associated with REM sleep abnormalities; treatment of Alzheimer's disease with cholinesterase inhibitors is accompanied by normalization of sleep patterns.

The biogenic amines dopamine, norepinephrine, and serotonin are inactivated during REM sleep and appear to have a permissive role. One theory of narcolepsy is that it is related to abnormal metabolism of the biogenic amines and thus defective monoaminergic control of cholinergic REM sleep mechanisms. This theory is consistent with clinical practice, namely, the use of psychostimulants, antidepressants, and dopamine agonists to control sleep attacks, cataplexy, and daytime somnolence in narcolepsy (123).

Reviews of narcolepsy seldom mention trauma as an etiologic consideration (124). There are a few reports of narcolepsy confirmed by sleep polysomnography secondary to brain tumors or multiple sclerosis involving the brainstem. Reports of posttraumatic, postanoxic, and postinfectious narcolepsy are rare but not unknown. They do not, as a rule, find an association with the HLA antigen (122). When narcolepsy occurs in a patient with TBI, the absence of HLA antigens may affirm the traumatic cause (125); their presence, conversely, suggests an interaction between trauma and genetic proclivity (126). In either event, when posttraumatic narcolepsy does occur, the onset may be weeks or months after injury.

Hypocretins

Hypocretin-1 and -2 are newly discovered neuropeptides that are processed from a common precursor molecule, preprohypocretin and are homologous with members of the secretin peptide family. Hypocretin-containing cells are located in the lateral hypothalamus and project widely to the entire neuraxis. The hypocretins function as neurotransmitters, with a dense pattern of innervation to other hypothalamic nuclei, the locus ceruleus, dorsal raphe nuclei, thalamus, and basal forebrain; in short, brain regions that are specifically occupied with the sleep-wake cycle (127–129).

The hypocretin neuropeptides appear to serve a number of physiologic functions that are germane to this discussion. Mutations in the hypocretin gene and other abnormalities related to the peptide cause narcolepsy in mice, dogs, and humans. Human narcoleptics have greatly reduced levels of hypocretin in their cerebrospinal fluid. It is possible that hypocretin cells drive cholinergic and monoaminergic activity across the sleep cycle (127,128).

The hypocretins are clearly involved in regulating the sleep-wake cycle and other physiologic systems including energy metabolism, hormone homeostasis, and cardiovascular activity. They are notably involved in the regulation of food intake. Thus, the association of hyperphagia and hypersomnia in the PWS and KLS is more than coincidental.

Sleep-Related Problems in Mentally Retarded People

High-quality, restorative sleep is the hallmark of well-balanced, rhythmic brain function, and disruptions of brain function almost always compromise the integrity of the sleep-wake cycle. Therefore, it is hardly surprising that mentally retarded people are prone to sleep disorders. As a rule, severely retarded people are more prone to sleep problems than mildly retarded people, autistic people who are retarded have more sleep problems than the nonautistic, and retarded people with behavior/emotional difficulties are much more prone to sleep disorders.

In one study, no fewer than 88% of a sample of retarded people with concomitant behavioral problems had significant sleep problems, and the presence of sleep problems was inversely correlated to IQ (130). Daytime irritability, stereotypy, hyperactivity, and self-injury are more common in retarded people who have disordered sleep (131).

The typical sleep problems that arise in retarded people include difficulty with sleep initiation, decreased total sleep time, decreased nocturnal sleep, frequent awakening, and early waking. Autistic people in particular may have extreme sleep latencies, a problem that may be aggravated by nocturnal rituals and increased anxiety at night. They are also prone to lengthy periods of night wakening, often accompanied by wandering or stereotyped behavior. They tend to wake up early in the morning, active if not refreshed. They seem to get by well enough with only a few hours of sleep. Autistic people who are mentally retarded seem to have more sleep-related problems than retarded people who are not autistic. Even a mild degree of MR is associated with sleep problems if the child is autistic, but this is rarely true of mildly retarded people who are not autistic. In addition, their sleep architecture tends to be immature and disorganized (132,133).

Two pathobehavioral syndromes are typically associated with abnormalities of sleep. PWS is associated with hypersomnia, excessive daytime sleepiness, and REM sleep onsets. Sleep-disordered breathing has only a limited role in the genesis of this problem and is not related to the HLA antigen (134).

Most people with Smith-Magenis syndrome have sleep problems including sleep initiation and maintenance, shortened sleep cycles, daytime somnolence, snoring, and enuresis. Most of them have to take some kind of medication to control sleep problems. Because they appear to have disturbed circadian secretion of melatonin, that substance is often recommended to improve sleep (133,135).

Indeed, just as trazodone and amitriptyline are favorite drugs for patients with BI, melatonin is popular among physicians who treat mentally retarded people with sleep disorders (136–138). I have never found a good explanation for this obscure aspect of clinical practice beyond historical accident. Smith-Magenis syndrome is the only MR syndrome that is thought to be associated with melatonin abnormalities. Theoretically, the various sensory and cognitive abnormalities associated with MR might "diminish the ability of these individuals to perceive and interpret the multitude of cues for synchronizing their sleep with the environment," and exogenous melatonin would compensate for their failure to generate an appropriate endogenous melatonin response (139). Whether or not that is the case, melatonin is safe and inexpensive, and if it works, so much the better. The usual dose is 2.5 to 10 mg qhs.

Sleep disturbance may also be a typical component of Williams syndrome (140), Angelman syndrome (141), and the Smith-Lemli-Opitz syndrome (142). Patients with Down's syndrome have abnormalities in REM sleep that resemble, to a degree, REM abnormalities in patients with dementia (133). They are also prone to central and obstructive sleep apnea, with significant effects on oxygen saturation (143). Sleep problems in Down's syndrome are more common in older patients with the beginnings of dementia and in severely retarded patients with Down's syndrome who are more prone to early dementia.

Sleep Reversal

Reversal of the normal 24-hour sleep-wake cycle almost always occurs in the presence of an encephalopathic condition. It is characteristic of trypanosomiasis and encephalitis lethargica, but North American physicians will encounter the problem most often in elderly patients with dementia or cerebrovascular disease who may sleep for much of the day but then are restless at night (144).

Sleep reversal is a rare problem in mentally retarded children but is more common in mentally retarded adults, especially those with autism. A typical scenario is a retarded person living at home with elderly parents who increasingly concede to their child's idiosyncratic sleep pattern until the household is turned upside-down. This kind of tyrannical behavior is best dealt with by out-of-home placement.

Intractable Insomnia

Physicians have a remarkable panoply of agents to induce sleep. As mentioned, trazodone, amitriptyline, and melatonin are used more than any other drugs for patients with BI and with MR who have insomnia. Other commonly used agents include tricyclics antidepressants such as doxepin, the new antidepressant mirtazapine, and all the benzodiazepines, especially the new, short-acting drugs zolpidem and zaleplon. There are also dietary supplements and herbal remedies such as tryptophan, kava kava, hydroxytryptophan, and valerian root.

Nevertheless, one occasionally meets with a case of severe insomnia that is refractory to treatment with the conventional agents. The patient is typically an autistic child who is also hyperactive, disorganized, and impulsive, a patient with TBI with headache or chronic pain, or a patient with dementia, stroke, or severe mental handicap who screams, or wanders at night. When such patients are referred to a neuropsychiatrist, it is usually after the attending physician has exhausted the usual therapeutic approaches.

The first step is to review the differential diagnosis, as already described. In such patients, medication is sometimes the culprit: drugs that should induce somnolence may, in encephalopathic patients, have a paradoxical effect. Anticonvulsants, mood stabilizers, antipsychotic drugs, antidepressants, analgetics all may, in some patients, actually induce insomnia or aggravate nocturnal agitation. One of the cardinal rules of medical practice is: "In fever of unknown origin, stop all medications." To paraphrase: in intractable insomnia, stop all medications.

The second step is to try to do a better job of treating the patient's diurnal difficulties: improved pain management, optimal anticonvulsant treatment, treatment for depression or anxiety states, and better control of hyperactivity. A more agreeable pattern of daytime activity with ample social contact and physical exertion may also help. It is always necessary to address the fundamentals of sleep hygiene as well. Simple environmental changes, such as a night-light or turning down the night staff's radio, may make a difference.

Of course, if steps one and two were likely to have worked, the patient would probably never have been referred in the first place. So what clever new idea is the neuropsychiatrist likely to come up with?

Clonidine is frequently used, especially in children with attention deficit/hyperactivity disorder who take stimulants. It is sometime useful for patients with posttraumatic stress disorder. The atypical antipsychotic drugs olanzapine and quetiapine in low doses are also hypnotics. Mirtazapine is another useful drug. Sometimes lithium is also at the hour of sleep. Sometimes psychostimulants or amantadine during the day will enhance sleeping at night. Cranial electrostimulation is another option (see Chapter 24).

Gamma-hydroxybutyrate is an illicit drug (the "date-rape" drug) that is supposed to be a strength enhancer, euphoriant, and aphrodisiac. It is a central nervous system depressant that may be lethal when combined with alcohol or other depressants. There is no medical indication for the drug, but there has been research in patients with narcolepsy. The idea is that it imparts a continuous night's sleep and thus yields relief from irresistible daytime sleep attacks (145). Research is underway on gamma-hydroxybutyrate for intractable insomnia in neurologic diseases.

DRUG TREATMENT FOR ORGANIC HYPERSOMNIA

The appropriate question is whether treatment for hypersomnia in patients with BI and MR is different from the normal therapeutic approaches to narcolepsy. The answer is not much.

Narcolepsy treatment involves three types of drugs: the psychostimulants, the antidepressants, and the novel agent modafinil. All the usual stimulants are effective for narcoleptic patients; perhaps pemoline is less effective, and perhaps the amphetamines are superior, but individual patient response usually guides one's choice of a stimulant drug.

Antidepressants that are noradrenergic, such as desipramine and venlafaxine, are probably used more for hypersomnia than the other antidepressants. Bupropion may work sometimes. The serotonergic antidepressants are not particularly good for narcolepsy. In fact, hypersomnia is sometimes a side effect. Antidepressants are combined with stimulants when necessary.

Hypersomnia has been treated with drugs that are noradrenergic or dopaminergic. Thus, in narcolepsy, the stimulants and adrenergic antidepressants are the drugs of choice or were until recently. One may use these drugs to treat organic hypersomnia as well and sometimes to good effect. Amantadine and dopamine agonist drugs are also used and may be combined with stimulants as well.

The hypersomnia of PWS and KLS is associated with a degree of mood instability, irritability, and aggressive behavior that sometimes calls for the introduction of a mood-stabilizing drug. We have examined the use of CBZ and lithium in both of these conditions. The conventional mood stabilizers, however, all carry with them the side effect of sedation. Lamotrigine appears to be the least sedating of the psychotropic anticonvulsants, and many patients describe it as an energizing drug. The extent to which it is effective as a substitute for CBZ, valproate, and lithium remains to be seen.

Modafinil

Modafinil is a new and unique wakefulness-promoting drug that is clearly different from the psychostimulants. In a number of different animal paradigms, modafinil seems to have few, if any, typical dopaminergic or noradrenergic effects. It does not stimulate dopamine release from the presynaptic neuron, cause stereotypy in rats, or block the dopamine uptake carrier. It does not bind to any known adrenergic receptors or inhibit spontaneous activity of norepinephrine or dopamine brainstem neurons. In short, it does not behave like an amphetamine, aside from promoting wakefulness and reducing the performance decrement that arises from sleep deprivation (146).

It seems to have fewer side effects than stimulants do and is not as likely to be abused. Even in its effect on wakefulness, it is different from amphetamine because it does not elicit a strong compensatory sleep response.

It is easier to say what modafinil does not do in terms of its neuropharmacologic effects than what it does. For example, it has no effects on melatonin secretion, cortisol, or growth hormone (147). It has been suggested that it facilitates arousal by decreasing γ-aminobutyric acid neurotransmission (148). It may even be neuroprotective; in cell cultures, it attenuates the effects of glutamate neurotoxicity (149).

Modafinil induces cFOS expression in the anterior hypothalamus, an area that is responsible for generating sleep-wake circadian rhythms in the paraventricular nucleus of the hypothalamus and in the amygdala. (In contrast, amphetamine and methylphenidate evoke cFOS immunoreactivity in the striatum and frontal cortex) (150). Perhaps the most interesting information about its mechanism of action is an activating effect that it has on hypocretin-containing neurons in the lateral hypothalamus (151,152).

If, in fact, modafinil has an effect on hypocretin, it may be interesting to test it in patients with PWS or KLS. It is clearly effective in narcolepsy. It seems to be good for promoting daytime wakefulness in conditions as diverse as Parkinson's disease, myotonic dystrophy, and sleep apnea (153–155). It is useful clinically as an augmenting agent in depression and a treatment for attention deficit/hyperactivity disorder (156,157). Obviously, its effects are not syndrome specific; the question is not about its clinical utility but rather the limits of its utility. These have not yet been fully measured.

Modafinil appears to be quite safe and well tolerated. The most common side effects in clinical trials have been headache, nausea, depression, nervousness, and insomnia. In my rather robust experience with the drug in various groups of patients, the major problems have been irritability and depression, which tend to develop after several weeks of treatment. In some patients, the benefits of the drug will be lost after some months.

Doses as high as 600 mg per day are well tolerated. Peak levels are reached in 2 to 4 hours, the half-life is 15 hours, and steady state is achieved in 2 to 4 days. It induces CYP2C19, CYP1A, and CYP3A, but no clinically significant drug interactions have been described thus far (158).

Modafinil deserves special attention as the first legitimate alternative to the psychostimulants for the problems of hypersomnia and hypoarousal and as the first therapeutic agent that may exert its effects by influencing hypocretin. It will almost certainly occupy an interesting niche in neuropsychiatry. Where precisely that niche will be is an open question, just as one wonders to what degree the problems of depression, irritability, and tachyphylaxis will limit its use.

COMPULSIVE WATER DRINKING

Disturbances in water and thirst regulation are not uncommon in the chronically mentally ill, patients with head injury, and the mentally retarded. Virtually all the research has been done in psychiatric patients, but the principles are the same for all three groups. Polydipsia may be the manifestation of a disease such as diabetes mellitus or diabetes insipidus (DI), a drug effect, the result of hypothalamic injury, or a compulsion or acquired habit—a peculiar form of addiction or self-stimulation.

It is a serious problem, whatever the patient group. Uncontrolled drinking can cause water intoxication, a potentially fatal event. The differential diagnosis is very important because management based on misdiagnosis can be disastrous. The drugs used frequently in retarded people and patients with head injuries, especially CBZ and lithium, can affect the regulation of salt and water balance.

Primary polydipsia refers to the ingestion of water in excess of that required to maintain normal water balance (159). Compulsive water drinking (CWD) refers to continuous or habitual drinking of excessive amounts of water, and psychogenic polydipsia refers to the consumption of extraordinary quantities over a short period of time (159,160).

Polydipsia is a common behavior that does not necessarily lead to intoxication because the kidneys can compensate by excreting large amounts of dilute urine. Compulsive drinkers may have low urinary specific gravity, but most of them do not develop severe hyponatremia. It is estimated, however, that one-fourth to one-half of the patients with psychogenic polydipsia do go on to develop water intoxication at one time or another (161).

Excessive drinking occurs in 3.3% to 17.5% of chronically mentally ill patients (162,163), but it is not specific to any particular diagnostic group. Most of the cases, however, are psychotic, and there may be an association between the encephalopathy that gives rise to schizophrenia and the inappropriate secretion of antidiuretic hormone [(ADH), vasopressin, or arginine vasopressin] (164,165). It has also been suggested that polydipsia is a hypothalamic manifestation of an underlying hyperdopaminergic state in psychotic patients (160). For example, adipsia can be induced in rats after chemical lesions to ascending dopaminergic pathways (166).

When compulsive drinking leads to water intoxication, the symptoms include headache, blurred vision, vomiting, diaphoresis, incoordination, irritability, and excitability. In severe intoxication, when water intake overwhelms renal output, hyponatremia develops. There is sudden dilution of body solutes, and the patient may exhibit muscle cramps, twitching, delirium, stupor, coma, and convulsions (167).

Excessive fluid intake may also be a symptom of DI, a disorder characterized by polyuria and secondary polydipsia. It is important to distinguish between CWD and DI because the management is quite different. Administration of ADH to a patient with CWD can lead to hyponatremia and signs of water intoxication; restriction of water to a patient with DI may lead to hypernatremia and serious dehydration (168).

DI may be neurogenic, by virtue of reduction of ADH production in the hypothalamus, or nephrogenic (NDI), a circumstance that arises when the distal tubule of the glomerulus is unresponsive to physiologic levels of ADH. Polydipsia in DI is a normal physiologic response to the primary metabolic derangement, so if the diagnosis is missed and fluid intake is restricted, the patient may develop a serious fluid and electrolyte imbalance (168).

DI is similar to CWD in that water consumption and urine output are excessively high and the concentration of the urine is low. In DI, however, serum sodium, blood urea nitrogen, and serum osmolality tend to be high in contrast to CWD (167).

Symptoms of nephrogenic DI may arise in patients who are treated with lithium, a drug that blocks the ADH receptor in the distal tubule. Lithium causes a NDI-type syndrome, with thirst, polydipsia, and polyuria, in a substantial number of patients who have blood levels in the therapeutic range. Fluid restriction is not appropriate in lithium-induced NDI.

Chlorpromazine, thioridazine, and other neuroleptics may also cause polydipsia through a direct hypothalamic effect, perhaps on dopaminergic neurons that govern thirst, drinking behavior, and ADH secretion (169). This may account for the side effect of enuresis nocturna.

DI may be caused by destructive events such as tumors or cerebral infection. DI has been described after TBI, in association with symptoms of rage, hyperphagia, and dementia and in association with lesions in the posterior hypothalamus (168).

The polar opposite of DI is the syndrome of inappropriate ADH secretion (SIADH) caused by ectopic production (e.g., oat cell carcinoma of the lung), Guillain-Barré, acute intermittent porphyria, central nervous system insults such as tumors, stroke, or TBI, or by drugs. SIADH is associated with elevated levels of ADH, increased urinary osmolality, and decreased serum osmolality and hyponatremia (161), whereas compulsive water drinkers tend to have dilute urine with low urine osmolality (167).

Inappropriate ADH secretion may, however, be seen in association with or as a consequence of CWD (170); for example, there is evidence of supersensitivity in the ADH receptor in psychiatric patients with CWD (171). This may be a reset secondary to a prolonged period of low ADH secretion to accommodate the chronic water load (172).

SIADH may be induced by treatment with anticonvulsants such as phenobarbital, phenytoin, or CBZ, or by neuroleptics (e.g., thiothixene, chlorpromazine, fluphenazine), or tricyclic antidepressants (e.g., amitriptyline) (170).

The effect of CBZ is not only to enhance the release of ADH from the neurohypophysis (173,174) but also to increase the sensitivity of adenyl cyclase in the distal tubule. Therefore, CBZ is an effective treatment for DI, although it has variable effects against lithium-induced NDI (175–177). On the other hand, it is not an effective treatment for primary NDI because its renal effect is relatively weak, and it is not effective for DI in patients with a total failure of ADH secretion (178).

The mechanism of direct CBZ effect on the posterior pituitary may lead to hyponatremia in patients on CBZ for epilepsy or for behavioral disorders (179). The effect is dose related (175). Hyponatremia may be the reason that some patients become irritable and aggressive on high doses of CBZ or even why some patients lose seizure control at high doses (180).

Treatment with thiazide diuretics has been associated with impaired free-water clearance and water intoxication in psychiatric patients with CWD (181). Thiazides are potentially lethal when they are used in patients who consume excessive amounts of water.

The treatment of compulsive water intoxication is restriction of fluid intake and attention to intrinsic or extrinsic factors that may be aggravating the situation. There are reports in the literature to support direct treatment either with propanolol (182) or demeclocycline, an antibiotic that induces a reversible NDI (183). Captopril, an inhibitor of the angiotensin I converting enzyme, blocks the formation of angiotensin II, a potent dipsogen; captopril has been reported to reduce polydipsia in at least some psychiatric patients with CWD (184).

CBZ, a drug that may cause SIADH, may be used to treat DI. CBZ may also reverse the effects of lithium-induced NDI (177). Lithium, conversely, may be used to treat SIADH. That would seem to make lithium and CBZ a natural combination. In fact, the combination can be neurotoxic. A delirious patient who has been on CBZ and lithium together probably does not have water intoxication but may well be neurotoxic from the drugs themselves (185,186).

REFERENCES

1. Mascari MJ, Gottlieb WMS, Rogan PK, et al. The frequency of uniparental disomy in Prader-Willi syndrome. *N Engl J Med* 1992;326:1599–1607.
2. Simonoff E, Bolton P, Rutter M. Genetic perspectives on mental retardation. In: Burack JA, Hodapp RM, Zigler E, eds. *Handbook of mental retardation and development*. Cambridge: Cambridge University Press,1998:41–79.
3. Holm VA, Pipes PL. Food and children with Prader-Willi syndrome. *Am J Dis Child* 1976;130:1063–1067.
4. Crnic KA, Sulzbacher S, Snow J, et al. Preventing mental retardation associated with gross obesity in the Prader-Willi syndrome. *Pediatrics* 1980;66:787–789.
5. Martin A, State M, Koenig K, et al. Prader-Willi syndrome. *Am J Psychiatry* 1998;155:1265–1273.
6. Goh K, Herman MA, Campbell RG, et al. Abnormal chromosome in Prader-Willi syndrome. *Clin Genet* 1984;26:597–601.
7. Wenger S, Rauch S, Hanchett J. Sister chromatid exchange analysis of the 15q11 region in Prader-Willi syndrome patients. *Hum Genet* 1989;83:111–114.
8. Strakowski SM, Butler MG. Paternal hydrocarbon exposure in Prader-Willi syndrome. *Lancet* 1987;2:1458.
9. Cassidy SB, Gainey AJ, Butler MG. Occupational hydrocarbon exposure among fathers of Prader-Willi syndrome patients with and without deletions of 15q. *Am J Hum Genet* 1989;44:806–810.
10. Akefeldt A, Anvret M, Grandell U, et al. Parental exposure to hydrocarbons in Prader-Willi syndrome. *Dev Med Child Neurol* 1995;37:1101–1109.
11. Gualtieri CT. *Neuropsychiatry and behavioral pharmacology*. Berlin: Springer-Verlag, 1990.
12. Hattori S, Mochio S, Kageyama A, et al. An autopsy case of Prader-Labhart-Willi syndrome. *No To Shinkei* 1985;37:1059–1066.
13. Hayashi M, Itoh M, Kabasawa Y, et al. A neuropathological study of a case of the Prader-Willi syndrome with an interstitial selection of the proximal long arm of chromosome 15. *Brain Dev* 1992;14:58–62.
14. Reske-Nielsen E, Lund E. Prader-Willi syndrome and central nervous system calcifications: chance or fundamentally related findings? *Clin Neuropathol* 1992; 11:6–10.
15. Swaab DF, Purba JS, Hofman MA. Alterations in the hypothalamic paraventricular nucleus and its oxytocin neurons (putative satiety cells) in Prader-Willi syndrome: a study of five cases. *J Clin Endocrinol Metab* 1995;80:573–579.
16. Bier DM, Kaplan SL, Havel RJ. The Prader-Willi syndrome: regulation of fat transport. *Diabetes* 1977;26: 874–881.
17. Bray GA, Dahms WT, Swerdloff RS, et al. The Prader-Willi syndrome: a study of 40 patients and a review of the literature. *Medicine* 1983;62:59–80.
18. Nardella MT, Sulzbacher SI, Worthington-Roberts BS. Activity levels of persons with Prader-Willi syndrome. *Am J Ment Defic* 1983;87:498–505.
19. Mitchell JE, Groat R. A placebo-controlled, double-blind study of amitriptyline in bulimia. *J Clin Psychopharmacol* 1984;4:186–191.
20. McElroy SL, Keck PE, Pope HG. Sodium valproate: its use in primary psychiatric disorders. *J Clin Psychopharmacol* 1987;7:16–24.
21. Akefeldt A, Ekman R, Gillberg C, et al. Cerebrospinal fluid monoamines in Prader-Willi syndrome. *Biol Psychiatry* 1998;44:1321–1328.
22. Herzog DB, Copeland PM. Eating disorders. *N Engl J Med* 1985;313:295–303.
23. Leibowitz SF. Noradrenergic function in the medial hypothalamus: potential relation to anorexia nervosa and bulimia. In: Pirke KM, Ploog D, eds. *The psy-*

chobiology of anorexia nervosa. Berlin: Springer-Verlag, 1984:35–45.
24. Ljungberg T, Ungerstedt U. Reinstatement of eating by dopamine agonists in aphagic dopamine denervated rats. *Physiol Behav* 1976;16:277–283.
25. Evans KR, Eikelboom R. Feeding induced by ventricular bromocriptine and amphetamine: a possible excitatory role for dopamine in eating behavior. *Behav Neurosci*1987;101:591–593.
26. Fuller RW, Wong DT. Fluoxetine: a serotonergic appetite suppressant drug. *Drug Dev Res* 1989;17:1–15.
27. Warnock JK, Clayton AH, Shaw HA, et al. Onset of menses in two adult patients with Prader-Willi syndrome treated with fluoxetine. *Psychopharmacol Bull* 1995;31:239–242.
28. Warnock JK, Kestenbaum T. Pharmacologic treatment of severe skin-picking behaviors in Prader-Willi syndrome: two case reports. *Arch Dermatol* 1992;128: 1623–1625.
29. Tu JB, Hartridge C, Izawa J. Psychopharmacogenetic aspects of Prader-Willi syndrome. *J Am Acad Child Psychiatry* 1992;31:1137–1140.
30. Durst R, Rubin-Jabotinsky K, Raskin S, et al. Risperidone in treating behavioural disturbances of Prader-Willi syndrome. *Acta Psychiatr Scand* 2000;102: 461–465.
31. Stein DJMB, Keating JBS, Zar HJMB, et al. A survey of the phenomenology and pharmacotherapy of compulsive and impulsive-aggressive symptoms in Prader-Willi syndrome. *J Neuropsychiatry Clin Neurosci* 1994;6:23–29.
32. Glenn M. Update on pharmacology: pharmacologic interventions in neuroendocrine disorders following traumatic brain injury, Part 1. *J Head Trauma Rehabil* 1988;3:87–90.
33. Pettigrew LC, Bieber F, Lettieri J, et al. Pharmacokinetics, pharmacodynamics, and safety of metrifonate in patients with Alzheimer's disease. *J Clin Pharmacol* 1998;38:236–245.
34. Keene J, Hope T. Natural history of hyperphagia and other eating changes in dementia. *Int J Geriatr Psychiatry* 1998;13:700–706.
35. Keene J, Hope T, Rogers P, et al. An investigation of satiety in ageing, dementia, and hyperphagia. *Int J Eat Dis* 1998;23:409–418.
36. Viola J, Ditzler T, Batzer W, et al. Pharmacological management of post-traumatic stress disorder: clinical summary of a five-year retrospective study, 1990–1995. *Mil Med* 1997;162:616–619.
37. Halmi KA. Basic biological overview of eating disorders. In: Bloom FE, Kupfer DJ, eds. *Psychopharmacology: the fourth generation of progress*, 4th ed. New York: Raven, 1995:1609–1616.
38. Morley JE, Levine AS. Stress-induced eating is mediated through endogenous opiates. *Science* 1980;209: 1259–1261.
39. Stapleton JM, Lind MD, Merriman VJ, et al. Naloxone inhibits diazepam-induced feeding in rats. *Life Sci* 1979;24:2421–2425.
40. Wolkowitz OM, Doran AR, Cohen MR, et al. Effect of naloxone on food consumption in obesity. *N Engl J Med* 1985;313:327.
41. Kyriakides M, Silverstone T, Jeffcoate W, et al. Effect of naloxone on hyperphagia in Prader-Willi syndrome. *Lancet* 1980;1:876–877.
42. Shapira N, Goldsmith T, McElroy S. Treatment of binge-eating disorder with topiramate: a clinical case series. *J Clin Psychiatry* 2000;61:368–372.
43. Walsh BT, Devlin MJ. Psychopharmacology of anorexia nervosa, bulimia nervosa and binge eating. In: Bloom FE, Kupfer DJ, eds. *Psychopharmacology: the fourth generation of progress*, 4th ed. New York: Raven, 1995:1581–1589.
44. Szarek B, Brandt D. A comparison of weight changes with fluoxetine, desipramine, and amitriptyline: a retrospective study of psychiatric inpatients. *J Nerv Ment Dis* 1993;181:702–704.
45. Fava M. Weight gain and antidepressants. *J Clin Psychiatry* 2000;61:37–41.
46. Rigler S, Webb M, Redford L, et al. Weight outcomes among antidepressant users in nursing facilities. *J Am Geriatr Soc* 2001;49:49–55.
47. Fava M, Judge R, Hoog S, et al. Fluoxetine versus sertraline and paroxetine in major depressive disorder: changes in weight with long-term treatment. *J Clin Psychiatry* 2000;61:863–867.
48. Taylor D, McAskill R. Atypical antipsychotics and weight gain—a systematic review. *Acta Psychiatr Scand* 2000;101:416–432.
49. Wetterling T. Bodyweight gain with atypical antipsychotics. A comparative review. *Drug Saf* 2001;24: 59–73.
50. Wirshing D, Wirshing W, Kysar L, et al. Novel antipsychotics: comparison of weight gain liabilities. *J Clin Psychiatry* 1999;60:358–363.
51. Lacruz A, Baptista T, de Mendoza S, et al. Antipsychotic drug-induced obesity in rats: correlation between leptin, insulin and body weight during sulpiride treatment. *Mol Psychiatry* 2000;5:70–76.
52. Goldstein L, Henderson D. Atypical antipsychotic agents and diabetes mellitus. *Prim Psychiatry* 2000;7: 65–68.
53. Morris G. Gabapentin. *Epilepsia* 1999;40:63–70.
54. Hogan R, Bertrand M, Deaton R, et al. Total percentage body weight changes during add-on therapy with tiagabine, carbamazepine and phenytoin. *Epilepsy Res* 2000;41:23–28.
55. Biton V, Mirza W, Montouris G, et al. Weight change associated with valproate and lamotrigine monotherapy in patients with epilepsy. *Neurology* 2000;56:172–177.
56. Kleine W. Periodische Schlafsucht Mschr Psychiatr. *Neurology* 1925;57:285.
57. Critchley M. The syndrome of hypersomnia and periodical megaphagia in the adult male (Kleine-Levin): what is its natural course? *Rev Neurol (Paris)* 1967; 116:647–650.
58. Mayer G, Leonhard E, Krieg J, et al. Endocrinological and polysomnographic findings in Kleine-Levin syndrome: no evidence for hypothalamic and circadian dysfunction. *Sleep* 1998;21:278–284.
59. Papacostas S, Hadjivasilis V. The Kleine-Levin syndrome. Report of a case and review of the literature. *Eur Psychiatry* 2000;15:231–235.
60. Lewis N. The psychoanalytic approach to the problems of children under 12 years of age. *Psychol Rev* 1926; 13:424–443.
61. Levin M. Periodic somnolence and morbid hunger: a new syndrome. *Brain* 1936;59:494.
62. Daniels L. Narcolepsy. *Medicine* 1934;13:1–122.
63. Powers PS, Gunderman R. Kleine-Levin syndrome as-

sociated with fire setting. *Am J Dis Child* 1978;132: 786–789.
64. Orlosky MJ. The Kleine-Levin syndrome: a review. *Psychosomatics* 1982;23:609–621.
65. Culebras A, Magana R. Neurologic disorders and sleep disturbances. *Semin Neurol* 1987;7:277–285.
66. Jurko MF, Andy OJ. Psychological changes correlated with thalamotomy site. *J Neurol Neurosurg Psychiatry* 1973;36:846–852.
67. Ranson S. Somnolence caused by hypothalamic lesions in the monkey. *Neurol Psychiatry* 1939;41:1–23.
68. Reeves AC, Blum D. Hyperphagia, rage, and dementia accompanying a ventro-median hypothalamic neoplasm. *Arch Neurol* 1969;20:616–624.
69. Mendez MF, Cummings JL, Benson F. Depression in epilepsy. *Arch Neurol* 1986;43:766–770.
70. Krahn DD, Mitchell JE. Case report of bulimia associated with increased intracranial pressure. *Am J Psychiatry* 1984;141:1099–1100.
71. Popoviciu L, Corfariu O. Clinical and polygraphic study of a case of Kleine-Levin-Critchley syndrome during a 24-hour period. *Rev Roumaine Neurol* 1972; 9:221–228.
72. Ferguson BG. Kleine-Levin syndrome: a case report. *J Child Psychol Psychiatry* 1986;27:275–278.
73. Goldberg MA. The treatment of Kleine-Levin syndrome with lithium. *Can J Psychiatry* 1983;28:491–493.
74. Thompson C, Obrecht R, Franey C, et al. Neuroendocrine rhythms in a patient with the Kleine-Levin syndrome. *Br J Psychiatry* 1985;147:440–443.
75. Merriman A. Kleine-Levin syndrome following acute viral encephalitis. *Biol Psychiatry* 1986;21:1301–1304.
76. Takrani LB, Cronin D. Kleine-Levin syndrome in a female patient. *Can Psychiatry Assoc J* 1976;21:315–318.
77. Carpenter S, Yassa R, Ochs R. A pathologic basis for Kleine-Levin syndrome. *Arch Neurol* 1982;39:25–28.
78. Gau SF, Soong WT, Liu HM, et al. Kleine-Levin syndrome in a boy with Prader-Willi syndrome. *Sleep* 1996;19:13–17.
79. Berthier ML, Santamaria J, Encabo H, et al. Recurrent hypersomnia in two adolescent males with Asperger's syndrome. *J Am Acad Child Psychiatry* 1992;31: 735–738.
80. Sagar RS, Khandelwal SK, Gupta S. Interepisodic morbidity in Kleine-Levin syndrome. *Br J Psychiatry* 1990;157:139–141.
81. Koerber RK, Torkelson R, Haven G, et al. Increased cerebrospinal fluid 5-hydroxytryptamine and 5-hydroxyindoleacetic acid in Kleine-Levin syndrome. *Neurology* 1984;34:1597–1600.
82. Fenzi F, Simonati A, Crosato F, et al. Clinical features of Kleine-Levin syndrome with localized encephalitis. *Neuropediatrics* 1993;24:292–295.
83. McGilchrist I, Goldstein LH, Jadresic D, et al. Thalamo-frontal psychosis. *Br J Psychiatry* 1993;163: 113–115.
84. Green LN, Cracco RQ. Kleine-Levin syndrome. A case with EEG evidence of periodic brain dysfunction. *Arch Neurol* 1970;22:166–175.
85. Garland H, Sumner D, Fourman P. The Kleine-Levin syndrome. Some further observations. *Neurology* 1965;15:1161–1167.
86. Lavie P, Gadoth N, Gordon CR, et al. Sleep patterns in Kleine-Levin syndrome. *Electroencephalogr Clin Neurophysiol* 1979;47:369–371.
87. Elian M, Bornstein B. The Kleine-Levin syndrome with intermittent abnormality in the EEG. *Electroencephalogr Clin Neurophysiol* 1969;27:601–604.
88. Thacore VR, Ahmed M, Oswald I. The EEG in a case of periodic hypersomnia. *Electroencephalogr Clin Neurophysiol* 1969;27:605–606.
89. Kupfer DJ, Heninger GR. REM activity as a correlate of mood changes throughout the night. Electroencephalographic sleep patterns in a patient with a 48-hour cyclic mood disorder. *Arch Gen Psychiatry* 1972; 27:368–373.
90. Chesson AL Jr, Levine SN, Kong LS, et al. Neuroendocrine evaluation in Kleine-Levin syndrome: evidence of reduced dopaminergic tone during periods of hypersomnolence. *Sleep* 1991;14:226–232.
91. Cuetter AC. Sleep apnea and the Kleine-Levin syndrome. *Mil Med* 1985;150:286–288.
92. Haas DC, Ross GS. Transient global amnesia triggered by mild head trauma. *Brain* 1986;109:251–257.
93. Gualtieri CT. *Neuropsychiatry and behavioral pharmacology*. Berlin: Springer-Verlag, 1990.
94. Ogura C, Okuma T, Nadazawa K, et al. Treatment of periodic somnolence with lithium carbonate [Letter]. *Arch Neurol* 1976;33:143.
95. Abe K. Lithium prophylaxis of periodic hypersomnia. *Br J Psychiatry* 1977;130:312–313.
96. Will RG, Young JP, Thomas DJ. Kleine-Levin syndrome: report of two cases with onset of symptoms precipitated by head trauma. *Br J Psychiatry* 1988;152: 410–412.
97. Lemire I. Review of Kleine-Levin syndrome: toward an integrated approach. *Can J Psychiatry* 1993;38: 277–284.
98. Pike M, Stores G. Kleine-Levin syndrome: a cause of diagnostic confusion. *Arch Dis Child* 1994;71:355–357.
99. Hawkins DR, Taub JM, Van de Castle RL. Extended sleep (hypersomnia) in young depressed patients. *Am J Psychiatry* 1985;142:905–910.
100. Strober M, Green J, Carlson G. Phenomenology and subtypes of major depressive disorder in adolescence. *J Affect Disord* 1981;3:281–290.
101. Bowden CL, Sarabia F. Diagnosing manic-depressive illness in adolescents. *Compr Psychiatry* 1980;21: 263–269.
102. Ballenger JC, Post RM. Carbamazepine in manic-depressive illness: a new treatment. *Am J Psychiatry* 1980;137:782–790.
103. Post RM, Uhde TW, Putnam FW, et al. Kindling and carbamazepine in affective illness. *J Nerv Ment Dis* 1982;170:717–729.
104. Kales A, Bixler EO, Vela-Bueno A, et al. Alprazolam: effects on sleep and withdrawal phenomena. *J Clin Pharmacol* 1987;27:508–515.
105. Jeffries JJ, Lefebvre A. Depression and mania associated with Kleine-Levin-Critchley syndrome. *Can Psychiatry Assoc J* 1973;18:439–444.
106. Roy-Byrne P, Uhde TW, Post RM, et al. Relationship of response to sleep deprivation and carbamazepine in depressed patients. *Acta Psychiatr Scand* 1984;69: 379–382.
107. Chouinard G, Annable L, Bradwejn J, et al. An early phase II clinical trial with followup of tomoxetine (LY139603) in the treatment of newly admitted depressed patients. *Psychopharmacol Bull* 1985;21:73–76.
108. Schou M. Lithium in the treatment of other psychiatric

and nonpsychiatric disorders. *Arch Gen Psychiatry* 1979;36:856–859.

109. Lena B. Lithium in child and adolescent psychiatry. *Arch Gen Psychiatry* 1979;36:854–855.
110. Wurthmann C, Hartung HP, Dengler W, et al. Kleine-Levin syndrome: the provocation of manic symptoms by an antidepressant and a therapeutic trial of carbamazepine. *Dtsch Med Wochenschr* 1989;114:1528–1531.
111. Krauthammer C, Klerman GL. Secondary mania: manic syndromes associated with antecedent physical illness or drugs. *Arch Gen Psychiatry* 1978;35:1333–1338.
112. Culebras A. Neuroanatomic and neurologic correlates of sleep disturbances. *Neurology* 1992;42:19–27.
113. Bliwise D. Sleep in normal aging and dementia. *Sleep* 1993;16:40–81.
114. Moe K, Vitiello M, Larsen L, et al. Symposium: cognitive processes and sleep disturbances: sleep/wake patterns in Alzheimer's disease: relationships with cognition and function. *J Sleep Res* 1995;4:15–20.
115. Cohen M, Oksenberg A, Snir D, et al. Temporally related changes of sleep complaints in traumatic brain injured patients. *J Neurol Neurosurg Psychiatry* 1992;55:313–315.
116. Beetar J, Guilmette T, Sparadeo F. Sleep and pain complaints in symptomatic traumatic brain injury and neurologic populations. *Arch Phys Med Rehabil* 1996;77:1298–1302.
117. Clinchot D, Bogner J, Mysiw W, et al. Defining sleep disturbance after brain injury. *Am J Phys Med Rehabil* 1998;77:291–295.
118. Tobe E, Schneider J, Mrozik T, et al. Persisting insomnia following traumatic brain injury. *J Neuropsychiatry Clin Neurosci* 1999;11:504–506.
119. Quinto C, Gellido C, Chokroverty S, et al. Posttraumatic delayed sleep phase syndrome. *Neurology* 2000;54:250–252.
120. Ivanhoe C, Lai J, Francisco G. Bruxism after brain injury: successful treatment with botulinum toxin-A. *Arch Phys Med Rehabil* 1997;78:1272–1273.
121. Guilleminault C, Faull KF, Miles L, et al. Posttraumatic excessive daytime sleepiness: a review of 20 patients. *Neurology* 1983;33:1584–1589.
122. Kramer R, Dinner D, Braun W, et al. HLA-DR2 and narcolepsy. *Arch Neurol* 1987;44:853–855.
123. Aldrich M. Narcolepsy. *Neurology* 1992;42:34–43.
124. Maccario M, Ruggles KH, Meriwether MW. Post-traumatic narcolepsy. *Mil Med* 1987;152:370–371.
125. Rivera VM, Meyer JS, Hata T, et al. Narcolepsy following hypoxic ischemia. *Ann Neurol* 1986;19:505–508.
126. Good JL, Barry E, Fishman PS. Posttraumatic narcolepsy: the complete syndrome with tissue typing. *J Neurosurg* 1989;71:765–767.
127. Sutcliffe J, de Lecca L. Novel neurotransmitters for sleep and energy homeostasis. *Results Probl Cell Differ* 1999;26:239–255.
128. Hungs M, Mignot E. Hypocretin/orexin, sleep and narcolepsy. *Bioessays* 2001;23:397–408.
129. Moore R, Abrahamson E, Van Den Pol A. The hypocretin neuron system: an arousal system in the human brain. *Arch Ital Biol* 2001;139:195–205.
130. Piazza C, Fisher W, Kahng S. Sleep patterns in children and young adults with mental retardation and severe behavior disorders. *Dev Med Child Neurol* 1996;38:335–344.
131. Brylewski J, Wiggs L. Sleep problems and daytime challenging behaviour in a community-based sample of adults with intellectual disability. *J Intellect Disabil Res* 1999;43:504–512.
132. Richdale A, Prior M. The sleep/wake rhythm in children with autism. *Eur Child Adolesc Psychiatry* 1995;4:175–186.
133. Diomedi M, Curatolo P, Scalise A, et al. Sleep abnormalities in mentally retarded autistic subjects: Down's syndrome with mental retardation and normal subjects. *Brain Dev* 1999;21:548–553.
134. Manni R, Politini L, Nobili L, et al. Hypersomnia in the Prader Willi syndrome: clinical-electrophysiological features and underlying factors. *Clin Neurophysiol* 2001;112:800–805.
135. Potocki L, Glaze D, Tan D, et al. Circadian rhythm abnormalities of melatonin in Smith-Magenis syndrome. *J Med Genet* 2000;37:428–433.
136. Akaboshi S, Inoue Y, Kubota N, et al. Case of a mentally retarded child with non-24 hour sleep-wake syndrome caused by deficiency of melatonin secretion. *Psychiatry Clin Neurosci* 2000;54:379–380.
137. Hayashi E. Effect of melatonin on sleep-wake rhythm: the sleep diary of an autistic male. *Psychiatry Clin Neurosci* 2000;54:383–384.
138. Pillar G, Shahar E, Peled N, et al. Melatonin improves sleep-wake patterns in psychomotor retarded children. *Pediatr Neurol* 2000;23:225–228.
139. Jan J, O'Donnell M. Use of melatonin in the treatment of paediatric sleep disorders. *J Pineal Res* 1996;21:193–199.
140. Einfeld S, Tonge B, Florio T. Behavioral and emotional disturbance in individuals with Williams syndrome. *Am J Ment Retard* 1997;102:45–53.
141. Summers J, Lynch P, Harris J, et al. A combined behavioral/pharmacological treatment of sleep-wake schedule disorder in Angelman syndrome. *Dev Behav Pediatr* 1992;13:284–287.
142. Tierney E, Nwokoro N, Kelley R. Behavioral phenotype of RSH/Smith-Lemli-Opitz syndrome. *Mental Retard Dev Disabil Res Rev* 2000;6:131–134.
143. Ferri R, Curzi-Dascalova L, Del Gracco S, et al. Respiratory patterns during sleep in Down's syndrome: importance of central apnoeas. *J Sleep Res* 1997;6:134–141.
144. Parkes J. The sleepy patient. *Lancet* 1977;1:990–993.
145. Broughton R, Mamelak M. The treatment of narcolepsy-cataplexy with nocturnal gamma-hydroxybutyrate. *Can J Neurol Sci* 1979;6:1–6.
146. Edgar D, Seidel W. Modafinil induces wakefulness without intensifying motor activity or subsequent rebound hypersomnolence in the rat. *J Pharmacol Exp Ther* 1997;283:757–769.
147. Brun J, Chamba G, Khalfallah Y, et al. Effect of modafinil on plasma melatonin, cortisol and growth hormone rhythms, rectal temperature and performance in healthy subjects during a 36 h sleep deprivation. *J Sleep Res* 1998;7:105–114.
148. Lin J, Hou Y, Jouvet M. Potential brain neuronal targets for amphetamine-methylphenidate-, and modafinil-induced wakefulness, evidenced by c-fos immunocytochemistry in the cat. *Neurobiology* 1996;93:14128–14133.
149. Antonelli T, Ferraro L, Hillion J, et al. Modafinil prevents glutamate cytotoxicity in cultured cortical neurons. *Neuroreport* 1998;9:4209–4213.

150. Engber T, Koury E, Dennis S, et al. Differential patterns of regional c-Fos induction in the rat brain by amphetamine and the novel wakefulness-promoting agent modafinil. *Neurosci Lett* 1998;241:95–98.
151. Chemelli R, Willie J, Sinton C, et al. Narcolepsy in orexin knockout mice: molecular genetics of sleep regulation. *Cell* 1999;98:437–451.
152. Scammell T, Estabrooke I, McCarthy M, et al. Hypothalamic arousal regions are activated during modafinil-induced wakefulness. *J Neurosci* 2000;20:8620–8628.
153. Damian M, Gerlach A, Schmidt F, et al. Modafinil for excessive daytime sleepiness in myotonic dystrophy. *Neurology* 2001;56:794–796.
154. Kingshott R, Vennelle M, Coleman E, et al. Randomized, double-blind, placebo-controlled crossover trial of modafinil in the treatment of residual excessive daytime sleepiness in the sleep apnea/hypopnea syndrome. *Am J Resp Crit Care Med* 2001;163:918–923.
155. Rabinstein A, Shulman L, Weiner W. Modafinil for the treatment of excessive daytime sleepiness in Parkinson's disease: a case report. *Parkinsonism Rel Disord* 2001;7:287–288.
156. Menza M, Kaufman K, Castellanos A. Modafinil augmentation of antidepressant treatment in depression. *J Clin Psychiatry* 2000;61:378–381.
157. Rugino T, Copley T. Effects of modafinil in children with attention-deficit/hyperactivity disorder: an open-label study. *J Am Acad Child Psychiatry* 2001;40:230–235.
158. McClellan K, Spencer C. Modafinil: a review of its pharmacology and clinical efficacy in the management of narcolepsy. *CNS Drugs* 1998;9:311–324.
159. Stevko RM, Balsley M, Segar EW. Primary polydipsia, compulsive water drinking. *J Pediatr* 1968;73:845–851.
160. Singh NN, Millichamp CJ. Pharmacological treatment of self-injurious behavior in mentally retarded persons. *J Autism Dev Disord* 1985;15:257–267.
161. Illowsky BP, Kirch DG. Polydipsia and hyponatremia in psychiatric patients. *Am J Psychiatry* 1988;145:675–683.
162. Jose CJ, Mehta S, Perez-Cruet J. The syndrome of inappropriate secretion of antidiuretic hormone. *Can J Psychiatry* 1979;24:225–231.
163. Blum A, Tempey FW, Lynch WJ. Somatic findings in patients with psychogenic polydipsia. *J Clin Psychiatry* 1983;44:55–56.
164. Hobson JA, English JT. Self-induced water intoxication. *Ann Intern Med* 1963;58:324–332.
165. Khamnei AK. Psychosis, inappropriate antidiuretic hormone secretion, and water intoxication. *Lancet* 1984;1:963.
166. Ungerstedt U. Adipsia and aphagia after 6-hydroxydopamine induced degeneration of the nigro-striatal dopamine system. *Acta Physiol Scand* 1971;367:95–122.
167. Singh S, Padi MH, Bullard H, et al. Water intoxication in psychiatric patients. *Br J Psychiatry* 1985;146:125–131.
168. Lishman WA. *Organic psychiatry, the psychological consequences of cerebral disorder,* 2nd ed. Oxford: Blackwell Scientific, 1987.
169. Smith WO, Clark ML. Self-induced water intoxication in schizophrenic patients. *Am J Psychiatry* 1980;137:1055–1060.
170. Ferrier IN. Water intoxication in patients with psychiatric illness. *BMJ* 1985;291:1594–1596.
171. Goldman MB, Luchins DJ, Robertson GL. Mechanisms of altered water metabolism in psychotic patients with polydipsia and hyponatremia. *N Engl J Med* 1988;318:397–403.
172. Hariprasad MK, Eisinger RP, Nadler IM, et al. Hyponatremia in psychogenic polydipsia. *Arch Intern Med* 1980;140:1639–1642.
173. Smith RB, Day E. The effects of cerebral electrotherapy on short-term impairment in alcoholic patients. *Int J Addict* 1977;12:575.
174. Thomas TH, Ball SG, Wales JK, et al. Effect of carbamazepine on plasma and urinary levels of 8-arginine vasopressin (AVP). *Clin Sci Mol Med* 1977;53:10.
175. Henry DA, Lawson DH, Reavey P, et al. Hyponatremia during carbamazepine treatment. *BMJ* 1977;1:83–84.
176. Braunhofer J, Zicha L. Eroffnet Tegretal neue Therapiemoglichkeiten bei bestimmen neurologischen und endokrinen Krankheitsbildern. *Med Welt* 1989;36:1875–1880.
177. Brooks SC, Lessin BE. Treatment of lithium-induced nephrogenic diabetes insipidus and schizoaffective psychosis with carbamazepine. *Am J Psychiatry* 1983;140:1077–1078.
178. Bonnici F. Antidiuretic effect of clofibrate and carbamazepine in diabetes insipidus: studies on free water clearance and response to a water load. *Clin Endocrinol* 1973;2:265–275.
179. Yassa R, Iskandar H, Nastase C. Propranolol in the treatment of tardive akathisia: a report of two cases. *J Clin Psychopharmacol* 1988;8:283–285.
180. Snead OC, Hosey LC. Exacerbation of seizures in children by carbamazepine. *N Engl J Med* 1985;313:916–921.
181. Day JO. Water intoxication in psychogenic water drinkers taking thiazide diuretics. *South Med J* 1977;70:572–575.
182. Shevitz SA, Jamieson RC, Petre WM. Compulsive water drinking treated with high dose propanolol. *J Nerv Ment Dis* 1980;168:246–248.
183. Nixon RA, Rothman JS, Chin W. Demeclocycline in the prophylaxis of self-induced water intoxication. *Am J Psychiatry* 1982;139:828–829.
184. Lawson WB, Williams B, Pasion R. Effects of captopril on psychosis and disturbed water regulation. *Psychopharmacol Bull* 1988;24:176–178.
185. Shukla S, Godwin CD, Long LEB, et al. Lithium-carbamazepine neurotoxicity and risk factors. *Am J Psychiatry* 1984;141:1604–1606.
186. Chaudry RP, Waters BGH. Lithium and carbamazepine interaction: possible neurotoxicity. *J Clin Psychiatry* 1983;44:30–31.

13

Disorders of the X and Y Chromosomes

SUMMARY

The sex chromosomes are uniquely involved in the genesis of mental retardation and for a very good reason. The sex chromosomes are unbalanced, and aberrant genes on the X cannot be compensated by the genes on the Y, which is sorely deficient in genetic material.

There is a good reason for that as well, as will be discussed, with respect to the evolution of intelligence. The development of brain capacity in the higher mammals was accompanied by a progressive deletion of genetic material from the Y chromosome. This, in turn, permitted genes on the X chromosome that encode for brain development to be expressed with greater vigor. Males, who possess an unbalanced X chromosome, express more behavioral and cognitive variability than females do. This, in turn, gives the process of sexual selection a wider scope of operation.

Because the unbalanced sex chromosomes generate a high degree of behavioral and cognitive variation, the cost has been a higher rate of mental retardation in males. More than 80 forms of mental retardation are linked to the X chromosome. The most important is fragile X syndrome (FXS), the second most common genetic cause of mental retardation.

The genesis of FXS lies in the amplification of a trinucleotide sequence, the CGG (cytosine guanine guanine) repeat. An excessive number of repeats inactivates the genetic region where the *FMR-1* gene resides, a gene that governs neuronal development. That the CGG repeat can be amplified from one generation to the next is not only interesting, it is ominous. Repeat amplification is like a genetic time bomb. The mechanism of repeat amplification has been discovered in other neurologic conditions. Its boundaries have not yet been measured.

Males with FXS are vulnerable to numerous emotional and behavioral problems, typically hyperactivity in childhood and emotional instability in adult life.

FXS is a "covert" disorder in the sense that the abnormality is not apparent in routine karyotyping. In contrast, the overt sex chromosome disorders, such as Turner's syndrome and Klinefelter's syndrome can be diagnosed with routine karyotyping. The behavioral problems associated with the overt sex chromosome disorders are less troublesome than those with FXS, but they are not trivial either.

SEX CHROMOSOME DISORDERS

Overt aberrations of the sex chromosomes occur in two to seven in 1,000 livebirths. Turner's syndrome, Klinefelter's syndrome, triple X (47,XXX), and double Y (47,XYY) account for the majority. Children with overt sex chromosome aberrations are prone to learning disorders and, to a lesser degree, behavioral/emotional problems (1).

FXS is a "covert" aberration because the abnormality is not apparent to routine cytogenetic study. It is more frequent than all of the other sex chromosome disorders put together. It is reliably associated with mental retardation and learning difficulties, and to a substantial degree, with behavior/emotional problems.

TURNER'S SYNDROME

Patients with Turner's syndrome have the morphologic appearance of females. They have cells with a single X chromosome, a deficiency of sex chromatin (Barr bodies). Almost all of them have a 45,X karyotype or else a mixture of such cells with normal female cells (hence, mosaics). The incidence is one in 5,000 livebirths (2,3). The dysmorphic features are short stature (50 to 60 in.), nuchal webbing, broad chest with widely spaced nipples, small mandible and receding chin, prominent auricles, abnormal nails, and pigmented moles. They have gonadal dysgenesis and internal female accessory organs that are infantile. They remain sexually immature at adolescence unless estrogen replacement therapy is instituted, in which case some secondary sexual characteristics develop. Growth hormone has been used to augment stature.

Most patients with Turner's syndrome have normal intelligence, although many have specific learning disabilities. Typically, their verbal IQ is higher than their performance IQ. Recent studies have focused on their relative weakness in visuospatial tasks; it has been suggested that space-form dysgnosia and a degree of dyscalculia may be characteristic elements of the syndrome (4). It was proposed that the function of the right cerebral hemisphere, particularly the parietal lobe, is selectively affected, but subsequent studies have failed to sustain the notion of a lateralized or a localized defect. That is consistent with the position that early aberrations in brain development have generalized rather than localized effects on brain functions in later life. Rather than manifesting an exaggerated female neuropsychological profile, girls with Turner's syndrome have deficits in cognitive abilities in which neither males nor females show superiority as a group. They appear to fall into a cognitively "neuter" category. This conceivably may be a failure of cerebral lateralization in the absence of an appropriate estrogenic milieu (5–7).

The physical and cognitive immaturity of girls with Turner's syndrome may be reflected in their behavior and psychosexual development. Traits of passivity, meekness, and overly compliant behavior are congruent with an immature personality; they may be at least partially correctable with replacement therapy (8,9).

Patients with Turner's syndrome are not prone to any particular neuropsychiatric disorder. Lishman (10) has opined that the lack of an X chromosome may be better than an extra X as far as mental health is concerned.

KLINEFELTER'S SYNDROME

One in 600 male infants is sex-chromatin positive, and almost all these children have the 47,XXY karyotype. Klinefelter's syndrome, however, is rarely diagnosed before puberty, when the XXY testis is determined to be small and undeveloped, and secondary sex characteristics are slow to develop, if they do at all. Testosterone levels do not reach adult levels, the ejaculate is aspermic and the patient is infertile. The typical XXY adult is tall, with gynecomastia and little face or body hair. The body build is eunuchoid (2,4). Intention tremors are not uncommon.

XXY males have a tendency toward dull mentality, although the syndrome is not incompatible with superior intelligence (11). Their average IQ is 10 to 15 points lower than their siblings, and 15% to 20% have IQs that are below 80 (3). Selective reduction of the verbal IQ has been reported. They are prone to speech and language problems and to reading and spelling disabilities. These difficulties have been attributed to left hemisphere involvement (12–14).

Behaviorally, XXY males are said to be "limited in their economic striving and in their sexual drive" (2). Some XXY men are said to have "disabling neurotic symptoms, marked by sexual and general inertia," and their rehabilitation is said to be "facilitated" by androgen treatment (15). Testosterone treatment for one boy with Klinefelter's syndrome led not only to sexual maturation but also to the reduction of aggressive behavior (16).

The behavioral phenotype of XXY males (like the XO females and XYY males) is not as stereotyped as it is for the pathobehavioral syndromes described in Chapters 11 and 12. It is possible to assert that boys with Klinefelter's syndrome are more prone to behavioral disturbance than girls with Turner's syndrome, but less so than boys with the XYY genotype, but group stereotypes are much less impressive than individual differences. XXY males tend to be immature, shy, timid, or insecure; stress intolerant or irritable; anergic or stubborn; or boastful, with poor judgment and a proclivity to "assertive" activities (3,17,18). Klinefelter (19) pointed out that most XXY patients "work regularly and lead normal lives except for their inability to procreate" and that "manic depressive psychosis, and schizophrenia seem not to occur more commonly in this syndrome than in controls." In fact, a high rate of affective psychoses and epileptic psychoses has been claimed (20–22) but also disputed (23). The incidence of anorexia nervosa and of FXS may be higher in XXY males than would be expected by chance association (24,25).

There is an "unascertained degree of association" between the XXY syndrome and increased incidence of criminal behavior. An approximate prevalence statistic for XXY men in maximum-security hospitals for defective delinquents is 1:150 (15).

The delinquent behavior of males with Klinefelter's syndrome has been described as asexual, perhaps because their indiscretions are not typified by passionate explosions of rage or defiance and because sexual misbehavior rarely goes beyond what a prepubescent boy might adventure. They are not unemotional and may be given to anxiety, depression, anger, aggression, and destructiveness. When they are given to conduct problems, however, they are exploratory, mischievous, and adventurous; they test the limits, as preadolescents do, rather than defy them, as adolescents do.

THE XYY MALE

The putative association between "ultramasculine" aggression and a supernumerary Y chromosome became quite popular after a paper was published in 1965 entitled "Aggressive Behavior, Mental Subnormality and the XXY Male." In this article, it was proposed that there was an excess of the **XYY karyotype** among very tall men in a Scottish institution for dangerous criminals (15). The prevalence of XYY was 3%, in contrast to an incidence of 1:840 in newborn males. Within 5 years, numerous incidence and prevalence studies on the occurrence and correlates of XYY were published, and the pooled data indicated that the prevalence of XYY karyotype among inmates of various penal and mental institutions, unselected for height, was 7:1,000, and the prevalence of XXY among inmates selected for tall stature (>6 ft) was 29:1,000 (26).

XYY syndrome is rarely detected during childhood, or even in adults, because the dysmorphic features (asymmetric, long facies, prominent glabella, large teeth and ears, pectus excavatum, long fingers) are subtle and not immediately attributable to a chromosomal abnormality. Behavioral problems, especially temper tantrums, defiance, and aggressive behavior are sometimes augmented by dull mentality (3,27). Antiandrogens have been suggested for treatment (15), but a follow-up study of XYY males thus treated was not encouraging (28).

Like XXY, the XYY male is not preordained to criminal behavior or to psychiatric disorder, and although intelligence is, on the average, low, neither syndrome is incompatible with normal or even superior intelligence. A supernumerary Y chromosome is more likely than a supernumerary X to predispose an individual to excessive, impulsive behavior. The XYY individual may be more prone to delinquent behavior and the XXY more prone to neurotic behavior, but the behavioral stereotype is by no means invariant (15). Individuals may be more likely differentiated based on dysmorphic features than their behavioral phenotype, and even those are comparatively weak.

XYY syndrome was, in its time, as fertile for idle theorizing as left and right brain and endogenous opiates were in theirs. XYY males were said to be "supermales" and their phenotype represented an exaggeration of typical male traits. One was expected to concede that violent aggression and criminal behavior were merely exaggerations of normal maleness, an idea that was as superficial as it was offensive. It was the subject of much public commentary, among the intelligentsia, at least.

In fact, the conceit was presaged by the French Dadaist Alfred Jarry who wrote a book called *The Supermale* in the years after World War I. After the supermale raced a Trans-Siberian Railroad train and won, he was challenged to make love to his girlfriend 100 times in a day. He won that bet, too. At midnight, though, she wanted him again; "This time," she said, "for love."

In fact, XYY supermales are not nearly so Olympian in their build or ability, and their motor coordination is usually a bit off (3). Despite Jarry's literary adumbrations, they are not hypersexual and when they show assaultive behavior, it is not usually of a sexual nature (15). Levels of testosterone and gonadotropin are not elevated prenatally or postnatally (26).

XO women are hypogonadal, as are XXY men, and, to a degree, their behavioral and/or cognitive phenotypes are consistent with decreased levels of circulating estrogen or testosterone. XXY men, however, are not hypergonadal, and when they exhibit aggressive and criminal behavior, it is not owing to supermale levels of androgen. Their aggression may actually be reduced by androgen replacement, and antiandrogens do not affect it (16,28).

FRAGILE X SYNDROME

In 1943, a pedigree of X-linked mental retardation was described by Martin and Bell (28a). In 1969, Lubs (29) described a "fragile site" on the long arm of the X chromosome in a family in which there were two retarded males and one unaffected female. A short time later, the association of a fragile X chromosome with mental retardation and macro-orchidism was described by Escalante et al. (30). FXS was soon established to be by far the most common X-linked cause of mental retardation (31). It accounts for no fewer than 10% of all cases of mental retardation (32). It is the second most common genetic cause of mental handicap and one of the most frequent single-gene disorders recognized in humans (33).

The discovery of the FXS is one of the signal developments in medical genetics and developmental medicine. The strong association between the syndrome and autism and affective disorders is equally important for neuropsychiatry. Since the discovery of the FMR-1 gene in 1991 and the elucidation of the peculiar genetics of the FXS, it has become clear that its real importance has yet to be measured.

The diagnosis of FXS was originally established by a special karyotyping technique that revealed the unstained or fragile sites by restricting folic acid and thymidine in the culture medium. The fragile sites were identified at Xq27.3. In 1991, the mutation responsible for FXS was delineated as an expansion of the trinucleotide sequence CGG within an evolutionarily conserved gene designated FMR-1. The CGG repeat is polymorphic in normal humans, ranging in size from six to 52 repeats. But in patients affected with the FXS, this trinucleotide sequence has undergone a remarkable expansion, to hundreds and sometimes thousands of CGG repeats. This expanded region of triplet repeats is, in fact, the fragile site itself (33). One can see it under a microscope.

When the number of CGG repeats in the *FMR1* gene exceeds approximately 230, the DNA of the entire local region of the gene is hypermethylated. This leads to inactivation of the *FMR-1* gene. As a result, in affected males, there is no detectable FMR-1 mRNA, and the encoded protein (FMRP) is not produced. The combination of trinucleotide repeat expansion and DNA hypermethylation is commonly referred to as a full mutation (33).

FMRP must have an effect on brain development because the lack of this protein results in the fragile X phenotype. In fact, detailed neuroanatomic studies in humans and rats show that FMRP is associated with the polysomes in dendrites and dendritic spines, suggesting that it plays a role in the translation of proteins related to dendritic function (34). Abnormalities of the dendritic tree are characteristic of FXS.

The dendrites in patients with FXS and in fragile X knockout mice are long and immature, features characteristic of early development or sensory deprivation. The fragile X protein is generated near synapses during neurotransmitter activation, suggesting that it plays a role in dendritic spine maturation or pruning and the alteration of synaptic structure (35,36).

In lymphocyte cultures, only approximately 50% of the cells have fragile sites. There is said to be instability of the CGG repeat, and mosaicism may occur. Mildly affected males may have this mosaic pattern. Alternatively, "higher functioning" patients with FXS may have borderline mutation size (200 to 300 repeats) (37,38).

Fragile X carriers have 50 to 230 triplet repeats (37). The intermediate level of expansion between normal and the abnormal full mutation is termed a premutation. Premutations are transcriptionally active and generate normal levels of FMRP. Premutations characterize male and female carriers who are unaffected.

The mutational mechanism by which the repeat segment is amplified is extraordinary. If the segment contains more than 50 repeats, it becomes unstable when transmitted. Fathers and mothers transmit premutation alleles to their offspring that are slightly different in size. Mothers transmit premutation alleles that are usually larger, and the premutation is susceptible to expansion to a full mutation in the offspring of female carriers. The more triplet repeats that are contained in the mother's premutation, the more likely it is that a full mutation will occur in her offspring. We do not understand why maternal premutations are more likely to expand when they are transmitted. Therefore, as the fragile X premutation is handed down from one generation to the next, there is a gradual accretion of trinucleotide repeats, greater numbers of affected offspring, and more severe manifestations of the condition (33). [The "law of anticipation" is decreasing age of onset or increasing disease severity in affected members of successive generations of a pedigree. There is some evidence that "anticipation" occurs in bipolar disorder and schizophrenia (39)].

The unusual mutational mechanism uncovered in FXS defines an entirely new mechanism by which genetic alterations result in clinically significant disease. Since the characterization of the fragile X mutation, no fewer than 20 genetic diseases, including Huntington's disease, Friedreich's ataxia, myotonic dystrophy, and Kennedy's disease, have been attributed to the process of trinucleotide repeat expansion (the exact repeat may be different as well as the gene it affects) (33). People with mild or asymptomatic forms of the diseases have genes that are functional but structurally unstable. They may gain or lose a few copies of a repeated unit with each round of DNA replication. If one such gene reaches a threshold length, however, a sudden cascade of further duplications takes place, and the disease is manifest.

Clinical Aspects of Fragile X Syndrome

The diagnosis of FXS should be suspected in males with mild to profound mental retardation who have a positive family history with an X-linked pattern. The family history may be positive for mental retardation, learning disabilities, or affective disorders. The syndrome cannot be diagnosed based on characteristic dysmorphic features. Individuals with FXS have dysmorphic features, including a long face with a prominent forehead, broad-based large nose, prognathism, and large, abnormally structured ears. Macro-orchidism is probably the most important dysmorphic feature, but it is not apparent until after puberty. The features are variable, however, so only approximately 60% of adult males have the classic triad (mental retardation, long face, megalotestes) (40). Therefore, they are unreliable for diagnostic purposes. A male with mental retardation and a familial neuropsychiatric history probably requires testing, whatever his physical appearance. The importance of testing and preventive screening cannot be denied because the carrier rate may be as high as one in 400 to 500 people (41).

Patients with FXS may have seizures (41%), dyskinesias (35%), or motor incoordination (59%) (42), but the neuropsychiatric manifestations are more impressive; The males are often hyperactive and may also be aggressive; autism and self-injurious behavior are not uncommon, and stereotypies are frequent concomitants (40,42,43). There are prominent deficits in short-term memory and sequencing and defective habituation to sensory stimuli (44,45). There is evidence for a decline in IQ scores from childhood to adult life (46) but no evidence of progressive dementia.

Not every male with FXS is retarded (47,48), although nonretarded males may be hyperactive and learning disabled (45). Conversely, not every female carrier is asymptomatic. Approximately 50% of the female carriers have been found to be borderline or mildly retarded, with a high frequency of psychiatric disturbance, especially psychosis and affective disorder (24,49,50). Male and female carriers of the premutation do not seem to have cognitive deficits, but most of the female carriers of the full mutation are known to be retarded. Full mutation carriers are also prone to learning disabilities, executive deficits on neuropsychological tests, depression, and schizotypal features (51).

Because the fragile marker at the q27 site is demonstrated in a folic acid–depleted environment, it seemed natural to experiment with folate treatment for children with FXS. Folate deficiency can cause a number of neuropsychiatric symptoms, and even though patients with FXS do not, as a rule, have folic acid deficiency, the experiment was not outlandish because folic acid treatment is said to improve the mood, drive, and sociability of patients with nonspecific psychiatric disorders. The doses used (5 to 10 mg) are a hundred times the dietary requirement, but folate is nontoxic even at high doses. The early reports of folic acid therapy were encouraging, with suppression of abnormal behavior, improved comportment and learning, and reduced aggression and stereotypy. The folate effect was likened to that of a psychostimulant. Subsequent experience and further studies have not been encouraging, however, although folate may still be given to young children with FXS, and many seem to respond (45,52–54).

The relative failure of folic acid as a treatment for people with FXS contrasts with the success of conventional psychiatric treatments. Children with FXS who are hyperactive and impulsive respond to stimulants, amantadine, or a combination of both. The α_2 agonists clonidine and guanfacine are frequently added to enhance the stimulant effect. Because so many children with FXS are temperamental, compulsive, or autistic, the serotonin reuptake inhibitors are also added to the mix. One of my colleagues refers to the "magic bullet" for children with FXS: a stimulant, an α_2 agonist, and a selective serotonin reuptake inhibitor.

The clinical presentation often changes with puberty, and the hyperactive, impulsive child with FXS may turn into an emotionally unstable, explosive, or aggressive adult. The magic bullet no longer seems to work very well. Fortunately, most such patients respond to a mood stabilizer, especially carbamazepine. Occasionally, combinations of mood stabilizers are necessary. Antipsychotic drugs may also be required, and not a few adults with FXS have psychotic symptoms.

It is my opinion that FXS responds better to psychotropic drug treatment than any other mental retardation phenotype, but it is the kind of psychopharmacology that is familiar to psychiatrists who work with the chronically mentally ill. Combinations of three, four, or five drugs may be needed, relapses are not uncommon, and drug adjustments are necessary as time goes on.

Serotonergic drugs such as paroxetine and buspirone are frequently used by female carriers with depression or anxiety.

SEX CHROMOSOMES AND THE EVOLUTION OF INTELLIGENCE

There is intense interest, among geneticists at least, in mental retardation syndromes that are linked to the X chromosome (XLMR). One reason is that there are so many of them. There are more than 80 different forms of XLMR, each one caused by a different mutant gene, each resulting in a characteristic (but not entirely unique) phenotype. X-linked genes contribute disproportionately to the sum of mental retardation syndromes, accounting for 10% to 20% or 25% to 50%, according to different authors (55,56). There may even be a concentration of *XLMR* gene loci in discrete areas of the X chromosome, an interesting if unproved idea (55,56). There is syndromal overlap. For example, cases have been described with the fragile X mutation but a Prader-Willi phenotype (57), Rett's syndrome (43), and Klinefelter's syndrome (58).

Organ system correlation with chromosomal abnormalities indicates an overrepresentation of X-linked genes in diseases of the sense organs, nerves, and brain (and a relative underrepresentation in structural and metabolic diseases) (59). Inactivation of a segment of the X chromosome, by any of a number of genetic mechanisms (e.g., pathologic assembly of repeats, microdeletion, aneuploidy) is reliably associated with learning difficulties and mental retardation.

Inactivation of segments of the X chromosome interferes with the normal development of the brain; therefore, genes that contribute to the normal development of the brain are on the X chromosome. Intellectual deficiency is the consequence of aberrations on the X chromosome; therefore, genes that contribute to the development of intelligence must be clustered there. X-linked genes contribute to the development of the brain and intelligence directly. Additionally, genes on the X chromosome may influence the brain and intelligence indirectly as regulators of gene expression on the autosomes. Because the genetic material of the X chromosome is well conserved across species, it is probably the latter mechanism that accounts for the X chromosome contribution to the development of intelligence.

Because so many of the XLMR syndromes have prominent neurobehavioral and affective characteristics, it is likely that many of the genes that regulate affective expression are also X linked. This is concordant with reports from the psychiatric literature on disorders, such as manic depression, that may occasionally be associated with loci on the X chromosome (60,61).

The XLMR syndromes, therefore, represent a series of natural experiments that hint at the nature of the genetic contribution to brain development, intelligence, behavioral aberration, and the vagaries of emotional expression. Very little can be said, however, of the nature of the contribution.

The literature gives ample attention to aberrations in gross brain development in the XLMR syndromes. That is to be expected because so many of the XLMR syndromes are associated with severe mental handicap. There is, however, no specific pattern to the neuropathology of the XLMR syndromes.

It is less well appreciated that genes that control the metabolism and the action of neurotransmitters have been identified on the X chromosome. This literature is less well developed, but, even at an early stage of observation, it indicates diverse neurochemical defects that do not follow a specific pattern.

For example, genes in close proximity to the fragile X locus are known to encode a subunit for the γ-aminobutyric acid receptor and for a neuronal antigen that exists in the cerebellum (44). The X chromosome is also the locus for at least one of the serotonin receptor genes (62), for the glycine receptor gene (63), and the glutamate receptor gene (64). Genes for glutamate dehydrogenase (which deaminates glutamate) and for synapsin (which is involved in neurotransmitter release from nerve terminals) are on the X chromosome (65,66). The genes for monoamine oxidase A and B are located next to each other in the p11.3–p11.4 region of the X chromosome (67). Brunner syndrome is an XLMR syndrome associated with mild mental retardation and impulsive, aggressive behavior (e.g., arson, attempted rape, exhibitionism) that characteristically occurs during discrete periods of several days during which diminished sleep and frequent night terrors also occur. The primary defect is in the structural gene for monoamine oxidase A and monoamine oxidase B on the short arm of the X chromosome (68,69).

Syndromes associated with Y chromosome aneuploidies (e.g., XYY, XXYY) are not, as a rule, associated with gross brain abnormalities or with high rates of learning disability. The observation, therefore, that a supernumerary Y contains a greater potential for behavioral instability finds no ready correlates on the anatomic level. That the aggressive behavior of XYY males represents an exaggeration of normal sexual behavioral dimorphism may find a basis in studies of mice, for which the agonistic behavior of offense is heritable. In some strains, genes for aggression are autosomal but are only expressed in the presence of androgen (70). Androgen sensitivity of certain organs is correlated with loci on the Y (71). In other strains, a gene locus on the Y chromosome has been directly implicated in agonistic aggression (72).

Both the X and the Y chromosomes contain "pseudoautosomal" regions on their distal short arms. Complete DNA sequence homology between the two chromosomes is found in this region and is believed to be important in mediating X-Y pairing in male meiosis (73). Loci on the pseudoautosomal region of the Y chromosome are correlated with attack behavior in mice (74,75). Crow (76) has theorized that there is a major predisposition to psychiatric illness, including psychosis, on the pseudoautosomal region of the Y chromosome, an area that is subject to a high rate of recombination and is thus likely to generate new mutations.

The Y chromosome has been linked to dopamine sensitivity in aggressive mice (74) and to decreased serotonin turnover in humans with the XYY genotype (77). Serotonergic treatment has been claimed to reduce aggression in XYY prisoners (77).

The clinical observation, therefore, of learning disability, aggressive behavior, affective disorder, and psychosis in patients with XXY, XYY, and FXS has its basis in genes on the X and Y chromosomes that mediate the development of intelligence, behavior, and emotional expression, influence the development of brain structures, and direct the actions of neurotransmitters and the sensitivity of tissues to the sex hormones. Beyond this general statement, the examples listed above should be taken only as dim perspectives on the actual molecular mechanisms that are at play.

The thrust of research is going to be in the direction of molecular mechanisms. There is new interest in the behavioral phenotypes and what they can tell us about the relationship between genes, brain, and behavior. That will be all to the good, but our chapter is not going to end with an encomium to the molecular basis of behavior. It is important to retain a sense of balance in the face of an avalanche of molecular data. It is important to remember that dissecting the sex chromosomes down is only one way to go. The other way is to consider their larger importance. They can tell us something about the evolution of intelligence and behavior.

The sex chromosomes have an evolutionary history. Much of the genetic material thereon has been conserved in the course of the descent of humans, but the evolution of the species has also been associated with a gradual loss of genetic material from the Y chromosome until only a few gene loci directly concerned with gonadal differentiation and a few genes on the pseudoautosomal region are left on it. Thus, the sexual selection that has driven mammalian evolution has been accompanied by conservation of genes on the X chromosome and progressive diminution in the genetic material of the Y chromosome.

Sexual reproduction was a signal event in the evolution of the higher species of plants and animals because it expanded the genetic diversity of organisms and thus afforded greater scope to natural selection. The evolution of sex dimorphic chromosomes has also been a signal event because it widened the potential for organismic diversity and thus afforded greater scope to the process of behavioral selection. As the autosomal contribution of the Y chromosome decreased, the diversity inherent in the genes of the X chromosome was allowed a greater degree of phenotypic expression, at least in the heterozygote. Thus, males were engineered to express a wider range of phenotypic diversity. In turn, females have a wider basis for choice. The mammalian male, therefore, is either a beneficiary or the victim of a mephistophelian bargain. He is either real good or real bad. If the former, he gets a lot of girlfriends.

If a deviant allele arises by mutation on the X chromosome that is advantageous to brain development, then the heterozygotic offspring enjoys the benefit undiminished by a normalizing dose of the homologous gene on the Y chromosome. In the evolution of higher animals, especially primates, this advantage has been expressed in the behavioral phenotypes of high intelligence, behavioral efficiency, and emotional stability. The reproductive advantage of such traits guarantees their reinvestment in succeeding generations. In contrast, low intelligence, behavioral instability, and erratic emotional expression confer a reproductive disadvantage that ultimately divests the species of deviant alleles that do not support the development of a healthy, more efficient brain.

Genetically determined mental retardation syndromes are most often X linked because genes for brain development and thus for behavior, emotional expression, and intelligence are clustered on the X chromosome. If an aberrant gene on the maternal X is not compensated by a normal gene on a paternal X, that is, if the paternal contribution is only a Y chromosome, then the aberrant gene on the X will be expressed in the phenotype of the resultant organism. Thus, the heterozygote will either suffer or profit from the expression of the aberrant gene.

The XLMR proband is clearly a victim of this faustian bargain. He suffers from the extreme manifestation of a deviant allele on the X chromosome that compromises the development of brain and cannot be moderated by a homologous gene derived from the paternal X.

Thus, the evolution of intelligence goes hand in glove with the evolution of what we, the beneficiaries of the process, naturally enough deem to be desirable behavioral and emotional attributes. Just as sexual selection drives the increasing complexity of new species, so behavioral selection drives the increasing complexity of new intelligence. The dimorphic sex chromosomes are the mediators of the evolution of intelligence.

Geneticists, like neuropsychiatrists, are impressed with the importance of the XLMR syndromes, just as seismologists are impressed with the importance of earthquakes. The strongest earthquake, however, is only a small hint of the inexorable movement of the tectonic plates. Thus, the XLMR syndromes and the sex chromosome aneuploidies are only surface tremors that hint at the immense laboratory of behavioral selection. The preponderance of males among mental retarded people is only a small and extreme example of the wider variability that males express in virtually every attribute that has to do with intelligence, behavior, and emotional response.

Males are the puppets of an unmoderated X chromosome. They react to the highs and lows of phenotypic expression. Females are the custodians of a balanced genotype and a moderate phenotype. They protect the good choices that evolution has conferred. As they make good choices in the dance of sexual selection, the genetic envelope is improved.

Lurking in that genetic envelope are abnormal alleles that possess the odd propensity of amplification as they are passed down from one generation to the next. Finally, as they are transmitted from mother to son, the accumulation of repeats exceeds the permissible threshold, an essential gene is inactivated, and a pathologic state ensues. FXS is only the first such condition that had been identified. Others have been identified, and more will be.

The predominance of FLMR among the genetic causes of mental retardation is entirely understandable within the framework of conventional genetics. FXS stands conventional genetics on its head. There seem to be dozens of genes on human DNA with repeat regions like those of FXS, and it is possible that at least some of them will be associated with diseases such as diabetes and schizophrenia, which are not transmitted by any known genetic mechanism. The origin of these fragile sites remains a mystery, however. Many cytogeneticists believe that fragile sites may represent the scars of chromosome translocations that have occurred during the evolution of species. It has been suggested that these sites contain small segments of telomeric DNA, where nonfunctional repeats occur normally, at the end of the DNA strand. There is also evidence of a "founder effect" in the fragile X mutation, a limited number of mutations that provided the origin of most of the present-day fragile X chromosomes. It is thought that it may take as long as 100 generations before a mutation in a normal allele results in a full mutation (78,79).

Thus, the gods visit the sins of the fathers, or at least their mutations, upon the children. If sexual selection conveys the impression of infinite perfectibility, by the discriminating taste of moderate females, the unveiling of fragile sites throughout the human genome suggests the accretion throughout the evolutionary process of hidden secrets. They erupt into bizarre pathology at unpredictable moments.

The accretion of repeats across the generations may just be a special event with no wider meaning beyond the pathologies that result. Or it may be meaningful on the wider canvas of natural selection in a new and different way. We shall occupy this question in Chapter 11.

REFERENCES

1. Hier D, Atkins L, Perlo V. Learning disorders and sex chromosome aberrations. *J Ment Defic Res* 1980;24: 17–26.
2. Gerald PS. Sex chromosome disorders. *N Engl J Med* 1976;294:706–708.
3. Smith DW, Jones KL. *Recognizable patterns of human malformation*, 3rd ed. Philadelphia: WB Saunders, 1982.
4. Money J. Two cytogenetic syndromes: psychologic comparisons 1. Intelligence and specific-factor quotients. *J Psychiatr Res* 1964;2:223–231.
5. Waber DP. Neuropsychological aspects of Turner's syndrome. *Dev Med Child Neurol* 1979;21:58–70.
6. McGlone J. Can spatial deficits in Turner's syndrome be explained by focal CNS dysfunction or atypical speech lateralization? *J Clin Exp Neuropsychol* 1985;7:375–394.
7. Nijhuis-van der Sanden R, Smits-Engelsman B, Eling P. Motor performance in girls with Turner syndrome. *Dev Med Child Neurol* 2000;42:685–690.
8. Rovet J, Holland J. Psychological aspects of the Canadian randomized controlled trial of human growth hormone and low-dose ethinyl oestradiol in children with Turner syndrome: The Canadian Growth Hormone Advisory Group. *Horm Res* 1993;39[Suppl 2]:60–64.
9. Ross JL, McCauley E, Roeltgen D, et al. Self-concept and behavior in adolescent girls with Turner syndrome: potential estrogen effects. *J Clin Endocrinol Metab* 1996;81:926–931.
10. Lishman WA. *Organic psychiatry, the psychological consequences of cerebral disorder*, 2nd ed. Oxford: Blackwell Scientific, 1987.
11. Money J. Two cytogenetic syndromes: psychologic comparisons 1. Intelligence and specific-factor quotients. *J Psychiatr Res* 1964;2:223–231.
12. Walzer S. X chromosome abnormalities and cognitive development: implications for understanding normal human development. *J Child Psychol Psychiatry* 1985; 26:177–184.
13. Patwardhan A, Eliez S, Bender B, et al. Brain morphology in Klinefelter syndrome: extra X chromosome and testosterone supplementation. *Neurology* 2000;54: 2218–2223.
14. Geschwind D, Boone K, Miller B, et al. Neurobehavioral phenotype of Klinefelter syndrome. *Mental Retard Dev Disabil Res Rev* 2000;6:107–116.
15. Jacobs PA, Brunton M, Melville MM, et al. Aggressive behavior, mental sub-normality and the XYY male. *Nature* 1965;208:1351–1352.
16. Sourial N, Fenton F. Testosterone treatment of an XXYY male presenting with aggression: a case report. Can J Psychiatry 1988;33:846–850.
17. Cinovsky K, Labady F, Koblik J. Psychologic follow-up of personality factors n the chromosomal anomaly of Klinefelter's syndrome. *Int Urol Nephrol* 1986;18: 99–103.
18. Singh TH, Rajkowa S. 49, XXXXY chromosome anomaly: an unusual variant of Klinefelter's syndrome. *Br J Psychiatry* 1986;148:209–210.

19. Klinefelter HF. Klinefelter's syndrome; historical background and development. *South Med J* 1986;79:1089–1093.
20. Mizukami K, Koizumi J, Shiraishi H, et al. A clinical case of Klinefelter's syndrome with various psychiatric symptoms. *Jpn J Psychiatry Neurol* 1989;43:639–644.
21. Miyamoto A, Kitawaki K, Koida H, et al. Klinefelter's syndrome and epileptic psychosis: a case report. *Jpn J Psychiatry Neurol* 1992;46:61–65.
22. Everman DB, Stoudemire A. Bipolar disorder associated with Klinefelter's syndrome and other chromosomal abnormalities. *Psychosomatics* 1994;35:35–40.
23. Inskip PD, Tarone RE, Hatch EE, et al. Cellular-telephone use and brain tumors. *N Engl J Med* 2001;344:79–86.
24. Fryns JP, Van den Berghe H. The concurrence of Klinefelter syndrome and fragile X syndrome. *Am J Med Genet* 1988;30:109–113.
25. el-Badri SM, Lewis MA. Anorexia nervosa associated with Klinefelter's syndrome. *Compr Psychiatry* 1991;32:317–319.
26. Sharma M, Meyer-Bahlburg H, Boon D, et al. Testosterone production by XYY subjects. *Steroids* 1975;26:175–180.
27. Gotz MJ, Johnstone EC, Ratcliffe SG. Criminality and antisocial behaviour in unselected men with sex chromosome abnormalities. *Psychol Med* 1999;29:953–962.
28. Wiedeking C, Money J, Walker P. Follow-up of 11 XYY males with impulsive and/or sex-offending behaviour. *Psychol Med* 1979;9:287–292.
28a. Martin JP, Bell J. A pedigree of mental defect showing sex linkage. *J Neurol Neurosurg Psychiatry* 1943;6:154–156.
29. Lubs HA. A marker X chromosome. *Am J Hum Genet* 1969;21:231–244.
30. Escalante H, Grunspun H, Frotarpassoa O. Severe sex-linked mental retardation. *J Genet Hum* 1971;19.
31. Opitz JM. Editorial comment: Brachmann-de Lange syndrome. *Am J Med Genet* 1985;22:89–102.
32. Rogers RC, Simensen RJ. Fragile X syndrome: a common etiology of mental retardation. *Am J Ment Defic* 1987;91:445–449.
33. Warren ST, Nelson DL. Advances in molecular analysis of fragile X syndrome. *JAMA* 1994;271:536–542.
34. Feng Y, Gutekunst C, Eberhart D, et al. Fragile X mental retardation protein: nucleocytoplasmic shuttling and association with somatodendritic ribosomes. *J Neurosci* 1997;17:1539–1547.
35. Irwin S, Swain R, Christmon C, et al. Evidence for altered fragile-X mental retardation protein expression in response to behavioral stimulation. *Neurobiol Learn Mem* 2000;74:87–93.
36. Irwin S, Patel B, Idupulapati M, et al. Abnormal dendritic spine characteristics in the temporal and visual cortices of patients with fragile-X syndrome: a quantitative examination. *Am J Med Genet* 2001;98:161–167.
37. Goldson E, Hagerman RJ. The fragile X syndrome. *Dev Med Child Neurol* 1992;34:822–832.
38. Berry-Kravis E, Hicar M, Ciurlionis R. Reduced cyclic AMP Production in fragile X syndrome: cytogenetic and molecular correlations. *Pediatr Res* 1995;38:638–643.
39. Margolis R, McInnis M, Rosenblatt A, et al. Trinucleotide repeat expansion and neuropsychiatric disease. *Arch Gen Psychiatry* 1999;56:1019–1031.
40. Fryns JP, Kleczkowska A, Kubien E, et al. Cytogenetic findings in moderate and severe mental retardation. *Acta Paediatr Scand Suppl* 1984;313:3–23.
41. Kathol RG, Wilcox JA, Turner RD, et al. Pharmacologic approaches to psychogenic polydipsia. *Prog Neuropsychopharmacol Biol Psychiatry* 1986;10:95–100.
42. Finelli PF, Pueschel SM, Padre-Mendoza T, et al. Neurological findings in patients with the fragile-X syndrome. *J Neurol Neurosurg Psychiatry* 1985;48:150–153.
43. Gillberg C, Wahlstrom J, Hagberg B. A "new" chromosome marker common to the Rett syndrome and infantile autism? The frequency of fragile sites at X p22 in 81 children with infantile autism, childhood psychosis and the Rett syndrome. *Brain Dev* 1985;7:365–367.
44. Reiss AL, Aylward E, Freund LS, et al. Neuroanatomy of fragile X syndrome: the posterior fossa. *Ann Neurol* 1991;29:26–32.
45. Hagerman RJ, Jackson III AW, Levitas A, et al. An analysis of autism in fifty males with the fragile X syndrome. *Am J Med Genet* 1986;23:359–374.
46. Lachiewicz AM, Gullion CM, Spiridigliozzi GA, et al. Declining IQs of young males with the fragile X syndrome. *Am J Ment Retard* 1987;92:272–278.
47. Gerald PS. X-linked mental retardation and the fragile-X syndrome. *Pediatrics* 1981;68:594–595.
48. Howard-Peebles PN, Friedman JM. Unaffected carrier males in families with fragile X syndrome. *Am J Hum Genet* 1985;37:956–964.
49. Knoll JH, Chudley AE, Gerrard JW. Fragile (X) X-linked mental retardation. II. Frequency and replication pattern of fragile (X)(q28) in heterozygotes. *Am J Hum Genet* 1984;36:640–645.
50. Reiss AL, Feinstein C, Rosenbaum KN. Autism associated with Williams syndrome. *J Pediatr* 1985;106:247–249.
51. Taylor A, Safanda JF, Fall MZ, et al. Molecular predictors of cognitive involvement in female carriers of fragile X syndrome. *JAMA* 1994;271:507–514.
52. Gillberg C, Wahlstrom J, Johansson R, et al. Folic acid as an adjunct in the treatment of children with the autism fragile-X syndrome (AFRAX). *Dev Med Child Neurol* 1986;28:624–627.
53. Rosenblatt DS, Duschenes EA, Hellstrom FV et al. Folic acid blinded trial in identical twins with fragile X syndrome. *Am J Hum Genet* 1985;37:543–552.
54. Aman MGP, Kern RAM. The efficacy of folic acid in fragile X syndrome and other developmental disabilities. *J Child Adolesc Psychopharmacol* 1990;1:285–295.
55. Neri G, Gurrieri F, Gal A, et al. XLMR genes: update 1990. *Am J Med Genet* 1990;38:186–189.
56. Kerr B, Turner G, Mulley J, et al. Non-specific X linked mental retardation. *J Med Genet* 1991;28:378–382.
57. de Vries B, Fryns J-P, Burler M, et al. Clinical and molecular studies in fragile X patients with a Prader-Willi-like phenotype. *J Med Genet* 1993;30:761–766.
58. Filippi G, Pecile V, Rinaldi A, et al. Fragile-X mutation and Klinefelter syndrome: a reappraisal. *Am J Med Genet* 1988;30:99–107.
59. Vogel F. Does the human X chromosome show evidence for clustering of genes with related functions? *J Hum Genet* 1969;17:475–477.
60. Baron M. Genes and psychosis: old wine in new bottles? *Acta Psychiatr Scand* 1995;92:81–86.
61. Mendlewicz J, Souery D. Heredity and manic-depressive psychosis. *Bull Acad Natl Med* 1995;179:755–764.
62. Ohta T, Ando K, Iwata T, et al. Treatment of persistent

sleep-wake schedule disorders in adolescents with methylcobalamin (vitamin B12). *Sleep* 1991;14: 414–418.
63. Derry JM, Barnard PJ. Mapping of the glycine receptor alpha 2-subunit gene and the GABAA alpha 3-subunit gene on the mouse X chromosome. *Genomics* 1991;10: 593–597.
64. McNamara JO, Eubanks JH, McPherson JK, et al. Chromosomal localization of human glutamate receptor genes. *J Neurosci* 1992;12:2555–2562.
65. Anagnou NP, Seuanez H, Modi W, et al. Chromosomal mapping of two members of the human glutamate dehydrogenase (GLUD) gene family to chromosomes 10q22.3–q23 and Xq22–23. *Hum Hered* 1993;43: 351–356.
66. Ferlini A, Ansaloni L, Nobile C, et al. Molecular analysis of the Rett syndrome using cDNA synapsin I as a probe. *Brain Dev* 1990;12:136–139.
67. Tivol EA, Shalish C, Schuback DE, et al. Mutational analysis of the human MAOA gene. *Am J Med Genet* 1996;67:92–97.
68. Brunner HG, Nelen MR, van Zandvoort P, et al. X-linked borderline mental retardation with prominent behavioral disturbance: phenotype, genetic localization, and evidence for disturbed monoamine metabolism. *Am J Hum Genet* 1993;52:1032–1039.
69. Cubells JF. An introductory overview of mutational analysis in psychiatric genetics. *Psychiatr Ann* 1997; 27:273–278.
70. Sandnabba NK. Selective breeding for isolation-induced intermale aggression in mice: associated responses and environmental influences. *Behav Genet* 1996;26:477–488.
71. Carlier M, Roubertoux PL, Kottler ML, et al. Y chromosome and aggression in strains of laboratory mice. *Behav Genet* 1990;20:137–156.
72. Maxson SC. Searching for candidate genes with effects on an agonistic behavior, offensive, in mice. *Behav Genet* 1996;26:471–476.
73. Ellison JW, Ramos C, Yen PH, et al. Structure and expression of the human pseudoautosomal gene XE7. *Hum Mol Genet* 1992;1:691–696.
74. Sluyter F, Bohus B, Beldhuis HJ, et al. Autosomal and Y chromosomal effects on the stereotyped response to apomorphine in wild house mice. *Pharmacol Biochem Behav* 1995;52:17–22.
75. Roubertoux PL, Carlier M, Degrelle H, et al. Co-segregation of intermale aggression with the pseudoautosomal region of the Y chromosome in mice. *Genetics* 1994;136:225–230.
76. Crow TJ. Sex chromosomes and psychosis. The case for a pseudoautosomal locus. *Br J Psychiatry* 1988;153: 675–683.
77. Bioulac B, Benezech M, Renaud B, et al. Serotonergic dysfunction in the 47, XYY syndrome. *Biol Psychiatry* 1980;15:917–923.
78. Jordan BR. Fragile X-linked mental retardation and the difficulties of reverse genetics. *Bioessays* 1991;13: 243–251.
79. Oostra BA, Halley DJJ. Complex behavior of simple repeats: the fragile X syndrome. *Pediatr Res* 1995;38: 629–637.

14
Autism

SUMMARY

What exactly is autism? It is a psychiatric diagnosis defined by major and minor symptoms, the most important being disordered communication and social relating. It resembles no other psychiatric disorder, and there is no specific psychiatric treatment for autism as such. It has the structure of a mental retardation syndrome, but not all autistic people are mentally retarded. It is probably a genetic syndrome, in the broad sense, but the genetics have not been worked out. There is known to be a familial association with the developmental language disorders. It is an encephalopathic syndrome to be sure. The "lesion" that causes autism, however, may be in the frontal, temporal, or parietal lobes, limbic cortex, cerebellum, or brainstem.

The genetics and neurochemistry of autism and the neuropsychology of the condition insofar as they are understood are reviewed and two anatomic models of autism are discussed in detail. The idea that autism is associated with cerebellar hypoplasia allows the reader to reflect on the complex functions of the cerebellum, an extremely compact and richly endowed organ that does much more than modulate motor behavior. The autism model I prefer is the Klüver-Bucy syndrome (KBS), an experimental preparation in monkeys that also occurs sometimes in patients with traumatic brain injuries. Children with brain injury who develop KBS symptoms during the recovery stage become extremely autistic over the long term.

Many esteemed investigators have tried to discover the "magic bullet" for autism. This is understandable; the children look so normal and so intelligent that one is certain there must be a key to unlock the secret of the condition and bring the children back. Perhaps this is why the parents of autistic children have been so vulnerable to fads, a few of which are discussed: fenfluramine, megavitamins, and secretin.

In fact, the psychopharmacology for autism is largely symptomatic and addresses emotional and behavioral problems that are concomitant with, but not central to, the condition. There are no magic keys to unlock the secret of autism, but several different drugs can diminish troublesome symptoms like repetitive behaviors, preoccupation with sameness, affective instability, aggression, and self-injury. Sometimes drugs can improve positive functions such as attention, communication, and learning. It is ironic, given the wealth of experiment and theorizing, that the most effective therapies for autistic people are no more than empirical and resemble rather closely the treatments used for other patients neuropsychiatric disorders.

AUTISM

Autism embraces a constellation of diverse attributes. Its borders are obscure, and it is not entirely clear where the center is. Beyond the behavioral definitions of the syndrome, there is little one can say for autism as a homogeneous or a biologically meaningful disorder. One can speak, therefore, about the medical treatment of autistic people, and some people do, but that has not been a fruitful approach to the problem.

The appropriate question is what one proposes to treat with a psychotropic drug, not autism certainly. That target is simply too broad, and that is why there has never been a drug effective for the treatment of autism. It is better to speak in terms of the specific behavioral and emotional problems that occur in people who happen to be autistic. These problems are familiar to neuropsychiatrists because they are not unique to autistic people. Treatments that address such problems are likely to be effective.

Autistic people are a diverse, heterogeneous group, by whatever dimension one may choose. Autistic individuals vary widely in clinical presentation, developmental level, etiologic factors, associated disorders, and prognosis. Autism may be genetic or acquired. If acquired, the cause may be infectious, traumatic, metabolic, structural, autoimmune, or some other undiscovered cause. The observed onset is usually during infancy, but autistic syndromes may arise in later childhood as a result of trauma, encephalitis, or seizures (e.g., Landau-Kleffner syndrome). Autistic people may be intellectually retarded, gifted, or somewhere in between. They may have seizures or not, they may be hyperactive or not, they may be verbal or not. They even vary in terms of the founding criterion, as it were—their capacity for interpersonal relatedness.

There is no element that is universal to the syndrome, no irreducible factor, no single point of departure. The deficit in communication is hopelessly broad and overlaps with other developmental dysphasias. The deficit in relatedness is the one element that is likely to improve when the child grows up (1,2). The very concept is shifting from the narrow perception of aloof autism to a wider one that includes a spectrum of conditions and even a broader, subclinical phenotype (3).

To understand autism with the idea of rendering treatment, one must appreciate its diversity, and disenthrall oneself from the idea that it is a unitary biologic entity. There is only the autistic individual with unique, individual requirements.

WHAT IS AUTISM?

What has been traditionally referred to as autism may be understood, not in terms of definitions, which are limiting, but in terms of models, which are potentially heuristic. Two models that can shed light on the medical treatment of autistic people are from developmental medicine and experimental neuropsychology. The first addresses the diversity of the syndrome and the second its specific features.

To build a model of understanding around a syndrome like autism, it is necessary to consider its structure, i.e., how autism resembles other conditions in psychiatry and neurology, and how it differs, especially in terms of etiologic factors, pathology, course, and response to treatment. In terms of the model from developmental medicine, it is suggested that the structure of autism is parallel, not to the functional psychiatric disorders, but to the structure of mental retardation.

For example, the cause of the disorder is not always known, but when it is known, it is a genetic, metabolic, toxic, hypoxic, infectious, or autoimmune insult to the brain. The same etiologic factors that cause mental retardation with autism in one individual can cause mental retardation without autism in another.

The onset of the disorder is, like mental retardation, in infancy. The course is static, i.e., not given to dramatic deterioration or improvement. Although autistic children are known to be extremely variable in behavioral and cognitive performance, the course of the disorder is not ordinarily given to relapses and remissions, with intervening periods of normal function, as are most of the psychiatric disorders.

Most autistic people are mentally retarded. The severity of their disorder parallels the severity of the mental handicap, and the prognosis is determined by the degree to which they are retarded, not the degree to which they are autistic (4). The prevalence of the disorder is highest in the most severely retarded. Not all autistic people are retarded, of course, but not all people with Down's syndrome are retarded either nor is everyone with Lesch-Nyhan, fragile X, or de Lange syndromes.

In terms of the developmental model, autism is a static encephalopathy. The spectrum of severity is relative to the extent of the causative encephalopathic event. Although there may be some unique neuropathic substrate to the syndrome, as explained later on, it is likely that the identification of neuropathic lesions will correlate better with the degree of mental handicap than with the degree of autism.

The psychopharmacology for autism also resembles the psychopharmacology for mental retardation. There is no drug treatment for mental retardation, but there are drugs to treat the psychiatric syndromes and target behaviors that occur in retarded individuals. The same is true for autistic individuals.

In terms of cause, neuropathology, course, treatment, and outcome, it is clear that autism has the structure of mental retardation. It is then a mental retardation variant, and this model accounts for the diversity of the syndrome.

The second model, from experimental neurology, should address the uniqueness of the syndrome. Autism, after all, may be a condition that is embedded in the study of mental retardation, but it is not identical to it. It is therefore necessary to consider the source of its distinctness. Is there a biologic element to account for its unique features?

There are four perspectives from which one might consider the unique attributes of the autistic condition: genetics, neurochemistry, neuropathology, and neuropsychology. Before we carry on with treatment issues, it is appropriate to address each of these dimensions.

Genetics

The risk of autism in a sibling of an affected child is approximately 3%, at least 50 times higher than the population rate (5,6). Monozygotic twins have a 36% concordance rate for diagnosed autism; the concordance rate is 82% for cognitive and social disabilities, more broadly defined. A famous twin study reported by Folstein and Rutter (7) in 1977 generated a "permissive" hypothesis of autism. They described a proclivity to dyslexia and developmental dysphasia in the families of autistic children on which was superimposed in the affected individual an encephalopathic insult. It was the latter that caused mental handicap, but the former that evoked the unique phenotype of autism. The model is important insofar as it describes an interaction between genetic proclivity and acquired lesion, but it does not suggest that autism is a genetic disorder in the sense that it has an established pattern of mendelian inheritance or is associated with a specific chromosomal abnormality or a specific gene. Distal 7q has emerged as a chromosomal region of interest, from autistic individuals with gross 7q abnormalities and from linkage and association data in families with language disorders (8). One suspects that the "autism gene," when and if it is identified, will code for a communication deficit and not for the condition *per se*.

There is genetic loading for autism, but it exists in the context of multifactorial causation (9).

Biochemistry

When one addresses the neurochemistry of a psychiatric disorder, it is customary to begin with two elements: a chemical alteration that reliably induces the condition and a chemical reversal that relieves the condition. For example, catecholamine depletion causes depression; effective antidepressants augment the central activity of the catecholamines, hence, the catecholamine hypothesis of depression. Amphetamine psychosis is caused by dopamine hyperactivity; antipsychotic drugs are antidopaminergic, hence, the dopamine hypothesis of schizophrenia. These venerable concepts are largely of historical interest, and the neurochemistry of depression and schizophrenia has proven to be vastly more complicated. In their time, however, the monoamine theories of depression and schizophrenia were compelling; in retrospect, they were heuristic and proved to be extremely productive.

The neurochemical theories of autism have been speculative rather than hypothetical. After all, no chemical alteration has been found to induce the condition, and no pharmacologic intervention has been found that relieves it. Nevertheless, it is useful to consider two theories that have received a great deal of attention over the years. One, the serotonin model, is based on no more than a serendipitous (albeit oft-repeated) observation. The other, the opioid hypothesis, is loosely derived from an animal model. Neither is compelling, at least in its current form, but both are interesting. Unlike the monoamine theories of depression and schizophrenia, they have not led to the development of effective treatments.

Serotonin

The neurochemical correlate that has been described most frequently, elevated peripheral levels of serotonin (10), is described as "one of the few enduring findings in all of psychiatric research," but its meaning is obscure. Blood serotonin levels are not correlated with serotonin levels in cerebrospinal fluid, and no central abnormality of serotonin metabolism or degradation has ever been detected in autistic people. Elevated blood serotonin has been proposed as a genetic marker for autism, but that, too, is a dubious contention because mentally handicapped people who are not autistic also have elevated levels of blood serotonin. It has been proposed that serotonin plays a trophic role in brain development and that an early defect in brain serotonin may disrupt the maturation of central nervous system (CNS) neurons, neuronal differentiation, and synaptogenesis (5). It is known that neurotransmitters in general, and the monoamines in particular, are involved in the regulation of neuronal outgrowth, plasticity, and survival. Neurotransmitters influence a wide spectrum of developmental processes before they are put to use in functional neuronal circuitries (11).

It is not easy to reconcile the known functions of central serotonin with the symptoms of autism (12). One possibility is that serotonin might play a role in the perception and filtering of sensory signals. In laboratory animals, increases (or decreases) in brain serotonin can disrupt synaptic connectivity in sensory cortical regions (13). Serotonin may play a role as well in social attachment. Hyperserotonemia (e.g., in laboratory animals) can reduce the drive for social attachment by inhibiting separation distress (6). Perhaps autistic children have an autoimmune disturbance directed against the serotonin receptor; cerebrospinal fluid antibodies to serotonin receptors have been reported in autistic children (5).

Elevation of whole blood serotonin is "the most robust and well replicated neurobiological abnormality in autism" (14). Hyperserotonemia, however, has been documented in association with severe mental retardation, chronic schizophrenia, and chronic neurologic diseases such as Huntington's chorea (15). Certainly drugs that influence serotonergic activity have a role to play in autistic patients; they have a role in other neuropsychiatric conditions as well.

Opioids

The discovery of the opioid receptor in the mammalian brain led to some wide-ranging speculations about what exactly the endogenous opiates were for (16). A series of very interesting experiments in rats led Panskepp (17) to hypothesize that endogenous opiates mediated the social bond. Love and opium, according to Panskepp, are both potent rewards and terribly addicting.

No one can argue with that proposition. There is room for doubt, however, about some of the inferential leaps that follow. Because autistic people have a profound deficit in social relating, scientists speculated that they might have abnormally high levels of endogenous opiates (17). According to this theory, the reason why autistic persons cannot respond to the rewarding climate of the social bond is because they produce all the endogenous rewards they need on their own. Hyperactivity of the endogenous opiate system could explain some, or most, of the symptoms of autism. The symptoms listed in Table 14.1 are characteristic of autistic children and adults; they are also observed in cases of opiate addiction, in humans, and in experimental animals (18).

TABLE 14.1. *Characteristics common to autism and opiate addiction*

Reduced socialization, aloofness
Reduced clinging in animals
Diminished crying
Repetitive stereotyped behaviors
Promotion of convulsive activity
Insensitivity to pain
Episodes of alternating hyperactivity/hypoactivity
Affective lability

Theoretically, opiate metabolism could be abnormal in autistic children by virtue of their genetic endowment, a problem of primary overproduction of endogenous opioids, deficient degradation, receptor sensitivity, or second messenger systems. Or it may constitute a developmental delay in the normal maturation of opioid systems or a secondary effect arising from stereotyped hyperactivity or repetitive self-injurious behavior (SIB). Other more elaborate schemes have been proposed, even linking opioid peptides to melatonin and serotonin (19). There is no shortage of candidate mechanisms to explain how opioids might be involved. Empirical data to support the theory, however, have not been nearly as compelling (18). The results of opiate-antagonist trials of naltrexone in autistic people, for example, have not been encouraging (20).

The question of naltrexone for SIB is dealt with in Chapter 15. The results of our research suggest that naltrexone is most effective after months of treatment. If that finding is at all relevant to autism, then the failure of naltrexone to alleviate the symptoms of the condition may be because the clinical trials have been short term.

Autism as a Metabolic Disease

Ramifications of the opioid theory have been insinuated into a couple of unlikely areas. Whether they speak to exciting new avenues for clinical investigation or simply to the feverish imagination of some autism investigators, is not for me to say, but elements of both have been manifest at one time or another.

It is been suggested that early, long-term overload of the CNS by opioids can arise from an exogenous source, possibly derived from incompletely digested dietary gluten and/or casein. The theory is one of deficient barriers, the fault lying in the bowel mucosa, in the blood-brain barrier, or in the failure of the intestinal and circulating peptidases that should convert opioids to innocuous metabolites (3).

Casein is a protein present in milk and gluten a protein that is present in wheat. From these dietary sources, a series of exomorphins are formed; they are broken down by intestinal peptidases. A failure at this point, e.g., a peptidase deficiency, or a defect in mucosal permeability could lead to increased systemic uptake of exomorphins and other food proteins and peptides (21). A defective mucosal barrier should be detected by higher levels of peptides in urine or by elevated levels of immunoglobulin A antibodies to food proteins in serum (22)

Perhaps food peptides that affect the CNS are involved in the pathophysiology of autism. Antibody reactivity to milk and wheat proteins may be higher in autistic children, compared to normal controls, and elimination of these foods from the diet is said to improve their behavioral symptoms (23).

It was within this context of innocent speculation that the "discovery" of secretin, a pancreatic hormone, met with extraordinary attention. In an obscure medical journal, a team of gastroenterologists reported that intravenous administration of secretin to three autistic children led to "a dramatic improvement in their behavior...[with] improved eye contact, alertness, and expansion of expressive language" (24). Soon after the article appeared, there were television appearances and dozens of newspaper and magazine articles. The small supply of secretin, heretofore used only for diagnostic purposes by gastroenterologists, was soon sold out. Entrepreneurs cornered the limited supply and offered vials of secretin for sale over the Internet.

The excitement subsided as parents and physicians learned that the benefits of secretin infusion were not as gratifying as they had heard on the television program "Good Morning America," and controlled studies have indicated no benefit from secretin infusion (25–27). If there is any benefit to secretin at all, it appears to be transient. The risk of periodic infusions of porcine pancreatic protein should not be minimized, but human synthetic secretin is now available. (On April 4, 2001, Repligen, a company that makes synthetic secretin, reported modest success in a placebo-controlled trial of secretin in 136 autistic children. The report was in the form of a press release.)

The secretin "affair" was a distraction from the central issue: whether something happening in the gut, occurring at a critical juncture, might have some impact on the early development of the CNS. The high rate of malabsorption syndromes in developmentally disabled children (e.g., Down's syndrome) strengthens one's suspicion that a connection exists (28,29). Whether it is epiphenomenal or causative is another question entirely.

Celiac disease is an inflammatory disease of the small intestine induced by cereal prolamins. It is a common, clinically heterogeneous disease, and the diagnosis is often overlooked. Patients with celiac disease have a lifelong intolerance to dietary gluten. The symptoms of the disease, protean as they are, are alleviated by a gluten-free diet. Screening tests for celiac disease look for antigliadin and antiendomysial antibodies (30,31). Celiac disease is said to be associated with an extraordinary range of psychiatric and neuropathologic conditions including depression, dyslexia, epilepsy, schizophreniform psychosis, cerebellar syndrome, brain atrophy, and dementia (22,32–36).

In a recent study of 12 children who had experienced severe developmental regression (most were autistic) accompanied by prominent gastrointestinal symptoms, there was indication of chronic intestinal inflammation and ileal lymphoid hyperplasia. It was suggested that exposure to measles virus, either wild-type or the attenuated form present in measles, mumps, rubella vaccine, was the triggering event (37,38). This report caused a stir, as one might expect, not over the suggestion that regression might be caused by bowel disease but rather over the idea that measles, mumps, rubella vaccine was the causative agent.

One presumes that the neuropsychiatric correlates of inflammatory bowel disease, if, indeed, they are real, may be related to a direct neuropathic effect of systemic food peptides or perhaps to an autoimmune reaction that they provoke. The relationship of inflammatory bowel disease to polyvalent measles vaccination is controversial to say the least. Its connection to autism is also speculative. Nevertheless, it is fertile ground for speculation. Whether harm will come of it or whether there will be a profound new understanding of the gut-brain axis, I cannot say.

THE NEUROPATHOLOGY OF AUTISM

Several possible neuropathologic sites have been suggested based on the clinical features of the disorder, and several different neuropathologic abnormalities have been described in the brains of autistic patients. The results of neuroimaging studies, functional neuroimaging, and autopsies have been tantalizing, if somewhat less than cohesive, and hardly given to a unified theory of the condition. Considering its clinical heterogeneity, however, one would only be surprised if they did. Autism has been variously proposed to be a disorder of the cerebral cortex (frontal, temporal, and parietal lobes), limbic cortex, basal ganglia, cerebellum, and brainstem. Recent research has focused on three particular regions of the brain: the cerebellum, temporal and limbic lobe structures, and cerebral cortex, and that is how the matter is addressed here, with the understanding that autism is not a single-lesion condition but rather the clinical manifestation of dysfunctions in several areas and on several levels. Clinically, autism is a multidimensional condition, the etiologic factors are many, and the neuropathology is disseminated rather than focal.

The Cerebellum in Autism

The first suggestions implicating cerebellar abnormalities in the pathophysiology of autism were put forward by Ornitz and Ritvo (39) during the 1970s based on clinical and neurophysiologic observations. The actual detection of structural abnormalities in the cerebellum was made much later based on histoanatomic observations of autopsy subjects (40,41). The microanatomic pathology comprised severe Purkinje neuron loss and neuron size reduction in the posterior vermis or vermal hypoplasia. The absence of concomitant gliosis seemed to indicate that neuronal loss must have occurred in early development. The idea developed from these studies that early loss of Purkinje cells disrupts the ontogeny of the cerebellar circuitry. Presumably, immature neurons persist, and a nonfunctional fetal pattern of circuitry is retained (5).

A series of neurodiagnostic studies indicated abnormalities of the cerebellar vermis and hemispheres (42). The results have not been uniformly replicated, and not everyone agrees that cerebellar hypoplasia is, in fact, specific to autism, or whether it is merely a manifestation of mental handicap, a primary event, or secondary to a primary lesion elsewhere in the CNS (43). Cerebellar pathology also occurs in nonautistic people who are mentally handicapped and in schizophrenics who are neither autistic nor mentally handicapped (44). That cerebellar hypoplasia is central or specific to autism, schizophrenia, or mental handicap is improbable; that it has an interesting role to play is likely. One cannot fail to be impressed with the fact that cerebellar abnormalities have been found in 16 quantitative magnetic resonance imaging (MRI) and autopsy studies from no fewer than nine independent research groups involving more than 240 autistic cases (45).

A role for cerebellar pathology in the genesis of autism is suggested by direct observations. and reinforced by three additional considerations: (i) there is a rationale for cerebellar vulnerability to brain insult in early life, (ii) the neuropsychology of the cerebellum is relevant to the clinical manifestations of autism, and (iii) the mechanism of corticocerebellar diaschisis links cerebellar pathology to events in the frontal and limbic cortices.

Cerebellar Vulnerability

Cerebellar vulnerability is probably a function of its protracted ontogenetic course. It has been suggested that brain structures whose development is protracted are more vulnerable to brain insult. Among the brain structures with such a developmental course, three stand out: the hippocampus, frontal cortex, and cerebellum. The neural makeup of the cerebellum is not complete at the time of birth, and the process of neural migration is longer in this organ than in other brain areas.

The vulnerability of cerebellar neurons is dramatically demonstrated in survivors of childhood leukemia who are treated with radiation and intrathecal chemotherapy before the age of 5 years. They show a pattern of macromorphologic changes in the cerebellum similar to that found in autism. The leukemia survivors experience a number of cognitive and social-emotional changes, but they do not display autistic features (46), which is not surprising because the timing of the insult is later than in autistic children.

The young child's cerebellum is vulnerable to the toxic effects of a number of infectious agents, as is known from studies of acute cerebellar ataxia (47).

Neuropsychology of the Cerebellum

Sherrington referred to the cerebellum as the head ganglion of the proprioceptive system, and the concept of the cerebellum as a modulator of motor function was dominant for the greater part of this century (47a). The cerebellum does participate in fine and gross motor control, and how it does this, through an elaborate system of cross connections to cortical and subcortical structures, is marvelous to contemplate. It seems to be responsible for patterning the sequence of contraction of agonist and antagonist muscles, and the timing of these sequences is faulted by cerebellar dysfunction. It monitors proprioceptive, cutaneous, and visual feedback, thus serving as a comparator between certain motor functions such as limb position and the engram of the position that is desired. The detection of mismatches can be involved in the coordination of movement and the adaption of movement to new situations as well as in motor learning (48). For the proper execution of such functions, the cerebellum is endowed with ample connections to the frontal neocortex. It also possesses a nerve cell population that exceeds the population of the cerebral cortex (49).

Elaborate as its motor functions may be, the concept of the cerebellum as a modulator of motor function is incomplete. Recent studies in animals and humans have concentrated on the role of the cerebellum in a variety of psychological functions such as language, learning and memory, emotional behavior, and complex motivated behaviors (40,50,51). This is no less than a throwback to the intuitions of Franz Joseph Gall, the Swiss neuroanatomist and impresario who founded phrenology. Gall proposed that the cerebellum was no less than the anatomic locus of sexual love (52).

The history of the cerebellum is even more interesting than that. During the course of human evolution as the brain enlarged, the cerebellum enlarged more dramatically than any other part of the brain except the cerebral cortex. The phylogenetically new parts of the cerebellum developed not in parallel with the cerebral cortex as a whole but specifically in parallel with the cerebral association areas (49). With millions of nerve fibers connecting the cerebellum to many parts of the forebrain and the brainstem, including all the lobes of the cerebral cortex, the cerebellum has developed as a participant in a number of higher functions. One presumes that its participation in nonmotor functions is characterized by the same role of a comparator or modulator.

Phylogenetically older areas of the cerebellum have outputs to the motor cortex and thus influence motor skills. By the same token, cerebellar outputs to the sensory system modulate the consistency of sensory input. It was the concept of perceptual inconstancy that led Ornitz and Ritvo to propose a cerebellar role in autism (39). Cerebellar outputs to the limbic system may modulate emotional behavior, and cerebellar outputs to cortical association areas may influence cognition and language (49). There is a growing body of behavioral observation from experimental animals and clinical subjects to support a cerebellar role in all these areas. In animals, the cerebellum is involved in learning, the production of classical conditioning responses, and long-term habituation. In humans, the cerebellum is involved in associative learning, and it appears to participate in the manifestations of intelligence on standard tests (44,53).

Courchesne et al. (42) emphasized a cerebellar link to attention. Cerebellar activity modulates brainstem, thalamic, hippocampal, and cerebral cortical responses to visual, auditory, and somatosensory stimulation. Animals with cerebellar lesions show perseverative behavior and fail to attend to appropriate distracters (51). The cerebellar vermis has extensive connections with structures that mediate arousal and attention, and cerebellar damage in humans can result in impairment in the ability to accurately and rapidly shift attention between and within sensory modalities. With a normal cerebellum, shifting the mental focus of attention is effortless, accurate, and timely, whereas when there is extensive damage, it is effortful, inaccurate, and poorly timed (42).

Corticocerebellar Diaschisis

The connections between the cerebellum and cortical brain structures are defined anatomically in terms of specific tracts such as the corticopontine-cerebellar connections. Equally pertinent to this discussion, it is defined pathophysiologically in terms of what is called crossed cerebellar diaschisis. The reader was introduced to von Monakow's concept of diaschisis during the discussion of traumatic brain injury in Chapter 4. Crossed cerebellar diaschisis is a well-recognized phenomenon that occurs after cerebral infarction. A focal supratentorial lesion interrupts corticopontocerebellar connections, causing deafferentation and transneural metabolic depression of the contralateral cerebellar hemisphere (54). Conversely, unilateral cerebellar infarctions have been noted to induce metabolic depression in contralateral basal ganglia and frontoparietal cortex (55).

Although the phenomenon has been documented by positron emission tomography and single photon emission computed tomography studies, its clinical significance is not fully understood. Nevertheless, clinical observations consistent with cerebellar impairment have been made in patients with supratentorial lesions and crossed cerebellar diaschisis (56,57). In adult patients with stroke, functional depression of the cerebellar metabolism is not necessarily associated with cerebellar atrophy, but it is interesting that in children with extensive cortical lesions, crossed cerebellar atrophy has been demonstrated on MRI (54).

If the primary pathologic event in the development of autism were a failure of cerebellar development, then diaschisis would induce remote functional changes in the frontal and limbic cortices and further compromise the development of cognitive, linguistic, social, and emotional functions. The cerebellum is vulnerable to brain insult and to developmental failure and participates to some degree in all the functional areas that are impaired in autistic people. But cerebellar atrophy might equally well be secondary to a primary lesion elsewhere in the cortex. After all, there are other areas of the brain that are equally or more vulnerable to perinatal insult than the cerebellum such as the medial temporal lobe and limbic and frontal cortex. Arguments from vulnerability and diaschisis do not necessarily mean that a cerebellar lesion is primary; it may be primary or secondary, or multiple lesions may arise from the same cause.

The participation of the cerebellum in the pathophysiology of autism is in all probability not as the site of a primary lesion but as one of the poles of an axis of derangement. Autism is a disorder of social and emotional behavior, cognitive impairment (in general) and linguistic impairment (in the particular), motoric peculiarities, and sensory integration. The rostral pole of this axis is in the frontal and medial temporal cortices; its caudal pole is in the brainstem and cerebellum. The neuroanatomy is not precise, but there is nothing about autism to indicate that it should be.

Cortical Structures

One would expect to find abnormalities of the cerebral cortex in patients with a disorder that is marked by deficits in information processing, social relatedness, language, and complex reasoning. It is no surprise then that several supratentorial abnormalities have been described in autistic patients including cortical volume gain (and loss), malformation of frontal lobe gyri, ventriculomegaly, thinning of the corpus callosum, hemispheric asymmetry, and abnormal glucose metabolism (5,45). Approximately 25% of autistic individuals have a larger than normal head circumference, a finding that is rare in mental retardation or language disorders. Thickening of the cerebral cortex (6) typically causes such megalencephaly. Haas et al. (45) proposed parietal-cerebellar dysfunction based on qualitative MRI studies and on specific neuropsychological deficits associated with parietal lobe dysfunction with spatial and attentional abilities.

Functional neuroimaging has indicated an imbalance in interregional and interhemispheric brain metabolism and blood flow as well as abnormalities in the anterior cingulate gyrus (58).

Temporal Lobe and Limbic Structures

Abnormalities in the limbic forebrain, albeit subtle and evident only after comparison with suitable controls, have provided the strongest correlation with the clinical features of the disorder. One of the earliest neurodiagnostic studies of autism using pneumoencephalography reported abnormalities of the medial temporal lobe (59). Subsequent computed tomography and MRI studies of this area were not consistent. More recent positron emission tomography studies, however, have revealed reduced volume and metabolic activity in the anterior cingulate gyrus and abnormalities of serotonin metabolism in the dentatothalamocortical pathway, remarkably consistent with an old hypothesis on the "localization" of autism by Maurer (60). A recent autopsy study of 19 autistic brains revealed structural and cellular pathology in the anterior cingulum, hippocampus, subiculum, entorhinal cortex, mammillary bodies, septal nuclei, and amygdala. Experimental lesions in these regions have produced deficits in memory, emotional expression, and other behaviors that resemble those seen in autistic individuals (40,43).

Klüver-Bucy Syndrome

KBS is a paradigm from the earliest days of experimental neurology. It retains at least a degree of relevance, especially in cases of young children who have had severe traumatic brain injuries. It is also a model for the temporal-limbic contribution to autism.

KBS is a monkey preparation with behavioral concomitants related to surgical resection of the temporal lobes, including the uncus, amygdala, and rostral hippocampus (61). Autistic people do not exhibit all the characteristics of KBS monkeys, of course, such as hyperphagia and hypersexuality, but neither are the neuropathic events that lead to autism as precise or anatomic. KBS monkeys are amnestic, and this feature does not necessarily characterize autistic people. Conversely, humans with acquired partial KBS are known to have severe communication deficits, a short attention span, distractibility, and echopraxia, and these are typical symptoms of autistic patients. The KBS model is supported by neuropathologic studies of autistic people who have demonstrated deep temporal lobe abnormalities (59) and by histoanatomic studies that indicate hippocampal and amygdaloid lesions (40).

The KBS model is not particularly helpful in directing pharmacologic intervention, although it is useful for the design of behavioral programs. In terms of psychopharmacology, the deep nuclei of the temporal lobe and rostral limbic lobe are so richly endowed with a host of neurotransmitter systems that it is not possible to base an argument for treatment on one particular neurotransmitter. What guides the psychopharmacology for autism is not a specific model such as KBS, but a broad overarching model such as mental retardation.

Brown and Schafer first observed KBS in 1888 in a rhesus monkey after the removal of both temporal lobes. The monkey had been fierce and aggressive, but after the operation he was placid and indifferent. There were some other peculiar behaviors:

> *He no longer seemed to understand the meaning of sounds, sights, and other impressions that reached him. Every object with which he came into contact, even those with which he was previously most familiar, appeared strange and were investigated with curiosity. Everything he endeavored to feel, taste, and smell and to carefully examine from every point of view. Food was devoured greedily, the head being dipped into the dish, instead of the food being conveyed to the mouth by the hands in the way usual with monkeys. Memory and intelligence seemed deficient (62).*

These were the important elements of a syndrome that Heinrich Klüver and Paul Bucy described in 1937: profound emotional changes in the direction of a placid temperament, psychic blindness (*Seelenblindheit*), hypermetamorphosis (exploratory behavior), and strong oral tendencies. They added hypersexuality as a feature of the syndrome but did not emphasize the loss of memory, an important element when KBS occurs in humans (61,63,64).

Much has been made of the question whether pure KBS does in fact occur in humans, although that is probably an irrelevant issue because KBS is a surgical preparation in laboratory monkeys. No surgical procedure in humans is likely to be so mutilatory and no pathologic event is likely to be so surgical to convey the full range of KBS. When extensive bilateral temporal lobectomies used to be done in humans, however, with removal of the medial surface to include the amygdala and anterior hippocampus, virtually all elements of KBS were observed (65).

The effects of viral infections of the CNS, such as herpes simplex encephalitis, may be localized to structures of the limbic cortices, owing perhaps to the unique antigenic property of the cells in that region (66). Herpes simplex encephalitis is sometimes associated with sequelae that resemble those of KBS (67–69). Cases of KBS have also been observed to follow brain trauma (70,71), toxic exposure (72), or dementia (71,73). KBS symptoms may be a transient correlate of coma recovery after traumatic brain injury (70).

The KBS has been proposed as a paradigm for the study of cognition. It has been observed, for example, that bilateral amygdalectomy impairs the capacity of the organism to establish sensory cross-modal associations. The psychic blindness and hypermetamorphosis that characterize KBS is really a failure of information received on one channel to register in a meaningful way on other sensory channels (74). A failure in the capacity to form cross-modal associations creates the necessity for constant sensory stimulation, especially by the near receptors (taste, touch, and smell). This represents an attempt to strengthen the engram that would normally be reinforced by parallel sensory systems. The cross-modal failure also weakens the capacity of the organism to grasp the wider meaning of events beyond their capacity to stimulate one sensory channel.

The memory impairment of KBS is the consequence of bilateral (not unilateral) temporal lobe ablation (75). Conjoint amygdaloid-hippocampal lesions are essential, it appears, to the development of dense amnesia (76,77). It is instructive to consider precisely what kind of memory is lost as a consequence of such lesions.

Lesions on the medial surface of the temporal lobes are associated with loss of declarative memory but not procedural memory (77). Declarative memory is the acquisition of new facts: what the name of a thing is, where it is hidden, its shape or color; procedural learning is the acquisition of new skills or procedures: how to do something. In the classic experiment, the dense amnestic cannot learn a simple word list, but he or she can acquire the skill for mirror writing.

The amygdala is also involved in social behavior. Autistic individuals fail to activate the amygdala when making "mentalistic inferences" from the facial expressions of other people (78). Animals with amygdala lesions have bizarre and inappropriate responses to social cues, a common feature of autism. When animals are lesioned in infancy, their avoidance of conspecifics is characterized by excess submissive behavior, also a finding in ethologic studies of avoidance behavior in autistic children. Animals with hippocampal lesions respond with perseveration when they are unable to solve a problem given to them, probably because of reduced ability to give up an inappropriate hypothesis or to focus their attention properly (60).

Understanding the psychology of KBS and other experimental preparations involving lesions to deep temporal nuclei may be an effective guide to behavioral and ecologic treatment for autistic patients, for example, and for patients with brain injury during the phase of coma recovery. The fact that declarative memory is impossible after bilateral injury to the amygdala and hippocampus suggests that behavioral treatments based on operant principles would tend to be minimally useful, whereas treatments that are based on principles of classic conditioning should be a better way to proceed. Operant conditioning, or learning from contingencies or consequences, is analogous to declarative memory and is therefore less suitable for the amnestic. Classic conditioning is based on the creation of associations by simple repetition; it is analogous to procedural learning and is thus more suitable for the patient with KBS.

The treatment of patients with KBS would require, therefore, structure and sameness, repetition and familiarity. The use of contingency systems to cope with undesirable target behaviors would be less effective than proactive efforts to guide behavior into enduring and familiar channels or habits. The essence of the education of patients with KBS should be in the acquisition of skills through constant repetition or repetition as many times as their stamina and attention span can abide. Efforts should be made to minimize the occurrence of novelty. Untoward behaviors in the face of novel circumstances should be understood to represent a physiologic, not a pathologic, response. The capacity to learn from novel events is not a characteristic of amnestics.

The treatment of patients with severe traumatic brain injuries or with severe developmental disabilities is based on learning or relearning. Learning in turn may be incremental, i.e., based on the introduction of new material, or repetitious, based on the invariance of the exercise. In fact, most learning involves both elements. For the sake of the paradigm, however, one should assume that the capacity for incremental learning requires an intact system for cross-modal association, and the functional anatomy of this system is in the nuclei of the medial temporal lobe. When this area has been damaged or ablated, one is left with the capacity only for learning by repetition, i.e., only with the ability to acquire procedures.

The therapeutic environment of such patients should be based on ecology not contingencies. It should be constructed like a finger exercise, and a finger exercise requires a keyboard that never changes. The expectation of flexibility is countertherapeutic.

Understanding the psychology of KBS permits us to understand the meaning of certain symptoms such as hyperactivity. In the context of such profound cognitive deficits, hyperactive/disorganized behavior in young autistic children, for example, must be considered physiologic, not pathologic. One should assume a failure to develop channels of understanding, by virtue of short-term memory loss, cross-modal failure, or both. There is a basic need to construct channels to bind and direct sensory input that the child is unable to satisfy. This in turn impedes the child's ability to inhibit behavior or to direct it in meaningful, consistent ways. The result is constant exploratory behavior. It is two things: in motive, a need to fill sensory channels that melt away even as they are formed; in result, a failure of behavioral direction along the course of such channels.

The Neuropsychology of Autism

To what degree do neuropathologic findings interleave with the observations of neuropsychologists who have studied the intricacies of the autistic mind in great detail and who have arrived at independent views of what represents the psychological core of the disorder?

The cognitive deficits of autistic children have generated a vast descriptive literature, for example, the observation that some cognitive functions are preserved while others are impaired. The extraordinary phenomenon of autistic savants is the best example of what has been termed "islets of ability." Memory deficits have also been described in autistic people, although not with consistency.

Attentional problems are probably central to the condition: distractibility and inability to concentrate in some patients and narrowing of attention, perseveration, and resistance to distraction in others. Usually both problems occur in the same patient. Patients with frontal lobe lesions also show this pattern of attentional dysfunction as do patients with attention deficit/hyperactivity disorder. It is curious to think that distractibility and hyperfocus might coexist, but it is explicable in terms of one's ability to shift attentional sets in response to appropriate environmental cues. It has been shown that autistic people are impaired in tasks that require rapid shifting of attention after a cue, either within or between modalities (42,79).

A relative inability to form abstract representations or ideas has long been considered one of the central cognitive features of autism. High-level autistic people usually do quite poorly on tests of frontal/executive ability that tax their capacity for abstraction. Verbal and nonverbal problem-solving deficits are prominent, even in autistic adults with average intelligence scores on standard tests (80). Most such tasks, however, entail the ability to shift attentional sets with flexibility, a skill that autistic people do not possess as a rule.

Communication failure has always been central to the definition of autism. So it is not surprising that abnormal language is a characteristic of the condition. As is the case with cognitive ability in general, language in autism shows both preserved and impaired functions. Their language deficits, however, are not typical of the developmental dysphasias, any more than their memory impairment is typical of global amnesia. They are given to abnormal, stilted prosody, idiosyncratic vocalizations, pronoun reversal, echolalia, neologisms, absence of figurative language, and so on. Lack of communication, however, rather than language, is characteristic of autism. Even autistic people with intact language skills have difficulty using it for intentional communication. Impairment in pragmatics—the mutuality of conversational speech—is a universal deficit in autistic people, and metalinguistic behaviors such as facial expression, tone-of-voice, and eye contact are notoriously deficient (79).

A theoretical link between cognitive skills and social functioning was presented by Leslie and Frith (81) who suggested that "metarepresentational deficits" impair the ability of autistic individuals to comprehend the mental states of others, i.e., they lack a theory of mind. The repertoire "of the autistic person's strange behavior can be better understood if we remember that he or she cannot mind-read the way most of us do" (79). In the same vein, it has been argued that the lack of social relatedness arises from a deficit in an inborn capacity to recognize and respond to the expression of emotional states in other people (82). Psychological studies have failed to support the theory of mind (83). Interestingly, however, a functional MRI study of several high-functioning autistic people showed significant differences (from normal controls) in the activity of cerebellar, mesolimbic, and temporal lobe cortical regions when processing facial expressions (84).

The neuropsychology of the cerebellum also indicates a degree of participation in functions that are relevant to autism, but the problem of specificity inheres. Children with cerebellar atrophy from radiation and chemotherapy are disturbed, to be sure, but they are not autistic. People with cerebellar agenesis are noted to have serious abnormalities, but they are not autistic either (85). Language may be impaired after cerebellar infarction, with a number of specific deficits such as agrammatism of spontaneous speech, but the peculiar linguistic defects of autistic people have not been described (86).

I can hardly do justice to the wealth of neuropsychological data that have accrued in the study of autistic patients or to the clever constructions that have been made in attempts to find coherence and meaning. Deficits in many key functions have been described, just as neuropathologic abnormalities are identified in many different structures and indeed as neurochemical aberrations are described in different systems. Interesting findings in one particular area promise to enlighten the central pathologic core of the condition; then they fail to be replicated. In most instances, this is because of the amazing degree of interindividual variation that is typical of virtually any sample of the autistic population.

PSYCHOPHARMACOLOGY FOR AUTISM

Having endured the foregoing discussion—far ranging as it is, but only skimming the surface of modern autism research—the reader is probably willing to concede that clinically autism is a multidimensional condition, etiologic factors are many, and the neuropathology is disseminated rather than focal. As we address, then, the problem of drug treatment for autistic children and adults, we must proceed carefully. There is no drug treatment specifically for autism. Drug treatment for autistic people addresses either conditions that are comorbid with autism, such as epilepsy or anxiety, or aimed at controlling symptoms that are related to autism, such as stereotypy or SIB.

The neuropathologic studies have done little to advance the cause of psychopharmacology. For example, on a neurochemical level, cerebellar activity is involved with glutamate, dopamine, norepinephrine, serotonin, γ-aminobutyric acid (GABA), and acetylcholine. There is no cerebellar neurotransmitter or cerebellar drug.

Neither has KBS been a useful paradigm for psychopharmacologists. In monkeys, the KBS preparation results in a partial deafferentation of excitatory projections to the amygdala, with attendant decreases in dopamine and serotonin and increases in norepinephrine (87). Such changes are not necessarily predictive of medication response. Carbamazepine, a prototypical temporal lobe drug, may be effective in controlling the agitation and assaultive behavior that often occur in humans with KBS (88). The other psychotropic anticonvulsants, the selective serotonin reuptake inhibitors (SSRIs), clonidine, and amantadine are possible alternatives, but drug treatment is really just trial and error (89). The wide swath of injury to brain regions endowed with multiple neurotransmitters militates against successful treatment for all or even most cases with any single drug.

Neither have the neuropsychological models contributed to a rational psychopharmacology for autism.

The attentional problems of autistic children are often treated with psychostimulants, but with little success. Their attentional deficits are not similar to those of patients with attention deficit/hyperactivity disorder. Their communication deficits, presumed weakness in making cross-modal associations or in abstract problem solving, or inability to "mind read" are not the kinds of neuropsychological problems that we are used to addressing pharmacologically. Theoretically, autistic people might respond to one or another of the new "memory" drugs—the cholinesterase inhibitors—but clinical trials have not been undertaken, and the anecdotal evidence to date is not encouraging.

The neurochemical models have been equally unproductive of useful treatments, at least so far. Thus, when drug treatment is applied, it is nothing if not empirical or symptomatic. It addresses the particular problems that autistic people have, not the problem of autism. It addresses the behavioral and emotional problems that autistic people have in common with other developmentally handicapped patients and not their unique attributes as autistic people.

Antipsychotic Drugs

At one time it was believed that autism was a form of infantile schizophrenia. It was reasonable, therefore, to treat autistic children with neuroleptic drugs. Low-potency neuroleptics such as chlorpromazine and thioridazine were found to be too sedating, but clinical trials of high-potency neuroleptics such as trifluoperazine, fluphenazine, and thiothixene were promising: "psychotic behavior" and hyperactivity were decreased, stereotypies were reduced, speech production improved, attention spans were longer, anergic children had more initiative, and withdrawn children were more "related" (90–92). This dramatic response to antipsychotic drugs seemed to affirm a connection between autism and schizophrenia.

Then haloperidol took center stage. It was a more potent neuroleptic, a virtually pure D_2 dopamine receptor antagonist. In autistic children, haloperidol was not only effective in controlling negative behaviors, but it was also said to improve discrimination learning (93) and the positive effects of behavioral therapy (94).

When the inevitable issue of tardive dyskinesia was finally raised, it was discovered that approximately 25% of autistic children on haloperidol developed early forms of tardive dyskinesia after only approximately 2 years of treatment (95). Then came the problems of neuroleptic malignant syndrome (96) and tardive akathisia (97). Within only a few years, the salience of neuroleptic drugs to the treatment of autistic people declined precipitously. Modern neuropsychiatrists tried to avoid such measures (98), and with a small degree of ingenuity, they hoped to achieve a good result with an alternative drug. The mood stabilizers, the new antidepressants, buspirone, clonidine, amantadine—physicians would try one or another, alone and in combination, hoping to achieve what was once so easy with haloperidol.

In fact, there was never a rationale for neuroleptic treatment in autism. Obviously, it is not a subtype of schizophrenia, and there is no compelling evidence for dopaminergic hyperactivity in the disorder. Nor did published studies of neuroleptics ever demonstrate more than short-term symptomatic improvement. Over the long term, higher doses were often necessary to achieve the same degree of behavioral control, and at higher doses, cognitive blunting and language suppression frequently outweighed the behavioral improvements. The frequent emergence of tardive akathisia after years of treatment was a major problem.

The alternative drugs, however, never achieved much success either. So when the atypical antipsychotic drugs were introduced, they came to be used more and more; today, risperidone is the most commonly prescribed psychotropic for autistic children in North America. The atypical drugs are discussed in greater detail below and again in Chapter 22.

Megavitamin Therapy

Orthomolecular treatment was introduced in the early 1950s by a few psychiatrists who added massive doses of various nutrients to the treatment regimens of their severely mentally ill patients. Orthomolecular treatment was defined as the treatment of disease by varying the concentrations of substances normally present in the human body. The idea was to correct molecular imbalance by administering the right nutrients, and their first notable contention was nicotinic acid for the treatment of schizophrenia.

In 1970, Linus Pauling, the only person ever to have won two unshared Nobel prizes, announced to an incredulous world that taking 1,000 mg of vitamin C every day reduced the occurrence of common colds. In another book he wrote in 1986, he said that megadoses of vitamins "can improve your general health...to increase your enjoyment of life and can help in controlling heart disease, cancer, and other diseases and in slowing down the process of aging (168,169)." Pauling died in 1994 at the age of 93.

In 1975, Turkel proposed the "U" series of dietary supplements for patients with Down's syndrome, and in 1981, Harrell and others reported to the National Academy of Sciences that a similar combination of high-dose vitamins and minerals increased the IQ of several mentally retarded children.

August bodies such as the National Institute of Mental Health and the American Academy of Pediatrics rejected most of the contentions made by the orthomolecular psychiatrists and deplored their methods as unscientific and potentially mischievous. A sound position at the time, I attest, having been (peripherally) involved in some of those deliberations myself. Perhaps not as sound at this time, however, as later discussion of vitamin E in the prevention of tardive dyskinesia, antioxidants in Down's syndrome, and various dietary supplements as "cognitive enhancers" shows.

So-called megavitamin therapy has been alive and well in the autism community since 1973, when Rimland first suggested that high doses of vitamin B_6 along with magnesium and other supplements led to cognitive and behavioral improvement in autistic children (170). No other such treatment has won more positive attention or has had the staying power. The glow has faded in recent years, but the whole episode deserves some attention, at least for a short diversion. The B vitamins in general, and B_6 in particular, should always be interesting to students of psychiatry.

Pyridoxine

Vitamin B_6, or pyridoxine, is widely distributed in foods, especially whole grains, meat, vegetables, and nuts. Dietary deficiency is rare, and the average daily intake is 2 to 4 mg, well in excess of the recommended intake (99,100). The metabolically active form of pyridoxine is pyridoxal phosphate (PLP), formed in the intestinal mucosa by phosphorylation and oxidation of pyridoxine. PLP is a coenzyme of numerous enzymes, e.g., decarboxylases and transaminases, most of which are involved in the metabolism of amino acids. PLP-dependent enzymes function in the synthesis of the neurotransmitters serotonin (tryptophan decarboxylase), epinephrine, norepinephrine (tyrosine carboxylase), and GABA (glutamate decarboxylase).

Deficiency or excess of B_6 can alter the metabolism of other B vitamins; B_6 deficiency may lead to vitamin C deficiency. Alcohol increases the turnover of pyridoxine, hydralazine and isoniazid are pyridoxine antagonists, and estrogens, including the oral contraceptives, seem to increase the requirement for B_6 (99). Pyridoxine deficiency can cause seizures or peripheral neuropathy.

Daily doses of 50 to 500 mg are believed to be helpful in the treatment of premenstrual syndrome, but it is not clear why. Because pyridoxine is a cofactor in the synthesis of dopamine and serotonin, it is said to have a positive effect on mood. Low levels of dopamine and serotonin lead to high levels of prolactin and aldosterone, thus explaining the fluid retention. Dopamine has an inhibitory effect on the secretion of prolactin, and estrogens decrease dopaminergic activity. Nobody is quite sure how B_6 works for premenstrual syndrome, but then its not clear that it does work. The results of controlled trials have not been impressive. Studies of pyridoxine in related conditions, such as depression associated with oral contraceptive use, suppression of lactation, postpartum depression, and emesis of pregnancy have not been impressive either (101–103).

Theoretically, pyridoxine suppresses prolactin (and stimulates growth hormone) because it enhances the synthesis of dopamine (104). However, it may also reverse the effects of L-dopa and has been used to treat the movement disorder that L-dopa sometimes causes (105). Actually, it attenuates the action of L-dopa by stimulating the peripheral decarboxylation of the drug to dopamine, which does not cross the blood-brain barrier. Whether pyridoxine really increases brain dopamine is questionable because dopa decarboxylase is not the rate-limiting enzyme for the synthesis of dopamine (106).

Pyridoxine-dependent epilepsy is a rare autosomal recessive disorder, associated with intractable seizures and a progressive encephalopathy leading to mental retardation (107). Lifelong treatment with pyridoxine is necessary to control the seizures. It is possible that a deficiency in glutamic acid decarboxylase, the enzyme that synthesizes GABA, may underlie the epileptic syndrome (108). Isoniazid overdose, which may also cause seizures, produces a decrease in brain GABA and may be treated with a single high dose of pyridoxine (109).

In B_6-dependent epilepsy, seizure control with the usual doses of pyridoxine (5 mg/kg) may not avert the development of mental retardation, but higher doses (10 mg/kg) may. The higher doses are more efficient at reducing brain levels of glutamate, an excitatory amino acid neurotransmitter (110). In cultured cells, pyridoxine reduces glutamate-induced neurotoxicity (111).

The peripheral neuropathy that occurs in cases of pyridoxine deficiency is illustrative of the role of vitamin B_6 in the synthesis of sphingomyelin (112). Pyridoxine is also used to treat the peripheral neuropathy associated with isoniazid or hydralazine. It is also used to treat carpal tunnel syndrome (200 mg/d) (113). It was surprising, therefore, to learn that megadoses of B_6 (2 to 6 g/d) caused a sensory neuropathy in seven otherwise healthy individuals who were taking the vitamin as a supplement (114). Sensory neuropathies have subsequently been reported in people who were taking much lower doses of B_6 (95,115). Sensory neuropathy has been described in no fewer than 40% of women taking pyridoxine in daily doses of 50 to 300 mg and with serum levels of B_6 above 18 ng/mL (116).

Apparently, the dorsal root ganglion cells are more vulnerable to the potential neurotoxicity of high doses of pyridoxine than the brain and spinal cord because pyridoxine does not cross the blood-brain barrier, whereas PLP, its active metabolite, does. If pyridoxine were to saturate PLP binding sites in dorsal root ganglion cells, it might even induce a relative PLP deficiency state that would be neurotoxic (112). High-dose pyridoxine neuropathy may be irreversible, but low-dose neuropathy is reversible (115,117).

Because pyridoxine is a cofactor in the synthesis of serotonin, administration of high doses of pyridoxine (500 to 1,000 mg/d) may increase brain levels of serotonin (118,119). The effect of B_6 on serotonin metabolism may be responsible for its putative effects for behavioral disorders in children (120), including attention deficit/hyperactivity disorder (121) and autism (122). Theoretically, it might also enhance the effects of serotonergic antidepressants (119).

In fact, the therapeutic utility of pyridoxine for premenstrual syndrome, carpal tunnel syndrome, behavioral disorders in children, or as augmentation for mood disorders is limited, if not dubious, despite the popularity of the vitamin and its ubiquity in various dietary supplement formulae. Is there a clinical rationale for B_6 supplementation beyond what is contained in the average multivitamin tablet or the average B complex tablet (<100 mg)?

The most vigorous arguments in favor of pyridoxine as a therapeutic agent have been raised by some of the autism people, led by Bernard Rimland, whose Autism Research Institute has been as much a source of solace and hope for the parents of autistic children as it has been a gadfly to the medical establishment. Rimland claimed that no fewer than 43% of autistic children have been helped by supplements containing pyridoxine and magnesium and that compared with various drug treatments (e.g., haloperidol, methylphenidate, diazepam), it had the most favorable ratio of benefit to side effects (122). The daily intake of pyridoxine by autistic children who were said to have responded to pyridoxine ranged from 75 to 3,000 mg (sic). The neurotoxicity of pyridoxine was ascribed to a relative deficiency of magnesium, folate, and perhaps other B vitamins induced by high-dose pyridoxine and is presumably preventable when additional supplements are taken with the B_6 (123).

The alleged benefits of pyridoxine in autism are said to occur in two dimensions: neurocognitive, e.g., improved communication and learning, and neurobehavioral, i.e., improvement in untoward behaviors such as hyperactivity and aggression. Indeed, there have been several double-blind studies published in reputable journals to support these contentions (122,124).

The recommendations on behalf of pyridoxine stem from a long line of articles in the medical, quasimedical, and lay press on behalf of various combinations of megavitamins for mentally handicapped children in general and people with Down's syndrome in particular (125–127). The reader is doubtless aware that attempts at replication have usually failed (128, 129). The mentally retarded, like the autistic, are still with us, and they are still as retarded and autistic as they were before. If pyridoxine or some other combinations of megavitamins are effective for some handicapped people, the effect is small indeed. Virtually every family I know who tried a megavitamin regimen gave it up long ago. Even the autism establishment seems to have moved on, to dimethyl glycine, to secretin, to blue-green algae, and other regimens.

Premenstrual syndrome, carpal tunnel syndrome, and treatment-refractory depression are still with us, despite vitamin B_6. One cannot really claim any specific neuropsychiatric benefit from high-dose vitamin B_6, and, especially when it is taken by itself, it can be neurotoxic.

Fenfluramine

Because high levels of the neurotransmitter serotonin were a consistent finding in studies of autistic people, it was natural to investigate the clinical efficacy of the serotonin antagonist fenfluramine, a diet pill and an atypical stimulant. In this vein, there had been unsuccessful trials of L-dopa (130) and lysergic acid diethylamide (of all things) (131), but not of Periactin (cyproheptadine) for some reason. What was interesting about fenfluramine was how quickly an uncontrolled clinical report grew to become a multicenter study. Critical judgment was suspended, it appeared, in the face of a rational treatment for autism. Fenfluramine was even said to double the IQ score of one autistic child (132). That contention alone should have raised some doubts.

As additional studies were reported, it became clear that fenfluramine was not very effective in the treatment of autism, although symptomatic improvement was seen in occasional cases. Whatever benefit fenfluramine did exert was independent of the patient's baseline serotonin levels, and the idea of a rational treatment fell by the boards. There were also troubling preclinical reports that suggested that fenfluramine, in clinically relevant doses, was neurotoxic (133).

Not many clinicians continued to prescribe fenfluramine to autistic children or adults after the initial fever passed, but the drug achieved notoriety when the *d*-isomer was combined with the amphetamine congener Ionamin (phentermine resin/lactose) for the treatment of obesity. What ensued was long-term treatment of many obese people for 2 years or more with this combination. This natural experiment was aborted because of side effects, primarily cardiac and pulmonary. Fenfluramine is gone now, but the neurotoxicity issue was never settled, at least in clinical populations. For the record, memory impairment was a not uncommon side effect of the Fen-Phen combination.

Serotonin antagonism at the 5-HT_{A2} receptor is a component of the action of atypical antipsychotics that may be relevant to their utility for the condition. On the other hand, no one can maintain that they are more effective for autism than the neuroleptics were, just that they are safer and better tolerated in the long term.

PSYCHOPHARMACOLOGY FOR AUTISTIC PEOPLE

If we accept the structure of autism as a variant of the static encephalopathies associated with mental retardation, the problem of psychopharmacology is more amenable to solution. Autism is an encephalopathy with various causes. The lesions are probably dispersed among the deep nuclei of the temporal lobe, especially the amygdala, septum, other limbic nuclei, and the frontal lobes. Cerebellar structures are probably also involved. In contrast to mental retardation, the encephalopathy of autism is more circumscribed. Rather than diffuse encephalopathy, in autism the lesions are variable in extent, which explains the wide range of cognitive dysfunction, and variable in location, which accounts for the diversity of its behavioral attributes.

Like mental retardation, autism may coexist with other neuropsychiatric syndromes such as epilepsy, Tourette's syndrome, intermittent explosive disorder, major affective disorder, and schizophrenia; that should not be surprising. All the neuropsychiatric disorders are known to overlap in some individuals: patients with Tourette's syndrome may be obsessional, epileptics may be explosive or psychotic, and schizophrenics get depressed. The ideal of perfectly discrete neuropsychiatric entities is counterintuitive and antiphysiologic. The brain is a conglomerate organ system, composed of many organs that live close together and are poorly insulated from the effects of one another. A hypoxic or viral insult to one small nucleus is likely to affect others nearby directly or indirectly through mechanisms such as kindling (134), diaschisis, or reciprocal inhibition or activation (135). The behavioral deficits that arise from such an insult will necessarily vary from person to person and from time to time, even within an individual's life span. Thus, an autistic child who is hyperactive and disorganized might develop a seizure disorder in adolescence, an explosive disorder in adult life, and then a case of early dementia.

That would be an extremely unfortunate autistic person, to be sure, but it is an illustrative case of how the practically minded neuropsychiatrist has to think, not in terms of autism but in terms of the behavioral or neuropsychiatric correlates of autism.

NEUROPSYCHIATRIC DISORDERS COMORBID WITH AUTISM

Epilepsy

Seizure disorders occur in at least one-third of all autistic people (136,137). Epilepsy may begin in infancy or during adolescence. The strong association between autism and epilepsy is one more piece of evidence in favor of an encephalopathic basis of the syndrome in the temporal and frontal lobes because these regions are much more likely to seize than the cerebellum, for example. The association should also raise one's suspicion when dealing with an autistic person who has severe behavioral problems that a psychotropic anticonvulsant may be the appropriate treatment.

The notion of subclinical epilepsy is too obscure to discuss in this chapter, but it is increasingly apparent that some nonspecific behavioral disorders have a paroxysmal structure that resembles epilepsy and that they may respond very well to antiepileptic drugs (138). Intermittent explosive disorder, with aggression, SIB, or both, may be a manifestation of subclinical epilepsy. That is an arguable point; the fact that such patients respond well to carbamazepine, valproate, or lamotrigine is not (139,140). Other clues to behavioral disorders that respond to the psychotropic anticonvulsants are disorders with wildly variable shifts in mood or behavior, rapid cyclers, nocturnal episodes, or extremely stereotyped behaviors. One sometimes hears the term organic affective disorder used to describe such patients.

Conversely, one sometimes sees autistic patients who had seizures early in life but who have been seizure free for many years and off drugs. Such patients might be referred with behavioral problems (e.g., aggressive behavior), SIB, or wildly variable mood and behavioral states. In these cases, it is usually a good idea to begin treatment with one of the psychotropic anticonvulsants. The idea is that the behavioral difficulties may be related in an obscure way to the same focus that at one time led to overt seizures.

Anxiety Disorders

It is my opinion that anxiety and clinical conditions related to anxiety are the most important psychiatric correlates of the autistic condition. In one's clinical experience with autistic people, the full range of anxiety variants are likely to be encountered: social anxiety, phobias, minor worries and repetitive questioning, anxious rumination and obsessions, somatic anxiety or hypochondriasis, panic attacks, agitation, and disorganizing agitation of psychotic dimensions. Anxiety symptoms in autistic people may be spontaneous or related to circumstances. They may come in response to an unexpected change or a demand that is impossible to satisfy. They may simply be pervasive or endogenous. Autistic symptoms, such as stereotypy and preoccupation with sameness, may be thought of as ways in which the autistic person attempts to "bind" anxiety. Angry outbursts, aggression, and self-injury may be manifestations of anxiety or panic.

The KBS model of autism predicts a degree of placidity or emotional detachment, and the latter is indeed frequently found in some autistic patients. As pointed out, however, KBS is an imperfect model of the autistic syndrome, and clinical examples of KBS (after head injury or encephalitis) are often associated with anxiety and agitation. Lesions of the amygdala and other deep temporal lobe nuclei and cerebellar lesions are often associated with anxiety. From the neuropsychological perspective, difficulties with communication, cross-modal association, perceptual inconstancy, and inability to shift attentional sets as circumstances demand may be expected to induce a state of dismay, frustration, mistrust, and anxiety. No anxiety state is quite as dramatic in all of psychiatry as that of an autistic child whose routine is interrupted or whose environment is changed.

It is unfortunate that more has not been written about the differential diagnosis of anxiety in autistic people. In a recent study of 44 children with pervasive developmental disorders, no fewer than 84% met full criteria for at least one anxiety disorder (141). School refusal, a childhood anxiety variant, is more common in autistic children compared with mentally retarded controls (142). In the families of autistic children, social phobia and obsessive-compulsive disorder (OCD) are highly prevalent (143–145).

It is sometimes hard to establish whether autistic individuals are anxious or prone to panic. Even autistic individuals with well-established verbal skills may lack the appropriate vocabulary or capacity for self-reflection to describe their inner state. The diagnosis is almost always inferential. In the past, autistic patients with anxiety or panic were said to be psychotic or agitated and were treated with neuroleptic drugs. Now clinicians are more likely to entertain the possibility that the patient may have an anxiety disorder and may use some of the usual treatments. In a recent review of psychopharmacologic treatments for autism, the following classes of drugs were said to be safe and effective, with the interesting caveat that "there are virtually no controlled data that support the efficacy of most of these drugs": benzodiazepines, beta-blockers, buspirone, guanfacine, and naltrexone, all of which are to some degree anxiolytic drugs (146). In an open-label study, the SSRI sertraline seemed good for "transition-associated anxiety" (147). Buspirone may be useful in low to moderate doses for retarded people who are autistic, anxious, aggressive, self-injurious, or disorganized (148,149).

One should never be surprised, then, when low to moderate doses of a long-acting anxiolytic drug such as oxazepam exercises a dramatic effect on an autistic individual who is emotionally unstable and prone to agitation, aggression, or running away. The success of the atypical antipsychotic drugs in autism may be related to their anxiolytic properties. Most interesting, however, are two new psychotropic anticonvulsants, gabapentin and tiagabine, two strongly GABAergic drugs that may be uniquely beneficial for some autistic people.

Obsessive-Compulsive Disorder

Of all the anxiety disorders, OCD may well be the most important psychiatric correlate of autism. Some autistic people are given to compulsive behaviors, rituals, and recurrent thoughts or ruminations. This may be especially true of high-level autistic people who are verbal and whose speech may return again and again to the same topics and phrases, often with a metallic, dysprosodic voice. Preoccupation with sameness is another autistic symptom that is sometimes interpreted as obsessional. Obsessional symptoms were discovered in almost all cases of autism in a study of 187 autistic adults (150). Tourette's syndrome, which many researchers believe is related to OCD, often coexists with autism-spectrum disorders (151). OCD and motor tics are frequently found in the families of autistic children (144).

Repetitive behaviors are not necessarily compulsions. The occurrence of pathologic repetition and cognitive rigidity is observed in a large number of neuropsychiatric syndromes: in autism and OCD certainly, and also in Tourette's syndrome. They also occur in less circumscribed conditions such as traumatic brain injury, chronic schizophrenia, dementia, and mental retardation.

Repetitive behavior encompasses a spectrum of behaviors including echolalia and echopraxia (speech and motor repetitions of another person's behavior), palilalia (the repetition of one's own utterances), mannerisms (goal-directed repetitive behaviors), stereotypy (nongoal directed repetitive behaviors performed in a uniform way), perseveration, compulsions, and ritualistic acts. Obsessions are forced or intrusive thoughts that are intense and repetitive and accompanied by a degree of discomfort, anxiety, or intensity. Cognitive rigidity is the inability to accommodate one's thinking to environmental feedback or to the exigencies of a novel situation (152).

Because repetitive behavior is one of the defining characteristics of autism, it is hardly surprising when almost all autistic patients are found to have obsessional symptoms. Whether autistic people are really obsessive-compulsive is the kind of question that nosologists like to argue about. Obviously, there are differences between the types of repetitive thoughts and behaviors of autistic people and obsessive-compulsive people (153). However, both conditions have been associated with abnormalities of the cingulate gyrus.

Whether the resemblance between autism and OCD is superficial or fundamental, the treatments overlap to a remarkable degree. There have been a few clinical trials of serotonergic antidepressants such as clomipramine and the SSRIs in autistic people with some considerable success (153–155). Published research, however, has not quite kept up with clinical practice, and among psychiatrists who treat autistic people, recourse to a serotonergic antidepressant is one of the most common remedies. The clinical response to these agents is similar to that of patients with OCD. Rituals and compulsive behaviors are reduced, anxiety, depression, and emotional instability are alleviated, the intensity of interpersonal reactions is diminished, and positive elements such as attention, productivity, and communication are increased. Aggression and SIB may also decrease. Like OCD, moderate to high doses are sometimes required, and sometimes combinations of serotonergic drugs work better than monotherapy. There does not seem to be a falloff in the drug effect as time goes by, and sometimes treatment may be successfully withdrawn after a couple of years. It is arguable that a serotonergic agent should be the first drug to try in an autistic person with compulsive behaviors, cognitive rigidity, or emotional instability.

Like OCD, autism treatment often requires the addition of other drugs to a serotonergic regimen, especially the mood stabilizers, buspirone, and the atypical antipsychotics. When the psychology of compulsive behavior is expressed in terms of tension reduction, one may reasonably expect that treatment with a serotonergic antidepressant will alleviate the discomfort that drives the behavior. If, conversely, compulsive behavior is a means to stem the anxiety that comes from a bewildering environment, because panic may be the consequence of interrupting a ritual, then treatment with a beta-blocker is indicated. (In high-level autistic people with panic attacks, a tricyclic antidepressant or benzodiazepine may also be considered.) Finally, there is the use of low-dose antipsychotics such as risperidone, olanzapine, or quetiapine, as one might consider for stereotypy, Tourette's syndrome, or SIB.

The prescription of serotonergics may be problematic, however, in developmentally handicapped individuals, especially autistic people. They seem to be particularly sensitive to SSRI-induced akathisia, disinhibition, or hypomania, and clomipramine may cause extreme irritability. The SSRIs may also cause vasodilation of the distal extremities or the auricles or severe diaphoresis.

Affective Disorders

Depression is the most common psychiatric complication of traumatic brain injury and stroke. Affective disorders are the most common psychiatric complication of mental retardation. Anxiety disorders are the main psychiatric correlate of autism. Depression and emotional instability in general, however, are by no means uncommon in autism. Despite the autistic person's "affective flattening," the "placidity" of the KBS model, and the autistic person's limited capacity for self-reflection, various types of depression are encountered.

How common is depression in autistic people? Not nearly as common as it is in the other groups listed above. It is said to be the most common comorbid state in high-level autistic adolescents and adults, at least in one small study (156). Autistic people who are depressed are found to have a higher incidence of depression in first-degree family members (157). Affective disorders are also known to occur at higher than expected rates in the families of autistic children who are not depressed (143–145,158,159). However, it is averred that "OCD, but not affective disorders, may index an underlying liability to autism" (144).

In my practice, I have seen autistic people who are prone to episodes of withdrawal and diminished interest in things, autistic people who are prone to episodes of severe emotional instability, and autistic people who are manic-depressive. I have seen autistic people who might have organic affective disorders, slow cyclers, and rapid cyclers, and they have responded well to conventional treatments with antidepressants or mood stabilizers. I have never encountered an autistic patient who was genuinely melancholic, but these days, with the new antidepressants used so widely, melancholia is not a common diagnosis in any group.

The structure of autism may well be that of a mental retardation variant, as mentioned previously, but the condition also has some unique attributes. A relatively lower vulnerability to affective disorders and a relatively higher vulnerability to anxiety disorders are not necessarily defining attributes of the autistic condition, but they seem to be characteristics.

Psychosis/Schizophrenia

We hardly ever use the term psychotic to describe the usual autistic symptoms (e.g., stereotypy, echolalia, self-stimulation, or preoccupation with sameness) or even the extremely disorganized behavior that characterizes some autistic children. The term is appropriate to apply to adults, especially high-level autistic adults who sometimes present with a manic or a schizophreniform psychosis and who may require the appropriate pharmacologic management. This is considered to be the simple coexistence of two neuropsychiatric conditions; there is no evidence that autistic people are any more prone to schizophrenia, for example, than any other group of developmentally impaired people (160,161). Conversely, schizophrenia may be overdiagnosed in autistic people with an affective psychosis or a severe panic disorder because their difficulties in communication and relating may resemble at least some of the characteristics of patients with schizophrenia.

TREATMENT FOR NONSPECIFIC SYMPTOMS OF AUTISM

Self-Injurious Behavior

SIB may be more common among autistic people than among retarded people in general, perhaps because of the unique frustration a communication-handicapped person has in dealing with the world. SIB, however, is a nonspecific symptom that does not differ in its presentation among autistic people from that in other mentally handicapped people who are not autistic. It may be constant (compulsive SIB), intermittent (paroxysmal SIB), or occasional (episodic SIB). Neither the topography nor the treatment of SIB is different in autistic people. As a rule, the therapeutic approach is the same as described in Chapters 15 and 16.

Aggression

The differential diagnosis of aggressive behavior in autistic patients is not different from that of SIB, and it is the same as in mentally retarded patients who are not autistic. In fact, many patients have aggression and SIB, and the treatments also overlap.

Three kinds of aggression occur in autistic people:

1. Affective aggression, which may be related to a seizure focus, an affective disorder, or a drug that lowers the threshold for irritability and explosiveness. Here, the usual treatments are mood stabilizers or anxiolytics.
2. Compulsive aggression, e.g., hitting, that is directed against a particular person (usually the primary caregiver) and occurs repetitively but unpredictably in the absence of irritability of an emotional explosion. One should try a serotonergic antidepressant first.
3. Aggression that occurs in the context of hyperactive/disorganized behavior and that may respond to amantadine or an atypical antipsychotic drug per the following discussion.

Abulia

The word abulia means lack of appetite, but it really refers to something else, as described in Chapter 7. Some autistic people seem to lack initiative and drive. They are content just to sit, and they have little inclination to involve themselves in activities or pastimes. When they do, it is without energy and enthusiasm. Their only verbal production (if they can talk) is to complain, whine, or demur.

This is an interesting problem and one that we occasionally encounter in patients with brain injury with lesions of the frontal convexity. It is also observed in patients with brain injury with striatal lesions, and the similarity to a cardinal feature of Parkinson's disease is probably not accidental. The success of antiparkinsonian drugs such as amantadine or bromocriptine is not that impressive, but they sometimes help.

Catatonia is sometimes observed in mentally retarded people, and some of the symptoms of catatonia, including posturing, immobility, and waxy flexibility, can overlap with abulia. In patients with psychiatric disorders, catatonia is more often a symptom of affective disorder than of schizophrenia (162). It is interesting, however, that treatment of catatonia often includes antiparkinsonian drugs (163).

Hyperactive/Disorganized Behavior

This is the one of the hardest problems to solve pharmacologically: hyperactivity, getting into everything, hypermetamorphosis, impulsive behavior, distractibility and short attention span, self-stimulation and stereotypy, emotional lability, and insomnia. This behavioral pattern is most frequent in retarded autistic children and in the past has been the occasion for treatment with neuroleptic drugs. That is a poor choice, but the problem is, what are the alternatives?

The answer is that there are quite a few alternatives, but they do not always work. Whether this is because of the nature of the behavioral disorder or the age of the patient, one cannot say, although it is my suspicion that the latter is very important. It is not uncommon for hyperactive/disorganized autistic children to improve substantially as they grow up. Alternatively, their behavioral problems may become more differentiated and thus more amenable to specific diagnosis and treatment.

The first approach is a differential diagnosis. One looks for some entree to treatment, much as one does for SIB, by examining the diagnostic alternatives—the possibility of an occult seizure disorder, a panic disorder, or a drug-induced syndrome—or by examining the treatment alternatives, or by focusing on explosive-aggressive behavior or SIB.

Stimulant drugs such as methylphenidate or amphetamine are among the most frequently prescribed treatments for autistic children, probably because they are the most common psychotropic drugs given to children, and the mention of motoric hyperactivity usually generates a stimulant prescription, especially from primary care physicians. Unfortunately, they usually do not help and often have behavioral toxicity, such as agitation or disorganization. They are indirect dopamine agonists and thus require an intact subcortical neuron to express a therapeutic effect. Because autism is, at least in part, a condition with subcortical pathology, the neural substrate that is necessary for an effective stimulant response is missing.

We have found that the excitatory amino acid antagonist amantadine is preferable to stimulants in patients with head injury who are agitated and disorganized (164) and that it works well in selected cases of hyperactive, disorganized autistic children (165). Amantadine may also be combined with a psychostimulant. It tends to augment the therapeutic effect and lessen toxicity.

When a problem is refractory to pharmacologic intervention, such as hyperactive/disorganized behavior in autistic children, one must examine the source of difficulty. The psychology of KBS would suggest that extreme degrees of exploratory behavior (hypermetamorphosis) are entirely expected, indeed physiologic, in an organism with profound derangements of sensory integration or memory. Thus, exploratory behavior would represent nothing more than a physiologic compensation for a structural deficit. Treatments aimed simply at the motor aspect of that compensation, such as the antipsychotics, will have only a limited effect. The direct-acting dopamine agonists are probably more physiologic because they are supposed to enhance cortical regulation of sensory and motor processes.

Hypervigilant/Hyperreactive Behavior

Some autistic people are intense, volatile, hypervigilant, and strongly reactive to any untoward stimuli. They may react to loud noises, crowds, exciting or unusual situations, or trivial events that would only upset an unusually sensitive individual. The reaction is usually intense: aggression, screaming, stereotypies, self-injury, or bolting. It is sometimes accompanied by symptoms of sympathetic hyperactivity: pupillary dilation, diaphoresis, tachycardia, tachypnea, or tremor.

This clinical condition is familiar to neuropsychiatrists. It is seen in during the agitated stage of coma recovery, in rare preictal states of terror, in the psychotic states of manics and schizophrenics, in agitated depression, and in panic disorders and severe anxiety. Its most enduring manifestation, however, is in the company of autistic individuals. In this group, it may be understood as an exaggeration of the preoccupation with sameness, a vulnerability to sensory overload, a panic attack, or a transient period of organic agitation.

The possibilities for pharmacologic management are as varied as the analogous states listed. Treatment may begin with a beta-blocker, or more likely of success, with an α_2 agonist. The usual antipanic treatments may be used, especially a potent benzodiazepine such as clonazepam, a long-acting benzodiazepine such as clorazepate, or one of the serotonergic antidepressants. Occasionally, one must resort to a mood stabilizer or an atypical antipsychotic. It is not uncommon to use drug combinations nor is it uncommon to achieve no more than a partial result.

The Reemergence of Antipsychotic Treatment

During the days when neuroleptics were the only antipsychotic drugs available, writers emphasized the difficulties of treating autistic people with drugs such as haloperidol: the drugs worked well, but only for a short time, higher doses were soon required for continued benefit, side effects such as tardive dyskinesia and tardive akathisia were quite common, and withdrawal from neuroleptic drugs often left the child worse off than before treatment. As a result, they believed that neuroleptic drugs were relatively contraindicated for autistic people.

The emergence of the new atypical antipsychotics has led physicians and parents to reconsider their reluctance to prescribe antipsychotic drugs to autistic people. There is not only the lower incidence of neurotoxic side effects with the newer drugs, but also what appears to be (but never proven) a superior clinical effect. As a result, treatment with drugs such as risperidone and olanzapine has become quite common for autistic people who are hyperactive/disorganized, aggressive, compulsive, self-injurious, or given to disabling stereotypies (166,167). The trend needs to be watched very closely and with an appropriate degree of doubt, but the results so far are mildly encouraging.

Ten years ago, in the face of the tardive dyskinesia/akathisia epidemic, prescribing a new neuroleptic drug was virtually abandoned in autistic patients who were hyperactive/disorganized or hypervigilant/hyperreactive. A host of different drug alternatives would be tried, in succession and in combination. Even the most creative approaches to drug treatment often failed. Thus, the arrival of the new atypical antipsychotics was greeted by clinicians with a sense of relief. Finally, there was something that worked as well as haloperidol once did, with fewer troublesome side effects and with (perhaps) more enduring effects. Informal surveys within the past year indicate that risperidone is the most commonly prescribed psychotropic drug for autistic people in North America.

It is interesting to reflect, after so much discussion about autism and its vicissitudes, that drug treatment has largely returned to where it was 50 years ago when Barbara Fish first began to study antipsychotic drugs for schizophrenic children. It would seem that all we have accomplished in the interval was to add the capacity for 5-HT_{2a} antagonism to the antipsychotic molecule.

AUTISM: A TREATMENT SUMMARY

That is a cynical point of view. The pharmacologic management of behavioral and emotional problems associated with autism has advanced well beyond an automatic recourse to antipsychotic drug treatment. The psychopharmacologist has a wealth of alternatives from which to choose, depending on the nature of the patient's difficulties, his or her age and developmental level, and comorbid conditions.

Hyperactivity drugs include all the stimulants, which are sometimes problematic to be sure, but their effects may be augmented and their side effects minimized by using amantadine, clonidine, or guanfacine.

Anxiety drugs include the benzodiazepines, which are underused in autistic people, beta-blockers, clonidine, guanfacine, and naltrexone. Gabapentin and tiagabine may well be the best of the lot, at least for autistic people.

Anticompulsive drugs, if one may coin a term, are primarily the serotonergic antidepressants. The similarities between autism and OCD may be fundamental or simply superficial. When repetitive thoughts or behaviors are problematic in autistic people, however, they may be treated just as one would treat people with OCD.

Mood-stabilizing drugs, especially the psychotropic antiepileptic drugs, have a wide range of clinical utility in autism that has not been fully explored.

Cognitive enhancers and neuroprotectant drugs, discussed at length in Chapter 25, represent a new and largely uncharted approach to the problem of autism.

Atypical antipsychotic drugs are always the fallback treatment for autistic people for hyperactivity, anxiety, repetitive behaviors, aggression, SIB, mood instability, and even cognitive enhancement. Their utility for so many autism-related behavioral difficulties suggests a specific action against some essential component of the autistic condition; their limited utility and the frequent development of tolerance to their clinical effects, however, suggest that their effect is nonspecific and far from whatever it is that comprises an essential element of autism.

REFERENCES

1. Wing L. The handicaps of autistic children—a comparative study. *J Child Psychol Psychiatry* 1969;10:1–40.
2. Wing L, Gould J. Severe impairments of social interaction and associated abnormalities in children: epidemiology and classification. *J Autism Dev Disord* 1979;9:11–30.
3. Berney TP. Autism—an evolving concept. *Br J Psychiatry* 2000;176:20–25.
4. Bartak L, Rutter M. Differences between mentally retarded and normally intelligent autistic children. *J Autism Child Schizophr* 1976;6:108–120.
5. Ciaranello AL, Ciaranello RD. The neurobiology of infantile autism. *Annu Rev Neurosci* 1995;18:101–128.
6. Trottier G, Srivastava LP, Walker CP. Etiology of infantile autism: a review of recent advances in genetic and neurobiological research. *J Psychiatry Neurosci* 1999;24:103–115.
7. Folstein S, Rutter M. Infantile autism: a genetic study of 21 twin pairs. *J Child Psychol Psychiatry* 1977;18:297–321.
8. Wassink T, Piven J. The molecular genetics of autism. *Curr Psychiatry Rep* 2000;2:170–175.
9. Le Couteur A, Bailey A, Goode S, et al. A broader phenotype of autism: the clinical spectrum in twins. *J Child Psychol Psychiatry* 1996;37:785–801.
10. Hanley HG, Stahl SM, Freedman DX. Hyperserotonemia and amine metabolites in autistic and retarded children. *Arch Gen Psychiatry* 1977;34:521–531.
11. Retz W, Kornhuber J, Riederer P. Neurotransmission and the ontogeny of human brain. *J Neural Transm* 1996;103:403–419.
12. Meltzer HY, Lowy MT. The serotonin hypothesis of depression. In: Meltzer HY, ed. *Psychopharmacology: the third generation of progress*. New York: Raven Press, 1987:513–526.
13. Chugani DC, Muzik O, Behen M, et al. Developmental changes in brain serotonin synthesis capacity in autistic and nonautistic children. *Ann Neurol* 1999;45:287–295.
14. Buitelaar J, Willemsen-Swinkels S. Autism: current theories regarding its pathogenesis and implications for rational pharmacotherapy. *Pediatr Drugs* 2000;2:67–81.
15. Cook E. Autism: review of neurochemical investigation. *Synapse* 1990;6:292–308.
16. Snyder SH. Opiate receptors in the brain. *N Engl J Med* 1977;296:266–271.
17. Panskepp JA. A neurochemical theory of autism. *Trends Neurosci* 1979;July:174–177.
18. Gillberg C. Endogenous opioids and opiate antagonists in autism: brief review of empirical findings and implications for clinicians. *Dev Med Child Neurol* 1995;37:239–245.
19. Chamberlain R, Herman B. A novel biochemical model linking dysfunctions in brain melatonin, proopiomelanocortin peptides, and serotonin in autism. *Biol Psychiatry* 1990;28:773–793.
20. Campbell M, Adams P, Small AM, et al. Naltrexone in infantile autism. *Psychopharmacol Bull* 1988;24:135–139.
21. Knivsberg A, Wiig K, Lind G, et al. Dietary intervention in autistic syndromes. *Brain Dysfunct* 1990;3:315–327.
22. Knivsberg A. Urine patterns, peptide levels and IgA/IgG antibodies to food proteins in children with dyslexia. *Pediatr Rehabil* 1997;1:25–33.
23. Lucarelli S, Frediani T, Zingoni A, et al. Food allergy and infantile autism. *Panminerva Med* 1995;37:137–141.
24. Horvath K, Stefanatos G, Sokolski KN, et al. Improved social and language skills after secretin administration in patients with autistic spectrum disorders. *J Assoc Acad Minor Phys* 1998;9:9–15.
25. Owley T, Steele E, Corsello C, et al. A double-blind, placebo-controlled trial of secretin for the treatment of autistic disorder. *Med Gen Med* 1999;Oct 6:E2.
26. Chez MG, Buchanan CP, Bagan BT, et al. Secretin and autism: a two-part clinical investigation. *J Autism Dev Disord* 2000;30:87–94.
27. Dunn-Geir J, Ho H, Auersperg E, et al. Effect of secretin on children with autism: a randomized controlled trial. *Dev Med Child Neurol* 2000;42:796–802.
28. Pueschel S, Romano C, Failla P, et al. A prevalence study of celiac disease in persons with Down syndrome residing in the United States of America. *Acta Paediatr* 1999;88:953–956.
29. Morris M, Yiannakou J, King A, et al. Coeliac disease and Down syndrome: associations not due to genetic linkage on chromosome 21. *Scand J Gastroenterol* 2000;35:177–180.
30. Catassi C, Fabiani E. The spectrum of coeliac disease in children. *Baillieres Clin Gastroenterol* 1997;11:485–507.
31. Reeves G, Burns C, Hall S, et al. The measurement of IgA and IgG transglutaminase antibodies in celiac disease: a comparison with current diagnostic methods. *Pathology* 2000;32:181–185.
32. Kristoferitsch W, Pointner H. Progressive cerebellar syndrome in adult coeliac disease. *J Neurol* 1987;234:116–118.
33. Collin P, Pirttila T, Nurmikko T, et al. Celiac disease, brain atrophy, and dementia. *Neurology* 1991;41:372–375.
34. Piatella L, Zamponi N, Cardinali C, et al. Endocranial calcifications, infantile celiac disease, and epilepsy. *Children Nerv Syst* 1993;9:172–175.
35. De Santis A, Addolorato G, Romito A, et al. Schizophrenic symptoms and SPECT abnormalities in a coeliac patient: regression after a gluten-free diet. *J Intern Med* 1997;242:421–423.
36. Corvaglia L, Catamo R, Pepe G, et al. Depression in adult untreated celiac subjects: diagnosis by the pediatrician. *Am J Gastroenterol* 1999;94:839–843.
37. Wakefield A, Murch S, Anthony A, et al. Ileal-lymphoid-nodular hyperplasia, non-specific colitis, and pervasive developmental disorder in children. *Lancet* 1998;351:637–641.
38. Kawashima H, Mori T, Kashiwagi Y, et al. Detection and sequencing of measles virus from peripheral mononuclear cells from patients with inflammatory bowel disease and autism. *Dig Dis Sci* 2000;45:723–729.

39. Ornitz E, Ritvo E. The syndrome of autism: a critical review. *Am J Psychiatry* 1976;133:609–621.
40. Bauman M, Kemper TL. Histoanatomic observations of the brain in early infantile autism. *Neurology* 1985;35:866–874.
41. Ritvo ER, Freeman BJ, Scheibel AB, et al. Lower Purkinje cell counts in the cerebella of four autistic subjects: initial findings of the UCLA-NSAC Autopsy Research Report. *Am J Physiol* 1986;143:862–866.
42. Courchesne EPD, Townsend J, Saitoh O. The brain in infantile autism: posterior fossa structures are abnormal. *Neurology* 1994;44:214–223.
43. Kemper TL, Bauman M. Neuropathology of infantile autism. *J Neuropathol Exp Neurol* 1998;57:645–652.
44. Martin P, Albers M. Cerebellum and schizophrenia: a selective review. *Schizophr Rev* 1995;21:241–251.
45. Haas RH, Townsend J, Courchesne EPD, et al. Neurologic abnormalities in infantile autism. *J Child Neurol* 1996;11:84–92.
46. Ciesielski KT, Knight JE. Cerebellar abnormality in autism: a nonspecific effect of early brain damage? *Acta Neurobiol Exp* 1994;54:151–154.
47. Connolly AM, Dodson WE, Prensky AL, et al. Course and outcome of acute cerebellar ataxia. *Ann Neurol* 1994;35:673–679.
47a. Sherrington CS. *The integrative action of the nervous system.* New York: Scribners, 1906.
48. Gilman S. Cerebellar control of movement. *Ann Neurol* 1994;353–354.
49. Leiner HC, Leiner AL, Dow RS. The human cerebrocerebellar system: its computing, cognitive and language skills. *Behav Brain Res* 1991;44:113–128.
50. Murakami JW, Courchesne E, Press GA, et al. Reduced cerebellar hemisphere size and its relationship to vermal hypoplasia in autism. *Arch Neurol* 1989;46: 689–694.
51. Bobee S, Mariette E, Tremblay-Leveau H, et al. Effects of early midline cerebellar lesion on cognitive and emotional functions in the rat. *Behav Brain Res* 2000;112:107–117.
52. Macklis RM, Macklis JD. Historical and phrenologic reflections on the nonmotor functions of the cerebellum: love under the tent? *Neurology* 1992;42:928–932.
53. Canavan AGM, Sprengelmeyer R, Diener H-C, et al. Conditional associative learning is impaired in cerebellar disease in humans. *Behav Neurosci* 1994;108: 475–485.
54. Infeld BMBF, Davis SM, Lichtenstein MMBF, et al. Crossed cerebellar diaschisis and brain recovery after stroke. *Stroke* 1995;26:90–95.
55. Botez JI, Leveille J, Lambert R, et al. Single photon emission computed tomography (SPECT) in cerebellar disease: cerebello-cerebral diaschisis. *Eur Neurol* 1991;31:405–412.
56. Di Piero V, Chollet F, Dolan RJ, et al. The functional nature of cerebellar diaschisis. *Stroke* 1990;21: 1365–1369.
57. Tanaka M, Kondo S, Hirai S, et al. Crossed cerebellar diaschisis accompanied by hemiataxia: a PET study. *J Neurol Neurosurg Psychiatry* 1992;55:121–125.
58. Deb S, Thompson B. Neuroimaging in autism. *Br J Psychiatry* 1998;173:299–302.
59. Hauser SL, Rosman NP. Pneumographic findings in the infantile autism syndrome. *Brain* 1975;98:667–688.
60. Maurer RG. Neuropsychology of autism. *Psychiatr Clin North Am* 1986;9:367–380.
61. Kl,ver H, Bucy KH. Preliminary analysis of functions of the temporal lobes in monkeys. *Arch Neurol Psychiatry* 1939;42:979–1000.
62. Brown S, Schafer EA. An investigation into the functions of the occipital and temporal lobes of the monkey's brain. *Philos Trans R Soc Lond B Biol Sci* 1988;179:303–327.
63. Klüver H, Bucy PC. "Psychic blindness" and other symptoms following temporal lobectomy in rhesus monkey. *Am J Physiol* 1937;119:352–353.
64. Klüver H, Bucy PC. An analysis of certain effects of bilateral temporal lobectomy in the rhesus monkey, with special reference to psychic blindness. *J Psychol* 1938;5:33–34.
65. Terzian H, Ore GD. Syndrome of Kl,ver and Bucy: reproduced in man by bilateral removal of the temporal lobes. *Neurology* 1955;5:373–380.
66. Levitt P. Monoclonal antibody to limbic system neurons. *Science* 1984;223:299–301.
67. Esiri MM. Herpes simplex encephalitis: an immunohistological study of the distribution of viral antigen within the brain. *J Neurol Sci* 1982;54:209–226.
68. Damasio AR, Van Hoesen GW. The limbic system and the localisation of herpes simplex encephalitis. *J Neurol Neurosurg Psychiatry* 1985;48:297–301.
69. Bakchine S, Chain F, Lhermitte F. Syndrome de Klüver-Bucy humain complet apres une encephalite a herpes simplex type 2. *Rev Neurol* 1986;142:126–132.
70. Gerstenbrand F, Aichner PF, Saltuari L. Klüver-Bucy syndrome in man: experiences with postraumatic cases. *Neurosci Biobehav Rev* 1983;7:413–417.
71. Lilly R, Cummings JL, Benson F, et al. The human Klüver-Bucy syndrome. *Neurology* 1983;33:1141–1145.
72. Sandson TA, Lilly RB, Sodkol M. Klüver-Bucy syndrome associated with delayed post-anoxic leucoencephalopathy following carbon monoxide poisoning. *J Neurol Neurosurg Psychiatry* 1988;51:156–157.
73. Cummings JL, Duchen LW. Klüver-Bucy dyndrome in Pick disease: clinical and pathologic correlations. *Neurology* 1981;31:1415–1422.
74. Murray EA, Mishkin M. Amygdalectomy impairs crossmodal association in monkeys. *Science* 1985; 228:604–605.
75. Scoville WB, Milner B. Loss of recent memory after bilateral hippocampal lesions. *J Neurol Neurosurg Psychiatry* 1957;20:11–21.
76. Mishkin M. Memory in monkeys severely impaired by combined but not by separate removal of amygdala and hippocampus. *Nature* 1978;275:297–298.
77. Zola-Morgan S, Squire LR, Mishkin M. The neuroanatomy of amnesia: amygdala-hippocampus versus temporal stem. *Science* 1982;218:1337–1339.
78. Baron-Cohen S, Ring HA, Bullmore ET, et al. The amygdala theory of autism. *Neurosci Biobehav Rev* 2000;24:355–364.
79. Happe F, Frith U. The neuropsychology of autism. *Brain* 1996;119:1377–1400.
80. Rumsey JM, Hamburger SD. Neuropsychological findings in high-functioning men with infantile autism, residual state. *J Clin Exp Neuropsychol* 1988; 10:201–221.
81. Leslie AM, Frith U. Metarepresentation and autism:

how not to lose one's marbles. *Cognition* 1987;27: 291–294.
82. Bailey AJ. Editorial: the biology of autism. *Psychol Med* 1993;23:7–11.
83. Waterhouse L, Modahl C, Fein D. Neurofunctional mechanisms in autism. *Psychol Rev* 1996;103:457–489.
84. Critchley HD, Daly DM, Bullmore ET, et al. The functional neuroanatomy of social behaviour: changes in cerebral blood flow when people with autistic disorder process facial expressions. *Brain* 2000;123:2203–2212.
85. Glickstein M. Cerebellar agenesis. *Brain* 1994;117: 1209–1212.
86. Silveri MC, Leggio MG, Molinari M. The cerebellum contributes to linguistic production: a case of agrammatic speech following a right cerebellar lesion. *Neurology* 1994;44:2047–2050.
87. Kling AS, Tachiki K, Lloyd R. Neurochemical correlates of the Klüver-Bucy syndrome by in vivo microdialysis in monkey. *Behav Brain Res* 1993;56:161–170.
88. Evans RW, Clay TH, Gualtieri CT. Carbamazepine in pediatric psychiatry. *J Am Acad Child Psychiatry* 1987; 26:2–8.
89. Slaughter J, Bobo W, Childers MK. Selective serotonin reuptake inhibitor treatment of post-traumatic Klüver-Bucy syndrome. *Brain Inj* 1999;13:59–62.
90. Wolpert A, Quintos A, White L, et al. Thiothixene and chlorprothixene in behavior disorders. *Curr Ther Res* 1968;10:566–569.
91. Campbell M, Fish B, Shapiro T, et al. Acute responses of schizophrenic children to a sedative and a "stimulating" neuroleptic: a pharmacologic yardstick. *Curr Ther Res* 1972;14:759–766.
92. Engelhardt DM, Polizos P, Waizer J, et al. A double-blind comparison of fluphenazine and haloperidol on outpatient schizophrenic children. *J Autism Child Schizophr* 1973;3:128–137.
93. Anderson LT, Campbell M, Grega DM, et al. Haloperidol in the treatment of infantile autism: effects on learning and behavioral symptoms. *Am J Psychiatry* 1984;141:1195–1202.
94. Campbell M, Anderson LT, Meier M, et al. A comparison of haloperidol and behavior therapy and their interaction in autistic children. *J Am Acad Child Psychiatry* 1978;17:640–655.
95. Perry R, Campbell M, Green WH, et al. Neuroleptic-related dyskinesias in autistic children: a prospective study. *Psychopharmacol Bull* 1985;21:140–143.
96. Guze BH, Baxter LR. Neuroleptic malignant syndrome. *N Engl J Med* 1985;313:163–166.
97. Barnes TRE, Braude WM. Akathisia variants and tardive dyskinesia. *Arch Gen Psychiatry* 1985;42:874–878.
98. Gualtieri CT, Barnhill LJ. Tardive dyskinesia in special populations. In: Wolf ME, Mosnaim AD, eds. *Tardive dyskinesia, biological mechanisms & clinical aspects*. Washington, DC: American Psychiatric Press, 1988: 137–154.
99. Mason P. Handbook of dietary supplements. Oxford: Blackwell Science, 1998.
100. Combs G. *The vitamins: fundamental aspects in nutrition and health*, 2nd ed. San Diego: Academic Press, 1998.
101. Livingston S. *Drug therapy for epilepsy*. Springfield, IL: Charles C Thomas, 1966.
102. Williams MJ, Harris RI, Dean BC. Controlled trial of pyridoxine in the premenstrual syndrome. *J Int Med Res* 1985;13:174–179.
103. Kleijnen J, Knipschild P. Ginkgo biloba for cerebral insufficiency. *Br J Clin Pharmacol* 1992;34:352–358.
104. Moretti C, Fabbri A, Gnessi L, et al. Pyridoxine (B6) suppresses the rise in prolactin and increases the rise in growth hormone induced by exercise. *N Engl J Med* 1982;307:444–445.
105. DeVeaugh-Geiss J, Manion L. High-dose pyridoxine in tardive dyskinesia. *J Clin Psychiatry* 1978;39:573–575.
106. Guilarte TR. Effect of vitamin B6 nutrition on the levels of dopamine, dopamine metabolites, dopa decarboxylase activity, tyrosine, and GABA in the developing rat corpus striatum. *Neurochem Res* 1989; 14:571–578.
107. Goutieres F, Aicardi J. Atypical presentations of pyridoxine-dependent seizures: A treatable cause of intractable epilepsy in infants. *Ann Neurol* 1985;17: 117–120.
108. Gospe SM Jr, Olin KL, Keen CL. Reduced GABA synthesis in pyridoxine-dependent seizures. *Lancet* 1994;343:1133–1134.
109. Wason S, Lacouture PG, Lovejoy FH Jr. Single high-dose pyridoxine treatment for isoniazid overdose. *JAMA* 1981;246:1102–1104.
110. Baumeister FA, Gsell W, Shin YS, et al. Glutamate in pyridoxine-dependent epilepsy: neurotoxic glutamate concentration in the cerebrospinal fluid and its normalization by pyridoxine. *Pediatrics* 1994;94:318–321.
111. Kaneda K, Kikuchi M, Kashii S, et al. Effects of B vitamins on glutamate-induced neurotoxicity in retinal cultures. *Eur J Pharmacol* 1997;322:259–264.
112. Rudman D, Williams PJ. Megadose vitamins. Use and misuse. *N Engl J Med* 1983;309:488–490.
113. Bernstein AL, Dinesen JS. Brief communication: effect of pharmacologic doses of vitamin B6 on carpal tunnel syndrome, electroencephalographic results and pain. *J Am Coll Nutr* 1993;12:73–76.
114. Schaumberg H, Kaplan J, Windebank A, et al. Sensory neuropathy from pyridoxine abuse. *N Engl J Med* 1983;309:445–448.
115. Dalton K, Dalton MJT. Characteristics of pyridoxine overdose neuropathy syndrome. *Acta Neurol Scand* 1987;76:8–11.
116. Wright G, Galloway L, Kim J, et al. Bupropion in the long-term treatment of cyclic mood disorders mood stabilizing effects. *J Clin Psychiatry* 1985;46:22–24.
117. Albin RL, Albers JW. Long-term follow-up of pyridoxine-induced acute sensory neuropathy-neuronopathy. *Neurology* 1990;40.
118. Dakshinamurti K, Sharma SK, Bonke D. Influence of B vitamins on binding properties of serotonin receptors in the CNS of rats. *Klin Wochenschr* 1990;68: 142–145.
119. Hartvig P, Lindner KJ, Bjurling P, et al. Pyridoxine effect on synthesis rate of serotonin in the monkey brain measured with positron emission tomography. *J Neural Transm* 1995;102:91–97.
120. Glazor W, Moore DC, Schooler NR, et al. Tardive dyskinesia: a discontinuation study. *Arch Gen Psychiatry* 1984;41:623–627.
121. Coleman M, Steinberg G, Tippett J, et al. A preliminary study of the effect of pyridoxine administration in a subgroup of hyperkinetic children: a double-blind

crossover comparison with methylphenidate. *Biol Psychiatry* 1979;14:741–751.
122. Rimland B. Controversies in the treatment of autistic children: vitamin and drug therapy. *J Child Neurol* 1988;3:68–72.
123. Rimland B. *Form letter regarding high dosage vitamin B6 and magnesium therapy for autism and related disorders*. San Diego: ICBR, 1989.
124. Martineau J, Barthelemy C, Roux S, et al. Electrophysiological effects of fenfluramine or combined vitamin B6 and magnesium on children with autistic behavior. *Dev Med Child Neurol* 1989;31:721–727.
125. Turkel H. Medical amelioration of Down's syndrome incorporating the orthomolecular approach. *Orthomol Psychiatry* 1975;4:102–115.
126. Harrell RF, Capp RH, Davis DR, et al. Can nutritional supplements help mentally retarded children? An exploratory study. *Proc Natl Acad Sci U S A* 1981;78: 574–578.
127. Boggs UR, Scheaf A, Santoro D, et al. The effect of nutrient supplements on the biological and psychological characteristics of low IQ, preschool children. *J Orthomol Psychiatry* 1985;14:98–127.
128. Smith GF, Spiker D, Peterson C, et al. Failure of vitamin/mineral supplementation in Down syndrome. *Lancet* 1983;41.
129. Menolascino FJ, Donaldson JY, Gallagher TF, et al. Vitamin supplements and purported learning enhancement in mentally retarded children. *J Nutr Sci Vitaminol* 1989;35:181–192.
130. Campbell M, Small AM, Collins PJ, et al. Levodopa and levoamphetamine: a crossover study in schizophrenic children. *Curr Ther Res* 1976;18:70–86.
131. Bender L, Cobrinik L, Faretra G, et al. The treatment of childhood schizophrenia with LSD and UML. In: Rinkel M, ed. *Biological treatment of mental illness*. New York: LC Page, 1966:84–92.
132. Geller E, Ritvo ER, Freeman BJ, et al. Preliminary observations on the effect of fenfluramine on blood serotonin and symptoms in three autistic children. *N Engl J Med* 1982;307:165–169.
133. Schuster CR, Lewis M, Seiden LS. Fenfluramine: neurotoxicity. *Psychopharmacol Bull* 1985;22:148–151.
134. Post RM, Putnam F, Contel NR, et al. Electroconvulsive seizures inhibit amygdala kindling: implications for mechanisms of action in affective illness. *Epilepsia* 1984;25:234–239.
135. Moscovitch M. Information processing and the cerebral hemispheres. In: Gazzaniga MS, ed. *Handbook of behavioral neurobiology: neuropsychology*. New York: Plenum,1979:379–446.
136. Deykin EY, Macmahon B. The incidence of seizures among children with autistic symptoms. *Am J Psychiatry* 1979;136:1310–1312.
137. Olsson I, Steffenburg S, Gillberg C. Epilepsy in autism and autisticlike conditions: a population based study. *Arch Neurol* 1988;45:666–668.
138. Monroe RR. Limbic ictus and atypical psychosis. *J Nerv Ment Dis* 1982;170:711–716.
139. McElroy SL, Keck PE, Pope HG. Sodium valproate: its use in primary psychiatric disorders. *J Clin Psychopharmacol* 1987;7:16–24.
140. Evans RW, Gualtieri CT, Patterson DR. Treatment of chronic closed head injury with psychostimulant drugs: a controlled case study and an appropriate evaluation procedure. *J Nerv Ment Dis* 1987;175:106–110.
141. Muris P, Steerneman P, Merckelbach H, et al. Comorbid anxiety symptoms in children with pervasive developmental disorders. *J Anxiety Disord* 1998;12:387–393.
142. Kurita H. School refusal in pervasive developmental development disorders. *J Autism Dev Disord* 1991;21: 1–15.
143. Smalley SL, McCracken J, Tanguay P. Autism, affective disorders, and social phobia. *Am J Med Genet* 1995;60:19–26.
144. Bolton PF, Pickles A, Murphy M, et al. Autism, affective and other psychiatric disorders: patterns of familial aggregation. *Psychol Med* 1998;28:385–395.
145. Piven J, Palmer P. Psychiatric disorder and the broad autism phenotype: evidence from a family study of multiple autism families. *Am J Psychiatry* 1999;156: 557–563.
146. Riddle MA, Bernstein GA, Cook EH, et al. Anxiolytics, adrenergic agents, and naltrexone. *J Am Acad Child Psychiatry* 1999;38:546–556.
147. Steingard RJ, Zimnitzky B, DeMaso DR, et al. Sertraline treatment of transition-associated anxiety and agitation in children with autistic disorder. *J Child Adolesc Psychopharmacol* 1997;7:9–15.
148. Ratey J, Sovner R, Mikkelsen E, et al. Buspirone therapy for maladaptive behavior and anxiety in developmentally disabled persons. *J Clin Psychiatry* 1989;50: 382–384.
149. McCormick LH. Treatment with buspirone in a patient with autism. *Arch Fam Med* 1997;6:368–370.
150. Kobayashi R, Murata T. Behavioral characteristics of 187 young adults with autism. *Psychiatry Clin Neurosci* 1998;52:383–390.
151. Kadesjo B, Gillberg C. Tourette's disorder: epidemiology and comorbidity in primary school children. *J Am Acad Child Psychiatry* 2000;39:548–555.
152. Ames D, Cummings JL, Wirshing WC, et al. Repetitive and compulsive behavior in frontal lobe degenerations. *J Neuropsychiatry Clin Neurosci* 1994;6:100–113.
153. McDougle CJ, Kresch LE, Posey DJ. Repetitive thoughts and behavior in pervasive developmental disorder: treatment with serotonin reuptake inhibitors. *J Autism Dev Disord* 2000;30:427–435.
154. Gordon C. A double-blind comparison of clomipramine, desipramine and placebo in the treatment of autistic disorders. *Arch Gen Psychiatry* 1993;50: 441–447.
155. McDougle CJM, Naylor STR, Cohen DJM, et al. A double-blind, placebo-controlled study of fluvoxamine in adult with autistic disorder. *Arch Gen Psychiatry* 1996;53:1001–1008.
156. Ghaziuddin M, Weidmer-Mikhail E, Ghaziuddin N. Comorbidity of Asperger syndrome: a preliminary report. *J Intellect Disabil Res* 1998;42:279–283.
157. Ghaziuddin M, Greden J. Depression in children with autism/pervasive developmental disorders: a case-control family history study. *J Autism Dev Disord* 1998; 28:111–115.
158. Gold N. Depression and social adjustment in siblings of boys with autism. *J Autism Dev Disord* 1993;23: 147–163.
159. Nasr A, Roy M. Association of a balanced chromosomal translocation (4; 12) (q21.3; q15), affective dis-

order and autism. *J Intellect Disabil Res* 2000;44: 170–174.
160. Green WH, Campbell M, Hardesty ASP, et al. A comparison of schizophrenic and autistic children. *J Am Acad Child Psychiatry* 1984;23:399–409.
161. Volkmar FR, Cohen DJ. Comorbid association of autism and schizophrenia. *Am J Psychiatry* 1991;148: 1705–1707.
162. Taylor MA, Abrams R. Catatonia prevalence and importance in the manic phase of manic depressive illness. *Arch Gen Psychiatry* 1977;34:1223–1225.
163. Baldessarini RJ. *Chemotherapy in psychiatry*. Cambridge: Harvard University Press, 1977.
164. Chandler MC, Barnhill JB, Gualtieri CT. Amantadine for the agitated head-injury patient. *Brain Inj* 1988; 2:309–311.
165. Chandler M, Barnhill LJ, Gualtieri CT. Amantadine: profile of use in the developmentally disabled. In: Ratey JJ, ed. *Mental retardation: developing pharmacotherapies*. Washington, DC: American Psychiatric Press, 1991:139–162.
166. McDougle CJ, Holmes JP, Carlson DC, et al. A double-blind, placebo-controlled study of risperidone in adults with autistic disorder and other pervasive developmental disorders. *Arch Gen Psychiatry* 1998;55: 633–641.
167. Potenza MN, Holmes JP, Kanes SJ, et al. Olanzapine treatment of children, adolescents, and adults with pervasive developmental disorders: an open-label pilot study. *J Clin Psychopharmacol* 1999;19:37–44.
168. Pauling L. Evolution and the need for ascorbic acid. Proceedings in the National Academy of Sciences 1970;67:1743–1748.
169. Pauling L, Moertel C. A proposition: megadoses of vitamin C are valuable in the treatment of cancer. *Nutritional Review* 1986;44:28–32.
170. Rimland B. Infantile autism: status of research. *Canadian Psychiatry Assoc J* 1974;19:130–135.

15
The Problem of Self-injurious Behavior

SUMMARY

Self-injurious behavior (SIB) is an extraordinary condition that can arise in diverse circumstances. It occurs most commonly, however, in mentally retarded people, in pathobehavioral syndromes such as Lesch-Nyhan syndrome (LNS) and de Lange syndrome, and in severely retarded people who are subjected to sensorimotor or environmental deprivation or chronic pain. It is not uncommon in patients with traumatic brain injury, especially during the unstable period of confusion and agitation that follows emergence from coma.

LNS is characterized by abnormal purine metabolism, cognitive impairment, dystonia, and self-mutilatory behavior (SMB). The genetics and neuropharmacology of LNS have been understood for many years. An animal model derived from this research is based on supersensitivity of the D_1 dopamine (DA) receptor. This model generated a series of clinical studies in patients with severe and refractory SIB. The mixed DA blocker fluphenazine (FPZ) was found to be successful in reducing or eliminating SIB in most cases, and the effect was sustained over long-term follow-up.

Not every self-injurious patient, however, responds to treatment with D_1 antagonists; other treatments and other models of SIB are also pertinent. SIB has been related to abnormalities in serotonin metabolism, and the mostly favorable experience with serotonergic drugs is reviewed here. SIB has also been related to abnormalities in the opiate system; it has been proposed that SIB is an autoaddiction, as it were, to endogenous opiates. Clinical experience with the opiate antagonist naltrexone has been mixed, but that may be because long-term treatment is necessary.

The neuropharmacologic models of SIB have been productive, at least to a degree, but it is important to recognize that SIB is not a unitary disorder. It can arise as a symptom of many different conditions including epilepsy, chronic pain, neuropathies, dysautonomia, and neurotoxic drug effects. The proper treatment of SIB should begin with a careful and wide-ranging differential diagnosis.

SELF-INJURIOUS BEHAVIOR

SIB is an extraordinary affliction of human behavior. The term refers to repetitive acts of physical violence directed against oneself. It occurs most commonly in mentally retarded people, in the past, as many as 14% of those who reside in institutions (1) and an equal number in community-based facilities (Phillips, unpublished, 1988).

Although most cases of SIB involve people who are mentally retarded, especially the severely retarded, it is not by any means restricted to retarded people. It occurs in the form of head banging as a developmental variant in normal infants, although it rarely causes tissue damage (2). It is not uncommon in the chronically mentally ill, especially schizophrenics and people with borderline personality disorder, although it is more likely to be paroxysmal and self-mutilatory in those patients (3). It was a ritual experience in certain primitive people (3), is common among incarcerated criminals, and occurs on occasion in present-day torture victims.

Caged animals sometimes engage in self-mutilation, for example, psittacine birds pluck their chest feathers and gouge their pectoral muscles if they are isolated and unhappy. Rhinos grind their noses against a wall, repetitively, compulsively, reducing their horns to mere nubs.

Therefore, SIB is not a rare occurrence by any means, but it is an extraordinary event whenever it occurs. It is one of those behaviors that affect caregivers as much as patients or even more. It is not only the pain, disfigurement, and horror it conveys; it is the vexing question of why such a thing should happen at all. What psychology can possibly explain it?

It is a vexing question indeed. One might as well ask where evil comes from or ponder the theodicy problem. I am hardly inclined to do either, at least in this chapter.

BACKGROUND

My introduction to the problem of SIB was 25 years ago with a group of behavioral psychologists at a nearby residential facility for mentally retarded people. They had an impressive program, and the staff was remarkably effective at reducing, even eliminating, SIB in many individuals, and they were not trivial cases. Most of the patients had spent years in restraints, wearing football helmets, face guards, and arm splints, and taking massive doses of sedating drugs.

At the time, it seemed that the best treatments for SIB were the various behavioral interventions such as contingent restraint, differential reinforcement, and overcorrection (4). There was very little in the way of effective pharmacotherapy for SIB. High doses of sedating neuroleptics were the prevailing treatment. Every year the doses were higher, and the effects of treatment were less impressive.

Conversely, successful behavior modification for severe SIB required an extraordinary investment of time and professional effort, and good behaviorists who could mount such efforts were always few. As a result, intensive behavioral treatment was available only to a minority of people with SIB. Restraint with helmets, handcuffs, or leather straps represented the usual treatment for most people with SIB. In the real world, away from research institutions, behavioral treatments were as heavy-handed as high-dose chlorpromazine. Aversive conditioning was often used.

As the years passed, the allure of intensive behavioral treatment for SIB waned. The treatment worked, but its expense was daunting, and the positive effects were often lost after the treatment ended. At the same time, there were stirrings of interest in the possibility of pharmacologic treatment. Anecdotal reports and small open trials were optimistic for a number of new and different treatments:

Lithium (5),
Tricyclic antidepressants (Hardy, unpublished, 1983),
5-Hydroxytryptophan (6),
Trazodone and tryptophan (7),
Beta-blockers (8),
L-dopa (9),
Selective serotonin reuptake inhibitors (10),
Naloxone and naltrexone (11).

Prospects for successful drug treatment seemed to be improving. Review articles on the psychopharmacology of SIB began to appear (12,13). Indeed, there were more review articles than controlled studies.

Perhaps the prospects looked better, but the actual state of pharmacotherapy was still risky. What worked for one patient did not work for very many others. No drug had any more than occasional success. Still, the anecdotal reports were cause for at least a degree of optimism. For the first time, some self-injurious individuals were responding to drug treatment that was not a high-dose, sedating neuroleptic. One hoped that treatment might move beyond trials that were merely empirical. Perhaps if there were a coherent theoretical model, one might make progress.

In 1984, a research group at the University of North Carolina with whom I had close ties was engaged in developing a theoretical model for SIB. Their model was based on studies of people with LNS, a syndrome that is associated with a grotesque form of compulsive mutilation (SMB). The fact that LNS was associated with a very specific biochemical derangement suggested that pharmacologic correction of an underlying deficit was not an unreasonable hope (14). In animal models, SMB could be elicited if the DA D_1 receptor were up-regulated or rendered "supersensitive." It was proposed that this pharmacologic model could explain the SMB of patients with LNS and possibly SIB in general.

It was reasonable, therefore, to pursue clinical trials of drugs that could block the D_1 receptor, and this we undertook to do with a modicum of success. Our studies of low-dose FPZ in severely self-injurious, mentally retarded individuals were the first controlled clinical trials of drug treatment for SIB, and the first studies to report success in long-term follow-up. The treatment, however, was clearly limited in efficacy, and many patients failed to respond at all. The experiments were only partially supportive of the D_1 model and only partially supportive of our hopes for a rational pharmacotherapy of SIB.

As years passed, we came to appreciate that the real problem was that SIB was being thought of as a unitary entity. The assumption that SIB is a unitary disorder was implicit to the D_1 model. We knew, of course, that SIB had many different causes but assumed that there was a common final pathway that was shared by all patients with SIB—a neurochemical end point, a single channel that mediated the behavioral stereotype. In retrospect, the idea was naive, but like most wrong-headed ideas, it had a perfectly reasonable argument behind it and some good did come from it.

Since our first clinical studies of FPZ in SIB, my colleagues and I have conducted clinical investigations based on the opiate model and the serotonin model. I have enjoyed a long and fruitful relationship with the Cornelia de Lange Syndrome Foundation, which is described in Chapter 16. Along the way, the hope that SIB is amenable to a unitary theory has been left behind. SIB, such as aggression, is not a disorder but a symptom. As such, it is the occasion for a differential diagnosis that embraces many different conditions and treatments.

Along the way, we also arrived at a system of pharmacotherapy for SIB that is less heavy-handed than it once was. At the same time, the incidence and prevalence of SIB seem to have decreased. Pharmacology was only a small part of that.

The DA D_1 theory of SIB was inspired by studies of LNS, which is a good starting point.

LESCH-NYHAN SYNDROME

LNS, an X-linked form of mental retardation, is an inborn error of purine metabolism marked by self-destructive behavior, spasticity, and mental deficiency. The specific biochemical defect is an inherited deficiency of the purine salvage enzyme hypoxanthine-guanine-phosphoribosyl transferase (HGPRT). This deficiency leads to an increase in the rate of purine biosynthesis and massive overproduction of uric acid. Elevated urate levels in LNS cause kidney stones and symptoms of gout (15,16). Allopurinol is used to diminish uric acid synthesis. It does not alleviate the devastating neurologic symptoms of LNS but does prevent the joint pain and neuropathy associated with accumulation of sodium urate crystals.

LNS was characterized as an X-linked recessive disorder in 1965. Genetic analysis of patients with LNS has shown that the syndrome is caused by mutations in the *HGPRT* gene, which resides on the long arm of the X chromosome. Mutations in the gene that encodes for HPGRT are associated with a spectrum of outcomes that range from hyperuricemia alone to hyperuricemia with profound neurologic and behavioral dysfunction. Patients with less severe clinical manifestations typically have mutations that permit some degree of residual enzyme function (17–19).

The syndrome is rare (approximately one in 100,000 livebirths). Children born with LNS appear normal at birth, but mental retardation and motor symptoms appear early in life. Motor delay develops between 3 to 6 months, often in association with frequent vomiting. Older patients typically show scissoring of the legs, increased deep tendon reflexes, and involuntary movements associated with spasticity and choreoathetosis; sometimes cerebral palsy is suspected. The motor impairment of children with LNS is profound, and they cannot sit or stand unaided. Indeed, the motor deficit is more severe than the deficit in intellectual development. Although many children with LNS are mild to moderately retarded (IQ of 40 to 80), others have normal intelligence (20,21). Because they are verbal, they can explain just how awful it is to self-injure; they do not like it.

The most striking aspects of LNS are SIB and aggression. Compulsive SIB is found in 85% of cases, with an average age of onset at 3.5 years. Patients as young as 2 years of age bite their fingers and lips, bang their heads and arms, or toss themselves about in attempts to cause injury, although finger and lip biting are common forms of self-injury, the number of ways self-injury can occur is limited only by the creativity of the patient and the availability of opportunities. It may increase in response to stress and usually decreases after age 12.

Patients with LNS experience pain in the same way as anyone else. Their ability to feel pain distinguishes LNS from conditions such as sensory neuropathy and familial dysautonomia, in which SIB occurs in the context of anesthesia. When children with LNS injure themselves, they cry out in pain. The children beg to be restrained in such a way that there is no possibility that they can injure themselves. They are only at ease when all possible opportunities for self-injury have been removed.

In addition, children with LNS are compelled to injure other people, often striking out, unprovoked and unexpectedly, at caretakers. Their aggression can be externally directed in attempts to harm others or it can be psychologically directed at themselves and others. Patients act in ways that bring harm to their self-esteem, their relationships with others, and their own self-interest. For example, it is not uncommon for a patient with LNS to try to alienate the people he or she cares about most or to deny him- or herself the simplest pleasure. For example, the child might say that he or she does not want a special treat, even though he or she is looking forward to it, or may deliberately give the wrong answers on a test.

They feel remorse for their behavior; indeed, their self-destructive behavior and aggression are pure compulsions: repetitive behaviors that are not only maladaptive but also completely against their will. They clearly do not want to harm themselves or others. They are, as a rule, highly social, have a good sense of humor, are keen observers of their surroundings, and care deeply for the people that they are close to. They feel deep regret for the interpersonal injuries that they have caused, distraught at not going on the class trip, or dejected after doing poorly on a test.

They are true contraries: what they do is exactly the opposite of what they want to do. They do not want to bite themselves, yet they do. They are appreciative of their caregivers, yet they strike out at them. They want to go on the outing, yet they succeed in getting left behind; they want to be pass the test, but they deliberately fail.

Treatment

At present, there is no treatment for the underlying enzymatic deficiency responsible for LNS. With allopurinol treatment, patients have an average life expectancy at least to the fourth decade. Without allopurinol and other treatments, life expectancy drops to less than 4 years.

Physical restraints and behavior management are essential to LNS treatment. Physical therapy is not notably helpful. Tooth extraction is a common way to manage biting of the fingers, lips, and cheeks. A parent survey by Anderson and Ernst (22) found that 60% of the patients had teeth extracted to prevent self-injury. Parents overwhelmingly endorse dental extraction as a way of managing self-biting. Their only regret was not having done it sooner to prevent tissue loss, particularly to the lips. All the patients expressed relief at having their teeth removed. (It is necessary to remove all the teeth. If you leave only a few molars, the patients will still manage to bite themselves. Dental guards can usually be thwarted.)

Patients with LNS should be monitored for depression. Depression has been observed in boys as young as 8 and seems to be the rule among the teenagers. Psychotherapy and antidepressant medications have been recommended.

All the drugs listed in the previous section have been tried in patients with LNS with mixed results. Anecdotal reports in recent years have supported risperidone (23), carbamazepine (24), gabapentin (25), and olanzapine (26). Parents have not tended to use any of these medications. According to surveys (22), the most commonly used medication for behavioral symptoms are the benzodiazepines. These antianxiety agents are thought to "take the edge off" a stressful period and help to calm the patient. Sedatives such as Benadryl and chloral hydrate are also used to give patients (and caregivers) a better night's sleep.

The reader will recognize a state of pharmacologic practice that is really quite rudimentary and rather at variance with the sophisticated investigations of the neuropharmacology of LNS. It is ironic that the study of LNS has been a fertile source for preclinical investigation, but a dry well when it comes to clinical prescription.

NEUROPHARMACOLOGIC MODELS OF SELF-INJURIOUS BEHAVIOR

The D_1 Dopamine Receptor Hypothesis

The DA D_1 receptor of SIB has five premises:

- Animal grooming behavior, arguably a nonpathologic precursor of SIB, is mediated by DA neurons.
- Manipulations of the DA system in animal models lead to SIB.
- Dopaminergic drugs can cause or aggravate SIB.
- Antidopaminergic drugs can arrest it.
- Abnormalities in LNS implicate DA.

We begin with LNS. LNS is a prototype for SIB. Its basis is a genetic deficit in the enzyme HGPRT. It is not entirely clear how the neurologic and behavioral characteristics of LNS are produced by an error in purine metabolism, but there is reason to believe that DA is involved (27,28).

In normal human beings, HGPRT activity is highest in brain tissue, especially in the basal ganglia. In brain tissue from patients with LNS, the activity of the enzyme is markedly reduced or absent (29). Volumetric studies of magnetic resonance imaging scans of patients with LNS show clear reductions in the size of the basal ganglia (30). Autopsy studies have not yet revealed specific neuropathologic abnormalities in LNS, but positron emission tomography studies have indicated significant reductions in DA transporters and DOPA uptake in the basal ganglia. Neurochemical studies have shown a substantial decrease in DA content in the basal ganglia. The prominence of extrapyramidal signs such as choreoathetosis and dystonia are consistent with DA dysfunction in the basal ganglia (17–19).

In fact, several neurotransmitter abnormalities have been reported in patients with LNS. These include abnormal adrenergic function peripherally and decreased serotonin turnover in the central nervous system (CNS). Castells et al. (31) reported a decrease in DA and serotonin metabolites in cerebrospinal fluid in a single patient. Lloyd et al. (14) reported significant regional decreases in DA metabolites in three postmortem LNS brains. Decreased levels of cerebrospinal fluid homovanillic acid and 5-HIAA were reported in four patients with LNS, with a rapid decline in the first 3 years of life (32).

The discovery of abnormal monoamine metabolism in LNS was heartening to neuropharmacologists who were able to induce SMB in animals by manipulating CNS monoamines with drugs such as caffeine (33), amphetamine (34), pemoline (34), and clonidine (35). The discovery that DA played an important role in LNS was especially interesting to Breese et al. (36). They had already established that neonatal treatment with 6-OHDA would selectively destroy DA-containing fibers in the rat. They were astounded to discover that when these animals were treated as adults with L-dopa, severe SMB occurred. The effect was dose dependent and was blocked by the DA D_1 blocker *cis*-flupenthixol but not by the DA D_2 antagonist haloperidol. This suggested to Breese et al. that a DA D_1 receptor supersensitivity state might be the pharmacologic basis of SMB in the neonatal 6-OHDA–treated rat (36). It was conceivable that in LNS, HGPRT deficiency was interfering in some way with the proper development of DA neurons in the basal ganglia (37).

Monkeys with ventromedial tegmental lesions of the brainstem inflicted when they were very young (2 to 3 years) have also been observed to develop SMB when they are challenged, as adults, with DA agonist drugs (Goldstein, unpublished, 1985). This, too, was attributed to sensitivity at the DA D_1 receptor. For example, when the monkeys with tegmental lesions were treated with DA D_1 blockers (FPZ, SCH 23390), the SMB was eliminated (Goldstein, unpublished, 1985).

The same group also reported success in controlling SIB in a 20-month-old patient with LNS with the D_1 blocker FPZ. They hypothesized a relationship between the specific enzyme deficit in LNS and DA receptor supersensitivity, perhaps related to the modulating effect of guanosine triphosphate on the activity state of DA receptors (Goldstein, unpublished, 1985).

Not all this information was available in 1984, when we began our clinical research activities with individuals with severe SIB at the Caswell Center, a large state residential facility in Kinston, NC, but the DA D_1 hypothesis was sufficiently compelling to warrant a preliminary trial. At the time, the only drug available in the United States to block the D_1 receptor was the mixed DA D_1/D_2 antagonist FPZ (38).

Testing the D_1 Model

The decision having been made to pursue clinical trials of FPZ, it was necessary to develop an appropriate method. It was necessary to sidestep many of the conventions that were current in psychopharmacology (39). If the purpose of the research were simply to test the D_1 hypothesis, one would design a controlled study to compare the effects of FPZ with the effects of a drug such as haloperidol, a relatively pure DA D_2 receptor antagonist, but there were competing considerations.

1. If there were a chance that the drug had any merit, its value should be tested immediately. Because FPZ was an approved drug and neuroleptic treatment was at the time quite common in individuals with SIB, there was really no obstacle to immediately examining its effects in the context of clinical treatment.
2. It was not acceptable to treat people with SIB in any drug protocol that would compromise the treatment programs that were already in place. A placebo-controlled study would impose an enormous burden on staff and subjects. Caring for people with severe SIB was already an enormous burden. Nothing should be done to jeopardize what little stability existed in their lives. It was hardly ethical to do so on behalf of a mere hypothesis and one that had virtually no support from clinical trials in human beings.
3. The more important question to address was not the DA D_1 hypothesis but the more fundamental question of whether this particular drug was potentially useful. If it worked, the D_1 hypothesis was supported but not confirmed; if it did not work, the hypothesis was not necessarily disconfirmed. At least we would know whether the treatment worked.
4. It was important to appraise the success of treatment over the long term. Other treatments, such as L-hydroxytryptamine, had been found to work for a short time but not in the long term. One would be ill advised to recommend treatment with a drug as troublesome as FPZ based on a short-term study. It is possible to blind a longitudinal study, but it is extremely expensive to do so.
5. There is the penicillin effect. We were "looking for penicillin," that is, a drug that would stop the problem of SIB when no other drug had previously been effective, a drug that would give more than a statistically significant result (e.g., episodes of head banging reduced by 50%, one-tailed test, $p < 0.05$), but rather a drug that would eliminate

the problem altogether. If FPZ were such a drug and if the effect were sustained, it should be readily apparent.

To begin, therefore, we selected six patients with severe SIB whom we had followed for a long time at the Caswell Center. They were all drug free, but that was because they had been treated before with a series of psychoactive drugs, including high-dose neuroleptics, with no success. These were people whose SIB had been sustained over many years. They were in restraints virtually all the time, they required one-on-one staff attention, or both. Two were blind from head punching or eye gouging, and all had significant tissue damage (40).

The initial design was A-B-A-B, which was our usual method for assessing psychoactive drug effects at the Center. Each condition was intended to last several months.

Five of the six patients responded dramatically to treatment with low doses of FPZ, from 2 to 8 mg per day. Higher doses tended to cause akathisia, with an attendant return of the SIB. One patient, who had been in restraints for no fewer than 32 years, was able to spend more than 90% of his waking hours out of restraints. In the other four, the results were almost as impressive. It looked like a "penicillin effect."

The effects were sustained over 16 to 24 months (mean, 21.4) of follow-up except in one case, an unfortunate young man who had previously blinded himself by persistent head punching. He developed tardive akathisia after 16 months on FPZ, and there was no way to recover the original beneficial effects. Now he spends most of his day in restraints, off medication, much as he was before.

The success of the first trial led to a change in plans. An A-B-A-B design was no longer feasible. We had the first A (drug-free baseline) and the first B (treatment with FPZ). Because no one wanted to withdraw such an effective treatment, the second A (a period of time off drug) was inconceivable.

Thus began a second series of nine retarded people with severe SIB treated with FPZ with the introduction of at least a degree of control. We introduced a placebo baseline of variable length before the drug was introduced under double-blind conditions. In this group, there were six responders. None responded to placebo. The beneficial effects of FPZ were again seen at very low doses and were sustained over a follow-up period that lasted for 8 to 23 months (mean, 15.3) (40). There was only one dropout for lost response after 6 months.

From the total group of 15 patients, therefore, four subjects were nonresponders, and 11 showed a very favorable response. One of the responders failed after 6 months and another after 16 months. The others showed no diminution of response over time. Because the doses were low, sedation was not a problem, and indeed the responders were more alert and attentive when they were on the drug. The only problem with treatment was the occurrence of extrapyramidal side effects (n = 4), especially akathisia (n = 3). The risk of tardive akathisia, of course, is something that looms over all patients who continue on FPZ. In the mentally retarded, it is a more important problem than tardive dyskinesia.

The (partial) DA D_1 receptor antagonist FPZ was effective, therefore, in at least nine of 16 retarded people who had severe SIB. They had not responded to other neuroleptics. Their baseline rates of SIB had been high for months of drug-free baseline, and there was no indication of positive effect during a placebo-controlled baseline period. The favorable effects of the drug were sustained over a prolonged follow-up period.

Higher doses of FPZ were not helpful. In most cases, higher doses were accompanied by symptoms of akathisia that actually made the SIB much worse, after an initial favorable response. In four cases, the patient was classified as a low-dose responder because titrating the FPZ dose downward led to significant improvement compared with baseline, placebo, and high-dose results.

Because FPZ is a DA antagonist at both the D_1 and D_2 receptors, one cannot really distinguish the exact mechanism of drug action in a clinical trial like this. Therapeutic response to FPZ in SIB may be a DA D_1 effect, a D_2 effect, a combined effect of blocking both receptors, or the result of some other action of the drug. There was no direct measure to address this question, short of positron emission tomography scanning with appropriately labeled ligands, but there were indirect measures of DA receptor activity. Extrapyramidal reactions and neuroleptic-induced hyperprolactinemia are believed to be the consequence of DA D_2 antagonism in the corpus striatum and hypothalamus, respectively.

Prolactin response to neuroleptics is believed to be mediated by the D_2 receptor, and DA D_1 receptor blockade is reported not to alter prolactin secretion (41). We measured prolactin levels while patients were on optimal therapeutic doses of FPZ, and as one might expect, most of the subjects had prolactin levels that were higher than normal baseline. However, two of the 11 responders on FPZ had morning venous prolactins less than 10, i.e., no neuroleptic-induced elevation. This suggests that a therapeutic response to FPZ occurred in at least two patients at a drug dose that did not yield a significant degree of DA D_2 receptor blockade. Neither of these patients experienced extrapyramidal side effects to FPZ, another indicator of DA D_2 receptor antagonism. It appeared, therefore, that DA D_2 receptor antagonism is not essential to the therapeutic effects of FPZ in SIB. DA receptor blockade at the D_1 receptor may therefore be the mechanism behind the therapeutic success of FPZ.

There have been incidental reports of low-dose FPZ in the treatment of retarded people with SIB, but no further clinical studies of the D_1 hypothesis. The treatment is still used on occasion, although it appears to have been superseded by some other new developments in the psychopharmacology of SIB, especially the atypical antipsychotics, the new antiepileptic drugs, the α_2 agonists, and the serotonergic antidepressants.

Is there a bottom-line to the D_1 hypothesis? Ironically, patients with LNS do not appear to respond very well to FPZ or to any other agent that blocks the D_1 receptor (e.g., clozapine) (24,42). The pure D_2 antagonist haloperidol is also thought to be effective in very low doses for SIB. It is an interesting theory, but it is in limbo. Perhaps it will be revived when a pure D_1 antagonist is available for clinical study.

The Opiate Hypothesis

In contrast to the several streams of evidence in support of the DA hypothesis of SIB, the origin of the opiate hypothesis of SIB was much simpler and more straightforward. Obviously, SIB has something to do with pain. The endogenous opiate system participates in the experience and modulation of pain. Therefore, endogenous opiates participate somehow in SIB.

Endogenous opiates or endorphins are released in the brain after painful stimulation. The chronic stimulation of endorphin receptors by repeated SIB was hypothesized to down-regulate the reactivity of these receptors and thus underlie an addiction to chronic painful stimulation. A simple, straightforward hypothesis and easily testable. If SIB were reinforced by the release of endorphins onto opiate receptors, then blocking those receptors may be expected to prevent the reinforcing consequences of the behavior and allow extinction to occur (11). The compulsive self-administration of painful stimuli, therefore, must speak to some kind of abnormality in the endogenous opiate system. With this rationale, Richardson and Zaleski (11) attempted the treatment of severe SIB in a 15-year-old retarded boy with the opiate antagonist naloxone, and the treatment, after a brief extinction burst, was successful.

The view that endogenous opiates may mediate or maintain SIB led to a long series of (inconclusive) experiments with the opiate antagonists naloxone and naltrexone (NLTX) (43–45). The animal literature would periodically report that NLTX was effective for conditions in animals characterized by stereotypic SIB, such as tail chasing or acral lick dermatitis. The clinical literature would present case reports from time to time, such as the patient with trichotillomania and obsessive-compulsive disorder whose hair-pulling behavior improved when NLTX (50 mg per day) was added to her regular dose of fluoxetine (46).

The idea that at least some SIB could be attributable to blunted nociception and maintained by the endorphin system was raised by Sandman et al. in 1993 (49). If it is correct, however, it holds for only a fraction of patients with SIB. The pain threshold of individuals who engage in SIB is really quite variable. Patients with LNS have a normal experience of pain. In others, the pain threshold appears to be quite low. Patients engage in self-injury to limbs that are deinnervated. SIB is common in people with congenital insensitivity to pain and familial dysautonomia, in which the perception of pain is aberrant. It may be difficult to infer precisely how a severely retarded and nonverbal individual experiences pain, but no one maintains that blunted nociception is a consistent feature.

Clinical Trials of the Opiate Hypothesis

The pharmacology of the opiate antagonists and the rationale for their use in the treatment of SIB have been reviewed on several occasions (47). The clinical studies of naloxone and NLTX in SIB have also been reviewed (47,48). To date, there are nine published studies of naloxone, comprising in total no more than 11 subjects. All were single-dose studies of intravenously administered medication. Beneficial effects were reported in seven of the nine studies.

There have been 22 published studies of NLTX, with a total of 110 subjects. The authors of these reports describe beneficial results in 59 subjects (54%). A more critical examination of the data by Aman (49) discovered unequivocal responders in 41% of the cases rereviewed. The effective dose of NLTX seems to range from 25 to 300 mg per day (47). In a controlled trial of NLTX in 24 institutionalized patients with SIB, 18 responded to treatment with NLTX with a reduction in SIB of at least 25% (49). In another controlled study of 32 institutionalized adults, the effects of NLTX (50 to 150 mg per day) were no better than those of placebo (50). None of the studies speaks of serious toxicity with naloxone or NLTX.

The prescription of NLTX is indeed experimental, but it appears to be safe, and a purported response rate in excess of 40% has encouraged its use. The widespread use of NLTX in clinical settings allowed my colleagues and me to examine the impact of NLTX treatment in a large population of mentally retarded individuals, the 10,000 residents of 13 state schools in Texas (51).

The idea was to conduct a retrospective review of all the residents of the Texas state schools who were self-injurious and who had been treated with NLTX over a 5-year period. SIB was operationally defined as the chronic infliction of bodily harm resulting in tissue damage occurring for at least 1 year. It included head banging, self-biting, hitting, scratching, kicking or gouging, hair pulling, and skin picking.

At the time. there were 13 state schools for the retarded in Texas, with a total population of more than 10,000. This population had previously been the subject of three epidemiologic studies of SIB (52,53). In 1986, 1,352 individuals with SIB were identified in the Texas state system (53). At that time, 38.8% were treated with psychoactive drugs, almost exclusively neuroleptics (53).

In January 1994, we contacted each of the state schools, asking them to identify every case of NLTX treatment for SIB over a 5-year period from 1/1/88 to 1/1/94. Of 13 state schools, 10 had residents who were self-injurious and who had been treated with NLTX during this period. The total number of subjects was 56. They all had been chronically self-injurious and had had prior drug treatment: 4.8 ± 2.6 prior psychoactive drugs.

According to the clinical impressions of the people who treated these subjects, 32 of the 56 patients who had been treated with NLTX were favorable responders and continued on NLTX. After we completed a blind review of the behavioral data that documented treatment response and eliminated possible confounds, we affirmed that 13 subjects had improved significantly when NLTX was added to their treatment regimen. Thus, 25% of the NLTX group were unequivocal responders.

Our data clearly supported a role for NLTX in the treatment of retarded people with severe and persistent SIB who had failed to respond favorably to other drug trials. Response was maintained over months of follow-up. In fact, we found something very curious about the NLTX response. The clinical improvement was incremental as time passed, even over 30 months of follow-up. In every case, the occurrence of SIB was less during the second half of the follow-up period than it was during the first half. During the first 6 months of treatment, SIB occurred at 71% of the baseline rate; during the second 6-month period, at 37%; during the third period, at 27%; during the fourth period, at 26%; and for the five subjects who had data from a fifth period, at 20%.

The published literature suggests that opiate antagonists may be a safe and effective treatment for SIB with a high rate of positive response (41% to 73%). In our study, treating clinicians reported a 57% response rate with NLTX. Although that figure is consistent with the literature, a blind review suggested that it was an optimistic estimate. A more systematic review indicated a response rate of 25%. Perhaps that figure is an underestimate.

Perhaps NLTX is an effective treatment for SIB in retarded people. If a substantial reduction in self-injury occurs in one of four patients, then the treatment may have some merit. It is also a safe treatment. Of the 56 patients treated with NLTX in our survey, during more than 2,000 patient-months of treatment, only one patient was withdrawn from treatment because of side effects.

If NLTX works by blocking the reinforcing effect of endogenous opiates, then the clinical response should be characterized by what behaviorists call an extinction burst, followed by a rapid decline in SIB. That was not observed in our data. It is conceivable that severely retarded individuals have a sluggish response to reinforcers or to their withdrawal and that it takes a long time for them to lose a habit of such long-standing intensity. Perhaps there is another mechanism.

NLTX may have anxiolytic effects and positive effects on learning. The delayed and incremental response to NLTX treatment may represent an indirect effect: a reduction in SIB might render the patient more amenable to behavioral and programmatic therapies already in place. It might be a direct effect of NLTX to improve memory and the capacity to learn from programming or to reduce the severity of the patient's stress response (54). Either effect would be associated with a gradual improvement over time. It may be, then, that NLTX is a good drug for SIB, but it may be that its short-term effects are less important than its long-term effects. It suggests that if one commits to a trial of NLTX, one should not abandon the effort for at least 6 months.

The Serotonin Hypothesis

Serotonergic neurons project from brainstem nuclei in the dorsal raphe to innervate cortical structures in the frontal lobes and subcortical structures in the striatum, hippocampus, and septum (55). Like the other monoamine neurotransmitters, serotonin seems to exercise a neuromodulatory or a neuroactivating effect on higher systems. Serotonin effects seem to be specifically devoted to the modulation of appetitive or vegetative functions such as sleep and waking, mood and pain, and water intake and sustenance (56).

The clinical meaning of such associations with serotonin metabolism has been developed with some success in the study of affective disorders (56,57). On a theoretical level, there is said to be to be a subcategory of affective illness that is primarily mediated by serotonin systems, and there is a practical benefit to be gained from the administration of a cascade of serotonergic antidepressants, including lithium and L-tryptophan, to some patients with refractory depression (58,59).

There is also an association, replicated on numerous occasions, with levels of the serotonin metabolite 5-HIAA in the cerebrospinal fluid of patients who attempt suicide (60,61). The connection, however, appears in patients from virtually every diagnostic group, and it does not seem to be a function of a depressive state so much as a tendency to impulsive, aggressive behavior. There is also a well-founded association between low levels of serotonin metabolism and aggressive behavior, exclusive of suicide (7,62).

Serotonin neurotransmission must have a role in obsessive-compulsive disorder because treatment usually involves a serotonergic antidepressant such as clomipramine or fluoxetine (63–65). The association is reinforced by studies of serotonin metabolites in patients with obsessive-compulsive disorder (65). Anorexia and bulimia nervosa are two other disorders that have also been linked to serotonin and may be treated successfully with the serotonergic antidepressants (66,67)

The role of serotonin in modulating aggressive behavior leads one to the consideration of developmental syndromes that are characterized by high rates of SIB. In LNS, there is evidence of decreased serotonin turnover in the CNS (31,32). Low levels of serotonin in the CNS may be associated with impulsive and aggressive behavior (62). Some conditions disposed to SIB such as Down's syndrome, autism, and de Lange syndrome are sometimes associated with low levels of serotonin (68). One study reported that patients with de Lange syndrome with low serotonin levels were more likely to have severe behavioral problems (69). O'Neal et al. (7) reported one patient with de Lange syndrome with SIB who had low levels of whole blood serotonin. Treatment with the serotonin reuptake blocker trazodone and the serotonin precursor L-tryptophan led to resolution of SIB and elevation of whole blood serotonin to normal levels (7).

What is common to patients with these disorders in addition to SIB is a degree of affective instability that is manifest clinically as dysphoria, irritability, emotional liability, and hyperreactivity to environmental stimuli. This phenotype of irritability, dysphoria, and affective instability is shared by children with phenylketonuria. Phenylketonuria has a hyposerotonergic component, as described in Chapter 11. Children with phenylketonuria, however, are not notably self-injurious.

Clinical Experience with Serotonergics

Although the rationale for serotonergic treatment of developmentally handicapped people with SIB is sound, the literature on this is limited. That is an example of research falling behind, rather than driving, clinical practice. The early reports of patients with LNS who responded to 5-hydroxytryptophan were never followed up, probably because the effects, although dramatic, were only temporary (6,9) An individual with de Lange syndrome and SIB who had low levels of whole blood serotonin responded well to the combination of L-tryptophan and trazodone (7). Subsequent papers describe treatment of SIB with trazodone (70), clomipramine (71,72), domperidone (73), fluoxetine (74–76), buspirone (77), and a tryptophan-rich diet (78). The reports are anecdotal and mostly uncontrolled. There have been no straight-up comparisons of any serotonergic with a high-potency neuroleptic or an opiate antagonist. Fluoxetine worked once in a naltrexone-resistant patient with SIB (75), and clomipramine was found to be better than desipramine for trichotillomania (71).

One of my most difficult patients with SIB was a profoundly retarded 4-year-old boy with Pierre-Robin syndrome who had a 3-year history of sleep disturbance, staying up all night, with progressive SIB, head banging, and head slapping. He was one of the most difficult patients with SIB whom I have ever encountered. He responded dramatically to the combination of L-tryptophan and fluoxetine. The response was sustained over 18 months of follow-up; it was lost on two occasions, when the tryptophan was withdrawn (10).

Most clinicians use serotonergics as first-line therapy for SIB despite the paucity of controlled trials. The drugs are quite safe and are appropriate to try for virtually any form of compulsive behavior, especially one with equal components of aggression and dysphoria. It is arguable that serotonergics represent at this time the treatment of choice for most cases of SIB.

One common problem in the serotonergic treatment of SIB, or any other behavioral problem in a retarded person, is the loss of effect after weeks or months of treatment. This problem is not unknown in patients with depression either, and in neither group is it well understood. It is presumably a form of tachyphylaxis, but it is not always possible to restore the therapeutic effect by increasing the dose or substituting a more potent or more selective serotonergic. One would do better to prevent its occurrence, and that may be done by augmenting the serotonergic with a serotonin precursor (e.g., tryptophan, 5-hydroxytryptophan) or with a serotonergic diet. The latter, developed by Gedye, entails the elimination of caffeine and the intake of large quantities of tropical fruits (banana, pineapple, papaya) or (more agreeably) passion fruit juice. Passion fruit juice is available as a component of most commercial guava nectars, especially in Anglo communities. The serotonergic diet is not associated with serotonin syndrome, but tryptophan combined with a selective serotonin reuptake inhibitor may be.

Clinicians choose serotonergics over high-potency neuroleptics because they are much safer and over NLTX because the effect is stronger and comes on sooner. They tend to start with relatively innocuous drugs such as trazodone, buspirone, and paroxetine. Fluoxetine, sertraline, and fluvoxamine are very good drugs, but they can be too activating for some retarded patients, and clomipramine can make children and retarded people quite irritable. Nevertheless, there is a widespread use of serotonergic drugs for retarded people in general and for patients with SIB in particular. Any one may be chosen, and combinations are frequently used. The only real problem with the serotonergic treatment is the very high doses of concomitant medications and precursors that are often necessary. Developmentally handicapped people, of all neuropsychiatric patients, require some of the highest doses of serotonergics.

Other Models of Self-injurious Behavior

There is also an adenosine hypothesis of SIB, which has evolved from an appreciation of the role of CNS purines, elevated in LNS, as neurotransmitters, neuromodulators, and regulators of receptor sensitivity, especially in relation to adenosine (79). Caffeine and theophylline can increase SIB in experimental animals (34,80); behavioral potency is related to the ability of these agents to block the adenosine receptor (81). Clonidine-induced self-mutilation in mice has been attributed to adenosine A_1 receptor blockade and may be inhibited by adenosine or by the adenosine agonist dipyridamole (82). Adenosine inhibits self-mutilation in the DA D_1 receptor supersensitive rats of Criswell et al. (83).

It is possible that some of the sedative properties of neuroleptic drugs are mediated by adenosine agonist effects (84). Carbamazepine, conversely, seems to be an adenosine antagonist (84). Dipyridamole is a commercially available drug with few side effects that is an adenosine agonist (85), but clinical trials of dipyridamole in patients with SIB in our program have not been impressive.

The γ-aminobutyric acid (GABA) hypothesis has been woven out of similar cloth. Muscimol, a GABA agonist, evokes intense stereotyped behavior including self-biting in laboratory animals (86), and the rat model of DA deficiency in LNS is more sensitive to SIB produced by muscimol (87). Caffeine inhibits the binding of diazepam to receptors, and diazepam also potentiates the adenosine effect in inhibiting the firing rates of neurons (79). GABA antagonists, however, do not necessarily suppress SIB (88). Most of our patients with SIB have at some time been treated with benzodiazepines with no benefit at all. Conversely, the new GABAergic drugs gabapentin and tiagabine may be useful for SIB.

The various neurochemical hypotheses have an intrinsic advantage because they lend themselves to empirical evaluation in clinical drug trials. Clinical trials based on neurochemical hypotheses, however, are predicated on the assumptions that SIB is a unitary condition and/or that it occupies a neurochemical "common final pathway." If, conversely, SIB is a symptom, not a disorder in its own right, then the clinical trials would indicate just what they have: some patients respond well to drug A, some to B, some to C, and so on.

The Differential Diagnosis of Self-injurious Behavior

For the clinician, it is necessary to describe SIB in terms of its behavioral topography and its overt clinical features; for example, head banging, occurring continuously, in circumstances of low stimulation, compulsive nail and cuticle picking, or paroxysmal explosions of rage and self-biting. It is also important to consider its possible operant properties; its psychological "function" as best we can infer it. Does it seem to serve the purpose of self-stimulation or tension reduction? Is it a response to pain, a form of attention seeking, or an attempt to communicate something? Behavioral psychologists are trained in the art of functional analysis to make sense of such things when the rest of us cannot.

If SIB is a symptom, the clinical approach requires a differential diagnosis. If SIB is the symptom, what is the disease? It is not always possible to answer that question because many cases are idiopathic, but it is a necessary starting point.

The differential diagnosis of SIB includes six broad categories:

1. Pathobehavioral syndromes,
2. Environmental stress or deprivation,
3. General medical causes,
4. Epilepsy and neurologic conditions,
5. Neuropsychiatric disorders,
6. Idiopathic SIB.

The etiologic factors of SIB are diverse. It may be associated with any of the pathobehavioral syndromes or nonspecific encephalopathies that cause mental retardation. The only mental retardation syndromes that are highly associated with SIB are LNS, de Lange syndrome, Smith-Lemli-Opitz syndrome, and Smith-Magenis syndrome. The mere diagnosis of a mental retardation syndrome such as fragile X syndrome, Down's syndrome, or autism is not sufficient to explain the occurrence of SIB (Table 15.1).

Before discussing the value of differential diagnosis, it is important to remember that the method cannot be applied to a patient in a confused and unstable system. It is not possible to attribute structure and pattern to a behavioral disorder that arises in the context of isolation, frustration, and dismay. A patient whose life is spent in such circumstances may only show a random and meaningless pattern of behavior, confronted as he or she may be by developmentally inappropriate expectations, by contingencies and consequences administered fitfully and unpredictably. Before one can posit some order to a behavior such as SIB, one must be assured that fundamental programmatic rules are addressed.

TABLE 15.1. *Mental retardation syndromes associated with self-injurious behavior*

Lesch-Nyhan syndrome	Common
de Lange syndrome	Common
Smith-Lemli-Opitz syndrome	Common
Smith-Magenis syndrome	Common
Lowe's syndrome	Occasional
Prader-Willi syndrome	Occasional
Fragile X syndrome	Unusual
Down's syndrome	Rare

It is hardly necessary to elaborate on what comprises a humane environment, a developmentally appropriate program, or an effective behavior management system. It is necessary to iterate, however, that to the degree such elements are absent from a patient's life, to that degree psychiatric diagnosis and treatment will be weak and ineffective. If one can ensure that these elements are operative, then neuropsychiatric diagnosis is possible and effective interventions can be undertaken.

The second element of the differential diagnosis, then, is to ensure that the patient's environment is not inhospitable, that he or she has an appropriate developmental and behavioral program administered by competent and humane professionals. Within this context, one is advised to collect baseline data on the occurrence of SIB and of related behavior problems using specific targets such as the number of self-injurious outbursts, the time in or out of restraints, and a more global measure of the patient's clinical condition such as the Self Injurious Behavior Questionnaire (Appendix). After the patient is followed for a period of time in a well-managed, developmentally appropriate program and a reliable data system is in place, it is possible to proceed with the functional analysis of behavior and a differential diagnosis.

General Medical Causes of Self-injurious Behavior

Any chronic painful condition can lead to SIB as an expression of pain and discomfort or an attempt to communicate the desire for relief. At various times, we have treated patients whose SIB was the consequence of undetected physical disorders such as headache, otitis, peptic ulcer disease, reflux esophagitis, endometriosis, premenstrual distress, menopause, and cystitis. When the medical disorder is brought under control, the SIB usually goes away.

Conversely, if SIB is the manifestation of a painful condition that is not treated soon enough, it is possible that it will become a habitual behavior sustained by its own dynamic. In such cases, alleviating the root cause may not correct the outcome. This is an old maxim from psychosomatic medicine: A psychosomatic symptom may have a psychological origin, but if it continues long enough, it achieves a degree of "autonomy," a life of its own.

Medical conditions such as reflux esophagitis and peripheral neuropathy are the likely origin of SIB in young patients with de Lange syndrome, as described in Chapter 16. Repeated self-injurious responses to such conditions are the sensitizing events that ultimately lead to the development of severe SIB when the patients get older.

Obviously, it is the physician's first responsibility to alleviate pain. In nonverbal patients, one may miss the opportunity to do so because the patients' ways of complaining are indirect and hard to interpret. It is important to mitigate pain, to the degree one is able to do so, because learned pain can become a habit.

Some drugs may cause SIB. The most common culprits are the sedative anticonvulsants phenobarbital, primidone, phenytoin, and ethosuximide. Other drugs that may cause SIB are the xanthines, theophylline, caffeine, and the neuroleptics, especially high-potency neuroleptics such as haloperidol, which can cause akathisia and dysphoria. The more potent selective serotonin reuptake inhibitors can actually induce compulsive SIB, and clomipramine can make some patients irritable and aggressive. Generally, any medication that can cause sedation, dysphoria, depression, irritability, or restlessness can cause or aggravate SIB.

Epilepsy and Other Neurologic Causes of Self-injurious Behavior

Mentally retarded people are prone to seizures, and many require long-term treatment with anticonvulsants. One can usually improve the quality of treatment for seizure disorders in retarded people by pursuing the goal of anticonvulsant monotherapy, withdrawing patients from anticonvulsants after their seizures have been under control for several years, or choosing anticonvulsants that are also psychotropic such as carbamazepine, valproic acid, lamotrigine, and gabapentin in preference to anticonvulsants that have behavioral toxicity such as phenytoin and barbiturates. Blood levels must be monitored periodically. Blood levels that are sufficient to control overt seizures may not control behavioral accompaniments of epilepsy such as aggression, disorganization, and SIB.

It is a prudent first step to attain optimal anticonvulsant therapy for patients with SIB who have a history of seizures, an active seizure disorder treated with phenytoin or a barbiturate, or, in some cases, who have no overt seizure history but a clearly defined record of paroxysmal SIB. Paroxysmal SIB may be considered a seizure equivalent or the manifestation of what psychiatrists call explosive disorder. In either event, the treatments overlap, and prescription of carbamazepine or valproic acid may be indicated.

SIB may also occur in connection with neuropathic conditions such as dysautonomia or after tissues are denervated and the sensation of pain is lost. In such cases, SIB is not paroxysmal but compulsive. Neurologic conditions such as neuropathy, migraine, phonophobia, or chronic pain may be sufficient to cause SIB.

Psychiatric Disorders

Retarded people are vulnerable to the full range of psychiatric disorders. This simple fact has been obscured in the past, when virtually any misbehavior that arose in a retarded person was treated with neuroleptics or dealt with by behavioral fundamentalists. It was impossible to differentiate among the major psychiatric diagnoses and the nonspecific behavior problems that are peculiar to retarded people. Now more attention is given to the issue of psychiatric diagnosis and treatment, and the benefits of conventional psychiatric treatments are many.

SIB may be a symptom of virtually any psychiatric disorder in a mentally retarded person. Because the major affective disorders and panic and anxiety disorders are probably their most common afflictions, antidepressants and mood-stabilizing drugs are the leading treatments. Affective psychoses are not uncommon in mentally retarded individuals. Tourette's syndrome is sometimes a cause of self-injury, as is the related condition obsessive-compulsive disorder. Schizophrenia is hard to diagnose (or nonexistent) in the severe to profoundly retarded people who are most likely to self-injure. Antipsychotic drug treatment for SIB is appropriate if the patient has Tourette's syndrome or an affective psychosis.

Idiopathic Self-injurious Behavior

Among the patients with SIB who have been referred to our clinic, only approximately one-half can be successfully diagnosed and treated according to the medical and neuropsychiatric paradigms discussed. Patients with the most severe SIB, especially very young children, do not seem to fit very well at all, nor do the chronic, refractory cases.

One may still encounter patients who typify the kind of SIB that we used to see all the time. They are usually severe to profoundly retarded and reside in a poor and degrading environment with little in the way of education or attachments. They have usually received long-term treatment with sedating medications (neuroleptics, anticonvulsants, or both). Their life has not been an accumulation of positive learning experiences but rather an accretion of negative responses under the guise of "behavioral management." For all practical purposes, self-injury is their life and personality. Even if they have long since been transferred to a more humane facility, the residua of years of neglect and suffering are reflected in their SIB.

As in young children, self-injury in such patients represents a primitive, undifferentiated behavior, one that is hard to codify or analyze. It exists largely as the absence of anything more positive, as an untoward habit that has developed a life of its own, independent of any pathologic event that may have caused or sustained it in the past.

Severe mental retardation is a manifestation of cortical underdevelopment. The executive, reflective, and modulatory capacities of the cerebral cortex are absent or dysfunctional. Their behavioral executor is the striatum, an organ that is much given to habit. They are creatures of habit, especially when they have never had the opportunity to learn any better. What begins as an innocent proclivity to scratch, pick, or bother a sore may grow into a habit and then to a compulsion.

Idiopathic SIB, therefore, refers to a behavioral pattern that is usually severe and compulsive. It may or may not be associated with dysphoria or emotional instability. It is far removed from and inexplicable in terms of any of the various etiologic factors described above. Because it occurs most frequently in young children and severely retarded people who have been largely deprived of training, we are compelled to think of it as a very low, undifferentiated form of behavior. This issue is discussed in Chapter 16.

REFERENCES

1. Schroeder SR, Mulick JA, Rojahn J. The definition, taxonomy, epidemiology, and ecology of self-injurious behavior. *J Autism Dev Disord* 1980;10:417–432.
2. Hoder EL, Cohen DJ. Repetitive behavior patterns of childhood. In: Levine M, Carey W, eds. *Developmental and behavioral pediatrics*. Philadelphia: WB Saunders, 1983:607–622.
3. Favazza AR. *Bodies under siege: self-mutilation in culture and psychiatry*. Baltimore: The Johns Hopkins University Press, 1987.
4. Singh NN. Current trends in the treatment of self-injurious behavior. *Adv Pediatr* 1981;28:377–440.
5. Sovner R, Hurley A. The management of chronic behavior disorders in mentally retarded adults with lithium carbonate. *J Nerv Ment Dis* 1981;169:191–195.
6. Mizuno T, Yugari Y. Prophylactic effect of L-5-hydroxytryptophan on self-mutilation in the Lesch-Nyhan syndrome. *Neuropediatrie* 1975;6:13–23.
7. O'Neal M, Page N, Adkins WN, et al. Tryptophan-trazodone treatment of aggressive behavior. *Lancet* 1986;2:859–869.
8. Ratey JJ, Mikkelsen EJ, Smith GB, et al. Beta-blockers in the severely and profoundly mentally retarded. *J Clin Psychopharmacol* 1986;6:103–107.
9. Nyhan WL, Johnson HG, Kaufman IA, et al. Serotonergic approaches to the modification of behavior in the Lesch-Nyhan syndrome. *Appl Res Ment Retard* 1980;1:25–40.
10. Gualtieri CT, Schroeder SR. Pharmacotherapy for self-injurious behavior: preliminary tests of the D1 hypothesis. *Prog Neuropsychopharmacol Biol* 1990;14[suppl]:S81–S107.
11. Richardson JW, Zaleski WA. Naloxone and self-mutilation. *Biol Psychiatry* 1983;18:99–101.
12. Singh NN, Millichamp CJ. Pharmacological treatment of self-injurious behavior in mentally retarded persons. *J Autism Dev Disord* 1985;15:257–267.
13. Farber JM. *Psychopharmacology of self-injurious behavior in mentally retarded persons*. National Center for the Study and Treatment of Head Injury, 1986:296–302.
14. Lloyd KG, Hornykiewicz O, Davidson L, et al. Biochemical evidence of dysfunction of brain neurotransmitters in the Lesch-Nyhan syndrome. *N Engl J Med* 1981;305:1106–1111.
15. Lesch M, Nyhan WL. A familial disorder of uric acid metabolism and central nervous system function. *Am J Med* 1964;36:561–570.
16. Wilson JM, Young AB, Kelly WN. Hypoxanthine-guanine phosphoribosyl-transferase deficiency: the molecular basis of the clinical syndromes. *N Engl J Med* 1983;309:900–910.
17. Ernst M, Zametkin A, Matochik J, et al. Presynaptic dopaminergic deficits in Lesch-Nyhan disease. *N Engl J Med* 1996;334:1568–1572.
18. Saito Y, Ito M, Hanaoka S, et al. Dopamine receptor upregulation in Lesch-Nyhan syndrome: a postmortem study. *Neuropediatrics* 1999;30:66–71.
19. Visser J, Bar P, Jinnah H. Lesch-Nyhan disease and the basal ganglia. *Brain Res Rev* 2000;32:449–475.
20. Matthews MK, Alter M, Sirken DH. Recognition of peduncular hallucinosis prompted by magnetic resonance images. *Neuropsychiatry Neuropsychol Behav Neurol* 1995;8:64–69.
21. Matthews W, Solan A, Barabas G, et al. Cognitive functioning in Lesch-Nyhan syndrome: a 4-year follow-up study. *Dev Med Child Neurol* 1999;41:260–262.
22. Anderson L, Ernst M. Self-injury in Lesch-Nyhan disease. *J Autism Dev Disord* 1994;24:67–81.
23. Allen S, Rice S. Risperidone antagonism of self-mutilation in a Lesch-Nyhan patient. *Prog Neuropsychopharmacol Biol* 1996;20:793–800.
24. Roach E, Delgado M, Anderson L, et al. Carbamazepine trial for Lesch-Nyhan self mutilation. *J Child Neurol* 1996;11:476–478.
25. McManaman J, Tam D. Gabapentin for self-injurious behavior in Lesch-Nyhan syndrome. *Pediatr Neurol* 1999;20:381–382.
26. Moy S, Knapp D, Breese G. Effect of olanzapine on functional responses from sensitized d(1)-dopamine receptors in rats with neonatal dopamine loss. *Neuropsychopharmacology* 2001;25:224–233.
27. Jinnah H, De Gregorio L, Harris J, et al. The spectrum of inherited mutations causing HPRT deficiency: 75 new cases and a review of 196 previously reported cases. *Mutat Res* 2000;463:309–326.
28. Puig J, Torres R, Mateos F, et al. The spectrum of hypoxanthine-guanine phosphoribosyltransferase (HPRT) deficiency. Clinical experience based on 22 patients from 18 Spanish families. *Medicine (Baltimore)* 2001;80:102–112.

29. Seegmiller JE, Rosenbloom FM, Kelly WN. Enzyme defect associated with a sex-linked human neurological disorder and excessive purine synthesis. *Science* 1967; 155:1682–1684.
30. Harris J, Lee R, Jinnah H, et al. Craniocerebral magnetic resonance imaging measurement and findings in Lesch-Nyhan syndrome. *Arch Neurol* 1998;55:547–553.
31. Castells S, Chakrabarti C, Winsberg BG, et al. Effects of L-5-hydroxytryptophan on monoamine and amino acids turnover in the Lesch-Nyhan syndrome. *J Autism Dev Disord* 1979;9:95–103.
32. Silverstein FS, Johnston MV, Hutchinson RJ, et al. Lesch-Nyhan syndrome: CSF neurotransmitter abnormalities. *Neurology* 1985;6:907–911.
33. Minana MD, Portoles M, Jorda A, et al. Lesch-Nyhan syndrome, caffeine model: increase of purine and pyrimidine enzymes in rat brain. *J Neurochem* 1984;43: 1556–1560.
34. Mueller K, Nyhan WL. Pharmacologic control of pemoline induced self-injurious behavior in rats. *Pharmacol Biochem Behav* 1982;16:957–963.
35. Mueller K, Nyhan WL. Clonidine potentiates drug induced self-injurious behavior in rats. *Pharmacol Biochem Behav* 1983;18:891–894.
36. Breese GR, Baumeister AA, McCown TJ, et al. Behavioral differences between neonatal and adult 6-hyroxydopamine-treated rats to dopamine agonists: relevance to neurological symptoms in clinical syndromes with reduced brain dopamine. *J Pharmacol Exp Ther* 1984; 231:343–354.
37. Yeh J, Zheng S, Howard B. Impaired differentiation of HPRT-deficient dopaminergic neurons: a possible mechanism underlying neuronal dysfunction in Lesch-Nyhan syndrome. *J Neurosci Res* 1998;53:78–85.
38. Seeman P. Brain dopamine receptors. *Psychol Rev* 1981;32:229–313.
39. Sprague R, Werry J. Methodology of psychopharmacological studies with the retarded. In: Ellis N, ed. *International review of research in mental retardation*. New York: Academic Press, 1971:148–219.
40. Gualtieri CT. The differential diagnosis of self-injurious behavior in mentally retarded people. *Psychopharmacol Bull* 1989;25:358–363.
41. Ioria LC, Barnett A, Leitz FH, et al. SCH 23390: a potent benzadiazepine antipsychotic with unique interactions on dopaminergic systems. *J Pharmacol Exp Ther* 1983;226:462–468.
42. Titeler M. In: Dekker M, ed. *Multiple dopamine receptors*. New York: Marcel Dekker, 1983:38–55.
43. Cataldo M, Harris J. The biological basis for self-injury in the mentally retarded. *Annu Interventions Dev Disabil* 1998;2:21–39.
44. Barron J, Sandman C. Paradoxical excitement to sedative-hypnotics in mentally retarded clients. *Am J Ment Defic* 1985;90:124–129.
45. Gillberg C. Endogenous opioids and opiate antagonists in autism: brief review of empirical findings and implications for clinicians. *Dev Med Child Neurol* 1995;37: 239–245.
46. Carrion VG. Naltrexone for the treatment of trichotillomania. *J Clin Psychopharmacol* 1995;15:444–445.
47. Ricketts R, Ellis C, Singh Y, et al. Opioid antagonists. II: clinical effects in the treatment of self-injury in individuals with developmental disabilities. *J Dev Phys Disabil* 1993;5:17–27.
48. Filla A, DeMichele G, Orefice G. A double-blind crossover trial of amantadine hydrochloride in Friedreich's ataxia. *Can J Neurol Sci* 1993;20:52–55.
49. Sandman C, Hetrick W, Taylor D, Barron J. Naltrexone reduces self-injury and improves learning. *Exp Clin Psychopharmacol* 1993;1:242–258.
50. Willemsen-Swenkels S, Bitelaar J, Nijof G, et al. Failure of naltrexone to reduce self-injurious and autistic behavior in mentally retarded adults. *Arch Gen Psychiatry* 1995;52:766–773.
51. Casner J, Weinheimer B, Gualtieri CT. Naltrexone and self-injury: a retrospective population study. *J Clin Psychopharmacol* 1996;16:389–394.
52. Griffin J, Williams D, Stark M, et al. Self-injurious behavior: a state-wide survey of the extent and circumstances. *J Appl Res Ment Retard* 1986;7:105–116.
53. Altmeyer B, Locke B, Griffin J, et al. Treatment strategies for self-injurious behavior in a large service-delivery network. *Am J Ment Defic* 1987;91:333–340.
54. Welch SP, Bass PP, Olson KG, et al. Morphine-induced modulation of calcitonin gene-related peptide levels. *Pharmacol Biochem Behav* 1992;43:1107–1116.
55. Molliver ME. Serotonergic neuronal systems: what their anatomic organization tells us about function. *J Clin Psychopharmacol* 1987;7:3.
56. Meltzer HY, Lowy MT. The serotonin hypothesis of depression. In: Meltzer HY, ed. *Psychopharmacology: the third generation of progress*. New York: Raven Press, 1987:513–526.
57. Van Praag HM. *Biogenic amines: new evidence of serotonin deficient depressions, in depressive disorders*. Stuttgart: FK Schattauer, 1978.
58. Hale AS, Proctor AW, Bridges PK. Clomipramine, tryptophan and lithium in combination for resistant endogenous depression: seven case studies. *Br J Psychiatry* 1987;151:213–217.
59. Blier P, De Montigny C, Chaput Y. Modifications of the serotonin systems by antidepressant treatments: implications for the therapeutic response in major depression. *J Clin Psychopharmacol* 1987;7:24.
60. Virkkunen M, De Jong J, Bartko J, et al. Psychobiological concomitants of history of suicide attempts among violent offenders and impulsive fire setters. *Arch Gen Psychiatry* 1989;46:604–606.
61. Arora RC, Meltzer HY. Serotonergic measures in the brains of suicide victims: 5-HT2 binding sites in the frontal cortex of suicide victims and control subjects. *Am J Psychiatry* 1989;146:730–736.
62. Eichelman B. Catecholamines and aggressive behavior. In: Usdin E, ed. *Neuroregulators and psychiatric disorders*. New York: Oxford University, 1977:146–150.
63. Insel TR, Murphy DL. The psychopharmacological treatment of obsessive-compulsive disorder: a review. *J Clin Psychopharmacol* 1981;1:304–311.
64. Rasmussen SA. Lithium and tryptophan augmentation in clomipramine-resistant obsessive-compulsive disorder. *Am J Psychiatry* 1984;141:1283–1285.
65. Zohar J, Mueller EA, Insel TR, et al. Serotonergic responsivity in obsessive-compulsive disorder. *Arch Gen Psychiatry* 1987;44:946.
66. Herzog DB, Copeland PM. Eating disorders. *N Engl J Med* 1985;313:295–303.
67. Goldbloom DS, Kennedy SH, Kaplan AS, et al. Anorexia nervosa and bulimia nervosa. *CMAJ* 1989; 140:1149–1153.

68. Coleman M. Serotonin & central nervous system syndromes of childhood: a review. *J Autism Child Schizophr* 1973;1:27–35.
69. Greenberg A, Coleman M. Depressed whole blood serotonin levels associated with behavioral abnormalities in the de Lange syndrome. *Pediatrics* 1973;51:720–724.
70. Gedye A. Trazodone reduced aggressive and self-injurious movements in a mentally handicapped male patient with autism. *J Clin Psychopharmacol* 1991;11:275–276.
71. Swedo SE, Rapoport JL, Cheslow DL, et al. High prevalence of obsessive-compulsive symptoms in patients with Sydenham's chorea. *Am J Psychiatry* 1989;146:246–249.
72. Lipinski JF Jr. Clomipramine in the treatment of self-mutilating behaviors. *N Engl J Med* 1991;324:1441–1442.
73. Russell JE, Gedye A. Self-injury, regurgitation, and antiemetics. *Lancet* 1989;1:225–226.
74. King BH. Fluoxetine reduced self-injurious behavior in an adolescent with mental retardation. *J Child Adolesc Psychopharmacol* 1991;1:321.
75. Bass JNM, Beltis JME. Therapeutic effect of fluoxetine on naltrexone-resistant self- injurious behavior in an adolescent with mental retardation. *J Child Adolesc Psychopharmacol* 1991;1:331.
76. Markowitz PIM. Effect of fluoxetine on self-injurious behavior in the developmentally disabled: a preliminary study. *J Clin Psychopharmacol* 1992;12:27–31.
77. Ricketts RWM, Goza ABM, Ellis CRM, et al. Clinical effects of buspirone on intractable self-injury in adults with mental retardation. *J Am Acad Child Psychiatry* 1994;33:270–276.
78. Gedye A. Dietary increase in serotonin reduces self-injurious behaviour in a Down's syndrome adult. *J Ment Defic Res* 1990;34.
79. Kopin I. Neurotransmitters & the Lesch-Nyhan syndrome. *N Engl J Med* 1981;305:1148–1150.
80. Nyhan WL. The Lesch-Nyhan syndrome. *Annu Rev Med* 1973;24:41–60.
81. Daly JW, Bruns RF, Snyder SM. Adenosine receptors in the central nervous system: relationship to the central actions of methylxanthines. *Life Sci* 1981;28:2083–2097.
82. Katsuragi T, Ushijima I, Furukawa T. The clonidine-induced self-injurious behavior of mice involves purinergic mechanisms. *Pharmacol Biochem Behav* 1984;20:943–946.
83. Criswell H, Breese GR, Mueller RA. Evidence for adenosine dopamine interactions in the LNS. *Soc Neurosci Abstr* 1986;12:1007.
84. Phillis JW. Chlorpromazine & trifluoperazine potentiate the action of adenosine on rat cerebral cortical neurons. *Gen Pharmacol* 1985;16:19–24.
85. Harker LA, Kadatz RA. Mechanism of action of dipyridamole. *Thromb Res* 1983;[Suppl IV]:39–46.
86. Frye GD, Baumeister AA, Crotty K, et al. Evaluation of the role of antinociception in self-injurious behavior following intranigral injection of muscimol. *Neuropharmacology* 1986;25:717–726.
87. Breese GR, Hulebak KL, Napier TC, et al. Enhanced muscimol-induced behavioral responses after 6-OHDA lesions: relevance to susceptibility for self-mutilation behavior in neonatally lesioned rats. *Psychopharmacology* 1987;91:356–362.
88. Sawynok J. Monoamines as mediators of the antinociceptive effect of baclofen. *Naunyn Schmiedebergs Arch Pharmacol* 1983;323:54–57.

16

Self-injurious Behavior II: The Cornelia de Lange Syndrome

SUMMARY

Cornelia de Lange syndrome (CDLS) is a pathobehavioral mental retardation syndrome characterized by dysmorphic facies and hirsutism, short stature, limb anomalies, and self-injurious behavior (SIB). More than 3,500 cases have been identified worldwide, and most of the clinical information about the syndrome has been generated by a particularly active parents' association that has chapters in several countries.

SIB in patients with CDLS tends to be reactive, in contrast to Lesch-Nyhan syndrome (LNS) in which it is compulsive. CDLS is associated with a number of painful physical anomalies including gastroesophageal (GE) reflex and peripheral neuropathy, and it is likely that self-injury develops in response to pain, perhaps as a means to "gate" it, as acupuncture does. From these origins, it can become habitual. Retarded people in general and patients with CDLS in particular are creatures of habit.

The pharmacologic management of SIB in CDLS is indirect. SIB will gradually come under control if intelligent steps are taken to control the painful physical conditions that are its cause. Drug intervention can aim to reduce patients' patterns of unusual emotional reactivity, impulsiveness or propensity to habit, or abnormal sleep-wake cycle. If one alleviates the uncomfortable and dismaying circumstances of their day-to-day lives, their SIB will gradually subside and will be replaced by more adaptive patterns of behavior.

SIB in LNS and CDLS is concentrated in children and adolescents. It tends to diminish as the patients grow up. This is also true of patients whose SIB is the result of sensorimotor deficits or dysautonomia. Severe SIB that persists into adult life is exceptional. SIB is a primitive, undifferentiated behavior that will subside if the patient is permitted to develop normal control systems. In the unfortunate cases in which SIB persists, it is usually the result of prolonged institutionalization or treatment with drugs that compromise development and learning. The improved living conditions of mentally handicapped individuals and improved teaching and medical care have together led to a general decline in the occurrence of SIB.

CORNELIA DE LANGE SYNDROME

CDLS (Brachmann-Cornelia de Lange syndrome) is a mental retardation syndrome characterized by short stature, hirsutism, and facial and skeletal anomalies (1–3). Cornelia Cornelia de Lange was a Dutch pediatrician, the first woman professor of medicine in Holland, an extraordinarily gifted individual and a hero of her people during World War II. She described the syndrome in 1933, but Brachmann, an Austrian physician, first described it in 1919.

CDLS is interesting by virtue of its association with a unique constellation of behavioral and temperamental attributes, most notably SIB.

THE CORNELIA CORNELIA DE LANGE SYNDROME FOUNDATION

Most of what we know about CDLS has been generated by the Cornelia Cornelia de Lange Syndrome Foundation (CCDLSF), a group that was organized in 1977 when a small group of families with children with CDLS met with a medical geneticist, Laird Jackson, and began to publish a newsletter. At the time, CDLS was an obscure genetic condition and thought to be extremely rare.

The parents' group grew, slowly at first, and then more rapidly. Families joined from around the United States and Canada and then the United Kingdom. The association began to attract the interest of professionals in various fields: geneticists at first, then a speech therapist, an educator, a pediatric dentist, a pediatric gastroenterologist. By 1988, when I was first invited to the annual meeting, there were more than 700 CDLS probands identified; 100 families attended the meeting. By then, it was the CCDLSF, with headquarters in Collinsville, CT, with the rudiments of an office, a staff, and a great deal of confidence and positive energy. Its mission was to support families and children with CDLS by sharing information and generating new knowledge about the condition by supporting the activities of professional investigators.

Alexis de Tocqueville observed that Americans, who are always dubious about the intrusions of government, have a unique proclivity to join voluntary associations. He was impressed by the spirit of cooperative, voluntary effort. That spirit imbues a number of organizations, developed for most of the mental retardation syndromes and modeled after the Association for Retarded Citizens. Because that organization has been so effective in influencing political and social policy, daughter organizations have been able to concentrate on supporting families and generating and disseminating knowledge. The CCDLSF is now international in scope, with branches in Europe, Australia, and Asia and biennial meetings that alternate from stateside to abroad. It represents 2,000 people with CDLS in the United States and 1,500 more in other countries. It has accomplished a great deal with very little help from the national institutes or eponymous foundations.

I have had the privilege of attending the CCDLSF meetings since 1988. People with CDLS are not the hopeless cases, behaviorally speaking, that we once believed, but they do have formidable neuropsychiatric problems, and the attention of psychiatrists, psychologists, and other behaviorists has always been appreciated. In 1989, the CCDLSF helped me to complete a survey of behavior in CDLS that assembled data from 138 probands. Important new information has accrued since then, our understanding of the syndrome and what drives its untoward behaviors has grown. Experience with CDLS has disconfirmed the old beliefs that CDLS is similar to LNS or that behavioral problems are inevitable. It has strengthened the conviction that SIB is not a unitary condition. It also taught a lesson about the accrual of knowledge. Accustomed as I had been to the academic way, with tight controls and research defined in terms of method rather than importance, it was a novel experience to be a naturalist and to do a field study.

THE SYNDROME

Patients with CDLS are small and hirsute, with characteristic dysmorphic features, developmental delays, and difficult behaviors. The phenotype is not invariant; it may change with age and may vary in relation to elements such as birth weight (Table 16.1).

CDLS is a genetic disorder but not especially heritable. It is sporadic, and the risk of recurrence within a sibship is rare. There are reports of monozygotic concordance and familial occurrence, but only if partial elements of the syndrome occur in family members (4–11). The similarities between CDLS and the phenotype of duplication 3q [dup (3q)] syndrome are interesting and 3q has been the focus of investigation for CDLS (12). The diagnosis is currently made on clinical grounds, based on morphologic features, and no genetic, biochemical, neurodiagnostic, or psychological measure can affirm the diagnosis.

The condition is not rare; the incidence is one in 10,000 to 30,000 livebirths (7,13).

Clinical Characteristics

Children and adults with CDLS are small and have distinctive facies and other dysmorphic features. It is not a difficult diagnosis to make based on physical characteristics alone. High-level children and adults

TABLE 16.1. *Cornelia de Lange syndrome*

Major characteristics
- Small size: low birth weight and length, growth retardation, microcephaly.
- Developmental delays: mental retardation ranging from mild to severe, learning and language disabilities.
- Behavior: self-injurious behavior, hyperactivity, repetitive behaviors, aggression.

Secondary characteristics
- Facies: synophrys; long eyelashes; upturned nose; thin, downturned lips; low-set ears; high arched or cleft palate.
- Hirsutism.
- Limbs: small hands and feet, clinodactyly, syndactyly of the toes, proximal thumb, missing portions of the upper limbs (usually the fingers, hands, and forearms), peripheral neuropathy.
- Neurosensory: hearing loss, absent tear ducts, blepharitis, ptosis, and extreme myopia.
- There are associated cardiac, gastrointestinal, and genital anomalies, such as ventriculoseptal defects, gastric reflux, peptic ulcer disease, cryptorchism, hypospadias. Most, but not all, of the identified cases are mentally retarded. Approximately 20% have seizures at some time in their lives.

with CDLS tend to be larger, with fewer dysmorphic features, except the characteristic synophrys (joined eyebrows) and mild hirsutism. In low-level children with CDLS, the upper limb abnormalities are quite striking.

They are prone to a number of medical and dental problems when they are children (3). Gastrointestinal difficulties are most prominent, most notably GE reflux. Reflux symptoms are extremely disturbing to these small, vulnerable children who hardly understand what is going on. They adopt strange and awkward positions to control the pain, especially lying prone on the floor and arching the back. For a long time, this was interpreted as a behavioral problem; in fact, it is almost always a symptom of GE reflux. Most children with CDLS are treated with H_2 blockers or proton pump inhibitors, with varying results. Almost all of them require a fundoplication; many need a feeding tube. (They may have serious problems with GE reflux, even if esophageal manometrics are normal and endoscopy does not reveal signs of esophagitis. We have a low threshold for recommending surgical correction.)

They are also given to head and neck problems such as otitis, bruxism, sinusitis, cataracts, dental crowding, dysplastic enamel, and retinal detachment; to respiratory problems such as asthma and frequent infections; to cardiac anomalies and genitourinary problems such as hypospadias, cryptorchism, and frequent urinary tract infections. All the conditions may be tricky to diagnose because the children are mostly nonverbal and do not readily consent to examination.

All these conditions are also the occasion of pain and discomfort, which aggravates the child's mental state and may contribute to the development of SIB. Most important in this regard is the problem of peripheral neuropathy, which we have only recently come to appreciate, which is discussed at some length here.

Myoclonus, the sudden and abrupt stimulation of a large group of coordinated muscles, is well known to occur in patients with CDLS. Sometimes it is perceived as a startle reaction, back arching, and sleep-onset myoclonus. Seizures, past or present, occur in approximately 20% of patients with CDLS. Virtually every seizure type has been reported. There does not seem to be a connection between the occurrence or nonoccurrence of seizures or any aspect of anticonvulsant treatment with behavioral problems or SIB. (Their seizures are not especially troublesome or difficult to treat. They do not usually persist past childhood.)

Sleep problems are very common: a variable sleep pattern, broken sleep, frequent awakening, insomnia, hypo- or hypersomnia, and sleep apnea. Eating problems are also common, as one might expect in children with reflux esophagitis, and other gastrointestinal conditions.

TABLE 16.2. *Behavioral problems in 138 children with Cornelia de Lange syndrome*

Behavioral problem	Number of children
Self-injurious behavior	88
Aggression	57
Hyperactivity	18
Oppositional-defiant behavior	14
Destructiveness	14
Temper tantrums	13
Anxious, easily upset	8
Irritable, dysphoric	7
Screaming	5
Withdrawal	5

Most children with CDLS are described by their parents and caretakers as affectionate. They tend to prefer sameness and routines and may be prone to repetitive behaviors, obsessions, and compulsions, autistic traits to be sure, but they are not autistic. They are frequently described as sensitive and easily frightened or startled.

Our initial survey of children with CDLS in 1989 asked about behavioral problems. SIB and aggression were the most commonly reported behavioral problems (Table 16.2).

Behavior in Cornelia de Lange Syndrome

It is appropriate to discuss the behavioral problems of children with CDLS in some detail. It is no less interesting than the better known behavioral phenotypes, but little has been written about it, and the old publications are outdated and misleading. The implacable self-mutilation and aggression that was once the behavioral stereotype of the patient with CDLS was, in retrospect, the result of institutional living and high doses of sedating neuroleptics and anticonvulsants (14–19).

Our long experience with patients with CDLS has mitigated that old view considerably. Although approximately two-thirds of them have behavioral problems, in most of them, the difficulties are entirely manageable in community settings, sometimes without drugs. They arise during the first decade, flourish (as it were) during the second, and then recede during the third. Adults with CDLS are usually mellow, pleasant, affectionate, and happy with life.

Personality

Children with CDLS are temperamental, to say the least, and prone to SIB and other behavioral problems when they are angry, frustrated, sick, or in pain, when demands are made on them, or when their routine is changed. Because they are temperamental, such occasions frequently arise.

Their temperaments are dysrhythmic, given to cycles of positive and negative affect and to irregularity in vegetative behaviors (e.g., eating and sleeping) and emotional response. They are also immature. What are perceived as behavioral problems, especially in the young patients with CDLS, are the kinds of behaviors that one associates with 2 year olds. What distinguishes children with CDLS from normal 2 year olds is that they are more temperamental, dysrhythmic, and hyperreactive.

Like very young children, they are affectionate and respond to warmth, gentle touch, and soothing stimuli and prefer routines and predictability. They are easy to frighten or startle and do not like loud noise or overstimulating environments.

They are hypersensitive, given to strong reactions to ordinary stimuli and prolonged reactions to stressors that are only transient. They are extremely sensitive to their physical environment.

Children and adults with CDLS are capable of a full range of emotional response, for better or worse. They are joyful, playful, and cheerful. They are most appreciative of human interactions, and their relationships are mutual and giving. They like to be happy, and the things that make them happy are what most young children enjoy.

Because they are temperamental, however, their moods can change quickly, even unpredictably. They can be extremely dysphoric, irritable, intolerant, and hard to satisfy. They are prone to anxiety but rarely depressed. They can have severe tantrums, with destruction, aggression, or self-injury.

People with CDLS have a few untoward personality characteristics. They can be impulsive, compulsive, or both. They can develop odd fixations, preoccupations, or obsessions. They are prone to repetitive behaviors and are creatures of habit. They can be stubborn, oppositional, provocative, or mischievous. However troublesome these traits are on a day-to-day basis, they are lovable and manage to inspire deep affection and loyalty in their families and caregivers.

Self-injurious Behavior

The behavioral problems to which children with CDLS are prone are reflective of their temperamental attributes, intellectual limitations, and physical characteristics. Their moods are variable, not consistent, as are their behavioral problems. The children (and the adults to a lesser degree) are given to good and bad times.

In the 1989 survey, SIB was the most commonly reported behavioral problem. Of 131 respondents to the survey, no fewer than 88 had current problems with SIB; 10 more had SIB in the past, and 33 reported none at all. SIB was reported to occur when the child was angry (53), frustrated (32), sick (30), when unreasonable demands were made (22), for attention (18), or in response to pain (8). Thus, the pattern of SIB was almost always perceived as reactive or occasional rather than constant in nature. Seventy-one of the respondents thought their children had a high pain threshold, 17 had a low pain threshold, and 29 had a normal pain threshold.

The most common forms of SIB were self-biting (27), hitting or slapping (20), hair pulling (15), head banging (11), picking (10), scratching (5), and gouging (5). Virtually every other form of SIB occurs sometimes: eye gouging, pulling at tissues, bruxism, rubbing, poking, cutting, and rectal digging. Gentle physical restraints by holding the child or applying soft ties, had been used for 34 of the subjects.

In terms of physical injury as a result of SIB, there were no reports of self-mutilation to the degree that one sees in LNS, nor have I ever seen such a case. Parents reported relatively mild injuries such as scratches (10), scars (9), bruises (8), bites (8), cuts (7), sores (5), infections (5), hair pulled out (4), two damaged tear ducts, and one broken nose. Not a trivial list, by any means, but not as severe as in LNS. (I have seen one patient with CDLS who was thought to be blind from self-induced injury. In fact, he had inverted eyelids and was blind from chronic corneal irritation. He probably pounded his eyes because they hurt so much.)

The difficult behaviors in patients with CDLS develop or grow more severe when the patients are adolescents. Parents were asked, therefore, when difficulties with SIB first developed and when the difficulties grew so severe that they sought professional consultation. The largest group of respondents reported that SIB first began at ages 2 to 4 years and that the problem of SIB became severe at ages 5 to 8. However, when parents and caretakers were asked to rate the subjects' behavior on the Self-injurious Behavior Questionnaire (SIBQ) (Appendix), a different picture emerged. The SIBQ scores for SIB and associated problems were highest in patients of ages 15 to 30.

Scores on the current status SIBQ were positively correlated with age for SIB ($r = 0.29$, $p = 0.002$), and the scores on the "at his worst" SIBQ were positively correlated with age for SIB ($r = 0.30$, $p = 0.001$). Although only a small amount of the variance in SIBQ scores could be attributed to age alone, the common lore appears to be correct. Although SIB begins during the first decade of life, behavioral problems increase as the children grow older, and they are at their worst during the second and third decades.

SIB in people with CDLS is reflective of their personality characteristics. They are temperamental and given to sudden mood changes. SIB usually occurs when they are in a bad mood for some reason. They are hypersensitive, and SIB usually occurs in reaction to some event. It may be an impulsive or compulsive response, for example, picking at a sore.

SIB is reflective of their cognitive limitations. It is much more likely to occur in severely retarded individuals and hardly ever is seen in people with CDLS of normal intelligence.

It is also reflective of their physical state. The occurrence of SIB in a young child with CDLS is usually related to a painful physical condition, such as GE reflux and sinusitis, or to limb pain caused by peripheral neuropathy. It is relatively mild, short-lived, and recedes after the painful condition is resolved. During puberty and adolescence, however, SIB is more likely to occur independently of an obvious physical stressor. It is a more serious problem, more sustained, and difficult to manage.

In adult life, the proclivity to SIB and other untoward behaviors is markedly reduced in most individuals. In some, however, they remain problematic. I was impressed in the past that most such individuals had been treated as children with high doses of neuroleptics or sedating anticonvulsants and had had multiple placements in residential facilities. Whether that was the cause or result of their severe, enduring behavioral problems, I cannot say. It was believed that enduring behavioral problems in adults with CDLS were wholly a function of tardive akathisia, anticonvulsant neurotoxicity, and the trauma of multiple, inept caregivers. That was true, for the most part, but it was also an overgeneralization. Some patients have enduring behavioral problems, including SIB, despite excellent care. Maybe it is not a matter of drug toxicity but the failure to find the right drugs.

The developmental trajectory of SIB in people with CDLS is this:

- A common, mild problem in childhood, usually related to an underlying painful condition,
- A common, severe problem in adolescence, generally independent of the child's physical state,
- Only rarely a severe and enduring problem in adults.

SIB in people with CDLS is reactive in the sense that it correlates with their affective state and painful medical conditions such as GE reflux. After the first decade, however, most of these medical conditions have resolved. The one continuing medical condition that they have, and probably the reason they are inclined to self-injure, is probably related to their underlying neurosensory problems.

Sensory Neuropathy

Several years ago, I had the opportunity to meet a pretty 16-year-old girl with CDLS who was a successful high school student. She was bright and had no behavioral or emotional problems. She was a self-assured young lady, not at all discomfited by the knowledge that she had a "mental retardation syndrome." I was able to talk to her for a long time. The only unusual problem that she had, she said, was burning pain in the soles of her feet.

Since then, I have always asked about painful sensations in the extremities when I evaluate a patient with CDLS. I have learned that most children with CDLS have similar problems. They say so if they can, or one infers that they do from their behavioral and emotional state. They hate to wear shoes, for example, and putting shoes on or keeping them on can be a major bone of contention. They stimulate their extremities in various ways, e.g., by locking them into tight places again and again, adopting odd and seemingly uncomfortable positions, or pinching, biting, or sucking them. Their arms and legs feel cold. They much prefer very warm or hot water. Livedo reticularis and Raynaud's phenomenon are not uncommon. You can calm them down by gently stroking their arms, sometimes by applying deep pressure. Mild analgesics such as acetaminophen or ibuprofen sometimes have a calming effect. These characteristics are virtually ubiquitous but are much more prominent in children with malformed arms and hands.

It is hardly an inferential leap to think that people with severe musculoskeletal malformations might also have abnormalities of the peripheral nerves, and supportive evidence is beginning to accumulate from histamine tests and nerve conduction velocity tests. At least a degree of improvement in difficult behaviors including SIB in people with CDLS who are treated with centrally acting antinociceptive drugs such as amitriptyline, trazodone, selective serotonin reuptake inhibitors, gabapentin, and tiagabine has been observed.

Inherited Polyneuropathies

There are several genetic syndromes that are characterized by focal or diffuse peripheral neuropathy involving motor, sensory, or autonomic nerves. They are not necessarily static but may evolve over the years, particularly during periods of rapid growth, for example, during adolescence. Some are associated with mental retardation (e.g., congenital insensitivity to pain, Refsum's disease, abetalipoproteinemia, familial dysautonomia).

It is possible that there is an element of sensory/autonomic polyneuropathy in CDLS. It does share some qualities with familial dysautonomia (Riley-Day syndrome): growth retardation, recurrent infections, impaired pain and temperature sensation with relative preservation of tactile and pressure sense, cold hands and feet, absence of overflow tearing, recurrent vomiting, sleep apnea, decreased peristalsis, and impaired gastric motility. Children with familial dysautonomia often require Nissen fundoplication to relieve their gastrointestinal difficulties and to prevent aspiration. Like children with CDLS, they sometimes require feeding tubes. They are also prone to mental retardation, emotional lability, and sometimes SIB. Intradermal histamine does not evoke a normal flare reaction.

Management of Behavioral and Emotional Problems in Cornelia de Lange Syndrome

Patients with CDLS are small and immature, and many of their behavioral problems, such as hyperactivity or "getting into everything," are explicable in terms of the exploratory behavior that one sees in normal children at age 2 or 3. Their problems with aggression, tantrums, destructiveness, provocative, mischievous, and oppositional behavior more closely resemble the problem behaviors of young children than those of neuropsychiatric patients.

Children with CDLS respond to psychoactive medications as very young children do, with a variable response to medications overall and a high risk of side effects and paradoxical responses.

SIB is not unknown in normal infants, and head banging, for example, is a problem that parents bring to their pediatrician. The appropriate management advice in such cases is to look for a medical condition that may be making the child uncomfortable, to find an alternative way to stimulate or comfort the child, to limit the damage the infant is able to do to himself with padding or soft restraints, and to avoid hysterical overreaction. The risk of ignoring SIB in such infants is that physical damage may occur or that the problem may turn from a transient event into a prolonged bad habit.

One should handle SIB in young patients with CDLS in almost exactly the same way. Look for a medical cause, such as otitis, esophagitis, urinary tract infections, neuropathy, or seizures. The children are particularly prone to painful medical conditions, such as GE reflux or neuropathic pain in their hands and feet. Find more appropriate ways to soothe or stimulate the child. Rely on redirection and soft restraint as primary methods of behavioral management. Examine the environment of the child to determine whether there are continuing stressors in his or her life that are provoking the SIB. Some children with CDLS have phonosensitivity or, less often, photosensitivity. Loud noises and bright light can be stressful to them. Stay away from psychoactive medications that are as likely to aggravate the problem as they are to improve it.

As a general rule, SIB in a child with CDLS is first the expression of pain, discomfort, frustration, or dismay. It is therefore an attempt to communicate or to resolve another problem. The appropriate treatment is exactly what the child would have you do, i.e., to get rid of the primary problem.

The observation that children with CDLS are temperamental, hypersensitive, and dysrhythmic also has practical implications.

The first implication is for prediction. It should be expected that most children with CDLS will have behavioral problems at some time, and one should be prepared to deal with those difficulties when they arise. Their management, unfortunately, is usually labor intensive, but there is no escaping that. When they are having a bad time, they require a lot of hands-on attention and management. Conversely, their untoward behaviors should be expected to resolve by themselves after a while. Bad times follow good times, but good times follow bad times. That should lend some encouragement at least to parents and teachers who have to endure the bad times to get to the good times. The arduous work of behavioral management will be rewarded, one may always expect, by a period of calm and compliance.

The second implication is for attribution. Although one must look for a physical or environmental stressor when a child begins to have behavioral problems, one must understand that there is not always a cause or precipitant. People who are hypersensitive and dysrhythmic may experience periods when their threshold is so low that even the normal stimuli of day-to-day life are intolerable grievances. It is as if the child wakes up with a hangover some mornings. The regular noises of the classroom may be jarring on such days, the failure of immediate gratification may be dealt with as if it were a major frustration, or a momentary lapse in normal interaction may be perceived as an intolerable slight. The child may just be in the mood for mischief. During such periods, it is futile to expect to find a clearly defined precipitant or even a satisfying explanation for the misbehavior.

The third implication is for prognosis. The temperamental attributes of children with CDLS lead one to expect that they may be vulnerable to pathologic transformation if their difficulties are not handled gently and appropriately early on. Children with CDLS are given to habits. They may begin to self-injure by rubbing or picking at a small lesion. Then it becomes a habit, with a feed-forward feature at that. The more the child picks, the longer his or her lesion will persist, and the more irritating it will be. Then the habit begins to generalize, and other forms of self-injury are recruited into the child's behavioral repertoire. Then its intentionality is expanded; self-injury is discovered to serve a useful purpose in controlling (or "gating") other forms of pain, controlling anxiety or frustration, or manipulating one's environment and the reactions of other people. Because they are temperamental and dysrhythmic, their pattern of self-injury will vary from day to day in frequency and severity. Some days it will seem to be associated with pain or dysphoria, and on other days it may be accompanied by laughter or a mischievous smile. This kind of variability will usually defy functional behavioral analysis.

If SIB is handled harshly, with aversives, for example, or by ignoring the child's distress or administering a drug that may cause sedation, dysphoria, or akathisia, then there is the risk of turning a minor, variable habit into a persistent pattern of pathologic behavior. The suggestion, then, is that SIB in CDLS represents a minor phenotype or a proclivity that may interact with circumstances in a particular way and thus become a major difficulty.

Conversely, because SIB is at least in part a function of the child's immaturity, one should expect that it will ultimately recede. The behavioral problems of patients with CDLS are recurrent but also self-limiting. If they are treated gently and without recourse to measures that carry their own risk of damage, they can be controlled and will not be permanently disabling.

Pharmacotherapy

The 1989 survey inquired whether medications had ever been used for SIB or other behavioral problems. The 138 respondents generated the following data:

Sixteen subjects had been treated with neuroleptics, but there were only three positive reactions, one only slight. In most cases, the behavior had grown much worse, or there were intolerable side effects such as dystonia.

Eleven subjects had been on psychostimulants, but drug treatment improved hyperactivity in only two of the 11, and in the others, it had either made the problem behaviors worse or caused anorexia, irritability, mood swings, or depression.

Thirteen were treated with sedative-hypnotics. One of four responded to chloral hydrate. The antihistaminics helped in two cases, benzodiazepines in one of five, and buspirone in one of two. Propanolol was tried twice and did not work well in either case. L-Tryptophan calmed one child and helped him to sleep better.

Seven had been treated with antidepressants. Three of five had done slightly better on imipramine, one subject had no effect on desipramine, and in one, fluoxetine helped at first and then the effect disappeared.

In seven subjects, anticonvulsants had been prescribed for behavioral problems independent of seizures. Carbamazepine and phenytoin had actually helped in three of these cases.

This survey, of course, was based on prescription practice during the 1980s. The data suggested that no medication or class of medications was predictably useful in alleviating SIB or other behavioral problems in patients with CDLS. Have matters improved at all since then?

Not much has improved, but some progress has been made. Here is what we have learned.

When we began our consultations with patients with CDLS through the foundation, my colleagues and I were cognizant of the three ways to develop effective drug therapy:

- Rational pharmacotherapy, i.e., drug treatment addressed to a known and specific pathophysiologic deficit. The best example in neuropsychiatry is L-dopa for Parkinson's disease. Because we do not know anything about the underlying neurochemical disturbance in the CDLS, this avenue was not open.
- Empirical pharmacotherapy, i.e., try it and see whether it works. This is what we tried to do with the 1989 survey. If a medication or class of medications seemed to work, one would follow the lead and explore the possibilities. The problem was that the survey yielded no good leads to follow.
- Intuitive pharmacotherapy. What are the symptoms that we are trying to treat, what tends to work for those symptoms in other mental retardation syndromes, and does it work in CDLS? This, in fact, is where we have been for the past 12 years.

Here is a simple example of intuitive pharmacotherapy: children with CDLS are dysrhythmic and their sleep patterns are often disturbed. Melatonin is often successful in retarded people with sleep disorders. Therefore, melatonin may be effective for children with CDLS with sleep disorders. In fact, most of the parents of children with CDLS who have tried melatonin report that it works quite well.

Trazodone is very good for insomnia in patients with brain injury but less effective in mentally retarded patients. Short-acting benzodiazepines are good sedatives for adults with insomnia, but they are not well tolerated by patients with brain injury and mental retardation. The same pattern holds true for CDLS. Trazodone may be helpful for sleep problems, but it is a second choice, after melatonin.

Another example of intuitive pharmacotherapy that holds promise is the use of the α_2-adrenergic drugs clonidine and guanfacine. They are often effective in young children who are hyperactive, impulsive, aggressive, temperamental, and compulsive and in patients with brain injury who are hypervigilant-hyperreactive. The α_2 agonists have been helpful in several children with CDLS for exactly these problems.

The α_2 agonists augment the therapeutic effects of stimulants in hyperactive children and mitigate some of their side effects. Amantadine serves the same purpose. Combining stimulant drugs with clonidine, guanfacine, and amantadine extends their utility to retarded children who are hyperactive but who would ordinarily have side effects if the stimulants were used by themselves. Children with fragile X syndrome are often treated with this combination therapy. The approach is also successful sometimes in hyperactive and impulsive children with CDLS.

The use of serotonergic drugs is another intuitive approach. There are several clinical characteristics of CDLS that serotonergic antidepressants might affect: emotional instability, dysphoria, anxiety, repetitive behaviors, sleep and appetite dysregulation, aggression, and SIB. They are also effective agents in cases of neuropathic pain. Selective serotonin reuptake inhibitors are often used for these indications in patients with fragile X syndrome and in other mentally retarded populations. They are also prescribed for patients with CDLS with at least a degree of success.

Low-dose tricyclic antidepressants (especially amitriptyline), trazodone, gabapentin, and tiagabine are also effective for chronic pain syndromes and neuropathic pain. They may also be effective in CDLS, perhaps for their behavior as mood stabilizers or anxiolytics or for their central antinociceptive effects. Carbamazepine or oxcarbazepine may serve the same purpose, but I am not aware of any positive responses to valproate.

It is my opinion that conventional neuroleptics are contraindicated for the treatment of patients with CDLS. There is very little evidence that they are helpful, and patients with CDLS may be at high risk to develop serious neuroleptic side effects such as tardive akathisia. It is likely that many of the severe cases of SIB in patients with CDLS reported in the literature are cases of tardive akathisia.

In the United States, conventional neuroleptics are rarely used, especially in the developmentally disabled. When physicians think an antipsychotic drug is indicated, they usually select one of the atypicals. No information has accrued about the atypical antipsychotics except risperidone. Low doses of risperidone have been used quite often, usually in adolescents with CDLS with severe SIB, hyperactivity, and aggression. Its therapeutic benefits have not been impressive, but there are occasional patients who seem to have improved. There have also been positive reports of olanzapine in self-injurious individuals.

In the clinical arena, pharmacotherapeutic research usually follows this progression: case reports → clinical series → controlled trials.

At this time, we are still accumulating case reports about drugs for the various behavioral problems associated with CDLS, but there is still not enough for a clinical series in any event. When a physician calls and asks for treatment recommendations, my colleagues and I are likely to suggest:

- Melatonin for sleep disorders,
- Clonidine or guanfacine for hyperactivity and impulsive behavior,
- Trazodone, amitriptyline, or a selective serotonin reuptake inhibitor for emotional instability, dysphoria, anxiety, repetitive behavioral disorders, aggression, and SIB,
- Gabapentin, tiagabine, or oxcarbazepine for the same indications.

THE MEANING OF SELF-INJURIOUS BEHAVIOR

I was once lecturing on the subject of SIB to a group of psychiatrists in Cincinnati. Someone asked a question that I could not answer. He asked: "Dr Gualtieri, why do your patients do this to themselves? What do they say about it?" It was a simple question, but I was nonplussed. I mumbled something to the effect that hardly any of my patients could talk, so I really could not say. He went on to announce that he had treated a number of borderline patients who engaged in self-mutilation, and they told him that they did it "so that they could feel." They said that "it made them experience the boundaries of their selves."

It is true that many psychiatrists, especially those of a psychoanalytic bent, have strong opinions about why their patients engage in self-injury. No two seem to share the same opinion, but the variety makes it interesting. Some of them think that self-injury enables the patient to feel the margins of his or her self, that it is an act of testing the boundaries of an uncertain personality, if you will. Others think that patients feel relief or diminished psychic pain when they self-mutilate; think about it as a form of autoacupuncture. The self-infliction of physical pain may give them control over psychic pain. I have heard psychiatrists say that self-injury is an act of aggression deflected from the "object" to the self. Torture victims are also said to have compulsive self-injury, what is referred to in some circles as "identification with the aggressor." Some of the ugliest self-injurious acts are committed by violent criminals in prison.

There is another school of psychologists who refer to themselves as behavioral analysts, and they too are given to strong opinions about why SIB occurs. They prefer to think of themselves as more empirical and less theoretical than the psychoanalysts, an opinion that may or may not be accurate. Like the psychoanalysts, they believe that human behavior is amenable to rational interpretation. Hence, the occurrence of self-injury is, to the behaviorist, an appropriate occasion for a functional analysis, i.e., a thoughtful dissection of the elements that generate, trigger, or sustain the behavior. The idea is that by manipulating one or another of those elements, one can alleviate the behavior itself. The function of SIB, to the behaviorist, varies from patient to patient. It may be an attempt to communicate, an expression of pain or dismay, an attention getter, a way to exert one's will, or a response pattern shaped over the years by the untoward responses of attendants.

Behind both of these viewpoints is the positivist conviction that even the most unlikely and senseless behavior is amenable to analysis and understanding. It is a conviction that one would expect to be shared by an author who writes a book about the pharmacologic modification of human behavior. The reader is therefore entitled to a modicum of surprise at my prejudice that the irrational and accidental play a far more impressive role in the lives of human beings—patients and others. The idea that human behavior is always given to rational interpretation is hopelessly naïve. My early experience with SIB did nothing to allay the prejudice.

Perhaps I was wrong. So I resolved soon after the lecture in Cincinnati to find out for myself why patients with SIB did what they did. I would ask them. The opportunity arose when I saw one of my mentally retarded patients at the Caswell Center, who had a long history of severe self-biting and who also happened to be quite verbal. I asked her, "Sue Carol, why do you bite yourself?" We were in a large conference room. The whole treatment team was there, and everyone felt, for some reason, that this was an important moment. We hung on her answer. I repeated the question, and she gave me one of her big smiles. Then she said: "Because I'm hungry." From that point, I resolved that people might indeed have a reason to self-injure, but it is never a very good one.

As I drove home from that consultation day at Caswell, I was thinking about the problem of SIB and how its meaning would always escape me. I thought about a patient with LNS at the Center who used to beg to be restrained from gouging his eye or tearing his lip. There were the young parents of a self-injurious child who had to take turns staying up all night to restrain him from beating himself. He was 4 years old. I had a patient who had died, not long before, severely demented. He had dementia pugilistica from 40 years of head banging. I had another patient who had been on very high doses of haloperidol and had been for years. The records were never explicit about why she was on such a high dose. We found out, after we lowered it: she liked to poke her hands through the window and lacerate her wrists on the fragments of glass. Was there any meaning to be found in stories like this? These autoviolations are so utter, they beg reason.

Thus occupied with lugubrious thoughts, driving across the long flat coastal plain, the story of Job entered my mind. The trials of Job, that is what it was—senseless, meaningless afflictions that we are never meant to understand.

Everyone is familiar with the story of Job. Most of us remember how it came about—a wager, of sorts, between God and Satan. As Job lay bereft, several friends came to visit and comfort him, I suppose. I had forgotten their names; I looked them up when I got home; they were Eliphaz the Temanite, Bildad the Shuhite, and Zophar the Naamathite.

Those three luminaries came to visit Job in his afflictions, and they wanted to help. Their way of doing this was to explain exactly why God was sending the trials his way: to make you stronger, Job. It is God's punishment for your transgressions, they told him. They must have thought that if they made sense of his travails, somehow the old man would be comforted. Job, of course, was not impressed [I have heard many such things: "Miserable comforters are ye all"—Job 16:2).]

During my years on the SIB project, I came to understand why old Job was so impatient with Eliphaz, Bildad, and Zophar and what they were telling him. In fact, they were making rationalizations. They were not very convincing; indeed, they did not make sense at all. Job knew that his transgressions were no more or less than any other person's. Why, then, was he being singled out? His trials were beyond understanding, and he knew it. Then, as you recall, the voice of God came out of the whirlwind and affirmed that his sufferings were, indeed, beyond man's understanding. "God thundereth marvelously with his voice; great things doeth he, which we cannot comprehend" (Job 37:5).

That is how I felt when I was young at least, and I guarded jealously my righteous indignation. SIB was a mystery and beyond my understanding. That is where things stayed for several years. I left the SIB project and spent the next few years working mainly with patients with traumatic brain injury (TBI).

People from the CDLS foundation, parents and professionals, kept on calling. I was an expert, and there was not any other psychiatrist who knew much about the condition. So I continued to consult with families and doctors from around the country, about little children who were usually quite sweet but who had the extraordinary propensity to beat themselves up. Every few days there was an e-mail to answer or a phone call to return. Talking to them about Job was not what they needed. Telling them what to do was what they needed.

I did not spend much time talking to them about the meaning of SIB. I just gave them small pieces of advice. Things they could do to alleviate the suffering, to control SIB, and to prevent it from getting out of hand. Avoid certain drugs. Improve the child's classroom experience as best you can. Deal with reflux and with other painful conditions. Try this drug or that one, but do not continue a drug if it does not work. Use gentle restraints and redirection, but do not ever submit to aversive conditioning. Try to keep things quiet, stable, and predictable. Avoid excessively noisy or stimulating environments, and try to keep the child at home. Do not move the child into a group home unless you are sure they can handle him or her; moving from one placement to another will have devastating effects. Above all, hang on. Be confident. If you do the right thing, the SIB will go away. It may get bad for a while, but it will go away. I had begun my work with patients with CDLS as a neuropharmacologist, and I found myself working like a naturalist. Now I was like an old country doctor, dispensing nostrums and good advice, recommending drugs that may not have done much good, but at least they did little harm.

Over the years, however, two very interesting things happened. The advice seemed to help. Attending the meetings every year, I met my old patients and discovered that they were doing well. I thought that all we had to offer was palliative treatment; that seemed to be enough. Doing very little turned out to be a great deal.

The other surprising thing was that as I told them what to do, they told me what it meant. The meaning of SIB, its purpose, its evolution, and its outcome—gradually they began to make sense of it for me. It was as if voices were coming out of the whirlwind again, but this time they were hundreds of children and their families and the doctors who looked after them. They were not indignant or angry but quiet, gentle, and reassuring. They said that this is what it is, this is what it means, and this is what you do about it.

SIB is, indeed, an affliction of jobian proportions, but it is comprehensible. Not in a simple cause-and effect model. It is a complex behavior and its roots are also complex. It begins in different ways, it is sustained or alleviated by different events, and it ends up in different places. It is not a unitary condition, the end product of a single gene or a single neurotransmitter. It is not the result of a linear chain of events. It is comprehensible, and it can be treated. This is what I think it is, and the meaning of it is tightly bound to what we should do for it.

SIB is not a complex behavior. On several occasions, SIB has been referred to as a complex behavior, and it is, but only in the sense that it recruits the agency of several domains in the central nervous system. It is a motor event of some complexity; it is amazing how the children can get around restraints, and a sensory event of even greater complexity. It is a sensory event of even greater complexity.

At the same time, the behavior is primitive and undifferentiated. We know that from the people who are prone to it: infants, children who are severely handicapped, children with profound sensory deficits, people with destabilizing mental conditions such as epilepsy and severe mental illness, patients with TBI as they emerge from coma, and violent prisoners. It arises in reaction to pain, isolation, and extreme stress.

Whatever function SIB may serve, it succeeds because pain is such an intense and transcendent experience. Violent behavior is always an inefficient means to an end, but it is effective in its own way. Without a better way to deal with pain, stress, anxiety, depression, or psychosis, SIB will do the job. Without a better way to communicate or organize one's environment, SIB will do it. As stated previously, people might have a reason to self-injure, but it is never a very good one. It is good enough for someone who has no other alternative.

SIB is genetically permissible. SIB is permissible within the normal genome of a higher animal. It is not a genetic freak. To freely choose pain or freely self-inflict it is ubiquitous. Everyone is familiar with the exquisite sensation of bothering a loose tooth or tearing a fingernail or a cuticle. There is the pain of athletic training, and there is religious mortification. Animals in captivity, especially psittacine birds, engage in self-mutilation. Fertility rituals and rites of initiation are often accompanied by the infliction of excruciating pain. The consumption of foods spiced heavily with capsicum is virtually ubiquitous among peoples who live in the hotter climes.

Individuals choose to experience self-induced pain for a variety of reasons. Their rationale might seem strange or even bizarre to others but not to the individual in question. Hot, spicy foods, for example, induce satiety in people who cannot afford a rich diet. Rigorous athletic training is rewarded by an exquisite sense of well-being, religious mortification confers a sense of ecstasy, and so on.

Controlled pain diminishes uncontrollable pain. Stimulating one class of nociceptive fibers "gates" the experience of pain emanating from another class of pain fibers. It is not counter to the "pleasure principle" but rather, an intelligent trade-off to substitute one form of pain for another. Therefore, the capacity to inflict pain on oneself is inherent. For most people, however, it is a circumscribed endeavor.

SIB is a low-level behavior that can be reproduced in lower creatures. SIB is a variant of very low level behaviors such as stereotypy, self-stimulation, and grooming—behaviors that are elicited in the lowest mammals when they are subjected to stress.

The nervous system requires stimulation, and it will self-stimulate if it has to. At the same time, the nervous system is resentful of overstimulation, and it has ways to reduce tension if it must. Stereotypy and perseverative behavior are arch examples of this in mentally retarded people, people with brain injury, mentally ill people, and normal people. It occurs in circumstances of low or high stimulation. In circumstances of low arousal, it aims to stimulate; in circumstances of high arousal, it aims to calm the organism. Pathologic SIB is a repetitive behavior that acts in precisely this way. Its locus is the reticular core of the central nervous system, from the brainstem to the orbitofrontal cortex. Its mediating neurohumors are norepinephrine and dopamine.

A second elemental behavior that gives rise to SIB is grooming, preening, caressing oneself, licking, rubbing, and even biting. It is universal among mammals, it is stereotyped, and it is a form of habit that occurs when the organism is bored or highly stimulated. It has the same humoral and anatomic basis as self-stimulation. It is also a repetitive behavior that is related to habit or compulsion. The self-mutilation that is induced in experimental animals by neonatal depletion of the dopaminergic neurons represents a pathologic exaggeration of grooming behavior. Grooming may be a form of self-stimulation or tension reduction.

A third element is habit, which is really just a magnification of stereotyped behavior, and compulsion, which is a magnification of habit. In Chapter 15, we discussed how proneness to habitual behavior is characteristic of the severely retarded. The localization of habit is subcortical, especially in the basal ganglia, and its primary mediating neurotransmitter is dopamine.

Pain experiences are dissociable. The experience of pain is a sensory or cognitive event ("I feel a sharp, stabbing pain in my finger") and an affective event ("Ouch. It hurts."). In normal people, the two elements are closely linked, if not locked together. In pathologic states, they may be dissociated, as they are in some patients with frontal lobe lesions who experience pain but do not react to it affectively. When patients with chronic pain were treated with orbital undercutting, a procedure that interrupted the connections between the frontal cortex and the thalamus, they were still cognizant of their painful condition, but it no longer bothered them. A contrasting event is thalamic dysesthesia in which the patient experiences normal sensations as excruciating pain. In cases of severe depression, the patient's very self-consciousness may be excruciatingly painful. We refer to that experience as anguish.

It was already pointed out that individuals with SIB seem to experience pain in different ways and that in some conditions (e.g., deafferentation), severe self-injury occurs without pain at any level. People with LNS perceive pain and react to it emotionally, just as anyone would. In some cases of SIB, however, the patient seems to experience the sensation of pain but not the negative emotional state that normally accompanies it. The physical perception of pain is one thing; the emotional experience of pain as "painful" is another thing entirely. The two events are dissociable. In this matrix of associations and dissociations between perception and reaction, the endogenous opiates and serotonin play a central role.

In the clinical presentations of SIB, there are only rarely pure types who represent a single, predominant element. Most cases represent different combinations and permutations. LNS is a pure example of compulsive SIB. Patients with LNS do not dissociate the experience of pain from the affective response; they do not like to hurt themselves. In CDLS, conversely, SIB does not seem to be experienced as a negative affective event. It is habitual, even compulsive, in some individuals and contains all four of the elementary features of SIB: stimulus modulation, habit, grooming, and pain/emotional self-control.

Mentally handicapped children who are deaf and blind are often given to SIB. The sensorially deprived individual is probably exercising the first element, a behavioral pattern that substitutes the experience of pain for the stimulation that normally resides in a sensory channel.

The retarded individual with a painful medical condition tries to gate the pain by a form of autoacupuncture. He or she perceives the self-induced pain, but it is not experienced as painful because it diminishes the intensity of some other source of pain. Controlled pain is thus substituted for uncontrollable pain.

SIB is occasionally met with in patients with TBI during the unstable phase of coma recovery. In this woeful condition, the personality is in an abject state, emotional responses are global and overwhelming, and the level of behavioral response is primitive and unpredictable. In this context, I think that SIB is recruited in the service of pain, rage, and fear. To the patient's confused state of mind, this intense, primitive behavior confers a degree of control. It alleviates confusion and emotional distress by allowing the patient to express and control it. Patients with the so-called borderline personality disorder engage in self-injury for similar reasons. They do it because physical pain alleviates psychic pain and, as our psychoanalyst in Cincinnati pointed out, to "feel the boundary of their selves."

SIB is a self-limiting condition. Neither patients with TBI nor the severely retarded are able to modulate extremes of emotional and behavioral response. Their capacity for self-regulation is clearly diminished. This is another element that contributes to the pathologic development of SIB: a failure in behavioral modulation, regulation, or self-control. In mentally retarded people, SIB usually begins gradually and then grows in intensity. Then it becomes habitual. It may have begun as a form of self-stimulation or as a measure to control pain, but as the years pass, it takes on an autonomy that is ultimately divorced from the original evocative agent. The patient loses control of the habitual behavior. It no longer serves its original purpose of self-stimulation or pain control, for example, but exists as an autonomous behavior, a bad habit, if you will.

This brings us to the crux of the argument. The most interesting thing about SIB, even in the severely retarded, is that those with SIB are able to gain control. It takes a while, but SIB does eventually diminish and finally disappear. We know that the natural course of SIB in people with LNS or CDLS is a gradual recession during the third decade of life. The behavior gradually fades away. As they grow up and if they stay healthy, their SIB will diminish and then disappear. This does not appear to be a treatment-related effect. It is not a drug effect, although the right drug can make it happen faster. It seems to be the natural course of the disorder. If we can understand how this happens, we will arrive at a better understanding of the meaning of SIB.

SIB is habitual. Whether it occurs often or seldom or compulsively or sporadically, it is a manifestation of a subcortical habit system. Habits are complex behaviors that exist to fulfill their own ends. They are divorced from motivation, intentionality, and ambition. They are solitary and nonmutual.

The people who are most prone to SIB are operating on a low level to begin with. They are severely retarded, brain injured, or mentally ill. They are prone to behavioral responses that are undifferentiated and to affective responses that are global and overwhelming. They are given to habitual behaviors that are unproductive and nonmutual.

Even the severely retarded are capable of developmental progress, just as patients with TBI ultimately recover from their transient state of confusion and agitation. During the course of development, and during TBI recovery, behavior grows increasingly more differentiated, and affective responses become less intense and more controlled. The arousal system becomes more modulated. The patient's level of confusion and dismay is gradually replaced by at least a measure of familiarity and comfort. The reaction to pain is improved, and the patient is less likely to resort to extreme measures to control it.

SIB subsides because the patient develops a behavioral and emotional repertoire that is stronger and more effective in accomplishing his or her goals. The patient is finally able to think in terms of goal-directed behavior. Undifferentiated behaviors are gradually replaced by differentiated behaviors, catastrophic emotional reactions by affective states that are better modulated.

During the course of normal development, a similar transition occurs and is related to the gradual encephalization of behavior and emotional response. During recovery from TBI, cortical control systems are gradually reestablished. One assumes that something similar happens in mentally retarded individuals as they grow up.

The way to control SIB, then, is to take a long-term approach to the problem. The way to overcome a primitive, undifferentiated pattern of behavior is to encourage the development of patterns that are more efficient and effective. It means giving the patient a learning environment that encourages development and maturation. It means treating conditions that interfere with development, such as chronic pain and discomfort, phonophobia, neuropathy, and dysautonomia. It means stabilizing the child's emotional environment by using psychotropic drugs judiciously. It involves controlling hyperarousal or hypoarousal with drugs or behavioral techniques. Sometimes it involves controlling the evolution of habitual behaviors into compulsive behaviors with drugs or behavioral techniques.

It also means avoiding circumstances, environments, management techniques, and drugs that compromise the developmental progress of the individual, impede cognitive development, or destabilize the patient's emotional state. Consigning retarded children to the bleak environments of large institutions and treating them with sedating anticonvulsants and high doses of neuroleptics do nothing to promote development and everything to impede it.

Several times in this chapter and the previous chapter, the horrible cases of people who spent their lifetime in physical restraints, people who engaged in SIB for 3ø0 years or more, and people who died because of complications from self-injury were discussed. The irony is that these patients did not suffer from lack of treatment. The problem is the treatment they got was heavy-handed and counterproductive.

In the previous chapter, we asserted that the prevalence and severity of SIB were declining. There are few data to support this contention beyond the clinical experience of my colleagues and myself. We know our patients and consult as much in facilities for the retarded as we did 20 years ago. There are still plenty of individuals with SIB out there, but it nothing like the SIB epidemic that it was in the past (one in eight). The patients whom we see are younger, the SIB is less severe, and when treatments are brought to bear, the problem recedes. The new drugs, administered in moderate doses, certainly seem to have made a difference. The biggest difference between 1981 and 2002, however, are the improvements in education and programmed care for retarded people. They are not institutionalized, and their medical needs are attended to. Their families and caretakers receive appropriate levels of support. Their lives are interesting and worthwhile.

In such circumstances, even the most severely handicapped individual can thrive, and even the most primitive behaviors will gradually be superseded by more differentiated and effective behaviors.

I think that I was right all along. SIB is a meaningless, irrational affliction. I was wrong, however, to rage against the wind. Job never did. He was patient, he kept the faith, and his trials passed.

REFERENCES

1. Cornelia de Lange C. Sur un type nouveau de de-degeneration (typus amstelodamensis). *Arch Med Enfant* 1933;36:713.
2. Cornelia de Lange C. Nouvelle observation du "typus amstelodamensis" et examen anatomopathologique de ce type. *Arch Med Enfant* 1938;41:193–203.
3. Hawley PP, Jackson LG, Kurnit DM. Sixty-four patients with Brachmann-Cornelia de Lange syndrome: a survey. *Am J Med Genet* 1985;20:453–459.
4. Choo PB, Bianchi GN. Brachmann-Cornelia de Lange syndrome: a report of four cases. *Aust Pediatr J* 1965;1:236.
5. Kroth H. Cornelia Cornelia de Lange Syndrome I bei Zwillingen (Amsterdamer Degenerationstyp). *Arch Kinderheilk* 1965;173:273–283.
6. Opitz JM. Editorial comments on the Brachmann-Cornelia de Lange syndrome. In: *Yearbook of pediatrics.* Chicago: Year Book, 1965:502–504.
7. Opitz JM. Editorial comment: Brachmann-Cornelia de Lange syndrome. *Am J Med Genet* 1985;22:89–102.
8. Kumar D, Blank CE, Griffiths BL. Cornelia Cornelia de Lange syndrome in several members of the same family. *J Med Genet* 1985;22:296–300.
9. Leavitt A, Nuhad D, Davis C. Cornelia Cornelia de Lange syndrome in a mother and daughter. *Clin Genet* 1985;28:157–161.
10. Robinson K, Wolfsberg E, Jones KL. Brachmann-Cornelia de Lange syndrome: evidence for autosomal dominant inheritance. *Am J Med Genet* 1985;22:109–115.
11. Bankier A, Haan E, Birrell R. Letter to the editor: familial occurrence of Brachmann-Cornelia de Lange syndrome. *Am J Med Genet* 1986;25:163–165.
12. Wilson GN, Dasouki M, Barr M. Further delineation of the dup(3q) syndrome. *Am J Med Genet* 1985;22: 117–123.
13. Beck B. Epidemiology of Cornelia Cornelia de Lange's syndrome. *Acta Paediatr Scand* 1976;65:631–638.
14. Bryson Y, Sakati N, Nyhan WL, et al. Self-mutilative behavior in the Cornelia Cornelia de Lange syndrome. *Am J Ment Defic* 1971;76:319–324.
15. Shear CS, Nyhan WL, Kirman BH, et al. Self-mutilative behavior as a feature of the Cornelia de Lange syndrome. *J Pediatr* 1971;78:506–509.
16. Greenberg A, Coleman M. Depressed whole blood serotonin levels associated with behavioral abnormalities in the Cornelia de Lange syndrome. *Pediatrics* 1973;51: 720–724.
17. Johnson HG, Ekman P, Friesen W, et al. A behavioral phenotype in the Cornelia de Lange syndrome. *Pediatr Res* 1976;10:843–850.
18. Andrasik F, Ollendick T, Turner SM, et al. Single case study: pharmacological treatment of aggressive behavior and emesis in the Cornelia Cornelia de Lange syndrome. *J Nerv Ment Dis* 1979;167:764–766.
19. Mueller K, Hsiao S. Pemoline-induced self-biting in rats and self-mutilation in the Cornelia de Lange syndrome. *Pharmacol Biochem Behav* 1980;13:627–631.

17
Epilepsy

SUMMARY

Seizures are common in people with brain injury and mental retardation, but that is not why the subject is raised here. Rather, we are concerned with matters related to seizures. Behavioral problems and emotional instability in neuropsychiatric patients can be preictal, ictal, or postictal. They can be the manifestations of a seizure disorder that is only partially treated or the result of anticonvulsant neurotoxicity. Epilepsy can be associated with intellectual decline, and one seizure syndrome, Landau-Kleffner syndrome (LKS), can cause aphasia and autism. The idea of an "epileptic personality" is probably overstated, but personality changes can occur in patients with temporal lobe seizures. Depression is a frequent complication of epilepsy.

Mentally retarded people, especially the severely retarded, are prone to epilepsy. When a retarded person with epilepsy is referred for a psychiatric consultation, one should first try to ensure that the patient is receiving optimal anticonvulsant treatment. A higher dose, or an alternative anticonvulsant, may alleviate the patient's psychiatric condition without having to resort to a psychotropic drug. This is referred to as the "primacy" of epilepsy.

Patients with brain injury are also prone to seizures, depending on the nature of the injury. Penetrating brain injuries are highly likely to cause posttraumatic seizures, closed head injuries less so. Seizures never occur consequent to concussion. Because patients with brain injury are so vulnerable to the neurotoxic effects of antiepileptic drugs, and the drugs themselves may impede the recovery process, "prophylactic" treatment is strongly discouraged.

Psychotropic drugs can raise or lower the seizure threshold or both. For example, moderate doses of stimulants or amantadine tend to raise the seizure threshold, but high doses can cause seizures. In fact, most of the psychotropic drugs have an ambiguous effect on the seizure threshold. Antidepressants, for example, are proconvulsant, but fluoxetine may possibly have anticonvulsant properties. The same may be true of lithium. The antipsychotic drugs, however, are mostly proconvulsant.

EPILEPSY

The prevalence of seizure disorders in mentally retarded people and people with dementia, with autism, brain injury, and stroke is much higher than it is in the general population. Their seizures, as a rule, are harder to control. They are more prone to the neurotoxic effects of antiepileptic drugs and the epileptogenic effects of psychotropic drugs. Their neurobehavioral difficulties respond selectively to the psychotropic anticonvulsants.

Therein lie areas of commonality. Of greater interest are the areas where differences are manifest.

SEIZURES AND MENTAL RETARDATION

Every type of seizure occurs in people who are mentally retarded, and some seizure disorders, such as infantile spasms and Lennox-Gastaut syndrome, occur only in mentally retarded people. Seizure disorders are very common in retarded people, and the prevalence of seizures correlates directly with the degree of mental handicap (1) (Table 17.1).

TABLE 17.1. *Prevalence of seizures by degree of mental handicap*

Population	Percentage with seizures
School-age children	0.7
IQ 50–70	3–6
Institutionalized children	19.5
IQ 35–49	23
IQ 20–34	28
IQ <20	50

By the age of 20, approximately one-half of the severe to profoundly mentally retarded population will have had a seizure, and in most large residential facilities for the mentally retarded, the prevalence of epilepsy is at least 50%.

There are three patterns to the co-occurrence of mental retardation, epilepsy, and psychiatric disorders:

1. The mild to moderately retarded, who do not have significant neuropathology as a rule, have seizures and psychiatric disorders just as the nonretarded do, and the regular associations apply, albeit to a more pronounced degree.
2. The profoundly retarded who also have severe sensorimotor impairments may have severe seizures that are only partially responsive to antiepileptic drug treatment. They are not, as a rule, prone to behavioral problems or recognizable psychiatric disorders.
3. There is a large number of people in between who are severely handicapped intellectually who also have epilepsy and behavioral disorders.

It is this last group that occupies our attention because most children with mental retardation and active epilepsy also have psychiatric disorders, more than 90% in one study from Sweden (2). Aggression, self-injury, hyperactivity, and intermittent agitation are the most common problems. The behaviors are not easily categorized using ordinary psychiatric classifications, and the interactions between seizures and behavior are highly idiosyncratic. In this group, drug effects on cognition, behavior, and seizures are hard to interpret or predict. The most common psychiatric diagnosis in mentally retarded children with epilepsy is autism (2,3).

Generalized convulsive seizures are the most common epileptic disorders in the general population of mentally retarded people, but in the more severely handicapped, partial seizures with or without secondary generalization tend to be the most frequent. Most retarded people tend to have mixed seizure types, and precise diagnosis, using the International Classification, for example, is only possible for one patient in three.

Seizures and Autism

The prevalence of seizures in autistic children is many times higher than the basal rate in the population, and every variant of epilepsy is represented (4). Children with autism usually have their first seizures in early childhood, but approximately one-third develops seizures for the first time in adolescence or early adult life (1).

Autistic regression is sometimes attributed to ictal or subictal events. Epilepsy or epileptiform electroencephalography (EEG) occurs in a significant minority of autistic children with a history of regression, but in a smaller minority without regression (5). LKS is the prototype. In this extraordinary condition, seizures of temporal lobe origin are associated with gradual loss of language ability. Autistic regression is sometimes the outcome of such activity (6,7).

LKS and the syndrome of continuous spike-and-wave complexes during slow-wave sleep are apparently related conditions characterized by developmental regression, especially the loss of the capacity for language, along with frequent, often generalized spike-and-wave complexes. The aberrant electrical activity can interfere with normal development, in particular the degeneration of unneeded synaptic connections by the process of programmed cell death or apoptosis. Thus, the formation of normal neural aggregates is thwarted, and normal development is impaired. If the temporoparietal cortex is primarily involved, language development is affected; if it is the frontal cortex, higher cognitive and integrative functions are affected. Aberrant electrical activity in the temporal cortex can also disrupt normal temporolimbic input to frontal lobe development (8).

LKS is comparatively rare, but autism is common. Is it possible that this peculiar epilepsy syndrome is more common than we think or that LKS variants exist and may account for more cases of autistic regression than we currently acknowledge? Not a trivial question because when LKS is diagnosed early, it is treatable and developmental regression may be reversed. If LKS were a frequent rather than a rare cause of autism, is it possible that vigorous antiepileptic treatment could prevent autism?

This line of reasoning is not too tortured for some in the autism community, especially parents of autistic children who seem to have developed normally and then in their second or third years, lose all language and sociability. Parents have asked whether the child's autistic regression might not have been prevented by the appropriate antiepileptic drug or possibly by a course of steroids. There is no easy answer to that question. In the absence of seizures or the typical EEG abnormalities of LKS, it is difficult to make any connection. The trick to preventive treatment, if there is any, is to catch the disorder early enough, recognizing the earliest signs of autistic regression, and then to make the appropriate diagnosis using EEG (9). It is difficult to catch the early signs of autistic regression. Even when one does, it is difficult to attribute relatively nonspecific developmental variations with autism.

A more pertinent issue is not whether epilepsy causes autism—it does, but not very often—but that the neuropathology that causes autism involves areas of the brain that are notably epileptogenic. The etiologic factors that cause neuropathology in autism are also prone to cultivate irritative foci. For example, many patients with autism and related communication disorders have deep temporal or frontal lobe lesions. The deep nuclei of the rostral cortex are vulnerable even to minor ischemic/hypoxic episodes at approximately the time of birth, and mesial temporal sclerosis is a common pathologic finding. This being the case, it is hardly surprising to find a high frequency of epilepsy and epileptiform disorders in autistic people. The incidence is easily as high as one in three, and complex-partial seizures are the most common type.

Autism is not a purely encephalopathic condition. There is evidence that it represents the superimposition of a nonspecific encephalopathic event on a substrate of communication handicap that is genetic in nature. One presumes that the tendency to seize is a function of the encephalopathic event. Epilepsy in autistic people, however, is not entirely related to brain lesions. Familial epilepsy occurs in autistic children who do not have organic antecedents or cerebral lesions (10). There is also a higher incidence of seizures in autistic people who are not mentally retarded.

When a patient with autism or a language handicap is seen in consultation for severe behavioral problems, the possibility of an epileptiform disorder should always be explored. In fact, psychotropic antiepileptic drugs such as carbamazepine and valproate are commonly used in autistic children for behavioral problems, and surveys indicate that care providers tend to be satisfied with the results (11).

POSTTRAUMATIC EPILEPSY

Seizures after brain injury are similar to seizures after stroke because they include immediate posttraumatic seizures, which have a relatively favorable prognosis, and delayed posttraumatic seizures, which usually signal the onset of posttraumatic epilepsy. The incidence of posttraumatic epilepsy is not much different from the incidence of poststroke epilepsy. Posttraumatic seizures, however, resemble more closely seizures that accompany mental retardation and differ from poststroke seizures in their frequent association with behavioral and emotional disorders and in the impact that ill-selected anticonvulsant treatment may have on neurocognitive function.

Within 5 years after closed head injury, the incidence of epilepsy is approximately 2% to 5%. Compared with population rates, the overall standardized incidence ratio is 3.1; after mild injuries, 1.5; moderate injuries, 2.9; and severe injuries, 17.0 (12). A considerably higher percentage of patients with penetrating injuries (compared with closed head injuries) develop seizures (13), and the cumulative incidence of epilepsy after wartime head injuries may be as high as 50% (14).

The risk of late posttraumatic seizures exceeds 30% in patients with severe head injuries and the following risk factors: penetrating brain injury, depressed skull fracture, intracerebral hematoma, subdural hematoma, and seizure within the first week after injury (15,16). Prolonged unconsciousness (posttraumatic amnesia lasting more than 24 hours) is sometimes listed as a risk factor. Without a focal lesion, it is probably not (17–19). Early seizures, occurring within the first week after injury, do not predict the development of subsequent epilepsy but increase its likelihood. There is preclinical evidence, however, that early seizures exercise a protective effect on the recovery process (20). Epileptiform EEG abnormalities are not predictive of posttraumatic epilepsy during the first year after injury but are more significant later on.

Other factors that increase the risk of posttraumatic epilepsy are persistent focal deficits, such as aphasia or hemiparesis, centroparietal or temporal location of the lesion, and age over 65 years (19,21). Although the onset of seizures is most often within 5 years of injury, later onset has been reported in a substantial number of patients (22). Children are more prone to posttraumatic epilepsy than adults, and the latency to epilepsy onset is longer (23).

Postnatal brain injury in children sufficient to cause mental retardation has the greatest likelihood of inducing epilepsy. The cumulative risk is no less than 53% at 5 years and 66% at 10 years after injury (24). Mesial temporal sclerosis after severe brain injury is often associated with severe and intractable seizures (25).

The occurrence of seizures after concussion is nil. In the Olmsted County study, mild brain injury was associated with a small increase in relative risk, but the definition of mild brain injury by the authors was more expansive than current usage allows (19). Motor and convulsive manifestations have been noted in relation to sports injury and given careful attention by video analysis. Tonic posturing and clonic movements are not uncommon when the victim is unconscious, or immediately thereafter, but they are not epileptic phenomena and the outcome is universally good (26).

Anticonvulsant prophylaxis of early posttraumatic seizures (during the first week after injury) is sometimes appropriate. Carbamazepine, phenytoin, and possibly valproate are acceptable treatments to reduce the incidence of early posttraumatic seizures. The rationale is that early seizures may cause secondary brain damage as a result of increased metabolic demands, increased intracranial pressure, and excess neurotransmitter release. Preventing early seizures, however, has no influence on the occurrence of late posttraumatic seizures (27,28).

Most studies do not support the use of anticonvulsant prophylaxis for late posttraumatic seizures (27–31). Anticonvulsant prophylaxis complicates the long-term management of patients with brain injury and may even retard the recovery process (32). It does no more than suppress seizures in the small number of patients with traumatic brain injury (TBI) who develop posttraumatic seizures while compromising recovery in the much larger number of patients who do not.

In some cases, a clinical decision in favor of anticonvulsant prophylaxis might be guided by the presence of significant risk factors (33,34). In a patient who is extremely likely to develop posttraumatic epilepsy, it may be justified to continue anticonvulsant therapy as if the patient did indeed have epilepsy, especially if the new occurrence of seizures would compromise some important aspect of his or her rehabilitation, for example, the ability to drive to work. One should never pretend that that is prophylaxis; call it instead anticipatory treatment. Clearly, there is no place for anticonvulsant prophylaxis for the patient who has sustained blunt trauma with no other element of risk. When such patients on phenytoin or another anticonvulsant for months or even years are seen in consultation, the beneficial effects of drug withdrawal can be dramatic. Memory deficits, fatigue, and depression may all vanish completely when the anticonvulsant is withdrawn.

Phenytoin is probably used more frequently for prophylaxis than any other anticonvulsant because it is begun in the neurosurgical intensive care unit where it can be given parenterally. If, however, a patient with brain injury must be on an anticonvulsant at all, carbamazepine and valproate are the recommended agents. Phenytoin does not make sense as a prophylactic drug because it is relatively weak against kindling. Carbamazepine and valproate may or may not be less neurotoxic than phenytoin in the short run but are indisputably better as psychotropics (35,36).

Some new anticonvulsants such as levetiracetam are reputed to be free-radical scavengers and antiperoxidants. Others such as valproate seem to promote neuroneogenesis. Should these considerations influence one's decision about anticonvulsant treatment in a patient with head injury (37)? Possibly they should, but there no studies yet to guide treatment.

Patients with brain injury who develop posttraumatic epilepsy have a poor prognosis. They are less likely to return to work and are more likely to experience late deterioration and even premature death (38–40). That is probably related to the severity of their brain injury rather than the seizures *per se* (41). Indeed, posttraumatic epilepsy need not require a lifetime commitment to anticonvulsant treatment (38). If a patient is seizure free for 5 years and the EEG is not active, it may be possible to withdraw the patient from antiepileptic drugs.

Posttraumatic epilepsy is not necessarily associated with behavioral or affective symptoms, but it often is. Patients with TBI with frontal or temporal lobe seizures may be especially prone to difficult behaviors that may not be brought under control even with optimal anticonvulsant therapy. The appropriate psychotropics are often needed for symptoms of depression, anxiety or panic, impulsiveness, aggression, or psychosis.

Seizures frequently enter the differential diagnosis of psychiatric conditions that arise in patients with brain injury, although it is not advisable to diagnose an incipient seizure disorder purely based on behavioral or emotional problems. Neuropsychiatric sequelae of brain injury are much more prevalent than posttraumatic epilepsy.

Seizures in Stroke and Dementia

Strokes are the most common cause of seizures in the elderly (42,43). They are estimated to occur in 5% to 10% of cases (44). Hemorrhagic strokes are the most likely to cause seizures, but thrombotic strokes, brain infarcts, lacunar infarcts, and transient ischemic attacks may also cause seizures (45–48). Simple partial seizures are the most common, followed by complex-partial seizures, and then generalized tonic-clonic seizures (45).

There is a distinction between early and late poststroke seizures. Early seizures tend to be focal motor, brief, and isolated and are easily controlled, usually with monotherapy. They are the result of acute local brain metabolic alteration induced by the cerebrovascular event. Once these derangements are reversed, the seizures disappear. Epilepsy does not usually result, but the risk is increased by virtue of an early seizure and increased further by early seizure recurrence (44,49). Long-term or prophylactic antiepileptic drug treatment is not usually necessary.

Prodromal seizures are often the initial sign of stroke (48,50). They generally occur within 48 hours of stroke onset (51).

Late seizures occur with increasing frequency over the years after stroke, especially if there is an irritative structural lesion or recurrent stroke. Late seizures are more likely to progress to poststroke epilepsy. The prevalence of poststroke epilepsy is 3% to 5% (49,52) or 6% to 8% (53), but in selected populations, it may be as high as 35% (54). Poststroke epilepsy is usually treatable with monotherapy (53).

Cortical strokes are more likely to be epileptogenic than subcortical strokes and bihemispheric strokes more than unilateral strokes (47). There are no "specific epileptogenic gyri" in the cerebral cortex (46).

Alzheimer's disease accounts for 7% of new seizures in people older than 60 (compared with 30% in stroke) (55). New-onset seizures occur in patients with Alzheimer's disease in approximately 10% of cases, 10 times the rate in a reference population. Nonepileptic myoclonus occurs in another 10% (56). Seizures are usually generalized and tonic-clonic. They occur when the dementia is advanced but rarely cause severe problems (57).

Late poststroke seizures may be associated with persistent worsening of the neurologic sequelae of stroke (58) but they are not usually associated with prominent affective or behavioral symptoms. The same appears to be true for epilepsy caused by dementia. This is probably an age-related phenomenon. Most patients having had a cerebrovascular accident and most patients with dementia are elderly, of course. Alzheimer's patients with dementia onset at a young age are more susceptible to seizures (59). When seizures develop in association with dementia in patients with Down's syndrome who are much younger, the behavioral correlates are much stronger, just as they are in mentally retarded people in general, people with autism, and patients with brain injury (60).

Seizures in elderly people are more often associated with "inhibitory" phenomena such as Todd's paralysis or transient confusional states (61,62). It is interesting that affective disorders occur with equal frequency among all these groups but that the behavioral and affective correlates of epilepsy are more likely to occur in the younger populations of patients with mental retardation and TBI. Their epilepsy, even without psychiatric complications, is harder to treat.

Intellectual Impairment and Brain Damage

Cognitive functioning can be affected for several days after a tonic-clonic or a complex-partial seizure. Seizures occurring at night leave a hangover effect on learning ability the next day. During the postictal state, patients experience confusion, amnesia, language dysfunction, blindness, paralysis, and even bulimia, but these episodes generally clear within 24 hours. However, in some patients, a prolonged postictal encephalopathy occurs, with symptoms that linger for days or weeks (63). This is especially notable in patients with brain injury or stroke when seizures occur during the course of recovery, and the recovery process is set back accordingly. It is possible that many of the behavioral problems that occur in retarded and/or autistic people with epilepsy are a function of a prolonged postictal encephalopathic state.

Transitory cognitive impairment refers to specific deficits in cognitive performance associated with subclinical epileptiform EEG discharges. The phenomenon has been extensively studied in children whose performance on psychometric tests is impaired when they display such discharges during testing (8).

Gradual deterioration of intellectual ability in patients with epilepsy was described in the era before anticonvulsant drugs (64). Mental deterioration in patients with epilepsy has been attributed to genetic proclivity, encephalopathic abnormalities acquired before the onset of seizures, epilepsy itself, and the neuropathologic sequelae of fits, psychosocial isolation, and overdose with sedative anticonvulsant drugs (65).

The IQ scores of patients with epilepsy are skewed to begin with. Mentally retarded patients are overrepresented, and intellectually above-average patients relatively underrepresented in populations of children with epilepsy and, to a lesser degree, in adults with epilepsy (66).

Epilepsy that is idiopathic or familial is less likely to be associated with mental regression or dementia than epilepsy associated with overt brain damage or conditions such as tuberous sclerosis or Parkinson's disease (66,67). Patients with epilepsy who are symptomatic are more likely to deteriorate cognitively than those who are idiopathic (65). The same factors that correlate with poor seizure prognosis are correlated with mental deterioration: age of onset, duration of the disorder, number of seizures, higher initial seizure frequency, poor response to anticonvulsant medication, and an excess of focal combined with generalized seizures (66,68).

It is not easy to distinguish epileptic dementia from anticonvulsant-induced dementia, nor is it always possible to exclude the other possible causes of dementia in a patient who has secondary epilepsy. For example, the frequent occurrence of dementia in World War II veterans with brain injuries and epilepsy was more likely the result of severe brain trauma than epilepsy (14).

It is widely accepted that there is an epileptic dementia associated with cerebral atrophy (69). How recurrent seizures lead to intellectual decline is not at all clear. It is known that seizures can, by themselves, provoke encephalopathic and metabolic changes in the brain, especially when they are frequent or prolonged (70–72).

Prolonged seizures in the young brain were originally thought to be less toxic than they are in the adult brain (73), but that may just be the consequence of the underlying pathology. Chronic epilepsy is sometimes associated with neuronal degeneration in the hippocampus, amygdala, and parahippocampal gyri. Excitotoxins stimulated by seizures can inhibit protein and DNA synthesis and growth cone expression (74). Even a single seizure can cause neuronal damage. Brain extracellular glutamate builds up to neurotoxic levels after a single partial seizure, and glutamate receptors are linked to various intracellular messenger systems that are implicated in oxygen radical production. Excitotoxicity and oxidative stress are candidate mechanisms for seizure-induced neurodegeneration (8,75). Untreated or undertreated epilepsy is not simply a random succession of seizures but rather a process in which frequent seizures cause neuronal damage and neurocognitive changes, such as memory impairment (76). This speaks not only to the importance of effective seizure control but also the importance of selecting an antiepileptic agent (for example, a glutamate inhibitor) that will address the underlying encephalopathic process. Neuroprotection, at least with respect to existing antiepileptic drugs, is largely a theoretical consideration, but there are hints that some antiepileptic drugs may be preferable to others. Phenytoin can decrease free-radical scavenger capacity, a mechanism that might account for phenytoin encephalopathy, which includes cerebellar deterioration and overt dementia. In contrast, antioxidant treatment may have beneficial effects for some neurodegenerative conditions of childhood associated with epilepsy (e.g., juvenile ceroid lipofuscinosis). Felbamate, vigabatrin, tiagabine, levetiracetam, and lamotrigine seem to be neuroprotective agents, at least *in vitro* (76,77).

The Primacy of Epilepsy

Because seizures are so common in people who are mentally retarded, people with autism, and in other encephalopathic populations, it is important to consider epilepsy in the differential diagnosis of virtually every psychiatric condition, especially one that is characterized by paroxysmal or cyclic sensory, motor, emotional, or behavioral events. Conversely, it is easy to go overboard and to overdiagnose epilepsy on the basis of equivocal data. Patients are thus subjected to intrusive and costly workups and unnecessary drug treatment. Attentional lapses, for example, are very common in children with autism. Transient sensorimotor phenomena frequently occur in patients with TBI and may easily be mistaken for partial seizures. Abnormal sensory phenomena may be migrainoid, not ictal. Periodic interruptions of behavior, such as the attentional lapses of autistic children, are not at all uncommon in any population of patients with brain injury. Seizures are rare, or even unheard of, in some encephalopathic states, such as postconcussion syndrome.

One may find it convenient to explain a behavioral aberration as a 'seizure equivalent', perhaps too convenient. 'Seizure equivalents' can be perceived anywhere by an observer who is so inclined. Kindling is another term that some psychiatrists have borrowed from epilepsy and used to explain a broad range of behavioral and emotional conditions. Just because a mental state change is abrupt and unanticipated does not mean that it is a 'seizure equivalent'. Just because a patient with a neuropsychiatric disorder responds to a psychotropic anticonvulsant does not mean that he or she has subclinical seizures any more than it means that he or she has a bipolar variant.

It is certainly true that interictal spikes are correlated with cognitive lapses, and psychiatric disorders and personality changes can develop during the interictal state. It is true that developmental regression occurs in LKS in the presence of epileptiform spikes but not necessarily overt seizures. However, terms such as seizure equivalents and subclinical seizures are of dubious utility, clinically speaking, and have little justification in the scientific literature.

I shall give short shrift to the thorny problem of 'seizure equivalents,' and advise the reader to do the same. It is better to concentrate one's energies on seizures that are really there. When the diagnosis is accurate, the treatment of epilepsy should always take precedence over the treatment of any concomitant behavioral or emotional problem. There is always a strong likelihood that when optimal anticonvulsant therapy is achieved, the psychiatric condition will improve as well. Thus, one might do well to consider an alternative antiepileptic drug in a patient whose seizures are well controlled but whose psychiatric symptoms are not. It is elegant practice, and sometimes attainable, to treat both conditions with one drug.

This is what is called the primacy of epilepsy. The presence of seizures in a patient with a neuropsychiatric condition, even a remote history of seizures, or epileptiform EEG, should always at least incline the physician toward the choice of a psychotropic anticonvulsant.

Conversely, treatment of concomitant psychiatric conditions may be expected to improve epilepsy control. Psychogenic seizures can arise in a patient whose epilepsy has been hitherto well controlled when a depression or psychosis develops. Appropriate treatment of the psychiatric disorder often brings the seizures back under control, even if the psychotropic drug that is chosen is one that (theoretically) lowers the seizure threshold.

NEUROPSYCHIATRIC CONDITIONS IN PATIENTS WITH EPILEPSY

Neuropsychiatric problems in patients with epilepsy may be related to the seizures themselves or the neuropathology that causes seizures. They can also be caused by anticonvulsant neurotoxicity.

Aberrant behavioral or emotional events may be ictal, preictal, or postictal phenomena. There is also an interictal syndrome that develops in some patients with epilepsy—changes in personality, behavior, emotional expression, or thinking that are somehow caused by the irritative focus or some other aspect of the disease.

Treatment-related difficulties may be the consequence of behavioral toxicity from anticonvulsant drugs or of partial or imperfect treatment. This problem is more important in patients who are mentally retarded and patients with brain injury than it is in the general population of patients with epilepsy. Anticonvulsants can cause impairment in cognition, or impaired cognition may be the result of epileptic activity that is only partially controlled. Anticonvulsant treatment may cause a psychiatric disorder in the patient: phenobarbital can cause hyperactivity, ethosuximide can cause depression, phenytoin can lead to dementia, valproate can make the patient anergic, and carbamazepine can sometimes make a patient aggressive. Conversely, continued behavioral problems in a patient with epilepsy can be the consequence of suboptimal anticonvulsant therapy.

It is not always possible to distinguish precisely which element is operative in a given patient. Sometimes one simply has to try different doses or different drugs. An antiepileptic drug may be sufficient to control ictal events but not paroxysmal outbursts of untoward behavior. The problem, then, is a function of the disease itself, but it is prolonged or aggravated by inadequate treatment. A psychiatric syndrome may be kindled in a patient with an epileptic focus who is treated with a drug that suppresses overt seizures ictus but not the irritative focus; the problem never would have arisen, theoretically at least, if the patient were treated with an anticonvulsant that had antikindling properties.

The third element to complicate one's interpretation of psychological events as they unfold in a patient with epilepsy is the influence of the underlying pathology that causes seizures as well as aberrant behavior. Thinking about epilepsy in this regard is like thinking about schizophrenia; as long as one is dealing only with the behavioral manifestations of an encephalopathic process and the process itself is poorly understood, cause-and-effect relationships will be hard to make.

That is why epilepsy is the most psychiatric of all the neurologic diseases and perhaps why it was once counted among the psychiatric diseases. Its core, a behavioral change that is correlated with an electrical event, is simply defined. Its ramifications, however, are protean, its boundaries are ambiguous, and its clinical manifestations are comprised of interwoven psychological, neuropathologic, and pharmacologic elements.

Personality

The list of personality traits attributed to individuals with epilepsy is limited only by one's industry in ferreting out fresh derogations (78). The idea that there is an epileptic personality is quaint but presumptuous. Epilepsy and personality are two broad and multifaceted constructs that can hardly be expected to unite in a single strain.

The idea that some patients with epilepsy are given to one or another of several nonpathologic personality traits is less ambitious and closer to the truth. The traits to which they are inclined are limited in number and thus amenable to empirical test. In patients with epilepsy with temporal lobe foci, for example, quantitative studies have demonstrated a profile of interictal changes in behavior (obsessiveness, circumstantiality), thought (religious and philosophical preoccupation), and affect (anger, emotionality, sadness) (79–81). Other traits attributed to the patient with temporal lobe epilepsy include interpersonal "stickiness," "viscosity," humorlessness, dependence, passivity, hypermoralism, personalization, and hyposexuality.

Whether these traits are a consequence of the epileptic process, the underlying temporal lobe lesion, or a synergy of the two is an open question. It is likely that they are not related to the convulsive process in its overt sense but rather to some specific aspect that has to do with the underlying focus. Such traits in patients with temporal lobe lesions who were not overtly epileptic have been noted on several occasions (82).

Nothing, however, in the literature should prepare the reader to expect an inevitable connection between temporal lobe foci and the personality traits in question or an absence of association, on occasion, with foci in other regions. It is a curious development that serious discussion of the psychiatric concomitants of temporal lobe epilepsy come at a time when epileptologists have abandoned the term and refer instead to complex-partial seizures or partial epilepsy and then refer to the specific focus, if it is known. It would be a singular event, indeed, if the research literature were unequivocal on behalf of a temporal lobe origin of all the traits attributed to that organ (83,84). We know that functions that are normally localized to a cortical region can be designated to another as the consequence of trauma, for example, and brain structures are insulated one from another only imperfectly. The effects of displacement of function, activation by contiguity, reciprocal inhibition, encephalization, kindling, and the development of mirror foci militate against any single-minded localization, especially to complex features such as personality traits.

There is said to be an unexpected frequency of dual personality and multiple personality in patients with complex-partial seizures, especially temporal lobe seizures (85–87). If it is difficult to draw a physiologic connection between epilepsy and any one personality type, it is daunting to make the link to more than one personality. Dissociative states and symptoms, however, are not unknown in patients with complex-partial epilepsy.

Depression

Emotions, as part of the epileptic experience, may be preictal, ictal, or postictal events. Fear, depression, pleasure, displeasure, and anger have all been documented as ictal manifestations (88). Depression as an interictal state, however, is an important issue in neuropsychiatry. Patients with epilepsy have more depressive characteristics on psychological tests; depression is a common reason for hospitalization, and people with epilepsy have a suicide rate that is five times higher than that of the general population (89).

Depression in patients with epilepsy is associated with vegetative features, but there seem to be fewer neurotic symptoms such as self-pity and brooding. Between major depressive episodes, patients with epilepsy are said to manifest a chronic dysthymic state, with more irritability, emotionality, and humorlessness than controls. Their affect is described as detached or distant rather than dysphoric (89). They may be prone to agitated depressive states with psychotic symptoms; alternatively, they may present as psychotic with strong affective symptoms (90).

It is appropriate to mention that studies of psychiatric patients with major affective disorders, unipolar and bipolar, reveal a high frequency of symptoms suggestive of temporal lobe epilepsy (91,92). No one has suggested that affective disorder is a variant of epilepsy or a manifestation of "subclinical epilepsy," but the pathophysiology of kindling might be an analog for the behavioral sensitization that occurs, for example, in the genesis of depression in response to chronic stress. The experimental model of behavioral sensitization is seen after chronic treatment with dopaminergic drugs such as apomorphine or cocaine, when the animal shows increasing hyperactivity or stereotypy to a subthreshold dose. The phenomenon occurs, of course, in the absence of an irritative focus, so it is not simply a variant of the kindling model; it seems to involve different neural systems, and the two processes are affected differentially by pharmacologic interventions (93). The theory suggests that recurrent affective disorder, cycling more rapidly and less related to external events as the years go by, is a function of behavioral sensitization.

Peculiar Behavior

The epilepsy literature has some good examples, such as giggle incontinence (94) and self-induced photosensitive absence seizures with orgasmic ictus (95). The range of phenomena that occur, especially in association with complex-partial seizures, is staggering. It is not always possible, therefore, to distinguish behavior related to ictus from behavior that is psychiatric simply on the basis of topography or whether it is associated with an identifiable provocation. That would be like differentiating between tardive dyskinesia and Huntington's chorea simply on the basis of the topography of the abnormal movements; it cannot be done. Sudden attacks of pain that flash from one part of the body to another may be associated with mesodiencephalic discharges (96). Painful auras preceding generalized seizures have been described (97). Although painful partial seizures are probably rare (98), central pain may be associated with lesions in the thalamus (99) and in the secondary sensory area (100). Fear and panic may be preictal, ictal, or postictal, but a seizure can make a person's hair stand up even without sensations of fear (pilomotor seizures) (101). Patients with complex-partial seizures of left temporal lobe origin may be more verbose than other patients with epilepsy (102). Patients with left temporal lobe epilepsy may also be given to hypergraphia (as Dostoyevsky was), but there is a converse form of epilepsy that is induced by writing (103) and a contrapositive that is induced by reading (104).

Forced thinking as an epileptic phenomenon may be confused with obsession, and the flood of ideas of epilepsy may be confused for the flight of ideas in mania. Seizures may be associated with hallucinations that are visual, auditory, vertiginous, olfactory, gustatory, somatosensory, or all of these (105).

Autoscopy is the sense that one can perceive oneself projected onto an external visual space. Macropsia and micropsia are sensations of perception through different ends of a telescope. *Déjà vu*, of course, is the sense that something new has happened before; *jamais vu* is the sense that something familiar is altogether new.

Frontal Lobe Epilepsy

Most, but not all, complex-partial seizures are of temporal lobe origin. The frontal lobes are the most common source for complex-partial seizures of extratemporal origin. Epileptologists are beginning to accept the idea that complex-partial seizures of frontal lobe origin show features of sufficient consistency to constitute a recognizable clinical syndrome (106).

In contrast to temporal lobe seizures, frontal lobe seizures are abrupt in onset and may last only for a few seconds, and patients tend to make prompt recoveries without a blunted postictal state. They are not usually associated with surface EEG abnormalities, and some authors have even suggested that intracranial EEG is essential for the diagnosis. Most interesting, however, especially to the psychiatrist, are the clinical manifestations of frontal lobe seizures. They include complicated automatisms, often with vigorous movements such as kicking and thrashing, finger-snapping, handclapping, shouts, obscenities, singing and humming, pelvic thrusting and genital manipulation, bouncing, groping, picking, chewing, lip smacking, and bizarre facial expressions (107–109). The motor behaviors and vocalizations often have an intense affective nature, sometimes with a sexual or aggressive quality. The absence of tonic-clonic movements, the occurrence of nonconvulsive status epilepticus characterized by inappropriate behavior, and the occurrence of seizures that are electroencephalographically silent may obscure the proper diagnosis. Many of the cardinal features of frontal lobe seizures are considered to be pathognomonic of hysterical pseudoseizures (106). In adults, many years may elapse before the condition is properly diagnosed.

Somatosensory manifestations occur in approximately one-half of the patients with frontal lobe seizures, and these, too, may be confusing to the physician, including such vague symptoms as oppression, electrical sensations in the head, sensations of body heat, and difficulty in controlling respiration. The patients may have visual or auditory aberrations, such as hallucinations, transient alterations in the perception of ambient brightness, blurred vision, a sensation of "resonating sounds," and the inability to recognize familiar objects, feelings of panic or dread, forced thoughts, echolalia, abnormal posturing and stereotypies, and the experience of being controlled. Patients may retain a degree of responsiveness during a seizure. The episodes may also be provoked by an emotional stimulus (110).

In short, virtually every element that leads the clinician to suspect that a patient experiencing seizures is, in fact, a hysteric or malingerer may be a characteristic feature of frontal lobe epilepsy. Neurodiagnostic studies may affirm the diagnosis of frontal lobe epilepsy, but normal studies do not, of themselves, disconfirm the diagnosis.

Failure to respond to appropriate treatment is sometimes the first hint that a patient with epilepsy may be less than he or she pretends to be. Malingered epilepsy rarely responds to anticonvulsant treatment. Frontal lobe epilepsy, however, does not always respond to antiepileptic drugs, and surgery is sometimes the only alternative. A Solomonic approach to differentiating between frontal lobe seizures and hysteria or malingering would be intracranial recording and extirpative surgery.

The second problem that is raised by the fact of frontal lobe seizures is the evaluation of retarded people with behavioral problems characterized, for example, by paroxysms of rage or panic, aggression or self-injury, stereotypies, posturing, attentional lapses.

Indeed, paroxysmal frontal lobe discharges have been held to account for autistic behavior (111) and for self-injurious and aggressive behavior in mentally retarded people (112,113). There may be some truth to these contentions, but it is impossible to anticipate the magnitude of the association or how the issue might be resolved with today's technology.

Intracranial leads and positron emission tomography scanning are available technologies, but one can hardly propose their routine use in the evaluation of large numbers of patients with head injury who may be concocting symptoms or the large numbers of mentally retarded people who are aggressive or self-injurious. One is usually guided by clinical judgment: whether the patient's pathology is likely to be associated with epilepsy and whether the patient's behavioral problems remit with antiepileptic therapy.

Neither represents a definitive test. It remains to be seen whether our renewed interest in frontal lobe epilepsy will lead to a net increase in misdiagnoses or to a net improvement in our ability to identify early cases and treat them properly.

Psychosis

In light of the extraordinary (yet very incomplete) list just given, it is not surprising that frank psychosis may also be an accompaniment of seizure disorders. It is, however, a relatively new idea, and there was a time when psychiatrists and neurologists thought that epilepsy and schizophrenia were incompatible or antagonistic diseases. That was the rationale for treating schizophrenic patients by making them seize.

The relationship between psychosis and epilepsy has several dimensions: the two disorders arising as disparate manifestations of an underlying lesion, psychosis as an ictal phenomenon such as generalized nonconvulsive status epilepticus, psychosis as a late manifestation of temporal lobe epilepsy, and psychosis as the consequence of anticonvulsant toxicity.

It is the psychosis of temporal lobe epilepsy that has received the most attention and for two good reasons. The late development of psychosis is consistent with a kindling model that obviously has broad import for the study of psychopathology in general (114, 115). The second compelling idea is that the schizophreniform psychosis of temporal lobe epilepsy is localized, relatively speaking, to the left hemisphere, whereas the psychosis of right temporal lesions is more likely to be affective (116).

The psychosis of temporal lobe epilepsy would be better termed temporal lobe psychosis because it has been observed in patients with temporal lesions and no overt seizures (82). It may also be termed late-onset psychosis because there is a delay of varying length between the initial insult or the first seizure and the development of psychosis. The psychosis is described as schizophreniform, but there are some key differences between temporal lobe psychosis and schizophrenia. The former is associated with many of the interictal personality traits of temporal lobe disease, especially cosmic preoccupation, hyperreligiosity, and paranoia. Demonic hallucinations are typical or thoughts that one is hearing the voice of God. Hallucinations may be transient or intermittent or may occur in spells, along with diminished mentation or perceptual abnormalities. The episodic nature of the symptoms may be the only clue to an epileptic origin. The patients may be given to sudden and abrupt changes in mood, and the moods may vary from ecstasy to profound depression or from laughter to crying or angry explosions. Suicide attempts are not uncommon (117).

Primary or schneiderian symptoms are usually more common than negative or deficit symptoms. In one's relationship with the patient, there is a sense that he or she is afflicted with psychotic symptoms but that the ego is intact and has not been submerged or subsumed by a pervasive psychotic process. When negative symptoms do arise in a person with temporal lobe psychosis, one must be aware of the possibility of a concurrent depression, and treatment with antidepressants may be necessary.

The treatment of temporal lobe psychosis requires a psychotropic anticonvulsant as an essential agent. There may only be a partial response, however, with reduction in emotional intensity or outbursts and elimination of spells. Persistent hallucinations, delusions, and paranoia may require the coadministration of low doses of a high-potency neuroleptic, especially fluphenazine or pimozide, which are least likely to lower the seizure threshold, or, better, an atypical antipsychotic. Centrencephalic epilepsy is associated with confusional psychosis (116,118) and should to be treated first with valproate.

The localization of temporal lobe psychosis, manic to the right and schizophrenic to the left, was introduced by Flor-Henry in 1969. In several studies, major and minor depressions have been attributed to posterior lesions in the right hemisphere (119). The literature, however, is not unanimous. There are also reports that depression occurs more frequently in patients with left hemisphere lesions (120–122).

Absence

One is trained to associate lapses in attention or daydreaming with petit mal or absence epilepsy, but that is not a particularly helpful approach for the practitioner who treats patients who are developmentally handicapped or patients with brain injury because they are always prone to lapses in attention and what appears to be daydreaming. The diagnosis of epilepsy should always be entertained in patients with severe disorders of attention, but in mental retardation, brain injury, and autism, attentional lapses are not usually ictal in nature.

The diagnosis of absence epilepsy is easier if there is complex absence, i.e., if the seizures are accompanied by mild clonic movements such as eye fluttering, mouth twitching, or movements of the upper extremity; changes in postural tone, especially head drooping or mild slumping; autonomic phenomena or urinary incontinence; or automatisms. It may be impossible to distinguish such cases from complex-partial seizures without EEG (123). Hyperventilation will evoke an absence seizure but not a complex-partial seizure (124).

The diagnostic ambiguity of frontal lobe epilepsy is visited again in pseudo-absence—sudden behavioral arrest without motor activity. Such events are associated with urinary incontinence, minimal gestural automatisms, humming, or other minor vocalization. They may be abortive and experienced as a vague sensation in the head or body, confused thinking, loss of thought control, doubling of thoughts, or an "idea void."

Nonconvulsive generalized status epilepticus (petit mal status) is a state lasting for 1 hour or longer with slowness in behavior and mentation, confusion, and sometimes stupor or coma. There is generalized epileptiform activity on EEG, continuous or nearly so with spike waves, polyspike waves, or more complex discharges (125). The duration may range from 12 hours to 4 days; the longest known attack was 31 days. The onset of the disorder may be at any age, and it is not an easy form of the disease to control. Naturally, the presentation can be confused with some of the psychiatric disorders. Conversely, it is not unusual for patients given to nonconvulsive generalized status to have severe psychiatric symptoms including psychosis (125).

Intermittent Explosive Disorder

Intermittent explosive disorder (episodic dyscontrol) refers to extreme emotional outbursts, with rage and sometimes violence, in patients who have no clearly defined cause, lesion, or psychiatric diagnosis. The evidence for an association with epilepsy is threefold: the common occurrence of such symptoms in patients with epilepsy, especially complex-partial epilepsy; the common finding of temporal lobe abnormalities on neurodiagnostic testing in patients without epilepsy with intermittent explosions; and the good response of explosive patients to carbamazepine and valproate.

The co-occurrence of violence with epilepsy has led naturally to controversy over whether to treat violent persons with amygdalotomy (126) or whether criminal violence may ever occur as a purely ictal event. The first idea has little empirical (or even theoretical) support. The second represents a crucial misunderstanding of epilepsy as well as the nature of personal responsibility for actions that are precipitated by an underlying cerebral disorder.

The idea that epilepsy is an all-or-none phenomenon is attractive and consistent with the electrical events that accompany ictus. It is inconsistent, however, with the fact that epilepsy may be partial and that complete loss of conscious control is not an invariant feature of the disease. A lesion that gives rise on occasion to seizures may on other occasions give rise to alternative manifestations—to paroxysms of behavior that are not really seizures at all.

The question of violent behavior as a correlate of epilepsy opens a serious line of reflection concerning personal responsibility for behavior that is potentially criminal in nature. This is the kind of question that is argued by experts in criminal proceedings. Strong convictions are sometimes expressed without support in the scientific literature. The arcane opinions of learned experts in such matters make one grateful for the wisdom of a jury of peers.

It is difficult to maintain that an act of ictal violence can occur in a patient who is not clearly given to overt seizures. It is also difficult to believe that a complex act of interpersonal violence could be a purely ictal event because the automatisms of complex-partial epilepsy are by definition fragmented, purposeless, and without definite and identifiable goals (127). It is also hard to distinguish between ictal violence and postictal or interictal violence, the latter being a relatively nonspecific aspect of a psychopathologic condition (128).

Aggression and self-injury are common behavioral problems in mentally retarded people with epilepsy. When such behaviors are related to epilepsy, in any of the different ways described, they are unplanned, explosive, relatively directionless, and quick to subside. Personal injury to the patient or a bystander may sometimes result.

PSYCHOTROPIC DRUGS AS PROCONVULSANTS AND ANTICONVULSANTS

Virtually all the psychoactive drugs can affect the seizure threshold if the dose is sufficiently high or if a change in dose is sufficiently abrupt. The effect is easier to detect if it is in the direction of lowering the seizure threshold because a drug-induced seizure is a notable event. The effect of any psychotropic drug, however, is probably less important than individual sensitivity. (The exceptions are clozapine and maprotiline.) One should never be surprised, therefore, if the introduction of a psychoactive drug is associated with a change in the clinical status of a patient with epilepsy. Even some of the anticonvulsants can cause seizures.

Psychoactive drugs alter the seizure threshold by (i) altering the metabolism or protein binding of an anticonvulsant, (ii) stabilizing the patient's psychological condition and thus improving the general stability of other systems, and (iii) exercising a direct effect on the mechanisms of epileptogenesis. Most of the known effects of psychotropics on the seizure threshold fall into the latter category.

The psychostimulants are, in many respects, prototypical in their biphasic effect on the seizure threshold. In high doses, they can cause seizures. Of all the recreational drugs, cocaine is the most likely to cause seizures. Seizures from amphetamine abuse are more likely in association with intravenous administration. In the low doses that are used for therapeutic purposes, however, stimulant-induced seizures are very rare. In fact, therapeutic doses of stimulants usually raise the seizure threshold and improve seizure control. In the past, amphetamine was routinely used along with anticonvulsants to counteract sedation (129).

Similarly, amantadine has been used as anticonvulsant, although higher doses have the opposite effect. If amantadine is used to treat patients with TBI in the coma-recovery phase, doses of 400 mg or more per day may cause seizures. The clinical benefit of amantadine in TBI is usually at 200 to 300 mg per day.

A patient with TBI who is taking amantadine should be advised against alcohol ingestion because the combination may lead to seizures. As a rule, the combination of two mildly proconvulsant drugs may cause a seizure, even if the doses of both are well below the ictal threshold.

Antidepressants and antipsychotic drugs are the psychoactive drugs most commonly associated with a lower seizure threshold (130). There is hardly any disagreement on that point. The incidence of seizures in people on tricyclic antidepressants is approximately 1% and approximately 1% to 2% in patients on neuroleptics (130). The incidence of seizures in patients with brain injury treated with tricyclic antidepressants may be as high as 19% (131). The important question is whether any particular drug in the class is more or less likely to carry the effect.

Maprotiline is probably the most likely antidepressant to induce a seizure (132). In the past, it was believed that amitriptyline was the least likely, although this information is based on just one preclinical study (133). It is a counterintuitive finding in light of the sedative and anticholinergic properties of amitriptyline and the results of clinical surveys (134). In one animal preparation, the proconvulsant effects of nine antidepressants were ranked, in descending order, as follows (135): amitriptyline → mianserin → imipramine → desipramine → viloxazine → maprotiline → zimelidine → clovoxamine → nomifensine = fluvoxamine.

Nomifensine (remember Merital?) was once marketed as an anticonvulsant antidepressant. The selective serotonin reuptake inhibitors as a group are thought to have a low seizure propensity; trazodone, moclobemide, and mirtazapine are said to be minimally proconvulsant (136).

The selective serotonin reuptake inhibitors are said to be the only antidepressants with a reliably synergistic effect with antiepileptic drugs. Fluoxetine has been shown to exert anticonvulsant effects in animal models of epilepsy. The anticonvulsant effect of fluoxetine is not specific to any particular seizure type and appears to be correlated with enhanced synaptic availability of serotonin (137). It has been suggested, based on animal studies, that fluoxetine and paroxetine (which have similar effects) may be the preferred drugs for patients with epilepsy who are depressed (138). I am not sure that fluoxetine, at any rate, has anticonvulsant properties. When combined with a mildly proconvulsant drug (e.g., tramadol, stimulants, amantadine, alcohol), seizures may occur.

Bupropion was withheld from the market for a while because of an apparent high frequency of generalized tonic-clonic seizures in some patient groups. This was a difficult problem to evaluate because virtually all the antidepressants are associated with occasional seizures; the association appears to be dose related (139). The incidence can only be estimated, although 0.5% to 1.0% is the usual range that is given for antidepressants in general. Bupropion's bad reputation in this regard, therefore, is hardly justified. The likelihood of a seizure with bupropion is only approximately 0.5% (140).

The manufacturer says that the incidence of seizures in patients treated with bupropion is four in 1,000. At doses higher than 450 mg per day, the risk of seizures may be higher. Seizures are said to be more likely to occur with bupropion if the patient has a predisposing factor, for example, a history of head trauma, drug or alcohol abuse, or concomitant treatment with other drugs that lower the seizure threshold. That is the kind of exculpatory language that finds its way into the *Physicians Desk Reference*. There is no empirical justification. In fact, bupropion is an excellent antidepressant for neuropsychiatric patients. The association between bupropion and seizures may simply turn out to be one of those spurious associations, such as carbamazepine and agranulocytosis, which clouds the reputation of a drug for years.

There is also some confusion about the epileptogenic potential of the neuroleptics. It was once believed that sedating neuroleptics were the most prone to lower the seizure threshold and the less sedating neuroleptics were less likely to provoke seizures. Chlorpromazine was the prime example. Thioridazine and mesoridazine, which are equally sedating, are not strongly proconvulsant (141). This may account for their frequent prescription for mentally retarded people.

In fact, more modern techniques suggest that haloperidol may be very likely to provoke seizures and that molindone, fluphenazine, and pimozide are preferred for patients who are prone to epilepsy (142). This is more in accord with my experience with children with epilepsy. In adults, it is not clear that the epileptogenic potential of any neuroleptic (except clozapine) has clinical significance. Among the atypical antipsychotics, clozapine is strongly proconvulsant, but the others (risperidone, olanzapine, quetiapine, ziprasidone) are probably comparable with the neuroleptics.

Lithium is supposed to be a drug that lowers the seizure threshold (143) but may have a beneficial effect for some patients with epilepsy (144). Lithium is not at all contraindicated in patients with epilepsy. The beta-blockers have a membrane-stabilizing effect and therefore are useful adjuncts to anticonvulsants in the treatment of epilepsy. The monoamine oxidase inhibitors are not thought to be proconvulsants. Buspirone does not affect the seizure threshold; in contrast to benzodiazepines, there is no risk of seizures if buspirone is abruptly withdrawn.

It is important to reiterate that appropriate psychopharmacology may always be expected to improve seizure control in a patient with epilepsy with a serious psychiatric disorder and that the risks inherent in a poorly treated psychiatric condition are almost always greater than the risk of a drug-induced seizure or two.

REFERENCES

1. Corbett JA. Psychiatric morbidity and mental retardation. In: James FE, Smith RP, eds. *Psychiatric illness & mental handicap*. London: Gaskell Press, 1979.
2. Steffenburg U, Steffenburg S. Epilepsy and other neuropsychiatric morbidity in mentally retarded children. In: Sillanpaa M, Gram L, Johannessen SI, et al., eds. *Epilepsy and mental retardation*. Petersfield, UK/ Philadelphia: Wrightson Biomedical, 1999:47–59.
3. Steffenburg S, Gillberg C, Steffenburg U. Psychiatric disorders in children and adolescents with mental retardation and active epilepsy. *Arch Neurol* 1996;53: 904–912.
4. Deykin EY, Macmahon B. The incidence of seizures among children with autistic symptoms. *Am J Psychiatry* 1979;136:1310–1312.
5. Tuchman RF, Rapin I. Regression in pervasive developmental disorders: seizures and epileptiform electroencephalogram correlates. *Pediatrics* 1997;99:560–566.
6. Deonna T, Ziegler A-L, Moura-Serra J, et al. Autistic regression in relation to limbic pathology and epilepsy: report of two cases. *Dev Med Child Neurol* 1993;35: 166–176.
7. Roulet Perez E, Davidoff V, Despland PA, et al. Mental and behavioural deterioration of children with epilepsy and CSWS: acquired epileptic frontal syndrome. *Dev Med Child Neurol* 1993;35:661–674.
8. Brown SW. Epilepsy dementia: intellectual deterioration as a consequence of epileptic seizures. In: Sillanpaa M, Gram L, Johannessen SI, et al., eds. *Epilepsy and mental retardation*. Petersfield, UK/Philadelphia: Wrightson Biomedical, 1999:115–134.
9. Berney TP. Autism—an evolving concept. *Br J Psychiatry* 2000;176:20–25.
10. Rossi PG, Parmeggiani A, Bach V, et al. EEG features and epilepsy in patients with autism. *Brain Dev* 1995; 17:169–174.
11. Aman MG, Van Bourgondien ME, Wolford PL, et al. Psychotropic and anticonvulsant drugs in subjects with autism: prevalence and patterns of use. *J Am Acad Child Psychiatry* 1995;34:1372–1681.
12. Annegers J, Hauser W, Coan S, et al. A population-based study of seizures after traumatic brain injuries. *N Engl J Med* 1998;338:20–24.
13. Epstein FM, Ward JD, Becker DP. Medical complications of head injury. In: Cooper PR, ed. *Head injury*, 2nd ed. Baltimore: Williams & Wilkins, 1987:390–421.
14. Weiss GHP, Salazar AN, Vance SC, et al. Predicting posttraumatic epilepsy in penetrating head injury. *Arch Neurol* 1986;43:771–773.
15. D'Alessandro R, Tinuper P, Ferrara R, et al. CT scan prediction of late post-traumatic epilepsy. *J Neurol Neurosurg Psychiatry* 1982;45:1153–1155.
16. Temkin N, Haglund M, Winn H. Causes, prevention,

and treatment of post-traumatic epilepsy. *New Horizons* 1995;3:518–522.
17. De Santis A, Sganzerla E, Spagnoli D, et al. Risk factors for late posttraumatic epilepsy. *Acta Neurochir Suppl (Wien)* 1992;55:64–67.
18. Asikainen I, Kaste M, Sarna S. Early and late posttraumatic seizures in traumatic brain injury rehabilitation patients: brain injury factors causing late seizures and influence of seizures on long-term outcome. *Epilepsia* 1999;40:584–589.
19. Annegers J, Coan S. The risks of epilepsy after traumatic brain injury. *Seizure* 2000;9:453–457.
20. Feeney DM, Bailey BY, Boyeson MG, et al. The effect of seizures on recovery of function following cortical contusion in the rat. *Brain Inj* 1987;1:27–32.
21. Feeney DM, Walker AE. The prediction of posttraumatic epilepsy: a mathematical approach. *Arch Neurol* 1979;36:8–12.
22. Salazar AM, Jabbari B, Vance SC, et al. Epilepsy after penetrating head injury. I. Clinical correlates: a report of the Vietnam Head Injury Study. *Neurology* 1985; 35:1406–1414.
23. Manaka S, Takahashi H, Sano K. The difference between children and adults in the onset of post-traumatic epilepsy. *Folia Psychiatr Neurol* 1981;35:301–304.
24. Goulden KJ, Shinnar S, Koller H, et al. Epilepsy in children with mental retardation: a cohort study. *Epilepsia* 1991;32:690–697.
25. Diaz-Arrastia R, Agostini M, Frol A, et al. Neurophysiologic and neuroradiologic features of intractable epilepsy after traumatic brain injury in adult. *Arch Neurol* 2000;57:1611–1616.
26. McCrory P, Berkovic S. Video analysis of acute motor and convulsive manifestations in sport-related concussion. *Neurology* 2000;54:1488–1491.
27. The Brain Trauma Foundation. The American Association of Neurological Surgeons. The Joint Section on Neurotrauma and Critical Care. Role of antiseizure prophylaxis following head injury. *J Neurotrauma* 2000;17:549–553.
28. Schierhout G, Roberts I. Anti-epileptic drugs for preventing seizures following acute traumatic brain injury. *Cochrane Database Syst Rev* 2000;2:CD000173.
29. Temkin NR, Dikmen SS, Wilensky AJ, et al. A randomized, double-blind study of phenytoin for the prevention of post-traumatic seizures. *N Engl J Med* 1990;323:497–502.
30. Jacobi G. Post-traumatic epilepsy. *Monatsschr Kinderheilkd* 1992;140:619–623.
31. Murri L, Arrigo A, Bonuccelli U, et al. Phenobarbital in the prophylaxis of late posttraumatic seizures. *Ital J Neurol Sci* 1992;13:755–760.
32. Dikmen SSP, Temkin NRP, Miller BM, et al. Neurobehavioral effects of phenytoin prophylaxis of posttraumatic seizures. *JAMA* 1991;265:1271–1277.
33. McQueen JK, Blackwood DHR, Harris P, et al. Low risk of late post-traumatic seizures following severe head injury: implications for clinical trials of prophylaxis. *J Neurol Neurosurg Psychiatry* 1983;46:899–904.
34. Young B, Rapp RP, Norton JA, et al. Failure of prophylactically administered phenytoin to prevent posttraumatic seizures in children. *Childs Brain* 1983;10: 185–192.
35. Smith KRM, Goulding PMP, Wilderman DR, et al. Neurobehavioral effects of phenytoin and carbamazepine in patients recovering from brain trauma: a comparative study. *Arch Neurol* 1994;51:653–660.
36. Dauch W, Schutze M, Guttinger M, et al. Post-traumatic seizure prevention—results of a survey of 127 neurosurgery clinics. *Zentralbl Neurochir* 1996;57: 190–195.
37. Iudice A, Murri L. Pharmacological prophylaxis of post-traumatic epilepsy. *Drugs* 2000;59:1091–1099.
38. Walker AE, Blumer D. The fate of World War II veterans with posttraumatic seizures. *Arch Neurol* 1989;46: 23–26.
39. Corkin S, Sullivan E, Carr F. Prognostic factors for life expectancy after penetrating head injury. *Arch Neurol* 1984;41:975–977.
40. Schwab K, Grafman J, Salazar A, et al. Residual impairments and work status 15 years after penetrating head injury: report from the Vietnam Head Injury Study. *Neurology* 1993;43:95–103.
41. Haltiner A, Temkin N, Winn H, et al. The impact of posttraumatic seizures on 1-year neuropsychological and psychosocial outcome of head injury. *J Int Neuropsychol Soc* 1996;2:494–504.
42. Luhdorf K, Jensen LK, Plesner AM. Etiology of seizures in the elderly. *Epilepsia* 1986;27:458–463.
43. Loiseau J, Loiseau P, Duche B, et al. A survey of epileptic disorders in southwest France: seizures in elderly patients. *Ann Neurol* 1990;27:232–237.
44. Asconape JJ, Penry JK. Poststroke seizures in the elderly. *Clin Geriatr Med* 1991;7:483–492.
45. Sung CY, Chu NS. Epileptic seizures in thrombotic stroke. *J Neurol* 1990;237:166–170.
46. Heuts-Van Raak EP, Boellaard A, De Krom MC, et al. Supratentorial brain infarcts in adult-onset seizures: The Maastricht Epilepsy Case Register. *Seizure* 1993; 2:221–227.
47. Lancman ME, Golimstok A, Norscini J, et al. Risk factors for developing seizures after a stroke. *Epilepsia* 1993;34:141–143.
48. Giroud M, Gras P, Fayolle H, et al. Early seizures after acute stroke: a study of 1,640 cases. *Epilepsia* 1996; 35:959–964.
49. So EL, Annegers JF, Hauser WA, et al. Population-based study of seizure disorder after cerebral infarction. *Neurology* 1996;46:350–355.
50. Shinton R, Gill J, Zezulka A, et al. The frequency of epilepsy preceding stroke. Case-control study in 230 patients. *Lancet* 1987;1:11-13.
51. Kilpatrick CJ, Davis SM, Tress BM, et al. Epileptic seizures in acute stroke. *Arch Neurol* 1990;47: 157–160.
52. Fratiglioni L, Grut M, Forsell Y, et al. Prevalence of Alzheimer's disease and other dementias in an elderly urban population: relationship with age, sex, and education. *Neurology* 1991;41:1886–1892.
53. Ryglewicz D. Epilepsy after stroke. *Neurol Neurochir Polska* 1992;26:83–89.
54. Kotila M, Waltimo O. Epilepsy after stroke. *Epilepsia* 1992;33:495–498.
55. Forsgren L, Bucht G, Eriksson S, et al. Incidence and clinical characterization of unprovoked seizures in adults: a prospective population-based study. *Epilepsia* 1996;37:224–229.
56. Hauser WA, Morris ML, Heston LL, et al. Seizures and myoclonus in patients with Alzheimer's disease. *Neurology* 1986;36:1226–1230.

57. McAreavey MJ, Ballinger BR, Fenton GW. Epileptic seizures in elderly patients with dementia. *Epilepsia* 1992;33:657–660.
58. Bogousslavsky JM, Martin RM, Regli FM, et al. Persistent worsening of stroke sequelae after delayed seizures. *Arch Neurol* 1992;49:385–388.
59. Mendez MF, Catanzaro P, Doss RC, et al. Seizures in Alzheimer's disease: clinicopathologic study. *J Geriatr Psychiatry Neurol* 1994;7:230–233.
60. McVicker RW, Shanks OE, McClelland RJ. Prevalence and associated features of epilepsy in adults with Downs syndrome. *Br J Psychiatry* 1994;164:528–532.
61. Godfrey JW, Roberts MA, Caird FI. Epileptic seizures in the elderly: II. Diagnostic problems. *Age Aging* 1982;11:29–34.
62. Lee H, Lerner AM. Transient inhibitory seizures mimicking crescendo TIAs. *Neurology* 1990;40:165–166.
63. Biton VM, Gates JRM, Sussman LdM. Prolonged postictal encephalopathy. *Neurology* 1990;40:963–966.
64. Reynolds J. *Epilepsy: its symptoms, treatment and relation to other chronic convulsive diseases*. London: Churchill, 1861.
65. Lennox WG, Lennox MA. *Epilepsy and related disorders*. London: J & A Churchill, 1960.
66. Tarter RE. Intellectual and adaptive functioning in epilepsy. *Dis Nerv Syst* 1972;33:763–770.
67. Ellenberg JH, Hirtz DG, Nelson KB. Do seizures in children cause intellectual deterioration? *N Engl J Med* 1986;314:1085–1088.
68. Brown SW, Reynolds EH. Cognitive impairment in epileptic patients. In: Reynolds EH, Trimble MR, eds. *Epilepsy and psychiatry*. Edinburgh: Churchill-Livingstone, 1981:147–164.
69. Lishman WA. *Organic psychiatry, the psychological consequences of cerebral disorder*, 2nd ed. Oxford: Blackwell Scientific Publications, 1987.
70. Meldrum BS, Brierley JB. Prolonged epileptic seizures in primates. *Arch Neurol* 1973;28:10–17.
71. Wasterlain CG. Effects of epileptic seizures on brain ribosomes: mechanism and relationship to cerebral energy metabolism. *J Neurochem* 1977;29:707–716.
72. Menini C, Meldrum BS, Riche D, et al. Sustained limbic seizures induced by intraamygdaloid kainic acid in the baboon: symptomatology and neuropathological consequences. *Ann Neurol* 1980;8:501–509.
73. Holmes GLM. The long-term effects of seizures on the developing brain: clinical and laboratory issues. *Brain Dev* 1991;13:393–409.
74. Wasterlain CG, Shirasaka Y. Seizures, brain damage and brain development. *Brain Dev* 1994;16:279–295.
75. Saukkonen A, Kalviainen R, Partanen K, et al. Do seizures cause neuronal damage? A MRI study in new diagnosed and chronic epilepsy. *Neuroreport* 1994;6: 219–223.
76. Kalviainen R, Pitkanen A. Prevention of seizure-induced neuronal damage and intellectual deterioration: experimental aspects and clinical implications. In: Sillanpaa M, Gram L, Johannessen SI, et al, eds. *Epilepsy and mental retardation*. Petersfield, UK/Philadelphia: Wrightson Biomedical, 1999:165–178.
77. Brodtkorb E. Treatment of epilepsy in patients with intellectual disabilities: general principles and particular problems. In: Sillanpaa M, Gram L, Johannessen SI, et al., eds. *Epilepsy and mental retardation*. Petersfield, UK/Philadelphia: 1999:74–89.
78. Stevens JR. Interictal clinical manifestations of complex partial seizures. *Adv Neurol* 1975;11:85–112.
79. Bear DM, Fedio P. Quantitative analysis of interictal behavior in temporal lobe epilepsy. *Arch Neurol* 1977; 34:454–467.
80. Hermann BP, Riel P. Interictal personality and behavioral traits in temporal lobe and generalized epilepsy. *Cortex* 1981;17:125–128.
81. Brandt J, Seidman LJ, Kohl D. Personality characteristics of epileptic patients: a controlled study of generalized and temporal lobe cases. *J Clin Exp Neuropsychol* 1985;7:25–38.
82. Barnhill LJ, Gualtieri CT. Late-onset psychosis after closed head injury. *Neuropsychiatry Neuropsychol Behav Neurol* 1989;2:211–218.
83. Mungas D. Interictal behavior abnormality in temporal lobe epilepsy. *Arch Gen Psychiatry* 1982;39:108–111.
84. Tucker DM, Novelly RA, Walker PJ. Hyperreligiosity in temporal lobe epilepsy: redefining the relationship. *J Nerv Ment Dis* 1987;175:181–184.
85. Benson F, Miller BL, Signer SF. Dual personality associated with epilepsy multiple personality and the illusion of possession. *Arch Neurol* 1986;43:471–474.
86. Schenk L, Bear D. Multiple personality and related dissociative phenomena in patients with temporal lobe epilepsy. *Am J Psychiatry* 1981;138:10:1311–1316.
87. Mesulam M-M. Dissociative states with abnormal temporal lobe EEG multiple personality and the illusion of possession. *Arch Neurol* 1981;38:176–181.
88. Hurwitz TA, Wada JA, Kosaka BD, et al. Cerebral organization of affect suggested by temporal lobe seizures. *Neurology* 1985;35:1335–1337.
89. Mendez MF, Cummings JL, Benson F. Depression in epilepsy. *Arch Neurol* 1986;43:766-770.
90. Betts TA. Depression, anxiety, and epilepsy. *Epilepsy Psychiatry* 1981;60–71.
91. Silberman EK, Post RM, Nurnberger J, et al. Transient sensory, cognitive and affective phenomena in affective illness: a comparison with complex partial epilepsy. *Br J Psychiatry* 1985;146:81–89.
92. Lewis DO, Feldman M, Greene M, et al. Psychomotor epileptic symptoms in six patients with bipolar mood disorders. *Am J Psychiatry* 1984;141:1583–1586.
93. Post RM, Uhde TW, Putnam FW, et al. Kindling and carbamazepine in affective illness. *J Nerv Ment Dis* 1982;170:717–729.
94. Rogers MP, Gittes RF, Dawson M, et al. Giggle incontinence. *JAMA* 1982;247:1446–1448.
95. Faught E, Falgout J, Nidiffer FD, et al. Self induced photosensitive absence seizures with ictal pleasure. *Arch Neurol* 1986;43:408–410.
96. Andy OJ, Jurko MF. Seizures and pain. *Clin Encephalogr* 1985;16:195–201.
97. Penfield W, Gage L. Cerebral localization of epileptic manifestations. *Arch Neurol Psychiatry* 1933;30: 709–727.
98. Trevathan E, Cascino G. Partial epilepsy presenting as focal paroxysmal pain. *Neurology* 1988;38:329–330.
99. Dejerine J, Roussy G. La syndrome thalamique. *Rev Neurol* 1906;14:521–532.
100. Biemond A. The conduction of pain above the level of thalamus opticus. *Arch Neurol Psychiatry* 1956; 75:231–244.
101. Brogna CG, Lee SI, Dreifuss FE. Pilomotor seizures magnetic resonance imaging and electroencephalo-

graphic localization of originating focus. *Arch Neurol* 1986;43:1085–1086.
102. Hoeppner JB, Garron DC, Wilson RS, et al. Epilepsy and verbosity. *Epilepsia* 1987;28:35–40.
103. Cirignotta F, Zucconi M, Mondini S, et al. Writing epilepsy. *Clin Encephalogr* 1986;17:21–23.
104. Kartsounis LD. Comprehension as the effective trigger in a case of primary reading epilepsy. *J Neurol Neurosurg Psychiatry* 1988;51:128–130.
105. Daly DD. Ictal clinical manifestations of complex partial seizures. *Adv Neurol* 1975;11:57–83.
106. Stores G, Zaiwalla Z, Bergel N. Frontal lobe complex partial seizures in children: a form of epilepsy at particular risk of misdiagnosis. *Dev Med Child Neurol* 1991;33:998–1009.
107. Waterman K, Purves SJ, Kosaka B, et al. An epileptic syndrome caused by mesial frontal lobe seizure foci. *Neurology* 1987;37:577–582.
108. Williamson PD, Spencer DD, Spencer SS, et al. Complex partial seizures of frontal lobe origin. *Ann Neurol* 1985;18:497–504.
109. Boone KB, Miller BL, Rosenbert L, et al. Neuropsychological and behavioral abnormalities in an adolescent with frontal lobe seizures. *Neurology* 1988;38:583–586.
110. Chauvel P, Kliemann F, Vignal JP, et al. *The clinical signs and symptoms of frontal lobe seizures*. New York: Raven Press, 1995.
111. Shinomiya M, Kawasaki Y, Yokota K, et al. Frontal EEG paroxysmal activity emerging in prepuberty and during puberty in autism. *Epilepsia* 1996;37:93.
112. Gedye A. Extreme self-injury attributed to frontal lobe seizures. *Am J Ment Retard* 1989;94:20–26.
113. Gedye A. Episodic rage and aggression attributed to frontal lobe seizures. *J Ment Defic Res* 1989;33: 369–379.
114. Waxman SG, Geschwind N. The interictal behavioral syndrome of temporal lobe epilepsy. *Arch Gen Psychiatry* 1975;32:1580–1586.
115. Stevens JR, Livermore A. Kindling of the mesolimbic dopamine system: animal model of psychosis. *Neurology* 1978;28:36–46.
116. Flor-Henry P. Psychosis and temporal lobe epilepsy. *Epilepsia* 1969;10:363–395.
117. Tucker GJ, Price TR, Johnson VB, et al. Phenomenology of temporal lobe dysfunction: a link to atypical psychosis—a series of cases. *J Nerv Ment Dis* 1986; 174:348–356.
118. Dongier S. Statistical study of clinical and electroencephalographic manifestations of 536 psychotic episodes occurring in 516 epileptics between clinical seizures. *Epilepsia Amsterdam* 1959;1:117–142.
119. Starkstein SE, Boston JDMA, Robinson RG. Mechanisms of mania after brain injury. *J Nerv Ment Dis* 1988;176:87–100.
120. Robinson RG, Kubos KL, Starr LB, et al. Mood changes in stroke patients: relationship to lesion location. *Compr Psychiatry* 1983;24:555–566.
121. Robinson RG, Szetela B. Mood change following left hemispheric brain injury. *Ann Neurol* 1981;9:447–453.
122. Starkstein SE, Robinson RG, Price TR. Comparison of patients with and without poststroke major depression matched for size and location of lesion. *Arch Gen Psychiatry* 1988;45:247–252.
123. Lockman LA. Absence seizures and variants. *Neurol Clin* 1985;3:19–29.
124. Adams DJ, Lueders H. Hyperventilation and 6-hour EEG recording in evaluation of absence seizures. *Neurology* 1981;31:1175–1177.
125. Guberman A, Cantu-Reyna G, Stuss D, et al. Nonconvulsive generalized status epilepticus: clinical features, neuropsychological testing, and long-term follow-up. *Neurology* 1986;36:1284–1291.
126. Mark VH, Ervin FR. *Violence and the brain*. New York: Harper & Row, 1970.
127. Delgado-Escueta AV, Kunze V, Waddell G, et al. Lapse of consciousness and automatisms in temporal lobe epilepsy: a videotape analysis. *Neurology* 1977;27: 144–155.
128. Delgado-Escueta AV, Mattson RH, King L. The nature of aggression during epileptic seizures. *N Engl J Med* 1981;305:711–716.
129. Livingston S. *Drug therapy for epilepsy*. Springfield, IL: Charles C Thomas, 1966.
130. Messing RO, Closson RG, Simon RP. Drug-induced seizures: a ten year experience. *Neurology* 1984;34: 1582–1586.
131. Wroblewski BAM, McColgan KL, Smith KR, et al. The incidence of seizures during the tricyclic antidepressant drug treatment in a brain-injured population. *J Clin Psychopharmacol* 1990;10:124–128.
132. Schwartz L, Swaminathan S. Maprotiline hydrochloride and convulsions: a case report. *Am J Psychiatry* 1982;139:243–244.
133. Clifford DB, Rutherford JL, Hicks FG, et al. Acute effects of antidepressants on hippocampal seizures. *Ann Neurol* 1985;18:692–697.
134. Thompson R, Huppert F, Trimble M. Anticonvulsant drugs, cognitive function and memory. *Acta Neurol Scand* 1980;80:75–81.
135. Krijzer F, Shelder M, Bradford D. Comparison of the (Pro) convulsive properties of fluvoxamine and clovoxamine with eight other antidepressants in an animal model. *Neuropsychobiology* 1984;12:249–254.
136. Curran S, de Pauw K. Selecting an antidepressant for use in a patient with epilepsy. Safety considerations. *Drug Saf* 1998;18:125–133.
137. Pasini A, Tortorella A, Gale K. Anticonvulsant effect of intranigral fluoxetine. *Brain Res* 1992;593:287–290.
138. Wada Y, Nakamura M, Hasegawa H, et al. Intra-hippocampal injection of 8-hydroxy-2-(di-n-propylamino)tetralin (8-OH-DPAT) inhibits partial and generalized seizures induced by kindling stimulation in cats. *Neurosci Lett* 1993;159:179–182.
139. Peck AW, Stern WC, Watkinson C. Incidence of seizures during treatment with tricyclic antidepressant drugs and bupropion. *J Clin Psychol* 1983;44:197–201.
140. Davidson J. Seizures and bupropion: a review. *J Clin Psychiatry* 1989;50:256–261.
141. Itil TM, Soldatos C. Epileptogenic side effects of psychotropic drugs. *JAMA* 1980;244:1460–1463.
142. Oliver AP, Luchins DJ, Wyatt RJ. Neuroleptic-induced seizures: an *in vitro* technique for assessing relative risk. *Arch Gen Psychiatry* 1982;39:206–209.
143. Brumback RA, Weinberg WA, Herjanic BL. Epileptiform activity in the electroencephalogram induced by lithium carbonate. *Pediatrics* 1975;56:831–834.
144. Jus A, Villeneuve A, Gautier J, et al. Some remarks on the influence of lithium carbonate on patients with temporal epilepsy. *Int J Clin Pharmacol* 1973;7: 67–74.

18

Psychostimulants, Dopamine Agonists, and Amantadine

The psychostimulants are the oldest psychotropic drugs in continuous use. They are the only drugs clearly demonstrated to have positive effects on cognitive performance in patients with cognitive impairment and in normal people. They also have positive effects on cortical recovery from stroke and brain injury in animal models and in patients. For these reasons, it is appropriate to address the neuropsychology and neuropharmacology of psychostimulant treatment in some detail.

It is well known that stimulants exercise beneficial short-term effects. The fact that they promote recovery from cortical injury suggests that they can also have long-term effects. The immediate effects of stimulant treatment are to enhance the activity of the monoamine neurotransmitters. Their long-term effects are more complicated and probably mediated by a genomic response. Here, then, is an appropriate place to describe the immediate-early genes (IEGs), or proto-oncogenes, that couple signals that are received at the cell surface into longer term alterations in the cell phenotype. Psychotropic drug effects on signal transduction and genomic activation are also discussed with respect to antidepressants, psychotropic anticonvulsants, and lithium.

Amantadine (AMT) was originally used in patients with brain injury because it was thought to be a dopamine (DA) agonist. It is not; it is a glutamate antagonist at the *N*-methyl-D-aspartate (NMDA) receptor. This raises interesting speculation about the nature of excitotoxicity and the therapeutic potential of drugs that can mitigate glutamatergic hyperactivity.

AMT is effective for agitated patients in coma recovery. It works much like a stimulant for patients with brain injury who are hypoaroused. It can also augment the effects of stimulant drugs or mitigate their toxic effects in children who are mentally retarded and autistic.

DA agonists such as L-dopa and bromocriptine (BCT) have also been used for states of hypoarousal after brain injury such as akinetic mutism.

PSYCHOSTIMULANTS

The psychostimulant drugs [methylphenidate (MPH), amphetamine (AMP), methamphetamine (m-AMP), and pemoline] are the oldest psychotropic drugs in continuous use. They were introduced as sympathomimetics in 1934 and have been used for disturbed children since 1937 (1). The conventional indications are attention deficit/hyperactivity disorder (ADHD), narcolepsy, and anergic depression in elderly people. The use of stimulants in neuropsychiatric patients, especially patients with traumatic brain injury (TBI) and stroke, is a relatively new development, but clinical practice is largely reflective of conventional usage.

1. Stimulants improve symptoms of inattention, distractibility, disorganization, hyperactivity, disinhibition, impulsiveness, and emotional lability in children and adults with ADHD. Many patients with TBI have similar symptoms and respond

equally well to low or moderate doses of stimulant drugs. This has been established in short term (2) and longer term studies (3).
2. Stimulants improve symptoms of hypersomnia, apathy, anergia, and hypoarousal in patients with narcolepsy, in patients with Kleine-Levin syndrome (4), and in senile apathy. Patients with TBI with similar symptoms often respond favorably to stimulants.
3. Stimulants are sometimes used for symptoms of fatigue, anergia, and depression in elderly people and may also be used to augment the effects of conventional antidepressants in patients with treatment-refractory depression. Stimulants are not very good as primary antidepressants as a rule, and depression is one of the potential complications of stimulant therapy. On the other hand, one should never be surprised when a depressed patient with TBI or stroke responds favorably to a stimulant but not to a conventional antidepressant. Stimulants are also used as antidepressants in the medically ill and patients with acquired immunodeficiency syndrome (4). There are occasional reports of clinical improvement in manic depressives and schizophrenics with stimulants. This is an odd case, indeed, because we know that stimulants can induce mania or psychosis in vulnerable individuals. Once again, one should never be surprised when a neuropsychiatric patient responds in an unexpected but favorable way to treatment with a stimulant.

The indications for stimulant treatment, therefore, in patients with TBI, stroke, and other neuropathic conditions are entirely within the range of conventional practice. They may be used for various groups of neuropsychiatric patients with chronic deficits in attention or arousal, fatigue, hypersomnolence, disinhibition, or depression. Stimulants may be used in stroke, multiple sclerosis, early dementia, and chronic fatigue syndrome.

What should interest the reader is not that stimulants have clinical utility, because that is intuitive, but rather why they work, what the dimensions of the stimulant response are, and what encephalopathic mechanisms are affected. There are also some practice guidelines to consider because stimulants are easy drugs to prescribe and easy to take—easy to a fault; serious difficulties may arise if they are not used properly.

Theoretical Aspects of the Stimulant Response

First, consider how stimulants work. This will be a long diversion, though, because there are several levels to consider.

Neuropsychological Effects

Stimulant drugs affect cognitive function in ways that clinicians may not appreciate. Their robust effects on attention, arousal, and fatigue have tended to obscure the equally strong influence that they have on learning and memory in animal models. The problem is that when the memory effect is studied in clinical populations, the results may be equivocal. Nevertheless, if appropriate doses are used and the patient population is young and healthy, careful research will usually affirm a positive effect on learning and memory. Stimulants were found to improve long-term memory in patients with ADHD and TBI, and the mechanism was direct, i.e., dissociated from medication effects on attention or fatigue (5,6).

The facilitation of long-term retention in animals when AMP is administered in appropriate doses is well documented. The central mechanism is now thought to be a direct effect on the consolidation of long-term memory traces. Facilitation of memory consolidation with AMP has been demonstrated in preclinical studies and in humans (7). AMP blocks amnesia induced by the protein synthesis inhibitors cycloheximide and acetoxycycloheximide (8). In studies of learning and memory in rats, enhancement by pemoline may be a function of enhancement of brain RNA polymerases (9).

Even a single dose of AMP promotes learning in laboratory animals, and the timing of the AMP dose is crucial, suggesting a consolidation effect (10). The critical timing of the AMP effect is consistent with a transcription process and the induction of primary response genes (11). Another theory is that stimulant-induced memory consolidation is a form of long-term potentiation (LTP) of synaptic transmission, a cognitive analog of what neuropharmacologists refer to as behavioral enhancement or sensitization. What stimulants do to enhance a course of training would this be to strengthen the hebbian net of synaptic efficiency. Low doses of stimulants are a form of intermittent treatment that supports sensitization, whereas high-dose treatment is associated with tolerance or long-term depression of the synaptic web.

The dose effect may explain why the memory effects of stimulants vary in human studies. It is not just a function of the specific clinical population, although stimulants never work reliably in elderly people, but rather of the doses chosen. Stimulant doses only slightly higher than the clinical optimum may actually impair memory and learning (12,13). The cognitive effects of stimulants have a much narrower therapeutic index than either their subjective or behavioral effects, and this can be problematic.

Stimulants are also known to improve perceptual-motor function in children with ADHD (14) and to improve fine motor speed, accuracy, and steadiness (15). In normal subjects, stimulants alleviate the perception of fatigue that accompanies strenuous exercise (16). These effects have also been reported in patients with TBI (17).

Reaction time and information-processing speed are also enhanced by stimulants in patients with ADHD and those with mild TBI. The availability of computer-based testing batteries such as the Neurobehavioral Evaluation System (NES) (18) makes this kind of information readily available in the clinician's office, and the fact that drugs such as MPH and AMP begin to work within 45 minutes permits the direct evaluation of neuropsychological effects with an inexpensive and convenient method. The narrow therapeutic index of stimulants with respect to neuropsychological parameters makes this kind of routine testing advisable.

It has been suggested that the stimulant effect on catecholaminergic neurotransmission is felt most strongly in rostral brain structures, especially in the frontal neocortex. Thus, the idea developed that psychostimulants are "frontal lobe drugs" (19). This concept may or may not be useful. At least one positron emission tomography study of patients with ADHD has demonstrated enhanced metabolism in frontal structures after a dose of MPH (20). Stimulants are useful for patients with TBI with frontal lobe deficits including diminished flexibility, inability to execute complex behavioral programs, poor planning, lack of initiative, poor impulse control, hyperactivity, and anergia.

It has been convenient to ascribe the stimulant effect in patients with TBI to the correction of deficits in monoaminergic neurotransmission that arise as a consequence of shear damage to axial brain structures, where the cell bodies of neurons that synthesize monoamines are concentrated. In the light of this rather simple formula, I once proposed that the administration of monoaminergic drugs such as the stimulants for patients with TBI was an example of "rational pharmacotherapy," i.e., drug therapy to correct a demonstrated and pathogenic neurochemical deficit (21).

Neurochemical Effects

The basic skeleton of AMP and its derivatives has a strong structural analogy with the catecholamines, which is important for understanding their mechanism of action. The stimulants influence the central nervous system (CNS) indirectly through interaction with central catecholaminergic [DA and norepinephrine (NE)] and indoleaminergic [serotonin (5-HT)] neurons (7).

The behavioral effects of the stimulants are generally ascribed to an increase in neurotransmitter activity at CNS monoamine receptors. This presumption is based primarily on the characterization of the behavioral effects of AMP. In preclinical studies, the two behavioral actions that are used most frequently as measures of the stimulant effects of AMP are locomotor activity and stereotypy. The effects of stimulants such as AMP on these parameters can be blocked by discrete lesions of catecholamine pathways, inhibition of catecholamine synthesis, and antagonists of catecholamine receptors (22).

Precisely how stimulants influence catecholamine concentrations at the synapse has always been unclear. The problem is not a lack of possibilities, but rather just the opposite. In different paradigms, AMP promotes the release of neurotransmitter into the synaptic cleft, blocks the reuptake transporter of catecholamines into the presynaptic neuron, inhibits the metabolism of catecholamines by monoamine oxidase, and binds directly to the postsynaptic catecholamine receptor. In clinically relevant doses, however, the primary action of AMP appears to be catecholamine release.

In neuropharmacologic studies, AMP is usually described as an indirect agonist of mesolimbic, mesocortical, and striatal DA secondary to drug-induced accelerative exchange diffusion (22). AMP and the other stimulants also induce comparable changes in the release/uptake of peripheral and CNS NE and 5-HT, although neuropharmacologists do not ordinarily consider these to be important effects. For example, prestimulant depletion of NE does not alter the behavioral effect of stimulants in most preclinical paradigms. It is entirely possible, however, that the focus on DA as the target of the stimulant effect is an artifact of neuropharmacologic paradigms that deal with relatively simple behaviors, such as rotation or stereotypy. In different species, different experimental preparations, and clinical practice, the stimulant effect on NE and 5-HT may be more salient (23).

Even in the rat, AMP has been shown to reverse stress-induced depletion of NE (24). The effect of AMP at the locus ceruleus is not dissimilar to that of desmethylimipramine, an NE reuptake inhibitor, and at NE nerve endings, AMP functions primarily as a reuptake inhibitor (22,25).

It is clear that stimulants such as AMP and MPH increase DA, NE, and 5-HT activity, perhaps by stimulating release or inhibiting reuptake. Which of these effects may be most meaningful clinically is an open question. It also appears that different psychostimulants in clinical use have different patterns of effect on DA, NE, and 5-HT.

The central stimulant effects of MPH are similar to those of AMP. They are both indirect catecholamine agonists, but MPH releases DA and NE from central, bound stores that are sensitive to reserpine, whereas AMP releases DA and NE from central, unbound newly formed stores sensitive to α-methylparatyrosine (26). MPH-induced release of DA may be primarily by exocytosis, whereas AMP-induced release is primarily by exchange diffusion (22). It has been suggested that MPH is a more purely dopaminergic drug than AMP (26), although MPH also reduces the firing rate of NE neurons in the locus ceruleus, just as AMP does (27). AMP and MPH also have different effects on the timing of neurotensin release. Neurotensin is a peptide that possesses modulatory effects on DA transmission (28).

Subtle differences in the biochemical mechanism may explain clinical differences between the isomers of AMP because d-AMP is approximately four to six times more potent that l-AMP with respect to various indices of DA (e.g., stereotypy), whereas the two isomers are approximately equal in their effects on NE mechanisms (e.g., locomotor hyperactivity) in the brain regions where NE is the primary catecholamine. The two isomers also differ in the time frame of their actions (29). m-AMP is equipotent to d-AMP on DA but more potent on NE (30).

It was once thought that d-AMP affected 5-HT to a greater degree than l-AMP (31), but more recent information suggests that the two isomers are equal in their effects. m-AMP, however, is much more potent on 5-HT than either d-AMP or l-AMP (30).

The actual differences among the AMP isomers and derivatives and MPH in clinical practice are hard to define, and the drugs behave similarly in most studies. Individual patients seem to prefer one drug over another, although there is no clear consistency to their preferences. It appears that the effects of MPH may be felt more strongly in cognitive dimensions of response, whereas AMP is more "activating" and more potent for temperamental symptoms such as irritability. The small differences among the clinically useful stimulants described in the preclinical literature may easily be overridden in the clinic by individual pharmacokinetic and pharmacodynamic differences. In cases in which the clinical response to a given psychostimulant is suboptimal, the literature provides a rationale for trying another. It may even be necessary to try all four [Ritalin (MPH), Dexedrine (dextroamphetamine, d-AMP), Adderal, and Desoxyn (m-AMP)] before one is entirely sure that the patient is a stimulant nonresponder.

Tolerance, Neurotoxicity, and Behavioral Sensitization

The early experience with psychostimulants was not with clinical issues but the problem of stimulant misuse. The epidemics of stimulant abuse that occurred in Japan and Sweden after World War II and in the United States during the 1960s were associated with widespread stimulant availability to the general public, often in over-the-counter preparations, and with no medical supervision. These unfortunate natural experiments generated two important observations about psychostimulant drugs. One was the rapid development of tolerance to the stimulant effects that the abusing population was most interested in: euphoria, activation, and anorexia. The second was the development of paranoid psychosis in some individuals.

The preclinical paradigm for the development of stimulant tolerance involves continuous infusion of AMP in high doses, which is associated with an initial increase and then a marked attenuation of behavioral indices of AMP response (32). This may be related to the ability of high-dose AMP to decrease the rate of synaptosomal DA synthesis (33). It may also speak to the neurotoxicity of AMP, its potential for damage by continuous overstimulation (34). Neither tolerance nor stimulant-induced neurotoxicity, however, occupies an important role in usual clinical practice except possibly in the case of long-term use of the atypical stimulant fenfluramine for autism or weight reduction (35).

Stimulant psychosis has been attributed to a peculiar effect of stimulant drugs—the occurrence of reverse tolerance or behavioral sensitization. An analog to this human tragedy is generated in preclinical experiments, when intermittent administration of AMP and other stimulants induces a state of reduced sensitivity to AMP-induced stereotypy (36). Repeated administration of AMP causes supersensitivity in the postsynaptic DA receptor site. In this way, AMP psychosis is comparable with the psychosis and dyskinesias caused by L-dopa (37). Intermittent stimulant treatment promotes a form of pharmacologic kindling (38). Behavioral sensitization to stimulants may be mediated by stimulation of excitatory amino acid (EAA) neurotransmission at the NMDA receptor (39) and may be blocked by NMDA antagonists (40). In the same vein, stimulant-induced neurotoxicity may also be a function of excitotoxicity and/or the excessive generation of oxygen free radicals.

Tolerance and neurotoxicity are high-dose phenomena, whereas behavioral sensitization and pharmacologic kindling are the result of intermittent, low-dose treatment. They are all illustrations of long-term neuronal change induced by stimulants. It is interesting to consider how short-term drugs, like stimulants, can induce long-term changes. The mechanisms that are thus brought to bear are relevant to the stimulant effect on memory consolidation and cortical recovery from stroke and TBI.

The Immediate-Early Response Genes

One of the more interesting aspects of the stimulant response is stimulation of IEGs (or primary response genes or proto-oncogenes). This is a relatively novel area that bears on the activity of other psychotropic drugs, as discussed in Chapters 19 and 20. It has no small bearing on the study of brain plasticity and drug effects on recovery from brain injury.

The IEGs are known as proto-oncogenes from the study of retroviruses that induce tumor development. Proto-oncogenes are cellular genes that normally govern cell division and proliferation, the generation of growth factors, and differentiation-inducing agents. They are active in the course of normal development. Because they have large areas of sequence identity with retroviral oncogenes, they are capable of reacting with retroviruses and will mutate as a result. The invading retrovirus thus changes the normal genomic direction of cell proliferation by turning proto-oncogenes toward tumor induction; thus, their name oncogenes.

Because they have a role in cell proliferation and differentiation, the detection of IEGs and their protein transcription factors in adult neurons was rather surprising at first (41–43). However, subsequent research has demonstrated that IEGs also play a role in the normal transmission of information within and between cells. In this role, the behavior of the IEGs is pertinent to neuropharmacology.

IEGs are sensitive to environmental signals and may be induced by growth factors, neuronal depolarization, and a number of other pharmacologic, electrical, and physiologic stimuli. The induction of IEGs thus represents a molecular mechanism by which adult neurons can adapt their phenotype over the long-term to environmental stimuli. Inducing IEGs is a mechanism for the conversion of ephemeral second messenger–mediated events into long-term cellular phenotypic alterations (41). They are thus hypothesized to act as third messengers, coupling cell-surface phenomena with the regulation of the "late-response genes" that are ultimately responsible for the cell's phenotypic long-term response to stimulation. The late-response genes induce long-term structural alterations in the neuron.

Drug effects on second messengers, so-called signal transduction, are discussed at some length in Chapters 19 and 20. Second messengers respond to events in the cellular environment and then stimulate expression of a small group of IEGs. These genes are the first targets of the signal transduction machinery of the cell, which is why they are sometimes called primary-response genes. They are activated by second messengers and then rapidly generate specific mRNA and proteins. The primary-response genes or IEGs couple short-term signals received at the cell surface with longer term alterations in the cell structure by generating transcription factors or DNA binding proteins. All this is accomplished within minutes. Two IEGs that have been the subject of recent investigation are *c-fos* and *c-jun* and the transcriptional proteins they generate are known as Fos and Jun.

Proteins generated by IEGs, such as Fos and Jun, play several roles in the signal transduction process: extracellular polypeptide messengers, cell-surface receptors, protein kinases, G proteins, and nuclear transcription factors. As nuclear transcription factors, they bind to DNA and thus regulate the expression of selected target genes. In different kinds of cells, the same transcription factors (such as Fos and Jun) generate unique kinds of cellular alterations. In the nervous system, the long-term responses of cells may contribute to phenomena such as differentiation, plasticity, learning, and regeneration (42).

The IEGs *c-fos* and *c-jun* and the proteins that they generate have provided useful markers to trace the effects of pharmacologic, electrical, and physiologic stimuli within the nervous system. It is appropriate to introduce the issue here because the activity of third messenger systems such as *c-fos* and *c-jun* is thought to mediate particular aspects of the psychostimulant response. For example, the psychostimulants AMP and cocaine are known to induce *c-fos* expression in the striatum, even after single-dose administration. This action is believed to be mediated by activation of the DA D_1 receptor.

The action of stimulant drugs on IEGs such as *c-fos* has not been of much interest to clinicians who study stimulant effects in patient populations to improve attention, memory, anergia, or somnolence in which drug effects are immediate; very low doses are used day after day for months at a time, and the clinical response is maintained unchanged over time. It has been of keen interest, however, to neuropharmacologists who study stimulants in different paradigms and who have always remarked on the changes that occur in the stimulant response over time. In some preparations, daily administration of stimulants leads to behavioral desensitization, whereas intermittent treatment causes increased sensitivity to the stimulant effect. The induction of IEGs is relevant to this phenomenon because daily stimulant treatment leads to a reduction in *c-fos* activity, and intermittent treatment actually increases *c-fos* activity (44).

It is always difficult to move from the preclinical study of stimulant effects in rats, which hardly even possess a cerebral cortex and in which extremely high dose studies are the norm, to the study of clinical effects of stimulants in human beings. However, the induction of IEGs by stimulants may be of particular interest to the understanding of drug-induced cortical recovery after stroke or TBI because the studies cited above indicate that even a single dose of AMP may enhance the recovery process. This raises the possibility that we are capable of doing two things with stimulants and by means of different mechanisms: improving deficit symptoms, such as inattention or hypoarousal, by stimulating the membrane receptor and inducing lasting changes in the structure and function of neurons by inducing the activity of IEGs. It is the latter effect that probably influences the rate of cortical recovery. It is unnerving, however, to think that these two actions might be mutually exclusive: that cortical recovery may be advanced by intermittent treatment while symptomatic relief is provided by a mode of treatment that is incompatible with structural alteration. I do not necessarily believe that this is true because symptomatic and cognitive improvement in TBI has only been demonstrated with very low doses of stimulants administered no more than twice daily. In fact, that is intermittent treatment.

The study of IEGs is relevant to other areas of psychopharmacology that are somewhat removed from this topic. For example, the neuroleptic haloperidol is a strong inducer of *c-fos* gene expression in the striatum, whereas clozapine is not (45). It is possible that this is related to the increased risk of extrapyramidal side effects with haloperidol compared with clozapine.

The study of IEGs has also been fertile ground for understanding encephalopathic mechanisms such as the hitherto mysterious process of kindling. Seizure activity results in increased *c-fos* gene expression in particular subsets of neurons (46). What is more interesting is that the subconvulsant electrical stimulus used to establish kindling also induces *c-fos* gene expression (41).

The expression of IEGs is stimulated by physiologic, pharmacologic, or electrical stimuli. It may also be stimulated by traumatic events. The most robust expression of IEGs does not, in fact, occur in the everyday activities of cells but rather when resting cells are suddenly and powerfully stimulated to undergo a rapid change in functional activity. In such circumstances, after trauma, for example, the IEGs may represent a kind of specialized rapid-response mechanism to alter the pattern of cellular gene expression (47).

Transient ischemia, cortical devascularization, and mechanical damage all are capable of inducing *c-fos* gene expression, even in areas not directly affected by the insult (48). Typically, CNS lesions are found to induce *c-fos* gene expression in the entire ipsilateral cortex (41). IEG expression in glia is detected around the margins of a lesion, an event that may be related to cellular proliferation after brain injury (43). Different patterns of IEG expression have been described in TBIs of varying severity (49), and IEG expression is more vigorous after trauma in young organisms (48). The discovery of IEG expression in brain areas that are remote from the actual site of injury suggests a molecular basis for the phenomenon of diaschisis (47).

These three items, however, suggest that induction of *c-fos* expression may be related to neuropathologic states as diverse as epilepsy, stroke, TBI, and tardive dyskinesia. Manipulating the third messenger system represented by IEGs may thus be an avenue to treat, control, or even prevent certain encephalopathic events. Someday, the pharmacologic manipulation of third messenger systems will be central to intelligent psychopharmacology; that is, unless we are doing it already.

The discussion of IEGs leads to an area that is dealt with at greater length in the section on AMT, an antagonist of EAA neurotransmission at the NMDA receptor channel. The EAA glutamate appears to provide one key mechanism for inducing *c-fos* expression, especially at the NMDA channel. NMDA receptors mediate *c-fos* expression in the hippocampus and in other brain regions (41); the NMDA response is, in fact, similar to the kind of *c-fos* induction by the experimental proconvulsant drug metrazole. Additionally, competitive and noncompetitive NMDA antagonists are capable of blocking metrazole-induced *c-fos* expression (42). Stimulant induction of *c-fos* can be blocked by pretreatment with the NMDA receptor antagonist MK-801 (50). Pharmacologic treatment with AMT, therefore, may actually be a way of undoing the excessive activation of IEGs that occurs after trauma. Cotreatment with AMT and a psychostimulant in patients with

TBI may actually protect patients from the potentially neurotoxic effects of psychostimulants. (Is this why mentally retarded children respond better to stimulants when they are combined with AMT?)

It grows increasingly apparent that the description of psychotropic drug effects in terms of unidirectional changes in synaptic concentrations of governing neurotransmitters such as DA or NE is only a part of what really happens. The clinician is actually manipulating a chain of extraneuronal and intraneuronal events, a series of dynamic and structural changes, the nature of which we understand only partially. The introduction of stimulant drugs and AMT singly or in combination, intermittently or continuously, to immature or adult organisms, in temporal proximity to a traumatic event or remote from it all represent variables with unknown effects on third messenger systems that govern the structure and function of neurons.

Clinical Aspects of Stimulant Treatment

Stimulants are comparatively easy to use, and positive effects, when they occur, are apparent within days or hours after an optimal dose is achieved. MPH (Ritalin) and d-AMP (Dexedrine) are the stimulants most frequently prescribed for ADHD, narcolepsy, Kleine-Levin syndrome, senile apathy, and probably also for TBI. Adderall is a long-acting variant of amphetamine that includes the l-isomer, thus resembling Benzedrine, which is no longer available in the United States. It is an old clinical belief that some patients with ADHD respond better to l-AMP than to d-AMP. m-AMP (Desoxyn) is the fourth option and a potent one. Pemoline (Cylert) is the fifth but not a terribly good one. It was never very effective clinically, although there were always a few patients who preferred it to the other stimulants. It is occasionally associated with serious hepatic toxicity.

Low doses of stimulant drugs are effective for virtually all the usual indications except narcolepsy (which is pharmacologically a case unto itself). There is the rare child with ADHD who requires high doses (i.e., >0.75 mg/kg two or three times daily), but most patients do perfectly well on low to moderate doses. What is remarkable about the clinical pharmacology of MPH and AMP is the consistency of dosing. Children with ADHD require MPH at doses of 0.2 to 0.6 mg/kg two or three times daily and AMP at doses of 0.1 to 0.4 mg/kg two or (less often) three times daily. The appropriate dose of m-AMP is slightly lower than that of AMP. As a rule, stimulant doses for adults are half those of children, and stimulant doses for elderly people are half again as low. It is not uncommon to treat an elderly person with 2.5 or 5.0 mg MPH in the morning. Recently, effective long acting-forms of MPH and of Adderall have become available. They are quite useful, much more so than the old forms of long-acting Ritalin or Dexedrine Spansules.

Appropriate stimulant dosing for TBI, stroke, depression, and other conditions is similar to that for ADHD. Measurement of stimulant blood levels does not improve clinical management.

One clue that the stimulant dose is too low is a short duration of action. Fatigue and irritability may also be low-dose effects. Doses that are slightly higher than the therapeutic optimum may have negative neuropsychological effects. More commonly, the patient experiences irritability, headache, dysphoria, or nervousness.

The optimal therapeutic dose remains stable over months or even years of treatment. Narcolepsy excluded, one rarely needs to increase the dose after the first few weeks of initial adjustment. If continued dose increases seem to be necessary, the problem may be drug abuse; more commonly, however, the patient is developing a major depression and is trying to mask the symptoms with stimulants. This is a dangerous situation because stimulants can aggravate the development of depression.

Stimulants are not hard to monitor for side effects; anorexia and insomnia are amenable to dose or dose-schedule adjustments; headache, dysphoria, irritability, "on-off," and rebound reactions usually respond to minor changes in prescription. The stimulant side-effect profile is, in fact, a model of clarity: acute toxic effects are clear and apparent and resolve quickly as soon as the drugs are withdrawn. Once the hurdle of initial sensitivity, however, is past, there is no long-term toxicity—no secret effect that will come along after months or years of treatment. Stimulants have the enormous advantage of being "digital" drugs; they either work or not, and when they do work, positive effects are readily apparent. Tolerance to stimulant effects does not usually occur in ADHD (51) or TBI, but it frequently does in narcolepsy and Kleine-Levin syndrome.

This is not to suggest that stimulants can be administered freely or they can be prescribed by inexperienced physicians. Stimulant therapy is perfectly safe in the hands of knowledgeable and responsible practitioners, but stimulants are complex drugs and acute toxicity is not an insignificant matter. Adults, for example, seem to be very sensitive to stimulants, and very low doses may be sufficient for a 70-kg man (52). Higher doses may cause cognitive overfixation, stereotyped thinking, perseveration, or palilalia. High doses may actually impair memory and clear thinking (12). A patient who is sensitive to stimulants may become anxious, disorganized, fearful, agitated, paranoid, or frankly psychotic. Somatosensory hallucinations (e.g., formication) may occur. Patients can develop increased spasticity, choreic and athetoid dyskinesias, and motor and phonic tics. Patients may become intensely dysphoric, irritable, and prone to rage attacks. Although stimulants may alleviate the symptoms of posttraumatic headache or enhance the effect of analgesic agents, they may also cause headache or precipitate migraine. This is not a trivial list by any means, and it speaks to the need for careful monitoring.

Side effects of stimulants also include agitation, disorientation, emotional lability, cognitive perseveration, increased spasticity, tremor, and dyskinesia, especially in patients with severe motor sequelae of TBI.

Although stimulant treatment can be stopped abruptly in patients with ADHD even after years of treatment with no withdrawal symptoms, patients with TBI seem to be different. In patients with TBI, abrupt discontinuation may lead to a withdrawal reaction, with symptoms of depression, anergia, or agitation. Thus, a clinical trial should never be undertaken lightly in a patient with TBI because the medication cannot be withdrawn suddenly without risking the additional problem of rebound depression. No patient with TBI should be treated with stimulants unless there is a physician experienced in the use of the drugs in close attendance and unless the patient and his or her family fully understand the attendant risks.

Research has not advanced to a point where it is possible to predict which patients with TBI should be treated with stimulant drugs. It is the author's clinical impression, however, that the best response occurs in relatively high level, mild to moderately impaired patients with relatively circumscribed deficits in attention, memory, organization, or initiative. More severely impaired subjects, especially those with severe motor impairment, seem less likely to respond and seem more prone to acute toxic effects and withdrawal reactions. This parallels the clinical experience of child psychiatrists and developmental physicians: children with ADHD are less likely to respond to stimulants if they have associated emotional, behavioral, or cognitive problems; mild to moderately retarded children are more likely to respond to stimulants than the severe to profoundly retarded, but they are less likely to respond than children of normal intelligence.

Stimulants do not have untoward reactions with other drugs except the sympathomimetics and monoamine oxidase inhibitors. They are commonly combined with antidepressants, beta-blockers, α_2 agonists, anticonvulsants, and antiparkinsonian drugs with no ill effects.

Combination therapy may be the result of two indications, e.g., carbamazepine for seizures and MPH for inattention and hypoarousal. Frequently, however, drugs are added to the stimulants to enhance the therapeutic effect, an augmentation strategy, or to diminish side effects. Stimulant combinations with AMT, bupropion, DA agonists, α_2 agonists, cyanocobalamin, and thyrotropin-releasing hormone may have synergistic effects on arousal, attention, memory, and disinhibition, the classic psychostimulant indications in TBI. Stimulant combinations with antidepressants, especially serotonergics, or α_2 agonists may be useful for obsessive-compulsive symptoms, tics, oppositional and negativistic behavior, irritability, and temper outbursts. Stimulants may augment antidepressants in refractory depression and thymoleptics for aggression and explosive behavior. The coadministration of a psychostimulant with AMT may alleviate the problem of stimulant toxicity while preserving or even augmenting the positive clinical effects. In this way, the benefits of stimulant therapy may be extended to moderately impaired patients with TBI or mentally handicapped individuals.

There is no absolute contraindication to stimulant therapy except perhaps in the case of patients with a history of stimulant abuse. Stimulants are likely to raise, not lower, the seizure threshold in patients with epilepsy, in spite of the warnng in the *Physicians Desk Reference* (53), although it is true that very high doses may be epileptogenic (54). When a stimulant is combined with another proconvulsant drug such as AMT or fluoxetine, however, there is a small increase in the risk of seizure.

In low doses, the cardiovascular effects of psychostimulants are minimal. Middle-aged or elderly patients, however, may develop tachycardia, hypertension, or arrhythmia in connection with stimulant treatment.

STIMULANT EFFECTS ON CORTICAL RECOVERY

That psychostimulants are beneficial for symptoms of inattention, abulia, and anergia in TBI is hardly controversial; one would be surprised if such were not the case. The idea that stimulants are the treatment of choice for depression after TBI requires a small degree of imagination, but it is not a staggering inferential leap. There is, however, a third area of speculation, and this does require the most critical scrutiny: the effect of stimulant drugs on the process of cortical recovery.

Neuropharmacologists study long-term stimulant effects (behavioral sensitization, pharmacologic kindling, neurotoxicity, consolidation of long-term memory), whereas clinicians think about stimulants in terms of their short-term effects. The idea that stimulant treatment may have an enduring effect is a novelty in clinical medicine. The best examples are the follow-up studies of children with ADHD, which have never shown convincing differences in outcome relative to drug treatment. Yet clinical studies indicate that children with ADHD, on average, usually require treatment with stimulants for no more than a couple of years. Clinical experience indicates that with appropriate treatment, they appear to mature and acquire more stable patterns of relating to their environment. They appear to do better after 1 or 2 years of stimulant treatment.

Children mature as a matter of course. The same pattern appears to hold for adults with ADHD, i.e., after 1 to 3 years of treatment, they acquire new habits and a new temperament, and drug treatment is no longer necessary.

There is evidence from studies of patients with TBI on stimulants (55). In a series of placebo-controlled studies, stimulants exercised cognitive, behavioral, and subjective effects that were sustained over months of follow-up. After the drugs were withdrawn after a year of treatment, however, there was no relapse to the premorbid condition. These were patients whose recovery before treatment had achieved a plateau. They were years postinjury. Stimulant treatment had lasting effects on their areas of deficit, and the effects were sustained, even after the drugs were discontinued. I speculated at the time that the drugs were having more than a symptomatic effect and were also influencing the trajectory of recovery.

The stimulant studies of patients with TBI have been aimed at the reduction of untoward behaviors (56,57), cognitive improvement (58), and subjective improvement (59). I am aware of only two controlled trials, one that is unequivocally positive in 15 patients (17) and one that is inconclusive (59). None of the TBI studies addresses the issue of stimulant-induced recovery directly.

Stimulant studies in patients with stroke often center on the problem of poststroke depression, for which MPH is found to be useful by itself or in conjunction with an antidepressant (60–64). In contrast to TBI, however, in stroke, there are at least a few reports of stimulant effects on recovery. Positive effects on recovery from aphasia were reported in six patients with stroke treated with AMP by Walker-Batson et al. (65). Positive effects on motor recovery were reported when AMP is combined with physical therapy (66–68).

None of the clinical studies in stroke or in TBI represents unequivocal and indisputable evidence. It is always hard to make specific attributions in a clinical study because stimulants have so many different actions. The stimulant effect may simply be an antidepressant effect or a nonspecific effect on general arousal or fatigue. The preclinical literature, however, is more salient and to the point.

Enduring recovery of function has been demonstrated in cats subjected to bilateral cortical ablations (69). Treatment with AMP, combined with visual experience, results in recovery of binocular depth perception. In rats, unilateral cortical ablation causes a motor deficit that is apparent when the animal has to traverse a narrow elevated beam (70). A single dose of d-AMP administered 24 hours after cortical ablation accelerates the rate of cortical recovery (71) as long as the drug is coupled with beam-walking experience. Postlesion treatment with AMP also enhances motor recovery in cats with unilateral or bilateral frontal cortex ablation (72).

The element that is common to both the clinical and preclinical studies of AMP-induced recovery is the requirement for cotraining, i.e., a drug combined with experience (training, therapy) exercises a positive effect when the drug alone does not. Brain plasticity, therefore, in a variety of paradigms in developing and adult animals, seems to require an optimal monoamine environment; conversely, the monoaminergic stimulants seem to require an optimal experiential environment (73). This suggests that the drug itself serves as a facilitator of the learning experience, an agent that renders the organism capable of capturing an experiential phenomenon in a meaningful way.

The pharmacologic mechanism of AMP-facilitated recovery is in all probability mediated by CNS noradrenergic, dopaminergic, or serotonergic neurons. Of these, NE is the most important. Coadministration of haloperidol in the beam-walking paradigm blocks the AMP response; haloperidol blocks DA and NE but not 5-HT (71). Intraventricular or cerebellar infusions of NE mimic the AMP effect, whereas infusions of DA do not. Antagonists or depleters of NE slow beam-walking recovery. The effect of MPH is less robust than that of AMP. Taken together, these findings suggest that stimulant-induced recovery is mediated by central NE. The effect of noradrenergic drugs on recovery is similar in traumatic cerebral contusion and cortical infarction models (74).

The stimulation of NE systems by AMP and other stimulants may correct the development of diaschisis, i.e., they attenuate the remote functional depression that follows brain injury, or it may facilitate the process of LTP, one of the synaptic bases for brain plasticity.

TBIs and strokes are known to cause dysfunction in brain areas remote from the primary insult. The resulting impaired regional blood flow and cerebral metabolism in these distant areas are referred to as cerebral diaschisis (75) or temporary functional deactivation of intact brain regions remote from the area of primary injury (76).

Unilateral cortical injury induced by suction ablation or weight-drop contusion evokes a widespread depression of cortical metabolism in the ipsilateral hemisphere. This metabolic depression may be attenuated by AMP and exaggerated by lesions to the locus ceruleus (77).

Experiments have demonstrated that injury-induced diaschisis can be blocked or reversed by noradrenergic drugs or intraventricular infusion of NE (77). Diaschisis is enhanced by lesions of the locus ceruleus (78). It has been suggested, therefore, that perturbations of NE activity may be a central event in the development of diaschisis (72,78). Conversely, the AMP effect on cortical recovery may be prevention or correction of injury-related metabolic depression.

LTP is one of the substrates for brain plasticity and memory formation in normal development and neuropsychopathology (79). Although the mechanisms responsible for the development and persistence of LTP are unknown, consideration is usually given to changes in synaptic strength, neosynaptogenesis, and use-dependent sprouting.

Changes in synaptic strength are believed to be the basis for learning and memory; neocortical neurons, for example, can display a sustained increase in synaptic efficacy after conditioning stimulation (80). In LTP, a brief tetanic stimulus to specific neural pathways produces an increase in synaptic responses that can last for days or weeks. The development of LTP is triggered by brief physiologic events, appears to be strengthened by repetition, and can persist indefinitely (81). If drugs such as AMP facilitate cortical recovery by enhancing the learning process, it is likely that LTP is at least one of the pertinent mechanisms.

If an optimal noradrenergic environment is necessary for the development of LTP in the service of recovery, a suboptimal NE environment may enhance the development of kindling, a potentially destructive variant of LTP.

The earliest stimulant studies of clinical effects on impulsive behavior and attention date from the 1930s (1). The earliest recognition of a stimulant effect on postural recovery in decorticate animals dates from the 1940s. Yet a half century has elapsed before the full range of stimulant effects has been appreciated in patients with stroke and brain injury. During that interval, and especially over the past 10 years, the basis for their effect has been developed in terms of the stimulation of monoamines, especially NE, the activation of IEGs to induce lasting phenotypic changes in the target neuron, the support of LTP, and the attenuation of diaschisis and kindling. The epidemics of psychostimulant abuse have prejudiced the medical community against a class of drugs whose full range of benefit is far more impressive than the conventional indications.

AMANTADINE

Neuropharmacology

AMT is water-soluble acid salt that can penetrate all cell membranes including those of the CNS. The usual indications are as an antiviral agent, for influenza A prophylaxis, for Parkinson's disease (PD), and for neuroleptic side effects, especially pseudoparkinsonism and the neuroleptic malignant syndrome. There is recent evidence of wider efficacy for a number of neuropsychiatric conditions.

The antiviral effects of AMT were first studied during the 1960s (82), and its efficacy in PD was discovered serendipitously when the drug was given for influenza prophylaxis to a woman with the disease (83). It is more or less equipotent to the anticholinergic drugs for patients with PD or neuroleptic-induced extrapyramidal symptoms with fewer side effects (84). Compared with benztropine, AMT does not impair memory in healthy volunteers who are young (85) or elderly (86).

The neuropsychiatric effects of AMT have been attributed to its effect on DA neurotransmission, but it was never really clear exactly what that effect was. In various models, AMT acts presynaptically to enhance DA release and inhibit DA reuptake (87). It has a direct, postsynaptic effect and may increase the density of postsynaptic DA receptors (87) or alter the conformation of the DA receptor (88). AMT antagonizes neuroleptic-induced prolactin secretion (89), indicating an effect on hypothalamic (or pituitary) DA receptors. It may even have a selective affinity for striatal DA receptors without affecting mesolimbic or mesocortical DA systems (88). The actions of AMT have been proposed to stem from a unique combination of presynaptic and postsynaptic effects, but no single action stood out from the others.

In fact, the doses of AMT used for successful antiparkinsonian therapy are unlikely to attain the high extraneuronal concentrations necessary to release DA in experimental preparations, diminishing the likelihood of a postsynaptic mechanism. By the same token, a presynaptic effect is rendered implausible by the fact that continued drug effects in animal preparations, even after synthesis, storage, and release of DA, are abolished (90).

The precise mechanism for AMT was unknown until recently when evidence accrued in favor of an effect as a glutamate receptor antagonist or, to be more specific, a noncompetitive antagonist of the NMDA receptor-ion channel (90). This is a plausible theory because an NMDA antagonist can influence parkinsonian symptoms in several ways: by countering the hyperactivity that is induced in glutamatergic pathways under conditions of DA deficiency, mitigating the excitotoxic damage of glutamatergic hyperactivity, or facilitating the effects of endogenous DA agonists.

The introduction of an alternative mechanism of action for AMT is sufficient to explain its unique position among the DA agonists. It is also an opportunity to discuss the EAA neurotransmitters and the problem of excitotoxicity.

Excitotoxicity in Disease and Therapeutics

Excitatory Amino Acid Neurotransmission

The relevance of the EAA systems to disease and therapeutics derives from (i) the physiologic basis of EAA transmission, (ii) the impact of EAA systems on other neurotransmitter systems such as DA, NE, 5-HT, and acetylcholine, and (iii) from the phenomenon of excitotoxicity. (see Chapter 4).

Most of the synapses that connect CNS neurons are excitatory and are believed to use the acidic amino acids L-glutamate and L-aspartate as neurotransmitters (91). These EAA neurotransmitters exist in high concentrations in every part of the brain and play a vital role in almost all brain processes (92). Aside from glutamate, aspartate, and perhaps homocysteate, we know little about the endogenous EAA transmitters. We are able, however, to dissect the nature of EAA neurotransmission on several distinct receptor sites, each of which can be activated in experimental preparations by a specific amino acid analogue. The best understood of these receptor classes is the NMDA type, so named because it is selectively activated by NMDA, a glutamate analogue that is not present in brain. Glutamate is the endogenous ligand with the highest affinity for the NMDA receptor (91).

Although glutamate exerts its diverse effects through pharmacologically distinct channels, both NMDA and non-NMDA receptors are present at the synapses involved, and transmission occurs through a coordinated effort of both (91,93). Fast synaptic excitatory neurotransmission is mediated by L-glutamate–gated ion channels mediated by AMPA-gated channels and by kainate. Excitatory transmission mediated by NMDA is slower and includes a calcium ion component. The NMDA receptors are especially important for their role in neuronal plasticity, LTP, kindling, and excitotoxicity (94). They are found primarily in the cerebral cortex (91).

Excitatory transmission at synapses that use NMDA receptors is different from the classic concept of transmission that is exemplified by the neuromuscular junction. At a classic synapse, the transmitter causes an increase in cation permeability and depolarizes the target cell in proportion to the net driving force of the ionic gradients. Usually, the number of channels opened by the neurotransmitter is independent of the membrane potential of the target cell. The NMDA-receptor channel complex is unusual because it is activated or gated by its neurotransmitters in a voltage-dependent manner and is permeable, not to sodium or potassium ions, but to calcium ions. The number of channels opened by the neurotransmitter increases as the target neuron is depolarized. The voltage dependence of the NMDA receptor functions therefore as a feed-forward mechanism that increases with depolarization.

Because the NMDA receptor depends on the level of target cell depolarization, determined by any variety of ancillary neurotransmitters or neuromodulators, NMDA activation is conditional or associative. It is, therefore, like the mythic hebbian synapse, a clear link between receptor activation and use-dependent regulation of synaptic activity. Activity-dependent processes of this nature may be presumed to mediate the temporal integration of neuronal activity, synaptic plasticity, or associative responses that account for learning, such as LTP. In fact, a substantial body of evidence exists to support a central role for the NMDA receptor in LTP (91).

The physiologic excitation of glutamate receptors generates a number of different intracellular signals (i.e., second messengers), including calcium, inositol phosphate, diacylglycerol, and arachidonic acid. These, in turn, activate a sequence of intracellular events such as the induction of early inducible genes encoding specific nuclear proteins (e.g., Fos, Jun), third messenger systems that activate specific gene expression programs. The coordination of specific genomic programs thus activated leads to the synthesis of proteins that are important in neuronal plasticity, LTP, the formation of synaptic spines, and the maintenance of appropriate synaptic connections during development and brain recovery (92).

The EAA neurotransmitters interact with the major neuromodulatory and inhibitory neurotransmitters, such as DA, and these interactions provide a new basis for studying the behavior of the centrally active drugs. For example, NMDA antagonist drugs tend to augment DA neurotransmission and compensate for the untoward consequences of DA deficiency states on the generation of excitotoxicity. The AA_2 EAA receptor participates in the activating effects of psychostimulant drugs (95), and the negative effects of tricyclic antidepressants on memory and learning may be mediated by blockade of the NMDA receptor (96). NMDA-receptor activation results in NE release in a synaptosome preparation (97). The activation of 5-HT_2 receptors facilitates neuronal depolarization by NMDA (98); the selective serotonin reuptake inhibitor sertraline will do the same, but not paroxetine (99). Ethanol tends to aggravate glutamate excitotoxicity, and this may account for the relative severity of TBI sequelae in patients who were intoxicated at the time of injury (100).

Excitotoxicity

In Chapter 4, glutamate, the principal excitatory neurotransmitter in the brain, was discussed. Two decades ago, glutamate was not as recognized as it is today as the natural neurotransmitter released at most excitatory synapses in the mammalian CNS and responsible for functions such as cognition, memory, movement, sensation, and neuronal plasticity. How excessive activation of the glutamate receptors causes neuronal injury or death and that there is only a small gradient between physiologic levels of glutamate and levels that may be toxic were also described. The possibility that excitotoxic cell death might contribute to the pathology of aging, stroke, PD, TBI, Alzheimer's disease, and other neurodegenerative conditions has aroused great interest, particularly as it opens the possibility of a therapeutic application of EAA antagonists (101).

The ambient concentrations of glutamate are very close to the concentration that can destroy neurons. There is a substantial reserve of glutamate that can leak out of damaged neurons, and neurons will die after only a few hours of exposure to excess glutamate. Furthermore, any condition that reduces the bioenergetics of the neuron may compromise the exquisite control mechanisms that hold the glutamate receptor in check, thereby allowing even physiologic concentrations of glutamate to induce an excitotoxic reaction (102). Excitotoxicity is clearly manifest in pathologic conditions such as PD, stroke, and TBI, but it may also be an active participant in the insidious degeneration that accompanies normal aging.

Hypoxic/ischemic and traumatic injury to the brain are attended by a massive outflow of EAAs, especially glutamate. During stroke and brain injury, glutamate accumulates in the cellular interstitium and acts persistently on receptors, a paroxysmal receptor occupation referred to as receptor abuse or excitotoxicity (92). It is not entirely clear how excessive excitation of NMDA receptors by abnormally high levels of glutamate leads to neuronal damage and death, but increased membrane permeability and abnormal sodium, chloride, and calcium influx are presumed to play a role (102). In neurodegenerative conditions such as PD, Huntington's chorea, and Alzheimer's' disease, excitotoxic damage may be the consequence of a pathologic chain of events that includes the generation of free radicals.

In PD, a deficit in DA function probably releases excitatory systems from inhibitory control, leading to paroxysmal or excitotoxic release of glutamate and thus to further neuronal damage and death. It also appears that many of the antiparkinsonian agents actually function as NMDA antagonists. For example, in 1989, the AMT analogue memantine, an antiparkinsonian and antispastic agent, was found to inhibit the binding of MK-801, an NMDA antagonist, to postmortem human brain homogenates (103). This finding and subsequent studies have indicated that the adamantanamine family of compounds, to which memantine and AMT both belong, possesses a micromolar affinity to one of the binding sites on the NMDA receptor and functions as noncompetitive receptor antagonists (90). In various animal models of focal brain hypoxia/ischemia, antagonists of the NMDA receptor, such as ketamine, memantine, or AMT, are found to exert neuroprotective effects (104,105).

In experimental studies of TBI, there is marked elevation of extracellular glutamate and aspartate adjacent to the trauma site, an increase that is proportional to the severity of injury and to the reduction in the cellular bioenergetic state (106). Cerebrospinal fluid levels of glutamate are elevated for days after severe TBI in humans (107). Thus, the idea has developed that glutamatergic excitotoxicity is central to the pathophysiology of TBI as it is after stroke. Treatment with NMDA antagonists has been found to limit the resultant neurologic dysfunction (106), although there is a therapeutic window of only a few hours after injury (or stroke) during which the treatment may be effective.

Excitotoxicity also plays a role in the neurotoxicity of psychostimulant drugs. The activating effects of psychostimulants are mediated, at least in part, by glutamate receptor activation at the AA_2 site (95), and glutamate antagonists alter the behavioral effects of acutely administered psychomotor stimulants. They also block the development of sensitization to the repeated administration of psychomotor stimulants in mesolimbic DA neurons (108). It also appears that NMDA receptor activation has a role to play in stimulant-induced DA and 5-HT neurotoxicity (109). NMDA antagonists have been found to attenuate dopaminergic neurotoxicity induced by m-AMP (110), and the neuroprotective effect of NMDA antagonists may occur by attenuating DA overflow (111).

The neurotoxic effects of repeated seizures and, indeed, the process of epileptogenesis have been attributed the behavior of the NMDA receptor complex (112,113). The NMDA effects of memantine and AMT may also underlie their dose-dependent anticonvulsant and proconvulsant effects because other noncompetitive NMDA antagonists such as phencyclidine and ketamine are known to exert anticonvulsant effects in some rodent models, whereas at higher doses, these drugs may induce seizures by themselves (114). It is also interesting that kindled rats are more susceptible to the proconvulsant effects of memantine than nonkindled rats, probably because of the altered involvement of NMDA receptors in synaptic transmission after kindling (114). In clinical practice, low doses of AMT tend to improve seizure control (115), but seizures may occur with higher doses, (e.g., >400 mg per day).

Recent *in vivo* studies described neurotoxic effects induced by competitive and noncompetitive NMDA receptor antagonists, a dose-dependent morphologic alteration in particular regional neurons characterized by multiple cytoplasmic vacuoles and that appears to be reversible (105). Although there are no clinical reports of neurotoxicity associated with prolonged use of AMT or memantine, exposure of cultured neurons to high concentrations of adamantanamines has produced irreversible toxic changes.

Amantadine: Clinical Applications

AMT is one of those drugs that have never found a secure home in neuropsychiatry. It is not very popular for PD or neuroleptic-induced extrapyramidal disorders, yet articles describing its potential utility for a number of different conditions continue to appear.

Patients with PD with symptoms of rigidity and akinesia are the ones most likely to respond to AMT (84). The drug has stimulating properties, and patients with PD report that they feel more lively and alert on the drug (116). The use of AMT in PD is limited, however, by its failure to work well for many patients and for a decline in clinical efficacy after a few months of treatment in the rest (116).

In the treatment of neuroleptic-induced extrapyramidal disorders, AMT is most effective for pseudoparkinsonism, bradykinesia, abulia, rigidity, and akinesia. It is relatively less effective for dystonia and akathisia (117–120). Its use as a neuroleptic companion is compromised by the occasional occurrence of behavioral toxicity, such as irritability, agitation, and exacerbation of psychosis. It may also be used to treat patients with neuroleptic malignant syndrome (121).

The activating properties of AMT have led to trials for patients with negative symptoms of schizophrenia (withdrawal, abulia, bradykinesia), and in this application, the drug has about as much success as the other DA agonists, that is to say, enough to write about, not enough to prescribe (122–124). AMT is occasionally effective in catatonia (125,126).

The results of clinical trials of AMT and memantine, a closely related derivative, in patients with dementia have not been encouraging (127,128). There have been occasional reports of reduced agitation and improved alertness in patients with dementia treated with AMT (129), but therapeutic effects have been compromised by the frequent occurrence of behavioral toxicity.

AMT is sometimes effective for fatigue and depression in multiple sclerosis (130,131). It does not seem to be effective for patients with Friedreich's ataxia (132) but may be effective for cases of ataxia associated with olivopontocerebellar degeneration, a syndrome that is associated with glutamate toxicity (133).

AMT may be a palliative treatment in tardive dyskinesia (134) and may facilitate detoxification in cocaine addicts (135). AMT is said to be effective for the treatment of one cerebral dysmaturation syndrome, nocturnal enuresis (136), but its effect in another, ADHD, is equivocal (137). Hardly anyone prescribes it for either.

None of these novel applications has excited a great deal of interest; positive studies tend to be small and tentative and often fail to replicate. It is only in TBI that AMT treatment seems to hold much promise.

Toxicity

AMT is a safe drug at least; at one time, it was administered to large numbers of elderly in nursing homes and children in orphanages as an influenza preventive (138,139). Behavioral toxicity has been the most important side effect, including insomnia, vivid dreams, anorexia, hallucinations, irritability, nervousness, agitation, disorganization, psychosis, hyperactivity, aggression, delirium, and depression. The symptoms remit when the dose is lowered or when the drug is discontinued.

Two peculiar side effects of AMT are livedo reticularis, a reticulated reddening of the distal extremities, and ankle edema. Livedo reticularis occurs in approximately 30% of patients with PD treated with AMT, but it is not nearly as frequent in patients with TBI or mental retardation, who tend to be much younger anyway. It has no pathologic significance except for the occasional occurrence of local irritation (140).

Schwab et al. (83,116) described seizures as a high-dose side effect of AMT, and I have observed the same association in clinical experience with patients with TBI. Conversely, DA agonists are usually associated with a higher seizure threshold, and there is one influential report that has claimed benefit for AMT in the treatment of refractory epilepsy in childhood (115).

Abrupt discontinuation of AMT in patients on neuroleptics may precipitate severe toxicity including neuroleptic malignant syndrome (141) and neuroleptic-induced catatonia (142).

AMT overdose is associated with cardiac arrhythmia (143). The interaction with phenelzine may cause severe hypertension (144).

Amantadine in Traumatic Brain Injury

My colleagues and I (145) started to use AMT in patients with brain injury in 1986 and reported our first successes a couple of years later. The reasoning behind it was (i) in TBI, one prefers to use agonist drugs rather than antagonists (such as the neuroleptics) because patients with TBI have reduced levels of the neurogoverning neurotransmitters DA, NE, and 5-HT; (ii) DA agonists such as the psychostimulants, L-dopa, and BCT work for some but not all patients with TBI; (iii) not all DA agonists are the same, therefore, it is worthwhile to experiment with other available drugs.

Our thinking was influenced by the belief that AMT was in fact a DA agonist. We were also influenced by the distinction between presynaptic agonists such as MPH and L-dopa and postsynaptic agonists such as BCT and lergotrile that had been drawn by Ross and Stewart (146) in their discussion of the treatment of a 36-year-old man with akinetic mutism from an anterior hypothalamic tumor. The patient responded to direct (postsynaptic) but not indirect (presynaptic) agonist drugs. For an indirect DA agonist to work, an intact presynaptic neuron is required. A patient with a brainstem lesion is only likely to respond to a direct DA agonist because the presynaptic neuron is damaged and resistant to the stimulation of an indirect agonist. The lesson drawn was terrifically appealing to my colleagues and me: pathologic anatomy could guide neuropharmacologic treatment and pathologic differences among patients could determine the selection of different neurochemical strategies.

It was an artful formulation with heuristic value and pertinence to clinical experience. The indirect agonist psychostimulants worked for relatively intact patients who had not had severe TBI or brainstem injuries. For patients with severe brain injuries, the direct agonists such as BCT were used to promote coma recovery. AMT, a drug that was presumably somewhere in between but closer to the latter, was used for patients who were recovering from coma. Further experience and new reports in the clinical literature supported the clinical observation, but the theoretical underpinnings were not quite as straightforward.

We originally reported a reduction of agitation and assaultive behavior with AMT treatment in two patients with frontotemporal lesions after closed head injury (145). They were young men whose difficulties arose during the transitional stage of coma recovery (Rancho Los Amigo stage IV). Severe aggression and agitation continued despite treatment with all the usual alternatives; AMT was tried in virtual desperation, and the response was swift and dramatic.

We followed this initial report with a clinical series of 30 patients with TBI in a rehabilitation hospital (Rebound in Nashville) (3). There were two types of patients: patients who were agitated during the course of coma recovery, like the two men described, and long-term patients with TBI who had had severe injuries, had recovered, but had persistent problems with abulia, anergia, negativism, disinhibition, oppositional behavior, and low arousal. The effects were similar in the two groups: more than half responded favorably, and only a few patients developed side effects such as irritability, insomnia, agitation, psychosis, edema, and seizures. The positive effects of AMT were sustained over months (and years) of follow-up.

For most patients with TBI, the symptoms of agitation during coma recovery are mild and transitory and may be dealt with behaviorally. For others, however, the symptoms can be severe: violence, wandering, negativism, severe agitation, screaming, sleep disturbance, and self-injurious behavior. In some unfortunate patients, these problems can persist for weeks or months. In such cases, psychotropic drugs are usually prescribed. However, no drug (e.g., carbamazepine, lithium, amitriptyline, propanolol) has achieved the success rate described for AMT—a success rate of more than 50%. Furthermore, treatment could continue for months, if necessary, without serious side effects (3). Other drugs are sometimes used, such as the neuroleptics and benzodiazepines, but their success was almost always short-lived, and they do little to enhance the trajectory of cortical recovery.

There are several possible treatment approaches to the long-term deficit symptoms of severe TBI (e.g., low arousal, negativism, disinhibition). Most, however, are in the ranks of the DA agonists: the stimulants and L-dopa most notably. They are good alternatives, but AMT is usually better. Its effects here reflect its utility in PD for symptoms of akinesia, abulia, rigidity, and low arousal. In some cases, combined treatments can be applied. Combinations such as AMT and MPH or AMT and L-dopa may be augmented further, either with nonspecific proarousal agents such as vitamin B_{12}, thyrotropin-releasing hormone, folate, or vitamin B_6 or with specific treatments such as serotonergics for emotionalism.

One advantage of AMT for patients with TBI, in contrast to the conventional psychotropic drugs, is that it is an easy drug to try. The dose range is narrow (100 to 400 mg per day), the onset of therapeutic action is relatively quick (4 days at each dose increment), the side-effect profile is favorable, monitoring is simple, and there are not a lot of troublesome drug interactions to worry about. AMT is not a sedating drug, and if behavioral toxicity develops, it is readily reversible when the drug is withdrawn.

There have been several subsequent reports from other centers that affirm our initial observations (147–153).

The successful treatment of posttraumatic syndromes with AMT is consistent with the theory that subcortical dopaminergic neurotransmission is severely impaired and that stimulation of striatal and cortical DA neurons will improve arousal and cognitive processing and thus reduce the occurrence of severe target behaviors such as agitation and assaultiveness. It is not clear, however, that AMT is doing this as a conventional DA agonist for the reasons listed above. Rather, it would seem that AMT is behaving as an NMDA antagonist. Its effects on DA transmission are neither direct nor indirect, in typical neuropharmacologic parlance, but rather oblique. As described above, an NMDA antagonist may stimulate dopaminergic neurons, may augment the actions of a DA agonist, or may mitigate the glutamatergic overactivity that attends a DA deficiency state. With AMT, one is modulating the effects of dopaminergic dysfunction and probably the effects of dysfunction in the other governing neurotransmitter systems as well.

Amantadine in Mentally Retarded Patients

It is one of the ironies of developmental medicine that the most severely hyperactive children respond poorly to psychostimulant drugs. Children, adolescents, and adults with ADHD respond well to stimulants such as MPH or AMP, but mentally retarded patients and patients with autisms who are hyperactive and disorganized respond poorly if at all. As in TBI, a stimulant may work extremely well for a few days, but then the effect is lost, or the patient becomes toxic, or both.

Having established a degree of success with AMT in some very difficult patients with TBI, my colleagues and I were encouraged to investigate its utility for two groups of developmentally handicapped patients: one group with symptoms of abulia, bradykinesia, and withdrawal and the other, a group whose behavioral difficulties we described as hyperactive-disorganized with symptoms of hyperactivity, impulsiveness, short attention span, aggression, screaming, agitation, noncompliance, destructiveness, emotional lability, and tantrums. The results of our initial clinical series with 28 patients were as gratifying as the experience with patients with TBI. Ten of the 28 patients responded very favorably to AMT, with a significant reduction in maladaptive behaviors and a clear improvement in functional parameters such as attention and communication; 11 more had positive but partial effects from the drug, and seven of the 28 failed to respond at all. The effects of AMT were apparent within days, toxicity was low, and the effects of treatment were sustained over months of follow-up (154). In a second series, we extended these findings to a small group of hyperactive retarded children with fragile X syndrome and observed that AMT could be successfully combined with stimulants when the benefits of each medication, individually administered, were only partial or short lived (155). These clinical observations have also been affirmed by clinicians around the country, although further publications and controlled trials have been slow to appear (156,157).

The therapeutic profile of AMT has thus expanded considerably with the inclusion of four patient groups who had not been previously considered: victims of head injury with symptoms of agitation and abulia and mentally handicapped individuals with analogous symptom pictures.

Some of the practical advantages of AMT treatment were mentioned previously, but it is appropriate to list a few more at this point. First, it is a digital, not an analogue drug; it either works or it does not, and when it does work, the effects are usually dramatic. It is not simply a mild tranquilizer that "takes the edge off" a troublesome behavior pattern. If the patient is not substantially improved, there is no reason to continue with the drug. Thus, there should be no difficulty in detecting the positive effects of treatment.

Second, therapeutic effects come quickly, within a matter of days, and dose increments, from 50 mg twice daily to a maximum of 400 mg daily, can be made at 4-day intervals. Thus, it should not take long before the effects are apparent.

Third, toxicity is overt, not covert, as it is for drugs such as the neuroleptics and phenytoin. The major side effects are behavioral toxicity and seizures. They are reversible when the drug is discontinued, and the drug may be discontinued abruptly if necessary.

Fourth, the drug is not sedating. It does not confer behavioral improvement at the expense of cognitive impairment. In fact, patients appear to be more alert and attentive in therapies of various types. Improvement is noted, not only in terms of symptom reduction but also in the improvement of adaptive behaviors, attention, and communication.

There is an occasional falloff in the AMT effect after a few months. In such cases, the original therapeutic effect may be recovered if the patient is given a brief respite from the drug.

There is a symmetry to these clinical explorations in patients with TBI and the developmentally handicapped. Children with ADHD who are well endowed intellectually respond well to stimulants; as one descends the ladder, however, the response lessens. Mildly retarded children respond less well to stimulants, moderately retarded children respond only on rare occasions, and severely retarded children do not respond at all. The degree of encephalopathic insult, then, measured in terms of intellectual capacity, predicts the success of treatment with psychostimulants. Yet, it is among the moderate and severely retarded that we find the greatest degree of AMT response. In TBI, stimulants are most useful for persistent symptoms of postconcussion syndrome or for patients with moderate to severe TBI who have made strong recoveries, whereas AMT is useful for similar symptoms in patients at a lower level of recovery.

The idea that indirect agonists require an intact presynaptic neuron is, in my opinion, still compelling. The idea that direct DA agonists such as BCT are the preferred treatment for patients with brainstem injuries is supported by an extensive literature. Where AMT fits in this paradigm is not somewhere in between but off to the side. As an antagonist of the NMDA-receptor channel, it seems to compensate for deficiencies in DA neurotransmission.

THE DOPAMINE AGONISTS

It was once suggested that L-dopa, AMT, piribedil, BCT, apomorphine, MPH, pemoline, and AMP represented a spectrum of drugs that act on the DA system but with different weightings of direct and indirect dopaminergic activity (158). The different clinical effects of DA agonists were therefore explained on the basis of differential actions on specific classes of DA receptors, e.g., excitatory and inhibitory receptors, pre- and postsynaptic receptors, D_1 and D_2 receptors (159).

Now we know that the clinical effects of stimulants are in large part mediated by NE and that AMT is an NMDA-receptor channel antagonist. Certainly, they also affect DA but are not DA agonists in the same sense as L-dopa, BCT, pergolide, and apomorphine. There is minimal overlap among the three classes of drugs in clinical treatment. For example, stimulants and AMT have limited utility in the treatment of PD. AMT and L-dopa have not been useful in ADHD (137,160). The antidepressant bupropion is also an effective treatment for patients with ADHD, and it was once thought to be a DA reuptake blocker (161). As will be seen, DA reuptake inhibition is not likely to explain its clinical effects.

It has been proposed that all the aforementioned drugs have therapeutic utility in the treatment of patients with TBI by virtue of their effects on DA. In studies using animal models, a number of different DA agonists (L-dopa, AMP, piribedil, apomorphine) led to a dramatic and apparently permanent abolition of the hyperreactivity or rage syndrome that results from surgical damage to the septal nuclei of the rat forebrain (162). Sensory inattention induced by DA lesions in rats is reversed by apomorphine, but the reversal is blocked by spiroperidol, a DA blocker (163). The DA agonists m-AMP and apomorphine facilitate recovery from septal and amygdaloid lesions in cats (164,165). Activation of DA appears to be important for functional sparing after cortical lesions in young rats, although NE and 5-HT activation also occurs (166). The interdependence of the biogenic amines may be more important than the action of DA alone; for example, developmental plasticity after DA lesions in neonatal rats leads to heterotypic sprouting of 5-HT fibers (167).

Several clinical reports of individual cases support the idea that DA agonists improve the state of patients with various types of brain injuries. It has been claimed that L-dopa promotes coma recovery (168). It has also been claimed that Sinemet (carbidopa) may advance the recovery process in patients with TBI who have reached a plateau in their recovery (169). Sadjapour et al. (unpublished, 1984) described the case of an 18-year-old man who had a left occipital lobectomy at age 9 because of an arteriovenous malformation. His residua included spastic right hemiparesis, bilateral spasticity, and expressive muteness. After treatment with Sinemet (25/100mg every 3 to 4 hours), the patient's motor function and expressive skills underwent a "remarkable transformation"; he was able to dress and feed himself, ambulate with assistance, and speak relatively fluently. Tremors and dysmetria were also improved. Clinical benefits were confirmed initially in a placebo comparison; they continued over 30 months of follow-up and were seen virtually every day when the patient experienced an "on-off" phenomenon.

A young woman with severe multifocal cerebral injuries, the result of TBI, and with severe dysarthria and motor impairment, experienced dramatic improvement in motor function and speech with L-dopa and BCT in succession (170).

BCT is a direct agonist at the DA receptor. Treatment with BCT has been reported to improve the level of arousal in one man with akinetic mutism (146), to alleviate symptoms of neglect in two patients with right hemisphere infarcts (171), and to improve symptoms of apathy and stereotyped behavior in a young woman with bilateral thalamic infarcts (172). BCT in doses of 25 to 70 mg daily improved the symptom of abulia in four patients, two with alcoholic encephalopathy, one with Wilson's disease, and one with a basal ganglia infarct (173).

The combination of BCT and morphine was successful in controlling diencephalic autonomic seizures in a young man with diffuse brain injuries (174). BCT also reversed the incapacitating effects of chronic portasystemic encephalopathy, a disorder that is believed to related to a defect in central DA neurotransmission (175).

Ross and Stewart (146) described a patient with akinetic mutism after surgical removal of a tumor from the anterior hypothalamus. He was apathetic, hypersomnolent, incontinent, and inattentive. Treatment with MPH and L-dopa was not successful, but lergotrile and BCT led to substantial improvement.

The preclinical literature and a few case reports once again support the utility of a class of dopaminergic drugs for neuropsychiatric patients with stroke or TBI. In this instance, however, the drugs are clearly dopaminergic, with few, if any, additional neurochemical actions, and demonstrated clinical utility in PD, a known DA-deficit condition.

SUMMARY

The clinical literature here is not notable for its methodologic sophistication or the size of its samples. The preclinical literature is scattered and obscure and never seems to venture very high up the evolutionary tree. There are no studies using monkeys, for example, let alone primates. So I am compelled to qualify my endorsements and to concede the weakness of my conclusions. They represent beliefs not conclusions, suggestions not recommendations.

Having made, therefore, an obligate apology to the purists and the therapeutic nihilists, I conclude with the following suggestions:

1. The psychostimulants, especially AMP and MPH, in low to moderate doses, are safe and effective for a variety of clinical symptoms after stroke and TBI, including (but not limited to) cognitive deficits in attention and memory, hypoarousal and somnolence, depression and disinhibition.
2. Stimulants may enhance recovery from stroke and TBI by attenuating negative processes such as diaschisis and kindling or by enhancing new learning and functional sparing. The stimulant effect may well be long-lived despite the short duration of drug action.
3. The stimulant effect on NE is probably central to both of these effects, although DA and 5-HT may also be involved.
4. Long-term treatment with stimulants is perfectly safe, but it is not always necessary. Treatment usually continues for a few weeks or a couple of years.
5. The action of stimulants overlaps with that of AMT and the DA agonists, but it is not identical. Stimulants are better for patients who have had milder injuries, or who have made good recoveries from severe injuries.
6. Stimulants may be successfully combined with AMT, DA agonists, antidepressants, and thymoleptics.
7. AMT is a unique drug, an NMDA antagonist whose actions on DA are indirect. It is an excellent drug for agitation during coma recovery and disinhibition, behavioral instability, abulia, and hypoarousal after severe TBI.

8. The DA agonists, L-dopa, BCT, pergolide, and lisuride may promote arousal and functional recovery in patients who have had severe injuries or subcortical strokes and may even facilitate recovery from akinetic mutism and coma.
9. The stimulants, AMT, and the DA agonists represent a class of drugs only if one is speaking very loosely, but no other class of drugs has ever been as successful for the clinical conditions that were addressed here. As we understand more about how these drugs work and how they influence the recovery process, the class will grow, new agents will be added, and our patients will get better.

REFERENCES

1. Bradley C. The behavior of children receiving Benzedrine. *Am J Psychiatry* 1937;94:587–590.
2. Evans RW, Gualtieri CT, Patterson DR. Treatment of chronic closed head injury with psychostimulant drugs: a controlled case study and an appropriate evaluation procedure. *J Nerv Ment Dis* 1987;175:106–110.
3. Gualtieri CT, Chandler M, Coons T, et al. Amantadine: a new clinical profile for traumatic brain injury. *Clin Neuropharmacol* 1989;12:258–270.
4. Orlosky MJ. The Kleine-Levin syndrome: a review. *Psychosomatics* 1982;23:609–621.
5. Evans RW, Amara I, Gualtieri CT. Methylphenidate and memory: dissociated effects in hyperactive children. *Psychopharmacolgy* 1986;90:211–216.
6. Evans KR, Eikelboom R. Feeding induced by ventricular bromocriptine and amphetamine: a possible excitatory role for dopamine in eating behavior. *Behav Neurosci* 1987;101:591–593.
7. Soetens E, D'Hooge R, Hueting JE. Amphetamine enhances human-memory consolidation. *Neurosci Lett* 1993;161:9–12.
8. Flood JF, Rosenzweig MR, Jarvik ME. Memory: modification of anisomycin-induced amnesia by stimulants and depressants. *Science* 1978;199:324–326.
9. Glasky AJ, Simon LN. Magnesium pemoline: enhancement of brain RNA polymerases. *Science* 1966; 151:702–703.
10. Haycock JW, Van Buskirk R, Gold PE. Effects on retention of posttraining amphetamine injections in mice: interaction with pretraining experience. *Psychopharmacology* 1977;54:21–24.
11. Nguyen PV, Abel T, Kandel ER. Requirement of a critical period of transcription for induction of a late phase of LTP. *Science* 1994;265:1104–1106.
12. Wetzel CD, Squire LR, Janowsky DS. Methylphenidate impairs learning and memory in normal adults. *Behav Neural Biol* 1981;31:413–424.
13. Sprague R, Sleator E. Methylphenidate in hyperkinetic children: differences in dose effects on learning and social behavior. *Science* 1977;198:1274–1276.
14. Golinko BE, Rennick PM, Lewis RF. Predicting stimulant effectiveness in hyperactive children with a repeatable neuropsychological battery. *Prog Neuropsychopharmacol* 1981;5:65–68.
15. Gualtieri CT, Hicks RE, Levitt J, et al. Methylphenidate & exercise: additive effects on motor performance, variable effects on the neuroendocrine response. *Neuropsychobiology* 1986;15:84–88.
16. Novack TA, Dillon MC, Jackson WT. Neurochemical mechanisms in brain injury and treatment: a review. *J Clin Exp Neuropsychol* 1996;18:685–706.
17. Gualtieri CT, Evans RW. Stimulant treatment for the neurobehavioral sequelae of traumatic brain injury. *Brain Inj* 1988;2:273–290.
18. Baker EL, Letz R, Fidler AT. A computer-administered neurobehavioral evaluation system for occupational and environmental epidemiology. *J Occup Med* 1985; 27:206–212.
19. Gualtieri CT, Hicks RE. Stimulants and neuroleptics in hyperactive children. *J Am Acad Child Adolesc Psychiatry* 1985;24:363–364.
20. Lou HC. Cerebral glucose metabolism in hyperactivity. *N Engl J Med* 1991;324:1216.
21. Gualtieri CT. The neuropharmacology of inadvertent drug effects in patients with traumatic brain injuries. *J Head Trauma Rehabil* 1990;5:32–40.
22. Kuczenski R. Biochemical actions of amphetamines and other stimulants. In: Creese I, ed. *Stimulants: neurochemical, behavioral & clinical perspectives*. New York: Raven Press, 1983:31–62.
23. Tessel RE. Noradrenergic processes in the behavioral actions of psychomotor stimulants. *Drug Dev Res* 1990;20:359–368.
24. Stone EP. Swim-stress-induced inactivity: relation to body temperature and brain norepinephrine and effects of *d*-amphetamine. *Psychosom Med* 1970;32:51–59.
25. Segal DS, Kuczenski R, Swick D. Audiogenic stress response: behavioral characteristics and underlying monoamine mechanisms. *J Neural Transm* 1989;75: 31–50.
26. Pechnick R, Janowsky DS, Judd L. Differential effects of methylphenidate and *d*-amphetamine on stereotyped behavior in the rat. *Psychopharmacology* 1979; 65:311–315.
27. Mathieu J-F, Ferron A, Dewar KM, et al. Acute and chronic effects of methylphenidate on cortical adrenoceptors in the rat. *Eur J Pharmacol* 1989;162:173–178.
28. During MJ, Bean AJ, Roth RH. Effects of CNS stimulants on the *in vivo* release of the colocalized transmitters, dopamine and neurotensin, from rat prefrontal cortex. *Neurosci Lett* 1992;140:129–133.
29. Segal DS. Behavioral characterization of d- and l-amphetamine: neurochemical implications. *Science* 1975; 190:475–477.
30. Kuczenski R, Segal DS, Cho AK, et al. Hippocampus norepinephrine, caudate dopamine and serotonin, and behavioral responses to the stereoisomers of amphetamine and methamphetamine. *J Neurosci* 1995;15: 1308–1317.
31. Lokiec F, Jacquot C, Rapin JR, et al. Effects of amphetamine on brain biogenic amines in isolated and aggregated rats. *Eur J Pharmacol* 1977;44:391–395.
32. Gately PF, Segal DS, Geyer MA. Sequential changes in behavior induced by continuous infusions of amphetamine in rats. *Psychopharmacology* 1987;91: 217–220.
33. Kuczenski R, Segal DS. Differential effects of D- and L-amphetamine and methylphenidate on rat striatal dopamine biosynthesis. *Eur J Pharmacol* 1975;30: 244–251.

34. Ellison G, Eison MS, Huberman HS, et al. Long-term changes in dopaminergic innervation of caudate nucleus after continuous amphetamine administration. *Science* 1978;201:276–278.
35. Gualtieri C. Fenfluramine and autism: a careful re-appraisal is in order. *J Pediatr* 1986;108:417–419.
36. Segal D, Weinberger S, Cahill J, et al. Multiple daily amphetamine administration: behavioral and neurochemical alterations. *Science* 1980;207:905–907.
37. Klawans HLM, Margolin DI. Amphetamine-induced dopaminergic hypersensitivity in guinea pigs. *Arch Gen Psychiatry* 1975;32:725.
38. Post RM, Kopanda RT. Cocaine, kindling and reverse tolerance. *Lancet* 1975;1:409–410.
39. Kalivas PW. Interactions between dopamine and excitatory amino acids in behavioral sensitization to psychostimulant. *Drug Alcohol Depend* 1995;37:95–100.
40. Itzhak Y. Modulation of the PCP/NMDA receptor complex and sigma binding sites by psychostimulants. *Neurotoxicol Teratol* 1994;16:363–368.
41. Morgan JI, Curran T. Stimulus-transcription coupling in the nervous system: involvement of the inducible proto-oncogenes fos and jun. *Annu Rev Neurosci* 1991;14:421–451.
42. Doucet JP, Squinto SP, Bazan NG. *Fos-Jun and the primary genomic response in the nervous system*. Totowa, NJ: The Humana Press, 1990.
43. Dragunow M, Hughes P. Differential expression of immediate-early proteins in non-nerve cells after focal brain injury. *Int J Dev Neurosci* 1993;11:249–255.
44. Norman AB, Lu SY, Klug JM, et al. Sensitization of *c-fos* expression in rat striatum following multiple challenges with D-amphetamine. *Brain Res* 1993;603: 125–128.
45. Robertson GS, Fibiger HC. Neuroleptics increase *c-fos* expression in the forebrain: contrasting effects of haloperidol and clozapine. *Neuroscience* 1992;46: 315–328.
46. Morgan JI, Cohen DR, Hempstead JL, et al. Mapping patterns of *c-fos* expression in the central nervous system after seizure. *Science* 1987;237:192–197.
47. Sagar SM. The molecular biology of brain ischemia: trendy genes in sick neurons. *Ann Neurol* 1993;33: 437–438.
48. Herrera DG, Figueiredo BF, Cuello AC. Differential regulation of *c-fos* expression after cortical brain injury during development. *Dev Brain Res* 1993;76: 79–85.
49. Phillips LL, Belardo ET. Expression of *c-fos* in the hippocampus following mild and moderate fluid percussion brain injury. *J Neurotrauma* 1992;9:323–333.
50. Cenci MA, Bjorklund A. Transection of corticostriatal afferents reduces amphetamine-and apomorphine-induced striatal fos expression and turning behaviour in unilaterally 6-hydroxydopamine-lesioned rats. *Eur J Neurosci* 1993;5:1062–1070.
51. Safer DJM, Allen RPP. Absence of tolerance to the behavioral effects of methylphenidate in hyperactive and inattentive children. *J Pediatr* 1989;115:1003–1008.
52. Gualtieri CT, Wargin W, Kanoy R, et al. Clinical studies of methylphenidate serum levels in children and adults. *J Am Acad Child Psychiatry* 1982;21:19–26.
53. Feldman H, Crumrine P, Handen BL, et al. Methylphenidate in children with seizures and attention-deficit disorder. *Am J Dis Child* 1989;143:1081–1086.
54. Alldredge BK, Lowenstein DH, Simon RP. Seizures associated with recreational drug abuse. *Neurology* 1989;39:1037–1039.
55. Gualtieri CT, Evans RW. Stimulant treatment for the neurobehavioral sequelae of traumatic brain injury. *Brain Inj* 1988;2:273–290.
56. Lipper S, Tuchman MM. Treatment of chronic post-traumatic organic brain syndrome with dextroamphetamine: first reported case. *J Nerv Ment Dis* 1976;162: 366–371.
57. Mooney GF, Haas LJ. Effect of methylphenidate on brain injury-related anger. *Arch Phys Med Rehabil* 1993;74:153–160.
58. Weinberg RM, Auerbach SH, Moore S. Pharmacologic treatment of cognitive deficits: a case study. *Brain Inj* 1987;1:57–59.
59. Speech TJ, Rao SM, Osmon DC, et al. A double-blind controlled study of methylphenidate treatment in closed head injury. *Brain Inj* 1993;7:333–338.
60. Lipsey JR, Pearlson GD, Robinson RG, et al. Nortriptyline treatment of post-stroke depression: a double blind study. *Lancet* 1984;11:297–300.
61. Masand P, Murray GB, Pickett P. Psychostimulants in post-stroke depression. *J Neuropsychiatry* 1990;23.
62. Lazarus LW, Winemiller DR, Lingam VR, et al. Efficacy and side effects of methylphenidate for poststroke depression. *J Clin Psychiatry* 1992;53:447–449.
63. Johnson ML, Roberts MD, Ross AR, et al. Methylphenidate in stroke patients with depression. *Am J Phys Med Rehabil* 1992;71:239–241.
64. Lazarus LW, Moberg PJ, Langsley PR, et al. Methylphenidate and nortriptyline in the treatment of post-stroke depression: a retrospective comparison. *Arch Phys Med Rehabil* 1994;75:403–406.
65. Walker-Batson D, Unwin H, Curtis S, et al. Use of amphetamine in the treatment of aphasia. *Restor Neurol Neurosci* 1992;4:47–50.
66. Davis JN, Crisostomo EA, Duncan P, et al. Amphetamine and physical therapy facilitate recovery of function from stroke: correlative animal and human studies. In: Raichle ME, Powers WJ, eds. *Cerebrovascular diseases*. New York: Raven Press, 1987:297–305.
67. Crisostomo EA, Duncan PW, Propst M, et al. Evidence that amphetamine with physical therapy promotes recovery of motor function in stroke patients. *Ann Neurol* 1988;23:94–97.
68. Bach-y-Rita P, Bjelke B. Lasting recovery of motor function, following brain damage, with a single dose of amphetamine combined with physical therapy; changes in gene expression. *Scand J Rehabil Med* 1991;23: 219–220.
69. Hovda DA, Feeney DM. Amphetamine with experience promotes recovery of locomotor function after unilateral frontal cortex injury in the cat. *Brain Res* 1984;298:358–361.
70. Goldstein LB, Davis JN. Clonidine impairs recovery of beam walking after a sensorimotor cortex lesion in the rat. *Brain Res* 1990;508:305–309.
71. Feeney DM, Gonzalez A, Law WA. Amphetamine, haloperidol and experience interact to affect rate of recovery after motor cortex surgery. *Science* 1982;217: 855–857.
72. Feeney DM, Sutton RL. Catecholamines and recovery of function after brain damage. In: Stein DG, Sabel BA, eds. *Pharmacological approaches to the treat-*

ment of brain and spinal cord injuries. New York: Plenum, 1988:121–142.
73. Exner M, Clark D. Subtle variations in living conditions influence behavioral response to d-amphetamine. *Neuroreport* 1993;4:1059–1062.
74. McGilchrist I, Goldstein LH, Jadresic D, et al. Thalamofrontal psychosis. *Br J Psychiatry* 1993;163:113–115.
75. von Monakow C. Diaschisis: localization in the cerebrum and functional impairment by cortical loci (1914). In: Pribram KH, ed. *Brain and behavior, volume I*. Baltimore: Penguin, 1969:27–36.
76. Feeney DM, Baron JC. Diaschisis. *Stroke* 1986;17: 817–830.
77. Dail WG, Feeney DM, Murray HM, et al. Responses to cortical injury: II. Widespread depression of the activity of an enzyme in cortex remote from the focal injury. *Brain Res* 1981;211:79–89.
78. Feeney DM, Sutton RL, Boyeson MG, et al. The locus coeruleus and cerebral metabolism: Recovery of function after cortical injury. *Physiol Psychol* 1985;13: 197–203.
79. Brinton RE. Neuromodulation: associative & nonlinear adaptation. *Brain Res Bull* 1990;24:651–658.
80. Sutor B, Hablitz JJ. Long-term potentiation in frontal cortex: role of NMDA-modulated polysynaptic excitatory pathways. *Neurosci Lett* 1989;97:111–117.
81. Lynch G, Baudry M. The biochemistry of memory: a new and specific hypothesis. *Science* 1984;224: 1057–1063.
82. Herrman EC, Grabliks J, Engle C, et al. Antiviral activity of l-adamantanamine (amantadine). *Proc Soc Exp Biol Med* 1960;103:625.
83. Schwab RS, England AC, Poskanzer DC, et al. Amantadine in the treatment of Parkinson's disease. *JAMA* 1969;208:1168–1170.
84. Harvey NS. Psychiatric disorders in Parkinsonism: 2. Organic cerebral states and drug reactions. *Psychosomatics* 1986;27:177–184.
85. Van Putten T, Gelenberg AJ, Lavori PW, et al. Anticholinergic effects on memory: benztropine vs. amantadine. *Psychopharmacol Bull* 1987;23:26–29.
86. McEvoy JP, McCue M, Spring B, et al. The effects of amantadine vs. trihexyphenidyl on memory in elderly normal volunteers. *Psychopharmacol Bull* 1987;23: 30–32.
87. Gianutsos G, Stewart C, Dunn JP. Pharmacological changes in dopaminergic systems induced by long-term administration of amantadine. *Eur J Pharmacol* 1985;110:357–361.
88. Allen R. Role of amantadine in the management of neuroleptic-induced extrapyramidal syndromes: overview and pharmacology. *Clin Neuropharmacol* 1983; 6:S64–S73.
89. Siever LJ. The effect of amantadine on prolactin levels and galactorrhea on neuroleptic-treated patients. *J Clin Psychopharmacol* 1981;1:2–7.
90. Starr MS, Starr BS. Locomotor effects of amantadine in the mouse are not those of a typical glutamate antagonist. *J Neural Transm* 1995;9:31–43.
91. Cotman CW, Bridges RJ, Taube JS, et al. The role of the NMDA receptor in central nervous system plasticity and pathology. *J NIH Res* 1989;1:65–74.
92. Manev H, Costa E, Wroblewski JT, et al. Abusive stimulation of excitatory amino acid receptors: a strategy to limit neurotoxicity. *FASEB J* 1990;4:2789–2797.
93. Daw NW, Stein PSG, Fox K. The role of NMDA receptors in information processing. *Annu Rev Neurosci* 1993;16:207–222.
94. Smirnova T, Stinnakre J, Mallet J. Characterization of a presynaptic glutamate receptor. *Science* 1993;262: 430–432.
95. Freed WJ, Cannon -Spoor HE. A possible role of AA2 excitatory amino acid receptors in the expression of stimulant drug effects. *Psychopharmacology* 1990; 101:456–464.
96. Watanabe Y, Saito H, Abe K. Tricyclic antidepressants block NMDA receptor-mediated synaptic responses and induction of long-term potentiation in rat hippocampal slices. *Neuropharmacology* 1993;32:179–486.
97. Montague PR, Gancayco CD, Winn MJ, et al. Role of NO production in NMDA receptor-mediated neurotransmitter release in cerebral cortex. *Science* 1994; 263:973–977.
98. Rahman S, Neuman RS. Activation of 5-HT2 receptors facilitates depolarization of neocortical neurons by N-methyl-D-aspartate. *Eur J Pharmacol* 1993;231: 347–354.
99. Bergeron R, Debonnel G, De Montigny C. Modification of the *N*-methyl-D-aspartate response by antidepressants or receptor ligands. *Eur J Pharmacol* 1993; 240:319–323.
100. Iorio KR, Tabakoff B, Hoffman PL. Glutamate-induced neurotoxicity is increased in cerebellar granule cells exposed chronically to ethanol. *Eur J Pharmacol* 1993;248:209–212.
101. Chapman AG, Durmuller N, Lees GJ, et al. Excitotoxicity of NMDA and kainic acid is modulated by nigrostriatal dopaminergic fibres. *Neurosci Lett* 1989; 107:256–260.
102. Olney JW. Excitatory transmitter neurotoxicity. *Neurobiol Aging* 1994;15:259–260.
103. Kornhuber J, Bormann J, Retz W, et al. Memantine displaces MK-801 at therapeutic concentrations in postmortem human frontal cortex. *Eur J Pharmacol* 1989; 166:589–590.
104. Ransom BR, Waxman SG, Davis PK. Anoxic injury of CNS white matter: protective effect of ketamine. *Neurology* 1990;40:1399–1403.
105. Kornhuber J, Weller M, Schoppmeyer K, et al. Amantadine and memantine are NMDA receptor antagonists with neuroprotective properties. *J Neural Transm* 1994; 43:91–104.
106. Faden AI, Demeduik P, Panter SS, et al. The role of excitatory amino acids and NMDA receptors in traumatic brain injury. *Science* 1989;244:798–800.
107. Baker AJ, Moulton R, MacMillian V, et al. Excitatory amino acids in cerebrospinal fluid following traumatic brain injury in humans. *J Neurosurg* 1993;79:369–372.
108. Witkin JM. Blockade of the locomotor stimulant effects of cocaine and methamphetamine by glutamate antagonists. *Life Sci* 1993;53:405–410.
109. Ohmori T, Koyama T, Muraki A, et al. Competitive and non-competitive *N*-methyl-D-aspartate antagonists protect dopaminergic and serotonergic neurotoxicity produced by methamphetamine in various brain regions. *J Neural Transm* 1993;92:97–106.
110. Sonsalla PK. The role of *N*-methyl-aspartate receptors in dopaminergic neuropathology produced by the amphetamines. *Drug Alcohol Depend* 1995;37:101–105.
111. Marshall JF, O'Dell SJ, Weihmuller FB. Dopamine-

glutamate interactions in methamphetamine-induced neurotoxicity. *J Neural Transm* 1993;91:241–254.

112. Stasheff SF, Anderson WW, Clark S, et al. NMDA antagonists differentiate epileptogenesis from seizure expression in an in vitro model. *Science* 1989;245: 648–651.
113. McDonald JW, Garofalo EA, Hood T. Altered excitatory and inhibitory amino acid receptor binding in hippocampus of patients with temporal lobe epilepsy. *Ann Neurol* 1991;29:529–541.
114. Loscher W, Honack D. High doses of memantine induced seizures in kindled but not in non-kindled rats. *Arch Pharmacol* 1990;341:476–481.
115. Shields WD, Lake JL, Chugani HT. Amantadine in the treatment of refractory epilepsy: an open trial in ten patients. *Neurology* 1985;35:579–581.
116. Schwab RS, Poskanzer DC, England AC, et al. Amantadine in Parkinson's disease. Review of more than two years experience. *JAMA* 1972;222:792–795.
117. Kelley JT, Abuzzahab FS. The antiparkinson properties of amantadine in drug-induced parkinsonism. *J Clin Pharmacol* 1971;11:211–214.
118. Ananth J, Sangani J, Noonan JPA. Amantadine therapy for drug induced extrapyramidal signs and depression. *Psychiatry J Univ Ottawa* 1977;1:27–33.
119. Gelenberg AJ, Mandel MR. Catatonic reactions to high-potency neuroleptic drugs. *Arch Gen Psychiatry* 1977;34:947–950.
120. Borison RL. Amantadine in the management of extrapyramidal side effects. *Clin Neuropharmacol* 1983; 6:557–563.
121. Lazarus A. Treating neuroleptic malignant syndrome. *Am J Psychiatry* 1984;141:1014–1015.
122. Angrist B, Rotrosen J, Gershon S. Differential effects of amphetamine and neuroleptics on negative vs. positive symptoms in schizophrenia. *Psychopharmacology* 1980;72:17–18.
123. Davidoff E, Reifenstein EC. Treatment of schizophrenia with sympathomimetic drugs: Benzedrine sulfate. *Psychiatr Q* 1939;127–144.
124. Kornetsky C. Hyporesponsivity of chronic schizophrenic patients to dextroamphetamine. *Arch Gen Psychiatry* 1976;33:1425–1428.
125. Baldessarini RJ. *Chemotherapy in psychiatry*. Cambridge: Harvard University Press, 1977.
126. Neppe VM. Management of catatonic stupor with L-DOPA. *Clin Neuropharmacol* 1988;11:90–91.
127. Reiser G, Binmoller FJ, Koch R. Memantine induced depolarization response in a neuronal cell line. *Brain Res* 1988;443:338–344.
128. Meldrum BS, Turski L, Schwarz M, et al. Anticonvulsant action of 1, 3-dimethyl-5-aminoadamantane. Pharmacological studies in rodents and baboon. *Naunyn Schmiedebergs Arch Pharmacol* 1986;332:93–97.
129. Muller HF, Dastoor DP, Klingner A, et al. Amantadine in senile dementia: electroencephalographic and clinical effects. *J Am Geriatr Soc* 1979;27:9–16.
130. Murray TJ. Amantadine therapy for fatigue in multiple sclerosis. *Can J Neurol Sci* 1985;12:251–254.
131. Cohen RA, Fisher M. Amantadine treatment of fatigue associated with multiple sclerosis. *Arch Neurol* 1989; 46:676–680.
132. Filla A, DeMichele G, Orefice G. A double-blind cross-over trial of amantadine hydrochloride in Friederich's ataxia. *Can J Neurol* Sci 1993;20:52–55.
133. Botez MI, Young SN, Botez T, et al. Treatment of heredo-degenerative ataxias with amantadine hydrochloride. *Can J Neurol Sci* 1991;18:307–311.
134. Allen R. Palliative treatment of tardive dyskinesia with a combination of amantadine-neuroleptic administration. *Biol Psychiatry* 1982;17:719–727.
135. Alterman AI, Droba M, Antelo RE. Amantadine may facilitate detoxification of cocaine addicts. *Drug Alcohol Depend* 1992;31:19–29.
136. Ambrosini PJ, Fried J. Preliminary report: amantadine hydrochloride in childhood enuresis. *Clin Psychopharmacol* 1984;4:223–235.
137. Mattes J. A pilot trial of amantadine in hyperactive children. *Psychol Bull* 1980;16:67.
138. MMWR. Antiviral agents for influenza A. *JAMA* 1987; 258:599–600.
139. Atkinson WL, Arden NH, Patriarca PA, et al. Amantadine prophylaxis during an institutional outbreak of type A (H1N1) influenza. *Arch Intern Med* 1986;146: 1751–1756.
140. Paulson GW, Brandt JT. Amantadine, livedo reticularis, and antiphospholipid antibodies. *Clin Neuropharmacol* 1995;18:466–467.
141. Hamburg P, Weilburg JB, Cassem NH, et al. Relapse of neuroleptic malignant syndrome with early discontinuation of amantadine therapy. *Compr Psychiatry* 1986; 27:272–275.
142. Brown CS, Wittkowsky AK, Bryant SG. Neuroleptic-induced catatonia after abrupt withdrawal of amantadine during neuroleptic therapy. *Pharmacotherapy* 1986;6:193–195.
143. Sartori M, Pratt CM, Young JB. Torsade de pointe malignant cardiac arrhythmia induced by amantadine poisoning. *Am J Med* 1984;77:388–391.
144. Jack RA, Daniel DG. Possible interaction between phenelzine and amantadine. *Arch Gen Psychiatry* 1984;41:726.
145. Chandler MC, Barnhill JB, Gualtieri CT. Amantadine for the agitated head-injury patient. *Brain Inj* 1988;2: 309–311.
146. Ross ED, Stewart RM. Akinetic mutism from hypothalamic damage: successful treatment with dopamine agonists. *Neurology* 1981;31:1435–1439.
147. Horiguchi J, Inami Y, Shoda T. Effects of long-term amantadine treatment on clinical symptoms and EEG of a patient in a vegetative state. *Clin Neuropharmacol* 1990;13:84–88.
148. Andersson S, Berstad J, Finset A, et al. Amantadine in cognitive failure in patients with traumatic brain injuries. *Tidsskr Nor Laegeforen* 1992;112:2070–2072.
149. Nickels JL, Schneider WN, Dombovy ML, et al. Clinical use of amantadine in brain injury rehabilitation. *Brain Inj* 1994;8:709–718.
150. Van Reekum R, Bayley M, Garner S. N of 1 study: amantadine for the amotivational syndrome in a patient with traumatic brain injury. *Brain Inj* 1995;9: 49–53.
151. Marin RS, Fogel BS, Hawkins J, et al. Apathy: a treatable syndrome. *J Neuropsychiatry Clin Neurosci* 1995; 7:23–30.
152. Kraus M, Maki P. Effect of amantadine hydrochloride on symptoms of frontal lobe dysfunction in brain injury: case studies and review. *J Neuropsychiatry Clin Neurosci* 1997;9:222–230.
153. Schneider W, Drew-Cates J, Wong T, et al. Cognitive

and behavioral efficacy of amantadine in acute traumatic brain injury: an initial double-blind placebo-controlled study. *Brain Inj* 1999;13:863–872.

154. Chandler M, Barnhill LJ, Gualtieri CT. Amantadine: profile of use in the developmentally disabled. In: Ratey JJ, ed. *Mental retardation: developing pharmacotherapies*. Washington, DC: American Psychiatric Press, 1991:139–162.
155. Gualtieri CT. Pharmacological interventions for cognitive and behavioral impairments. In: Finlayson MAJ, Garner S, eds. *Brain injury rehabilitation: clinical considerations*. Baltimore: Williams & Wilkins, 1993: 264–278.
156. King B, Wright D, Snape M, et al. Case series: amantadine open-label treatment of impulsive and aggressive behavior in hospitalized children with developmental disabilities. *J Am Acad Child Psychiatry* 2001; 40:654–657.
157. King B, Wright D, Handen B, et al. Double-blind, placebo-controlled study of amantadine hydrochloride in the treatment of children with autistic disorder. *J Am Acad Child Psychiatry* 2001;40:658–665.
158. Schneiden H, Cox B. A comparison between amantadine and bromocriptine using the stereotyped behavior response test (SBR) in the rat. *Eur J Pharmacol* 1976; 39:133–141.
159. Gianutsos G, Moore KE. Differential behavioral and biochemical effects of four dopaminergic agonists. *Psychopharmacology* 1980;68:139–146.
160. Langer DH, Rapoport JL, Brown GL, et al. Behavioral effects of carbidopa-levodopa in hyperactive boys. *J Am Acad Child Psychiatry* 1982;21:10–18.
161. Clay TH, Gualtieri TC, Gullion C. Clinical and neuropsychological effects of the novel antidepressant, bupropion. *Psychopharmacol Bull* 1988;24:143–148.
162. Marotta RF, Potegal M, Glusman M, et al. Dopamine agonists induce recovery from surgically-induced septal rage. *Nature* 1977;269:513–515.
163. Marshall JF, Gotthelf T. Sensory inattention in rats with 6-hydroxydropamine-induced degeneration of ascending dopaminergic neurons: apomorphine-induced reversal of deficits. *Exp Neurol* 1979;65:398–411.
164. Maeda H, Maki S. Dopaminergic facilitation of recovery from amygdaloid lesions which affect hypothalamic defensive attack in cats. *Brain Res* 1986;363:135–140.
165. Maeda H, Maki S. Dopamine agonists produce functional recovery from septal lesions which affect hypothalamic defensive attack in cats. *Brain Res* 1987;407: 381–385.
166. de Brabander JM, van Eden CG, de Bruin JPC, et al. Monoamine concentrations in rat prefrontal cortex and other mesolimbocortical structures in response to partial neonatal lesions of the medial prefrontal cortex. *Brain Res* 1993;601:20–27.
167. Takeuchi Y, Sawada T, Jenner P. Plasticity in dopamine-depleted neonates. *Brain Dysfunct* 1991;4:93–103.
168. Bareggi SR, Porta M, Selenati A, et al. Homovanillic acid and 5-hyydroxyindole-acetic acid in the CSF of patients after a severe head injury. I. Lumbar CSF concentration in chronic brain post-traumatic syndromes. *Eur Neurol* 1975;13:528–544.
169. Lal S, Merbtiz CP, Grip JC. Modification of function in head-injured patients with Sinemet. *Brain Inj* 1988; 2:225–233.
170. Liebson E, Walsh MJ Jankowiak J, et al. Pharmacotherapy for posttraumatic dysarthria. *Neuropsychiatry Neuropsychol Behav Neurol* 1994;7:122–124.
171. Fleet WS, Valenstein E, Watson RT, et al. Dopamine agonist therapy for neglect in humans. *Neurology* 1987; 37:1765–1770.
172. Catsman-Berrevoets CE, van Harskamp F. Compulsive pre-sleep behavior and apathy due to bilateral thalamic stroke: response to bromocriptine. *Neurology* 1988;38: 647–649.
173. Barrett K. Treating organic abulia with bromocriptine and lisuride: four case studies. *J Neurol Neurosurg Psychiatry* 1991;54:718–721.
174. Bullard DE. Diencephalic seizures: responsiveness to bromocriptine and morphine. *Ann Neurol* 1987;21: 609–611.
175. Morgan MY, Jakobovits A, Elithorn A, et al. Successful use of bromocriptine in the treatment of a patient with chronic portasystemic encephalopathy. *N Engl J Med* 1977;296:793–794.

19

Antidepressants

SUMMARY

The modern antidepressants are broad-spectrum psychotropic drugs. They are effective for the wide range of depression and anxiety disorders, even in patients with neuropsychiatric disorders. They are also effective for chronic pain, headache, aggression, self-injurious behavior, and other conditions that are well beyond even an expanded concept of depression or anxiety. In fact, their wide range of clinical efficacy reflects the diverse activity of the noradrenergic and serotonergic systems they affect.

Antidepressant drugs are a good example of how drugs affect, not psychiatric disorders, but rather the complex functional systems that underlie the disorders. Affective regulation, appetite, pain regulation, cognition, and circadian and seasonal rhythms are complex systems that are amenable to the influence of antidepressant drugs. I argue that antidepressants do not exercise categorical effects on depression and anxiety but rather dimensional effects. They restore the equilibrium of complex functional systems by altering the activity of the governing neurotransmitters.

Antidepressants are the most widely prescribed psychotropic drugs worldwide. They are prescribed for schoolchildren and patients with cognitive impairment. They are prescribed for high-functioning adults who make their living by their wits and sometimes for comparatively trivial indications. It is not reassuring, then, that the long-term cognitive effects of antidepressants have not been addressed more systematically. It is troubling to learn that long-term treatment, even with the new and improved antidepressants, can cause memory impairment, anergia, and an amotivational state. The difficulty of studying the neuropsychological effects of drugs such as the antidepressants is addressed. The important issue of an antidepressant effect on brain plasticity is also considered.

The individual antidepressants are also discussed. The relative merits of the new antidepressants have been the subject of furious competition among the manufacturers, I try to give the issue disinterested treatment. The selective serotonin reuptake inhibitors (SSRIs) are sometimes associated with drug interactions, which may or may not be clinically important. The SSRIs also have a peculiar pattern of side effects.

To round out the discussion, the tricyclic antidepressants and the monoamine oxidase inhibitors (MAOIs) are discussed. Their usefulness in modern neuropsychiatry is limited, and for good reason. The monoamine oxidase B inhibitor deprenyl (Selegiline), however, is known to be protective in Parkinson's disease (PD). It is the only drug ever seriously advanced as something that can increase the life span.

THEORY OF ANTIDEPRESSANTS

Depression is a disease, a psychiatric disorder characterized by particular signs and symptoms, with identifiable subtypes and a more or less predictable course. The cause is related to genetic proclivity and environmental stressors. The pathogenesis is related to abnormalities in the governing neurotransmitters, particularly the monoamines. It is effectively treated by drugs that influence the metabolism of serotonin (5-HT) and norepinephrine (NE).

This explanation is an oversimplification, but it captures the essence of conventional thinking and has guided the development of a large, diverse, and productive family of antidepressants. The antidepressant drugs are heterogeneous, to be sure—different in structure, pharmacologic activity, and historical background, but they are all effective, more or less equally effective, for the different kinds of depression and all act on the metabolism of NE, 5-HT, or both.

The discovery that effective treatments for psychiatric disorders such as depression and schizophrenia had in common a rather specific neuropharmacologic effect led psychiatrists to hope that they might reconstruct the pathogenesis of the disorders in terms of those effects, "reverse engineering," if you will, applied to biologic systems—thus, the "dopamine (DA) theory" of schizophrenia and the "catecholamine theory" of depression.

Neuropharmacologic theories of depression originally focused on the catecholamines, especially NE. From the beginning, the tricyclic antidepressants (TCAs), especially the secondary TCAs, were known to be inhibitors of NE reuptake. It was appreciated that noradrenergic transmission participated in arousal, stress modulation, and emotional response. Catecholamine depletion by drugs such as reserpine induced a state of psychomotor retardation that was not unlike depression. Thus, it was suggested that some, if not all, depressive states were caused by a functional deficiency of NE in the central nervous system (CNS) (1,2).

It was also appreciated, however, that the TCAs inhibited reuptake of 5-HT and NE. Therefore, there were interesting discussions about the relative attributes of NE and 5-HT depressions (1). The consensus, however, was that it was better to affect both NE and 5-HT metabolism; the nonselectivity of the TCAs and the MAOIs represented a therapeutic advantage. Drugs that selectively influenced only one neurotransmitter system were thought to be less efficacious.

As years passed, more evidence accrued for a serotonergic role in the pathogenesis and treatment of depression. Finally, antidepressants appeared that were specific to serotonergic neurotransmission. As the reader knows, they met with no small degree of success. Clearly, 5-HT was relevant both to depression and antidepression. 5-HT systems participate in functions that are disturbed in depression, such as sleep, appetite, pain tolerance, sexuality, and aggression. Indeed, virtually every effective antidepressant has some effect on enhancing serotonergic neurotransmission. (The exception, of course, is tianeptine, a perfectly good French antidepressant that is one more Gallic contrary. It is an enhancer of 5-HT uptake that decreases brain extracellular 5-HT (3–6). How that one works in depression, and it does as well as imipramine (IMI), I leave to others to explain. It is not available in the United States.)

This discussion is deliberately oversimplified. It makes no allusion to theories of depression that incorporate the neurotransmitters DA and acetylcholine, the various humors and neuropeptides, or the fact that depression treatment sometimes requires somatic therapies that are not overtly noradrenergic or serotonergic. It says nothing about the functional significance of receptor subtypes or the actions of antidepressants and mood stabilizers on second messenger systems and gene expression. It is presented in this manner mainly to set the historical and conceptual context. The point is that conceptualizing depression and antidepression within a narrow framework has been a productive way to deal with a complex problem. Psychiatrists have always understood that depression is not a discrete disorder and that antidepressant treatment is not specific. However, it has been useful, heuristic, as they say, to act as if they were.

When one addresses the use of antidepressant drugs in neuropsychiatry, however, it is necessary to go beyond depression and antidepression within a narrow framework. The antidepressants are so widely used in neuropsychiatry for so many indications and in so many different ways that one should think of them as broad-spectrum psychotropic drugs. With that in mind, it is better to conceptualize their effects, not in terms of nosologic specificity, but in terms of specific biologic functions.

To explain, the psychobiologic processes that are influenced by serotonergic neurons are not specific to depression, anxiety, or any particular psychiatric disorder, nor are the psychobiologic processes that are influenced by the neurotransmitter NE specific to any particular psychiatric disorder. Dysfunction of 5-HT systems has been implicated in disorders as diverse as obsessive-compulsive disorder (OCD), eating disorders, seasonal affective disorder, alcoholism, chronic pain, schizophrenia, headache, autism, and Tourette's syndrome. Dysfunction of NE systems has been implicated in attention deficit/hyperactivity disorder (ADHD), posttraumatic stress disorder, anxiety, PD, and Alzheimer's disease. This extraordinary degree of syndromal overlap is reflective of the wide range of clinical utility of the antidepressant drugs (7).

To explain further, preclinical studies that define a drug's pharmacologic activity tend to emphasize isolated aspects of neurotransmitter function. That is what *in vitro* experiments are set up to do. That kind of circumscribed view of what a drug does to a particular receptor, transporter, or enzyme, however, is not necessarily reflective of what the drug does in the intact organism. *In vivo*, the activity of 5-HT, for example, cannot be readily separated from that of other neurotransmitters such as NE, DA, γ-aminobutyric acid, and the excitatory amino acids. *In vivo*, cerebral functions are the result of the convergent actions of many different neurotransmitters. For example, excitability in the human cortex is regulated by acetylcholine, γ-aminobutyric acid, NE, histamine, purines, and 5-HT. Each of these neurotransmitters may produce more than one postsynaptic signal in the same neuron, and more than one neurotransmitter may induce the same change in postsynaptic neurons. This kind of overlap is not necessarily redundant. Rather, it provides a mechanism for the fine tuning of complex adaptations to multiple kinds of input. The interactions among various 5-HT subsystems and between 5-HT and other neurotransmitters make it possible for 5-HT to contribute to the regulation of many core functions that are disrupted in depression, including mood, anxiety, arousal, vigilance, irritability, cognition, circadian, and seasonal rhythms (8).

Antidepressants work by enhancing the metabolism of 5-HT and/or NE. They also exercise downstream effects on other neurotransmitters, neuropeptides, second messengers, genes, and the dynamics of receptor molecules. In so doing, they have wide-ranging effects. They change the behavior of neuronal systems and thus the behavior of core functions that govern the expression of mood and the experience of anxiety. They also influence arousal, vigilance, irritability, cognition, and circadian and seasonal rhythms. One should say, then, that their effects are exercised not against depression *per se*, but against the core functions that go awry in depression. In other psychiatric conditions, the same core functions go awry, and the antidepressants work as well there, too.

When we say that the antidepressants are broad-spectrum psychotropic drugs, we mean this: whether their pharmacology is specific, whether they are serotonergic, noradrenergic, or both, they are effective for a wide range of clinical conditions that may or may not be related to depression or anxiety (Table 19.1). Indeed, the extraordinary diversity of their clinical actions makes it impossible to argue that antidepressants possess nosologic specificity, just as the wide-spread impact of their neurochemical effects makes it impossible to argue that they are neuropharmacologically specific.

TABLE 19.1. *Wide range of antidepressant action*

Related conditions	Unrelated conditions
Major depression	Attention deficit/ hyperactivity disorder
Chronic dysthymia	Autism
Explosive disorder	Chronic pain
Bipolar II disorder	Headache
Generalized anxiety disorder	Tourette's syndrome
Panic disorder	Smoking cessation
Social anxiety disorder	Paraphilias
Posttraumatic stress disorder	Self-injurious behavior
Premenstrual syndrome	Aggression
Obsessive-compulsive disorder	Organic hyperphagia
	Oppositional-defiant disorder
	Emotional incontinence

Depression and antidepression, therefore, are only special cases in the broad spectrum of activity that is inherent in this class of drugs. Their general effect seems to be to restore equilibrium to the disordered brain by manipulating the activity of the governing neurotransmitters. Their specific effects are felt, not against psychiatric disorders, but against core functions that are dysfunctional in the various neuropsychiatric disorders.

This point will be less obscure if we consider examples of the antidepressant effect in neuropsychiatry as it is directed against specific core functions.

The best example of a pure mood disorder is emotional incontinence, the pathologic laughing or (more commonly) crying that occurs in patients with brain injuries, stroke, or dementia. Pathologic crying is especially disturbing to patients because it arises in response to the most trivial event, watching a television commercial, for example, and sometimes it is entirely unprovoked. "Incontinence" is a good word for it. Patients are as embarrassed as they would be if they had wet their pants. It is utterly disconnected from the patient's underlying affective state, i.e., it does not occur because the patients are depressed down deep inside. It is not a motor program divorced from feeling, like the pathologic laughter or crying that occurs in pseudobulbar palsy or Angelman syndrome. The patient with poststroke emotionalism feels genuinely sad during his or her outburst, if but for a moment.

Emotional incontinence is effectively treated by antidepressants but only by serotonergic antidepressants such as amitriptyline (AMI), fluoxetine (FXT), or trazodone (TRZ). Noradrenergic antidepressants and psychostimulants have no effect on emotionalism.

The antidepressant effect on mood in cases of emotional incontinence represents a pure and specific effect. The dysphoric mood that overtakes a patient with stroke or traumatic brain injury (TBI) with pathologic crying is dissociated from any clinical element that is normally associated with depression: environmental stressors or precipitants, a genetic proclivity to depression, a cognitive set that is negative or pessimistic, or allied symptoms such as low energy, circadian dysregulation, vegetative changes. Antidepressants are highly effective for the condition, but only the serotonergic antidepressants.

Anxiety is commonly encountered in neuropsychiatric patients. In patients with stroke, TBI, or Alzheimer's disease, virtually all the anxiety disorders may co-occur, but generalized anxiety and obsessive rumination are most common. In my opinion, however, the best example of anxiety in a neuropsychiatric population is the case of autism. In addition to generalized anxiety and obsessive rumination, people with autism have anxiety attacks, episodes of disorganizing agitation, and agoraphobia. They try to "bind" anxiety by repetitive behaviors, rituals, compulsions, preoccupation with sameness, repetitive speech, perseveration, and stereotypies.

Anxiety symptoms in people with autism and in others with neuropsychiatric disorders are often effectively treated with serotonergic antidepressants. In contrast, noradrenergic antidepressants and stimulants tend to make anxiety symptoms much worse.

Repetitive behaviors include stereotypies, tics and mannerisms, compulsions, and perseveration. They occur most frequently in people with severe developmental disabilities, autism, and Tourette's syndrome. Repetitive behaviors often seem to be a means to control anxiety in the face of what is perceived as a threatening environment. Yet they frequently occur in patients who do not seem to be experiencing anxiety and in environments that are safe, predictable, and not excessively stimulating.

In mentally retarded people, aggression and self-injurious behavior sometimes occur as stereotyped, unemotional events. They are sometimes said to be compulsive in nature, but they are not like the compulsions of patients with OCD, behavioral events that are intended to control or mitigate anxiety.

Repetitive behaviors in neuropsychiatric patients respond reasonably well to serotonergic antidepressants whether they are associated with anxiety or not. Adrenergic drugs tend to make them worse.

Another core function that is part of depression and effectively treated with antidepressant drugs is pain. Patients with anguished depression describe their experience as painful or excruciating, a condition that an observer can readily appreciate. Depression aggravates the painful response to physical conditions, and chronic physical pain almost always leads to depression.

The pattern already remarked on holds true in this instance as well. Antidepressants are effective treatments for some kinds of pain, even when it is not associated with depression or anxiety. Serotonergic antidepressants are frequently used for the treatment of headache, peripheral neuropathy, and central pain syndromes such as thalamic dysesthesia. Doses well below the usual antidepressant dose are often sufficient. The pattern of use overlaps with the antiepileptic drugs, which are also used for headache and chronic pain. Noradrenergic antidepressants are not useful for pain treatment as a rule.

In all these examples, emotional incontinence, anxiety, pain, and repetitive behaviors, the success of serotonergic antidepressants does not require an underlying depression or anxiety disorder. The drug is operating on core functions, all of which may be dysfunctional in cases of depression or anxiety, but at a level that is more fundamental than the psychiatric disorders themselves. The same pattern is true for core functions that respond to noradrenergic antidepressants.

Cognitive symptoms are, of course, characteristic of depression and anxiety disorders. These may be cognitive impairments such as inattention, cloudy thinking, or poor memory or cognitive sets that are pathologic. The pessimism and hopelessness of a severely depressed individual are an example of a pathologic cognitive set.

Negativism is a pathologic cognitive set that is occasionally encountered in patients with frontal lobe lesions, especially of the convexity. A patient is said to be negativistic if he or she greets the normal activities and intrusions of day-to-day life with reluctance, pessimism, hostility, or an attitude of opposition. Conceptually, it is a state of inertia. It arises because the normal executive functions of the frontal lobes—initiative, motivation, and flexibility—are impaired. It is difficult to treat pharmacologically because there is not drug that can restore a patient's executive capacity. When one can alleviate the problem with a drug, for example, in a patient with TBI, it tends to be a noradrenergic antidepressant, a psychostimulant, or a DA agonist.

Anergia, fatigue, and impersistence are also states of inertia that may be seen in patients with frontal lobe lesions or subcortical pathology. Motor slowing, sluggish response to stimuli or rewards, and prolonged information processing are related problems. The core functions that underlie these symptoms are related to the executive functions of the frontal lobes or to a generalized arousal system. Dopaminergic and noradrenergic neurons modulate arousal and activation at the subcortical level and in the frontal lobes. Dopaminergic drugs and noradrenergic antidepressants are sometimes effective for such problems, whatever the causative pathology. Serotonergic drugs, in contrast, sometimes aggravate the symptoms. Fatigue, anergia, and insouciance are SSRI side effects.

Anhedonia is a cardinal symptom of depression. Abulia is the neuropsychiatric equivalent. Abulia is another frontal lobe syndrome that is treated with dopaminergic or adrenergic but not serotonergic drugs.

The sleep-wake cycle, the secretion of endocrine hormones, and levels of mood, activity, and cognitive performance are all governed by circadian rhythms that are driven by a central pacemaker located in the suprachiasmatic nuclei of the anterior hypothalamus and influenced by events in the external environment. Circadian dysrhythmia is a major component of the mood disorders. Disruption of the sleep-wake cycle is a cardinal symptom of the depression, and sleep deprivation, of all things, has a potent antidepressant effect. Some forms of bipolar disorder demonstrate diurnal cycling, and there is seasonal affective disorder, which is dependent on ambient light exposure. There are even theories of mood disorders that posit a primary causative role to circadian rhythm disturbance. Antidepressants have a variable effect on the circadian clock, although improvement in the sleep-wake cycle is essential to the antidepressant response. Desipramine (DMI) and moclobemide (a reversible MAOI) regularize the circadian clock in animal paradigms (9).

Circadian dysrhythmia is also characteristic of neuropsychiatric patients in general. Perhaps the most cogent examples are children with autism or severe mental retardation in which sleep disorders are common, to say the least, and often associated with severe diurnal behavior problems (Chapter 12). It is possible to argue that a mentally retarded person with irregular sleep and self-injurious behavior has a "depressive equivalent." One would have heard that argument rather frequently years ago, but a better way to understand the problem is to suggest that such a person has a circadian dysrhythmia, i.e., that that is the genesis of his or her self-injurious behavior and that if he or she were not retarded and the primary problem were allowed to develop in a brain of regular capacity, the result would be a mood disorder.

In all these examples, the success of noradrenergic and dopaminergic drugs does not require an underlying depression or anxiety disorder. The drugs operate on core functions, all of which are seen in cases of depression or anxiety, but at a level that is more fundamental than a fully differentiated psychiatric disorder.

Antidepressants are not nosologically specific but are broad-spectrum psychotropic drugs. Antidepression and anxiolysis are their overt clinical effects. Enhancement of NE and 5-HT neurotransmission is their overt neurochemical effects. Interposed between the initiating neurochemical events and the clinical outcome, however, is a cascade of secondary events, effects on second messengers, gene transcription, protein synthesis, and receptor dynamics. The behavior of neural systems is amended, and core functions are thus improved. Only then are the clinical effects manifest.

COGNITIVE EFFECTS

What we know as cognition is something that is itself comprised of core functions. Intelligence is a feature of cognition that is comprised of working memory and attention, coordination of goal-directed cognitive processes, and inhibition of goal-irrelevant processes. Information-processing speed is a feature of neural networks that contributes to (or subtracts from) intelligence. Two other features are efficiency and reliability.

Attention and memory, for example, may be core functions that comprise intelligence, but they too may be broken down into constituent functions that are more basic to cognition. Attention, for example, is a multifaceted function. Attention may refer to scanning attention, sustained attention (concentration), vigilance, freedom from distractibility, and the ability to shift attentional sets flexibly and appropriately. It is a function of the arousal system in the brainstem and an executive system that resides in the frontal cortex. On a neurochemical level, it responds to the activity of neurons that secrete NE and DA.

Every cognitive function can thus be deconstructed to more fundamental cognitive elements, neurophysiologic elements, and cellular and molecular events. The further down the chain one moves, the functional systems prove to be less differentiated. That means they are less specifically connected to the cognitive function that was originally at issue and more generally associated with a number of different cognitive functions. Arousal and processing speed, for example, underlie virtually every aspect of cognitive performance. Psychomotor speed is essential to good performance on virtually every neuropsychological test. The efficiency with which neural nets are mobilized to address a cognitive task will determine performance, whatever the task and cognitive function.

Depression is associated with cognitive dysfunction at virtually every level of analysis. The conscious thinking of a depressed person is dominated by morbid or pessimistic content—a negative cognitive set. Depression in elderly people strips the intellect itself—the condition known as pseudodementia. Depression is associated with deficits in attention, memory, and psychomotor speed. The simplest cognitive tasks are difficult to do, and the patient fatigues easily. The arousal system is either hyperactive or underactive. Effective antidepressant treatment alleviates cognitive dysfunction at every level.

After this discussion, the cognitive effects of antidepressants in terms of the various constituents of cognitive performance are examined. For example, antidepressants sometimes cause memory dysfunction. When that happens, it may be because they alter the subject's motivation to do well on a neurologic test, because the subject is less attentive, or because psychomotor speed is reduced. A drug can interfere with the encoding of short-term memory in the hippocampus, especially if it is an anticholinergic drug, or it may interfere with long-term potentiation and the laying down of long-term memory traces. A drug that reduces arousal or processing speed can compromise the subject's performance on memory tests.

It has not been possible to dissect the cognitive effects of antidepressants with any such degree of precision, and there are several reasons for this. First, the cognitive effects of antidepressants, for better or worse, are not especially robust. Their cognitive effects vary with the drug in question and the dose, and they interact with patient-related variables such as age, premorbid cognitive status, and pathologic condition.

When antidepressants have positive effects on cognitive performance, it is most often an indirect effect limited to the reversal of the primary condition. When a patient with depression (or anxiety) is treated with an effective antidepressant, performance on neuropsychological measures improves, but only as the primary condition is brought under control. The antidepressant drug effect on cognition is indirect. It is similar to the effect of an antipyretic or hypoglycemic drug. Patients with fever and patients with poorly controlled diabetes do poorly on cognitive tests. When fever is controlled or when blood sugar returns to normal levels, cognitive performance improves. Aspirin and sulfonylureas are not cognitive enhancers.

Antidepressants are not cognitive enhancers either. They improve cognitive performance, but only if cognitive performance is impaired by virtue of depression or anxiety. In normal people, and patients with primary cognitive disorders, they have no such effect. In most circumstances, they are cognitively neutral, and in some circumstances they impair cognition.

Compare the antidepressants as a class with the psychostimulants. Stimulants improve attention, memory, reaction time, information-processing speed, fine and gross motor coordination, endurance, and energy. They have a robust effect that is demonstrable in cognitively impaired patients and in normal people. The antidepressants have no such effect. At best, they exercise no effect at all on any of these functions, and sometimes they exercise a negative effect.

In some clinical circumstances, the therapeutic effects of stimulants and antidepressants overlap. In these conditions, however, careful analysis indicates a clear divergence in the nature of their clinical effects.

One example is ADHD. It is usually treated with psychostimulants, but the following antidepressants are also effective: DMI, bupropion (BP), venlafaxine (VFX), and atomoxetine. They all are noradrenergic antidepressants. A careful examination of the relative benefits of stimulants and antidepressants in ADHD indicates that their benefits are divergent. The stimulants are much better for symptoms of inattention, distractibility, disorganization, lack of focus, and procrastination. The antidepressants are better for temperamental and impulsive behavior problems that are also symptoms of the condition. That is why stimulants continue to be the mainstay of ADHD treatment despite their myriad problems and side effects. That is why university students with ADHD almost invariably prefer a stimulant to an antidepressant. The latter simply do not have the same beneficial effect on concentration.

Another example is postconcussion syndrome. Antidepressants are frequently prescribed for postconcussion symptoms such as irritability, depression, headache, and insomnia. For these symptoms, serotonergic antidepressants tend to work very well, but they do not work well for postconcussion symptoms such as fatigue, inattention, and memory impairment. For these problems, stimulants are effective and antidepressants are not.

Considering their diverse neurochemical effects, different antidepressants should have markedly different effects on cognition. For example, antidepressants whose actions are primarily noradrenergic tend to be memory neutral, but the serotonergics (and lithium) tend to cause mild memory impairment as a side effect. Antidepressants with strong anticholinergic properties, especially the TCAs, are notorious for causing memory impairment, especially in elderly patients. TCAs such AMI and doxepin (DOX) are especially problematic in patients with TBI.

The relative anticholinergic potencies of commercially available TCAs are (in descending order): AMI → DOX → protriptyline → IMI → nortriptyline → DMI (10).

This list is important for physicians who treat neuropsychiatric patients because anticholinergic drugs have negative effects on memory and motor performance (11). Thus, nortriptyline and DMI are better choices for the patient with TBI than more anticholinergic TCAs such as AMI, DOX, or IMI. On theoretical grounds, one is led to prefer secondary amines because they are less anticholinergic. In individual cases, however, such theoretical differences are less salient; there may be clinical success with a tertiary amine TCA, and behavioral improvement may occur without overt evidence of cognitive/motor compromise (12,13).

One would expect, if anything, that antidepressants with potent noradrenergic effects should be cognitive enhancers. NE neurotransmission is an essential component of the arousal system and has a facilitatory role in long-term potentiation. BP, in particular, has small but positive neurocognitive effects, but DMI and VFX do not (14).

5-HT systems participate in cognitive activity by modulating information processing, sensory processing, and motor output. The popularity of the SSRIs, in fact, has been at least partially attributable to the fact that they are less likely to cause cognitive blunting than the TCAs, which they have largely supplanted. Nevertheless, memory impairment has always been recognized as a side effect of SSRI treatment.

Is this a serious problem? It is probably not in the short term. Conversely, patients who take SSRIs or other antidepressants for several years and who are doing well in terms of their primary condition sometimes report mild cognitive impairments in memory and the ability to concentrate or reduced initiative, energy, and motivation. It is possible that tolerance to the antidepressant or anxiolytic effect is responsible for the problem but not likely. The effect is reported by sophisticated patients who know their primary condition well and who appreciate that the new problem is different from the depression that they encountered before. Furthermore, when the antidepressant is discontinued, cognitive impairment improves, and they feel sharper and more energetic (at least until their original problem with depression or anxiety returns). It is not obvious that any one of the various new antidepressants is more or less likely than another to cause this problem.

Theoretically, at least, in the neuropsychological laboratory, acute treatment with SSRIs has negative effects of attention and memory. In one study, the relative neurotoxicity of antidepressants was expressed in terms of rank order with respect to a series of cognitive tasks including critical flicker fusion, choice reaction time, tracking error, and sedation (the lower the rank order, the less behavioral toxicity) (15).

The information presented in Table 19.2 is interesting but should not be taken as canonical. It is an example of the kind of work that ought to be done on this important class of psychotropic drugs but only rarely has been. Our information base on the neurocognitive effects of antidepressant drugs is no less than woeful, a sorry state of affairs to be sure. After all, the drugs are prescribed for schoolchildren, the elderly, and patients with cognitive impairment, not to mention professional people who make their living by their wits.

The cognitive toxicity of antidepressants is not usually a problem in clinical practice because the therapeutic benefits usually overshadow the theoretical risk of impairment. Short-term memory and attention problems can be dealt with by choosing an alternative antidepressant. Cognitive problems associated with long-term treatment appear to be reversible, at least on the basis of our studies to date. There is no reason to believe that we are presiding over a tragedy such as tardive dyskinesia. Nevertheless, annual evaluation of the cognitive status of patients on long-term antidepressant treatment, perhaps with one of the computerized batteries mentioned, is probably not a bad idea.

TABLE 19.2. *Relative neurotoxicity of antidepressants*

Antidepressant	Relative neurotoxicity
Trazodone	10.8
Fluoxetine	8.6
Fluvoxamine	7.6
Desipramine	7.0
Paroxetine	5.6
Bupropion	5.4
Sertraline	4.0

EFFECTS ON BRAIN PLASTICITY

If the effects of antidepressants on cognition are ambiguous, their effects on brain plasticity have been utterly obscure. That antidepressants influence neural events that contribute to the plasticity of brain has recently attained a degree of prominence in the research literature and for good reason.

- New theories of depression have proposed pathophysiologic mechanisms involving the regulation of synaptic connectivity and neuronal atrophy in response to chronic stress (16,17). Loss of cell volume in some brain structures is demonstrated in imaging studies of patients with chronic depression (18).
- Complementary theories of antidepression propose that antidepressant treatment can block or reverse stress-induced atrophy of hippocampal neurons, increasing cell survival and function (19).
- The action of antidepressant drugs, such as FXT, affects intracellular transduction pathways and neurotrophic factors, thus changing the electrophysiologic and morphologic properties of neurons (20). They also modulate glutamate neurotoxicity (21).
- Lithium has been found to increase neuroneogenesis in the hippocampus of adult rodents and the new cells are neurons, progenitor cells, and glia. (22). It has been reported that gray matter volume increased in patients with bipolar affective disorder who had been treated with lithium for 4 weeks (23).
- Neuroprotective actions against apoptosis and glutamate excitotoxicity have been attributed to lithium and valproate (24,25). In rats, lithium pretreatment reduces neurologic deficits caused by ischemia (26).
- Electrically induced seizures, similar to those used in the treatment of severe depression, stimulate the expression of neurotrophic factors and sprouting of hippocampal neurons in laboratory animals (27).
- In preclinical studies of TBI, enhancing the activity of various neurotransmitters, such as DA and NE, promotes recovery of function. Perturbations of NE activity are a central event in the development of diaschisis and can be blocked or reversed by noradrenergic drugs such as amphetamine or DMI. Clinical studies on TBI and stroke recovery are supportive (28–31).

It is intuitive that drugs with long-standing effects on mood and behavior might do so by altering the structure and function of neural elements. That antidepressants change the structure of the monoamine synapse has been appreciated for a long time (32). To amplify that knowledge and understand its mechanism and implications have taken many years.

The basis of the catecholamine theory of depression was the observation that NE depletion was associated with a state of depression and lethargy. Antidepressants were effective because they increased synaptic monoamine concentrations, thus, a self-contained unit. From the very beginning, however, it was clear that the activity of antidepressants was not simply a function of NE and 5-HT reuptake blockade. Psychostimulants also increase synaptic concentration of monoamines but are not very good antidepressants. They reverse the state of lethargy, anergia, and lassitude associated with brain injury, stroke, and neurodegenerative disease but do not control depression.

Another problem with the theory was that antidepressant drugs increase synaptic monoamines after a single dose, but the therapeutic effect in depression is not manifest, as a rule, until the patient has been treated for at least 2 or 3 weeks. Clearly, something else is going on between the initial monoaminergic stimulus and the therapeutic response.

The initial stimulus of an antidepressant drug is exercised at NE and 5-HT receptors, all of which happen to be G protein–linked receptors. That means they transduce neurotransmitter signals to the cell interior by activating G proteins. G proteins can alter membrane excitability by changing K^+ and Ca^{2+} ion channels and can also generate second messengers within the neuron. Among these second messengers are protein kinases—enzymes that produce protein phosphorylation. Phosphorylation alters the sensitivity of receptors, the responsiveness of ion channels, and the activity of enzymes that synthesize neurotransmitters. Protein kinases can also enter the cell nucleus where they phosphorylate nuclear proteins (transcription factors) and regulate gene expression.

One presumes that somewhere in the cascade of cell membrane effects, intracellular changes, and gene regulation, events transpire that are somehow meaningful to the resolution of depression or, to be more precise, to altering the core functions that have gone awry in the clinical condition known as depression. Exactly what those events are, however, we do not know. The essential point is, however, that antidepression is ultimately a function of neuronal adaptation— plasticity, if you will.

Therefore, antidepressants change the function of neural systems by changing their structure. The next question is whether this kind of plasticity effect is relevant to the clinical circumstances of neuropsychiatric patients. All the antidepressants and mood stabilizers have at least some measure of structural or ultrastructural impact. What does that mean in terms of their effect on recovery from brain injury? What does it mean with respect to antidepressant treatment for children or people who are aging or elderly? This is not a trivial issue by any means, considering how often antidepressants are given to patients with brain injury and stroke, children, and the elderly. There are three possibilities:

- They may have a positive effect. Perhaps they actually promote recovery and development and prevent age-related deterioration. After all, it is arguable that they "optimize" the monoamine environment of the brain. It is also arguable that depression is a neurodegenerative disease.
- They may be neutral, meaning that no effect at all on brain plasticity beyond the benefit of treating the primary condition. This is what most neuropsychiatrists believe; physicians who treat cognitively impaired patients have no inhibitions against prescribing antidepressants.
- They may have a negative effect, but that is not likely. They do cause cognitive impairment in some patients. In Chapter 2, brain plasticity after perinatal brain damage was discussed. It is true that structural adjustments to neuronal injury can sometimes be counterproductive. Neuronal plasticity is not always a positive event.

It is not possible to address this question directly despite its importance because there is no base of evidence. The issue is just beginning to come into focus.

ANTIDEPRESSANT DRUGS

Antidepressant drugs may be classified in different ways. They may be defined structurally (e.g., tricyclics, tetracyclics), pharmacologically (e.g., MAOIs, SSRIs), or even historically (e.g., the new antidepressants). They have been a class for almost 50 years. They are a heterogeneous group, and their therapeutic domain is always expanding. They are the most frequently prescribed psychotropic medications; in 1997, no fewer than three of the top 10 prescription drugs in the United States were antidepressants.

There are two reasons for the extraordinary and growing popularity of this class of medication. The first is obvious: mood disorders and anxiety disorders, the usual targets of antidepressant prescription, are the most common psychiatric conditions. It is arguable that most people at some time in their lives will be afflicted with at least a mild form of depression or anxiety. Whether they chose to deal with the problem pharmacologically is a matter of personal choice, social custom, and physician preference. Increasingly, choice, custom, and clinical practice favor one or another of the new antidepressants.

The second reason is their wide range of clinical utility, as described above and as amplified in the next few sections. However one chooses to frame the argument, the popularity of antidepressants is really a phenomenon of the SSRIs.

SELECTIVE SEROTONIN REUPTAKE INHIBITORS

As evidence accrued for a serotonergic role in the pathogenesis and treatment of affective disorders, research laboratories undertook to search for more potent inhibitors of 5-HT reuptake. Fluvoxamine (FVX) was synthesized in 1973 and registered in Switzerland in 1983. FXT, a substituted propylamine, was first described in 1974 and approved by the U.S. Food and Drug Administration in 1988. Within only a few years, SSRIs became the most frequently prescribed antidepressants worldwide (33,34).

The spectrum of clinical efficacy of the SSRIs is similar to that of the TCAs. There is no evidence that they are more effective than other classes of antidepressants, but they are no less effective either. What accounts for their amazing popularity is patient acceptance. They are far more agreeable to take than the older antidepressants, largely free of troublesome side effects such as orthostatic hypotension, dry mouth, urinary retention, blurred vision, and weight gain. Nor are they associated with catastrophic side effects such as fatal overdose or hypertensive crisis. (5-HT syndrome is something to worry about with the SSRIs, but it is not a common problem, at least in severe form. Suicidality is discussed in later sections.) They are "clean" drugs, free of the antimuscarinic, antihistaminic, and anti–α-adrenergic activity that account for the many unwanted actions of the TCAs and that contribute little to their therapeutic usefulness (35).

The SSRIs are perfectly good antidepressants, although there certainly are patients with depression who are resistant to SSRIs and respond better to other antidepressants. What is impressive about the SSRIs is their broad spectrum of clinical utility: they are effective for all the anxiety disorders including panic disorder, posttraumatic stress disorder, and OCD. They are also useful for the treatment of Tourette's syndrome, obesity, paraphilia, alcoholism, posttraumatic stress disorder, and the negative symptoms of schizophrenia.

The SSRIs are commonly prescribed for an even broader range of problems associated with neuropsychiatric disorders. They are effective for virtually all the organic affective disorders, including poststroke emotionalism. Other applications include central pain syndromes, thalamic dysesthesia, and self-injurious behavior. They are effective for obsessions and compulsive behaviors in autistic and mentally retarded people and sometimes for aggression. In patients with brain injury, SSRIs are prescribed for irritability and depression in postconcussion syndrome and for emotional incontinence after severe TBI.

The Relative Merits of the Serotonergic Antidepressants

Five SSRIs are available in the United States at the time that this is written. They are, in order of introduction in the United States, FXT, sertraline (STR), paroxetine (PXT), FVX, and citalopram. They are equal as antidepressants and all seem to have the same wide spectrum of clinical efficacy and the same side effects, and none has been found to be fatal in overdose. How, then, does one decide which to prescribe?

The answer is usually the secondary issues related to side effects or pharmacokinetics. The latter issue is rule governed, the former is not. With respect to adverse effects, the response to SSRIs is almost entirely idiosyncratic. For example, a patient may be allergic to one SSRI but not to the others because the SSRIs are grouped together in terms of their neurochemical effects and not their chemical structure.

It is true that FXT has been implicated in more catastrophic reactions than the other SSRIs, ranging from suicide and death by overdose to bleeding diathesis, neuroleptic malignant syndrome, and phospholipidosis. Whether these side effects are really unique to FXT is unlikely. Their seeming association with FXT may be entirely a function of the much greater exposure that the drug has had.

Patients may experience activation on one SSRI and not another. All the drugs in this class can produce activation or sedation, and the effect might be desirable or undesirable. Patients on a SSRI usually appreciate the burst of energy they get from the drug or the mild disinhibition; they usually do not appreciate the drug-induced insomnia, hypomania, or akathisia. STR is the likeliest one to cause disinhibition, especially in children. FXT and citalopram (CTP) may be more activating than paroxetine (PXT) and FVX. All the SSRIs can cause insomnia or excessive somnolence and can all lead to vivid dreams, which may be enjoyable and cinematic or morbid, violent, and disturbing. It is likely that PXT is the most anxiolytic of all the SSRIs.

Their effects on sexuality and appetite are also variable. It is known that FXT can suppress appetite, especially in high doses. It is possible, but unproved, that PXT is the likeliest to induce hyperphagia and weight gain. All the SSRIs are less likely than the TCAs to cause weight gain. Anyone on an SSRI is capable of gaining weight, usually by eating a lot, and the comparative data are neither incriminating nor exculpatory for any individual antidepressant. CTP is said to be less likely to suppress sexual desire than the others, and FXT may be more likely to delay ejaculation, but any SSRI can cause sexual dysfunction, and, again, data do not support one over another. All of them can cause hypersexuality or priapism but never very often (36,37).

They can all cause extrapyramidal reactions, especially akathisia, but also myoclonus, tremor, and choreoathetosis. FXT may be the most likely to induce akathisia or even tardive dyskinesia–like movements (38). Increased CNS 5-HT levels may lead to an imbalance of 5-HT and DA and a relative hypodopaminergic state. This is probably the cause of extrapyramidal symptoms (EPS) caused by SSRIs. All the SSRIs have been implicated in the development of neuroleptic malignant syndrome (39,40), as have VFX, nefazodone (NFZ), and the TCAs.

They all are capable of reducing tics associated with stimulant treatment or with Tourette's syndrome, but none seems to have the advantage. They are probably equally effective for the treatment of OCD.

They all have a long half-life, although the half-life of FXT is so long it has been referred to as a "depot antidepressant." Dosing with any SSRI is seldom necessary more often than once per day. There is a FXT preparation that is dosed weekly and works well enough.

It may be that STR is the SSRI most likely to lose its effect after months of treatment. It is clear that PXT is the likeliest to induce withdrawal symptoms (especially dizziness) (41).

No one SSRI has achieved distinction over the others. They all have advantages and disadvantages and are all excellent drugs. Table 19.3 gives my preferences.

Pharmacology of the Serotonergic Antidepressants

All the new antidepressants are well absorbed with bioavailability values of 60% to 100%. Systemic availability of less than 100% suggests incomplete absorption. In fact, it reflects uptake of a drug into hepatocytes during the first pass through the liver, when a portion of the dose is transformed into metabolites.

All the new antidepressants achieve maximum concentration within 6 to 8 hours after a single oral dose. The SSRIs are absorbed more slowly than the

TABLE 19.3. *Relative merits and demerits of the SSRIs*

Fluoxetine
Pro: Extremely long half-life, high doses for compulsive hyperphagia, activating
Con: Inhibits CP2D6, CP2C9, CP34A; akathisia; some bad publicity years ago
Paroxetine
Pro: No active metabolites, the best anxiolytic SSRI
Con: Inhibits CP2D6, withdrawal syndrome, occasional hyperphagia
Sertraline
Pro: Activating
Con: Inhibits CP34A, behavioral disinhibition, tolerance may develop
Fluvoxamine
Pro: No active metabolites, good for some refractory patients
Con: Inhibits CP2D6, CP1A2, CP2C9
Citalopram
Pro: Fewer sexual side effects, little effect on cytochrome P-450 isoenzymes
Con: Perhaps less effective than the other SSRIs

SSRI, selective serotonin reuptake inhibitor.

other antidepressants, but the effect is probably not clinically significant.

The new antidepressants are all extensively metabolized, and typically only 1% to 10% of an oral dose is excreted unchanged in the urine. Only FVX and PXT are without pharmacologically active metabolites. Active metabolites of FXT and VFX contribute substantially to the therapeutic and/or adverse-effect profile. Because formed metabolites have a half-life that is equal to or greater than that of the parent compound, they contribute to the time required to achieve steady state or complete elimination. Time to steady state is usually four to five times the elimination half-life of the drug; the elimination half-life of norfluoxetine, the active metabolite of FXT, is 4 to 16 days. Thus, 16 to 80 days are required before FXT and its metabolite are completely clear (42). This may be important when treatment with a MAOI follows FXT withdrawal. This is not likely to be a common event. Most of the time, the long half-life of FXT and norfluoxetine is a distinct advantage.

The correlations found between plasma concentration of the newer antidepressants and therapeutic response or adverse effects have not supported routine plasma concentration monitoring.

Drug Interactions

The major drug toxic effect of the serotonergic antidepressants is the possibility of 5-HT syndrome, which comprises a number of symptoms including mental state changes (agitation, confusion, disorientation, drunkenness, restlessness, coma), motor system changes (myoclonus, rigidity, hyperreflexia, tremor, incoordination), and autonomic instability (fever, nausea, diaphoresis, headache, shivering, tachycardia, tachypnea, blood pressure changes, pupillary dilation). 5-HT syndrome is rarely associated with seizures, opisthotonos, oculogyric crisis, disseminated intravascular coagulation, myoglobinuria, renal failure, hyperthermia, cardiac arrhythmia, and death. The symptoms may resemble neuroleptic malignant syndrome, presumably because a sudden increase in brain 5-HT is capable of inducing an acute hypodopaminergic state (43).

5-HT syndrome usually arises within hours or days of initiating an untoward drug combination or of raising the dose of one of the offending agents. The syndrome typically develops when a serotonergic antidepressant is combined with a MAOI or if the interval between treatments is too short. It may occur when serotonergics are used in combination with L-tryptophan or hydroxytryptophan or with drugs as diverse as meperidine, carbamazepine, dextromethorphan, nortriptyline, sumatriptan, and pentazocine (43).

The SSRIs are also capable of inhibiting the hepatic metabolism of some drugs, usually by inhibiting the cytochrome P-450 isoenzyme systems in hepatic microsomes (15).

The Cytochrome P-450 System

Most drugs undergo their first metabolic steps in the liver, often involving oxidation. This is true of all the psychotropic drugs except lithium and gabapentin. Only recently, however, have we come to understand that the cytochrome P-450 isoenzyme system is responsible for the biotransformation of most drugs. The cytochrome P-450 system is a family of more than 30 proteins that catalyze the oxidative metabolism of drugs and other chemicals. Each enzyme displays a certain specificity for a biotransformation reaction, with some overlap among the substances that each can degrade. Because the antidepressants are metabolized by isoenzymes of the cytochrome P-450 system, they may participate in drug-drug interactions by competitive enzyme inhibition. Sometimes a drug can inhibit an isoform that is different from the one that is used in its own metabolism.

The cytochrome 2D6 enzyme is responsible for the biotransformation of many drugs including some of the antipsychotics, antidepressants, beta-blockers, antiarrhythmics, dextromethorphan, and carbamazepine. All the SSRIs are capable of inhibiting this enzyme. Their effect on 2D6 is expressed by the inhibition constant (normalized to the K_i of FXT) (15,44) (Table 19.4).

Inhibition of CYP2D6 can lead to an increase in plasma levels of drugs that are metabolized by this isoform such as the TCAs. As a result, the effect of combining certain SSRIs with TCAs, antipsychotics, and carbamazepine is highly variable and unpredictable for patient outcome (15,42,45).

The cytochrome 3A4 enzyme mediates demethylation of TCAs, some of the benzodiazepines, carbamazepine, and some other widely used drugs. Interactions involving 3A4 substrates and inhibitors have been life threatening. STR, FXT, and NFZ may also inhibit this enzyme, and there is one report of cardiac arrhythmia when FXT was added to terfenadine. VFX and the TCAs do not inhibit this isoform. Cotreatment of STR, FXT, or NFZ with carbamazepine may increase the concentration of the latter. NFZ increases the half-life of triazolam threefold (42). Grapefruit juice also is an inhibitor of the 3A4 enzyme.

FVX is a potent inhibitor of cytochrome 1A2, which may lead to clinically significant interactions with drugs metabolized by this system including theophylline, phenytoin, and haloperidol (42). Clozapine is metabolized by 1A2, and its plasma levels may be increased by coadministration of FVX.

Cytochrome 2C9 may be inhibited by STR and thus inhibit the metabolism of its substrates, diazepam, some of the tertiary amine TCAs, phenytoin, warfarin, and tolbutamide. FVX and FXT may also be inhibitors of this system (42).

Drug-drug interactions involving the SSRIs have been the object of heated discussion. That is not surprising because competition for market share has been so intense and there are so few meaningful differences among them. Many of the drug-drug interactions described in the literature and this chapter are theoretical or based on single case reports. It is very hard to keep up with literature in this area. Physicians have increasingly relied on computerized drug-interaction profiles to guide their prescription practice.

TABLE 19.4. *Relative affinities for CP2D6*

Fluvoxamine	8.7
Sertraline	5.7
Citalopram	5.1
Fluoxetine	1.0
Paroxetine	0.80

The Curious Side Effects of Serotonergic Drugs

The common side effects of the SSRIs are nausea, nervousness, insomnia, headache, drowsiness, hyposexuality, diaphoresis, and diarrhea (Ayd, 1988) , but it is really quite remarkable how seldom side effects occur with most of the SSRIs, especially at the ordinary therapeutic doses. Difficulties with one SSRI do not necessarily predict difficulty with another, except for patients with anxiety or panic disorder who may develop akathisia at miniscule doses of all the SSRIs. They are all free of anticholinergic side effects (except perhaps PXT) and have no cardiovascular side effects such as arrhythmia or orthostasis.

The SSRIs all have the infuriating habit of inducing side effects that are polar opposites such as somnolence and insomnia, anorexia and hyperphagia, activation and anergia, hypersexual disinhibition and decreased libido, mood stabilization and hypomania, and antidepression and suicidality. There is no class of drugs with such a pattern of side effects. It makes one feel foolish sometimes trying to explain this to patients. In fact, there is a good explanation.

Although the SSRIs are, indeed, selective for 5-HT over NE reuptake, they act nonselectively at all the multiple 5-HT receptor subtypes. That is, they enhance the availability of 5-HT throughout the CNS and cause all the 5-HT receptor subtypes to be stimulated. The perfectly idiosyncratic pattern of SSRI side effects is almost certainly a pharmacodynamic problem, the result of eccentric effects at receptor subtypes that may be more or less sensitive in a given individual. True 5-HT receptor subtype selectivity has only been achieved by another class of drugs, which is described in a later section (The Triazolopiridines) and in Chapter 22, but not by the SSRIs (33,46).

One may speculate that FXT, as a cationic amphiphilic drug, can lead to intracellular accumulation of phospholipids. This is more than a theoretical risk, but its clinical significance may not be so important. It does cause phospholipidosis in animals, however, and there are at least a couple of case reports of pulmonary phospholipidosis in humans (47).

The bleeding diathesis associated with FXT (or with all SSRIs?) manifested by bruising is a rare problem that has not been traced to any abnormality in platelet aggregation, hemostasis, or coagulation profile (48–50). It may be related to capillary fragility, and it is reversed by vitamin C.

There are no clinical laboratory tests that seem to be affected by SSRI treatment. No deaths have been reported thus far from overdose with SSRIs alone. Overdoses of FXT have resulted in death, but rarely when it was the only drug ingested (35,51). Doses of FXT in the range of 1 to 3 g have been noted to cause seizures, blurred vision, tachycardia, emesis, and ST segment depression (52).

Sudden withdrawal from a SSRI may lead to rebound headache or even migraine or severe dizziness. The physical symptoms of SSRI withdrawal may be quite severe and may require long and gradual taper. It is much more disturbing, however, to observe a dramatic increase in symptoms of anxiety or depression in a patient withdrawn from a SSRI, even in excess of what the patient experienced before treatment. Patients who have become accustomed over the years to a relatively mild dysthymia with drug treatment should be warned about the possibility of rebound depression.

Tolerance to the effects of SSRIs has not been reported in the literature but is a phenomenon that is met with quite frequently in clinical practice. It is not uncommon for an initial antidepressant or antiobsessional effect to be diminished or lost entirely after weeks or months of treatment. It is possible that STR is the worst in this regard. Adjusting the dose does not always correct the problem.

No discussion of SSRI side effects is complete without allusion to red ear syndrome, conceivably a manifestation of thalamic irritation or a migraine equivalent (53).

Fluoxetine and Suicide

The description of intense suicidal preoccupation in six patients on FXT (54) led to a furor in the medical and lay press. Although the hysteria has died down, the issue has not yet been resolved satisfactorily. Most psychiatrists have been reassured by the obligate panel of experts. Their meta-analysis of large numbers of depressives in clinical trials demonstrated no statistically significant increase in suicide in patients treated with FXT compared with other antidepressants (55). Most generalists were reassured by the availability of SSRIs that were not named Prozac.

It is well known that suicide is likely to occur in depressed people after they have begun antidepressant treatment, when they are more active and energetic but before they have fully recovered from the dangerous subjective state of depression. A severely depressed patient may simply be too depressed to take untoward action; when he or she has more energy and initiative, he or she is more dangerous. Because FXT is such a good antidepressant and is given to so many people, it is possible that the observation of compulsive suicidality is only a spurious exaggeration of something that is a calculated risk in all antidepressant treatment. It is also likely that psychiatrists select modern antidepressants, which are not fatal in overdose, for patients who are potentially suicidal.

It is also possible that the special proclivity of SSRIs to side effects such as akathisia, disinhibition, and violent dreams may make an excessive contribution to compulsive or impulsive suicidality. One should not expect short-term clinical trials to detect a relatively rare side effect that may simply contribute to the dropout statistic. Compulsive suicidality is an occasional side effect of antidepressants in general and SSRIs in particular. Is FXT more likely to elicit this side effect? We do not know. There is evidence that it may be (56) and evidence that it is not (55). It does have a rapid onset on action, strong activating properties, and a proclivity to induce the side effect of akathisia (57,58). It does appear that SSRIs are more likely to induce deliberate self-harm than the older antidepressants; of course, they are more dangerous in overdose (59).

In 2000, the U.K. Medicines Control Agency called for suicide warnings to be added to SSRI package inserts:

> Whilst the reporting rate of suicidal behavior for all SSRIs has been low in recent years, there continue to be anecdotal case reports of suicidal behavior associated with fluoxetine. Prescribers and patients should be aware that it is general clinical experience that the risk of suicide may increase in the early stages of treatment with any antidepressant. Patients thought to be at risk should be carefully monitored (Reuters, 10/18/2000).

Their Wide Range of Clinical Utility

As described in the beginning of this section, there is a host of psychiatric indications for the serotonergic antidepressants. The SSRIs are safely administered to children and elderly people for all the usual psychiatric indications.

Their range of clinical utility is no less wide in neuropsychiatry where the serotonergic drugs have achieved a degree of prominence for many conditions. In mental retardation and autism, they are used for various states characterized by emotional dysregulation, compulsive behavior, aggression, and self-injury. FXT may only have limited benefit as an appetite suppressant or weight-loss drug in the general population, but it is one of the few treatments that is ever effective for organic bulimia (or hyperphagia).

Physicians have begun to use the serotonergic drugs, especially the SSRIs, for a number of central pain syndromes including fibromyalgia and thalamic dysesthesia. FXT may prove to be the drug of choice for poststroke emotionalism and poststroke depression (60). The spectrum of activity of SSRIs for patients with TBI is equal to its use in other clinical populations, and we have no experience of special sensitivity in this population to the side effects of SSRIs (61).

THE TRIAZOLOPYRIDINES TRAZODONE AND NEFAZODONE

Trazodone

TRZ is a phenylpiperazine derivative of triazolopyridine. It was the first representative of a unique class of antidepressant drugs. It has been used in Europe since 1974 and in the United States since 1982.

TRZ is said to be a competitive inhibitor of 5-HT reuptake into the synaptosome, with little effect on the uptake of NE or DA. It is less potent than clomipramine in terms of 5-HT reuptake but more selective in terms of effect on other monoamine neurotransmitters (62). Although selective blockade of 5-HT reuptake is the most commonly discussed mechanism of action for TRZ, that may not be the pertinent drug effect. In fact, TRZ is an order of magnitude less potent than FXT, and no more potent than DMI in terms of 5-HT reuptake blockade. Certainly, the clinical effects of TRZ do not closely resemble those of the SSRIs. TRZ is less effective than the SSRIs as an antidepressant and less effective for panic but better as an anxiolytic, at least for some patients. It has different effects on sleep, body weight, sexuality, and prolactin secretion (63).

It has been shown that TRZ is much more potent in blocking 5-HT receptors than blocking 5-HT reuptake. It is 25 to 330 times more potent in blocking the 5-HT receptor, whereas the SSRIs are approximately 15 times more potent in blocking 5-HT reuptake. It has been suggested that TRZ works as an antidepressant by antagonizing the 5-HT_{1A}, 5-HT_{1C}, and 5-HT_2 receptors (63).

TRZ is an antidepressant, and the primary indication is treatment of unipolar depression. It may be good for depression with anxiety or severe insomnia. Because it is serotonergic, it is also considered an alternative treatment for neuropsychiatric disorders that are customarily treated by other serotonergic antidepressants. An example is OCD, although FXT and clomipramine are usually better choices. Some patients with OCD, however, develop akathisia on FXT and clomipramine and thus are better treated with TRZ. AMI and FXT are prescribed for patients with chronic pain and/or dysesthesia of thalamic origin; TRZ is another alternative.

One's real interest in TRZ is in the neuropsychiatry clinic. It is the drug most commonly used for patients with brain injury with agitated depression and patients with postconcussion syndrome with severe insomnia. TRZ has been effective in the treatment of sleep apnea associated with olivopontocerebellar degeneration (64). It has also been effective in two severe cases of essential tremor that failed to respond to propanolol (65). It may be used as an alternative serotonergic for autistic or mentally retarded people with dysphoria, dysregulation of mood, insomnia, aggression, and self-injurious behavior.

The singular advantage of TRZ is its relative lack of cardiovascular and anticholinergic side effects, which makes it a good choice, for example, for the depressed geriatric patient (66,67). It is, however, very sedating. This might be an advantage for patients with severe insomnia, but excessive daytime sedation is its major limitation.

Sedation is the most common psychological side effect of TRZ, but there have been reports of delirium (68) and mania (69). It may increase the libido (70). There was one report of women who took TRZ and experienced spontaneous orgasm whenever they yawned (70a).

The catastrophic side effect of TRZ is priapism. Some of the reported cases had reported abnormal or unusual erections before priapism developed; patients on TRZ should be advised to discontinue the medication if this occurs (71). It was once used for the treatment of erectile incompetence.

The most common symptoms of TRZ overdose are drowsiness, ataxia, nausea/vomiting, and dry mouth. In some cases, CNS depression may progress to coma, but this is more likely if TRZ is taken with alcohol or other CNS depressant drugs. There have been no reported cases of death from TRZ overdose (72).

TRZ has fallen from favor among psychiatrists because as an antidepressant, it is terribly idiosyncratic and sedation is often intolerable. Its use in general psychiatry is almost entirely as a sedative or an antidepressant augmenter. It remains a favorite, however, among neuropsychiatrists who treat patients with TBI, especially for insomnia.

Nefazodone

NFZ is chemically similar to TRZ, with similar effects at the 5-HT receptor but less activity as an α_1-adrenergic antagonist (hence, less priapism). It may also be less sedating than TRZ. When NFZ is given chronically, it down-regulates both β-adrenergic and $5\text{-}HT_2$ receptors; the theory is that $5\text{-}HT_2$ receptors exercise an inhibitory influence on central $5\text{-}HT_{1A}$ receptor-mediated function and that $5\text{-}HT_{1A}$ activity may be important in conferring antidepressant potential. Like TRZ, it is devoid of monoamine oxidase, anticholinergic, and antihistamine activity and has no known cardiotoxicity (73). In animal models, it has mild analgesic activity. Whether it is more effective than AMI for the treatment of various pain conditions (migraine, neuropathy, chronic pain) remains to be seen.

NFZ inhibits the cytochrome CYP3A4 isoenzyme and thus may decrease the metabolism of triazolam, alprazolam, and digoxin.

NFZ is an effective antidepressant that is well tolerated, with less sedation than TRZ and fewer sexual side effects than TRZ or the SSRIs. It is less likely to cause sexual dysfunction than even the noradrenergic antidepressants. It is an excellent antidepressant but is not as useful as TRZ for the treatment of insomnia in neuropsychiatric patients.

THE AMINOKETONE BUPROPION

BP is a unique antidepressant (a phenylaminoketone or monocyclic phenylbutylamine). It works perfectly well for depression and ADHD. How it works is, however, a bit of a mystery. The chemical structure of BP bears some resemblance to that of amphetamine and other central stimulants, and it is a good treatment for ADHD but does not have amphetamine-like abuse potential (74). At high doses, BP is apparently a DA reuptake inhibitor; for that reason, it was said to be a "dopaminergic antidepressant" (75).

BP is not a MAOI, an anticholinergic, an antihistaminic, or a blocker of the α-adrenergic receptors. It is not an inhibitor of the reuptake of 5-HT or NE (76). In doses that are clinically relevant, however, it reduces the firing rate of neurons in the locus ceruleus, probably through some sort of interaction with intracellular NE (77). It may, therefore, be considered a noradrenergic antidepressant.

BP has several advantages over the TCAs: it has no anticholinergic side effects, it does not cause tachycardia or orthostatic hypotension (78), there is no tendency to weight gain, it does not have an additive depressant effect with alcohol, and it is not lethal in circumstances of overdose (76). It does not have an adverse effect on memory or motor performance. Indeed, it may improve neuropsychological performance in some patients (79).

It also has an advantage over the SSRIs in terms of its side effects. It is not likely to affect sexuality except for the better and is not given to extrapyramidal side effects such as akathisia. It is good for ADHD, whereas the SSRIs are not. The problem is that it is not quite as good for depression, and it is hardly ever effective for anxiety or panic.

The efficacy of BP in depression is said to be equal to that of the other antidepressants, and it is, when it works, but it does not always work. There is a class of people with depression who respond extremely well to BP and they are fortunate indeed. The positive effects of the drug seem to endure, even over years of treatment, and there are few, if any, long-term side effects. There are not many such patients, however, to make BP a good first-choice drug for depression in the general population. Conversely, it is not a bad choice to add to a SSRI for antidepressant augmentation.

BP is also an effective treatment for patients with ADHD; in these patients, positive behavioral effects may be complemented by positive effects on attention, memory, and motor performance (79).

BP may be an effective prophylaxis against cyclic mood disorders (80,81). It may be particularly good for patients who are called bipolar II, which is mostly depression with occasional periods of hypomania.

The side-effect profile is quite favorable. Skin rash occurs in approximately 3% of patients. There are no associated laboratory or electroencephalographic changes (76,82). Death owing to overdose is a rare occurrence (83). The major side effects are neuropsychiatric. BP may evoke vivid dreams, increased emotionality, increased intensity of sensory experience, and alteration of time perception (84). Some of the subjective effects may be positive, such as the feeling of improved attention and memory (84), but subjective side effects that are really bothersome are nervousness, agitation, and excitement, even to the point of frank psychosis (85).

Bupropion and Seizures

BP was withheld from the market because of an apparent high frequency of generalized tonic-clonic seizures in some patient groups. This was a difficult problem to evaluate because virtually all the antidepressants have been associated with occasional seizures; the association appears to be dose related (86). The incidence can only be estimated, although 0.5% to 1.0% is the usual range given. It is not clear that any existing antidepressant is better than another for the patient who is prone to seizures, although some clinicians have recommended DOX and others,

AMI. We have already alluded to the possible antiepileptic effects of the SSRIs.

The manufacturer says that the incidence of seizures in patients treated with BP is four in 1,000, which is in the same range as all the other antidepressants, except maprotiline. At doses greater than 450 mg per day, the risk of seizures may be higher. Seizures are said to be more likely to occur with BP if the patient has a predisposing factor, for example, a history of head trauma, drug or alcohol abuse, or concomitant treatment with other drugs that lower the seizure threshold, but that is conjecture. The association between BP and seizures may simply turn out to be one of those spurious associations, such as carbamazepine and agranulocytosis that cloud the reputation of a drug for years. That is a shame because BP is in all other respects an ideal antidepressant for patients with head injury and for other neuropathic groups such as patients with dementia and PD.

It should be remembered that psychostimulants and DA agonists such as amantadine in high doses may also occasionally cause seizures. That has never prevented their prescription to patients with brain injury, mental retardation, or even epilepsy for that matter. The problem of seizures at high doses does not limit the clinical utility of a drug at moderate doses. By the same token, moderate doses of BP are usually perfectly safe.

VENLAFAXINE

During the 1970s, some people believed that the nonselectivity of the TCAs and MAOIs represented a therapeutic advantage and that drugs that selectively influenced a particular neurotransmitter system would be less efficacious. That opinion tended to diminish after the successful introduction of the SSRIs, but it has revived recently, and many clinicians believe that VFX, by virtue of its combined effect, is superior to the SSRIs. Compared with the SSRIs, VFX is more likely to induce remission from depression rather than just clinical improvement (87).

VFX is a structurally novel (bicyclic) antidepressant with potent monoamine reuptake-blocking effects. It inhibits the reuptake of 5-HT, NE, and DA, in that order. Like the SSRIs, it has no appreciable anticholinergic, antihistaminic, or MAO inhibition effects. Because its effects on 5-HT and NE are equivalent to those of IMI, without the usual TCA side effects, it should be the ideal antidepressant: a drug whose side-effect profile is as benign as that of the SSRIs but whose effectiveness for severe depression is the equal of that of the best TCAs.

VFX has not been as popular as the SSRIs, mainly because of the occurrence of severe and even debilitating nausea and/or abdominal pain when treatment is initiated. This unfortunate side effect was almost entirely a consequence of the high initial doses (e.g., 75 mg daily or twice per day) originally recommended by the manufacturer. If treatment is begun with low doses (e.g., 12.5 or 18.75 mg per day), the patient adjusts to the gastrointestinal effects of the drug, and therapeutic doses (as high as 450 mg per day) can be attained (88). More recently, the introduction of an extended-release version of the compound has lessened the problem of gastrointestinal toxicity to a considerable degree. The therapeutic utility of VFX and its popularity expanded accordingly. Dose titration is still a good idea.

Is it true that antidepressants that inhibit monoamine reuptake nonselectively, such as VFX and the TCAs, are more effective than the SSRIs for severe depression? Yes, that may true. If VFX is a more potent antidepressant, should it not be everyone's first-choice drug? Perhaps, although titration to therapeutic levels tends to counterweigh one of the essential advantages of the new antidepressants: a rapid onset of antidepressant action.

If the pharmacologic profile of VFX is similar to that of IMI, then it should prove to be useful treatment for ADHD or an alternative to psychostimulants for patients with TBI, with narcolepsy, and with post-stroke depression. In fact, it is almost as good for ADHD as BP is, although it does not rival the stimulants. In clinical practice, it is no better for patients with BI (or worse for that matter) than any other antidepressant.

Seizures or death from overdose are rare events (89,90). It is a CYP2D6 inhibitor but much less so than PXT or FXT. It does not seem to affect the other CYP450 isoforms. Sustained hypertension is an occasional, dose-related side effect.

MIRTAZAPINE

Mirtazapine is a tetracyclic antidepressant with a unique pharmacologic profile: an antagonist of the (presynaptic) α_2 adrenoreceptor, which causes an increase in NE release and, indirectly, release of 5-HT. Its clinical profile should resemble that of VFX, therefore, and the TCAs, although it is not anticholinergic at all (91). It is generally well tolerated, but it can be an extremely sedating drug. It has a low propensity to cause seizures but may cause neutropenia; how frequently, one cannot say, but blood monitoring may be necessary, at least until the issue is settled (92). It is very sedating and is used as a hypnotic sometimes.

If mirtazapine were in fact a noradrenergic antidepressant, it should have the same spectrum of utility in neuropsychiatry as BP and VFX. If that were true, one would expect it to be good for ADHD, but it does not seem to be, at least for most patients with ADHD. It is occasionally useful, however, for children and developmentally handicapped adults with hyperactivity and impulsive behavior, especially when accompanied by sleep disturbance. It causes weight gain, but even that may be an advantage in some young patients and in patients with depression who are cachectic.

THE TRICYCLIC ANTIDEPRESSANTS

The TCAs are like phenytoin: inexpensive, effective, and indispensable for some cases. Like phenytoin and the MAOIs, however, they have been superseded by a new generation of drugs. IMI is the standard by which new antidepressants are judged; AMI is the standard against which analgesic antidepressants are judged. No new antidepressant has been proven more effective than the TCAs, but they are not without fault.

The TCAs are composed of two groups: the tertiary or the dimethylated amines (IMI, AMI, DOX, clomipramine) and the secondary or monomethylated amines (DMI, nortriptyline, protriptyline). You can tell the difference by holding a tablet up to the light and counting the number of methyl groups on the side chain. This structural difference confers special pharmacologic effects. Tertiary amines, for example, are more potent blockers of NE reuptake (93). It is possible that this structural difference accounts for the relative potency of tertiary amine TCAs in agitated depressives because it confers a sedative effect.

The sedating effects of a given TCA may also be a function of its anticholinergic and antihistaminic properties. The relative antihistaminic potencies of the TCAs are (in descending order): DOX → AMI → nortriptyline → IMI → protriptyline → DMI (10).

On this count, then, DMI ought to be the first-choice drug for depressed patients with TBI when sedation is not a desired effect. In patients with TBI, it hardly ever is. Usually, however, the new antidepressants are less sedating and have less cognitive toxicity than any of the TCAs. DOX or AMI might be a good choice for the depressed patient with TBI with severe insomnia; in some instances, the importance of restful sleep may outweigh the theoretical disadvantage of negative memory and motor effects. Usually, TRZ is a better choice. One advantage of AMI is that it is said to be the TCA that is least likely to lower the seizure threshold (94), which may or may not be true. Here again, the SSRIs seem to hold an advantage.

All the TCAs are toxic in overdose situations. In an adult, as little as 800 mg IMI, for example, can be fatal; suicide is always a risk in patients with TBI, and the TCAs are the most lethal of all psychoactive drugs. At various times in the past 30 years, TCAs have been among the leading drugs to cause death by poisoning. The danger of TCA use in elderly patients, in whom orthostasis can lead to broken hips, cannot be underestimated.

The one unequivocal indication for TCAs is for refractory depression, after a trial of new antidepressants has failed, alone and in combination (e.g., a SSRI with BP) and after the usual augmentation strategies have also failed. Their efficacy for anxiety and panic disorders has not diminished over the years, and they continue to be used by patients who cannot tolerate the SSRIs or benzodiazepines. When success is achieved, then, with moderate doses of a TCA, one remembers why, at one time, these agents were so popular.

DMI continues to be used in the treatment of ADHD, although its popularity has declined since the reports of sudden cardiac death in children. The association may be spurious, but there is a lingering fear that DMI may be more cardiotoxic than the other TCAs. Very low doses of AMI are still used by neurologists and neurosurgeons for neuropathic pain, a harmless if not exactly cutting edge practice. Clomipramine remains an effective agent for patients with OCD who have failed at various combinations of serotonergic therapy with the newer agents.

In almost every domain, then, the TCAs are second- or third-choice drugs. They will never become extinct, but in psychiatry they are being prescribed less. In fact, it is likely that more TCAs are prescribed by neurologists and other physicians who treat patients with chronic pain and migraine than by psychiatrists.

It is not clear why TCAs, or antidepressants in general, are effective for chronic pain or why the doses that seem to be effective are much lower than those required to treat depression. There is also AMI, a drug that psychiatrists hardly ever prescribe any more but that widely thought to be the antidepressant of choice for pain. The SSRIs and TRZ are also used for chronic pain, but AMI is still the favorite.

AMI is as effective as the SSRIs and TRZ for the treatment of emotional incontinence after stroke and TBI or in dementia, but anticholinergic side effects limit its usefulness.

THE MONOAMINE OXIDASE INHIBITORS

The MAOI antidepressants began with iproniazid, which caused euphoria in patients with tuberculosis, an effect that was at first attributed to improvement in their disease. Kline's suggestion that iproniazid was, in fact, an antidepressant was a landmark in psychiatry; previously, the only effective antidepressant treatment had been electroconvulsant therapy (94a). Iproniazid was subsequently withdrawn because of hepatotoxicity but was succeeded by isocarboxazid and phenelzine.

During the 1960s, the "cheese reaction" became apparent. MAOIs inhibit intestinal MAO, and the consumption of tyramine-rich foods (Chianti, beer, aged cheese, broad beans) could lead to hypertensive crisis. Physicians were more inclined to prescribe TCAs, and patients were reluctant to forgo delicacies such as dried figs and broad beans. That may have represented an excess of zeal, however, because tyramine-induced hypertensive crisis is not a common sequela to MAOI treatment, and the drugs are effective antidepressants with stimulant-like effects and hardly any known negative neuropsychological effects (95). They are barely anticholinergic (96) and may be particularly useful in the atypical depressions that patients with TBI experience (97). They are especially effective for the anergic depressions that occur in patients with bipolar disorder (98). They are among the most effective treatments for panic and phobic disorders, and the combination of a MAOI and a TCA used to be prescribed for refractory depression. Conversely, Saran (99) did not have much success in depressed patients with TBI treated with the MAOI phenelzine.

The MAOI phenelzine was at one time proposed for patients with a form of atypical depression known as hysteroid dysphoria. This term referred mainly to female patients with histrionic character traits who experience depressions that are usually precipitated by rejections, especially the loss of romantic attachment, and whose depressive episodes are characterized by a tendency to oversleep or spend more time in bed, overeat, or crave sweets (especially chocolate), a sense of inertia or leaden paralysis, and a labile mood that improves temporarily when they get attention or praise (100). Many of these young women would, by today's standards, be termed adults with ADHD and would be treated with a stimulant and a SSRI. In fact, many of the original clinical indications for the MAO have been occupied by the psychostimulants or the SSRIs, just as they were a generation ago by the TCAs.

Representatives of this class of antidepressants include phenelzine (Nardil), tranylcypromine (Parnate, Eutonyl), and isocarboxazid (Marplan). All these are competitive inhibitors of MAO-A, so patients who take them are vulnerable to the "cheese effect." Deprenyl is an inhibitor of MAO-B, and moclobemide is a reversible MAOI, so patients who take them do not have to worry about the dangers of cheese, figs, or broad beans. MOAIs should not be used in combination with SSRIs, stimulants, or carbamazepine or with sympathomimetic or TCA drugs.

Deprenyl or Selegiline

The new name is selegiline, but for a long time it was called L-deprenyl and is still called that by some. It has been used in the United States, but it has been used in Europe since 1985 as an adjunct in the treatment of PD and as an antidepressant. It is a MAOI, a selective and irreversible inhibitor of MAO-B. Because this is the primary enzyme that metabolizes DA in the brain, treatment with deprenyl increases the availability of endogenous and exogenous DA, thus, its antiparkinsonian and antidepressant effects.

Because deprenyl is an inhibitor only of MAO-B, it is free of the "cheese effect," the sympathetic crisis produced by ingestion of tyramine, L-dopa, or other amines (101). That is a function of antagonism of MAO-A, which is located primarily in the periphery (i.e., outside the brain, especially in the gut) and which catabolizes 5-HT, NE, and tyramine. Because deprenyl is only an MAO-A inhibitor at high doses, the risk of hypertensive crisis is small, except perhaps in overdose situations.

Deprenyl was synthesized and developed in Hungary as a novel MAOI antidepressant. When L-dopa was introduced, people began to use deprenyl as a supplementary treatment for PD (101).

Maximum plasma levels are achieved within 30 to 120 minutes after oral administration, and a decline in platelet MAO-B activity is apparent in most subjects after 2 hours. The elimination half-life averages 39 hours, and after the drug is discontinued, MAO-B activity returns to baseline levels in 2 or 3 weeks (101). Because of the long half-life, a once-daily dose is possible, and the usual dose is 5 mg in the morning or twice daily. Inhibition of MAO-A probably does not begin until a dose of 40 mg per day has been achieved (101,102). It is not at effective antidepressant, however, until doses of 40 mg or higher per day are attained (103).

Deprenyl is metabolized to amphetamine and methamphetamine, although it is not believed that its therapeutic effects are related to the amphetamine metabolites. The toxicity profile is quite favorable, with no observed cardiovascular effects such as orthostatic hypotension. Peptic ulcer disease may be reactivated by deprenyl, and mild and usually transient elevations of hepatic enzymes have been noted.

The importance of deprenyl is more than its adjunctive behavior with L-dopa and its unique status as a safe MAOI antidepressant. There have been reports to suggest that it may prolong the life of patients with advanced PD and that it may delay the need to initiate treatment with L-dopa in patients with the beginning symptoms of PD. It may delay the death of striatal dopaminergic neurons. The experimental model was a unique experiment of nature—the development of PD in a group of heroin addicts who had been exposed to the neurotoxic contaminant. The conversion of *N*-methyl-4-phenyl-1,2,3,6-tetrahydropyridine to a neurotoxic metabolite, 1-methyl-4-phenylpridinium ion (MPP+), is blocked by MAOIs including deprenyl. The idea grew that striatal death may be delayed in patients with PD by preventing the formation of pyridinium species (104).

The alternative is the oxidation hypothesis: oxidation of DA by MAO results in the formation of oxygen-derived species such as hydrogen peroxide and hydroxyl radicals that can be toxic to dopaminergic neurons. As neurons die, turnover of DA is increased in the neurons that remain, and there is even more production of neurotoxic oxygen radicals. Deprenyl is thought to be prophylactic in PD because it moderates oxidative stress by preventing the oxidation of DA by MAO-B. This may have some importance in the physiology of normal aging, a process that is associated with an inexorable depletion of dopaminergic neurons even in the absence of PD. Indeed, deprenyl has been discovered to prolong the life span of laboratory rats that do not have PD (101,104).

If deprenyl does exercise some sort of prophylactic effect in PD or if it does attenuate one of the natural degenerative processes associated with aging, one should ask whether it can also be useful in slowing the course of deterioration in other neurodegenerative conditions such as Alzheimer's disease. There have been reports of symptomatic improvement in patients with Alzheimer's disease treated with deprenyl over the short term (102), so it is not unreasonable to test the hypothesis in longer term trials.

Clinical experience with deprenyl has not been as favorable, as the literature might suggest. It does not seem to be used much by patients with PD, and there has not been an increase in the use of deprenyl among other types of neuropsychiatric patients. Deprenyl is at least an alternative dopaminergic drug for patients with TBI, and the possible indications are the same as they are for the other dopaminergic drugs, stimulants, and antidepressants. It may also be used for other conditions, such as ADHD and narcolepsy, for which stimulants are normally prescribed. It certainly is an alternative, but I am not aware of many neuropsychiatrists who use it very often. It may not be a very good alternative.

Moclobemide

Moclobemide is a benzamide derivative that is structurally unrelated to any of the classic MAOIs. It is a preferential and reversible inhibitor of MAO-A that is virtually devoid of any of the major problems (hepatotoxicity, "cheese effect," orthostatic hypotension) associated with the other irreversible MAO-A inhibitors. Because it is reversibly bound to MAO, the drug is displaced from its binding site in the intestine by ingested, indirectly sympathomimetic amines such as tyramine, thus avoiding the initiation of the hypertensive crisis. The classic MAOIs are irreversible in that body concentrations of MAO do not return to normal until 2 weeks after the end of treatment, until new enzyme is synthesized. During this period, new drugs, such as the TCAs, cannot be introduced (105,106).

Moclobemide has little, if any, cognitive toxicity, even in elderly patients (107). It is not supposed to inhibit sexual function and is even said to enhance it (108).

At doses of 150 to 400 mg per day, it is as effective an antidepressant as the SSRIs with fewer side effects than the TCAs. It is said to be good for anergic depression and atypical depression, but it may be less anxiolytic than the classic MAOI antidepressants. It may prove to be a good alternative to the psychostimulants for ADHD or TBI. Moclobemide and deprenyl are probably the only MAOIs with a future in neuropsychiatry.

It is possible to combine moclobemide with another antidepressant or stimulant or with other drugs (e.g., dextromethorphan), but there is also the risk of 5-HT syndrome (109).

REFERENCES

1. Maas J. Biogenic amines and depression: biochemical and pharmacological separation of two types of depression. *Arch Gen Psychiatry* 1975;32:1357–1361.
2. Harley C. A role for norepinephrine in arousal, emotion and learning?: Limbic modulation by norepinephrine and the Kety hypothesis. *Prog Neuropsychopharmacol Biol Biol Psychiatry* 1987;11:419–458.
3. Dalta KP, Curzon G. Behavioural and neurochemical evidence for the decrease of brain extracellular 5-HT

by the antidepressant drug tianeptine. *Neuropharmacology* 1993;32:839–845.
4. Wilde MI, Benfield P. Tianeptine. A review of its pharmacodynamic and pharmacokinetic properties, and therapeutic efficacy in depression and coexisting anxiety and depression. *Drugs* 1995;49:411–439.
5. Marinesco S, Poncet L, Debilly G, et al. Effects of tianeptine, sertraline and clomipramine on brain serotonin metabolism: a voltametric approach in the rat. *Brain Res* 1996;736:82–90.
6. Ginestet D. Efficacy of tianeptine in major depressive disorders with or without melancholia. *Eur Neuropsychopharmacol* 1997;7:S341–S345.
7. Dubovsky S. Beyond the serotonin reuptake inhibitors: rationales for the development of new serotonergic agents. *J Clin Psychiatry* 1994;55:34–44.
8. Dubovsky S, Thomas M. Serotonergic mechanisms and current and future psychiatric practice. *J Clin Psychiatry* 1995;56:38–48.
9. Wirz-Justice A. Biological rhythms in mood disorders. In: Bloom FE, Kupfer DJ, eds. *Psychopharmacology: the fourth generation of progress*. New York: Raven Press, 1995:999–1017.
10. Richelson E. Tricyclic antidepressants and neurotransmitter receptors. *Psychiatr Ann* 1979;9:16–31.
11. Wetzel CD, Squire LR, Janowsky DS. Methylphenidate impairs learning and memory in normal adults. *Behav Neural Biol* 1981;31:413–424.
12. Jackson RD, Corrigan JD, Arnett JA. Amitriptyline for agitation in head injury. *Arch Phys Med Rehabil* 1985; 66:180–181.
13. Marcopulos B, Graves R. Antidepressant effect on memory in depressed older persons. *J Clin Exp Neuropsychol* 1990;12:655–663.
14. Nathan P, Sitaram G, Stough C, et al. Serotonin, noradrenaline and cognitive function: a preliminary investigation of the acute pharmacodynamic effects of a serotonin versus a serotonin and noradrenaline reuptake inhibitor. *Behav Pharmacol* 2000;11:639–642.
15. Goodnick PJ. Pharmacokinetic optimisation of therapy with newer antidepressants. *Clin Pharmacokinet* 1994; 27:307–330.
16. Duman R, Malberg J, Nakagawa S, et al. Neuronal plasticity and survival in mood disorders. *Biol Psychiatry* 2000;48:732–739.
17. Reid IC, Stewart C. How antidepressants work: New perspectives on the pathophysiology of depressive disorder. *Br J Psychiatry* 2001;178:299–303.
18. Duman R, Heninger GR, Nestler E. A molecular and cellular theory of depression. *Arch Gen Psychiatry* 1997;54:597–606.
19. Duman R, Malberg J, Thome J. Neural plasticity to stress and antidepressant treatment. *Biol Psychiatry* 1999;46:1181–1191.
20. Stewart CA, Reid IC. Repeated ECS and fluoxetine administration have equivalent effects on hippocampal synaptic plasticity. *Psychopharmacology* 2000;148: 217–223.
21. Abakumova O, Podobed OV, Tsvetkova TA, et al. Modulation of glutamate neurotoxicity in the transformed cell culture by monoamine oxidase inhibitors, clorgyline and deprenyl. *J Neural Transm Suppl* 1998;52:91.
22. Manji H, Moore G, Chen G. Clinical and preclinical evidence for the neurotrophic effects of mood stabilizers: implications for the pathophysiology and treatment of manic-depressive illness. *Biol Psychiatry* 2000; 48:740–754.
23. Collins S, Moore R, McQuay H, et al. Antidepressants and anticonvulsants for diabetic neuropathy and postherpetic neuralgia: a quantitative systematic review. *J Pain Symptom Manage* 2000;20:449–458.
24. Chen RW, Chuang DM. Long term lithium treatment suppresses p53 and Bax expression but increases Bcl-2 expression. A prominent role in neuroprotection against excitotoxicity. *J Biol Chem* 1999;274:6039–6042.
25. Li R, El-Mallahk RS. A novel evidence of different mechanisms of lithium and valproate neuroprotective action on human SY5Y neuroblastoma cells: caspase-3 dependency. *Neurosci Lett* 2000;294:147–150.
26. Nonaka S, Hough C, Chuang D. Chronic lithium treatment robustly protects neurons in the central nervous system against excitotoxicity by inhibiting N-methyl-D-aspartate receptor-mediated calcium influx. *Proc Natl Acad Sci U S A* 1998;95:2642–2647.
27. Duman R, Vaidya V. Molecular and cellular actions of chronic electroconvulsive seizures. *J ECT* 1998;14: 181–193.
28. Dail WG, Feeney DM, Murray HM, et al. Responses to cortical injury: II. Widespread depression of the activity of an enzyme in cortex remote from the focal injury. *Brain Res* 1981;211:79–89.
29. Feeney DM, Sutton RL. Catecholamines and recovery of function after brain damage. In: Stein DG, Sabel BA, eds. *Pharmacological approaches to the treatment of brain and spinal cord injuries*. New York: Plenum, 1988:121–142.
30. Boyeson MG, Harmon RL. Effects of trazodone and desipramine on motor recovery in brain-injured rats. *Am J Phys Med Rehabil* 1993;72:286–293.
31. Goldstein L, Henderson D. Atypical antipsychotic agents and diabetes mellitus. *Prim Psychiatry* 2000; 7:65–68.
32. Peroutka SJ, Snyder SH. Long-term antidepressant treatment decreases spiroperidol-labeled serotonin receptor binding. *Science* 1980;210:88–90.
33. Stahl S. Serotonergic mechanisms and the new antidepressants. *Psychol Med* 1993;23:281–285.
34. Wong DT, Bymaster FP, Engleman EA. Prozac (fluoxetine, Lilly 110140), the first selective serotonin uptake inhibitor and an antidepressant drug: twenty years since its first publication. *Life Sci* 1995;57:411–441.
35. Hollister L, Claghorn J. New antidepressants. *Annu Rev Pharmacol Toxicol* 1993;32:165–177.
36. Sussman N, Ginsberg D. Rethinking side effects of the selective serotonin reuptake inhibitors: sexual dysfunction and weight gain. *Psychiatr Ann* 1998;28: 89–97.
37. Harvey B, Bouwer C. Neuropharmacology of paradoxic weight gain with selective serotonin reuptake inhibitors. *Clin Neuropharmacol* 2000;23:90–97.
38. Dubovsky SL, Thomas M. Tardive dyskinesia associated with fluoxetine. *Psychiatry Serv* 1996;47:991–993.
39. Halman M, Goldbloom DS. Fluoxetine and neuroleptic malignant syndrome. *Biol Psychiatry* 1990;28: 518–521.
40. Assion H, Heinemann F, Laux G. Neuroleptic malignant syndrome under treatment with antidepressants? A critical review. *Eur Arch Psychiatry Clin Neurosci* 1998;248:231–239.
41. Hindmarch I, Kimber S, Cockle S. Abrupt and brief

discontinuation of antidepressant treatment: effects on cognitive function and psychomotor performance. *Int Clin Psychopharmacol* 2000;15:305–318.
42. DeVane CLPD. Pharmacokinetics of the newer antidepressants: clinical relevance. *Am J Med* 1994;97: 13S–23S.
43. Bodner RA, Lynch T, Lewis L, et al. Serotonin syndrome. *Neurology* 1995;45:219–223.
44. Harvey A, Preskorn S. Interactions of serotonin reuptake inhibitors with tricylcic antidepressants. *Arch Gen Psychiatry* 1995;52:783–785.
45. Preskorn S. Targeted pharmacotherapy in depression management: comparative pharmacokinetics of fluoxetine, paroxetine and sertraline. *Int Clin Psychopharmacol* 1994;9:13–19.
46. Gualtieri CTM. The functional neuroanatomy of psychiatric treatments. *Psychiatr Clin North Am* 1991; 14:113–124.
47. Gonzalez-Rothi RJ, Zander D, Ros PR. Fluoxetine hydrochloride (Prozac)-induced pulmonary disease. *Chest* 1995;107:1763–1765.
48. Berk M, Jacobson BF, Hurly E. Fluoxetine and hemostasis function: a pilot study. *J Clin Psychiatry* 1995; 56:14–16.
49. Pai VB, Kelly MW. Bruising associated with the use of fluoxetine. *Ann Pharmacother* 1996;30:786–788.
50. Alderman CP, Seshadri P, Ben-Tovim DI. Effects of serotonin reuptake inhibitors on hemostasis. *Ann Pharmacother* 1996;30:1232–1234.
51. Kincaid RL, McMullin MM, Crookham SB, et al. Report of a fluoxetine fatality. *J Anal Toxicol* 1990;14: 327–329.
52. Somni RW, Crismon ML, Bowden CL. Fluoxetine: a serotonin-specific, second generation antidepressant. *Pharmacotherapy* 1987;7:1–15.
53. Lance J. The red ear syndrome. *Neurology* 1996;47: 617–620.
54. Teicher MH, Glod CRNMSCS, Cole JO. Emergence of intense suicidal preoccupation during fluoxetine treatment. *Am J Psychiatry* 1990;147:207–210.
55. FDA. Antidepressants update. *Talk Paper* 1991;T91–64.
56. Jick SS, Dean AD, Jick S. Antidepressants and suicide. *BMJ* 1995;310:215–218.
57. Power AC, Cowen PJ. Fluoxetine and suicidal behaviour: some clinical and theoretical aspects of a controversy. *Br J Psychiatry* 1992;161:735–741.
58. Crundwell JK. Fluoxetine and suicidal ideation—a review of the literature. *Int J Neurosci* 1993;68:73–84.
59. Donovan S, Clayton A, Beeharry M, et al. Deliberate self-harm and antidepressant drugs. Investigation of a possible link. *Br J Psychiatry* 2000;177:551–556.
60. Wiart L, Petit H, Joseph P, et al. Fluoxetine in early poststroke depression: a double-blind placebo-controlled study. *Stroke* 2000;31:1829–1832.
61. Cassidy JW. Fluoxetine: a new serotonergically active antidepressant. *J Head Trauma Rehabil* 1989;4:67–70.
62. Riblet LA, Gatewood CF, Mayol RF. Comparative effects of trazodone and tricyclic antidepressants on uptake of selected neurotransmitters by isolated rat brain synaptosomes. *Psychopharmacology* 1979;63:99–101.
63. Marek GJ, McDougle CJ, Price LH, et al. A comparison of trazodone and fluoxetine: implications for a serotonergic mechanism of antidepressant action. *Psychopharmacology* 1992;109:2–11.
64. Salazar-Grueso EF, Rosenberg RS, Roos RP. Sleep apnea in olivopontocerebellar degeneration: treatment with trazodone. *Ann Neurol* 1988;23:399–401.
65. McLeod NA, White LE. Trazodone in essential tremor. *JAMA* 1986;256:2675–2676.
66. Gerner R, Estabrook W, Steuer J, et al. Treatment of geriatric depression with trazadone, imipramine, and placebo: a double-blind study. *J Clin Psychiatry* 1980; 41:216–220.
67. Gershon S. Comparative side effect profiles of trazodone and imipramine; special reference to the geriatric population. *Psychopathology* 1984;17:39–50.
68. Damlouji NF, Ferguson JM. Trazodone-induced delirium in bulimic patients. *Am J Psychiatry* 1984;141: 434.
69. Warren M, Bick PA. Two case reports of trazodone-induced mania. *Am J Psychiatry* 1984;141:1103.
70. Gartrell N. Increased libido in women receiving trazodone. *Am J Psychiatry* 1986;143:781–782.
70a. Purcell P, Ghurye R. Trazodone and spontaneous orgasms in an elderly postmenopausal woman: a case report. *J Clin Psychopharmacol* 1995;15:293–295.
71. Hayes PE, Kristoff CA. Adverse reactions to five new antidepressants. *Clin Pharm* 1986;5:471–480.
72. Coccaro EF, Siever LJ. Second generation antidepressants: a comparative review. *J Clin Pharmacol* 1985; 25:241–260.
73. D'Amico MFMS, Roberts DL, Robinson DS, et al. Placebo-controlled dose-ranging trial designs in phase II development of nefazodone. *Psychopharmacol Bull* 1990;26:147–149.
74. Griffin JD, Carranza J, Griffith C, et al. Bupropion: clinical assay for amphetamine-like abuse potential. *J Clin Psychiatry* 1983;44:206–208.
75. Dufresne RL, Weber SS, Becker RE. Bupropion hydrochloride. *Drug Intell Clin Pharm* 1984;18:957–964.
76. Stern WC, Harto-Truax N, van Wyck Fleet J, et al. Clinical profile of the novel antidepressant bupropion. In: Costa E, Racagni G, eds. *Typical and atypical antidepressants: clinical practice.* New York: Raven Press, 1982.
77. Cooper BR, Wang CM, Cox RF, et al. Evidence that the acute behavioral and electrophysiological effects of bupropion (Wellbutrin) are mediated by a noradrenergic mechanism. *Neuropsychopharmacology* 1994; 11:133–141.
78. Chouinard G, Annable L, Langlois R. Absence of orthostatic hypotension in depressed patients treated with bupropion. *Prog Neuropsychopharmacol* 1981;5: 483–490.
79. Clay TH, Gualtieri TC, Gullion C. Clinical and neuropsychological effects of the novel antidepressant, bupropion. *Psychopharmacol Bull* 1988;24:143–148.
80. Wright G, Galloway L, Kim J, et al. Bupropion in the long-term treatment of cyclic mood disorders mood stabilizing effects. *J Clin Psychiatry* 1985;46:22–24.
81. Shopsin B. Bupropion's prophylactic efficacy in bipolar affective illness. *J Clin Psychiatry* 1983;44:163–169.
82. van Wyck Fleet J, Manberg PJ, Miller LL, et al. Overview of clinically significant adverse reactions to bupropion. *J Clin Psychiatry* 1983;44:191–195.
83. Harris CR, Gualtieri J, Stark G. Fatal bupropion overdose. *J Toxicol Clin Toxicol* 1997;35:321–324.
84. Becker RE, Dufresne RL. Perceptual changes with bupropion, a novel antidepressant. *Am J Psychiatry* 1982;139:1200.

85. Golden RN, James SP, Sherer MA, et al. Psychoses associated with bupropion treatment. *Am J Psychiatry* 1985;142:1459.
86. Peck AW, Stern WC, Watkinson C. Incidence of seizures during treatment with tricyclic antidepressant drugs and bupropion. *J Clin Psychol* 1983;44:197–201.
87. Thase M, Entsuah A, Rudolph R. Remission rates during treatment with venlafaxine or selective serotonin reuptake inhibitors. *Br J Psychiatry* 2001;178:234–241.
88. Salzman C. New drug review; venlafaxine (Effexor). *J Pract Psychiatry Behav Health* 1995:107–108.
89. Long C, Crifasi J, Maginn D, et al. Comparison of analytical methods in the determination of two venlafaxine fatalities. *J Anal Toxicol* 1997;21:166–169.
90. Klatsky AL, Armstrong MA, Friedman GD. Red wine, white wine, liquor, beer, and risk for coronary artery disease hospitalization. *Am J Cardiol* 1997;80:416–420.
91. Mullin J, Lodge A, Bennie E, et al. A multicenter double-blind, amitriptyline-controlled study of mirtazapine in patients with major depression. *J Psychopharmacol* 1996;10:235–240.
92. Burrows GD, Kremer CME. Mirtazapine: clinical advantages in the treatment of depression. *J Clin Psychopharmacol* 1997;17:34S–39S.
93. Svensson TH. Feedback inhibition of brain noradrenaline neurons by tricyclic antidepressants: L-receptor mediation. *Science* 1978;202:1089–1091.
94. Clifford DB, Rutherford JL, Hicks FG, et al. Acute effects of antidepressants on hippocampal seizures. *Ann Neurol* 1985;18:692–697.
94a. Healy D. Pioneers in psychopharmacology. *Int J Neuropsychopharmacol* 1998;1:191–194.
95. Zametkin A. Treatment of hyperactive children with monoamine oxidase inhibitors. I. Clinical efficacy. *Arch Gen Psychiatry* 1985;42:962–966.
96. Comfort A. Phenelzine therapy: the doctor, the patient, and the wine and cheese party. *J Oper Psychiatry* 1982;13:37–40.
97. Robinson DS, Nies A, Ravaris CL, et al. Clinical pharmacology of phenelzine. *Arch Gen Psychiatry* 1978;35:629–635.
98. Himmelhoch JM, Thase ME, Mallinger AG, et al. Tranylcypromine versus imipramine in anergic bipolar depression. *Am J Psychiatry* 1991;148:910–916.
99. Saran AS. Depression after minor closed head injury: role of dexamethasone suppression test and antidepressants. *J Clin Psychiatry* 1985;46:335–338.
100. Kayser A, Robinson DS, Nies A, et al. Response to phenelzine among depressed patients with features of hysteroid dysphoria. *Am J Psychiatry* 1985;142:486–488.
101. Sonsalla PK, Golbe LI. Deprenyl as prophylaxis against Parkinson's disease. *Clin Neuropharmacol* 1988;11:500–511.
102. Tariot PN, Cohen RM, Sunderland T, et al. L-Deprenyl in Alzheimer's disease. *Arch Gen Psychiatry* 1987;44:427–433.
103. Quitkin FM, Liebowitz MR, Stewart JW, et al. L-Deprenyl in atypical depressives. *Arch Gen Psychiatry* 1984;41:777–781.
104. Tetrud JW, Langston JW. The effect of deprenyl (selegiline) on the natural history of Parkinson's disease. *Science* 1989;245:519–522.
105. Freeman MP, Stoll AL. Mood stabilizer combinations: a review of safety and efficacy. *Am J Psychiatry* 1998;155:12–21.
106. Lecrubier Y. Risk-benefit assessment of newer versus older monoamine oxidase (MAO) inhibitors. *Drug Saf* 1994;10:292–300.
107. Hindmarch I, Kerr JS, Fairweather DB. The effects of moclobemide on psychomotor performance and cognitive function in the elderly. *Dementia* 1992;3:355–359.
108. Reynaert C, Parent M, Mirel J, et al. Moclobemide versus fluoxetine for a major depressive episode. *Psychopharmacology* 1995;118:183–187.
109. Singer PP, Jones GR. An uncommon fatality due to moclobemide and paroxetine. *J Anal Toxicol* 1997;21:518–520.

20

The Psychotropic Effects of Antiepileptic Drugs

SUMMARY

Twenty years ago, no one would have predicted the current importance of antiepileptic drugs (AEDs) in psychiatry. Now they are routinely prescribed for affective disorders, aggression, chronic pain, headache, and a host of other problems. They, too, are broad-spectrum psychotropics.

All the AEDs have multiple actions, and their therapeutic value is a reflection of combined or diverse effects. They allow the neuronal cell membrane to maintain its stability in the face of an irritative focus or destabilizing event. They do so by affecting the channels that mediate ion transport across the cell membrane or affecting neurotransmitters like γ-aminobutyric acid (GABA) or glutamate.

In the neuropsychiatric disorders, however, more attention has been addressed to their actions on signal transduction pathways, where their effects are similar but not identical to the unique psychotropic drug, lithium. Because their effects are overlapping as well as divergent, lithium, carbamazepine, and valproate can be used interchangeably, alternatively, or synergistically.

In this chapter, we discuss the individual AEDs and their neuropsychiatric indications. Carbamazepine and its new, improved congener, oxcarbazepine, are a signal to discuss drug interactions with the anticonvulsants as well as the problem of kindling. The discussion of valproate introduces a couple of obscure but important issues. One is the amino acid carnitine, which mediates fatty acid transport across the mitochondrial membrane. AED-induced carnitine deficiency can have neurotoxic consequences. Valproate (and some other psychotropic drugs) can have unusual effects on hair.

Anticonvulsants are widely used for the treatment of chronic pain. Here, gabapentin is the exemplar.

ANTIEPILEPTIC DRUGS

"Clinically, DPH (i.e., phenytoin) has a calming effect on the overactive brain... [it] is effective with extremes of mood ranging from depression to the hyperexcitable state" (Dreyfuss Foundation).

Anticonvulsant pharmacology began with the serendipitous discovery that two central nervous system (CNS) depressants that were used as sedatives for patients with mental illness, bromide salts and later phenobarbital, could also control seizures (1). For more than 100 years, anticonvulsant and psychiatric pharmacology evolved along similar lines, sometimes diverging, sometimes intersecting. In recent years, there has been a remarkable convergence.

Bromides and barbiturates have had their day, of course. Clearly, they were troublesome drugs, and as new treatments evolved, psychiatrists and neurologists alike abandoned them. Nevertheless, as recently as 1972, controlled studies indicated that phenobarbital was effective for the "relief of psychoneurotic conditions" (2), and in 1999, it was reported that primidone, a derivative of phenobarbital, was effective for patients with bipolar disorder who were refractory to other treatments (3).

The discovery of phenytoin was far from accidental. It was developed by Merritt and Putnam in 1938, the result of systematic investigation of drugs to control electrically induced convulsions in animals and one of the first instances of rational pharmacotherapy development in the history of medicine. Soon thereafter, physicians learned that phenytoin was a potent psychotropic drug as well, and effective for behavioral conditions refractory other treatments, e.g., affective disorders, aggression in schizophrenia, behavior disorders in mentally retarded people. Phenytoin, however, was never very popular among psychiatrists. In fact, a successful encounter with that drug led the financier Dreyfuss to publish a monograph subtitled *An Extraordinary Treatment That Has Been Overlooked.*

The older AEDs have long since been supplanted by modern drugs for the treatment of seizures that are at least as effective and much less prone to untoward effects. The older anticonvulsants like phenobarbital, primidone, and phenytoin were notorious for the problem of neurotoxicity, especially in mentally handicapped people. In residential institutions, retarded people with difficult seizure disorders were invariably treated with the combination of phenytoin and phenobarbital. Their seizures were controlled but usually at the expense of dysphoria, cognitive blunting, and behavioral problems.

Psychopharmacologists were slow to appreciate the therapeutic potential of the new AEDs. Carbamazepine, for example, was the first anticonvulsant drug to achieve prominence as a psychotropic. It was introduced as an anticonvulsant in Europe in 1962, and its beneficial effects for trigeminal neuralgia were first noted at that time. In 1968, it was approved in the United States for neuralgia, and in 1974, it won labeling approval as an anticonvulsant for adults.

For a long time, however, carbamazepine was considered only second-line treatment for seizures. This was based on what turned out to be exaggerated fears of its effect on hematopoiesis. Ultimately, serious and fatal hematopoietic disturbances associated with carbamazepine (e.g., thrombocytopenia, agranulocytosis, aplastic anemia) proved quite rare (4,5). The recommendation for serial blood count monitoring was dropped, and the drug became a first-line therapy for adults and children with seizure disorders.

Physicians who prescribed carbamazepine as an anticonvulsant soon noted that it often led to improvement in behavioral problems such as aggression and hyperactivity. From 1970 to 1978, there were no fewer than 40 published reports of beneficial carbamazepine effects on mood and behavior in patients with epilepsy (6,7).

The first pure psychiatric application of the drug, however, came from Japan, when Takezaki and Hanaoka (8) reported that it was effective for patients with bipolar affective disorder. Ironically, the Japanese were interested in carbamazepine because of their exaggerated fears of lithium toxicity; at the time, lithium was not available in Japan. Further investigations were pursued in Japan (9–11). Finally, in the United States, Ballenger and Post (7) published the first controlled study of carbamazepine for patients with bipolar disorder and related its efficacy to the kindling model of epileptogenesis. In only a few years, it became one of the established treatments for manic depression and has been widely used ever since.

The history of valproic acid is an uncanny parallel to that of carbamazepine: anticonvulsant properties discovered in 1963 (12), release in the United States in 1978, widespread fears of catastrophic hepatotoxicity soon thereafter, and then an explosion of prescription 10 years later, first as an anticonvulsant and then as a psychotropic. In 1995, it became the first anticonvulsant to win U.S. Food and Drug Administration (FDA) approval as a psychotropic drug for the treatment of bipolar affective disorder.

The utility of carbamazepine and valproic acid for patients whose psychiatric conditions were poorly controlled by traditional agents has led to an explosion of interest among psychopharmacologists in the new AEDs as they are introduced, lately in growing numbers. The long run-in that carbamazepine and valproate endured is no longer the case. Lamotrigine, gabapentin, tiagabine, and topiramate are as popular among psychiatrists today as they are among epileptologists.

The psychotropic anticonvulsants comprise a distinct category of drugs for the treatment of severe psychiatric disorders: certainly, for patients with bipolar disorder and people with refractory affective disorders but also for explosive disorder or "episodic dyscontrol" and periodic aggressive behavior associated with schizophrenia, brain injury, mental handicap, and the antisocial personality disorder. They are frequently used for agitation in the wide range of neuropsychiatric conditions including dementia, stroke, and coma recovery. Their clinical utility is hardly circumscribed by the fact that, as a class, they are clumsily named (mood stabilizers, thymoleptics, psychotropics, AEDs, psychotropic AEDs, and psychotropic anticonvulsants). This small point is reflective of the more serious problem: that no one is sure precisely how or why they work so well.

THE ANTICONVULSANT MECHANISM OF ACTION

"It is clear that AEDs (anti-epileptic drugs) are powerful psychotropic drugs...they have a powerful influence on excitatory and inhibitory processes within the brain" (13). AEDs are powerful psychotropics, and they are effective for a wide range of emotional and behavioral problems in neuropsychiatric patients. There is no compelling explanation for this fortuitous happenstance. In the clinical literature, one encounters vague references to their neuromodulatory effect or their action to stabilize the neuronal cell membrane. In the theoretical literature, there is a great deal of specific information about their actions and speculation about how they might be clinically relevant, but no definitive explanation has emerged. In this regard, as in so many others, they resemble lithium, another drug that has an extraordinary range of biologic activity but no agreed-on mechanism of action.

If their mechanism is obscure in the treatment of psychiatric conditions, it is only a bit more enlightened with respect to their action in controlling seizures. Here, again, a wealth of specific information exists, and some overarching principles as well, but also a good deal of ambiguity. Almost all the AEDs seem to have multiple actions, and this complicates the understanding of their anticonvulsant spectra. How much each separate mechanism contributes to the overall anticonvulsant effects of these different drugs is controversial (Table 20.1) (14).

When Merritt and Putnam (15) developed the first modern anticonvulsant phenytoin, their research rested on two foundations: an appreciation of the structural composition of the known barbiturate anticonvulsants, which gave them an idea of what anticonvulsant should look like, and a useful animal model, the maximal electroshock model, which allowed them to screen potential new compounds for anticonvulsant activity (16). Understanding the action of anticonvulsants was beyond their grasp. An anticonvulsant was a compound that borrowed the cyclic structure of phenobarbital and that was "effective in preventing electrically induced convulsive seizures in cats" (15).

AEDs are no longer defined in terms of their chemical structure. Valproate, for example, bears little resemblance to the major anticonvulsants phenytoin and carbamazepine, although all three have effects in animal models and a clinical spectrum of activity that overlaps to a considerable degree. Today, AEDs are described in terms of their effect on specific seizure types. Their mechanism of action is understood in terms of the cellular and molecular processes that govern neuronal excitability. Particular attention is addressed to the four ion channels that mediate the transport of sodium, calcium, chloride, and potassium across the neuronal cell membrane.

It is known that an epileptic event is marked by what is called a paroxysmal depolarizing shift, a sustained movement of the neuronal resting potential above threshold for 10 to 50 times the duration of a normal action potential. The excitability of an epilep-

TABLE 20.1. *Anticonvulsant mechanisms of action (14)*

Antiepileptic drug	Na^+ channel blockade	T-type Ca^{2+} channel blockade	Non–T type Ca^{2+} channel blockade	GABA-mimetic drugs	Antiglutamate action
Phenytoin	+++		+	+	
Primidone	++		+	++	++
Carbamazepine	+++			+	+
Oxcarbazepine	+++		+		+
Valproate	++	+		++	+
Ethosuccimide		+++			
Clonazepam	+		+	+++	
Lamotrigine	+++				+
Vigabatrin				+++	
Tiagabine				+++	
Gabapentin	+			++	+
Felbamate	+		+	+	++
Topiramate	++			++	++

+++, well-documented effect believed to account for a major part of the drug's anticonvulsant effects; ++, effect probably of clinical significance; +, effect only tentatively characterized or seen only at supratherapeutic concentrations.

tic neuron is determined by the four ion channels. Positive charge is carried into the cell, first through Na^+ channels and then through Ca^{2+} channels. Calcium entry into the cell produces a proportional degree of K^+ channel opening, which serves to terminate the paroxysmal depolarizing shift and induces a prolonged a quiescent state of afterhyperpolarization of the cell membrane. Failure of the calcium-dependent potassium current leads to a state of sustained high-frequency repetitive firing, propagation of the paroxysmal event, and the induction of seizure (16).

Anticonvulsant activity may be conceptualized in terms of a drug's activity on depolarizing Na^+ and Ca^{2+} channels or on repolarizing K^+ and Cl^- channels. It may also be defined in terms of receptors that are linked to those channels [e.g., *N*-methyl-D-aspartate (NMDA), AMPA] or the endogenous ligand to those receptors (e.g., GABA, glutamate). Within this scheme, the AEDs fall into four broad categories:

- Phenytoin and carbamazepine are prototypical anticonvulsants that inactivate voltage-dependent Na^+ channels. They display in common the ability to block sustained repetitive firing and therefore reduce neuronal excitability. Activity in this model is predictive of the ability to protect against partial and secondarily generalized seizures. Valproate and the new anticonvulsants oxcarbazepine, felbamate, gabapentin, lamotrigine, and topiramate share this effect (1).
- Ethosuximide suppresses generalized spike-wave epilepsy of the absence type. It acts by inhibiting Ca^{2+} conductance across low threshold ("T-type") channels. Valproate is effective against absence seizures and may also inhibit activity at the T-type calcium channel.
- Benzodiazepine and barbiturate anticonvulsants interact with the $GABA_A$ receptor. Activation of $GABA_A$ receptors results in membrane hyperpolarization secondary to inward chloride flux. Felbamate also interacts with the $GABA_A$ receptor, and other AEDs, notably valproate, gabapentin, primidone, vigabatrin, tiagabine, and topiramate influence chloride influx by increasing the availability of GABA (1).
- Glutamate antagonism is the fourth mechanism of anticonvulsant activity. Glutamate is the principal fast excitatory transmitter ion the brain; aspartate is another. Sustained repetitive firing may be decreased by compounds that are glutamate or aspartate antagonists. Glutamate induces neuronal excitation at three different postsynaptic receptors: the NMDA receptor, the AMPA receptor, and the kainate receptor. An epileptiform pattern of activity can be induced by glutamate acting at the NMDA receptor; glutamate acting at the AMPA or kainate receptors leads to sustained depolarization of the membrane potential with a maintained increase in the neuronal firing rate (17–19). In addition to valproate, antiglutaminergic drugs include primidone, carbamazepine/oxcarbazepine, felbamate, gabapentin, lamotrigine, and topiramate.

Current thinking is that all AEDs, old and new, have their principal actions on these four classes of ion channels and their related NMDA, AMPA, and $GABA_A$ receptors. Not all the drugs affect all the mechanisms. Different drug profiles, then, might account for different patterns of anticonvulsant activity, side effects, and efficacy for neuropsychiatric disorders. Drugs that delay the recovery from inactivation of sodium channels decrease sustained repetitive firing and are efficacious in blocking partial and generalized tonic-clonic seizures. Drugs that block T-type calcium channels are effective against generalized absence seizures. GABAergic drugs ought to be efficacious against all types of seizures. One presumes that it is "a combination of the mechanisms of action of a drug, in some critical proportion, (that may) be what determines its potency," (19). By the same token, combination therapy with anticonvulsant drugs might be more rational and more effective if they are chosen based on complementary or synergistic mechanisms (19).

AEDs are effective because they allow the neuronal cell membrane to retain its stability in the face of a pathologic event or condition that seeks to destabilize the cell. The actions cited above are widely accepted as explanatory; they are heuristic and drive present efforts to develop new AEDs. Are they sufficiently well developed to explain all the idiosyncrasies of seizure management? Clearly they are not. Do they have any bearing on the neuropsychiatric actions of the drugs? That remains to be seen.

At least some psychiatrists have proposed that the sedating or activating effects of AEDs might be related broadly to two of the mechanisms cited above. Drugs that act predominantly by enhancing inhibitory GABAergic tone (barbiturates, benzodiazepines, valproate, gabapentin, tiagabine, and vigabatrin) then would be relatively sedating, associated with side effects such as fatigue, cognitive blunting, and weight gain, as well as antimanic and anxiolytic effects. Drugs whose action was predominantly to attenuate glutamatergic excitatory neurotransmission (e.g., felbamate, lamotrigine) would be associated with activation, weight loss, and anxiogenic and antidepressant effects (20). It is an intelligent proposal, but it is not likely that the preponderance of the psychiatric and psychological effects of these remarkable drugs can be captured simply in terms of two mechanisms of action.

To understand the psychiatric effects of valproate and carbamazepine, the appropriate basis for comparison is lithium, which they resemble more than any other psychotropic drug. The new anticonvulsants seem more or less to follow this pattern as well. It is appropriate then to compare the actions of valproate and carbamazepine with those of lithium. If a common ground were found to exist, one could conceivably reverse-engineer an explanation for the pathogenesis of bipolar affective disorder. In fact, there are several potential mechanisms that might account for their common effects in the treatment of neuropsychiatric disorders.

THE ACTIONS OF LITHIUM COMPARED WITH THOSE OF THE PSYCHOTROPIC ANTICONVULSANTS

Long before the lithium ion was conceived to have a psychotropic effect, it was used as a salt substitute for cardiac patients. It is odd to think of a day when people had a salt cellar full of lithium on their kitchen table, but the idea of lithium as a substitute for sodium contributed to no small degree to the first, tentative theories of its psychotropic effect. It was thought that lithium, by substituting for Na^{2+} in the interstitial fluid, could stabilize neuronal cell membranes and thus alter the properties of excitable tissue.

Something like that does occur, but the process is a little more complicated. The action of the lithium ion, like the classic neurotransmitters, is not simply to enhance or suppress postsynaptic potentials. Rather, it influences many different aspects of the target neuron's behavior by affecting a complex network of intracellular messenger systems. To the neuron, lithium represents an extracellular signal, but its signal is transmitted to a number of intracellular sites by means of a species of membrane proteins known as G-protein coupling factors. Thus begins a process known as signal transduction. G proteins couple receptors on the cell membrane to ion channels across the lipid bilayer and from there to second messenger pathways within the cell. The second messengers have diverse physiologic effects within the cell and generate cascades of intracellular messengers. In most cases, these cascades involve changes in protein phosphorylation (21).

Inositol lipids play a major role in intracellular signaling as precursors of second messengers, which in turn mobilize intracellular calcium and thus trigger a spectrum of synaptic events. The lithium ion can influence this cascade of intracellular events by inhibiting the final dephosphorylation step of inositol synthesis. At therapeutically relevant concentrations, it is an inhibitor of inositol monophosphatase, which plays a major role in the recycling of inositol phosphates. By interfering with phosphoinositol metabolism, lithium has multiple targets for limiting neuronal overactivity (22,23). Berridge (22) proposed that inositol depletion was an obligate physiologic consequence of lithium's action. Lithium also exerts significant effects on the cyclic adenosine 3′,5′-monophosphate second messenger system and on protein kinase C, another intracellular mediator of receptor-generated signals (24).

Lithium is an effective treatment for acute mania, bipolar affective disorder, and some types of depression. It is not likely to achieve all these effects by controlling a single neurotransmitter system. Because it is likely that multiple interacting and overlapping systems are involved in the regulation of mood and affect, a drug such as lithium (or valproate or carbamazepine) is likely to have a broad spectrum of effects on multiple systems. Signal transduction pathways, such as G proteins, and second messenger systems, such as phosphoinositide, adenyl cyclase, and protein kinase C, are attractive candidates to explain its efficacy for a broad range of affective conditions (23,24).

What lithium does then can be conceptualized as the regulation of signal transduction. It modulates the intracellular cascade of responses to neuronal excitation to maintain homeostatic regulation within the cell and to modulate the genetic expression of proteins that are critical to synaptic function (24). One can think of lithium as being able to mute overactive pathways through actions on adenylate cyclase or phosphoinositol turnover, which might be differentially activated in mania and depression. A regulatory or homeostatic effect on second messenger systems can explain the biphasic action of lithium against both mania and depression (23).

The lithium effect on second messenger systems is shared by the psychotropic anticonvulsants valproate and carbamazepine. In fact, all three drugs appear to exercise a multiplicity of effects on different signal transduction components, effects that overlap to a degree but that also diverge. This pattern of overlapping and divergent actions is the same pattern noted in the previous section with respect to the myriad of antiepileptic actions. In both instances, we have drugs that can be used interchangeably: lithium and carbamazepine are both quite good for manic depression, carbamazepine and valproate are both good for generalized tonic-clonic seizures, or they can be used alternatively—if one does not work, the other might. They can be used synergistically—two drugs together may work better than either one by itself. As stated before: not all the drugs affect all the mechanisms; different drug profiles then might account for different patterns of anticonvulsant activity, side effects, and efficacy for neuropsychiatric disorders. One assumes that it is "a combination of the mechanisms of action of a drug, in some critical proportion, (that may) be what determines its potency" (19).

Therefore, we find that valproate and lithium both bring about a strikingly similar reduction in protein kinase C isoenzymes, an effect that is apparently not shared by carbamazepine (25,26). Lithium and valproate have similar effects on G-protein signal transduction, and carbamazepine does not (27).

Carbamazepine and lithium inhibit the phosphorylation of inositol. Valproate may or may not share this effect (28,29). Lithium tends to blunt the cyclic adenosine 3′,5′-monophosphate signal transduction pathway, but valproate does not (30).

The complexity of the interactions between lithium, valproate, and carbamazepine and signal transduction pathways begs a simple, unitary explanation for their psychotropic effects. Their effects in other candidate systems are no less complex, ambiguous, or obscure. Carbamazepine up-regulates adenosine receptors (electroconvulsive therapy does also), but lithium does not (23). All three drugs increase GABA turnover, but, as we have seen, the GABAergic effects of valproate may be less important than was believed at one time. The interactions of the three drugs with the monoamine neurotransmitters also follow the pattern of overlapping and divergent effects.

The same is true with respect to their effect on excitatory neurotransmission. Extracellular glutamate induces neuronal excitation, and glutamate inhibition plays a role in the antiepileptic effects of several drugs, including valproate and carbamazepine. In some circumstances, lithium stimulates glutamate release, probably by inhibiting reuptake (31). This may account for the proconvulsant effects of lithium, as well as its excitotoxic effects, which usually occur at supratherapeutic levels. Raising extracellular glutamate should be an effect that differentiates lithium from the psychotropic anticonvulsants, but then in some paradigms, valproate does the same thing—a counterintuitive observation, to say the least (32). Stimulating glutamate acutely, and at high doses, however, may not be an appropriate reflection of what lithium (or valproate) really does to excitatory neurotransmission. In a chronic treatment paradigm, lithium actually serves to stabilize glutamate uptake to a degree that modulation of glutamate receptor hyperactivity has been proposed as a component of its efficacy in the treatment of manic depression (33,34).

Lithium is potentially neurotoxic, but at therapeutic levels, it is actually neuroprotective. In this regard as well, its action is reflective of the psychotropic AEDs. Regulation of glutamate excitotoxicity is one example of a neuroprotective mechanism that is shared by lithium and valproate (35). There is, however, a deeper layer to the mechanism of neuroprotection, beyond the action of drugs at a neurotransmitter level (glutamate), at the receptor level (NMDA, AMPA, kainate), past the ion channels and the second messenger systems. Downstream from the signal transduction pathways, the action of drugs such as lithium and valproate are ultimately felt at the genomic level. They affect gene expression, for example, *fos* mRNA, a so-called "master switch" that turns on a wave of specific neuronal genes. Through *fos* and other immediate-acting genes, lithium and valproate can modulate the genetic expression of specific proteins involved in synaptic expression in the brain (24).

B-cell lymphoma protein-2 (bcl-2) is an antiapoptotic and neurotrophic protein in the brain. Expression of bcl-2 has been shown to protect neurons from a variety of insults *in vivo* and *in vitro*. bcl-2 enhances the regeneration of axons in the mammalian CNS, promotes neural outgrowth, and increases axonal growth rate (36). One remarkable effect of lithium and valproate is to increase the expression of bcl-2 in various brain regions, including the frontal cortex, hippocampus, and striatum. They increase the expression of this cytoprotective protein in a robust, dose-dependent manner and at therapeutic concentrations (37–39).

The idea that lithium might be neuroprotective is not surprising. Clinicians are all too aware of the drug's narrow therapeutic index and the frequent occurrence of neurotoxic side effects in lithium-treated patients, including tremor, dystonia, ataxia, and cognitive blunting. In appropriate circumstances, however, lithium mitigates glutamate-induced excitotoxicity, and, at the genomic level, it evokes the overexpression of the cytoprotective protein bcl-2.

What does this mean? Does it mean that taking lithium for a long time is all right or that it is something that everybody ought to do because it prevents neurodegeneration, as gingko biloba or vitamin E is supposed to do? Does it mean that taking lithium along with a conventional neuroleptic will reduce the risk of developing tardive dyskinesia? Not too long ago, in fact, people thought that might be true. In 1978, it was reported that cotreatment with lithium prevented haloperidol-induced dopamine supersensitivity in rat striatum (40,41). There was a flourish of research activity around the prevention and treatment of tardive dyskinesia with lithium; the results were uniformly negative (42,43).

If clinicians might be doubtful about the suggestion that lithium is, indeed, neuroneoprotective, they are entitled to greet the next proposal with incredulity: neuroneogenesis may be stimulated by lithium—to be precise, the birth and development of new functional neurons in adult animals (44). Lithium, in therapeutic concentrations, has been found to increase neuroneogenesis in the hippocampus of adult rodents, presumably because of its effect on bcl-2 (36). The new cells appear to be neurons, progenitor cells, and glia. Furthermore, based on three-dimensional magnetic resonance imaging, it was reported that gray matter volume increased in a group of patients with bipolar affective disorder who had been treated with lithium for 4 weeks (26).

These findings are made in the context of recent discoveries that chronic mood disorders are associated with reduction in regional CNS volume and neuronal and glial cell atrophy or loss, especially in the hippocampus, and that administration of a variety of antidepressants also increases hippocampal neurogenesis (45). Thus, antidepressants and mood stabilizers seem to exert neurotrophic/neuroprotective effects, and this action may be clinically meaningful, at least with respect to the pathogenesis and treatment of affective disorders.

The idea that anticonvulsant drugs are effective for treating bipolar disorder has always been counterintuitive, to say the least. Lithium and, indeed, all the antidepressants are proconvulsant, not anticonvulsant. Depression is frequently comorbid with epilepsy, but bipolar disorder is not (46). Most impressive is the fact that electrically induced seizures are and always have been the most effective treatment available for severe depression as well as acute mania. Why are AEDs effective for the treatment of conditions that may also be treated by inducing seizures?

It is perhaps because the outcome of seizures and of AEDs is ultimately the same: the expression of endogenous anticonvulsant substances. Epileptologists have long suspected that seizures, occurring naturally or in response to electroconvulsive therapy, might generate an endogenous anticonvulsant. Adenosine and galanin are two candidates for that role (47,48). At the genomic level, electrically induced seizures, similar to those used in the treatment of severe depression, stimulate the expression of neurotrophic factors and sprouting of hippocampal neurons in laboratory animals (49). It appears likely that electroconvulsive therapy, lithium, and the psychotropic AEDs exercise a meaningful influence on the dynamics of gene transcription and especially the expression of neurotrophic and activator proteins (50).

It is appropriate to consider the actions of AEDs in epilepsy in terms of their effects on conductance across ion channels and the actions of lithium in terms of signal transduction pathways. Those mechanisms are, in all probability, necessary to their therapeutic effects. They are probably not sufficient to explain their effects. It is probably true that "a combination of the mechanisms of action of a drug, in some critical proportion, [may] be what determines its potency" (19). The actual mechanisms of these drugs include some novel actions that are only now coming into perspective.

LITHIUM, VALPROATE, AND CARBAMAZEPINE

The combination of mechanisms described in the most cursory terms form the basis of therapeutic effects that are remarkably similar among three chemically dissimilar drugs. Lithium, valproate, and carbamazepine are all effective by themselves in the treatment of acute mania, controlling bipolar disorder in the long term, the prophylaxis of recurrent unipolar depression, and the control of affective disorder variants such as intermittent explosive disorder. By themselves, they are comparatively weak antidepressants, but they are all effective as antidepressant augmenters in cases of refractory depression. They represent three legitimate alternatives for all these conditions. One will work in cases in which the others do not. Two together may sometimes work better than one; one is less secure in proposing that three together may work better than two (51–53).

It is commonly held that approximately 80% of patients with bipolar disorder respond favorably to lithium. However, this high response rate is not borne out in controlled studies, which have indicated a relatively high failure rate, and good outcomes in fewer than half of patients with bipolar disorder receiving long-term treatment (54). When data from controlled studies are pooled, 68% of patients with acute mania experienced a complete or partial response to lithium (53). Controlled studies with carbamazepine in acute mania show an overall response rate of 61%; it is almost as effective as lithium (or neuroleptics) and better tolerated (54). For valproate, the pooled response rate from controlled studies is 54%. For prophylaxis of bipolar disorder, the overall rate of lithium response is 66% compared with 63% for carbamazepine and 64% for valproate (52,54). For all practical purposes, the three drugs are equally effective for acute mania and bipolar prophylaxis. Data for other indications, e.g., recurrent unipolar depression, depression augmentation, explosive disorder, are less well developed, but one supposes that the three drugs are equivalent there as well.

Individual patients tolerate one of the three better than they will tolerate another, but, in general, their side effect profiles are equally troublesome, if different in nature, one from another. Alone among the psychoactive drugs, serial blood-level monitoring is an essential component of the standard of care.

In neuropsychiatric patients, for example, mentally retarded people or patients with brain injuries, stroke, or dementia, they are essential treatments. Affective instability is the most frequent and most debilitating component of the psychiatric problems that are evoked by these neuropathologic conditions, and achieving stability of mood is thus a major goal of psychiatric treatment. Thus, it is not unlikely that a retarded person who is explosive and aggressive would be treated with valproate; if that same patient were referred to another physician, the choice of carbamazepine might be made, with equal confidence that the drug was going to work. By the same token, combinations of mood stabilizers might be prescribed in refractory cases.

Beyond the idiosyncrasies of patient response, where differences are inevitable among any three drugs, are there meaningful clinical differences? Is there a way to choose one over the other or is the most enlightened clinical choice just as good as a coin toss? Patient tolerability is one good criterion. Although in terms of potential side effects, the three drugs are equal; in terms of likely side effects, valproate is probably the best and lithium the worst. Oxcarbazepine, the new analogue of carbamazepine, is tolerated better than its parent and may prove to be as well tolerated (or better) as valproate.

Because lithium has such a narrow therapeutic window, the incidence of neurotoxic side effects is high. The new information cited above about neuroprotection and neurogenesis, however, suggests that lithium (or valproate) might be preferred for neuropsychiatric patients. This aspect of comparative pharmacology, however, is too novel and undeveloped to form a sound basis for clinical choice. For example, in one paradigm (nuclear chromatin condensation), carbamazepine/oxcarbazepine seems to be relatively neurotoxic (55), and in another (regulation of oxidant stress), carbamazepine is clearly superior to valproate (56). We simply have no idea how to incorporate these preclinical observations into our clinical decision making.

Poor lithium response is associated with a number of clinical features: dysphoric mania, rapid cycling, lack of family history of primary affective disorder, comorbid substance abuse, more than three affective episodes before treatment, and a particular kind of affective episode sequence (depression-mania-well interval as opposed to mania-depression-well interval). Valproate and carbamazepine are more effective than lithium in cases of dysphoric mania and rapid cycling. They are also superior for patients without a family history of affective disorder. It is believed that the response for hereditary mood disorders is better with lithium, and for nonhereditary mood disorders, it is better with carbamazepine and valproate. It is also believed that organic mood disorders respond well to carbamazepine and valproate and poorly to lithium (54).

In an earlier monograph, it was suggested that carbamazepine was a "temporal lobe drug" and was the preferred treatment for patients with partial complex seizures arising from a temporal focus or for explosive patients with a temporal lobe focus on electroencephalography (EEG) (288). Indeed, in kindling studies, carbamazepine is superior to other anticonvulsants in inhibiting full-blown amygdala-kindled seizures and their underlying excitability (57). Lithium, as one would expect, is not effective against kindled seizures, but valproate is (58,59).

It would seem, then, that our theoretical physician treating a retarded person who was explosive and aggressive might choose valproate or carbamazepine with equal assurance, but lithium only with temerity. Unless, of course, he or she believed that lithium-induced neuroneogenesis was indeed a clinically meaningful outcome.

With respect to the newer AEDs, the so-called third generation of anticonvulsants, an Expert Consensus Guideline recommended them only as second-line therapies for severe affective disorders, i.e., to be used when lithium, carbamazepine, and valproate have failed or were contraindicated (51).

What Is Kindling?

"Similarly, it can be argued that the phenomenon described in the present note is analogous to learning. At the very least, it is a relatively permanent change in behavior that depends on repeated experience" (60).

What is kindling and does it have to do with anything? Kindling is an experimental paradigm for seizure generation that has a lot to do with how seizures get started in relation to a source of irritation. Imaginative scientists have proposed that it has something to do with learning in general, psychopathology in particular, and especially the actions of mood-stabilizing drugs (Table 20.2).

A kindling experiment begins with a series of intermittent subictal electrical stimuli administered to a particular region of the brain. At first, the current has no effect, but after a while, it elicits an afterdischarge. With repeated stimuli, the afterdischarge grows and becomes more extensive and prolonged until ultimately a generalized seizure occurs. The propensity to seize, thus induced, is more or less permanent. This is the kindling effect, and the most productive areas for kindled seizures are deep limbic structures, especially the amygdala and hippocampus, and frontal cortex (61–63).

The experimental paradigm is reflective of a normal physiologic process:

> *Some patients who seem to have made a good recovery from head injury become epileptic at some later date. An "incubation" period elapses between the causative brain trauma and the first epileptic attack, and the underlying process may require months or even years to reach fruition...such pathological events need not imply the emergence of new and uniquely different properties of neural tissue, but more likely imply particular variations on normal physiological mechanisms (61).*

Thus, an irritative focus, traumatic in origin, can ultimately kindle seizures after an "incubation" period lasting several years and induce a persistent state of posttraumatic epilepsy.

The physiologic basis for kindled seizures seems to reflect the process of normal learning. The neural changes that underlie kindling were soon found to parallel many aspects of long-term memory formation. Both kindling and memory result from neural activation and are relatively permanent, involve brain areas considered important for motivation and reinforcement, require the synthesis of proteins, result from repeated experience, and require some period of neural processing (64). The similarities (and differences) between kindling and long-term potentiation have been the subject of some discussion (65).

Early work with continuous subictal amygdala stimulation in laboratory animals had induced behavioral changes and epileptiform activity that was long lasting but would ultimately recede after the stimulation was withdrawn (66). In contrast, electrical stimulation in the kindling model was intermittent and generated a propensity to seizure that was permanent. The parallel to behavioral experiments in which continuous reinforcement induces short-term behavioral change and intermittent reinforcement leads to lasting change was not lost on investigators nor were the facts that the kindling phenomenon was modulated by monoamines (depletion of dopamine, norepinephrine, and serotonin) and accelerated the development of kindled seizures; that the kindling process led to a gradual depletion of dopamine, norepinephrine, and serotonin (67), and that the brain regions most susceptible to kindling are those associated with learning and emotional expression (68).

Clinically, the kindling model seemed most relevant to three overlapping conditions: posttraumatic epilepsy, temporal lobe epilepsy, and frontal epilepsy, three seizure disorders with a diverse range of

TABLE 20.2. *Potential psychotropic actions of the mood-stabilizing drugs*

Mechanism of action	Lithium	Valproic acid	Carbamazepine	Lamotrigine	Gabapentin	Tiagabine	Zonisamide	Topiramate
Signal transduction	+	+	+					
Phosphoinositol inhibition	+	+/–	+					
Cyclic adenosine 3′, 5′-monophosphate	+	—						
Protein kinase C	+	+	—					
G proteins	+	+	—					
Antikindling	—	+	+			+		
Neuroprotection	+	+	+	+		+	+	
Neurononeogenesis	+							
BCL-2 protein	+	+						
GABAergic	+	+/–	+		+	+	+	+
Antiglutaminergic	+	+	+	+	+			+
Adenosine agonist	—		+					

+, established effect; +/–, ambiguous effect; —, no effect. An empty box indicates that data are not available.

psychopathologic correlates. Pharmacologically, the two anticonvulsants that are most potent in suppressing kindled seizures are carbamazepine and valproate (59,69). It was inevitable, then, that kindling would be put forth as a model for some forms of psychopathology. Thus, it could be said that there was an analogous relationship between the progression of amygdaloid kindling and the natural course of affective disorders, from minor to major episodes and from triggered to spontaneous episodes. The course of bipolar disorder, untreated over a lifetime, is typically associated with manic and depressive episodes of greater severity, frequency, and duration (57).

Modified kindling leads to interictal behavioral and emotional changes in laboratory animals. Thus, interictal changes in behavior may result from amygdala-kindled seizures (70–72).

The kindling process leads to morphologic rearrangements of synaptic connections in the dentate gyrus in laboratory animals, and similar changes have been noted in patients with long-standing complex-partial seizures. Epileptogenesis in general and kindling in particular are mediated by gene expression and synaptic plasticity. Cells are damaged and lost, and new, aberrant axonal sprouting contributes to the hyperexcitability of epileptic brain tissue. Limbic permeability is a term to describe the degree of propagation that occurs between limbic system structures and their output fields; apparently, its output may be measured not only in terms of ictus but also emotional and behavioral events (63,71,73).

The kindling model, however, is only directly pertinent to the interictal personality and behavioral changes that occur with particular forms of epilepsy. It has been entertained as the source for a number of nonepileptic psychiatric conditions including depression and anxiety, bipolar disorder, and posttraumatic stress disorder. It is claimed that "all established mood stabilizers also exhibit antikindling effects" (74). That may or may not be the case. A more conservative view is that the kindling process involves gene expression and synaptic plasticity, that the physiology of learning and the development of psychopathology are mediated by similar processes, and the fact that antikindling drugs are also mood stabilizers speaks to some continuity at the level of gene expression and synaptic plasticity.

CARBAMAZEPINE AND OXCARBAZEPINE

Carbamazepine is a tricyclic compound with a steric structure that resembles that of imipramine, chlorpromazine, and maprotiline (75,76). It also shares structural features with the anticonvulsants phenytoin, clonazepam, and phenobarbital (77). In structure as well as function, it has a psychotropic and anticonvulsant pedigree.

One of the main metabolites of carbamazepine is the 10,11-epoxide, which is also active as an anticonvulsant but contributes disproportionately to the clinical toxicity of the parent compound. Conversely, oxcarbazepine, a dihydroketo analogue of carbamazepine, has an efficacy profile similar, if not identical to, the original drug, but it does not generate an epoxide metabolite and therefore is much better tolerated than carbamazepine (78,79). Essentially, it is carbamazepine with fewer side effects and the convenience of twice daily dosing. (Carbamazepine and oxcarbazepine are chemically quite similar, but hypersensitivity reactions to carbamazepine, such as skin rash, are not an absolute contraindication to trying oxcarbazepine. Start with a very low dose, such as 150 mg per day, and titrate slowly upward. This may avoid the side effect of rash.)

Carbamazepine as a Psychotropic

Soon after carbamazepine came into use, it was repeatedly observed that it had a beneficial effect on epileptic patients beyond the control of seizures. There was an increase in "psychic tempo" in patients with the "epileptic personality," with improvement in attention, concentration, and perseverance (6). Physicians described activation and stabilization, normalization of confused or paranoid episodes, relief from periodic depressions, increased alertness and initiative, decreased "sluggishness of thought and stickiness of personality," and a decrease in emotional overswings. Affective symptoms, emotional instability, and aggressive outbursts were particularly affected (80).

The use of carbamazepine as an alternative to lithium in the treatment of bipolar affective disorder was first undertaken in Japan. It was found to exercise a prophylactic effect (11) as well as direct effects in acute mania (10). Subsequent investigations established that it was effective for patients who failed to respond to lithium, was synergistic with lithium for patients who failed to respond to either drug alone, and effective in cases of schizoaffective disorder (81). Like lithium, it can prevent the reoccurrence of periodic unipolar depressions and it can also be used as an antidepressant augmenter for refractory depression (82,83).

The psychotherapeutic effects of carbamazepine are not, however, limited to affective disorders. It is an effective adjunct in the treatment of some subgroups of schizophrenics (84–88). It is an essential part of the treatment of late-onset psychosis after brain injury and in the related psychosis that sometimes accompanies temporal lobe epilepsy (89).

Like valproate and lithium, carbamazepine is effective in the treatment of the episodic dyscontrol syndrome (intermittent explosive disorder), but the literature on this point is largely anecdotal. Although many of these patients have neurodiagnostic evidence of temporal lobe lesions, such as epileptiform EEG, the presence of such a finding is not necessary to justify a trial of carbamazepine. Like valproate and lithium, it has even been used, albeit with less success, for patients whose aggressive behavior is thought to be "predatory" rather than "affective," i.e., patients with antisocial personality disorder and children with conduct disorder.

Finally, carbamazepine, like lithium and valproate, has always been a reasonable choice for treating virtually any severe behavioral disorder that occurs in a child, mentally retarded person, or patient with brain injury. A global statement like this is not likely to find specific support in the research literature, but it is supported by the weight of clinical experience. One would like to say that the disorders that are most likely to respond to these drugs are characterized by extreme emotional variability, behavioral disorganization, or paroxysmal outbursts, but the list of odd patients who seem to do well on carbamazepine, for example, after all else has failed includes a number who defy any attempt at predictive grouping.

Clinical Pharmacology

It is clinical lore that the "psychotropic effects of carbamazepine may appear after months of treatment, but may also be evident after only a few days" (77). The psychiatric literature, however, supports a carbamazepine effect within a few days (7,84,90–92). Initial improvement with carbamazepine may diminish within the first 2 weeks of treatment owing to enzyme autoinduction and lowered serum levels. Oxcarbazepine is not given to microsomal autoinduction (79).

No correlation has yet been drawn between serum levels of carbamazepine and therapeutic response in psychiatric conditions (80). Therefore, the guideline of 4 to 12 mg/L is only an approximation, and some patients do well at 3 to 4 mg/L, whereas others require serum levels as high as 16. In this regard, carbamazepine seems to have established a pattern that the later generation of psychotropic anticonvulsants followed: valproate, gabapentin, lamotrigine, and topiramate may all be used for a variety of psychiatric conditions, but psychiatric patients may respond to doses that are much lower than are commonly used to treat epilepsy. (Very occasionally, higher doses are needed. For example, in the case of a retarded person whose seizures are well controlled at a low serum level but whose difficult behaviors persist, raising the anticonvulsant dose may bring both problems under control with one drug.)

The importance of serum level monitoring for carbamazepine and indeed for all psychotropic anticonvulsants is mainly a way to guarantee that the full range of therapeutic opportunity has been explored. In the long run, serum levels relative to a fixed maintenance dose may change if the hepatic metabolism of carbamazepine slows down with age, as it does in the transition from childhood to adolescence and in elderly patients, or if the patient begins a drug or is withdrawn from a drug that interferes with carbamazepine metabolism. Carbamazepine induces the enzymes of its own metabolism, but serum levels should stabilize within a couple of weeks after treatment has begun.

Begin with a test dose, for example, 200 mg twice daily for an adult or 100 mg twice daily for a child weighing less than 40 kg. After 3 days, increase to a schedule of three times daily, and then change doses and monitor blood levels at the appropriate intervals. The reason for the low-dose interval is that some people simply cannot take carbamazepine. Approximately 5% of patients treated with carbamazepine must discontinue treatment because of toxic reactions (5). Skin reactions, nausea and vomiting, irritability, dyskinesia, and agitation may be early side effects that one can detect during a test-dose interval.

The recent availability of extended-release carbamazepine has liberated many patients from the necessity of frequent daily doses; we have had patients who responded favorably to carbamazepine four times daily but not to three times daily dosing. Not everyone enjoys the same benefit from the extended-release formulation, however, and some patients prefer the old-fashioned brand.

Another annoying problem in clinical management is the patient who is inadvertently switched from Novartis' Tegretol to a generic brand of carbamazepine. It is one of the few drugs for which the proprietary brand is sometimes preferable to the generic (93–95).

Oxcarbazepine is a twice-daily drug, therapeutically identical to carbamazepine but better tolerated. At first, it was not the custom to switch patients who were well maintained on carbamazepine to its new congener, but new starts were always with oxcarbazepine. As experience with the new drug developed, we discovered that patients almost always did better on oxcarbazepine, and this seems to be true even of patients who had no signs of overt carbamazepine toxicity. Therefore, it may not be a bad idea to switch patients over even if they are stable. Dosing begins at 150 mg twice daily. The usually antiepileptic dose is 900 to 1,200 mg per day, but doses as high as 3,000 mg per day have been used (96).

Toxicity

In terms of behavior toxicity, carbamazepine compares favorably with the old-line anticonvulsants, but that does not mean it is free of adverse behavioral effects. In fact, a substantial proportion of patients will have serious behavioral problems from carbamazepine. These are not, as a rule, in the direction of blunting, as with phenytoin, or disinhibition, as with the barbiturates, or depression, as with ethosuximide. Sometimes the behavioral toxicity of carbamazepine is like that of the tricyclic antidepressants: sedation, fatigue, hyperphagia, disorganization, agitation, delirium, hallucinations, and psychosis (97). More commonly, however, the side effects are stimulant-like: irritability, aggressiveness, dysphoria, restlessness, and emotional lability (80).

If a patient develops behavioral toxicity with the first few doses of carbamazepine, it is usually futile to raise the dose in search of a therapeutic window. Such action is likely only to make the problem worse. This is also true of the other psychotropic anticonvulsants.

The following dyskinetic movements have been described in connection with carbamazepine: tics, dystonia, orofacial dyskinesia, myoclonic jerks, ballismus, asterixis, and choreoathetosis (80). Carbamazepine usually aggravates tardive dyskinesia and akathisia. It is not helpful in the treatment of tics or Tourette's syndrome, although it does seem to be effective for rheumatic chorea (98).

Carbamazepine can cause seizures or can aggravate a seizure disorder, especially at high serum levels (i.e., >8 ng/mL). Patients who are prone to absences, have a spike-and-wave pattern on EEG, or have juvenile myoclonus are likelier to seize on carbamazepine (99–101). Oxcarbazepine is likely to do the same.

Cognitive impairment is a rare but serious side effect of carbamazepine. Much was made of the relative safety of carbamazepine in terms of memory performance, for example, especially when it was compared with the older anticonvulsants. It does not appear, however, to compare quite so favorably with the newer anticonvulsants, but sedation or cognitive blunting may occur with any anticonvulsant, new or old, especially in susceptible individuals.

Anticonvulsant Drug Interactions

Combinations of AEDs sometimes work better than a single drug alone. The use of combinations has long been a mainstay of seizure management; it is increasingly important for the management of neuropsychiatric disorders, as new anticonvulsants come on line, and used to augment existing medication regimens for patients whose response has been less than complete.

AED combinations should be chosen rationally or as intelligently as the state of the art allows. Some combinations are more likely to be synergistic than others, and some are more likely to be subtractive or even dangerous. Drug interactions, therefore, might happen for the better or worse. With respect to this class of drugs, it is a vexing problem because we know so little about their exact mechanisms of action. They are frequently prescribed for patients with severe conditions who may require combinations of four or more psychotropic drugs; the potential for harm is thus exponentially increased.

With respect to synergistic drug interactions in patients with generalized tonic-clonic or partial seizures, the following mechanistic combinations may be useful:

1. the combination of a sodium channel blocker with a GABAergic drug ,
2. combining two GABAergic drugs,
3. combining an AMPA antagonist with a NMDA antagonist.

For seizure management, combinations such as carbamazepine/valproate, valproate/lamotrigine, and carbamazepine/topiramate may be promising, whereas phenytoin/carbamazepine and carbamazepine/lamotrigine are not. These suggestions are based on animal studies and clinical reports (19). Carbamazepine and lamotrigine have similar mechanisms of action, and no particular benefit accrues from combining the two, at least for seizures. Their side effects also are additive; severe toxicity may occur if lamotrigine is added to the regimen of a patient who is already taking high doses of carbamazepine (102).

There is no comparable literature on combinations for patients with affective disorder, nor do the actions listed above necessarily relate to the psychotropic effects of anticonvulsant drugs, which remain clouded in the obscurity of second messenger systems, gene expression, and synaptic plasticity. As a result, psychiatrists are more familiar with a literature that addresses drug interactions that are counterproductive or even dangerous. Carbamazepine is a major contributor to this litany of therapeutic pitfalls.

Carbamazepine (like the older anticonvulsants phenytoin, phenobarbital, and primidone) is a broad-spectrum inducer of hepatic microsomal enzymes, the cytochrome P-450 isoenzymes. The clearance of drugs whose catabolism is mediated by cytochrome P-450 may be markedly increased by carbamazepine; many of these are psychotropic drugs. Cotreatment with carbamazepine then is likely to reduce the serum concentrations of virtually all the antipsychotic drugs, the benzodiazepines, and the tricyclic antidepressants in addition to the anticonvulsants valproate, topiramate, tiagabine, and zonisamide, and other drugs such as warfarin, theophylline, corticosteroids, oral contraceptives, propanolol, digoxin, and many others (103–109).

Carbamazepine does not influence the metabolism of the selective serotonin reuptake inhibitors, but several of the selective serotonin reuptake inhibitor antidepressants (e.g., fluoxetine, paroxetine, fluvoxamine) are potent inhibitors of the isoenzyme cytochrome P-50 2D6; theoretically at least, they may cause an increase in carbamazepine serum levels. Important clinical interactions, however, may not be predictable based on microsomal enzyme effects. They may rely instead on pharmacodynamic interactions, which are more difficult to anticipate. For example, the combination of fluoxetine and carbamazepine has been associated with the serotonin syndrome, the combination of carbamazepine and clozapine with neuroleptic malignant syndrome, and the combination of carbamazepine and lithium with severe neurotoxicity (103,110).

Drugs that inhibit the cytochrome P isoenzyme 3A4 may interfere with carbamazepine metabolism and increase serum concentrations. These include verapamil, diltiazem, danazol, propoxyphene, cimetidine, isoniazid, nicotinamide, St. John's wort, protease inhibitors, and macrolide antibiotics. It is not clear that the selective serotonin reuptake inhibitors fluoxetine, fluvoxamine, and paroxetine interact with carbamazepine, although they are 3A4 inhibitors (111). Grapefruit juice is a 3A4 inhibitor, and it does interact (112). Valproate does not inhibit 3A4 but does inhibit epoxide hydrolase, thus inhibiting clearance of carbamazepine epoxide, which is responsible for many of the toxic effects of carbamazepine. The combination of oxcarbazepine and valproate, therefore, represents a safer alternative.

Compared with carbamazepine, valproate is a much "cleaner" drug but not entirely free of troublesome interactions. Valproate inhibits cytochrome P2C isoenzymes; lamotrigine is particularly sensitive to inhibition by valproate, and the incidence of serious rashes is much higher in patients who receive the combination. It can increase both free and bound diazepam levels. Salicylates and nonsteroidal anti-inflammatory drugs can displace valproate from plasma proteins and thus cause inadvertent valproate toxicity.

The new anticonvulsants are cleaner still. Gabapentin, of course, is the paragon of this group of drugs. It is not metabolized at all but excreted unchanged by the kidney; thus, it has no known drug interactions. Tiagabine, zonisamide, and levetiracetam do not seem to be enzyme inducers. Lamotrigine, as we have seen, is given to a number of interactions with AEDs, and therapeutic drug monitoring is recommended (113). Oxcarbazepine is much less likely than carbamazepine to induce pharmacokinetic interactions and is unaffected by 3A4 inhibitors (109).

VALPROIC ACID

Clinical experience indicates that valproate and carbamazepine, as psychotropics, are more or less venerable than the experience with carbamazepine, clinical experience indicates that the two drugs are more or less interchangeable, and only the patient's idiosyncratic reaction will decide which is the better choice. The fact that valproate has won FDA labeling for bipolar disorder, and the manufacturers of carbamazepine have never even tried to get it, does not alter their therapeutic equivalence. Valproate is better tolerated than carbamazepine but is no better than oxcarbazepine. It is more likely to have teratogenic effects than either drug.

Valproate (or valproic acid) is a simple molecule, dipropylacetic acid, similar to naturally occurring fatty acids and chemically different from traditional anticonvulsant drugs. It was first synthesized in 1881, but its antiepileptic properties were not appreciated until 1963, when it was being used as an organic solvent for various compounds that were potential anticonvulsants. It was marketed in France in 1967 and in the United States in 1975.

Valproate was originally promoted as a drug that was more effective in controlling generalized rather than focal seizures (114), and this has led to the unfortunate surmise that it is never effective for focal or complex-partial seizure disorders; nothing could be further from the truth (115). It was first used as an alternative to ethosuximide, tridione, and other drugs for absence seizures, but now it is considered a useful alternative to carbamazepine, especially for refractory seizures of many types (116,117). As a beginning point for treatment, however, most epileptologists believe that valproate is the first choice for patients with absence fits, or a spike-and-wave pattern on EEG; carbamazepine is preferred for complex-partial seizures and fits that arise from a temporal lobe focus (118).

The major concern over valproate administration has been hepatotoxicity, which may be catastrophic. Fatal hepatotoxicity occurs in the first 6 months of therapy but appears to be concentrated in children, especially young children (less than 2 years old), and when valproate is used in conjunction with other AEDs. Valproate can cause pancreatitis. [Could this be a problem if valproate is given with a dibenzodiazepine (clozapine, olanzapine, quetiapine)?] The most common side effects are gastrointestinal: nausea, vomiting, and indigestion. Anorexia may be a troublesome effect; weight gain is another (119).

The other side effects of valproate are thrombocytopenia, which may occur even after years of treatment, and inhibition of platelet aggregation. The CNS side effects are usually in the direction of stimulation: insomnia, agitation, excitement, hyperactivity, and disorganization. Occasionally, however, a patient will be sedated on valproate. Valproate has been reported to have negative effects on psychological measures like finger tapping, visual-motor performance, and reaction time and attention (120,121).

Like carbamazepine, valproate was noted early on to improve some of the psychiatric problems of patients with epilepsy. In 1966, Lambert and colleagues (122) discovered antimanic properties for the anticonvulsant dipropylacetamide, which is metabolized rapidly to valproate, and in 1980 Emrich et al (289). described successful treatment of manic patients with valproate who had failed to respond to lithium. The development of valproate as an antimanic drug has been summarized on several occasions (51–54).

It is presumed that the psychotropic effects of valproate for bipolar disorder, schizophrenia, and severe behavioral disorders characterized by emotional instability are related to its properties as a $GABA_A$ agonist. In theory, at least, a GABAergic drug may down-regulate the dopamine receptor, for example, in the mesoprefrontal tracts (123). Valproate is structurally similar to GABA (124), and its anticonvulsant effects were initially attributed to an effect on GABA neurotransmission. It inhibits the degradative enzyme GABA transaminase, activates the biosynthetic enzyme glutamic acid decarboxylase, and raises the whole-brain GABA concentration. Thus, it potentiates GABA-mediated inhibition, but it does so only at doses and concentrations that are higher than those achieved in patients with epilepsy.

GABAergic effects are insufficient to explain the anticonvulsant action of valproate. It is also capable of inhibiting spike generation independent of the GABAergic system (124). Like phenytoin and carbamazepine, it blocks voltage-gated Na^+ channels (125) but once again at supratherapeutic concentrations. Valproate affects brain levels of glutamic acid and aspartic acid and inhibits NMDA-evoked depolarizations (20,126). Nevertheless, the precise and relevant mechanism of valproate remains obscure (1).

In 1995, the FDA approved valproate for the treatment of acute mania, its first psychiatric indication. It is currently one of the most frequently prescribed drugs by psychiatrists for patients with severe mental illness, affective disorders, and schizophrenia (127). It has been recommended for mood disorders in mentally retarded children (128) and for posttraumatic seizures and agitation associated with coma recovery in patients with brain injuries (129,130).

As often happens with new drugs, valproate looked awfully good when it was first introduced. When physicians compared it with drugs such as phenytoin, carbamazepine, and lithium, they found that it was tolerated better in most patients and that sedation, motor impairment, and cognitive deficits were less likely to occur. Because it has become a mainstream drug in neuropsychiatry, virtually a first-choice drug for most severe affective conditions, its image has been tarnished a little. Sedation, motor impairment, and cognitive blunting can indeed occur in patients on valproate, especially after long-term treatment.

Years ago, a neuropsychiatrist could do well with patients with brain injury; the patients would present months after the trauma reporting sedation, motor impairment, or cognitive slowing. In those days, most of them were on phenytoin, prescribed as anticonvulsant prophylaxis by their assiduous neurosurgeons who recommended they stay on the drug for a year or two. Almost all of them improved when the phenytoin was withdrawn. A similar situation occurs these days in patients with affective disorder who come for a second opinion, after years of treatment with no more than a partial response and with complaints of cognitive slowing, and continued treatment on valproate. The patient will often improve after the valproate is withdrawn. Physicians sometimes forget that long-term valproate can cause blunting, slowness, and weight gain.

Reversible dementia and apparent brain atrophy are rare but serious side effects of long-term treatment with valproate (131). Chorea may also be a long-term side effect (132). As more and more psychiatric patients are treated with valproate, there will be ample opportunity to evaluate its long-term toxicity.

Carnitine

Encephalopathy and hepatotoxicity associated with valproate treatment have been related to carnitine deficiency.

Carnitine is an amino acid derivative and an essential factor in the transport of fatty acids across the mitochondrial membrane, where beta-oxidation takes place. Patients with carnitine deficiency have impaired ketogenesis and enhanced beta-oxidation and may develop hepatocerebral dysfunction reminiscent of Reye's syndrome; in fact, children with Reye's syndrome are often found to be carnitine deficient. Valproate-induced encephalopathy is also associated with carnitine deficiency. Valproate tends to increase carnitine excretion (133–135). It is more likely to do so when combined with other anticonvulsants (a circumstance that in children increases the risk of hepatotoxicity); phenytoin, carbamazepine, and phenobarbital can also reduce carnitine but not to the degree that valproate does (136,137).

There are no controlled studies to indicate that carnitine supplementation prevents valproate-induced hepatoencephalopathy, but the few limited studies available suggest that carnitine supplements result in subjective and objective improvements, correlated with increased serum carnitine, in patients treated with valproate. Supplementation has been advised in appropriate circumstances (138).

Carnitine is thought to be cardioprotective and is sometimes recommended for elderly cardiac patients. It may be neuroprotective, and its association with acetylcholine metabolism has led to trials for patients with dementia (139,140). Carnitine deficiency is found on Lowe's syndrome (i.e., mental retardation, congenital cataracts, and renal tubular dysfunction) and possibly in autism (141,142). There are people in the autism community who think that carnitine supplementation is helpful.

Should carnitine supplementation be given to patients on valproate who develop problems with cognitive blunting? Not an outlandish idea, at least if their serum carnitine levels are low. Is it a "tonic" for patients with autism or Lowe's syndrome; there is no evidence to support that view.

Drugs and Hair

"I'd rather be a bald rooster than a hairy capon" as one of my patients said, a young man who developed a severe mood disorder after closed head injury. He responded equally well to lithium and valproate; with the former, however, he had sexual dysfunction and with the latter, alopecia.

Drug-induced alopecia is probably more common than physicians realize, and the mood stabilizers, valproate, lithium, and carbamazepine are the most frequent inducers of hair loss or even changes in texture and color. Valproate is particularly troublesome. The frequency of alopecia with valproate may be as high as 12%, and hair-texture changes, including increased waviness, curliness, and thinning, may occur in another 11%. It is no small surprise to the patient whose hair changes color or gets curly after being on valproate.

Hair loss, thinning, or increased straightness occurs with lithium, almost as frequently as valproate. Lithium has a high rate of dermatologic side effects. It is necessary to check the patient's thyroid status; lithium-induced hypothyroidism can cause hair loss or dry skin. Hair loss may occur with carbamazepine but much less frequently (143).

Drug-induced hair loss may be dose related or related to the duration of treatment. Lowering the dose may solve the problem. When the drug is discontinued, the problem usually corrects itself.

The mechanism may be related to depletion of trace minerals, especially selenium, zinc, or copper (144); supplements may or may not correct the problem. High doses of selenium, however, may cause hair loss.

Other drugs that may cause alopecia are haloperidol, olanzapine, and risperidone but not the other antipsychotic drugs and clonazepam but not the other benzodiazepines; buspirone and most antidepressants can as well (143).

Drug-induced alopecia is not a trivial problem. It may be the reason for noncompliance.

CLONAZEPAM

Clonazepam was originally approved in 1976 as an anticonvulsant for absence attacks, infantile spasms, petit mal variant, myoclonic seizures, and akinetic seizures. It is one of two benzodiazepines that have been demonstrated effective orally as an anticonvulsant (nitrazepam is the other). Clonazepam suppresses seizure activity in many animal models and suppresses many types of paroxysmal activity on EEG; generalized EEG abnormalities are more readily suppressed than focal abnormalities. Clonazepam often limits the spread of discharge from a focal lesion while not suppressing the primary focus. These observations may be explained by the ability of benzodiazepines to enhance polysynaptic inhibitory processes at all levels of the CNS (145).

Clonazepam does not have any special toxicity beyond that which the benzodiazepines have as a class. In fact, it has been said to be the safest drug alternative for the treatment of mania (146). What is special about the side effects of clonazepam is largely a function of the patient population for whom it is prescribed. Sedation, weakness, and fatigue are problems with clonazepam in adults with anxiety or affective disorders, but behavioral and emotional disturbances are more common in children, and the rate of behavioral toxicity has ranged from 2% to 52% in various studies (145). Young patients on clonazepam may become irritable, dysphoric, aggressive, violent, noncompliant, and hyperactive. This is the typical manifestation of behavioral disinhibition that has always limited the use of benzodiazepines, for example, in the treatment of patients with traumatic brain injury; children with serious epilepsy do not seem to be much different.

The frequency of this behavioral toxicity, coupled with the problem of tolerance to the anticonvulsant effects of the drug in approximately one-third of patients (145), has limited the use of clonazepam as an anticonvulsant to only the particular patients, and the particular seizure disorders, where it is uniquely effective. In contrast to carbamazepine and valproate, clonazepam has never been an anticonvulsant that impressed with its favorable psychological profile.

In fact, it was Chouinard (146), when examining the effects of treating mania with serotonergic drugs such as tryptophan combined with lithium, who selected clonazepam by virtue of its ability to stimulate serotonin synthesis. His group described acute antimanic effects with clonazepam and then a wider range of clinical effects, for example, in nonspecific agitation, steroid psychosis, tricyclic-induced mania, neuroleptic-induced somnambulism, atypical psychosis, and the schizophrenia-like psychosis of epilepsy. He proposed that clonazepam was an acute antipsychotic, the first legitimate alternative to the neuroleptics for acute management of the severely disturbed patient. Chouinard's work has been replicated (147–151).

Investigators found that clonazepam was an effective drug for panic disorder by virtue of comparison with alprazolam, a high-potency benzodiazepine with a short half-life; clonazepam was a high-potency benzodiazepine with a longer half-life, so the problem of rebound was not likely to be much of a problem. Its subsequent efficacy for panic disorder was reported by Fontaine (152), Beaudry et al. (153), and Pollack et al. (154). Tolerance to the antipanic effects of the drug does not seem to develop, and the effective dose is low (0.25 to 6.0 mg per day) (154).

Not only is clonazepam a reasonable substitute for the class of drugs that appear to cause tardive dyskinesia, but it also seems to be an occasional treatment for tardive dyskinesia (155). It appears to provide some symptomatic relief for selected patients, perhaps until the problem resolves itself. Whether it is better than other benzodiazepines in this regard, one cannot say. It is also prescribed as one of the only effective treatments for tardive akathisia, but that is not to say that it is especially effective in this regard (156). It has been effective also for Meige's syndrome, a form of idiopathic tardive dyskinesia (Goldstein, unpublished work, 1986). The idea is that the benzodiazepines, as GABA-mimetic drugs, inhibit striatal dopaminergic hyperactivity.

Is Clonazepam Different from the Other Benzodiazepines?

Clonazepam is popular among psychiatrists for two reasons: it has an intermediate duration of action, not so long as to accumulate, not so short as to cause withdrawal and has no active metabolites. Thus, it escapes the problems that inhere to long-acting benzodiazepines such as diazepam and chlordiazepoxide or short-acting ones such as triazolam and alprazolam. Lorazepam is another high-potency benzodiazepine with the same advantages as clonazepam.

Clonazepam was chosen as a potential antimanic drug because of its putative serotonergic effects; lorazepam is at least as effective as clonazepam for acute mania (54).

Clonazepam was first developed as an anticonvulsant and approved for absence, myoclonic, and akinetic seizures in 1976. That clonazepam and nitrazepam are effective oral anticonvulsants has been attributed to the fact that they are 7-nitro derivatives, a configuration that increases their potency (146). In fact, all the 1,4-benzodiazepines, including clorazepate, diazepam, and midazolam, have antiepileptic properties. Their principal molecular target is the postsynaptic $GABA_A$ receptor; activating this receptor results in membrane hyperpolarization secondary to inward chloride flux (1).

Clonazepam is a potent benzodiazepine that is antiepileptic and antimanic, but it is not unique.

ACETAZOLAMIDE

Acetazolamide has been used as an adjunctive antiepileptic since 1953, usually for cases or refractory partial or generalized seizures. It is an inhibitor of carbonic anhydrase, an enzyme that catalyzes the hydration of carbon dioxide and the dehydration of carbonic acid. Inhibition of carbonic anhydrase leads to an increase in CO_2 accumulation in neurons, changes in neuronal and interstitial fluid pH, lower concentrations of K^+ in the cellular interstitium, and thus a decrease in neuronal excitability. It is also a diuretic that promotes the renal loss of carbonate ion, a decrease in the concentration of bicarbonate in the extracellular fluid, and metabolic acidosis (1).

Tolerance may develop to the anticonvulsant effects of acetazolamide, but it can be used as an intermittent treatment for the prevention of catamenial seizures. Prescribing the drug for 2 weeks on and 2 weeks off seems to prevent the development of tolerance (157).

In the eye, it reduces the secretion of aqueous humor and causes the intraocular pressure to fall, which accounts for its use in the treatment of glaucoma. Carbonic anhydrase regulates potassium concentration in the vestibular endolymph; thus, acetazolamide has been used successfully for disabling vertigo (158). It has been effective for cases of hereditary paroxysmal ataxia and premenstrual periodic paralysis (159) and also for sleep apnea (160).

Acetazolamide is sometimes prescribed to prevent altitude sickness. It can also prevent the neuropsychological decompensation that accompanies the syndrome (161). One side effect of the drug is dysgeusia for beer, of all things; think twice, therefore, before you recommend it to a patient who is off on a ski holiday.

An interesting report by Hiroshi et al. (162) describes a small number of patients with atypical psychosis who responded to acetazolamide treatment. The rationale for the study was that the acetazolamide had effect of ion flux across the neuronal membrane similar to that of lithium. The best results were observed in patients who had periodic psychosis that coincided with the menstrual cycle, which is consistent with its use in catamenial epilepsy. Other reports suggest benefit for acute mania (163) and refractory bipolar disorder (164).

Acetazolamide has a favorable toxicity profile, and the dose range is narrow (250 to 1,000 mg per day). It may be added to carbamazepine or valproate in the event of partial response to the primary drug. Whether this strategy is also useful for the treatment of psychiatric disorders remains to be seen, but it is not an outlandish idea to pursue.

One of my more difficult cases was a retarded preadolescent girl with complex partial seizures and severe aggressive and self-injurious behavior. The seizures were only partially controlled with phenobarbital and phenytoin, but the behavioral problems were severe. Changing to carbamazepine led to a substantial improvement in behavior, but there were still frequent lapses in seizure control.

After years of behavioral difficulty, she entered menarche, and her seizure pattern and the pattern of misbehavior changed dramatically. Both seizures and aggression began to cluster around her menstrual periods, and before each period she would become particularly dysphoric. Cotreatment with acetazolamide led to a dramatic improvement in seizure and behavioral control, and the effect was sustained over prolonged follow-up.

Such a case is particularly given to a trial of acetazolamide for its diuretic effects, its action to enhance brain levels of carbamazepine, and its known effects on catamenial seizures.

GABAPENTIN

Gabapentin was approved in 1994 as an "add-on" treatment for partial seizures.

It was designed as a cyclic GABA analogue to mimic the steric conformation of GABA. As a centrally active GABA agonist, it should have therapeutic potential as an anticonvulsant. It is effective for partial and generalized tonic-clonic seizures but does not bind to the GABA receptor, although it does seem to increase GABA levels in the brain (165,166). Its action seems to be related to binding to a specific protein that is only found on neurons in the CNS.

Because it is a small molecule, like an amino acid, gabapentin is eliminated entirely by urinary excretion. (It is one of the few psychiatric drugs that are not metabolized by the liver. Lithium is another.) It is not protein bound or metabolized and neither induces nor inhibits hepatic enzymes. Therefore, it does not interact with other anticonvulsants or any other class of drug studied to date (167).

Gabapentin also appears to be a safe drug, with no hematopoietic or hepatic toxicity even at the very high doses that are sometimes used (168). Routine laboratory testing is not necessary. Its main side effects are CNS related: somnolence, dizziness, ataxia, fatigue, and nystagmus. It may cause involuntary choreiform movements in neurologically impaired patients (169).

Gabapentin has also been reported to cause agitation in patients with brain injury (170) and hyperactivity, aggression, tantrums, and oppositional-defiant behavior in children (171,172). Conversely, it has been used successfully to treat agitation in neuropsychiatric patients (173). Low doses of gabapentin are effective for elderly patients with agitation and dementia or refractory mood disorders (174). In low doses (50 to 400 mg), gabapentin has positive neuropsychological effects, not unlike a stimulant, on concentration, memory, and reaction time (175). Higher doses are associated with loss of concentration.

It has been proven effective for social phobia and is sometimes effective for severe panic disorder (176). In our practice, we have used the drug, with a degree of success, in autistic and retarded patients with ruminative anxiety. Gabapentin has anxiolytic effects in various animal models and decreases ratings of anxiety in patients with epilepsy (53).

Like all the new anticonvulsants, gabapentin was applied to the problem of mood stabilization, especially in refractory patients with bipolar disorder, unipolar depression, and organic affective disorders. There have been several encouraging reports in the literature (177–180). In our practice, we have used gabapentin with a degree of success in patients with neuropsychiatric conditions with ruminative anxiety but have not been impressed with it for refractory affective disorders.

Gabapentin may be useful for tinnitus (181).

Withdrawal from gabapentin may induce severe dizziness and other symptoms.

The action of gabapentin seems to be new and unique. It is a specific ligand for a member of the system L transporter family of brain cell membranes that provide a means of exchange for amino acids such as glycine and glutamate (170,182).

ANTICONVULSANTS FOR CHRONIC PAIN

Anticonvulsants have been used in pain management since the 1960s. The clinical impression is that they are useful for neuropathic pain, especially if the pain is described as lancinating or burning. Carbamazepine has been the drug of choice for trigeminal neuralgia, a prototypical "central pain" disorder, followed by phenytoin and valproate (183).

Anticonvulsants have continued to be a mainstay of pain treatment, and in clinical practice, their use has never been limited to neuropathic pain, central pain, or pain with particular subjective qualities. Rather, they have been used as the antidepressants have been used, for the wide range of chronic pain syndromes, irrespective of cause, and especially in conditions in which the etiology is unknown. It is ironic that such a venerable clinical practice has had little support from placebo-controlled studies or head-to-head comparisons with alternative treatments (184).

Anticonvulsants best documented for chronic pain are carbamazepine, clonazepam, and valproate (185). The newer anticonvulsants, especially gabapentin, seem to be equally useful or equally useless, as the case may be (186).

Gabapentin is already used quite widely for a number of different pain syndromes including neuropathy, migraine, reflex sympathetic dystrophy, facial neuralgia, radiculopathy, radiation myelopathy, and pain associated with tetraplegia (170,187,188). The doses may be quite high, often well above the recommended anticonvulsant dose (e.g., 4 to 6 g per day) (189). It has achieved a degree of popularity among physicians who treat chronic pain. Painful conditions, such as restless legs syndrome, seem to respond quite favorably to gabapentin.

Controlled studies have indicated good potential for lamotrigine to modulate and control neuropathic pain. Topiramate and tiagabine also have potential, at least based on animal models (190).

Lamotrigine

The development of lamotrigine originated with the observation that folate could induce seizures in experimental animals and that some anticonvulsants, notably phenobarbital, primidone, and phenytoin, reduced folate levels. Therefore, antifolate activity might be related to anticonvulsant activity. Lamotrigine was developed as an antifolate anticonvulsant; it proved to be an effective AED, but not by virtue of its antifolate activity. Presumably, its anticonvulsant activity is at the voltage-dependent Na channels, thus stabilizing the neuronal membrane and inhibiting the release of the excitatory neurotransmitters glutamate and aspartate (165). This mechanism, however, may not be sufficient to explain its broad range of clinical efficacy (191), and lamotrigine is found to modulate potassium and calcium currents, among other effects (192).

Lamotrigine is a triazine molecule, structurally unrelated to the other anticonvulsants. It is effective for various seizure types, especially generalized seizures. In mentally retarded patients, it is good for generalized epilepsies, complex partial seizures, and mixed seizures after brain injury (96). The half-life is 25 to 38 hours, and therefore it has the potential advantage of once-daily administration (193,194). It has little cognitive or behavioral toxicity compared with phenytoin, phenobarbital, and carbamazepine (195). Indeed, in early trials of the drug, patients with epilepsy were said to improve in "mood and mastery" (196). In retarded people, when lamotrigine was added to an antiepileptic regimen, it had impressive behavioral effects (less lethargy, decreased hyperactivity, improved social interactions, more appropriate speech, less irritability); only occasionally were its behavioral effects negative (irritability, overarousal, mania, screaming, tantrums, increased stereotypies, and hyperactivity) (197).

Lamotrigine is prone to the usual anticonvulsant side effects, such as fatigue, dizziness, and ataxia, but not to a great degree, and it is unusually well tolerated by patients. It may occasionally cause diplopia. The rash that it causes, however, is a problem. The FDA estimates that potentially life-threatening skin reactions occur in one of 50 to 100 children (compared with one in 1,000 adults) treated with lamotrigine. They are more likely to occur in patients cotreated with valproic acid. The skin reaction may progress to Stevens-Johnson syndrome, and fatalities have occurred. Theoretically, slow introduction of a very low dose of lamotrigine reduces the risk of severe reaction. Physicians are reminded in a boxed warning that the drug is not indicated in patients younger than 16 years of age (198).

Clinical reports beginning in 1994 suggested that lamotrigine was effective for affective disorder. Clinical surveys and controlled studies have affirmed its utility, especially for bipolar disorder and refractory depression (199–202), and the manufacturer is seeking a psychiatric indication. It has already won favor among psychiatrists who treat patients with refractory mood disorders. Very low doses (e.g., 25 mg twice daily) may be effective, although the usual dose is around 200 mg daily, and high doses (400 to 1,000 mg daily) are sometimes (but rarely) necessary. The value of monitoring serum levels is not established. A tentative target range of 1 to 4 mg/L has been proposed, although some patients with epilepsy have tolerated and benefited from levels higher than 10 mg/L.

The interaction between lamotrigine and valproate is poor because the two drugs appear to be synergistic in the treatment of epilepsy. The actions of the two drugs are complementary, one being a glutamate inhibitor, the other GABAergic. They may well have been synergistic, also, in the treatment of mood disorders (203). In contrast, lamotrigine and carbamazepine are both sodium channel blockers and serotonin reuptake inhibitors; theoretically, at least, no benefit should accrue from their combination (204,205).

Rett's syndrome is a mental retardation syndrome associated with autistic behaviors and progressive deterioration. Because an excess of glutamate is thought to play a role in the pathogenesis of Rett's syndrome, lamotrigine has been proposed as a potential treatment. In four girls with the syndrome, it improved their activities of daily living but not the frequency of their seizures (96,169). It is thought to be a relatively neuroprotective AED (206). For example, it improves neurologic outcome in experimental animals subjected to cerebral hypoxia (207).

Zonisamide

Zonisamide is a sulfonamide derivative developed in Japan with broad-spectrum antiepileptic activity against partial and generalized seizures (208). It has been commercially available in Japan since 1989. The mechanism of action is not clear but may involve blockade of sodium and T-type calcium channels, modulation of GABA and dopamine, and inhibition of carbonic anhydrase (53,96,209). Its half-life in single-dose studies is 52 to 60 hours (210).

Zonisamide is "structurally similar to serotonin" and has a pharmacologic profile that is very similar to carbamazepine. It was found to be effective in an open trial of patients with acute manic bipolar disorder (211). It is also a dopaminergic drug, and psychotic episodes have been noted (212,213).

Zonisamide has the following properties, which may make it interesting to neuropsychiatrists: it reduces cerebral damage after transient focal ischemia in rats (214) and is a free-radical scavenger (215). Leukopenia and renal stones are troublesome side effects.

Topiramate

Topiramate is a potent, broad-spectrum AED. It is approved in the United Kingdom "for the add-on treatment of patients whose partial seizures, with or without secondary generalization, are inadequately controlled." It was approved by the FDA at the end of 1996. It has a favorable toxicity profile, few interactions with other AEDs (216), and a twice-daily dosing schedule with a narrow therapeutic range (200 to 1,000 mg per day) and no need for therapeutic monitoring (217). It is structurally distinct from the other AEDs, but its action resembles that of all the known AEDs: it blocks the voltage-dependent sodium channels (as phenytoin and carbamazepine do), enhances GABAergic transmission (as valproate and the benzodiazepines do), inhibits carbonic anhydrase (as acetazolamide does), and blocks the excitatory amino acid neurotransmitters glutamate and aspartate (as the barbiturates do) (218).

It is said to have mild CNS side effects: somnolence, mental slowing, fatigue, dizziness, ataxia, and irritability (219). It needs to be introduced slowly to minimize these effects (Kerr, 1998) (290), although gradual titration may not prevent their occurrence. It is associated with a high rate of psychiatric side effects including depression and psychosis (220,221).

These may arise early in treatment or after months or years. Nevertheless, it has been proposed as a mood stabilizer for patients with refractory affective disorder (53,222). Many neurologists have been using topiramate for headache and chronic pain.

The starting dose in adults with epilepsy is 25 mg daily, increasing to 100 mg in two divided daily doses. Most patients respond to 400 mg daily or less, although doses as high as 1,600 mg per day may be used (96).

The most interesting effect of this drug is weight loss (223); ordinarily, anticonvulsants, mood stabilizers, and antidepressants are expected to stimulate weight gain. In contrast, topiramate has been found to significantly reduce body weight in patients with seizures. The mechanism is not known, and although it is not a potent anorectic, in animal studies, it both reduces food intake and increases energy expenditure (224). The results of clinical trials in bulimia nervosa and organic hyperphagia are eagerly awaited; my experience, thus far, is encouraging.

Tiagabine

Tiagabine is a structural modification of nipecotic acid, a substance that has been used for some years by basic researchers as a GABA reuptake inhibitor (225). It is a selective GABA reuptake inhibitor that is effective as an add-on for patients with refractory partial epilepsy (226). It does not seem to affect the hepatic metabolism of other AEDs, but it has a short half-life, which may require two to four daily doses. It also appears to be an antikindling drug that is effective for temporal lobe epilepsy (227). It is safe and well tolerated (228). Most of its side effects are CNS related (dizziness, weakness, fatigue, nervousness, depression, emotional lability, and tremor), and it may actually evoke partial status epilepticus (226,229). It appears to be safe and effective in mentally handicapped patients and does not appear to have cognitive toxicity (230,231).

The usual antiepileptic dose is 30 to 70 g daily, divided into two to four doses (96).

We have only suggestions that tiagabine might be a useful drug in neuropsychiatry: a mood-stabilizing effect in several patients with bipolar disorder (53, 232), and, in experimental animals, an antinociceptive effect (233), a neuronal-protective effect (234), and a protective effect against haloperidol-induced dyskinesia (235).

Tiagabine, like gabapentin, may sometimes be dramatically effective for neuropsychiatric patients with severe anxiety, e.g., children with autism.

Vigabatrin

Vigabatrin, formerly γ-vinyl GABA, was designed to be an inhibitor of GABA transaminase, the rate-limiting metabolic enzyme for GABA. It is a useful drug for some childhood forms of epilepsy, including infantile spasms and seizures associated with Lennox-Gastaut syndrome, for which little good therapy currently exists (194), and refractory epilepsy in mentally retarded people (236).

There is a significant incidence of psychiatric disorders with vigabatrin, such as depression, aggression, and psychosis, the latter occurring in 3% to 6% of patients in the British studies (194,237). It does not seem to possess cognitive neurotoxicity (238). Approval was delayed because of microvacuolization of the white matter of rodents and dogs, an effect that was said to be species specific and not pertinent to the treatment of humans (239). One side effect that may well be is constriction of the visual fields (169).

In one study of vigabatrin in mentally retarded patients with severe behavioral problems, treatment was associated with improvement in stereotypies, impulsiveness, and mood instability (240).

Felbamate

Felbamate is a dicarbamate that is structurally similar to meprobamate, an old tranquilizer that was notorious for inducing withdrawal seizures. Its mechanism of action may be at the GABA receptor, the voltage-dependent Na channel, or the glycine site of the NMDA receptor (165).

Felbamate was introduced as a broad-spectrum anticonvulsant that was particularly effective for Lennox-Gastaut seizures. It was said to be remarkably free of side effects, and it was, except for gastrointestinal upset at higher doses. In fact, even that effect could be put to productive use as one of the very few treatments for organic bulimia.

Then 10 cases of aplastic anemia developed in patients on felbamate. By 1995, there had been 32 cases with 10 fatalities and eight cases of hepatic failure with four fatalities. There had been no hint of any such side effects during the preapproval trials. Felbamate remains on the market, but its only current indication is for refractory encephalopathic epilepsies (241).

NEUROCOGNITIVE EFFECTS

Years ago, when I reviewed the neuropsychological effects of carbamazepine, the weight of the literature supported the idea that it was superior to phenytoin and barbiturate anticonvulsants in a broad swath of neurocognitive measures (80). In controlled studies, investigators had established that the sedating anticonvulsants, or, as some called them, "archaic anticonvulsants," influenced performance on tasks requiring attention, memory, and motor concentration in a negative way (242–245). It was also possible to demonstrate that increased serum levels were associated with proportionate decrements in performance (246,247). Therefore, if carbamazepine were compared with phenytoin, primidone, or clonazepam, it would usually be found to improve the patient's neuropsychological test profile. There was no question that it was less toxic than the barbiturates and phenytoin, but the issue is more complicated than that.

One issue is the population under study. When one considers the cognitive and motor effects of an anticonvulsant, it is essential to consider the type of patients using it. A group of highly intelligent children with benign familial epilepsy, for example, may have sufficient psychological reserve to render the negative cognitive effects of phenytoin or phenobarbital imperceptible. Such patients will do well, despite a drug that has the potential to hinder performance, just as they do well in the face of other forms of adversity. The negative cognitive and motor effects of a drug are best studied in a population with compromised function. Their cognitive reserve is limited, and they are more likely to feel the negative effects of a sedating anticonvulsant and to benefit from the substitution of a drug such as carbamazepine.

A second problem is that epilepsy by itself may be associated with blunting of motor performance, cognitive ability, or other aspects of personality. It may be difficult to dissociate drug effects in patients with epilepsy from the psychological effects of the disease for which the drugs were originally prescribed. The assessment measures that are used in such studies have neither been designed for nor standardized on patients with epilepsy, who represent a clinically diverse and heterogeneous population, let alone patients with brain injury or mental retardation with epilepsy. The measures of attention, memory, motor performance, and processing speed that are most commonly used are also known to be negatively affected in epileptic populations not receiving drugs (246–248).

The weight of the literature was indeed supportive of the idea that carbamazepine was superior to phenytoin and barbiturate anticonvulsants in measures of attention, alertness, reflectiveness-impulsivity, visual scanning, and cognitive flexibility; in memory for words and pictures and immediate and delayed recall; and in measures of motor speed, motor accuracy, and constructional praxis. Over the past few years, however, the picture has grown less clear. Timed tests are now known to be more sensitive to drug effects than untimed tests, and it is possible that the negative cognitive effects of certain anticonvulsants are solely attributable to a subtle effect on the speed of motor response (249). Thompson (250), for example, maintained that the memory effect of anticonvulsants is entirely a function of their effect on attention and information processing speed.

The long-term effects of phenytoin, compared with those of carbamazepine, are "few and restricted mainly to some visually guided motor functions" (251), which could be the result of cerebellar effects. In another study, the negative cognitive effects of phenytoin compared with carbamazepine were attributable to excessively high phenytoin levels, and when that was taken into account, the neuropsychological differences disappeared. Although the study of anticonvulsant prophylaxis in patients with head injury established a negative effect for phenytoin (252), in a study that compared carbamazepine with phenytoin in patients recovering from brain injury, both drugs had negative cognitive effects (253).

When carbamazepine was compared with valproate, no difference was found between the two drugs on memory tasks (254). In patients who had a craniotomy, valproate and phenytoin were equally well tolerated (255). When patients were withdrawn from therapeutic levels of phenytoin, carbamazepine, and valproate, they all improved in simple motor skills, and there was no significant difference among the three (256).

The recent literature, therefore, has been less negative when it comes to phenytoin and tends to emphasize that phenytoin, valproate, nor carbamazepine is a benign drug, from the neuropsychological point of view. My belief is that phenytoin is, in practice, more problematic than the others, but one must concede that the literature is equivocal on the matter.

What about the new anticonvulsant drugs? One has the right to expect that third-generation anticonvulsants are less toxic than the old ones, just as the selective serotonin reuptake inhibitors are better tolerated than the tricyclic antidepressants, and the "atypicals" are better tolerated than the older antipsychotic drugs. Neuropsychological evaluation has accompanied the new AEDs to the marketplace, and, as one might expect, it tends to be favorable, although one cannot be sanguine about the results until they are reported based on wider clinical experience by disinterested investigators.

All the findings reported below are from studies of patients with epilepsy (unless otherwise indicated):

Lamotrigine: No objective cognitive effects on neuropsychological tests (257,258), positive effects on quality of life and patient perceptions when compared with phenytoin and carbamazepine (257).

Tiagabine: Positive changes on neuropsychological tests except at the highest doses (259), no evidence of untoward interaction with ethanol or triazolam in healthy volunteers (260,261).

Gabapentin: Improvement in some neuropsychological measures, no evidence of impairment on any measures, and much superior to carbamazepine (262); no effect on neurocognitive measures; improved adjustment and mood (263,264).

Vigabatrin: Overall, studies show no detrimental effects or improved function (265), no detrimental effects on the Luria-Nebraska neuropsychological battery (266), "a tendency for improvement on most tests of cognitive function and mood" (267), no negative cognitive effects when used as an add-on (268).

Zonisamide: Early treatment effects on learning and memory at therapeutic levels, but tolerance seems to develop to the cognitive effects (269).

Levetiracetam: No negative cognitive effects when used as an add-on (270).

Then there is topiramate; a drug that has such promise as a psychotropic, but significant cognitive and behavioral effects:

Significant declines on measures of attention and fluency, acutely, and after several weeks of treatment with topiramate; there were no such effects with gabapentin or lamotrigine (219). In one series, 41% of patients were forced to discontinue the drug because of side effects, most often "cognitive dulling" (Dooley et al., 1999). In another, "the majority of the side effects were related to behavioral and cognitive difficulties" (271). In yet another, 47% discontinued treatment with topiramate because of side effects, especially weight loss, fatigue, behavioral, and cognitive problems (272). In a fourth study, five of 80 patients developed psychotic reactions (273).

It may be that gradual introduction of the drug and small dose increments can minimize the occurrence of cognitive toxicity with topiramate (274).

TERATOGENIC EFFECTS

A good deal more is known about the teratogenic effects of AEDs when the drugs are used for epilepsy; one extrapolates from the epilepsy data in making recommendations *vis-à-vis* neuropsychiatric treatment. This is not entirely sound because epilepsy itself is associated with difficult pregnancies and deliveries and with fetal malformations unrelated to AED treatment (275). But it is the best one can do.

As recently as 1980, phenobarbital was recommended as the anticonvulsant of choice for women with epilepsy who were pregnant or contemplating a pregnancy; the evidence is clear, however, that both phenobarbital and phenytoin are associated with higher risk of birth defects. In fact, exposure *in utero* both to phenobarbital and phenytoin has subsequently been related to significant cognitive deficits (276,277).

Then, the consensus was that carbamazepine was the safest AED for pregnant women, and it may well be. There is an incidence of minor dysmorphic features and a small risk of spina bifida, but nothing like there was with the older anticonvulsants and valproate (278). A "carbamazepine syndrome," associated with mild mental retardation, may be related to increased concentrations of the epoxide metabolite in women who are deficient in the enzyme epoxide hydrolase, another reason to prefer oxcarbazepine (279).

Valproate, conversely, is in a class by itself (280). When it was first introduced, it was considered quite safe, but soon there were reports of neural tube defects. In 1982, a study in Britain indicated a 5% occurrence rate of spina bifida and 15% occurrence of other structural defects including cardiovascular, orofacial, urogenital, and digital defects (280,281). Such extraordinary rates may have been the consequence of anticonvulsant polypharmacy and the lack of folate supplementation, both of which increase the risk of fetal damage.

It is currently believed that the risk of spina bifida with valproate monotherapy is 1% to 2%; for carbamazepine, the risk is, at most, 0.5% to 1% (282). The most recent surveys indicate that carbamazepine is not quite as innocent as was once believed but that valproate is clearly more teratogenic (283–285). Because valproate is such a popular psychiatric drug, special measures will be necessary to reduce fetal risk (286).

Therefore, all the established anticonvulsants are known teratogens. What about the new ones? The animal data are promising, but clinical data have not accrued yet, and one will have to wait and see (287).

REFERENCES

1. Rho J, Sankar R. The pharmacologic basis of antiepileptic drug action. *Epilepsia* 1999;40:1471–1483.
2. Uhlenhuth EH, Stephens JH, Dim BH, et al. Diphenylhydantoin and phenobarbital in the relief of psychoneurotic symptoms. A controlled comparison. *Psychopharmacologia* 1972;27:67–84.
3. Schaffer L, Schaffer C, Caretto J. The use of primidone in the treatment of refractory bipolar disorder. *Ann Clin Psychiatry* 1999;11:61–66.

4. Schain RJ, Ward JW, Guthrie D. Carbamazepine as an anticonvulsant in children. *Neurology* 1977;63: 476–480.
5. Schmidt D. *Adverse effects of antiepileptic drugs*. New York: Raven Press, 1982.
6. Dalby MA. Antiepileptic and psychotropic effect of carbamazepine in the treatment of psychomotor epilepsy. *Epilepsia* 1971;12:325–334.
7. Ballenger JC, Post RM. Therapeutic effects of carbamazepine in affective illness: a preliminary report. *Commun Psychopharmacol* 1978;2:159–175.
8. Takezaki H, Hanaoka M. The use of carbamazepine in the control of manic-depressive psychosis and other manic depressive states. *Seishin Igaku* 1971;13: 173–183.
9. Okuma T, Kishimoto A, Inoue K. Anti-manic and prophylactic effects of carbamazepine on manic-depressive psychosis: a preliminary report. *Folia Psychiatr Neurol Japon* 1973;27:283–297.
10. Okuma T, Kishimoto A, Inoue K. Anti-manic and prophylactic effects of carbamazepine on manic-depressive psychosis. *Seishin Igaku* 1975;17:617–630.
11. Okuma T, Inanaga K, Otsuki S. Comparison of the antimanic efficacy of carbamazepine and chlorpromazine: a double-blind controlled study. *Psychopharmacology* 1979;66:211–217.
12. Meunier G, Carraz G, Meunier Y. Pharmacodynamic properties of N-dipropylacetic acid. *Therapie* 1963;18: 435–438.
13. Fenwick PB. Antiepileptic drugs and their psychotropic effects. *Epilepsia* 1992;33:S33–S36.
14. Deckers C, Czuczwar S, Hekser Y, et al. Selection of antiepileptic drug polytherapy based on mechanisms of action: the evidence reviewed. *Epilepsia* 2000;41: 1364–1374.
15. Merritt HH PT. Sodium diphenyl hydantoinate in the treatment of convulsive disorders. *JAMA* 1938;111: 1068.
16. Bleck T, Klawans H. Convulsive disorders: mechanisms of epilepsy and anticonvulsant action. *Clin Neuropharmacol* 1990;13:121–128.
17. Meldrum B. Excitatory amino acid transmitters in epilepsy. *Epilepsia* 1991;32:s1–s3.
18. Rogawski M, Donevan S. AMPA receptors in epilepsy and as targets for antiepileptic drugs. *Adv Neurol* 1999;79:947–963.
19. Deckers C, Czuczwar S, Hekser Y, et al. Selection of antiepileptic drug polytherapy based on mechanisms of action: the evidence reviewed. *Epilepsia* 2000;41: 1364–1374.
20. Ketter T, Post R, Theodore W. Positive and negative psychiatric effects of antiepileptic drugs in patients with seizure disorders. *Neurology* 1999;53:s53–s67.
21. Duman R, Nestler E. Signal transduction pathways for catecholamine receptors. In: Bloom F, Kupfer D, eds. *Psychopharmacology: the fourth generation of progress*. New York: Raven Press, 1995:303–320.
22. Berridge MJ. Inositol trisphosphate, calcium, lithium, and cell signaling. *JAMA* 1989;262:1834–1841.
23. Post R, Weiss S, Chuang D. Mechanisms of action of anticonvulsants in affective disorders: comparisons with lithium. *J Clin Psychopharmacol* 1992;12:s23–s35.
24. Manji H, Potter W, Lenox R. Signal transduction pathways. *Arch Gen Psychiatry* 1995;52:531–543.
25. Lenox R, McNamara R, Watterson J, et al. Myristoylated alanine-rich C kinase substrate (MARCKS): a molecular target for the therapeutic action of mood stabilizers in the brain? *J Clin Psychiatry* 1996;57: 23–31.
26. Manji H, Bebchuk J, Moore G, et al. Modulation of CNS signal transduction pathways and gene expression by mood-stabilizing agents: therapeutic implications. *J Clin Psychiatry* 1999;60:27–39.
27. Bowden C. New concepts in mood stabilization: evidence for the effectiveness of valproate and lamotrigine. *Neuropsychopharmacology* 1998;19:194–199.
28. Vadnal R, Parthasarathy R. Myo-inositol monophosphatase: diverse effects of lithium, carbamazepine, and valproate. *Neuropsychopharmacology* 1995;12: 277–285.
29. O'Donnell T, Rotzinger S, Nakashima T, et al. Chronic lithium and sodium valproate both decrease the concentration of myo-inositol and increase the concentration of inositol monophosphates in rat brain. *Brain Res* 2000;880:84–91.
30. Wang J, Asghari V, Rockel C, et al. Cyclic AMP responsive element binding protein phosphorylation and DNA binding is decreased by chronic lithium but not valproate treatment of SH-SY5Y neuroblastoma cells. *Neuroscience* 1999;91:771–776.
31. Dixon J, Hokin L. Lithium acutely inhibits and chronically up-regulates and stabilizes glutamate uptake by presynaptic nerve endings in mouse cerebral cortex. *Proc Natl Acad Sci U S A* 1998;95:8363–8368.
32. Dixon J, Hokin L. The antibipolar drug valproate mimics lithium in stimulating glutamate release and inositol 1,4,5-trisphosphate accumulation in brain cortex slices but not accumulation of inositol monophosphates and bisphosphates. *Proc Natl Acad Sci U S A* 1997;94:4757–4760.
33. Nonaka S, Hough C, Chuang D. Chronic lithium treatment robustly protects neurons in the central nervous system against excitotoxicity by inhibiting N-methyl-D-aspartate receptor-mediated calcium influx. *Proc Natl Acad Sci U S A* 1998;95:2642–2647.
34. Karkanias N, Papke R. Subtype-specific effects of lithium on glutamate receptor function. *J Neurophysiol* 1999;81:1506 1512.
35. Mora A, Gonzalez-Polo R, Fuentes J, et al. Different mechanisms of protection against apoptosis by valproate and Li+. *Eur J Biochem* 1999;266:886–891.
36. Chen G, Rajkowska G, Du F, et al. Enhancement of hippocampal neurogenesis by lithium. *J Neurochem* 2000;75:1729–1734.
37. Manji H, Moore G, Chen G. Lithium at 50: have the neuroprotective effects of this unique cation been overlooked? *Biol Psychiatry* 1999;46:929–940.
38. Manji H, Moore G, Chen G. Clinical and preclinical evidence for the neurotrophic effects of mood stabilizers: implications for the pathophysiology and treatment of manic-depressive illness. *Biol Psychiatry* 2000;48:740–754.
39. Chen RW, Chuang DM. Long term lithium treatment suppresses p53 and Bax expression but increases Bcl-2 expression. A prominent role in neuroprotection against excitotoxicity. *J Biol Chem* 1999;274:6039–6042.
40. Pert A, Rosenblatt J, Sivit C, et al. Long-term treatment with lithium prevents the development of dopamine receptor supersensitivity. *Science* 1978;201:171–173.
41. Sternberg D, Bowers M Jr, Heninger G, et al. Lithium

prevents adaption of brain dopamine systems to haloperidol in schizophrenic patients. *Psychiatry Res* 1983; 10:79–86.
42. Licht R, Larsen J, Smith D, et al. Effect of chronic lithium treatment with or without haloperidol on number and sizes of neurons in rat neocortex. *Psychopharmacology (Berl)* 1994;115:371–374.
43. McGrath J, Soares K. Miscellaneous treatments for neuroleptic-induced tardive dyskinesia. *Cochrane Database Syst Rev* 2000;2:459.
44. Biebl M, Cooper CM, Winkler J, et al. Analysis of neurogenesis and programmed cell death reveals a self- renewing capacity in the adult rat brain. *Neurosci Lett* 2000;291:17–20.
45. Duman R, Malberg J, Nakagawa S, et al. Neuronal plasticity and survival in mood disorders. *Biol Psychiatry* 2000;48:732–739.
46. Barry J, Huynh N, Lembke A. Depression in individuals with epilepsy. *Curr Treatment Options Neurol* 2000;2:571–585.
47. Berman R, Fredholm B, Aden U, et al. Evidence for increased dorsal hippocampal adenosine release and metabolism during pharmacologically induced seizures in rats. *Brain Res* 2000;872:44–53.
48. Mazarati A, Hohmann J, Bacon A, et al. Modulation of hippocampal excitability and seizures by galanin. *J Neurosci* 2000;20:6276–6281.
49. Duman R, Vaidya V. Molecular and cellular actions of chronic electroconvulsive seizures. *J ECT* 1998;14: 181–193.
50. Hope BT, Kelz MB, Duman RS, et al. Chronic electroconvulsive seizure (ECS) treatment results in expression of a long-lasting AP-1 complex in brain with altered composition and characteristics. *J Neurosci* 1994;14:4318–4328.
51. Sachs G, Printz D, Kahn D, et al. The Expert Consensus Guideline Series: medication treatment of bipolar disorder. *Postgrad Med* 2000;1–104.
52. Sachs G, Thase M. Bipolar disorder therapeutics: maintenance treatment. *Biol Psychiatry* 2000;48:573–581.
53. McElroy S, Keck P. Pharmacologic agents for the treatment of acute bipolar mania. *Biol Psychiatry* 2000;48: 539–557.
54. Dunn R, Frye M, Kimbrell T, et al. The efficacy and use of anticonvulsants in mood disorders. *Clin Neuropharmacol* 1998;21:215–235.
55. Ambrosio A, Silva A, Araujo I, et al. Neurotoxic/neuroprotective profile of carbamazepine, oxcarbazepine and two new putative antiepileptic drugs, BIA 2-093 and BIA 2-024. *Eur J Pharmacol* 2000;406:191–201.
56. Yuksel A, Cengiz M, Seven M, et al. Erythrocyte glutathione, glutathione peroxidase, superoxide dismutase and serum lipid peroxidation in epileptic children with valproate and carbamazepine monotherapy. *J Basic Clin Physiol Pharmacol* 2000;11:73–81.
57. Post R, Denicoff K, Frye M, et al. A history of the use of anticonvulsants as mood stabilizers in the last two decades of the 20th century. *Neuropsychobiology* 1998; 38:152–166.
58. Silver J, Shin C, McNamara J. Antiepileptogenic effects of conventional anticonvulsants in the kindling model of epilepsy. *Ann Neurol* 1991;29:356–363.
59. Weiss S, Post R, Sohn E, et al. Cross-tolerance between carbamazepine and valproate on amygdala-kindled seizures. *Epilepsy Res* 1993;16:37–44.
60. Goddard V. Development of epileptic seizures through brain stimulation at low intensity. *Nature* 1967;214: 1020–1021.
61. Goddard G, McIntyre D, Leech C. A permanent change in brain function resulting from daily electrical stimulation. *Exp Neurol* 1969;25:295–330.
62. Wake A, Wada J. Frontal cortical kindling in cats. *Can J Neurol Sci* 1975;493–499.
63. Westbrook G. Seizures and epilepsy. In: Kandel E, Schwartz J, Jessell T, eds. *Principles of neural science*, 4th ed. New York: McGraw-Hill, 2000:910–935.
64. Rogers IO, Jackson W. The effect of hypophysectomy, ACTH fragments and thalamic lesions upon kindled epilepsy. *Brain Res* 1987;403:96–104.
65. Cain D. Long-term potentiation and kindling: how similar are the mechanisms? *Trends Neurosci* 1989;12: 6–10.
66. Alonso-DeFlorida F, Delgado J. Lasting behavioral EEG changes in cats induced by prolonged stimulation of amygdala. *Am J Physiol* 1958;193:223–229.
67. Lewis J, Westerberg V, Corcoran M. Monoaminergic correlates of kindling. *Brain Res* 1987;403:205–212.
68. Hiyoshi T, Matsuda M, Wada J. Centrally induced feline emotional behavior and limbic kindling. *Epilepsia* 1990;31:259–269.
69. Albright P, Burnham W. Development of a new pharmacological seizure model: effects of anticonvulsants on cortical and amygdala-kindled seizures in the rat. *Epilepsia* 1980;21:681–689.
70. Adamec R. Does kindling model anything clinically relevant? *Biol Psychiatry* 1990;27:249–279.
71. Helfer V, Deransart C, Marescaux C, et al. Amygdala kindling in the rat: anxiogenic-like consequences. *Neuroscience* 1996;73:971–978.
72. Kalynchuk L. Long-term amygdala kindling in rats as a model for the study of interictal emotionality in temporal lobe epilepsy. *Neurosci Biobehav Rev* 2000;24: 691–704.
73. Trimble M. *The psychoses of epilepsy*. New York: Raven Press, 1991.
74. Stoll A, Severus W. Mood stabilizers: shared mechanisms of action at postsynaptic signal-transduction and kindling processes. *Harv Rev Psychiatry* 1996;4:77–89.
75. Post RM, Uhde TW, Putnam FW, et al. Kindling and carbamazepine in affective illness. *J Nerv Ment Dis* 1982;170:717–729.
76. Rodin EA. Carbamazepine (Tegretol). In: Brown TR, Feldman RG, eds. *Epilepsy diagnosis and management*. Boston: Little Brown, 1983:203–214.
77. Dalby MA. Behavioral effects of carbamazepine. In: Penry JK, Daly DD, eds. *Complex partial seizures and their treatment*. New York: Raven Press, 1975:331–344.
78. Farago F. Trigeminal neuralgia: its treatment with two new carbamazepine analogues. *Eur Neurol* 1987;26: 73–83.
79. Tecoma E. Oxcarbazepine. *Epilepsia* 1999;40:s37–s46.
80. Evans RW, Gualtieri CT. Carbamazepine: a neuropsychological and psychiatric profile. *Clin Neuropharmacol* 1985;8:221–241.
81. Nolen WA. Carbamazepine, a possible adjunct of alternative to lithium in bipolar disorder. *Psychiatr Scand* 1983;67:218–225.
82. Post RM, Uhde TW, Ballenger JC. Efficacy of carbamazepine in affective disorders: implications for underlying physiological and biochemical substrates. In:

Emrich HM, Okuma T, Muller AA, eds. *Anticonvulsants in affective disorders*. Amsterdam: Elsevier Science, 1984:93–115.

83. Stuppaeck C, Barnas C, Miller C, et al. Carbamazepine in the prophylaxis of mood disorders. *J Clin Psychopharmacol* 1990;10:39–42.
84. DeVogelaer J. Carbamazepine in the treatment of psychotic and behavior disorders. *Acta Psychiatr Belg* 1981;81:532–541.
85. Hakola HPA, Laulumaa VA. Carbamazepine in treatment of violent schizophrenics. *Lancet* 1982;8285:1358.
86. Neppe VM. Carbamazepine as adjunctive treatment in nonepileptic chronic inpatients with EEG temporal lobe abnormalities. *J Clin Psychiatry* 1983;44:326–331.
87. Luchins DJ. Carbamazepine for the violent psychiatric patient. *Lancet* 1983;1:766.
88. Klein E, Bental E, Lerer B, et al. Carbamazepine and haloperidol vs. placebo and haloperidol in excited psychoses. *Arch Gen Psychiatry* 1984;41:165–170.
89. Barnhill LJ, Gualtieri CT. Late-onset psychosis after closed head injury. *Neuropsychiatry Neuropsychol Behav Neurol* 1989;2:211–218.
90. Hooshmand H, Sepdham T, Vries JK. Klüver-Bucy syndrome, successful treatment with carbamazepine. *JAMA* 1974;229:1782.
91. Lutz EG. Alternative drug treatments in Gilles de la Tourette's syndrome. *Am J Psychiatry* 1977;134:98–99.
92. Moss GR, James CR. Carbamazepine and lithium carbonate synergism in mania. *Arch Gen Psychiatry* 1983;40:588.
93. Oles K, Gal P. Bioequivalency revisited: Epitol versus Tegretol. *Neurology* 1993;43:2435–2436.
94. Gilman J, Alvarez L, Duchowny M. Carbamazepine toxicity resulting from generic substitution. *Neurology* 1993;43:2696–2697.
95. Besag F. Is generic prescribing acceptable in epilepsy? *Drug Saf* 2000;23:173–182.
96. Sorensen T. New antiepileptic drugs. In: Sillanpaa M, Gram L, Johannessen SI, et al, eds. *Epilepsy and mental retardation*. Petersfield, UK/Philadelphia: Wrightson Biomedical, 1999:91–104.
97. Silverstein FS, Parrish MA, Johnston MV. Adverse behavioral reactions in children treated with carbamazepine. *J Pediatr* 1982;101:785–787.
98. Harel L, Zecharia A, Straussberg R, et al. Successful treatment of rheumatic chorea with carbamazepine. *Pediatr Neurol* 2000;23:147–151.
99. Snead OC, Hosey LC. Exacerbation of seizures in children by carbamazepine. *N Engl J Med* 1985;313:916–921.
100. Genton P, Gelisse P, Thomas P, et al. Do carbamazepine and phenytoin aggravate juvenile myoclonic epilepsy? *Neurology* 2000;55:1106–1109.
101. Osorio I, Reed R, Peltzer J. Refractory idiopathic absence status epilepticus: a probable paradoxical effect of phenytoin and carbamazepine. *Epilepsia* 2000;41:887–894.
102. Besag F, Berry D, Pool F, et al. Carbamazepine toxicity with lamotrigine: pharmacokinetic or pharmacodynamic interaction? *Epilepsia* 1998;39:183–187.
103. Ketter T, Post R, Worthington K. Principles of clinically important drug interactions with carbamazepine. Part II. *J Clin Psychopharmacol* 1991;11:306.
104. Ketter T, Post R, Worthington K. Principles of clinically important drug interactions with carbamazepine. Part I. *J Clin Psychopharmacol* 1991;11:198–203.
105. Leinonen E, Lillsunde P, Laukkanen V, et al. Effects of carbamazepine on serum antidepressant concentrations in psychiatric patients. *J Clin Psychopharmacol* 1991;11:313–318.
106. Monaco F, Cicolin A. Interactions between anticonvulsant and psychoactive drugs. *Epilepsia* 1999;40:s71–s76.
107. Spina E, Avenoso A, Facciola G, et al. Relationship between plasma concentrations of clozapine and norclozapine and therapeutic response in patients with schizophrenia resistant to conventional neuroleptics. *Psychopharmacology (Berl)* 2000;148:83–89.
108. Sayal KS, Duncan-McConnell DA, McConnell HW, et al. Psychotropic interactions with warfarin. *Acta Psychiatr Scand* 2000;102:250–255.
109. French J, Gidal B. Antiepileptic drug interactions. *Epilepsia* 2000;41:s30–s36.
110. Shukla S, Godwin CD, Long LEB, et al. Lithium-carbamazepine neurotoxicity and risk factors. *Am J Psychiatry* 1984;141:1604–1606.
111. Sproule B, Naranjo C, Brenmer K, et al. Selective serotonin reuptake inhibitors and CNS drug interactions. A critical review of the evidence. *Clin Pharmacokinet* 1997;33:454–471.
112. Garg S, Kumar N, Bhargava V, et al. Effect of grapefruit juice on carbamazepine bioavailability in patients with epilepsy. *Clin Pharmacol Ther* 1998;64:286–288.
113. Bottiger Y, Svensson J, Stahle L. Lamotrigine drug interactions in a TDM material. *Ther Drug Monit* 1999;21:171–174.
114. Lewis JR. Valproic acid (Depakene): a new anticonvulsant agent. *JAMA* 1978;240:2190–2192.
115. Turnbull DM, Howel D, Rawlins MD, et al. Which drug for the adult epileptic patient: phenytoin or valproate? *BMJ* 1985;290:815–819.
116. Barnes SE, Bower BD. Sodium valproate in the treatment of intractable childhood epilepsy. *Dev Med Child Neurol* 1975;17:175–182.
117. Mattson R, Cramer J, Collins J, et al. A comparison of valproate with carbamazepine for the treatment of complex partial seizures and secondarily generalized tonic-clonic seizures in adults. *N Engl J Med* 1992;327:765–771.
118. Marson A, Williamson P, Hutton J, et al. Carbamazepine versus valproate monotherapy for epilepsy. *Cochrane Database Syst Rev* 2000;3:30.
119. Wilder B, Karas B, Penry J, et al. Gastrointestinal tolerance of divalproex sodium. *Neurology* 1983;33:808–811.
120. Sommerbeck KW, Theilgaard A, Rasmussen KE, et al. Valproate sodium: evaluation of so-called psychotropic effect. A controlled study. *Epilepsia* 1977;18:159–167.
121. Gallassi R, Morreale A, Lorusso S, et al. Cognitive effects of valproate. *Epilepsy Res* 1990;5:164.
122. Lambert P-A, Carraz G, Borselli S, et al. Action neuro-psychotrope d'un nouvel anti-epileptique: le diamide. *Ann Med Psychol* 1966;1:707–710.
123. Wassef AA, Dott SG, Harris A, et al. Critical review of GABA-ergic drugs in the treatment of schizophrenia. *J Clin Psychopharmacol* 1999;19:222–232.
124. Buchhalter JR, Dichter MA. Effects of valproic acid in cultured mammalian neurons. *Neurology* 1986;36:259–262.

125. White H. Clinical significance of animal seizure models and mechanism of action studies of potential antiepileptic drugs. *Epilepsia* 1997;38:s9–s17.
126. Slevin JT, Ferrara LP. Chronic valproic acid therapy and synaptic markers of amino acid neurotransmission. *Neurology* 1985;35:728–731.
127. Winterer G, Hermann W. Valproate and the symptomatic treatment of schizophrenia spectrum patients. *Pharmacopsychiatry* 2000;33:182–188.
128. Kastner T, Friedman D, Plummer A, et al. Valproic acid for the treatment of children with mental retardation and mood symptomatology. *Pediatrics* 1990;86:467–472.
129. Yang L, Benardo L. Valproate prevents epileptiform activity after trauma in an in vitro model in neocortical slices. *Epilepsia* 2000;41:1507–1513.
130. Chatham Showalter PE, Kimmel DN. Agitated symptom response to divalproex following acute brain injury. *J Neuropsychiatry Clin Neurosci* 2000;12:395–397.
131. Papazian O, Canizales E, Alfonso I, et al. Reversible dementia and apparent brain atrophy during valproate therapy. *Ann Neurol* 1995;38:687–691.
132. Lancman M, Asconape J, Penry J. Choreiform movements associated with the use of valproate. *Arch Neurol* 1994;51:702–704.
133. Triggs W, Bohan T, Lin S, et al. Valproate-induced coma with ketosis and carnitine insufficiency. *Arch Neurol* 1990;47:1131–1133.
134. Opala G, Winter S, Vance C, et al. The effect of valproic acid on plasma carnitine levels. *Am J Dis Child* 1991;145:999–1001.
135. Camina M, Rozas I, Gomez M, et al. Short-term effects of administration of anticonvulsant drugs on free carnitine and acylcarnitine in mouse serum and tissues. *Br J Pharmacol* 1991;103:1183.
136. Hug G, McGraw C, Bates S, et al. Reduction of serum carnitine concentrations during anticonvulsant therapy with phenobarbital, valproic acid, phenytoin, and carbamazepine in children. *J Pediatr* 1991;119:799–802.
137. Campistol J, Chavez B, Vilaseca M, et al. Antiepileptic drugs and carnitine. *Rev Neurol* 2000;30:s105–s109.
138. Raskind J, El-Chaar G. The role of carnitine supplementation during valproic acid therapy. *Ann Pharmacother* 2000;34:630–638.
139. Igisu H, Matsuoka M, Iryo Y. Protection of the brain by carnitine. *Sangyo Eiseigaku Zasshi* 1995;37:75–82.
140. Combs G. *The vitamins: fundamental aspects in nutrition and health*, 2nd ed. San Diego: Academic Press, 1998.
141. Charnas L, Bernardini I, Rader D, et al. Clinical and laboratory findings in the oculocerebrorenal syndrome of Lowe, with special reference to growth and renal function. *N Engl J Med* 1991;324:1318–1325.
142. Lombard J. Autism: a mitochondrial disorder? *Med Hypotheses* 1998;50:497–500.
143. Mercke Y, Sheng H, Khan T, et al. Hair loss in psychopharmacology. *Ann Clin Psychiatry* 2000;12:35–42.
144. Hurd RW, Van Rinsvelt HA, Wilder BJ, et al. Selenium, zinc and copper changes with valproic acid: possible relation to drug side effects. *Neurology* 1984; 34:1393–1395.
145. Browne TR. Clonazepam. *N Engl J Med* 1978;299: 812–816.
146. Chouinard G. Antimanic effects of clonazepam. *Psychosomatics* 1985;26:7–12.
147. Victor BS, Link NA, Binder RL, et al. Use of clonazepam in mania and schizoaffective disorders. *Am J Psychiatry* 1984;141:1111–1112.
148. Freinhar JP, Alvarez WH. Use of clonazepam in two cases of acute mania. *J Clin Psychiatry* 1985;46:29.
149. Freinhar JP. Clonazepam treatment of a mentally retarded woman. *Am J Psychiatry* 1985;142.
150. Freinhar JP, Alvarez WA. Clonazepam: a novel therapeutic adjunct. *Int J Psychiatry Med* 1985;15:321–328.
151. Aronson TA, Shukla S, Hirschowitz J. Clonazepam treatment of five lithium-refractory patients with bipolar disorder. *Am J Psychiatry* 1989;146:77.
152. Fontaine R. Clonazepam for panic disorders and agitation. *Psychosomatics* 1985;26:13–18.
153. Beaudry P, Fontaine R, Chouinard G, et al. Clonazepam in the treatment of patients with recurrent panic attacks. *J Clin Psychiatry* 1986;47:83–85.
154. Pollack MH, Tesar GE, Rosenbaum JF, et al. Clonazepam in the treatment of panic disorder and agoraphobia: a one-year follow-up. *J Clin Psychopharmacol* 1986;6:302–304.
155. Bobruff A, Gardos G, Tarsy D, et al. Clonazepam and phenobarbital in tardive dyskinesia. *Am J Psychiatry* 1981;138:189.
156. Kutcher S, Williamson P, MacKenzie S, et al. Successful clonazepam treatment of neuroleptic-induced akathisia in older adolescents and young adults: a double-blind, placebo-controlled study. *J Clin Psychopharmacol* 1989;9:403.
157. Reiss W, Oles K. Acetazolamide in the treatment of seizure. *Ann Pharmacother* 1996;30:514–519.
158. Hester RB, III, Farris BK. Acetazolamide in the treatment of abnormal oculovestibular Response. *Am J Ophthalmol* 1991;III:215–220.
159. Sarova-Pinhas I, Brajam J, Shalev A. Premenstrual periodic paralysis. *J Neurol* 1981;44:1162–1164.
160. Inoue Y, Takata K, Sakamoto I, et al. Clinical efficacy and indication of acetazolamide treatment on sleep apnea syndrome. *Psychiatry Clin Neurosci* 1999;53: 321–322.
161. White AJ. Cognitive impairment of acute mountain sickness and acetazolamide. *Aviat Space Environ Med* 1984;July:598–602.
162. Hiroshi I, Hidebumi H, Kaoru H, et al. Antipsychotic and prophylactic effects of acetazolamide (Diamox) on atypical psychosis. *Folia Psychiatr Neurol Japon* 1984;38:425–436.
163. Brandt C, Grunze H, Normann C, et al. Acetazolamide in the treatment of acute mania. A case report. *Neuropsychobiology* 1998;38:202–203.
164. Hayes S. Acetazolamide in bipolar affective disorders. *Ann Clin Psychiatry* 1994;6:91–98.
165. Macdonald RL, Kelly KM. Mechanisms of action of currently prescribed and newly developed antiepileptic drugs. *Epilepsia* 1994;35:S41–S50.
166. Petroff OACM, Rothman DLP, Behar KLP, et al. The effect of gabapentin on brain gamma-aminobutyric acid in patients with epilepsy. *Ann Neurol* 1996;39: 95–99.
167. Leiderman DB. Gabapentin as add-on therapy for refractory partial epilepsy: results of five placebo-controlled trials. *Epilepsia* 1994;35:S74–S76.
168. The U.S. Gabapentin Study Group. The long-term safety and efficacy of gabapentin (Neurontin) as add-on therapy in drug-resistant partial epilepsy. *Epilepsy Res* 1994;18:67–73.

169. Brodtkorb E. Treatment of epilepsy in patients with intellectual disabilities: general principles and particular problems. In: Sillanpaa M, Gram L, Johannessen SI, et al., eds. *Epilepsy and mental retardation*. Petersfield, UK/Philadelphia: 1999:74–89.
170. Childers MK, Holland D. Psychomotor agitation following gabapentin use in brain injury. *Brain Inj* 1997; 11:537–540.
171. Lee DO, Steingard FJ, Cesena M, et al. Behavioral side effects of gabapentin in children. *Epilepsia* 1996;37: 87–89.
172. Wolf SM, Shinnar S, Kang H, et al. Gabapentin toxicity in children manifesting as behavioral changes. *Epilepsia* 1996;36:1203–1205.
173. Roane D, Feinberg T, Meckler L, et al. Treatment of dementia-associated agitation with gabapentin. *J Neuropsychiatry Clin Neurosci* 2000;12:40–43.
174. Sheldon L. Gabapentin in geriatric psychiatry patients. *Can J Psychiatry* 1998;43:422–423.
175. Saletu B, Grunberger J, Linzmayer L. Evaluation of encephalatrophic and psychotropic properties of gabapentin in man by pharmaco-EEG and psychometry. *Int J Clin Pharmacol* 1986;24:362–373.
176. Pande AC, Davidson JRT, Jefferson JW, et al. Treatment of social phobia with gabapentin: a placebo-controlled study. *J Clin Psychopharmacol* 1999;19:341–348.
177. Ghaemi S. Gabapentin treatment of mood disorders: a preliminary study. *J Clin Psychiatry* 1998;59:426–429.
178. Knoll J. Clinical experience using gabapentin adjunctively in patients with a history of mania or hypomania. *J Affect Disord* 1998;49:229–233.
179. Cabras PL, Hardoy MJ, Hardoy MC, et al. Clinical experience with gabapentin in patients with bipolar or schizoaffective disorder: results of an open-label study. *J Clin Psychiatry* 1999;60:245–248.
180. Letterman L, Markowitz JS. Gabapentin: a review of published experience in the treatment of bipolar disorder and other psychiatric conditions. *Pharmacotherapy* 1999;19:565–572.
181. Zapp J. Gabapentin for the treatment of tinnitus: a case report. *Ear Nose Throat J* 2001;80:114–116.
182. Taylor CP. Emerging perspectives on the mechanism of action of gabapentin. *Neurology* 1994,44.S10–S16.
183. McQuay H, Carroll D, Jadad A, et al. Anticonvulsant drugs for management of pain: a systematic review. *BMJ* 1995;311:1047–1052.
184. Collins S, Moore R, McQuay H, et al. Antidepressants and anticonvulsants for diabetic neuropathy and postherpetic neuralgia: a quantitative systematic review. *J Pain Symptom Manage* 2000;20:449–458.
185. Covington E. Nonanalgesic pharmacotherapy of pain. Symposium 119—chronic pain: multidisciplinary approaches educational objectives for this symposium, 1997.
186. Wiffen P, Collins S, McQuay H, et al. Anticonvulsant drugs for acute and chronic pain. *Cochrane Database Syst Rev* 2000;3:1133
187. Backonja M, Beydoun A, Edwards KR, et al. Gabapentin for the symptomatic treatment of painful neuropathy in patients with diabetes mellitus. *JAMA* 1998;280:1831–1836.
188. Solaro C, Messmer Uccelli M, et al. Low-dose gabapentin combined with either lamotrigine or carbamazepine can be useful therapies for trigeminal neuralgia in multiple sclerosis. *Eur Neurol* 2000;44:45–48.
189. Herranz J. Current data on gabapentin. *Rev Neurol* 2000;30:s125–s131.
190. Tremont-Lukats I, Megeff C, Backonja M. Anticonvulsants for neuropathic pain syndromes: mechanisms of action and place in therapy. *Drugs* 2000;60:1029–1052.
191. Culy C, Goa K. Lamotrigine. A review of its use in childhood epilepsy. *Pediatr Drugs* 2000;2:299–330.
192. Grunze H, von Wegerer J, Greene R, et al. Modulation of calcium and potassium currents by lamotrigine. *Neuropsychobiology* 1998;38:131–138.
193. Weilburg JB, Mesulam MM, Weintraub S, et al. Focal striatal abnormalities in a patient with obsessive-compulsive disorder. *Arch Neurol* 1989;46:233–235.
194. Fisher RSM. Emerging antiepileptic drugs. *Neurology* 1993;43:S12–S20.
195. Gillham R, Kane K, Bryant-Comstock L, et al. A double-blind comparison of lamotrigine and carbamazepine in newly diagnosed epilepsy with health-related quality of life as an outcome measure. *Seizure* 2000;9:375–379.
196. Smith D, Chadwick D, Baker G, et al. Seizure severity and the quality of life. *Epilepsia* 1993;34:S31–S35.
197. Ettinger AB, Weisbrot DM, Saracco J, et al. Positive and negative psychotropic effects of lamotrigine in patients with epilepsy and mental retardation. *Epilepsia* 1998;39:874–877.
198. FDA. Summaries of "Dear Health Professional" letters & other safety notifications. *FDA Med Bull* 1997;27: 6–7.
199. Bowden CL, Swann AC, Calabrese JR, et al. Maintenance clinical trials in bipolar disorder: design implications of the divalproex-lithium-placebo study. *Psychopharmacol Bull* 1997;33:693–699.
200. Fatemi S, Rapport D, Calabrese J, et al. Lamotrigine in rapid-cycling bipolar disorder. *J Clin Psychiatry* 1997; 58:522–527.
201. Kotler M, Matar M. Lamotrigine in the treatment of resistant bipolar disorder. *Clin Neuropharmacol* 1998; 21:65–67.
202. Suppes T, Brown E, McElroy S, et al. Lamotrigine for the treatment of bipolar disorder: a clinical case series. *J Affect Disord* 1999;53:95–98.
203. Sills GJ, Carswell A, Brodie MJ. Dose-response relationships with nimodipine against electroshock seizures in mice. *Epilepsia* 1994;35:437–442.
204. Waldmeier PC, Baumann PA, Wicki P, et al. Similar potency of carbamazepine, oxcarbazepine, and lamotrigine in inhibiting the release of glutamate and other neurotransmitters. *Neurology* 1995;45:1907–1913.
205. Southam E, Kirkby D, Higgins GA, et al. Lamotrigine inhibits monoamine uptake in vitro and modulates 5-hydroxytryptamine uptake in rats. *Eur J Pharmacol* 1998;358:19–24.
206. Kalviainen R, Pitkanen A. Prevention of seizure-induced neuronal damage and intellectual deterioration: experimental aspects and clinical implications. In: Sillanpaa M, Gram L, Johannessen SI, et al., eds. *Epilepsy and mental retardation*. Petersfield, UK/Philadelphia: Wrightson Biomedical, 1999:165–178.
207. Anttila V, Rimpilainen J, Pokela M, et al. Lamotrigine improves cerebral outcome after hypothermic circulatory arrest: a study in a chronic porcine model. *J Thorac Cardiovasc Surg* 2000;120:247–255.
208. Iinuma K, Minami T, Cho K, et al. Long-term effects of zonisamide in the treatment of epilepsy in children

with intellectual disability. *J Intellect Disabil Res* 1998;42:68–73.
209. Mimaki T. Clinical pharmacology and therapeutic drug monitoring of zonisamide. *Ther Drug Monit* 1998;20:593–597.
210. Kochak GM, Page JG, Buchanan RA, et al. Steady-state pharmacokinetics of zonisamide, an antiepileptic agent for treatment of refractory complex partial seizures. *J Clin Pharmacol* 1998;38:166–171.
211. Kanba S, Yagi G, Kamijima K, et al. The first open study of zonisamide, a novel anticonvulsant, shows efficacy in mania. *Prog Neuropsychopharmacol Biol Psychiatry* 1994;18:707–715.
212. Okada M, Kaneko S, Hirano T, et al. Effects of zonisamide on dopaminergic system. *Epilepsy Res* 1995; 22:193–205.
213. Miyamoto T, Kohsaka M, Koyama T. Psychotic episodes during zonisamide treatment. *Seizure* 2000; 9:65–70.
214. Minato H, Kikuta C, Fujitani B, et al. Protective effect of zonisamide, an antiepileptic drug, against transient focal cerebral ischemia with middle cerebral artery occlusion-reperfusion in rats. *Epilepsia* 1997;38:975–980.
215. Mori A, Noda Y, Packer L. The anticonvulsant zonisamide scavenges free radicals. *Epilepsy Res* 1998;30: 153–158.
216. Bourgeois B. Drug interaction profile of topiramate. *Epilepsia* 1996;37:S14–S17.
217. Faught E, Wilder BJ, Ramsay RE, et al. Topiramate placebo-controlled dose ranging trial in refractory partial epilepsy using 200-, 400-, and 600-mg daily dosages. Topiramate YD Study Group. *Neurology* 1996; 46:1684–1690.
218. Shank RP, Gardocki JF, Vaught JL, et al. Topiramate: preclinical evaluation of structurally novel anticonvulsant. *Epilepsia* 1994;35:450–460.
219. Martin R, Kuzniecky R, Ho S, et al. Cognitive effects of topiramate, gabapentin, and lamotrigine in healthy young adults. *Neurology* 1999;52:321–327.
220. Tartara A, Sartori I, Manni R, et al. Efficacy and safety of topiramate in refractory epilepsy: a long-term prospective trial. *Ital J Neurol Sci* 1996;17:429–432.
221. Crawford P. An audit of topiramate use in a general neurology clinic. *Seizure* 1998;7:207–211.
222. Marcotte D. Use of topiramate, a new anti-epileptic as a mood stabilizer. *J Affect Disord* 1998;50:245–251.
223. Gordon A, Price LH. Mood stabilization and weight loss with topiramate. *Am J Psychiatry* 1999;156:968–969.
224. Richard D, Ferland J, Lalonde J, et al. Influence of topiramate in the regulation of energy balance. *Nutrition* 2000;16:961–966.
225. Loiseau P. New drug treatments in epilepsy. *Eur Neurol* 1994;34:4–10.
226. Adkins JC, Noble S. Tiagabine. A review of its pharmacodynamic and pharmacokinetic properties and therapeutic potential in the management of epilepsy. *Drugs* 1998;55:437–460.
227. Morimoto K, Sato H, Yamamoto Y, et al. Antiepileptic effects of tiagabine, a selective GABA uptake inhibitor, in the rat kindling model of temporal lobe epilepsy. *Epilepsia* 1997;38:966–974.
228. Leppik IE, Gram L, Deaton R, et al. Safety of tiagabine: summary of 53 trials. *Epilepsy Res* 1999;33: 235–246.
229. Trinka E, Moroder T, Nagler M, et al. Clinical and EEG findings in complex partial status epilepticus with tiagabine. *Seizure* 1999;8:41–44.
230. Dodrill CB, Arnett JL, Sommerville KW, et al. Cognitive and quality of life effects of differing dosages of tiagabine in epilepsy. *Neurology* 1997;48:1025–1031.
231. Kalviainen R. Tiagabine: a new therapeutic option for people with intellectual disability and partial epilepsy. *J Intellect Disabil Res* 1998;42:63–67.
232. Kaufman KR. Adjunctive tiagabine treatment of psychiatric disorders: three cases. *Ann Clin Psychiatry* 2000;10:181–184.
233. Ipponi A, Lamberti C, Medica A, et al. Tiagabine antinociception in rodents depends on GABA(B) receptor activation: parallel antinociception testing and medial thalamus GABA microdialysis. *Eur J Pharmacol* 1999;368:205–211.
234. Halonen T, Nissinen J, Jansen JA, et al. Tiagabine prevents seizures, neuronal damage and memory impairment in experimental status epilepticus. *Eur J Pharmacol* 1996;299:69–81.
235. Gao XM, Kakigi T, Friedman MB, et al. Tiagabine inhibits haloperidol-induced oral dyskinesias in rats. *J Neural Transm* 1994;95:63–69.
236. Matilainen R, Pitkanen A, Ruutiainen T, et al. Vigabatrin in epilepsy in mentally retarded patients. *Br J Clin Pharmacol* 1989;27:113S–118S.
237. Sander JW, Hart YM, Trimble MR, et al. Vigabatrin and psychosis. *J Neurol Neurosurg Psychiatry* 1991;54:435–439.
238. Gillham RA, Blacklaw J, McKee PJW, et al. Effect of vigabatrin on sedation and cognitive function in patients with refractory epilepsy. *J Neurol Neurosurg Psychiatry* 1993;45:1271–1275.
239. Mumford JP, Cannon DJ. Vigabatrin. *Epilepsia* 1994;35:525–528.
240. Veggiotti P, De Agostini G, Muzio C, et al. Vigabatrin use in psychotic epileptic patients: report of a prospective pilot study. *Acta Neurol Scand* 1999;99:142–146.
241. Brodie MJ, Pellock JM. Taming the brain storms: felbamate updated. *Lancet* 1995;346:918–919.
242. Livingston S. *Drug therapy for epilepsy*. Springfield, IL: Charles C Thomas, 1966.
243. Smith WL, Lowrey JB. The effects of diphenylhydantoin on mental abilities in the elderly. *J Am Geriatr Soc* 1975;23:207–211.
244. Stores G, Hart J, Piran N. Inattentiveness in school children with epilepsy. *Epilepsia* 1978;19:169–175.
245. Delaney R, Rosen AT, Mattson RH, et al. Memory function in focal epilepsy: a comparison of non-surgical unilateral temporal lobe and frontal lobe samples. *Cortex* 1980;16:103–107.
246. Matthews CG, Harley JP. Differential psychological test performances in toxic and nontoxic adult epileptics. *Neurology* 1975;25:184–188.
247. Thompson R, Huppert F, Trimble M. Anticonvulsant drugs, cognitive function and memory. *Acta Neurol Scand* 1980;80:75–81.
248. Loiseau P, Strube E, Broustet D, et al. Learning impairment in epileptic patients. *Epilepsia* 1983;24:183–192.
249. Dodrill CB. Problems in the assessment of cognitive effects of antiepileptic drugs. *Epilepsia* 1992;33: S29–S32.
250. Thompson PJ. Antiepileptic drugs and memory. *Epilepsia* 1992;33:S37–S40.
251. Pulliainen V, Jokelainen M. Comparing the cognitive

effects of phenytoin and carbamazepine in long-term monotherapy: a two-year follow-up. *Epilepsia* 1995; 36:1195–1202.
252. Dikmen SSP, Temkin NRP, Miller BM, et al. Neurobehavioral effects of phenytoin prophylaxis of posttraumatic seizures. *JAMA* 1991;265:1271–1277.
253. Smith K, Goulding P, Wilderman D, et al. Neurobehavioral effects of phenytoin and carbamazepine in patients recovering from brain trauma: a comparative study. *Arch Neurol* 1994;51:660.
254. Butlin AT, Wolfendale L, Danta G. The effects of anticonvulsants on memory function in epileptic patients: preliminary findings. *Clin Exp Neurol* 1980;17:79–84.
255. Beenen L, Lindeboom J, Kasteleijn-Nolst Trenite D, et al. Comparative double blind clinical trial of phenytoin and sodium valproate as anticonvulsant prophylaxis after craniotomy: efficacy, tolerability, and cognitive effects. *J Neurol Neurosurg Psychiatry* 1999;67:474–480.
256. Duncan JS, Shorvon SD, Trimble MR. Effects of removal of phenytoin, carbamazepine, and valproate on cognitive function. *Epilepsia* 1990;31:584–591.
257. Meador K, Baker G. Behavioral and cognitive effects of lamotrigine. *J Child Neurol* 1997;12:s44–s47.
258. Marciani M, Stanzione P, Mattia D, et al. Lamotrigine add-on therapy in focal epilepsy: electroencephalographic and neuropsychological evaluation. *Clin Neuropharmacol* 1998;21:41–47.
259. Dodrill C, Arnett J, Shu V, et al. Effects of tiagabine monotherapy on abilities, adjustment, and mood. *Epilepsia* 1998;39:33–42.
260. Richens A, Marshall R, Dirach J, et al. Absence of interaction between tiagabine, a new antiepileptic drug, and the benzodiazepine triazolam. *Drug Metab Drug Interact* 1998;14:159–177.
261. Kastberg H, Jansen J, Cole G, et al. Tiagabine: absence of kinetic or dynamic interactions with ethanol. *Drug Metab Drug Interact* 1998;14:259–273.
262. Meador K, Loring D, Ray P, et al. Differential cognitive effects of carbamazepine and gabapentin. *Epilepsia* 1999;40:1279–1285.
263. Leach J, Girvan J, Paul A, et al. Gabapentin and cognition: a double blind, dose ranging, placebo controlled study in refractory epilepsy. *J Neurol Neurosurg Psychiatry* 1997;62:372–376.
264. Dodrill C, Arnett J, Hayes A, et al. Cognitive abilities and adjustment with gabapentin: results of a multisite study. *Epilepsy Res* 1999;35:109–121.
265. Monaco F. Cognitive effects of vigabatrin: a review. *Neurology* 1996;47:s6–s11.
266. Monaco F, Torta R, Cicolin A, et al. Lack of association between vigabatrin and impaired cognition. *J Intern Med Res* 1997;25:296–301.
267. Guberman A, Bruni J. Long-term open multicentre, add-on trial of vigabatrin in adult resistant partial epilepsy. The Canadian Vigabatrin Study Group. *Seizure* 2000;9:112–118.
268. Provinciali L, Bartolini M, Mari F, et al. Influence of vigabatrin on cognitive performances and behaviour in patients with drug-resistant epilepsy. *Acta Neurol Scand* 1996;94:12–18.
269. Berent S, Sackellares J, Giordani B, et al. Zonisamide (CI-912) and cognition: results from preliminary study. *Epilepsia* 1987;28:61–67.
270. Neyens L, Alpherts W, Aldenkamp A. Cognitive effects of a new pyrrolidine derivative (levetiracetam) in patients with epilepsy. *Prog Neuropsychopharmacol Biol Psychiatry* 1995;19:411–419.
271. Mohamed K, Appleton R, Rosenbloom L. Efficacy and tolerability of topiramate in childhood and adolescent epilepsy: a clinical experience. *Seizure* 2000;9:137–141.
272. Svendsen T, Johannessen S, Nakken K. Topiramate—a new antiepileptic agent. *Tidsskr Nor Laegeforen* 2000; 120:1536-1538.
273. Khan A, Faught E, Gilliam F, et al. Acute psychotic symptoms induced by topiramate. *Seizure* 1999;8: 235–237.
274. Aldenkamp A, Baker G, Mulder O, et al. A multicenter, randomized clinical study to evaluate the effect on cognitive function of topiramate compared with valproate as add-on therapy to carbamazepine in patients with partial-onset seizures. *Epilepsia* 2000;41:1167–1178.
275. Stumpf D. Anticonvulsant use during pregnancy. *Clin Ther* 1985;7:258–264.
276. Scolnik D, Nulman I, Rovet J, et al. Neurodevelopment of children exposed *in utero* to phenytoin and carbamazepine monotherapy. *JAMA* 1994;271:767–770.
277. Reinisch J, Sanders S, Mortensen E, et al. *In utero* exposure to phenobarbital and intelligence deficits in adult men. *JAMA* 1995;274:1518–1525.
278. Vestermark V. Teratogenicity of carbamazepine: a review of the literature. *Dev Brain Dysfunct* 1993;6: 266–278.
279. Ornoy A, Cohen E. Outcome of children born to epileptic mothers treated with carbamazepine during pregnancy. *Arch Dis Child* 1996;75:517–520.
280. Koch S, Losche G, Jager-Roman E, et al. Major and minor birth malformations and antiepileptic drugs. *Neurology* 1992;42:83–88.
281. Paulson R, Sucheston M, Hayes T, et al. Teratogenic effects of valproate in the CD-1 mouse fetus. *Arch Neurol* 1985;42:980–983.
282. Lindhout D, Omtzigt J. Pregnancy and the risk of teratogenicity. *Epilepsia* 1992;33:s41–s48.
283. Samren E, van Duijn C, Koch S, et al. Maternal use of antiepileptic drugs and the risk of major congenital malformations: a joint European prospective study of human teratogenesis associated with maternal epilepsy. *Epilepsia* 1997;38:981–990.
284. Arpino C, Brescianini S, Robert E, et al. Teratogenic effects of antiepileptic drugs: use of an international database on malformations and drug exposure. *Epilepsia* 2000;41:1436–1443.
285. Moore S, Turnpenny P, Quinn A, et al. A clinical study of 57 children with fetal anticonvulsant syndromes. *J Med Genet* 2000;37:489–497.
286. Kennedy D, Koren G. Valproic acid use in psychiatry: issues in treating women of reproductive age. *J Psychiatry Neurosci* 1998;23:223–228.
287. Morrell M. The new antiepileptic drugs and women: efficacy, reproductive health, pregnancy, and fetal outcome. *Epilepsia* 1996;37:34–44.
288. Gualtieri CT. *Neuropsychiatry & behavioral pharmacology*. Berlin: Springer-Verlag, 1990.
289. Enrich HM, von Zerssen D, Kissling W, et al. Effect of sodium valproate on mania. The GABA-hypothesis of affective disorders. *Arch Psychiatr Nervenkr* 1980; 229:1–16.
290. Kerr MP. Topiramate uses in people with an intellectual disability who have epilepsy. *J of Intellectual Disability Research* 1998;42:74–79.

21
Lithium Salts

SUMMARY

After the long and rambling discussions of the previous chapter, is there anything left that one can say about lithium? Yes, there is, and not only its peculiar history and the quaint stories people tell about the curative value of lithium springs.

The use of lithium in patients with brain injury introduces the important issue of posttraumatic bipolar disorder. The success of lithium in patients with mental retardation reflects the prevalence of affective instability syndromes in that population. Lithium is also the first psychotropic drug to have been systematically investigated for the treatment or prevention of aggression.

LITHIUM SALTS

> *Prefrontal leukotomy has been performed recently on restless and psychopathic mental defectives in an attempt to control their restless impulses and ungovernable tempers. It is likely that lithium medication would be effective in such cases and would be much preferred to leukotomy (1).*

Natural spring waters containing lithium were reputedly used by the ancient Greeks as a treatment of ill humor and excitement. In the nineteenth century, lithium salts were added to patent medicine formulations, perhaps for their mild sedating properties. Lithium bromide was used as an anticonvulsant ["In epilepsy it is the best of all bromides" (Squires quoted in ref. 1)]. In the Southern states, there are several towns named Lithium Springs, old country towns where people would go to "take the cure." Lithium urate is quite soluble, and therefore, lithium salts were prescribed for the treatment of gout.

During the 1940s, lithium chloride was marketed as a salt substitute. It is a monovalent cation that resides just above sodium on the periodic table of the elements and shares some characteristics with sodium and potassium. Patients with cardiac disease would actually flavor their food with the its salty crystals, and a few deaths resulted. This experience probably contributed to the initial skepticism that greeted the idea that lithium was a psychotropic drug. Despite the signal work of the Australian John Cade and then the work of Poul Christian Basstrup and Mogens Schou in Denmark in the 1950s, lithium was not approved by the U.S. Food and Drug Administration until 1970, for the treatment of acute mania, and not until 1974 for prophylaxis in manic depression.

Cade had been looking for toxic nitrogenous substances in the urine of patients with mental disorders to test in guinea pigs. With lithium carbonate, the animals became lethargic and unresponsive (1). Although "it may seem a long distance from lethargy in guinea pigs to the excitement of psychotics," Cade gave lithium carbonate to 16 patients with chronic psychosis and reported remarkable results, especially in those with manic depression. This inferential leap still leaves one breathless. It led to the lithium era, one of the most important chapters in the history of psychiatry. Cade's genius was inspired not only by his experiments in lower animals. He cited as support for his findings that "the waters of certain wells (with) special virtue in the treatment of mental illness.... Very likely proportional to the lithium content of the waters." [As recently as 1994, it was suggested that "a statistically significant inverse correlation [exists] between mental hospital admissions, homicides, rapes and drug-related crimes and the lithium concentration in drinking water" (2).]

The old lithium springs are forgotten now; there are just quiet old country towns where no one goes to take the waters. The world's supply of lithium is mined just outside of Gastonia, NC, but there is not even an outlet shop at the plant. The stores nearby sell bottled tea laced with ginseng and gotu kola, not lithium bromide or lithium urate. No one still believes that lithium in the water supply has special virtue for mental illness. If there were enough lithium in the water supply to generate even a low therapeutic blood level, it would be grossly unpalatable. [Lithium elixir is singularly foul, and patients hate it. It is a hard taste to disguise. Shepherds out West use lithium, incidentally, to protect their sheep against predation by coyotes. They lace a fresh kill with lithium salts; when the coyote returns to enjoy his lamb, the horrid taste of lithium gives him a taste aversion that lasts forever (3).]

Lithium is indicated for the treatment of acute mania and the prophylaxis of manic and depressive episodes in patients with bipolar disorder. Its prophylactic effect is also felt in recurrent unipolar depression (4). The drug is also useful for people with severe mood swings; patients who are "cyclothymic," but not given to extremes of mania or depression. It augments the treatment of depression in patients who are refractory to antidepressant treatment (5) and in patients with obsessive-compulsive disorder who are refractory to the effects of serotonergic antidepressants (6).

Lithium is also effective for aggression. Its antiaggressive effects have been well documented and are equally impressive in studies of laboratory animals and in humans. In clinical populations, lithium has a relatively specific effect against aggressive behavior, not only in patients with affective disorders or intermittent explosive disorder but in aggressive patients with schizophrenia and in patients with dementia, traumatic brain injury (TBI), mental retardation, and Huntington's chorea. It is almost as effective in patients whose aggressive behavior is predatory rather than pathologic or temperamental, e.g., patients with antisocial personality disorder and children with conduct disorder. In animals, lithium reduces aggression in pathologic models, such as electroshock-induced aggression, as well as in predatory animals.

The use of lithium among patients with neuropsychiatric disorders is largely reflective of its use in the wider population of patients with mental illness: as a primary treatment for bipolar disorder and an alternative treatment for any other condition that is characterized by severe emotional instability or aggression. The use of lithium in patients with neuropsychiatric disorders, however, highlights a few issues that are especially important, if not unique, to these patients.

NEUROTOXICITY

I raised the issue of lithium-induced neuroprotection and neurononeogenesis with a measure of skepticism. It is not that the idea is absurd or that the research findings in laboratory animals and clinical samples are without merit but rather that they seem to fly in the face of long clinical experience with the drug. Patients as a group do not especially like taking lithium. In comparative studies, patients with bipolar disorders usually prefer carbamazepine or valproate; they associate lithium with tremor, sedation, cognitive blunting, memory, and motor impairment. Indeed, these are well-known side effects of the drug when optimal blood levels are exceeded. They may also occur at therapeutic blood levels. Lithium is sometimes associated with severe neurotoxic reactions, e.g., dystonia, and even these may occur at low levels.

One might expect that patients with neuropsychiatric conditions by virtue of their preexisting neuropathology or diminished cerebral reserve would be more susceptible to the neurotoxic effects of lithium. There is evidence to suggest this may be true (7). Even if the neurocognitive problems encountered with lithium, however, were magnified in patients with neuropathic conditions, they are far from benign in any class of patient. What always matters is the patient's individual susceptibility, not his or her cognitive status at baseline. In general, its cognitive toxicity is problematic.

Although some neuropsychological studies have reported no deficits in patients treated with lithium, most have reported impaired performance (8–10). Negative effects have been noted in digit symbol and trails in normal subjects (11); in tactual performance, finger tapping, block design, and digit symbol, trails, form board, and verbal comparison in patients with psychoses (12); in short-term memory in patients with depression (13,14); and in aggressive children (15). After lithium treatment is discontinued or when patients are switched to an alternative mood stabilizer, such as valproate, their cognitive status usually improves (16,17). Lithium can be sedating in both normal subjects and patients (18).

Such effects would ordinarily be troublesome for patients with head injury or mental retardation, but then lithium is rarely prescribed for any such patients unless they have severe and disabling behavioral problems or emotional instability, against which a modicum of impairment, if it occurred, would be an acceptable price to pay.

In patients with neuropsychiatric disorders, lithium has two advantages: it is a digital, not an analog, drug;

i.e., it tends to work either very well or not at all. It is rarely difficult to decide whether a lithium trial has been successful, especially if therapeutic blood levels are maintained, and as long as the positive effects of drug treatment, over several months in some cases, are allowed to unfold.

The second advantage of lithium is its unique toxicity profile. A low therapeutic index is sometimes thought to be a disadvantage, but a drug that makes the patient sick when toxic levels are approached has some real advantages for monitoring. High (but not dangerous) levels of lithium are associated with nausea, vomiting, diarrhea, irritability or sedation, and tremor or muscle rigidity. When this occurs, the medication can be stopped until the blood concentration falls to a safer level, and serious toxicity can be averted. A simple examination for hyperreflexia will usually reveal mildly elevated lithium levels. Conversely, tremor, polyuria, and polydipsia are side effects that occur within the therapeutic range. Although lithium toxicity can be catastrophic, it can be avoided by exercising the most elementary precautions.

The long-term studies of lithium have tended to concentrate on renal effects, which have probably been overstated (19), and thyroid effects, which need to be dealt with. Lithium-induced hypothyroidism is particularly common in people with mental retardation for reasons that are not apparent to me.

Extended periods of lithium intoxication can cause a persistent encephalopathy with dementia, extrapyramidal signs, or both. Less well appreciated is a syndrome of weakness, anergia, and memory impairment that sometimes occurs in patients on long-term lithium treatment. A similar effect is also seen with some antidepressants and with valproate. When it arises, it is usually necessary to find an alternative drug (17). Long-term studies of patients taking lithium however do not indicate that this syndrome is common (20). To confound the issue further, the clinical course of bipolar disorder by itself may be correlated with deterioration in neuropsychological performance (21). (In this study, 25 patients with bipolar disorders in the euthymic state were found to have cognitive dysfunction. The number of months that the patients had been manic or depressed was negatively correlated with their performance on neuropsychological tests. Memory and frontal/executive systems were selectively impaired, presumably the result of their illness and not the result of lithium treatment.)

Lithium is said to lower the seizure threshold (22), and it may, at supertherapeutic levels. At therapeutic blood levels, lithium treatment can actually raise the seizure threshold (23). In patients with epilepsy who have psychiatric disorders for which lithium may be indicated, carbamazepine and valproate are obvious choices, but lithium is not contraindicated.

LITHIUM COMPARED TO THE PSYCHOTROPIC ANTICONVULSANTS

For all practical purposes, lithium, carbamazepine/oxcarbazepine, and valproate are equivalent treatments for most psychiatric indications. When is it appropriate to choose one and not another?

The clinical features that are said to diminish the likelihood of a favorable lithium response in patients with bipolar disorder are salient only to a small degree in patients with neuropsychiatric conditions. These include dysphoric mania, rapid cycling, lack of family history of primary affective disorder, comorbid substance abuse, more than three affective episodes before treatment, and a particular kind of affective episode sequence (depression-mania-well interval as opposed to mania-depression-well interval). Valproate and carbamazepine are clearly more effective than lithium in cases of dysphoric mania and rapid cycling; both conditions are relatively common in patients with brain injury and mental retardation.

It is believed that the response for familial mood disorders is better with lithium and for acquired mood disorders better with carbamazepine and valproate. It is also believed that organic mood disorders respond well to carbamazepine and valproate and poorly to lithium (24). This, together with the neurotoxicity problem, has generally made lithium a second-choice alternative for patients with brain injury or mental retardation. So be it; there is not likely ever to be a head-to-head comparison to decide the issue.

BIPOLAR DISORDER FOLLOWING BRAIN INJURY

Depression is an extremely common problem in epilepsy, brain injury, and stroke, but in all these neuropathic conditions, bipolar affective disorder is relatively uncommon. Nevertheless, manic depression may arise *de novo* in all three conditions, in patients who were predisposed, for example, by virtue of family history. After TBIs, especially lesions to the orbitomedial frontal lobes, a rather impressive and persistent manic syndrome may develop, sometimes referred to as secondary mania (25,26). In people with brain injury and mental retardation, bipolar variants, such as mixed mania, schizophreniform symptoms, dysphoric mania, and rapid cycling are the rule rather than the exception (27–29).

Robinson et al. (30) prefer to use lithium for poststroke mania and consider carbamazepine and valproate to be secondary treatments. Bakchine et al. (26), conversely, proposed clonidine for persistent mania after brain injury. My colleagues and I used to prefer the psychotropic antiepileptic drugs, but currently, we are more likely to use an atypical antipsychotic.

AFFECTIVE INSTABILITY IN PATIENTS WITH MENTAL RETARDATION

Patients with mental retardation are prone to a wide range of psychiatric disorders, and most of them have been discussed in detail already. It is appropriate to reiterate, however, the degree to which emotional instability characterizes the neurobehavioral correlates of mental handicap. Sudden and extreme changes in mood, angry outbursts, good and bad days, or periods of cheerfulness or placidity punctuated by emotional overreactions or intervals or irritability and dysphoria—all these complicate the lives of some persons with mental retardation. The diagnosis of organic affective disorder or atypical bipolar disorder is often given to such problems. Antidepressants, atypical antipsychotics, and mood-stabilizing drugs are the most common interventions.

When a mood stabilizer is indicated, the choice may be lithium, carbamazepine/oxcarbazepine, or valproate, with reasonable assurance that one is likely to be as effective as another. The facts that epilepsy is so common in the severely retarded and that bipolar disorder, when it occurs, is likely to be manifestly atypical, usually incline the decision in the direction of one of the psychotropic anticonvulsants.

Nevertheless, in people with mental retardation, as in other classes of patients, success may be found with lithium when no other drug has been successful and in unusual conditions in which a likely response can hardly be predicted (31).

LITHIUM FOR AGGRESSION

The pharmacotherapy of aggressive behavior includes a number of drugs discussed throughout this volume. The serotonergic antidepressants have been especially prominent in this direction for the past several years, but lithium was the first specific antiaggression drug, followed by carbamazepine and then valproate.

Lithium was the first psychotropic drug found to possess specific antiaggression properties, originally in people with mental retardation (32) and then in violent prisoners (33). Lithium reduces territorial aggression in mice and hamsters (34); it can induce Siamese fighting fish to live together harmoniously in the same tank. Isolation-induced aggression and footshock-induced aggression decreases in lithium-treated rats (35), and the hyperaggressive and hypersexual behavior of cats and rats treated with p-chlorophenylalanine is inhibited by lithium in doses that do not inhibit motor activity (35). Lithium has reduced aggressive behavior in assaultive prisoners (36), aggressive mentally retarded people (37), and self-injurious mentally retarded people (38).

The site and mode of therapeutic action of lithium for aggression or for any of its psychiatric indications are unknown. The antiaggression is not necessarily mediated by mood stabilization; it is seen in animals and in people, whose aggressive behavior is instrumental rather than temperamental. Neurotransmitter effects linked to suppression of aggression include prostaglandin E_1 synthesis inhibition, enhanced reuptake of serotonin and norepinephrine, and a functional decrease in presynaptic dopamine. Lithium may also decrease dopamine and norepinephrine effects at postsynaptic receptors. It even may interfere with testosterone synthesis (39). In terms of a mode of action against aggression, however, the fact that its effects are, again, more or less equivalent to those of the anticonvulsants requires that a common mechanism be sought. This probably resides, as we have seen, in second messenger systems, gene expression, and synaptic plasticity.

LITHIUM FOR BRAIN INJURY

There are no controlled studies of lithium in patients with TBI, but there is an extensive anecdotal literature on its use in patient classes with organic brain syndromes of various types. Successful lithium trials were reported in four adults with severe TBI and aggressive and self-injurious behavior (40,41); in organic brain syndromes of "diverse etiology" (including TBI) characterized by affective instability (42); in one patient with TBI with agitation, confusion, and belligerence (43); and in one patient who became hypomanic after cerebrovascular accident and surgical trauma to the temporal lobe (44). In an open trial of lithium in 10 patients with TBI with "severe, unremitting, aggressive, combative or self-destructive behavior or severe affective instability," five had a dramatic response and one had a moderate response (45). The same research group reported good results with valproate in five patients with similar clinical problems who had failed on lithium, with "a lower propensity towards sedation and cognitive impairment" (46).

When should lithium be considered in a patient with TBI? When there is a traditional psychiatric indication and when other, less sedating drugs have failed. Not necessarily for classical affective disorders because these are not very common in patients with TBI, rather for its secondary indications, for conditions characterized by extremes of emotional instability, such as explosions of rage or violence. Lithium is one of the best of the antidepressant augmenters for refractory unipolar depression, but it is not quite as useful in patients with TBI who need augmentation. My colleagues and I tend to use a stimulant, a dopamine agonist, or a psychotropic antiepileptic drug first. For secondary mania associated with frontal lobe lesions, in our experience, an atypical antipsychotic usually works better.

LITHIUM INTERACTIONS

Lithium clearance is decreased by nonsteroidal antiinflammatory drugs, tetracycline, thiazide diuretics, and furosemide, but increased by verapamil, theophylline, and acetazolamide (47). Lithium can increase the likelihood of toxicity related to fluoxetine and carbamazepine, probably a pharmacodynamic interaction.

TERATOGENICITY

Lithium passes freely across the placental membrane, and the concentration in breast milk is one-third to one-half of maternal serum levels. Fetotoxicity was originally related to cardiac organogenesis (48,49). More recent reviews suggest that it is not a strong teratogen (50–53). It is probably less teratogenic than valproate, more or less the same as carbamazepine.

REFERENCES

1. Cade JFJ. Lithium salts in the treatment of psychotic excitement. *Med J Aust* 1949;36:349–352.
2. Schrauzer GH, De Vroey E. Effects of nutritional lithium supplementation on mood; a placebo-controlled study with former drug users. *Biol Trace Elem Res* 1994;40:89–101.
3. Smith DF. *Lithium and animal behavior*. Montreal: Eden Press, 1977.
4. Gerbino L, Oleshansky M, Gershon SI. Clinical use and mode of action of lithium. In: Lipton MA, Dimascio A, Killiam KF, eds. *Psychopharmacology: a generation of progress*. New York: Raven Press, 1978:1261–1275.
5. Heninger GR, Charney DS, Sternberg DE. Lithium carbonate augmentation of antidepressant treatment: an effective prescription for treatment—refractory depression. *Arch Gen Psychiatry* 1983;40:1335–1342.
6. Rasmussen SA. Lithium and tryptophan augmentation in clomipramine—resistant obsessive-compulsive disorder. *Am J Psychiatry* 1984;141:1283–1285.
7. Bell A, Cole A, Eccleston D, et al. Lithium neurotoxicity at normal therapeutic levels. *Br J Psychiatry* 1993; 162:689–692.
8. Henry GM, Weingartner H, Murphy DL. Influence of affective states and psychoactive drugs on verbal learning and memory. *Am J Psychiatry* 1973;130:966–971.
9. Ananth J, Ghadirian A, Engelsmann F. Lithium and memory: a review. *Can J Psychiatry* 1987;32:312–316.
10. Honig A, Arts B, Ponds R, et al. Lithium induced cognitive side-effects in bipolar disorder: a qualitative analysis and implications for daily practice. *Int Clin Psychopharmacol* 1999;14:167–171.
11. Judd LL, Hubbard B, Janowsky DS, et al. The effect of lithium carbonate on the cognitive functions of normal subjects. *Arch Gen Psychiatry* 1977;34:335–357.
12. Friedman MJ, Culver CM, Ferrell RB. On the safety of long-term treatment with lithium. *Am J Psychiatry* 1977;134:1123–1126.
13. Kusumo KS, Vaugn M. Effect of lithium salts on memory. *Br J Psychiatry* 1977;131:453–457.
14. Christodoulo GN, Kokkevi A, Lykouras EP. Effects of lithium on memory. *Am J Psychiatry* 1981;138:847–848.
15. Platt JE, Campbell M, Green MH. Effects of lithium carbonate and haloperidol on cognition in aggressive hospitalized school-age children. *J Clin Psychopharmacol* 1981;1:8–13.
16. Kocsis J, Shaw E, Stokes P, et al. Neuropsychologic effects of lithium discontinuation. *J Clin Psychopharmacol* 1993;13:268–276.
17. Stoll A, Locke C, Vuckovic A, et al. Lithium-associated cognitive and functional deficits reduced by a switch to divalproex sodium: a case series. *J Clin Psychiatry* 1996;57:356–359.
18. Reisberg B, Gershon S. Side effects associated with lithium therapy. *Arch Gen Psychiatry* 1979;36:879–887.
19. Jenner FA. Lithium and the question of kidney damage. *Arch Gen Psychiatry* 1979;36:888–890.
20. Mauri M, Laini V, Scalvini M, et al. Lithium safety in the prophylaxis of bipolar disorders: a study with plasma levels. *Eur Rev Med Pharmacol Sci* 1999;2:63–69.
21. Van Gorp WG, Altshuler L, Theberge DC, et al. Cognitive impairment in euthymic bipolar patients with and without prior alcohol dependence. A preliminary study. *Arch Gen Psychiatry* 1998;55:41–46.
22. Brumback RA, Weinberg WA, Herjanic BL. Epileptiform activity in the electroencephalogram induced by lithium carbonate. *Pediatrics* 1975;56:831–834.
23. Jus A, Villeneuve A, Gautier J, et al. Some remarks on the influence of lithium carbonate on patients with temporal epilepsy. *Int J Clin Pharmacol* 1973;7:67–74.
24. Dunn R, Frye M, Kimbrell T, et al. The efficacy and use of anticonvulsants in mood disorders. *Clin Neuropharmacol* 1998;21:215–235.
25. Krauthammer C, Klerman GL. Secondary mania: manic syndromes associated with antecedent physical illness or drugs. *Arch Gen Psychiatry* 1978;35:1333–1338.
26. Bakchine S, Lacomblez L, Benoit N, et al. Manic-like state after bilateral orbitofrontal and right temporoparietal injury: efficacy of clonidine. *Neurology* 1989;39: 777–781.
27. Bamrah J, Johnson J. Bipolar affective disorder following head injury. *Br J Psychiatry* 1991;158:117–119.
28. Jan J, Abroms I, Freeman R, et al. Rapid cycling in se-

verely multidisabled children: a form of bipolar affective disorder? *Pediatr Neurol* 1994;10:34–39.
29. Vanstraelen M, Tyrer S. Rapid cycling bipolar affective disorder in people with intellectual disability: a systematic review. *J Intellect Disabil Res* 1999;43:349–359.
30. Robinson RG, Starr LB, Kubos KL, et al. A two-year longitudinal study of post-stroke mood disorders: findings during the initial evaluation. *Stroke* 1983;14:736–741.
31. Fahs H, Beauquier-Maccotta B. Preventive role of lithium in self-injurious behavior: a case report. *Encephale* 1999;25:175–178.
32. Dostal T, Zvolsky P. Antiaggressive effect of lithium salts in severe mentally retarded adolescents. *Int Pharmacopsychiatry* 1970;5:203–207.
33. Sheard M. Effect of lithium on human aggression. *Nature* 1971;230:113–114.
34. Weischer ML. Uber die Antigressive Wirkung von Lithium. *Psychopharmacologia*1969;15:245–254.
35. Sheard MH. Effect of lithium on footshock aggression in rats. *Nature* 1970;228:284–285.
36. Sheard MH. Effect in the treatment of aggression. *J Nerv Ment Dis* 1975;160:108–118.
37. Worrall EP, Moody JP, Naylor GJ. Lithium in nonmanic depressives: antiaggressive effect and red blood cell lithium values. *Br J Psychiatry* 1975;126:464–468.
38. Cooper AF, Fowlie HC. Control of gross self-mutilation with lithium carbonate. *Br J Psychiatry* 1973;22:370–371.
39. Jefferson JW, Greist JH, Ackerman DL. *Lithium encyclopedia for clinical practice*. Washington, DC: APA Press, 1983.
40. Rosenbaum AH, Barry MJ. Positive therapeutic response to lithium in hypomania secondary to organic brain syndrome. *Am J Psychiatry* 1975;132:1072–1073.
41. Bellus S, Stewart D, Vergo J, et al. The use of lithium in the treatment of aggressive behaviours with two brain-injured individuals in a state psychiatric hospital. *Brain Inj* 1996;10:849–860.
42. Hale MS, Donaldson JO. Lithium carbonate in the treatment of organic brain syndrome. *J Nerv Ment Dis* 1982; 170:362–365.
43. Haas JF, Cope DN. Neuropharmacologic management of behavior sequelae in head injury: a case report. *Arch Phys Med Rehabil* 1985;66:472–474.
44. Levine LS, Glen MB, Wroblewski B, et al. Use of lithium carbonate and comprehensive behavioral treatment in two severely brain-injured patients. 1986.
45. Glenn M, Wroblewski B, Parziale J, et al. Lithium carbonate for aggressive behavior or affective instability in ten brain-injured patients. *Am J Phys Med Rehabil* 1989;68:221–226.
46. Wroblewski B, Joseph A, Kupfer J, et al. Effectiveness of valproic acid on destructive and aggressive behaviours in patients with acquired brain injury. *Brain Inj* 1997;11:37–47.
47. Ananth J, Johnson K. Psychotropic and medical drug interactions. *Psychother Psychosom* 1992;58:178–196.
48. Schou M, Amdisen A. Lithium and pregnancy-III, lithium ingestion by children breast-fed by women on lithium treatment. *BMJ* 1973;2:138.
49. Schou M. What happened later to the lithium babies? A follow-up study of children born without malformations. *Acta Psychol* 1976;54:193–197.
50. Leonard A, Hantson P, Gerber G. Mutagenicity, carcinogenicity and teratogenicity of lithium compounds. *Mutat Res* 1995;339:131–137.
51. Kucera V. Is lithium a teratogen? *Cas Lek Cesk* 1996; 135:726–728.
52. Altshuler L, Cohen L, Szuba M, et al. Pharmacologic management of psychiatric illness during pregnancy: dilemmas and guidelines. *Am J Psychiatry* 1996;153: 592–606.
53. Lanczik M, Knoche M, Fritze J. Psychopharmacotherapy during pregnancy and lactation. 1: pregnancy. *Nervenarzt* 1998;69:1–9.

22

Anxiolytics and Antipsychotics

SUMMARY

What exactly is an atypical antipsychotic drug? In pharmacologic terms, it is a serotonin (5-HT_{2A}) antagonist with weak effects on the D_2 dopamine receptor. In clinical terms, it is an antipsychotic drug that does not raise serum prolactin and has a low rate of acute and chronic extrapyramidal side effects. One clinical test for atypicality is whether the drug is tolerated by patients with Parkinson's disease who are also psychotic. In fact, atypicality is a not a categorical statement but a dimension.

The five atypical antipsychotic drugs currently available in the United States are more or less equally effective for schizophrenia. Clozapine is more equal than the others. They differ in their clinical effects, much as the conventional antipsychotics were different, depending on the idiosyncrasies of patient response. Where they differ most, however, is in their side-effect profiles. Clozapine, olanzapine, and quetiapine are associated with weight gain, hyperlipidemia, and type II diabetes; ziprasidone with QTc prolongation; and risperidone with extrapyramidal side effects.

The old neuroleptic drugs were never popular among neuropsychiatrists; not only because of the high rates of extrapyramidal side effects but also because of their negative effects on cognitive performance and the important observation that they retard recovery in experimental brain injury paradigms. That the neuroleptics are less effective than the atypical antipsychotic drugs is still a matter of debate. The atypical antipsychotic drugs are better tolerated by patients. Their effects on cognition and brain plasticity are still obscure.

Metoclopramide is a dopamine antagonist that is used to promote gastric motility. For that indication, it is often prescribed for patients with neuropsychiatric conditions. Metoclopramide, however, can cause depression, cognitive blunting, akathisia, and tardive dyskinesia. From the psychiatrist's perspective, there should be better ways to improve gastrointestinal function.

The benzodiazepines (BZs) have never been very popular in neuropsychiatry either. They can cause irritability, cognitive impairment, and disinhibition, but these side effects are probably overstated. I have argued that anxiety disorders tend to be underdiagnosed in neuropsychiatric patients. There is ample room for the BZs, especially for people with mental retardation.

Buspirone, conversely, has always been favored by neuropsychiatrists, partly because of its tolerability and mainly because of its usefulness as an augmenter to the antidepressants and mood stabilizers.

TRANQUILIZERS

Their old name was tranquilizers, major and minor. You hardly hear it anymore. It is an archaic term, impossibly optimistic and utterly sweet. The idea that a drug might induce a state of tranquillity seems quaint now, but it speaks to a time when psychopharmacology was a marvelous thing. There was no little harm that came from the wonder drugs of the 1950s and 1960s, but it rose from a surfeit of enthusiasm that is entirely understandable.

The tranquilizers are better now, tamed, as it were, and more focused. They have had a checkered history, but they are finding new therapeutic roles in the special populations.

ATYPICAL ANTIPSYCHOTIC DRUGS

In the United States, first-time prescription of an antipsychotic drug for a patient with schizophrenia is usually for one of the new atypical antipsychotics. In other countries, where more constraint is exercised on pharmaceutical expenditure, the atypical antipsychotic drugs are still used, but as second-choice drugs, when the conventional neuroleptic drugs have failed or after side effects have supervened. That is probably a false economy. If it is true that the atypical antipsychotic drugs provide superior efficacy, fewer side effects, and the prospect of better compliance, their greatest impact may be when they are used early in the course of the illness (1).

The degree to which the atypical antipsychotic drugs are clinically superior to the conventional neuroleptic drugs, at least for schizophrenia, has been the subject of much recent discussion. There is no question that clozapine has a unique level of efficacy; for the other drugs, the data are less secure. They all have a lower incidence of extrapyramidal side effects, however, and patients do prefer them (2,3).

The atypical antipsychotic drugs are defined by several criteria: (i) they have a greatly reduced incidence of acute and chronic extrapyramidal side effects and (ii) they do not raise serum prolactin levels (4). Both of these criteria speak to a relative weakness of dopamine antagonism at the D_2 receptor site. Weakness at D_2 is demonstrated in binding studies by the fact that they produce weaker catalepsy in rodents and also by the fact that they are well tolerated by patients with Parkinson's disease who are psychotic (5). The third defining criterion is blockade of the 5-HT_{2A} receptor. The addition of 5-HT_{2A} antagonism was thought to broaden the therapeutic activity of the atypical antipsychotics, maintaining control of positive symptoms of schizophrenia while improving negative or deficit symptoms and attenuating the severity of extrapyramidal side effects including tardive dyskinesia. Weak antagonism at D_2 combined with strong antagonism at 5-HT_{2A} was originally thought to be the essential characteristic of an atypical antipsychotic drug (5). Their alternative name is 5-HT/dopamine antagonists (SDAs).

There are other elements at play, however. The novel antipsychotic drugs differ among themselves in the degree of limbic versus striatal inhibition of dopamine function they possess. Clozapine and sertindole are the most limbic selective, followed by quetiapine, ziprasidone, olanzapine, and remoxipride. Risperidone has a preferential striatal profile that is similar to that of haloperidol (6), and it is the most harmful one of the group when it comes to extrapyramidal side effects (7). The activity of clozapine at the dopamine D_4 receptor may be important (8) as well as its activity at adrenergic and muscarinic receptors (9). There are so many aspects to these new agents that it is difficult at this point to say what exactly comprises atypicality beyond the defining criteria listed previously. Perhaps it is better to conceptualize atypicality as dimensional rather than categorical (10).

Clozapine

Clozapine is the prototypical atypical antipsychotic. It was discovered in 1960 and first became available for general use in Europe in 1975. Its use was sharply curtailed when a number of clozapine-treated patients developed agranulocytosis, and several fatalities occurred. It was not completely withdrawn from use, however, probably because it was observed from the beginning to be a superior antipsychotic drug for some patients with schizophrenia (11) and because of its favorable profile with respect to extrapyramidal side effects and tardive dyskinesia (12,13). Use of the drug was revived in 1989, after research clearly documented its superiority for a large segment of the population with schizophrenia (14). It was only available, however, within the constraints of a controlled monitoring system that clearly lessened the occurrence of severe hematologic side effects but also added inordinately to the cost of treatment.

The neuropharmacologic actions of clozapine are far ranging, and it is speculative to attribute its unique actions to any particular action. It is more likely that the differential effects of antipsychotic drugs in general and clozapine in particular are related to the interactions of their various receptor effects. It exhibits a relatively high affinity for the newly discovered dopamine D_4 receptor and a lower affinity for D_1 and D_2 receptors. It has high affinity for the 5-HT_{2A}, α_1-adrenergic and muscarinic M_1 receptors. It is a potent anticholinergic drug and a glutamate antagonist. 5-HT antagonism is thought to play a role in the success of clozapine for negative symptoms and for its reduced motor effects (15,16).

Agranulocytosis caused by clozapine is said to occur in 1% to 2% of treated patients. The monitoring system may reduce the rate by half, which is considerably higher, however, than any other antipsychotic drug (17). Sedation and weight gain are troublesome side effects, occurring equally with olanzapine and quetiapine, but less so with risperidone and ziprasidone. Seizures have been said to occur in 10% of clozapine-treated patients, which is almost certainly an exaggeration. Cotreatment with valproate is a common strategy.

Fluoxetine and fluvoxamine impede the metabolism of clozapine, raising serum levels substantially. One way to reduce the cost of clozapine prescription is to cotreat the patient with a very low dose of fluoxetine.

Clozapine is clinically effective for patients with neuropsychiatric conditions, and there are anecdotal reports of success in people with mental retardation and patients with traumatic brain injury (TBI) with psychosis and/or aggression, in patients with Parkinson's disease who develop psychosis, in patients with Huntington's chorea, and for some movement disorders such as tardive dyskinesia but also spasmodic torticollis (18–20). It is said to reduce limbic system kindling, a peculiar observation for such a strongly proconvulsant drug (21). The ability to reduce kindling may be a common feature of drugs that are effective for bipolar disorder; indeed, clozapine alone may be an effective treatment for bipolar disorder (22).

Among patients with schizophrenia, risperidone and olanzapine are prescribed more frequently than clozapine because they are usually as effective and their safety profile is much better. Nevertheless, as has always been the case with antipsychotic drugs, there are patients who respond better to clozapine than to any other drug. That is probably also true of patients with mental retardation and patients with brain injury, but in those groups, the newer atypical antipsychotic drugs are used much more than clozapine. As better alternatives are generated, the unique importance of clozapine is likely to fade.

Risperidone

Risperidone is the number one antipsychotic in the United States and it probably deserves to be. It may not be as dramatically effective for the refractory patient as clozapine is and it may be slightly more prone to extrapyramidal toxicity, but the two are broadly comparable (23). It is much safer than clozapine, with no greater tendency to catastrophic side effects than are any of the conventional neuroleptic drugs. The effective dose range is quite narrow. The draconian measures that guide clozapine monitoring are irrelevant to risperidone. It is not only prescribed for neuroleptic-refractory patients; American psychiatrists use it as the antipsychotic of choice.

The popularity of risperidone has begun to counteract the neuroleptic phobia that gripped the profession a few years ago, which is good and bad. It is good because patients who need them again have an appropriate level of access to antipsychotic drugs and because risperidone is probably safer than the conventional neuroleptics, at least in terms of tardive dyskinesia. It is bad because prescription of antipsychotic drugs is creeping up in the same patient groups who experienced its overprescription not too long ago and because risperidone may cause tardive extrapyramidal side effects (24).

The tendency of risperidone to induce extrapyramidal side effects, tardive dyskinesia, and even neuroleptic malignant syndrome is low compared with the conventional neuroleptic drugs and high compared with the other SDAs (7,25,26). However, D_2 blockade is a more prominent effect at higher doses of risperidone. Because most patients with neuropsychiatric disorders who need an antipsychotic drug respond to relatively low doses, the danger of extrapyramidal side effects is not great and is more than counterbalanced by its therapeutic utility. Risperidone has been effective in patients with TBI who are psychotic, in mentally retarded patients who are impulsive and aggressive, in patients with Parkinson's disease who are psychotic, in patients with dementia who are agitated, and in patients with Huntington's chorea (27–30).

Because risperidone was the first SDA available for routine prescription, without weekly complete blood counts and other monitoring, it has been used quite widely in facilities for mentally retarded people. Usually, it is substituted for an existing neuroleptic drug. The results have been quite favorable; it is rare that a patient will not tolerate the substitution. Simon et al. (31) were the first to report success with risperidone substitution. In our own clinical surveys, risperidone substitution has been associated with clinical improvement, or at least clinical stability, and frequently with resolution of neuroleptic side effects, most notably tardive akathisia.

Olanzapine, Quetiapine, and Ziprasidone

Olanzapine is a thienobenzodiazepine that has a receptor-binding profile similar to that of clozapine (32). It has thus far passed all the obligate tests required of a new atypical antipsychotic drug: it is at least as effective as haloperidol in the treatment of schizophrenia (33), more effective than conventional neuroleptics for patients with refractory schizophrenia (34), and useful for patients with psychosis with Parkinson's disease (35). For all practical purposes, it is risperidone with a slightly greater proclivity to sedation and weight gain and less tendency to extrapyramidal side effects (36). Rats cannot tell the difference between olanzapine and clozapine (37).

Quetiapine is a dibenzothiazepine derivative with a strong affinity for 5-HT_{2A} and a weak affinity for dopamine D_2 receptors. It has the same degree of limbic selectivity as clozapine (6) but is much less anticholinergic (38). It is as effective as conventional neuroleptics in the treatment of patients with schizophrenia (38,39). It is not likely to cause extrapyramidal side effects but may cause weight gain and sedation.

Gelenberg (40) says that "clinicians we know who have tried quetiapine in difficult to treat patients with chronic psychotic disorders have not been impressed with its efficacy." My experience with quetiapine in difficult to treat patients has been more positive thus far. Successful treatment with quetiapine requires much higher doses than the manufacturer recommended at first.

The latest addition to the atypical antipsychotic drugs is ziprasidone, a novel molecule with a relatively high ratio of 5-HT_{2A} to D_2 blockade, a moderate tendency to block norepinephrine and 5-HT reuptake, and unique agonist effects at the 5-HT_{1A} receptor. Thus, it has some of the pharmacologic properties of venlafaxine, imipramine, buspirone, and gepirone. It has lower affinity for muscarinic receptors than does clozapine or olanzapine. Its neurochemical "pedigree," then, is rather interesting and suggests that it might be a useful drug (41).

It does appear to be effective for patients with schizophrenia and schizoaffective disorder, with a low liability for motor side effects and, even more important, weight gain. It is, however, associated with QTc prolongation, and the physician is reminded of that in a black box in the package insert.

Comparing the Atypical Antipsychotic Drugs

Physicians and patients have many options when it comes to the treatment with antidepressants, mood stabilizers, and now antipsychotic drugs. In each category, there are so many good ones, how is one to choose? In each category, therapeutic efficacy is more or less equal, and the decision is usually made based on the side effects, possible drug interactions, and patient compliance.

It would appear that clozapine is a uniquely valuable drug in the treatment of patients with schizophrenia and that pattern may extend into other patient categories, including patients with neuropsychiatric disorders. Even if the danger of agranulocytosis were not so onerous, clozapine would still be a troublesome drug, if not for its proclivity to induce seizures, then certainly for its tendency to induce hyperphagia and weight gain.

Weight gain and other attendant problems, type II diabetes, and severe hyperlipidemia are significant problems with the atypical neuroleptic drugs, especially clozapine, olanzapine, and quetiapine. Obesity was a problem with the older neuroleptic drugs but not haloperidol; the phenothiazines were also associated with modest increases in serum triglycerides but not to the extreme degree observed recently (serum triglycerides >600 mg/dL) with clozapine, olanzapine, and quetiapine (42).

That clozapine, olanzapine, and quetiapine are structurally related dibenzodiazepines may account for their unique effects on serum lipid levels and their prominent effects on hyperphagia and weight gain. With respect to SDA-induced obesity, the drugs may be ranked as follows (43–45): clozapine → olanzapine → quetiapine → risperidone → ziprasidone.

The mechanism of SDA-induced hyperphagia is still obscure, although there are several candidate theories, and it is possible that multiple mechanisms are involved. The relative affinities of the atypical antipsychotic drugs for the histamine H_1 receptor, and the ratio of their 5-HT_{2A} affinities are robust correlates of the clinical findings (43). Atypical antipsychotic drugs that antagonize the 5-HT_{2A} receptor may decrease the responsiveness of pancreatic beta cells to blood sugar levels or they may have in some instances a direct toxic effect on the pancreatic islet beta cell (46).

If ziprasidone is unrelated to weight gain but equally effective for its clinical indications, it will be a welcome addition. The data thus far are encouraging, but one will have to be patient; it is still a very new drug. In the meantime, one is left with the problem of QT prolongation, and ziprasidone, after thioridazine, mesoridazine, and pimozide, seems to have the greatest proclivity in this direction.

The degree to which QT prolongation will be a problem with ziprasidone is not known. In the past, there were cases of sudden death reported in patients on thioridazine, but no such catastrophic consequences have been reported with ziprasidone. Routine electrocardiographic monitoring has not been recommended for patients on that drug, but it should not be prescribed for a patient with a congenitally prolonged QT interval, bradycardia, hypokalemia, or hypomagnesemia or a patient who is taking a diuretic, a tricyclic antidepressant, or any other drug that also may prolong the QT (47,48).

It is hard to measure the value of an antipsychotic drug relative to its peers until years have elapsed. Because the patients are likely to be treated long term, physicians will have time to compare the clinical effects of different ones. We may even discover that low-dose antipsychotic combinations are needed in some patients who are refractory to treatment.

NEUROLEPTICS

The prejudice against the use of conventional neuroleptic drugs in patients with neuropsychiatric disorders was never ill-founded. They were overused in residential facilities for the mentally retarded and in nursing homes for the elderly. The tardive dyskinesia epidemic was a regrettable chapter in the early history of psychopharmacology. During the 1950s, soon after they were introduced, several psychologists observed their blunting effects. Neuroleptic treatment was referred to as a "chemical lobotomy" (49,50).

The conventional neuroleptics, potent blockers of the dopamine D_2 receptor, are widely believed to compromise the recovery process for patients with TBI. This belief is an extrapolation from the preclinical studies of Feeney et al. (51), who demonstrated a slower rate of cortical recovery from experimental TBI in cats when they were treated with haloperidol. Presumably, this is related to deficits in dopaminergic neurotransmission, which have a role in the pathophysiology of TBI. Dopaminergic neurons are relatively stress sensitive. Their number and efficiency decline naturally with aging, and that decline may be aggravated by trauma or toxic exposure. Drugs such as haloperidol used to be prescribed quite frequently for patients with TBI in the agitated postcoma state, but only at the expense of retarding their cognitive and motor recovery. These observations were entirely in accord with human and animal studies of neuroleptic-induced anhedonia (52), dysphoria (53), and cognitive and motor impairment (54). Thus, in the treatment of patients with brain injury, it is believed that neuroleptics are relatively contraindicated.

The idea is that the D_2 blockers are antithetical to an optimal monoamine environment, a condition necessary for brain plasticity and that was addressed in Chapters 4 and 18. In those chapters, the ample preclinical evidence, the studies of patients with TBI and stroke, which are supportive if not confirmatory, were reviewed. Studies that show psychostimulants enhance recovery from TBI and stroke are consistent, as are preclinical observations that dopamine antagonists retard the recovery process. It is convincing to clinicians, who frequently observe an acceleration of functional recovery when patients with TBI or stroke are withdrawn from neuroleptic drugs (55). The paradigm suggests that stimulants and related drugs are rational pharmacotherapy for stroke and TBI and that neuroleptic therapy by extension is irrational.

The wider neurotoxicity of the neuroleptics, especially in people with mental retardation and those with autism, is dealt with extensively in Chapter 23. Patients with preexisting brain injury, acquired or congenital, are thought to be more vulnerable to the toxic effects of neuroleptics. Preexisting brain damage is sometimes listed as a risk factor for tardive dyskinesia. The clinical evidence is equivocal on this point, but the research is suggestive (56).

Neuropsychiatrists, therefore, have developed an affinity for drugs that are capable of enhancing cognitive/motor performance and promoting neuronal plasticity. These are the stimulants, *N*-methyl-D-aspartate antagonists such as amantadine, cholinesterase inhibitors such as donepezil, vitamin E, clonidine, deprenyl, and nimodipine. Although a positive effect is not invariant, or even predictable, for each drug, there is a clinical situation or an experimental paradigm that would seem to demonstrate a neuroprotective or a neurohabilitative effect. With respect to brain plasticity, therefore, they are "good drugs."

In contrast, the new antidepressants, buspirone, and the thymoleptic drugs are thought to have no effect, for better or worse, in terms of neuroprotection or neural recovery. The effectiveness of tricyclic antidepressants and BZs is marginal. These drugs are thought to be neutral with respect to brain plasticity.

The neuroleptic drugs, then, with clearly defined patterns of neurotoxicity in several different paradigms are necessarily "bad drugs" for the patient with a neuropsychiatric disorder. At least that is the prevailing wisdom, and I must take at least some responsibility for the eminence of that point of view.

If neuroleptic drugs do in fact impede cortical recovery in patients with TBI, can they ever be a good thing for young retarded people, those with autism, or those with epilepsy who are psychotic? If they are so likely to cause tardive dyskinesia and tardive akathisia in retarded people, if they are so damaging to the basal ganglia, could they possibly be good to prescribe for patients with TBI? If their negative effects on cognition and motor performance are so prominent, are they ever an appropriate treatment for people whose psychiatric symptoms arise in the context of preexisting cognitive and motor impairments?

Extrapolating from preclinical studies and research in other populations has been the métier of psychopharmacologic practice in neuropsychiatry. Because there is so little controlled research directed at the unique problems of special populations, one relies on theoretical considerations and clinical extrapolations. Because the latter are compelling, perfectly competent practitioners may agonize over the decision to prescribe a neuroleptic drug for a patient with brain injury or with mental retardation. Sometimes our preoccupation with neuroleptic toxicity militates against sound judgment.

I mentioned the psychologists who studied neuroleptic drugs during the 1950s and remarked on their blunting effects. The same researchers, however, were unable to demonstrate reliably a negative neuroleptic effect on neuropsychological performance in patients with schizophrenia. In fact, patients with schizophrenia always tend to test better when they are on antipsychotic drugs. This is not a surprising result, however, because the dramatic effects of neuroleptics on the disease itself far outweigh the relatively small cognitive effects (not to mention theoretical concerns over brain plasticity). Patients who are psychotic who respond to neuroleptics are able to focus their attention and to cooperate with testing in ways that untreated patients can never do. In fact, low-dose neuroleptics may actually enhance cognitive performance, for example, in attentional tasks (57); this is probably a presynaptic stimulant-like effect (58).

Perhaps the conventional neuroleptics are relatively contraindicated for patients with neuropsychiatric disorders. Sometimes, however, they happen to be necessary. When they are necessary, the urgency and severity of the clinical situation are far more important that the theoretical risk of a recovery effect or a negative neurocognitive effect.

Neuroleptic drugs are unsurpassed for the treatment of acute psychosis, hallucinosis, paranoia, agitation, disorganization, or assaultiveness in patients with a wide range of mental disorders. They have the undisputed value of rapid and reliable tranquilization. They are easy to use and come in all the necessary preparations, their side effects are well known, their results are predictable, and they are inexpensive. In patients with neuropsychiatric disorders, therefore, in whom there are several sound indications for acute neuroleptic treatment, it is specious to state that such treatment is irrational or counterproductive.

The problem in neuropsychiatry is that the short-term benefits of neuroleptic treatment segue into long-term treatment of limited utility. The following is a typical neuroleptic drug scenario for patients with TBI. A patient is treated with intramuscular and then oral haloperidol to control agitation and assaultiveness during emergence from coma. The drug is continued for months after the patient is discharged. Then the patient appears for evaluation at a rehabilitation facility and is anergic, depressed, and apathetic with fine and gross motor coordination problems and deficits in attention, memory, and emotional control. The neuroleptic drug is withdrawn, and there is immediate improvement.

This is a typical sequence of events for a mentally retarded person: any one of a number of antipsychotic drugs is selected to treat outbursts of temper, agitation, and aggression. Low doses have a beneficial effect for a while. Then the target behaviors recur, the dose is increased, and improvement follows, but it is not as dramatic as before. After a few more dose increases, the patient is on a high dose of a neuroleptic drug, but the effectiveness is limited. His or her behavior is as difficult as it was before the neuroleptic drug was prescribed. When attempts are made to lower the dose or to withdraw the drug entirely, the behaviors grow worse.

A similar train of events usually attends the prescription of high-potency neuroleptics such as haloperidol for children with autism who are hyperactive/disorganized and for the elderly in nursing homes who are easily upset and emotionally unstable.

In all the special populations, there are legitimate indications for long-term treatment with neuroleptic drugs. They are schizophreniform psychosis, various types of affective psychoses, movement disorders such as Tourette's syndrome, and some of the personality disorders that are associated with an extreme degree of emotional instability and impulsive, aggressive, or self-destructive behavior. In the special populations, like the "normal" populations, low to moderate doses are usually sufficient, and cotreatment with mood-stabilizing drugs may reduce the requisite neuroleptic load or eliminate the need for neuroleptic drugs. All the populations are equally prone to catastrophic neuroleptic toxicity, such as the neuroleptic malignant syndrome. Different groups are more or less vulnerable to the tardive syndromes, but risk management is amenable to careful monitoring, and vitamin E may exercise a protective influence. A small degree of cognitive blunting or motor impairment may be a necessary concomitant of neuroleptic treatment, but it is more than balanced by the therapeutic effects of the drugs in the face of devastating psychopathology.

The psychosis of temporal lobe epilepsy and compulsive self-injury is indications for long-term therapy in special populations. For the following problems, however, brief treatment courses are usually sufficient: immediate posttraumatic psychosis, peduncular hallucinosis, and the syndrome of huntingtonian movements, disorganization, and agitation that occasionally occurs during coma recovery after TBI.

In mentally retarded people, withdrawal from neuroleptic drugs can be an exorbitant and prolonged and compounded by the problem of tardive akathisia. In patients with TBI, prior neuroleptic exposure is not usually so intense, and therefore drug withdrawal is somewhat easier. The usual course is to gradually taper the neuroleptic drug dose after the patient's emotional state has been stable for a few weeks. Neuroleptics should usually be tapered, not withdrawn abruptly; abrupt withdrawal from neuroleptics may precipitate seizures (59) and can also be the occasion of prompt relapse of severe behavioral problems. Stepwise reduction by 25% decrements over 4 to 8 weeks usually averts such problems.

There are low- and high-potency neuroleptic drugs. The low-potency neuroleptics are thioridazine and chlorpromazine; they tend to be sedating, and thioridazine in particular is a strongly anticholinergic neuroleptic. It also appears that the neuroleptic chlorpromazine may impair short-term memory at doses less than those required to cause motor impairment (60). Such drugs probably should be avoided in patients with TBI. The high-potency neuroleptics are less sedating and are preferred when a neuroleptic is required. Representatives of this class include fluphenazine, trifluoperazine, and haloperidol. Haloperidol, however, commonly causes dysphoria. High-potency neuroleptics are more likely to cause acute extrapyramidal reactions and neuroleptic malignant syndrome. In fact, these fine distinctions are probably anachronistic. Most new patients, including patients with neuropsychiatric disorders, are treated first with an atypical antipsychotic drug.

Neuroleptics can lower the seizure threshold. Pimozide and fluphenazine are the two neuroleptics least likely to do so, and haloperidol and thioridazine are among those most likely to lower the seizure threshold (59,61) as well as clozapine.

Clozapine is not a neuroleptic drug. It is an antipsychotic drug, but, like risperidone, olanzapine, quetiapine, and ziprasidone, it does not deserve the appellation of neuroleptic. Extrapyramidal effects are neither intrinsic nor necessary to their clinical use. This brings us back to where we started, to the atypical antipsychotics.

The atypical antipsychotic drugs have changed psychopharmacology for severe mental illness in the same way that the psychotropic anticonvulsants have changed the treatment of severe affective disorders and the selective 5-HT reuptake inhibitors have changed treatment of virtually everything else. Because the risk of acute extrapyramidal side effects, tardive dyskinesia, akathisia, and neuroleptic-induced dysphoria is very low for the atypical antipsychotic drugs, they have moved a step higher on the neuropsychiatrist's hierarchy of preferred agents. At least with respect to the treatment of psychosis and agitation, they have moved a step higher than bad but sometimes necessary.

In the treatment of patients with neuropsychiatric disorders, however, one is necessarily interested in the cognitive effects of a given drug and its potential effects on brain plasticity. The conventional neuroleptics clearly leave a great deal to be desired with respect to the former dimension. With respect to cognitive effects, the atypical antipsychotic drugs are clearly superior. Studies in patients with chronic schizophrenia, elderly patients, and patients with bipolar disorder clearly indicate superior performance on neuropsychological tests when atypical antipsychotic drugs are substituted for conventional antipsychotic drugs (62–65).

The cognitive effects of different atypical antipsychotic drugs are different, probably related to their differential effects on acetylcholine and 5-HT$_2$ receptors. Clozapine improves attention, verbal fluency, and some types of executive function, but not memory; risperidone has consistently positive effects on working memory, attention, and executive function, but not verbal learning or memory; olanzapine improves verbal learning and memory, fluency, and executive function, but not attention, working memory, visual learning, or memory (65).

The neuroleptic effect on brain plasticity is unequivocally negative. The clinical manifestations of tardive dyskinesia are probably related to ultrastructural and synaptic changes in the caudate nucleus (66). Dopamine antagonists decrease synaptic density in the prefrontal cortex and induce long-term depression in the midbrain (67,68). In rats, even short-term administration of haloperidol decreases the activity of neurotrophic factors that support dopaminergic neurons during development and mediate synaptic and morphologic plasticity in numerous regions of the adult central nervous system (69). Less is known about the comparative effects of atypical antipsychotic drugs, although their reliance on dopamine antagonism is less profound. In fact, in some models, they are known to increase dopaminergic activity, for example, in the frontal cortex. When risperidone was substituted for haloperidol in a small group of patients with schizophrenia, for example, functional activation of the prefrontal, motor, and parietal cortex increased dramatically (70). Clozapine is less likely than conventional neuroleptics to induce neuropathologic changes in the caudate (66).

In terms of their cognitive effects and their influence on brain plasticity, the conventional neuroleptic drugs are, in my opinion, bad, and the atypical antipsychotic drugs are at least neutral. The experimental data on which these judgments are based are indirect and derivative, but they are reflective of clinical operations: for the first time in years, antipsychotic drugs (atypicals, to be sure) are being routinely prescribed for patients with TBI with severe agitation, mentally retarded people who are aggressive, and children with autism who are hyperactive and disorganized.

Am I entirely comfortable with this development? It certainly has enhanced the short-term practice. Perhaps, it will enhance the long-term outcome of the patients as much as it helps in the short term, but the medical literature is hardly enlightening on this point. Clinical trials, even of long-term medications like the antipsychotics, are based on treatment courses that run for weeks or months.

Metoclopramide

Metoclopramide is a special case, a dopamine antagonist that is not supposed to be a psychoactive drug; in fact, as a treatment for psychosis, it is an utter failure. As an inadvertent cause of typical neuroleptic toxicity, like akathisia or tardive dyskinesia, it is a complete success.

Metoclopramide is a procainamide derivative, the first of a new class of dopamine antagonists with pronounced effects on the gastrointestinal tract (altered motility and antiemetic effects) (71). It is prescribed for patients with TBI in a coma to alleviate some of the problems attendant with gastrostomy and gastric tube feeding, such as esophageal reflux and gastric distention because it decreases gastric emptying time. It is important to remember, however, that metoclopramide is also a centrally acting dopamine blocker, with particular affinity to the D_2 receptor; that it is in essence an neuroleptic with all the problems that drugs of this class may hold for patients with TBI, e.g., extrapyramidal effects, tardive dyskinesia, sedation, and possibly delayed or diminished recovery (72).

Cisapride was a novel agent unrelated to metoclopramide and that had no central nervous system effects. It was as effective in promoting gastric emptying and gut motility and was always preferred to metoclopramide. Then it fell victim to the QTc problem and is no longer available.

BUSPIRONE

Buspirone was introduced as an anxiolytic, but it is an azaspirodecanedione, not a BZ. It is said to be as effective as diazepam as an anxiolytic, but it is nonsedating and nonaddictive and does not seem to have any unfavorable neuropsychological effects. Its effect is not additive or synergistic with alcohol, overdose is not lethal (73,74), and it is not a respiratory depressant (75) or muscle relaxant.

Buspirone is an anxiolytic and is prescribed by physicians who are concerned with the potential toxicity of BZs and antidepressants, the alternative treatments for generalized anxiety disorder. Because the onset of action is over a few weeks, however, it is not the same as taking a Valium or a drink of whiskey. That kind of delay is not well tolerated by patients with anxiety who tend to worry about such things. It may be more acceptable to patients who have never taken benzodiazepines before, and have not been conditioned to seek immediate relief from anxiety.

Buspirone has a different kind of effect on anxiety, and its mechanism of action is, indeed, different from that of the BZs. It does not exert an anxiolytic effect by directly occupying the BZ receptor, although it may exert an indirect effect at this locus (76). There may be a γ-aminobutyric acid antagonist (GABA) aspect to its action, in contrast to the BZs, which are GABA-mimetic (77).

Buspirone does have pharmacologic effects on 5-HT, norepinephrine, and dopamine systems, although the nature of these effects and their relationship to the clinical actions of the drug are still not clear. It increases the activity of noradrenergic neurons that originate in the locus ceruleus, an event that is consistent with the absence of sedation or psychomotor impairment but hard to reconcile with its action as an anxiolytic (76).

It is a specific dopamine antagonist at the presynaptic receptor and has some postsynaptic dopamine blocking effects, such as reduction of apomorphine-induced stereotypy (77). It also increases the firing rate of midbrain dopamine neurons and is capable of reversing neuroleptic-induced catalepsy with more potency than amantadine (78).

In fact, the action of buspirone allows us to consider the clinical importance of drugs that exercise specific 5-HT receptors. Buspirone and its structural analogues gepirone and ipsapirone are 5-HT agonists at the 5-HT_{1A} receptor (78) and reduce 5-HT turnover by inhibiting the firing rate of 5-HT neurons in the dorsal raphe. They decrease striatal 5-HT concentration and the number of 5-HT binding sites in the frontal cortex (77). It is possible that the effect of buspirone in reducing neuroleptic-induced catalepsy is a function of its anti–5-HT effect, in contrast to the selective 5-HT reuptake inhibitors, which induce a hypodopaminergic state and can cause extrapyramidal side effects such as akathisia. In some patients, buspirone can improve akathisia associated with TBI.

Little, if anything, is known about buspirone and brain plasticity. In one paradigm, 5-HT_{1A} agonist pretreatment attenuated ethanol-induced neurotoxicity (79).

The ambiguity of its neurochemical profile is a measure of one's clinical uncertainty about what exactly buspirone is good for. No doubt it is an effective treatment for generalized anxiety disorder, and its many advantages over the BZs guarantee its place in the formulary of useful psychotropic drugs. Its neuropsychiatric indications, however, may be much broader, and it may prove to be a very important drug for some clinical problems that so far have been resistant to pharmacotherapy.

Buspirone has been effective in the treatment of agitation associated with dementia (80) and head injury (81); this is a therapeutic effect that comes on almost immediately, in contrast to the 2-week latency of its anxiolytic effects. It has been reported to be effective in controlling aggression, self-injurious behavior, and psychosis in patients with mental retardation (82,83), and aggression and hyperactivity in patients with autism (84). It is one of the first drugs prescribed for aggressive behavior in patients who are developmentally handicapped. It does not always work, but a therapeutic trial is easy and trouble free, and when it does work, the effect never wanes.

We have had positive effects in the treatment of akathisia, anxiety, and depression after head injury, and it appears to be particularly effective in relatively intact patients with temporal lobe symptoms such as somatic preoccupation, hypochondriasis, nervousness, and the peculiar kind of turgid self-concern one learns to associate with temporal lobe lesions. It is particularly effective as an augmenter to lithium, valproate, or carbamazepine in aggressive patients with brain injury. Its positive effects on agitation during the coma-recovery phase after TBI are not especially impressive, but occasionally (sometimes rarely) it works when nothing else does.

Buspirone is commonly used by psychiatrists as an antidepressant augmenter and as adjunctive treatment for obsessive-compulsive disorder. It is useful for children with attention deficit/hyperactivity disorder who are anxious, temperamental, or oppositional.

Considering the extremely favorable side-effect profile of buspirone, the possibility of positive effects on neuropsychological performance, and its general profile as a stimulator of monoaminergic activity, it should be an important compound to investigate further for patients with TBI. It works quickly, the dose range is narrow, and the initiation of treatment does not require intensive medical monitoring, as do carbamazepine, lithium, and the beta-blockers. We need to discover which patients buspirone will benefit and exactly how it works.

Because we have claimed that the side effects of buspirone are very mild, it is necessary to add that they may be intolerable. Because the benefit of drug treatment comes on slowly and usually after a latency of several weeks and the side effects come on early, people will stop taking the drug, saying that "it didn't work, and it made me light-headed (or, dizzy)" (the two most common side effects). The others are headache, nervousness, diarrhea, paresthesia, excitation, and sweating/clamminess (85). The side effects of dizziness, lightheadedness, and headache limit its appeal to some patients with postconcussion syndrome.

BENZODIAZEPINES

BZs do not have a strong history of prescription for special populations because they are a troublesome class of drugs and never seem to have worked very well. Occasionally a patient with TBI who had insomnia, agitation, or anxiety or panic did well on one of the BZs without any subsequent difficulties, but this is rare. BZs tend to impair memory (86–88) and may be disinhibiting, like alcohol and the barbiturates (89). This may account for why they are rarely preferred drugs for TBI. Neither problem represents an invariant effect, and there is no need to take that occasional patient who responds to a BZ off the drug simply because of a theoretical side effect. [Preclinical studies suggest that GABAergic drugs may actually improve recovery from brain injury (90).]

Moreover, taking the patient off the drug may not be that easy. BZ withdrawal has proven to be the major difficulty of long-term treatment rebound anxiety or panic, restlessness, insomnia, apprehension, dizziness, nausea, tremor, and seizures (91). It is difficult to know what is rebound from preexisting symptoms and what is new and entirely withdrawal induced.

BZ withdrawal may be very important, however, in a patient who shows signs of depression, psychomotor retardation, cognitive or motor impairment, or failure to progress satisfactorily in therapy. Depression, anergia, and lack of motivation are some of the most troubling side effects of prolonged treatment. They may be more likely to occur in patients on long-acting BZs because the drugs will tend to accumulate, especially in elderly patients or patients on concomitant therapy with cimetidine (92).

There are several BZs from which to choose. The various compounds are usually differentiated based on metabolism, whether psychologically active metabolites are formed from the parent compound, and the half-life of the drug. The reason why clonazepam and lorazepam are currently favored as acute anxiolytics is that they have no active metabolites whose metabolism and elimination may be extremely slow. The elimination of lorazepam and clonazepam is intermediate, neither fast, like triazolam, nor slow, like diazepam or chlordiazepoxide. Thus, there is not the danger one faces with diazepam, for example, of gradual accumulation over time or with triazolam, for example, of early morning insomnia or rebound anxiety (93). Lorazepam also has the advantage of prompt and reliable action with intramuscular injection (94). Clonazepam has the special advantages of antimanic activity and antiepileptic activity in the oral form.

Alprazolam is equal to diazepam as an anxiolytic and to imipramine as an antidepressant and antipanic drug. For a short while, it was the perfect drug and a mainstay of outpatient psychiatric treatment. Then it turned out to be even more difficult to be withdrawn from than the other BZs, with the problems of rebound panic, nocturnal panic, a unique withdrawal syndrome, and occasionally seizures (95,96).

The other new BZ was triazolam, a sedative with an amazingly short onset of action and a short duration of action that rendered it free of morning hangovers. Short-acting BZs such as triazolam and alprazolam, however, may be more likely to induce rebound symptoms because they are eliminated quickly; longer acting BZs, eliminated more slowly, may be less likely to cause rebound (97). There have also been reports of transient global amnesia with triazolam, especially when it is taken with alcohol (98).

Both alprazolam and triazolam have been associated with severe disorganizing side effects such as depression (96), mania (99), and paroxysmal excitement (100). The clinical problem is similar to akathisia with neuroleptics. It is too easy for the clinician to mistake BZ-induced excitement or agitation for a recurrent symptom of what the drug was originally prescribed for; therefore, the dose is increased, the problem grows worse, the patient is finally judged to be psychotic, and a neuroleptic is prescribed. It is the kind of vicious circle that leads to unnecessary hospitalization, misdiagnosis, and long-term treatment for an iatrogenic disease.

There is a small role for BZs in patients with TBI, especially for patients with associated cervical injuries and patients with spasticity. Diazepam, which is a particularly good muscle relaxant, may be very good for posttraumatic headaches. Midazolam, a parenteral BZ for anesthesia induction, is used occasionally to control acute behavioral outbursts (101).

In the past, BZs were discouraged in mentally retarded populations, ostensibly because of their disinhibiting effects and the occasional dysphoria that occurs with their use in the long term. The experience with clonazepam, often used as an anticonvulsant, was discouraging. Patients were unduly sedated, irritability was a problem, and tolerance to the anticonvulsant effects developed (102).

In fact, BZs have not been used very much in the mentally retarded because people tend to forget that those with mental retardation are prone to anxiety or panic just as normal people are. The occurrence of aggression, self-injury, screaming, insomnia, or angry outbursts in mentally retarded people is rarely attributed to anxiety, but it may be. The indications for BZ in those with mental retardation conform rather closely with the general indications for their use. It is likely that they are underused.

REFERENCES

1. Lieberman JA. Atypical antipsychotic drugs as a first-line treatment of schizophrenia: a rationale and hypothesis. *J Clin Psychiatry* 1996;57:68–71.
2. Kennedy E, Song F, Hunter R, et al. Risperidone versus typical antipsychotic medication for schizophrenia. *Cochrane Database Sys Rev* 2000.
3. Chakos M, Lieberman J, Hoffman E, et al. Effectiveness of second-generation antipsychotics in patients with treatment-resistant schizophrenia: a review and meta-analysis of randomized trials. *Am J Psychiatry* 2001;158:518–526.
4. Kinon BJ, Leiberman JA. Mechanisms of action of atypical antipsychotic drugs: a critical analysis. *Psychopharmacology* 1996;124:2–34.
5. Meltzer HY, Matsubara S, Lee J-C. Classification of typical and typical antipsychotic drugs on the basis of dopamine D-1, D-2 and serotonin2 pKi values. *J Pharmacol Exp Ther* 1989;251:238–246.
6. Arnt J, Skarsfeldt T. Do novel antipsychotics have similar pharmacologic characteristics? A review of the evidence. *Neuropsychopharmacology* 1998;18:63–101.
7. Knable MB, Heinz A, Raedler T, et al. Extrapyramidal side effects with risperidone and haloperidol at comparable D2 receptor occupancy levels. *Psychiatry Res* 1997;75:91–101.
8. Seeman P, Corbett R, Van Tol HH. Atypical neuroleptics have low affinity for dopamine D2 receptors or are selective for D4 receptors. *Neuropsychopharmacology* 1997;16:93–110.
9. Meltzer HY. Role of serotonin in the action of atypical antipsychotic drugs. *Clin Neurosci* 1995;3:64–75.
10. Stip E. Novel antipsychotics: issues and controversies. Typicality of atypical antipsychotics. *J Psychiatry Neurosci* 2000;25:137–153.
11. Gerlach J, Koppelhus P, Helweg E, et al. Clozapine and haloperidol in a single-blind cross-over trial: therapeutic and biochemical aspects in the treatment of schizophrenia. *Acta Psychiatr Scand* 1974;50:410–424.
12. Gerlach J, Thorsen K, Fog R. Extrapyramidal reactions

and amine metabolites in cerebrospinal fluid during haloperidol and clozapine treatment of schizophrenic patients. *Psychopharmacologia* 1975;40:341–350.
13. Bablenis E, Weber SS, Wagner RL. Clozapine: a novel antipsychotic agent. *Ann Pharmacother* 1989;23: 109–115.
14. Kane J, Honigfeld G, Singer J, et al. Clozaril Collaborative Study Group. Clozapine for the treatment-resistant schizophrenic. *Arch Gen Psychiatry* 1988;45: 789–796.
15. Lidsky TI, Yablonsky-Alter E, Banerjee SP, et al. Antiglutamatergic effects of clozapine. *Neurosci Lett* 1993; 163:155–158.
16. Brunello NP, Masotto CP, Steardo LM, et al. New insights into the biology of schizophrenia through the mechanism of action of clozapine. *Neuropsychopharmacology* 1995;13:177–213.
17. Alvir JMJ, Lieberman JAM, Safferman AZM, et al. Clozapine-induced agranulocytosis. *N Engl J Med* 1993;329:162–167.
18. Sajatovic MM, Verbanac PM, Ramirez LFM, et al. Clozapine treatment of psychiatric symptoms resistant to neuroleptic treatment in patients with Huntington's chorea. *Neurology* 1991;41:156.
19. Sajatovic M, Ramirez LF, Kenny JT, et al. The use of clozapine in borderline-intellectual-functioning and mentally retarded schizophrenic patients. *Compr Psychiatry* 1994;35:29–33.
20. Rubin M, Langa A. Clozapine, mental retardation and severe psychiatric illness: clinical response in the first year. *Harv Rev Psychiatry*, 1995;3:293–294.
21. Graham SR, Kokkinidis L. Clozapine inhibits limbic system kindling: implications for antipsychotic action. *Brain Res Bull* 1993;30:597–605.
22. Tohen M, Zarate CA Jr. Antipsychotic agents and bipolar disorder. *J Clin Psychiatry* 1998;59:38–48.
23. Bondolfi G, Dufour H, Patris M. Risperidone versus clozapine in treatment-resistant chronic schizophrenia: a randomized, double-blind study. *Am J Psychiatry* 1998;155:499–504.
24. Chouinard GM, Jones BM, Remington GM, et al. A Canadian multicenter placebo-controlled study of fixed doses of risperidone and haloperidol in the treatment of chronic schizophrenic patients. *J Clin Psychopharmacol* 1993;13:25–40.
25. Bajjoka I, Patel T, O'Sullivan T. Risperidone-induced neuroleptic malignant syndrome. *Ann Emerg Med* 1997;30:698–700.
26. Gutierrez-Esteinou R, Grebb JA. Risperidone: an analysis of the first three years in general use. *Int Clin Psychopharmacol* 1997;4:3–10.
27. Borre RV, Vermote R, Buttiens M, et al. Risperidone as add-on therapy in behavioural disturbances in mental retardation: a double-blind placebo-controlled crossover study. *Acta Psychiatr Scand* 1993;87:167–171.
28. Furmaga KMP, DeLeon OAM, Sinha SBM, et al. Risperidone in the treatment of patients with refractory psychosis due to brain injury. American Psychiatric Association 148th Annual Meeting, 1995.
29. Reveley MA, Dursun SM, Andrews H. A comparative trial use of sulpiride and risperidone in Huntington's disease: a pilot study. *J Psychopharmacol* 1996;10: 162–165.
30. Workman RH Jr, Orengo CA, Bakey AA, et al. The use of risperidone for psychosis and agitation in demented patients with Parkinson's disease. *J Neuropsychiatry Clin Neurosci* 1997;9:594–597.
31. Simon EW, Blubaugh KM, Pippidis M. Substituting traditional antipsychotics with risperidone for individuals with mental retardation. *Ment Retard* 1996;34:3 59–366.
32. Robertson GS, Fibiger HC. Effects of olanzapine on regional c-fos expression in rat forebrain. *Neuropsychopharmacology*, 1996;14:105–110.
33. Kando JC, Shepski JC, Satterlee W, et al. Olanzapine: a new antipsychotic agent with efficacy in the management of schizophrenia. *Ann Pharmacother* 1997; 31:1325–1334.
34. Martin J, Gomez J, Garcia-Bernardo E, et al. Olanzapine in treatment-refractory schizophrenia: results of an open label study. *J Clin Psychiatry* 1997;58:479–483.
35. Wolters ECM, Jansen ENHM, Tuynman-Qua HGM, et al. Olanzapine in the treatment of dopaminomimetic psychosis in patients with Parkinson's disease. *Neurology* 1996;47:1085–1087.
36. Tran P, Hamilton S, Kuntz A, et al. Double-blind comparison of olanzapine versus risperidone in the treatment of schizophrenia and other psychotic disorders. *J Clin Psychopharmacol* 1997;17:407–418.
37. Porter JH, Strong SE. Discriminative stimulus control with olanzapine: generalization to the atypical antipsychotic clozapine. *Psychopharmacology* 1996;128: 216–219.
38. Small J, Hirsch S, Arvanitis L, et al. Quetiapine in patients with schizophrenia. *Arch Gen Psychiatry* 1998; 54:549–557.
39. Peuskens J, Link CG. A comparison of quetiapine and chlorpromazine in the treatment of schizophrenia. *Acta Psychiatr Scand* 1997;96:265–273.
40. Gelenberg A. Quetiapine (Seroquel): another 'atypical neuroleptic'. *Biol Ther Psychiatry Newslett* 1998;21: 1–2.
41. Daniel D, Zimbroff D, Potkin S, et al. Ziprasidone 80 mg/day and 160 mg/day in the acute exacerbation of schizophrenia and schizoaffective disorder: a 6-week placebo-controlled trial. *Neuropsychopharmacology* 1999;24:491–505.
42. Meyer J. Novel antipsychotics and severe hyperlipidemia. *J Clin Psychopharmacol* 2001;21:374.
43. Wirshing D, Wirshing W, Kysar L, et al. Novel antipsychotics: comparison of weight gain liabilities. *J Clin Psychiatry* 1999;60:358–363.
44. Taylor D, McAskill R. Atypical antipsychotics and weight gain—a systematic review. *Acta Psychiatr Scand* 2000;101:416–432.
45. Wetterling T. Bodyweight gain with atypical antipsychotics. A comparative review. *Drug Saf* 2001;24: 59–73.
46. Goldstein L, Henderson D. Atypical antipsychotic agents and diabetes mellitus. *Prim Psychiatry* 2000;7: 65–68.
47. Buckley N, Sanders P. Cardiovascular adverse effects of antipsychotic drugs. *Drug Saf* 2000;23:215–228.
48. Gury C, Canceil O, Iaria P. Antipsychotic drugs and cardiovascular safety: current studies of prolonged QT interval and risk of ventricular arrhythmia. *Encephale* 2000;26:62–72.
49. Porteus SD. Maze test reactions after chlorpromazine. *J Consult Psychol* 1957;18:2–8.
50. Daston PG. Effects of two phenothiazine drugs on

concentrative attention span of chronic schizophrenics. *J Clin Psychol* 1959;15:106–109.
51. Feeney DM, Gonzalez A, Law WA. Amphetamine, haloperidol and experience interact to affect rate of recovery after motor cortex surgery. *Science* 1982;217: 855–857.
52. Wise RA. Neuroleptics and operant behavior: the anhedonia hypothesis. *Behav Brain Sci* 1982;5:39–87.
53. Caine ED, Polinski RJ. Haloperidol-induced dysphoria in patients with Tourette syndrome. *Am J Psychiatry* 1979;136:1216–1217.
54. Killian GA, Holzman PS, Davis JM, et al. Effects of psychotropic medication on selected cognitive and perceptual measures. *J Abnorm Psychol* 1984;93: 58–70.
55. Stanislav S. Cognitive effects of antipsychotic agents in persons with traumatic brain injury. *Brain Inj* 1997; 11:335–341.
56. Kane JM, Smith JM. Tardive dyskinesia, prevalence and risk factors. *Arch Gen Psychiatry* 1982;39:473–481.
57. Gualtieri CT, Hicks RE. Stimulants and neuroleptics in hyperactive children. *J Am Acad Child Adolesc Psychiatry* 1985;24:363–364.
58. Gualtieri CT, Patterson DR. Neuroleptic-induced tics. *Am J Psychiatry* 1986;143:1176–1177.
59. Itil TM, Soldatos C. Epileptogenic side effects of psychotropic drugs. *JAMA* 1980;244:1460–1463.
60. Johnson FN. Psychoactive drugs and stimulus analysis: III. Adjustment of behavioral measures for drug-induced memory effects and state dependence: the case of chlorpromazine. *Int J Neurosci* 1983;20: 25–32.
61. Oliver AP, Luchins DJ, Wyatt RJ. Neuroleptic-induced seizures: an in vitro technique for assessing relative risk. *Arch Gen Psychiatry* 1982;39:206–209.
62. Reinares M, Martinez-Aran A, Colom F, et al. Long-term effects of the treatment with risperidone versus conventional neuroleptics on the neuropsychological performance of euthymic bipolar patients. *Acta Esp Psiquiatr* 2000;28:231–238.
63. Byerly M, Weber M, Brooks D, et al. Antipsychotic medications and the elderly: effects on cognition and implications for use. *Drugs Aging* 2001;18:45–61.
64. Cuesta M, Peralta V, Varzuela A. Effects of olanzapine and other antipsychotics on cognitive function in chronic schizophrenia: a longitudinal study. *Schizophr Res* 2001;48:17–28.
65. Meltzer H, McGurk S. The effects of clozapine, risperidone, and olanzapine on cognitive function in schizophrenia. *Schizophr Bull* 1999;25:233–255.
66. Harrison P. The neuropathological effects of antipsychotic drugs. *Schizophr Res* 1999;40:87–99.
67. Sugahara M, Shiraishi H. Synaptic density of the prefrontal cortex regulated by dopamine instead of serotonin in rats. *Brain Res* 1998;814:143–156.
68. Thomas M, Malenka R, Bonci A. Modulation of long-term depression by dopamine in the mesolimbic system. *J Neurosci* 2000;20:5581–5586.
69. Dawson N, Hamid E, Egan M, et al. Changes in the pattern of brain-derived neurotrophic factor immunoreactivity in the rat brain after acute and subchronic haloperidol treatment. *Synapse* 2001;39:70–81.
70. Honey G, Bullmore E, Soni W, et al. Differences in frontal cortical activation by a working memory task after substitution of risperidone for typical antipsychotic drugs in patients with schizophrenia. *Proc Natl Acad Sci U S A* 1999;96:13432–13437.
71. Harrington RA, Hamilton CW, Brogden RN, et al. *Drugs* 1983;25:451–494.
72. Albibi R, McCallum RW. Metoclopramide: pharmacology and clinical application. *Ann Intern Med* 1983; 98:86–95.
73. Kastenholz KV, Crismon ML. Buspirone, a novel nonbenzodiazepine anxiolytic. *Clin Pharm* 1984;3: 600–607.
74. Staughan JL, Conradie EA. Buspirone—frontrunner of a new genre of anxiolytics. *South Am Med J* 1988; 75:441–444.
75. Garner SJ, Eldridge FL, Wagner PG, et al. Buspirone, an anxiolytic drug that stimulates respiration. *Am Rev Respir Dis* 1989;139:946–950.
76. Skolnick P, Paul SM, Weissman BA. Preclinical pharmacology of buspirone hydrochloride. *Pharmacotherapy* 1984;4:308–314.
77. Eison AS, Temple DL. Buspirone: review of its pharmacology and current perspectives on its mechanisms of action. *Am J Med* 1986;80:1–9.
78. Goa KL, Ward A. Buspirone: a preliminary review of its pharmacological properties and therapeutic efficacy as an anxiolytic. *Drugs* 1986;32:114–129.
79. Eriksen J, Gillespie R, Druse M. Effects of in utero ethanol exposure and maternal treatment with a 5-HT(1A) agonist on S100B-containing glial cells. *Brain Res Dev Brain Res* 2000;121:133–143.
80. Colenda CC. Buspirone in treatment of agitated demented patient. *Lancet* 1988;1:1169.
81. Levine AM. Buspirone and agitation in head injury. *Brain Inj* 1988;2:165–167.
82. Ratey J, Sovner R, Mikkelsen E, et al. Buspirone therapy for maladaptive behavior and anxiety in developmentally disabled persons. *J Clin Psychiatry* 1989;50: 382–384.
83. Sovner R, Parnell-Sovner N. Use of buspirone in the treatment of schizophrenia. *J Clin Psychopharmacol* 1989;9:61–62.
84. Realmuto GM, August GJ, Garfinkel BD. Clinical effect of buspirone in autistic children. *J Clin Psychopharmacol* 1989;9:122–124.
85. Newton RE, Marunycz JD, Alderdice MT, et al. Review of the side-effect profile of buspirone. *Am J Med* 1986;80:17–21.
86. Jounela AJ, Lilja M. Interactions between beta-blockers and clonidine. *Ann Clin Res* 1984;16:181–182.
87. Tinklenberg JR, Taylor JL. Assessments of drug effects on human memory functions. In: Squires LR, Butters N, eds. *Neuropsychology of memory*. New York: Guilford Press, 1984:213–223.
88. Romney DM, Angus WR. A brief review of the effects of diazepam on memory. *Psychopharmacol Bull* 1984; 20:313–316.
89. Gualtieri CT, Evans RW. Stimulant treatment for the neurobehavioral sequelae of traumatic brain injury. *Brain Inj* 1988;2:273–290.
90. O'Dell D, Gibson C, Wilson M, et al. Positive and negative modulation of the GABA(A) receptor and outcome after traumatic brain injury in rats. *Brain Res* 2000;861:325–332.
91. Power AC, Cowen PJ. Fluoxetine and suicidal behav-

iour: some clinical and theoretical aspects of a controversy. *Br J Psychiatry* 1992;161:735–741.

92. Greenblatt DJ, Abernethy DR, Morse DS, et al. Clinical importance of the interaction of diazepam and cimetidine. *N Engl J Med* 1984;310:1639–1643.
93. Greenblatt DJ, Shader RI, Abernethy DR. Drug therapy: current status of benzodiazepines. *N Engl J Med* 1983;309:354–358.
94. Greenblatt DJ, Shader RI. Drug therapy: prazepam and lorazepam, two new benzodiazepines. *N Engl J Med* 1978;299:1342–1344.
95. Breier A, Charney DS, Nelson JC. Seizures induced by abrupt discontinuation of alprazolam. *Am J Psychiatry* 1984;141:1606–1607.
96. Lydiard RB, Laraia MT, Ballenger JC, et al. Emergence of depressive symptoms in patients receiving alprazolam for panic disorder. *Am J Psychiatry* 1987;144:664.
97. Noyes R, Clancy J, Coryell WH, et al. A withdrawal syndrome after abrupt discontinuation of alprazolam. *Am J Psychiatry* 1985;142:114.
98. Morris HH, Estes ML. Traveler's amnesia. Transient global amnesia secondary to triazolam. *JAMA* 1987; 258:945–946.
99. Pecknold JC, Fleury D. Alprazolam-induced manic episode in two patients with panic disorder. *Am J Psychiatry* 1986;143:652.
100. Strahan A, Rosenthal J, Kaswan M, et al. Three case reports of acute paroxysmal excitement associated with alprazolam treatment. *Am J Psychiatry* 1985;142:859.
101. Wroblewski BA, Joseph AB. The use of intramuscular midazolam for acute seizure cessation or behavioral emergencies in patients with traumatic brain injury. *Clin Neuropharmacol* 1992;15:44–49.
102. Isojarvi J, Tokola R. Benzodiazepines in the treatment of epilepsy in people with intellectual disability. *J Intellect Disabil Res* 1998;42:80–92.

23

Tardive Dyskinesia and Tardive Akathisia

SUMMARY

Do the tardive syndromes deserve a chapter of their own? Are they not just relics of the bad old days when neuroleptics were used indiscriminately in nursing homes and institutions for the mentally retarded? The epidemic of tardive diskinesia a generation ago was a blight on the history of psychopharmacology, but what pertinence does it have today?

It is appropriate to reflect on historical matters, and the history of tardive dyskinesia (TD) illuminates two points that I have tried to make on several occasions: first, psychotropic drugs are safe and easy to use but can be dangerous and require careful medical follow-up. Second, the long-term effects of psychotropic drugs deserve careful study because toxicity may not be apparent until years have passed. Whether a drug is prone to long-term side effects is never evident in the short-term studies needed to win drug approval.

This chapter is more than an exercise in historical reflection. The neuroleptics are still prescribed, and even the atypical antipsychotics can occasionally cause tardive syndromes. Therefore, several clinical issues such as the vexing problem of tardive akathisia (TDAK), the little-appreciated problem of tardive pain, and the possibility of a behavioral analog of TD are discussed. This last issue is another opportunity to consider the neuropsychology of the basal ganglia.

The epidemiology of the tardive syndromes indicates that a number of treatment-related and patient-related variables predispose to the condition. Patients with neuropsychiatric disorders in general and mentally retarded patients in particular appear to be more vulnerable to the neurotoxic effects of the old antipsychotic drugs. Malignant TD, conversely, is more common in patients with affective disorders.

When one considers the pathophysiology of TD, the problem of oxidant stress is raised again. The evidence base may be shallow, but the theory is compelling. For that reason, one may be inclined to recommend antioxidant supplements to patients who are on long-term antipsychotic drug treatment. Because several other psychotropics are also capable of generating a free-radical burden, it is reasonable to propose antioxidants for patients in general who require long-term drug treatment. Will this issue ever be addressed in controlled studies? As previously stated, long-term studies of drug toxicity, or the prevention of it, are rarely, if ever, done.

NEUROLEPTIC DRUGS

The neuroleptic drugs were so-called by Delay (1955) because he believed that their antipsychotic action was necessarily correlated with a tendency to produce extrapyramidal side effects (EPS). The term is now reserved for the old antipsychotic drugs; the new atypicals are equally effective with a low propensity for EPS. They are much less likely to cause the most serious EPS, TD. For this and other reasons, they have won most of the antipsychotic market, and the problem of

TD has receded accordingly, but it is not extinct, by any means, and in some parts of the world, it continues to be a vexing problem. It merits our attention as much for its historical importance as for its clinical salience.

My familiarity with the issue stems from a series of studies done in the late 1970s that demonstrated TD and related disorders had achieved alarming dimensions in children and mentally retarded people. In those unenlightened days, it was not uncommon to prescribe neuroleptics for children with relatively minor behavioral problems such as attention deficit/hyperactivity disorder. As for mentally retarded people, if they were living in institutions, most of them were taking neuroleptics, usually at high doses and for long periods of time. In 1968, the national rate of neuroleptic prescription for retarded people was approximately 50% (1) and approximately the same in 1978 (2). It fell to approximately 30% in 1985 (3). It is now less than 20%. This reflected patterns of psychiatric care in the general population in which neuroleptics were routinely used for anxiety disorders and affective disorders during the 1960s and 1970s, and then their use declined.

The first descriptions of TD date from the mid-1950s (4,5), and complaints that the side effect was potentially dangerous came soon after (6), but little attention was paid. The problem was that continued neuroleptic treatment tends to obscure the characteristic dyskinetic movements and patients with schizophrenia are prone to abnormal grimaces and posturing as part of the condition. Institutional psychiatrists were oppressed by the job of day-to-day management of many desperate patients. They were much more impressed by the therapeutic utility of the new drugs, and justifiably so, than they were by what seemed to be at the time a minor side effect. Looking back, we can afford to shake our heads because we have learned from their mistakes.

The first report of TD in mentally retarded people on long-term neuroleptic treatment was published in 1975 (7), and there were several subsequent reports over the next few years (8,9). This was no less than 20 years after the disorder was first described by European psychiatrists, but it was contemporary with the development of serious concern about TD among American psychiatrists.

It was not until the publication of the APA Task Force Report in 1979 that medical concern was directed to the problem of TD, even for the mentally ill. Five years later, the problem gained widespread publicity, as lawsuits began to multiply, and even the public media began to address the issue. TD became a major issue for physicians who treated chronic mentally ill patients, administrators and makers of public policy, and research scientists in psychiatry and neuropharmacology. The development of an antipsychotic drug that did not cause TD became a prime focus of psychopharmacologic research.

It is possible that recognition of TD as a serious, potentially debilitating side effect of neuroleptic treatment was responsible for the dramatic decrease in neuroleptic prescription for retarded people that occurred during the 1980s (10), although other factors also played a role (e.g., the community movement, widespread skepticism of the medical model, renewed emphasis on behavioral and developmental programming, new attention to alternative pharmacologic treatments). Nevertheless, the problem of TD was a red flag around which adherents rallied to reduce the unnecessary prescription of neuroleptic drugs and to improve programmatic treatments for retarded people. It was certainly the specter of TD that led general psychiatrists to be more judicious in their use of neuroleptic drugs and child psychiatrists to abjure their use almost entirely.

TD began to be perceived as a hazard to the public health. It was widely held that neuroleptics were relatively contraindicated in mentally retarded people, children, patients with brain injury, and the elderly. Regulations at the state and federal levels reinforced those clinical beliefs. When neuroleptic prescription was considered for a patient who was not overtly schizophrenic, the treatment decision was made with great care. Written informed consent and formal TD monitoring systems came to be the standard of care. Drug withdrawal trials or gradual dose reductions were mandated at appropriate intervals to test for occult or covert TD and to determine whether continued drug treatment was necessary. It was generally accepted that any patient whose behavioral problems were so severe as to warrant neuroleptic prescription should also have a concomitant behavioral program.

Although this enlightened approach was associated with a substantial diminution in the problem of TD in special populations, even before the new antipsychotics were introduced, it was not without problems of its own. The judicious use of antipsychotic drugs was interpreted by some to mean nonuse. The pendulum was swinging too far in the other direction. This was especially true for the mentally retarded and nursing home elderly, for whom it was difficult for physicians to prescribe a neuroleptic for patients who needed it. Lawsuits, largely spurious, were filed against physicians who prescribed conventional neuroleptics, under any circumstances, if any side effect ensued at all. Many patients who might have benefited from a neuroleptic were thus deprived of a therapeutic opportunity.

Since the atypicals have been introduced, attitudes have relaxed considerably. The new drugs are much safer, monitoring requirements are less stringent, and regulatory bodies are less critical of their use. Consequently, the use of antipsychotic drugs in the mentally retarded, the elderly, children, and patients with brain injuries has rebounded. Ironically, the transfer of large numbers of retarded individuals from institutions into the community has been associated with a dramatic increase in antipsychotic prescription. This also reflects general psychiatric practice, in which the atypicals are increasingly used for severe anxiety disorders (e.g., posttraumatic stress disorder, obsessive-compulsive disorder) and treatment-refractory affective disorders.

Nevertheless, TD remains a problem, especially in mentally retarded people who may well be especially vulnerable to the side effect. Even atypical antipsychotic drugs may sometimes cause the disorder. Thus, TD remains a continuing problem, even in the face of convenient solutions. It is also a prototypical movement disorder, around which a number of interesting neuropsychiatric problems are concentrated.

It is appropriate to refer to the tardive syndromes because TD is only one of a number of related conditions associated with long-term antipsychotic treatment. In addition to TD, there is TDAK, tardive dystonia, tardive pain, tardive Tourette's syndrome, and a behavioral analog of TD that has been controversial, which will be discussed in this chapter.

SERIOUS SIDE EFFECTS OF NEUROLEPTIC DRUGS

Tardive Dyskinesia

Estimates of TD prevalence published in the psychiatric literature have varied a great deal, largely as a consequence of idiosyncrasies in measurement and definition. The average prevalence of TD based on 33 studies reported from 1970 to 1979 was 24% (11), but the true rate varies, depending on the clinical population: from 12% among outpatients in a Department of Veterans Affairs clinic to 13% in an acute psychiatric hospital to 36% in a state hospital to 67% among state hospital patients older than 65 years of age. The cumulative incidence of TD in patients with psychiatric disorders is said to be approximately 5% at 1 year, 10% at 2 years, 15% at 3 years, and 19% at 4 years (12). There is said to be a 40% cumulative rate of TD in adult patients with psychiatric disorders after 8 years of exposure to neuroleptic drugs (13). With every year of treatment, it would appear that the rate of TD increases by 5% until it reaches asymptote at approximately 67%. Does that mean that one-third of patients is immune to neuroleptic toxicity? Perhaps it does.

In fact, it is hard to be confident in the numbers generated in studies of patients who have not been withdrawn from neuroleptic drug treatment because maintenance neuroleptic treatment tends to mask the presence of the disorder. Therefore, any prevalence estimate will necessarily be influenced by the patient's medication status. A true prevalence rate can only be determined from the study of drug-free patients, and this is not done very often in studies of patients with psychiatric disorders. In one survey of patients who had no signs of TD as long as they were taking neuroleptics, new signs of TD emerged in no fewer than 34% when the neuroleptics were subsequently withdrawn (12).

The problem is illustrated by the changing prevalence of TD in mentally retarded populations. In a study by Paulson et al. (7), the prevalence was 20%, but most patients who were surveyed were still on neuroleptics. In two other surveys, conducted on the heels of medication withdrawal, the prevalence was much higher: persistent TD (34% to 45%) and transient withdrawal dyskinesia (29%) (9,14).

Epidemiologic studies of TD and related disorders are also complicated by the existence of spontaneous dyskinesias, i.e., choreic, athetoid, and tic-like movements that seem to occur quite naturally without medication in the elderly, patients with chronic schizophrenia, and mentally retarded individuals. There is a 4% rate of mild involuntary movements in healthy elderly volunteers (11), but a much higher rate, approaching 40%, in the elderly with dementia (15).

One cannot argue that the estimate of TD occurrence in people with mental retardation is inflated because they are given to a wide range of abnormal movements, even in the absence of neuroleptic treatment. The assessment of dyskinetic movements in people with severe to profound retardation may be problematic because they are prone to a number of abnormal movements and the patients may not cooperate with the examination procedure. Conversely, Kalachnik et al. (9) arrived at a true prevalence rate for TD by subtracting the basal rate of dyskinesia in drug-free controls.

In a unique prospective study of haloperidol treatment for children with autism, most of whom were mentally retarded, the incidence of TD after 6 to 30 months of follow-up was 25% (16). The dyskinesias that arose were transient, however, as one might expect in young patients treated with low doses of a neuroleptic for a relatively short period. Conversely, the fact that an early form of TD arose in one-fourth of treated patients within the span of 30 months suggests, to me at least, that neuroleptics are relatively contraindicated in this group.

In the face of such extraordinary figures, one is compelled to warn patients on long-term neuroleptic treatment that the development of TD is a likely event. Conversely, it is also appropriate to assure patients that TD can be prevented by judicious use of neuroleptic drugs and by careful and knowledgeable medical supervision. It has been suggested that even patients with chronic psychotic disorders can be maintained on neuroleptic doses that are 10% to 20% of those in common use (17). After all, the highest rates of TD are found in public institutions for the mentally ill and mentally handicapped, where drugs have been used in lieu of programming and medical supervision is sometimes less than optimal. If neuroleptics are used in low-to-moderate doses, even for a sustained period, the level of risk is probably acceptable. If the novel antipsychotics are used, in preference to the conventional neuroleptics, whenever they are effective, the risk of TD is even lower, and the annual incidence is much lower than 5%.

The issue of TD prevalence, however, obscures a more important issue: the need to distinguish between the prevalence of severe and debilitating cases of TD and those that are relatively mild and persistent cases and those that will only last a few months or a year or two. Prevalence rates from 25% to 33% should ordinarily be cause for alarm. If only a few of those cases, however, are severe and persistent and most are mild or self-limiting, then the problem is manageable. If severe cases can be prevented by careful monitoring, then physicians will have the right to reassure patients and their families.

Conversely, if severe and persistent cases comprise a significant fraction of the population of patients with TD, then draconian measures will be required to reduce neuroleptic prescription. Most psychiatrists would say that severe cases are only a minority of patients with TD, and I have never argued with that contention. When the issue is put to the test, however, severe TD variants have been observed in more than one-fifth of all diagnosed TD cases (18).

Tardive Dyskinesia Variants

The typical case of TD is characterized by irregular choreoathetoid movements occurring predominantly in the buccal-lingual-masticatory musculature and distal extremities. It is the most common manifestation of the syndrome (93% of TD cases). Tardive dystonia is characterized by sustained contractions of skeletal musculature; it has been found to account for 26% of all TD cases referred to a movement disorder clinic. TDAK is estimated to comprise 18% of TD cases. Tardive Tourette's syndrome is characterized by motor and phonic tics (5% of cases) (18). Tardive pain syndrome is a curious phenomenon and is described below.

Extrapyramidal Reactions

TD is a late extrapyramidal syndrome associated with neuroleptic treatment, as distinguished from the early EPS. These, of course, are pseudoparkinsonism, acute dystonia, akathisia, akinesia (19), and aphonia (20). In fact, the term neuroleptic was coined because it was thought that the therapeutic action of antipsychotic drugs was necessarily correlated with their tendency to produce EPS. (Clozapine, risperidone, olanzapine, quetiapine, and ziprasidone should be called antipsychotics because they are less prone to produce EPS; they defy the correlation.)

Neuroleptic Malignant Syndrome

Neuroleptic malignant syndrome (NMS) is a devastating, sometimes fatal neuroleptic side effect arising early in treatment, especially with high-potency drugs. The symptoms are muscular ("lead-pipe") rigidity, mental state changes (e.g., delirium), and autonomic changes (e.g., hyperthermia, hypertension, tachycardia), accompanied by elevation of the whole blood cell count and serum creatine phosphokinase. If the disorder is not recognized promptly and proper treatment measures are not instituted immediately, the patient may die of renal failure. Treatment is neuroleptic withdrawal, fluid replacement, and dantrolene or dopamine agonists (e.g., bromocriptine). It is said that NMS occurs in 1% to 2% of neuroleptic-treated patients and that 10% to 20% of cases are fatal (21). That estimate is probably too high, but there is no denying that increased familiarity with this extraordinary syndrome leads to increased recognition.

Although NMS is most likely to occur early in treatment, it may arise at any point, even when the patient is on a stable maintenance dose (22). Risk factors include a state of psychomotor agitation before neuroleptic treatment, high doses of neuroleptics that are increased rapidly, and intramuscular administration (23). Other risk factors are the use of high-potency neuroleptics and patient-related variables, such as a dehydrated or physically exhausted state or a history of neuroleptic toxicity. It is incredible that a side effect so severe and presumably so common went unrecognized for so many years (24).

NMS is a major problem for nursing personnel because the keys to successful treatment are early recognition and a high index of suspicion. Any patient on neuroleptic treatment with rigidity and mental state changes should be reported to the attending physician immediately as a medical emergency, and neuroleptics should be withheld until an examination can be done and the appropriate laboratory tests can be done. Dealing with NMS requires special training for nurses who care for patients on neuroleptic treatment and careful monitoring by physicians who are familiar with the syndrome. NMS, more than any movement disorder, should limit the widepread use of neuroleptics. Neuroleptics are not routine treatments to be administered by primary care physicians with no special training in psychopharmacology.

The atypical antipsychotic drugs are much less likely to cause NMS.

Tardive Akathisia

Akathisia is a Greek word that means "not to sit still." (In fact, the Greek word is *kathisia*, which refers to the act of sitting, and akathisia is a neologism.) The word describes the subjective state of motor restlessness and dysphoria that occurs in many clinical conditions. It was first adopted by Haskovec (25) to refer to patients whose problems were hysterical in origin. Later, Bing (26) described akathisia in patients with postencephalitic parkinsonism. Since then, akathisia has been considered a disease of the basal ganglia (27).

Soon after the introduction of neuroleptic drugs, clinicians noted patients who had symptoms of restlessness and dysphoria (4,28,29). The term neuroleptic-induced akathisia (NIA) joined pseudoparkinsonism and dystonia in the trio of acute extrapyramidal reactions caused by neuroleptic drugs. The prevalence of NIA has been estimated at approximately 20%, although the figure may be as high as 45% (30).

Early reports of NIA also included descriptions of patients whose symptoms arose only after several years of neuroleptic treatment and co-occurred with symptoms of TD (6,28,31,32). In 1977, Simpson suggested that late-onset NIA was persistent, even after neuroleptic withdrawal, and that it was virtually untreatable. In 1983, Munetz and Cornes introduced the term TDAK: "an akathisia-like syndrome (characterized by) late onset, treatment resistance, and potential irreversibility despite discontinuance of neuroleptics." The overt symptoms of TDAK are indistinguishable from those of NIA, and the direct examination of the patient yields the same findings. The symptoms of patients with TDAK, of course, tend to increase when the neuroleptic dose is lowered, whereas the symptoms of patients with NIA tend to improve.

TDAK was further described in a series of clinical reports (33–37), and it was operationally defined in a systematic study by Barnes and Braude (30). The prevalence of TDAK was reported to be 18% in patients referred for evaluation at a TD clinic (18) and 6% to 14% in mentally retarded patients treated with neuroleptics (38,39).

TDAK is a relatively common and severe problem, causing distress to the patient and demanding a great deal of attention by physicians and direct care personnel. Because akathisia is a state of restless, dysphoric hyperactivity, it may also be the occasion of secondary behavioral problems, a "setting event" for the occurrence of difficult behaviors such as aggression (40) or self-injury (41). The emergence of what are referred to as target behaviors (e.g., disorganization, agitation, aggression, hyperactivity, self-injurious behavior) in the circumstances of neuroleptic withdrawal might represent the recurrence of a preneuroleptic psychiatric condition or alternatively the manifestation of TDAK. The diagnostic and therapeutic dilemma is daunting.

People with akathisia are miserable. They feel as if they were crawling out of their skin, and they have to pace constantly just to win a small degree of relief. They are irritable, unhappy, and emotionally unstable. They are so unhappy and find it so hard to understand what is happening to them that they may erupt in explosions of aggressive, destructive, or self-injurious behavior. They may be described as hyperactive, disorganized, or psychotic. In other words, they may develop, as a consequence of long-term neuroleptic treatment, persistent symptoms that are identical to the problem behaviors for which neuroleptics were originally prescribed.

Dysphoria, Anxiety, and Pain

Several other unpleasant subjective states may also occur in association with neuroleptic treatment, occurring as side effects of acute treatment, as tardive syndromes, occurring in association with better known EPS such as akathisia, or standing alone. One example is neuroleptic-induced dysphoria (without motor restlessness), especially with haloperidol, which can also cause anxiety and even overt panic attacks (42). Acutely treated patients may also complain of painful sensations (43). These are usually described as poorly localized, intermittent, aching sensations involving all four limbs symmetrically and sparing the head and ventral torso. Complaints of pain tend to be more frequent in patients who also have pseudoparkinsonism or akathisia (44). Oral and genital pain have been described as a tardive syndrome, said to be an example of pure cognitive akathisia (45). Analogously, patients with postencephalitic or idiopathic parkinsonism experience distressing and ill-defined sensations, commonly referred to as primary sensory symptoms (46). The lesson is that "all the side effects of neuroleptics have already been described between 1920 and 1935 as a sequela of (von Economo) encephalitis" (47).

The sensation of pain as an EPS of neuroleptic treatment illuminates the role of opioid drugs (codeine, propoxyphene, nitrous oxide), which seem to be effective for NIA but not for TDAK. This may have to do with the presence of opiate receptors on presynaptic dopaminergic neurons and on neurons that carry the postsynaptic dopamine receptors (48). The striatum contains high concentrations of both dopamine and opioid receptors, and the number of opioid binding sites is reduced after denervation of dopaminergic neurons (49).

Restless Legs Syndrome

Patients with restless legs syndrome also improve when they are treated with low doses of opiates (48). The syndrome was first described by Ekbom who described restless movements of the legs arising spontaneously in some people especially in the elderly and especially at night (50). The condition is autosomal dominant, but it may also be manifest as a variant of NIA or TDAK.

The symptoms of restless legs syndrome include painful paresthesias of the legs, especially in the calves, occurring at rest. The patient finds relief only by moving his or her lower extremities. Because the problem is most intense at night, the patient experiences severe insomnia and all the secondary problems that arise from it. The paresthesias are often described as burning or a deep ache.

It is interesting that virtually all the treatments recommended for NIA and TDAK have also been useful (on occasion) for cases of restless legs syndrome, most notably, carbamazepine, vitamin E, folate, beta-blockers, benzodiazepines, clonidine, and tryptophan (51). The opiates, then, are hardly unique. None of these treatments, however, is uniformly effective. Recently, gabapentin has come to be one of the most successful treatments for restless legs syndrome. It may also be useful for NIA and TDAK.

Treatment

Akathisia, acute or tardive, is often treated with beta-blockers (52–54) or clonidine (54,55). The frequent success of such drugs in the treatment of akathisia suggests an effect of chronic neuroleptic blockade on noradrenergic neurotransmission. Neuroleptics are known to increase cerebrospinal fluid and brain levels of norepinephrine; the mechanism may be presynaptic dopamine blockade, a neuroleptic effect that has been determined to increase norepinephrine release, at least in laboratory animals (56).

Lorazepam or clonazepam may also be used, with only occasional success; benzodiazepines may even be used in conjunction with beta-blockers. There have been reports of successful treatment with amantadine (57), which I have been unable to confirm, and with buspirone (58), which we have. Gabapentin and tiagabine are other alternatives.

As in severe cases of TD, the only effective treatment may well be reinstitution of neuroleptics. In the past, atypical neuroleptics such as molindone or thioridazine were recommended, but not any more. They never worked very well, and the pharmacologic treatment of TDAK was for a very long time as unsuccessful as Paulson et al. (7) suggested in 1975. Since clozapine, however, the clinical picture has changed dramatically, and since the other atypical antipsychotics were introduced, it has improved even more. Today, one recommends the introduction of an atypical antipsychotic in the usual doses and then a very gradual withdrawal.

Tardive Akathisia in the Mentally Handicapped

Because neuroleptic drugs have been prescribed quite often for mentally retarded adults (1,2), there has been a strong movement in recent years to reduce unnecessary or excessive neuroleptic drug use. In many clinical facilities, however, the reduction of neuroleptic prescription has led to the unmasking of neuroleptic side effects such as TD and TDAK (39). In 1993, I reported the results of a longitudinal study of TDAK and its behavioral concomitants (59). The study was undertaken at a large residential facility for the mentally handicapped. Of a population of 356, no fewer than 180 residents had been treated long term with neuroleptic drugs. TDAK was diagnosed in 25 patients (14% of the population at risk).

Three years after the patients with TDAK were first identified, I found that 10 patients (40%) succeeded in remaining neuroleptic free. Their clinical status was unstable at first, but it gradually improved. Symptoms of akathisia and target behaviors had abated, and there was no need for continued neuroleptic treatment. Fifteen patients (60%) had to remain on neuroleptics, despite the TDAK, because of severe behavioral problems that could not be controlled by alternative interventions.

One year later, the original 10 patients remained stable and neuroleptic free. The other 15 continued on neuroleptics, albeit on comparatively lower doses. With selective concomitant treatment (e.g., beta-blockers, benzodiazepines) or substitution of novel antipsychotics, they also stabilized, with no further progression of TDAK (59).

It was encouraging that a substantial number of retarded people with TDAK could be successfully withdrawn from neuroleptic drugs and that their symptoms gradually abated. It was discouraging that three-fifths of the group could never be withdrawn from the offending agents, but at least TDAK was not progressive as long as their management was judicious.

The problem of TDAK generates difficult clinical situations that seem to be unique to patients who are mentally retarded and patients with brain injury. Many are patients who never respond very well to neuroleptics to begin with but who grow much worse after they are withdrawn. Their behavior deteriorated sharply after the neuroleptic dose is lowered beyond a certain point, but they remain difficult and hard to manage even after the dose is returned to what had earlier been a therapeutic level. Their TD symptoms are accompanied by high levels of hyperactivity and restlessness; they are extremely dysphoric when neuroleptics are withdrawn and seem to be manageable with any pharmacologic agent. The problem is usually TDAK, and the only reasonable solution is to switch to an atypical antipsychotic drug and then gradually lower the dose.

A Behavioral Analog of Tardive Dyskinesia

For a long time, my colleagues and I were preoccupied with the possibility of a behavioral analog of TD (60). It was an important question that seemed to beg solution. If neuroleptics were prescribed for people who were cognitively impaired and behaviorally unstable to begin with, how could one know whether cognitive impairment or behavioral instability, emerging after neuroleptic withdrawal, was in fact the result of drug treatment.

In 1979, Davis and Rosenberg raised the question of a limbic equivalent of TD, that is, behavioral toxicity as a consequence of neuroleptic-induced changes in mesolimbic dopamine receptors. In the same year, investigators reported more intellectual deterioration in neuroleptic-treated patients with TD than in non-TD controls (61). Two questions were then posed: Could neuroleptic treatment lead to behavioral deterioration, and could neuroleptics cause dementia? In other words, whether higher cortical functions might be damaged, much in the same way that motor control systems were damaged. You can imagine the excitement and dismay this question raised. It was a difficult point to prove one way or the other.

Cases of supersensitivity psychosis were described by Chouinard and Jones (62) (who coined the term), Sale and Kristall (63), and Caine et al. (64). These were neuroleptic-treated patients who developed a dramatic, rapid-onset psychosis as soon as neuroleptics were withdrawn. The psychosis was held to be a consequence of neuroleptic treatment, not simply the reemergence of a preexisting disorder. The psychiatric community has not found this contention particularly believable (12), although it would be imprudent to dismiss it.

There is near unanimity, however, on the issue of dementia because virtually every study that has researched the issue has found an association between TD and signs of dementia or so-called negative symptoms of schizophrenia. When patients with TD are compared with similar patients who do not have TD, clear evidence of cognitive dysfunction is almost invariably demonstrated in the TD group (65–74). What is at issue is how to account for the finding. The usual explanation is that patients with preexisting neuropsychological deficits are more vulnerable to the neurotoxic effects of neuroleptic drugs. The alternative explanation is that neuroleptics cause cognitive decline in some patients, that neuroleptic treatment may cause subcortical dementia (73) or frontal lobe syndrome (66). This idea is supported by a recent positron emission tomography study that demonstrated long-term neuroleptic effects on brain glucose metabolism in patients with schizophrenia in the direction of decreased metabolism in the frontal lobes (hypofrontality) and enhanced metabolism in the corpus striatum (75). Neither alternative is attractive to physicians who treat patients who are retarded, elderly patients who are demented, or patients with head injury. Either encephalopathy is a risk factor for the development of TD or it is a risk inherent to long-term neuroleptic treatment.

Because TDAK has been clearly established as one of the tardive syndromes attributed to neuroleptic treatment, the arguments over a behavioral or cognitive analog to TD can be considered settled (10). Stahl (76), for example, suggested that TDAK is both a movement disorder and a mental disorder because it has both objective and subjective components. In other words, TDAK is a movement disorder with a psychological dimension. As discussed previously, it may manifest itself as a purely subjective state without the movement disorder.

Akathisia, like TD, and all the hyperkinetic movement disorders are manifestation symptoms of basal ganglia disease. Postmortem studies (77,78) and magnetic resonance imaging studies (79,80) have demonstrated basal ganglia lesions in patients with TD, especially in the caudate nucleus. Lesions of the basal ganglia may evoke movements that are indistinguishable from TD.

Parkinson's disease (PD), Huntington's chorea (HC), and Wilson's disease (WD) are progressive diseases of the basal ganglia that are very similar to TD. Akathisia, for example, is a symptom of PD and choreoathetosis is a symptom of HC and WD. Although persistent TDAK and TD appear to be static not progressive encephalopathies, their similarity to the major diseases of the basal ganglia goes deeper than the surface manifestations of akathisia and dyskinesia.

The issue is especially relevant to the putative cognitive and behavioral analogs of TD. PD, for example, is associated with depression and dementia (81–83). HC and WD are associated with affective instability, psychosis, and dementia (84–88). If behavioral instability and intellectual impairment are inevitably a part of PD, HC, and WD, should they not also occur in TD?

Patients with PD, HC, and WD also have neuropathologic changes in cortical structures, and therefore it is not possible to attribute all the cognitive and behavioral elements of those conditions to lesions in the basal ganglia. Conversely, intellectual impairment has been noted in patients with PD with lesions in the subcortical nuclei but not in the cortex (89) and in patients with PD after *N*-methyl-4-phenyl-1,2,3,6-tetrahydropyridine exposure, who had neither cortical lesions nor motor impairment (90). In WD, the severity of neuropsychological impairment is correlated with abnormalities in the basal ganglia but not in the cortex or cerebellum (91). We also know that circumscribed lesions in the basal ganglia are sometimes associated with significant psychiatric conditions (92, 93) or neuropsychological deficits (94–97).

The basal ganglia may be the "dark basement" of the brain, but they are not without intelligence of their own. The basal ganglia do participate in, and may even regulate, some intellectual activities, particularly those involving complex or sequential motor activities (81). The corpus striatum subserves a number of frontal lobe functions in the juvenile primate (98). The frontal lobes are richly connected with areas in the neostriatum (99). Neostriatal lesions mimic the effects of frontal lesions (100,101) and lesions in either the frontal lobes or neostriatum disturb and slow down neural activities throughout the frontostriatal circuit (99). Even more compelling, the mosaic of deficits caused by lesions of the frontal lobes is reflected by similar deficits caused by lesions in striatal areas to which the frontal cortex projects (102–104).

One may surmise, therefore, that affective instability and intellectual impairment may be the consequence of neuropathology at the level of the basal ganglia. Because TD is the result of neurotoxicity in the basal ganglia, some patients with TD may be expected to have behavioral and cognitive deficits as well. TDAK is one manifestation of that effect. There are probably others.

Is This Really Tardive Akathisia?

The emergence of troublesome behaviors, accompanied by dysphoria and restlessness, when a retarded person is withdrawn from neuroleptic medication, is sufficient to suggest the diagnosis of TDAK, especially when the patient has concomitant signs of drug-induced neurotoxicity (i.e., TD). Conversely, as previously mentioned, the diagnostic problem is daunting because the diagnosis is no more than presumptive, and the alternative construction is that the patient is simply manifesting the reemergence of the problem behaviors that led physicians to prescribe neuroleptics in the first place. Retarded children who are hyperactive, aggressive, and easily agitated are likely to be given a strong psychotropic drug. When that drug is withdrawn, is it any surprise that they are again hyperactive and dysphoric?

There is a theoretical answer to that question, as described in the foregoing section. There is unfortunately no direct clinical measure to decide the issue in the individual case. In practice, one may be told that a patient with presumed TDAK was, in fact, "just like that" before neuroleptics were ever prescribed. In contrast, one does see young patients who are retarded and autistic who are restless, impulsive, irritable, and emotionally unstable. They are like that, never having been treated with neuroleptic drugs.

The difference is that for the past 10 or 15 years "children like that" have not been treated with neuroleptics in high doses. They have been treated with serotonergics, or amantadine, or α_2 agonists, or mood stabilizers—drugs that are more specific for the organic affective disorders, which is what we usually deal with. Never having been exposed to neuroleptics, their outcomes have been much more sanguine; when the drugs are withdrawn, they do not revert to their original pattern of hyperactive, disorganized behavior.

Long-term treatment of retarded people with neuroleptics may cause TDAK. Alternatively, long-term treatment may have another kind of neurotoxic effect—interfering with learning and preventing development in an already compromised brain. The reemergence of difficult behaviors after the withdrawal of neuroleptics may represent the failure of the development of cognitive systems that lend control to a primitive, undifferentiated state of irritability and hyperreactivity.

The atypical antipsychotics are less neurotoxic, and the few cognitive studies that have been done to date do not indicate impairment of function. Developmental studies have not been undertaken. We assume that, like the new antidepressants, the atypical antipsychotics are at least neutral with respect to cognitive performance and brain development. That is, of course, no more than an assumption. As the drugs are used more often in handicapped children, we will have an opportunity to test its validity.

RISK FACTORS FOR TARDIVE DYSKINESIA

Patient-Related Risk Factors

Three patient-related risk factors seem to be associated with increased risk for TD: age, gender, and affective disorder. A fourth, preexisting brain damage may be also be associated, although the data are by no means definitive. As a general rule, a risk factor that is linked to a higher likelihood of developing TD will also be linked to severity and to persistence.

The risk factor most consistently identified with the development of TD and severe persistent TD is age. Elderly patients are more prone to the disorder, an effect that is probably independent of cumulative neuroleptic dose or the duration of neuroleptic exposure (12,105). It is possible that this association is related to the age-related decline in dopamine neurons in the striatum, an idea that is strengthened by the spontaneous occurrence of buccal-lingual dyskinesias in elderly patients who have never taken neuroleptic drugs (70).

It appears that females are at greater risk than males to develop TD and severe forms of the disorder are likelier to occur in females (11). This may speak to estrogen-related dopamine sensitivity (106). Nicotine can also sensitize the dopamine receptor, and therefore tobacco addiction must be counted among the risk factors for TD (107). Cannabis may also predispose to TD and possibly alcohol (108,109).

Clinical lore holds to the ironic contention that TD is more likely to occur in patients who do not respond particularly well to neuroleptic treatment, but whether this is related to high-dose treatment, frequent dose changes, conjunctive treatment, or some other factor is not known. It may be that the neuroleptic nonresponders are people with affective disorders.

It appears that patients with affective disorders are peculiarly vulnerable to malignant TD (110). This is very important for the treatment of mentally retarded people, among whom affective disorders tend to be underdiagnosed, and it may explain why the tardive syndromes have been so troublesome in this population.

Whether preexisting brain damage may actually predispose to TD or severe and persistent TD is not known, although it is an important question for practitioners who deal with patients with mental retardation, dementia, or neurobehavioral sequelae of traumatic brain injury (111). Neuroleptics have always been frequently prescribed for these groups (10).

Treatment-Related Risk Factors

Several factors related to treatment with neuroleptic drugs have been associated with increased risk of TD, but only one, early development of EPS, has gained wide acceptance on the basis of controlled experiments.

Results from the New York Longitudinal Study suggest that patients who develop TD are more likely to have EPS early in their treatment (112). The association does not appear to be related to treatment with selected neuroleptics with a low proclivity for EPS; rather, patients who are prone to early EPS are at greater risk for TD by virtue of some unique pharmacodynamic tendency (113).

If concomitant anticholinergic treatment is associated with TD at all, the effect is probably mediated by the occurrence of early EPS. That is, patients who develop early EPS are more likely to receive anticholinergics; the former confers risk, not the latter.

One would think that neuroleptic dose has something to do with the development of TD, but the clinical literature is equivocal. Cumulative neuroleptic dose was found to be associated with severe TD in one study of mentally retarded patients (114), but not in studies of patients with schizophrenia and other psychiatric disorders. It is likely that there is no linear association between cumulative dose and TD but that a minimum cumulative dose is necessary to evoke the phenotype in patients who are vulnerable to TD by virtue of other risk factors. The importance of idiosyncrasy cannot be minimized because some patients have been known to develop TD after short-term treatment with very low neuroleptic doses, whereas others seem to be free of the disorder even after years of high-dose treatment.

Until clozapine, there was never a particular neuroleptic that was more or less likely to cause TD. Other serious side effects, such as agranulocytosis and hepatotoxicity, are more likely with the low-potency neuroleptics thioridazine and chlorpromazine, and those drugs exhibit more cytotoxicity in tissue cultures (115). Among the conventional neuroleptics, however, there is no rank order.

An appreciation of TD risk factors is essential to clinical treatment because it allows the physician to recognize cases that require very careful monitoring, more frequent neuroleptic withdrawals or at least dose reductions, and a more aggressive approach to identifying pharmacologic alternatives. The informed consent process should address the patient's individual vulnerability to TD. To reiterate, established risk factors for neuroleptic-induced TD are advanced age, female gender, smoking, affective disorder, early EPS, and possibly brain damage and cumulative neuroleptic dose.

Protective Factors

What may be done to reduce the likelihood of a tardive syndrome? Reduce the number of patients who are exposed to neuroleptic drugs, maintain patients on long-term treatment on a minimum effective dose, and use the novel antipsychotics instead of the conventional neuroleptics. The neuroleptics have joined the ranks of "archaic" drugs, which include the sedating anticonvulsants and tricyclic antidepressants. Nevertheless, there are still occasions when the prescription of an archaic drug is necessary, and sometimes, high-dose neuroleptics are necessary for patients with severe affective disorders, even older female patients who drink, toke, and smoke.

In the history of psychopharmacology, several possible protectants have been proposed, for example, lithium and amantadine. None has worked. So it was hardly surprising that psychiatrists greeted with skepticism the news that various megavitamin combinations actually exerted a protective effect. One formula, arrived at empirically, contained niacin, pyridoxine, ascorbate, and vitamin E (116).

The free-radical theory of cytotoxicity that was current among neurologists who study PD led to a series of trials of vitamin E that were for the most part disappointing. At the same time, however, it was suggested that the neuroleptics might be cytotoxic because by increasing catecholamine turnover and metabolism, there should necessarily be increased production of highly reactive free radicals (117). The theory was supported by the findings that patients with TD had higher levels of thiobarbituric acid–reactive substances, an indicator of lipid peroxidation (i.e., free-radical damage to body fats) (117,118) and that vitamin E (with or without selenium) prevented the development of TD in dopamine-hypersensitive rats (119,120). Clinical studies of patients with TD have actually demonstrated reduction in AIMS scores when they are treated with vitamin E in doses as high as 1,600 IU per day (121–124).

There is no reason why neuroleptic-treated patients should not take concomitant vitamin E, perhaps with some of the other free-radical scavengers such as selenium. It seems to be the psychopharmacologic equivalent of one baby aspirin every other day.

BIOLOGICAL MECHANISMS

The prevailing view of the pathophysiology of TD is that chronic blockade of striatal D_2-dopamine receptors leads to a state of denervation supersensitivity and that the abnormal movements are a manifestation of dopamine hypersensitivity (125). Support for this idea comes from animal studies in rats, cats, and primates in which chronic neuroleptic administration is known to increase the number and density of striatal dopamine binding sites (126), to elicit behaviors such as gnawing or rotation that are mediated by dopamine (127), and to cause choreoathetoid movements that are typical of TD (128). The abnormal movements of TD are topographically identical to dyskinesias that characterize other hyperdopaminergic states: HC, Tourette's syndrome, and L-dopa–induced dyskinesias (129).

The dopamine supersensitivity hypothesis is not sufficient to explain the phenomenon, however. For example, the dyskinesias that arise in animal models of TD are early onset and readily reversible. With prolonged neuroleptic administration, the dopamine receptor hypersensitivity actually disappears (130). In human postmortem studies, patients with TD are not invariably found to have D_1 or D_2 hypersensitivity (131), nor do they show cerebrospinal fluid or neuroendocrine indices of dopamine sensitivity (130). The supersensitivity hypothesis may underlie the occurrence of transient or withdrawal dyskinesias, but the pathophysiology of persistent unremitting TD is unknown (132).

If receptor supersensitivity cannot account for cases of severe and persistent TD, then it is necessary to consider alternative hypotheses. The facts that the disorder can be irreversible, refractory to treatment, and occasionally associated with continued deterioration even after drug withdrawal (133) lead inevitably to the idea that neuroleptics may exercise, in some patients at least, a cytotoxic effect. This may conceivably be a cytotoxic metabolite, perhaps a selective product of neuroleptic metabolism in patients vulnerable to severe TD. Alternatively, TD may be the consequence of oxidative stress. The neuroleptics are, comparatively speaking, metabolically active compounds and strong free-radical generators. Neuroleptic drugs increase the turnover and metabolism of dopamine, with the formation of dopamine quinines and hydrogen peroxide. Long-term exposure to neuroleptics in animals increases manganese and iron, which are free-radical catalysts, in the central nervous system (134). Neuroleptic treatment has been found to retard recovery from brain injury in rats (135).

Neuroleptic blockade of presynaptic dopamine D_2 receptors increases the synaptic release of aspartate and glutamate in the striatum. Persistent activation of glutaminergic ionotropic receptors causes neuronal degeneration, an effect that is mediated by increased oxygen free-radical generation and oxidative damage to the cell membrane, cellular proteins, and DNA. Markers for enhanced excitatory neurotransmission have been discovered in the central nervous system of patients with schizophrenia with TD (136). This represents a cogent rationale for the use of antioxidants, especially vitamin E, for the prevention and possible treatment of TD. As a preventive agent, vitamin E is promising, at least on theoretical grounds; as a treatment measure, especially in advanced cases, it may not be effective (134).

Dopamine neurons are remarkably stress sensitive and that is why parkinsonian symptoms are so common, even with normal aging. Occasional reports of postmortem findings in patients with TD have demonstrated neuronal degeneration in the substantia nigra (77) and caudate nucleus atrophy (78,137). Nielson and Lyon (138) observed cell death in the corpus striatum of rats given neuroleptics long term.

DIAGNOSIS

The diagnosis of TD requires more than the simple administration of a rating scale like the AIMS or the DISCUS. Those are only screening instruments and are useful because they can be reliably administered by a nonphysician and because they raise the level of staff consciousness concerning TD. They are complements to the neurologic examination and the process of differential diagnosis, not a substitute for it.

The first step in diagnosis requires a thorough description of the patient's abnormal movements, including a topographic analysis of the distribution of dyskinesia and an accurate description of its nature. The topographic categories are orofacial, buccal-lingual-masticatory, truncal (or axial), centrifugal (i.e., involving the extremities), and holokinetic (i.e., all over). The different types of dyskinesia are choreoathetoid, dystonic, myoclonic, ballistic, and tic-like movements (so-called tardive Tourette's syndrome).

Topography and dyskinesia interact in relatively predictable patterns. Choreiform movements are often centrifugal, whereas dystonic movements are more commonly axial in distribution. The area of distribution is significant because severe TD may sometimes have a total body distribution and thus render the patient incapacitated by virtue of holokinetic movements. Movements that are circumscribed in area are not as likely to be incapacitating unless they are dystonic or involve the oropharyngeal or respiratory musculature. These elements are essential for determining the severity of TD and may also aid in the prediction of outcome. Severe and persistent TD is most often associated with mixed types of movements with a generalized distribution or with dystonic movements with a more local distribution.

The next step involves the process of differential diagnosis. The topography and classification of dyskinesia do not establish diagnosis. Indeed, many other movement disorders may resemble TD. Stereotypies and manneristic behaviors are common in patients with severe mental retardation and autism. These movements may be suppressed by neuroleptics and reemerge when the drug is reduced in dose or discontinued entirely. Such movements are usually more complex than those seen in TD and are usually stereotyped in quality. Nevertheless, TD coinciding with stereotypies may pose a diagnostic problem.

The differential diagnosis of TD includes Tourette's syndrome, choreoathetosis attendant on cerebral palsy, HC, WD, and other disorders of the basal ganglia; Hallervorden-Spatz syndrome (dystonia); familial dystonia and chorea; ballistic movements related to vascular disease; and other drug-induced dyskinesias, e.g., those related to phenytoin (139), carbamazepine (140), valproate, tricyclic antidepressants, or stimulants. Dyskinesias may arise spontaneously in elderly patients or patients with dementia. Idiopathic calcification of the basal ganglia is associated with dyskinesia and other neuropsychiatric symptoms (141,142).

Other causes of movement disorder include Sydenham's chorea, systemic lupus erythematosus, and some encephalitides. Disturbance in thyroid and parathyroid function may be associated with dyskinesia (113). The differential diagnosis of dystonia has been addressed most recently by Burke et al. (143).

The evaluation of a patient with possible TD may involve a series of steps to exclude alternative causes of dyskinesia, especially treatable conditions such as WD. A family history is very important. Laboratory diagnosis may rule out infectious, endocrine, metabolic, and degenerative disorders. Appropriate studies include a toxic drug screen, serum electrolytes, sedimentation level, ASO titers, thyroid and parathyroid studies, serum ceruloplasmin, lupus erythematosis (LE) prep, and antinuclear antibodies. Appropriate neurodiagnostic studies include computed tomography or magnetic resonance imaging, at least in selected cases. Calcification of the basal ganglia, iron deposition in the globus pallidus, or degeneration of the caudate and other subcortical structures may provide etiopathogenic evidence that can influence clinical decisions.

The differential diagnosis is important, but a thorough neurodiagnostic evaluation is not necessary for most cases of TD. The most important diagnostic element is a history of toxic exposure (to neuroleptics or other dopamine blockers such as metaclopramide) and a high index of suspicion on the part of the treating physician. A patient with dyskinesia and a history of neuroleptic exposure has TD until proven otherwise.

TREATMENT

It is not easy to discuss the treatment of TD because no treatment is reliably effective. The basic treatment is to withdraw neuroleptics, keep the patient drug free, and wait for the disorder to remit. If antipsychotics cannot be withdrawn, substitute a novel antipsychotic. There is reason to believe that clozapine may be an effective treatment for the tardive syndromes. Vitamin E is the third treatment alternative.

Patients with choreiform TD may respond to drugs that influence γ-aminobutyric acid (GABA) neurotransmission such as clonazepam, baclofen, or valproic acid (144). The timing of treatment may be important because some patients with TD progress to a severe dystonic form of the disorder that is usually resistant to pharmacologic treatment (110). Drugs that deplete presynaptic dopamine such as reserpine or tetrabenzamine may be helpful, but they can exacerbate affective illness in vulnerable patients (145,146). Patient response to acetylcholine agonists is variable. Physostigmine provocation has been advocated as a screening procedure to identify patients who will respond to cholinergic precursors (147,148). Clinically, acetylcholine agonist treatment approaches have been disappointing, and side effects have limited their utility (149).

Tardive dystonia differs clinically from idiopathic forms of dystonia, yet it may respond to similar treatments. In dystonia, physostigmine tends to increase the severity of abnormal movements. Anticholinergic drugs have been helpful, but their clinical utility is limited by the occurrence of memory impairment, agitation, and delirium (150). Dopamine-depleting drugs may be helpful in 10% to 12% of patients with dystonia (150). Dopamine agonists such as L-dopa and amantadine may be effective in a similar percentage of patients with dystonia (129). The use of GABAergic drugs has been of limited benefit.

THE COURSE OF THE DISORDER

It is a mistake to classify TD as irreversible because patients with chronic TD may experience remission even after several years. It is better to classify TD as transient or persistent and specify precisely how long the movement disorder has in fact persisted.

What proportion of patients has TD that remits after only a few weeks or a few months, and what proportion persists for years? Although these are important questions, they cannot be answered based on direct research. The persistence of TD may be masked by continued neuroleptic treatment, and most TD studies in populations with psychiatric disorders have been done in patients with schizophrenia who are treated with neuroleptics even after TD is diagnosed.

In elderly patients, TD is usually a persistent disorder, whereas in studies of children treated with neuroleptics, the remission rate is very high (16,151). Although persistent cases are not unknown, they are rare (8). There is an age-dependent decrease in dopamine neurotransmission that may interact with neuroleptic neurotoxicity to cause severe and persistent forms of TD in elderly patients, and this same element could conceivably confer a measure of protection to young people (70). Children usually are treated with low doses of neuroleptics for shorter periods, and they metabolize drugs more efficiently. The relative persistence rates for TD in young and elderly patients may be a pharmacodynamic phenomenon or it may simply be related to prescription habits.

It is possible that even transient TD in early life may set the stage for neurodegenerative changes in later years, admittedly a speculation but one based on some established models of the evolution of neuropsychiatric disorders: postencephalitic parkinsonism, the late neuropathic sequelae of poliomyelitis, late-onset psychosis after traumatic brain injury, and the putative kindling psychosis of temporal lobe epilepsy (10). These are all models of early central nervous system insult followed by late deterioration in function. It is possible that some patients who have had transient TD in early life will develop encephalopathic changes when they are old.

This is another example of cerebral reserve, a concept that was introduced in Chapter 6 in the discussion of postconcussion effects. It is said that the dopamine system is particularly vulnerable to the effects of insult; postencephalitic parkinsonism, post–*N*-methyl-D-aspartate parkinsonism, and TD are three concrete examples. In the first case, it is youthful exposure to the virus that leads to parkinsonism in middle age. We have no way of knowing whether exposure to neuroleptics in childhood may have a similar effect. TD in children tends to be transient; they have so many extra neurons, even in the dopamine system, that it is hard to confirm the possibility of a late effect, but it is possible, and with time, we may find out.

In mentally retarded people, one of our studies reported TD in 25 of 38 individuals who were withdrawn from neuroleptic treatment, but 13 of 25 had transient TD that remitted within only a few weeks (152). A subsequent study of a subgroup of that original sample who returned to neuroleptic treatment and who were withdrawn from neuroleptics a second time 3 years later demonstrated progressive TD in five patients and TD that had actually decreased in severity in four patients; the former had been treated with high doses of neuroleptics, the latter group with low doses (10). Although this was only a small study, it suggests that patients with TD may continue on neuroleptics if they absolutely have to, as long as the doses are kept low.

Paulson et al. (7) reexamined a group of mentally retarded people 4 years after a neuroleptic withdrawal trial and found that six (of 15) had persistent TD with no change in severity, five had more severe TD, and four had actually improved.

If one can surmise anything from these small studies, it is that TD is persistent in some substantial fraction (one-third or two-thirds) of mentally retarded patients who have the disorder, that persistence is to be measured in years, but that remission may occur with time and judicious management. How do these conjectures correspond with the results of TD research in other patient groups?

The research data from studies of adults with schizophrenia are contradictory and hard to interpret. In one study of patients with TD maintained off neuroleptics, no appreciable symptom reduction was noted after 12 months (153). In another, Yassa et al. (154) reported a 2-year follow-up: 66% of the patients with TD showed no change, 18% improved, and 16% grew worse over time. In a 5-year follow-up study by Chouinard et al. (155), the annual, remission rate in patients with TD was 5.5%; this was outweighed by an incidence rate for new cases of 8.4%. In contrast, there have been several reports suggesting that TD remits far more often than it persists (130,156–159), even if neuroleptic treatment is continued. Exactly how substantial the fraction is then of those who have persistent TD remains an area of surmise.

Well-controlled epidemiologic studies of the course of TD are extremely difficult to do because the recruitment of a large number of subjects will necessarily include patients on psychoactive drugs that may influence the course of the disorder, patients who will drop out for one reason or another, and patients with degenerative central nervous system disorders. As a consequence, research attention is turning in the direction of case-control strategies. It is assumed that at least some patients will have long-term persistent TD and that others will remit. The relative proportions are irrelevant; the key to the strategy is accurate assignment to one group or the other. The next step is to identify clinical elements that are associated with persistence and to replicate the finding. This is the difficult part. First, clinical elements from the medical history will be hard to discover, especially in patients with chronic TD who are institutionalized. Second, subject variance will make a successful replication difficult. The strategy, however, is important; if reliable information is attainable, it can be used to guide programs for TD prevention.

A first attempt at this strategy was published by Gardos and Casey (110). They found that generalized dystonic and athetoid movements characterized a more malignant and persistent form of TD. They also reported that patients with severe and persistent TD displayed a variety of axial and centrifugal movements, with buccal-lingual-masticatory choreoathetosis early in the clinical course and a gradual evolution to dystonia as the disorder progressed. Males were more commonly affected with severe and persistent TD, and the duration of treatment was relatively short (less than 1 year). Gardos and Casey concluded that patients who develop severe and persistent TD have a unique vulnerability to neuroleptic-induced movement disorders and that this could be defined in terms of the TD risk factors discussed earlier, especially age, early EPS, and affective disorder.

Malignant Tardive Dyskinesia

The severity of TD is defined in terms of persistence, the nature of the dyskinesia, and the degree to which it afflicts the patient's behavior and compromises the activities of daily life. The disagreement over relative rates of persistence is mirrored in controversies about relative severity or whether patients with TD are even bothered by their disorder. There is little to be gained from a reiteration of these arguments.

The consensus developing among psychopharmacologists is that TD may sometimes be a malignant disorder, rapid in onset and extreme in its consequences. It seems that some patients are uniquely vulnerable to severe and persistent TD, they can develop the disorder after only a brief course of low-dose neuroleptic treatment, their TD is extraordinarily debilitating, and dystonia and akathisia are its likeliest manifestations. Patients with so-called malignant TD tend to have affective disorders to begin with (110). They are often young, and their disorder is persistent and refractory to treatment. They are rarely if ever anosognosic for the condition. This is a very serious problem (143).

There are only estimates of the relative prevalence of severe forms of TD. The most recent survey, based on 100 TD cases seen at a movement disorder clinic that were probably a seriously afflicted group to begin with, reported 23 severe manifestations of the disorder: persistent bruxism (one case), masseter or lingual hypertrophy (three cases), sustained involuntary tongue protrusion (six cases), incomprehensible speech arising from dysarthria (two cases), spasmodic dysphonia (two cases), anterior cervical spondylolisthesis (one case), palatal dyskinesia with secondary sinus pain (one case), respiratory stridor with laryngospasm (two cases), and disabling dystonic posturing (five cases) (18).

Neuroleptic Nonresponders

It is important to remember that there are even some patients with schizophrenia whose condition grows worse with neuroleptic treatment. In rare cases, psychosis may even occur as an effect of neuroleptic treatment (160). Neuroleptics can cause dysphoria (161), panic (162), phobia (163), and depression (164). Although acute behavioral toxicity to neuroleptic treatment may not be common, it is by no means uncommon. Not only may some patients fail to respond to neuroleptic treatment, but some patients, even those diagnosed with schizophrenia, may actually grow worse with the drugs.

REFERENCES

1. Lipman RS. The use of psychopharmacological agents in residential facilities for the retarded. In: Menolascino F, ed. *Psychiatric approaches to mental retardation*. New York: Basic Books, 1970:387.
2. Sprague RL, Baxley GB. Drugs used in the management of behavior in mental retardation. In: Wortis J, ed. *Mental retardation & developmental disabilities*. New York: Brunner Mazel, 1978.
3. Hill BK, Balow EA, Bruinincks RH. *A national study of prescribed drugs in institutions and community residential facilities for mentally retarded people*. Minneapolis: University of Minnesota, 1983.
4. Steck H. Le syndrome extrapyramidal et diencephalique au cours des traitements au largactil et au serpasil. *Ann Med Psychol* 1954;112:737–743.
5. Schonecker M. Ein eigentomliches Syndrom in oralen Bereich bei Megaphenapplikation. *Neruenarzt* 1957;28.
6. Uhrbrand L, Faurbye A. Reversible and irreversible dyskinesia after treatment with perphenazine, chlorpromazine, reserpine, and electroconvulsive therapy. *Psychopharmacologia* 1960;1:408–418.
7. Paulson GW, Rizvi CA, Crane GE. Tardive dyskinesia as a possible sequelae of long-term therapy with phenothiazines. *Clin Pediatr* 1975;14:953–955.
8. Gualtieri CT, Hawk B. Tardive dyskinesia and other drug-induced movement disorders among handicapped children and youth. *J Appl Res Ment Retard* 1980;1:55–69.
9. Kalachnik JE, Harder SR, Kidd-Nielsen P, et al. Persistent tardive dyskinesia in randomly assigned neuroleptic reduction, neuroleptic nonreduction, and no-neuroleptic history groups: preliminary results. *Psychopharmacol Bull* 1984;20:27–31.
10. Gualtieri CT, Barnhill LJ. Tardive dyskinesia in special populations. In: Wolf ME, Mosnaim AD, eds. *Tardive dyskinesia, biological mechanisms & clinical aspects*. Washington, DC: American Psychiatric Press, 1988: 137–154.
11. Kane JM, Smith JM. Tardive dyskinesia, prevalence and risk factors. *Arch Gen Psychiatry* 1982;39:473–481.
12. APA Task Force on Tardive Dyskinesia. *Tardive dyskinesia: a task force report of the American Psychiatric Association*. Washington, DC: American Psychiatric Association, 1992.
13. Saltz BL, Kane JM, Woerner MG, et al. Prospective study of tardive dyskinesia in the elderly. *Psychopharmacol Bull* 1989;25:52–56.
14. Gualtieri CT, Schroeder SR, Hicks RE, et al. Tardive dyskinesia in young mentally retarded individuals. *Arch Gen Psychiatry* 1986;43:335–340.
15. Delwaide PJ, Desseilles J. Spontaneous buccolinguofacial dyskinesia in the elderly. *Acta Neurol Scand* 1977;56:256–262.
16. Perry R, Campbell M, Green WH, et al. Neuroleptic-related dyskinesias in autistic children: a prospective study. *Psychopharmacol Bull* 1985;21:140–143.
17. Baldessarini RJ. Clinical and epidemiologic aspects of tardive dyskinesia. *J Clin Psychiatry* 1985;46:8–13.
18. Davis RJ, Cummings JL. Clinical variants of tardive dyskinesia. *Neuropsychiatry Neuropsychol Behav Neurol* 1988;1:31–38.
19. Rifkin A, Quitkin F, Klein DF. Akinesia: a poorly recognized drug-induced extrapyramidal behavioral disorder. *Arch Gen Psychiatry* 1975;32:672–674.
20. Behrman S. Mutism induced by phenothiazines. *Br J Psychiatry* 1972;121:599–604.
21. Keck PE, Pope HG, McElroy SL. Frequency and presentation of neuroleptic malignant syndrome: a

prospective study. *Am J Psychiatry* 1987;144: 1344–1346.
22. Guze BH, Baxter LR. Neuroleptic malignant syndrome. *N Engl J Med* 1985;313:163–166.
23. Keck PE, Pope HG, Cohen BM, et al. Risk factors for neuroleptic malignant syndrome. *Arch Gen Psychiatry* 1989;46:914–921.
24. Levenson JL. Neuroleptic malignant syndrome. *Am J Psychiatry* 1985;142:1137–1145.
25. Haskovec L. Akathisie. *Arch Boheme Med Clin* 1902; 3:193–200.
26. Bing R. Uber Einige Bemerkenswerte Begleiterscheinungen der Exrapyramidalen Rigiditat (Akathesie–Mikrographie–Kinesia paradoxica). *Schweiz Med Wochenschr* 1923;53:167–171.
27. Bing R. *Textbook of nervous diseases*, 5th ed. London: Henry Kimpton Press, 1939.
28. Ayd FJ. A survey of drug-induced extrapyramidal reactions. *JAMA* 1961;175:1054–1060.
29. Kruse W. Persistent muscular restlessness after phenothiazine medication: report of 3 cases. *Am J Psychiatry* 1960;117:152–153.
30. Barnes TRE, Braude WM. Akathisia variants and tardive dyskinesia. *Arch Gen Psychiatry* 1985;42:874–878.
31. Demars JCA. Neuromuscular effects of long-term phenothiazine medication, electroconvulsive therapy and leukotomy. *J Nerv Ment Dis* 1966;143:73–79.
32. Faurbye A, Rasch P-J, Petersen PB. Neurological symptoms in pharmacotherapy of psychosis. *Acta Psychiatr Scand* 1964;40:10–27.
33. Brandon S, McClelland MA, Protheroe C. A study of facial dyskinesia in a mental hospital population. *Br J Psychiatry* 1971;118:171–184.
34. Chouinard G, Annable L, Ross-Chouinard A. Fluphenazine enanthate and fluphenazine decanoate in the treatment of schizophrenic outpatients: extrapyramidal symptoms and therapeutic effect. *Am J Psychiatry* 1982;139:312–318.
35. Kennedy PF, Hershon HI, McGuire RJ. Extrapyramidal disorders after prolonged phenothiazine therapy. *Br J Psychiatry* 1971;118:509–518.
36. Mukherjee S, Rosen AM, Cardenas C, et al. Tardive dyskinesia in psychiatric outpatients. *Arch Gen Psychiatry* 1982;39:466–469.
37. Wojcik JD, Gelenberg AJ, LaBrie RA, et al. Prevalence of tardive dyskinesia in an outpatient population. *Compr Psychiatry* 1980;21:370–380.
38. Ganesh S, Rao JM, Cowie VA. Akathisia in neuroleptic medicated mentally handicapped subjects. *J Ment Defic Res* 1989;33:323–329.
39. Gualtieri CT. *Neuropsychiatry and behavioral pharmacology*. Berlin: Springer-Verlag, 1990.
40. Keckich WA. Neuroleptics. Violence as a manifestation of akathisia. *JAMA* 1978;240:2185.
41. Drake RE, Ehrlich J. Suicide attempts associated with akathisia. *Am J Psychiatry* 1985;142:499–501.
42. Mikkelsen E, Detlor J, Cohen D. School avoidance and social phobia triggered by haloperidol in patients with Tourette's disorder. *Am J Psychiatry* 1981;138:1572.
43. Carter G. The abrupt withdrawal of antiparkinsonian drugs in mentally handicapped patients. *Br J Psychiatry* 1983;142:166–168.
44. Decina P, Caracci G, Harrison K, et al. *Painful sensory symptoms in neuroleptic-induced extrapyramidal syndromes*. New York, 1990.
45. Ford BM, Greene PM, Fahn SM. Oral and genital tardive pain syndromes. *Neurology* 1994;44:2115–2119.
46. Koller WC. Sensory symptoms in Parkinson's disease. *Neurology* 1984;34:957–959.
47. Deniker P. From chlorpromazine to tardive dyskinesia (brief history of the neuroleptics). *Psychiatry J Univ Ottawa* 1989;14:253–259.
48. Walters A, Hening W, Chokroverty S, et al. Opioid responsiveness in patients with neuroleptic-induced akathisia. *Mov Disord* 1986;1:119–127.
49. Ebadi M, Srinivasan SK. Pathogenesis, prevention, and treatment of neuroleptic-induced movement disorders. *Pharmacol Rev* 1995;47:575–604.
50. Ekbom DA. Asthenia crurum paraesthetica ("irritable legs"). *Acta Med Scand* 1944;118:197–209.
51. Walters AS, Hening W. Clinical presentation and neuropharmacology of restless legs syndrome. *Clin Neuropharmacol* 1987;10:225–237.
52. Yassa R, Iskandar H, Nastase C. Propranolol in the treatment of tardive akathisia: a report of two cases. *J Clin Psychopharmacol* 1988;8:283–285.
53. Ratey JJ, Sorgi P, Polakoff S. Nadolol as a treatment for akathisia. *Am J Psychiatry* 1985;142:640.
54. Zubenko GS, Cohen BM, Lipinski JF, et al. Use of clonidine in the treatment of akathisia. *Psychiatry Res* 1984;13:253–259.
55. Adler L, Angrist B, Peselow E, et al. Clonidine in neuroleptic-induced akathisia. *Am J Psychiatry* 1987;144: 235–236.
56. De Keyser J, Ebinger G, Herregodts P. Pathophysiology of akathisia. *Lancet* 1987;2:336.
57. Borison RL, Diamond BI. Treatment of extra-pyramidal side effects: amantadine versus benzotropine. *World J Psychosynthesis* 1984;16:40–43.
58. D'Mello DA, McNeil JA, Harris W. Buspirone suppression of neuroleptic-induced akathisia: multiple case reports. *J Clin Psychopharmacol* 1989;9:151–152.
59. Gualtieri CT. The problem of tardive akathisia. *Brain Cognition* 1993;23:102–109.
60. Gualtieri CT, Guimond M. Tardive dyskinesia and the behavioral consequences of chronic neuroleptic treatment. *Dev Med Child Neurol* 1981;23:255–259.
61. Famuyiwa OO, Eccleston D, Donaldson AA, et al. Tardive dyskinesia and dementia. *Br J Psychiatry* 1979; 135:500–504.
62. Chouinard G, Jones BD. Neuroleptic-induced supersensitivity psychosis: clinical and pharmacologic characteristics. *Am J Psychiatry* 1980;137:16–21.
63. Sale I, Kristall H. Schizophrenia following withdrawal from chronic phenothiazine administration: a case report. *Aust N Z J Psychiatry* 1978;12:73–75.
64. Caine ED, Margolin DI, Brown GL, et al. Gilles de la Tourette's syndrome, tardive dyskinesia and psychosis in an adolescent. *Am J Psychiatry* 1978;135:241–243.
65. Edwards H. The significance of brain damage in persistent oral dyskinesia. *Br J Psychiatry* 1970;116:271–275.
66. Wilson IC, Garbutt JC, Lanier CF, et al. Is there a tardive dysmentia? *Schizophr Bull* 1983;9:187–192.
67. Struve FA, Willner WA. Cognitive dysfunction and tardive dyskinesia. *Br J Psychiatry* 1983;143:597–600.
68. Wolf ME, Ryan JJ, Mosnaim AD. Cognitive functions in tardive dyskinesia. *Psychol Med* 1983;13:671–674.
69. Collerton D, Fairbairn A, Britton P. Cognitive performance of medicated schizophrenics with tardive dyskinesia. *Psychol Med* 1985;15:311–315.

70. Waddington JL, Youssef HA, Mooloy AG, et al. Association of intellectual impairment, negative symptoms, and aging with tardive dyskinesia: clinical and animal studies. *J Clin Psychiatry* 1985;46:29–33.
71. Wegner JT, Catalano F, Gibralter J, et al. Schizophrenics with tardive dyskinesia. *Arch Gen Psychiatry* 1985; 42:860–865.
72. Thomas P, McGuire R. Orofacial dyskinesia, cognitive function and medication. *Br J Psychiatry* 1986;149: 216–220.
73. Gilleard CJ, Vaddad KS. Mood, memory, and performance and the severity of tardive dyskinesia. *Percept Mot Skills* 1986;63:1037–1038.
74. Goldberg E. Akinesia, tardive dysmentia, and frontal lobe disorder in schizophrenia. *Schizophr Bull* 1985; 11:255–263.
75. Szechtman H, Nahmias C, Garnett ES, et al. Effect of neuroleptics on altered cerebral glucose metabolism in schizophrenia. *Arch Gen Psychiatry* 1988;45: 523–532.
76. Stahl SM. Akathisia and tardive dyskinesia: changing concepts. *Arch Gen Psychiatry* 1985;42:915–917.
77. Christensen E, Miller JE, Faurbye A. Neuropathological investigation of 28 brains from patients with dyskinesia. *Acta Psychiatr Scand* 1970;46:14–23.
78. Hunter R, Blackwood W, Smith MC, et al. Neuropathological findings in three cases of persistent dyskinesia following phenothiazine medication. *J Neurol Sci* 1968;7:263–273.
79. Bartzokis G, Garber HJ, Marder SR, et al. MRI in tardive dyskinesia: shortened left caudate T2. *Biol Psychiatry* 1990;28:1027–1036.
80. Mion CC, Andreasen NC, Arndt S, et al. MRI abnormalities in tardive dyskinesia. *Psychiatry Res Neuroimag* 1991;40:157–166.
81. Mayeux R, Stern Y. Intellectual dysfunction and dementia in Parkinson's disease. In: Mayeux R, Rosen WG, eds. *The dementias*. New York: Raven Press, 1983:211–227.
82. Mayeux R, Stern Y, Rosen J, et al. Depression, intellectual impairment and Parkinson disease. *Neurology* 1981;31:645–650.
83. Taylor AE, Saint-Cyr JA, Lang AE, et al. Parkinson's disease and depression: a critical re-evaluation. *Brain* 1986;109:279–292.
84. Brandt J, Strauss ME, Larus J, et al. Clinical correlates of dementia and disability in Huntington's disease. *J Clin Neuropsychol* 1984;6:401–412.
85. Dening TR, Berrios GE. Wilson's disease: psychiatric symptoms in 195 cases. *Arch Gen Psychiatry* 1989;46: 1126–1134.
86. Folstein SE, Leigh J, Parhad IM, et al. The diagnosis of Huntington's disease. *Neurology* 1986;36:1279–1283.
87. Sax DS, O'Donnell B, Butters N, et al. Computed tomographic, neurologic, and neuropsychological correlates of Huntington's disease. *Int J Neurosci* 1983; 18:21–36.
88. Starosta-Rubinstein S, Young AB, Kluin K, et al. Clinical assessment of 31 patients with Wilson's disease: correlations with structural changes on magnetic resonance imaging. *Arch Neurol* 1987;44:365–370.
89. Chui HC, Mortimer JA, Slager U, et al. Pathologic correlates of dementia in Parkinson's disease. *Arch Neurol* 1986;43:991–995.
90. Stern Y, Tetrud JW, Martin WRW, et al. Cognitive change following MPTP exposure. *Neurology* 1990; 40:261–264.
91. Medalia A, Isaacs-Glaberman K, Scheinberg H. Neuropsychological impairment in Wilson's disease. *Arch Neurol* 1988;45:502–504.
92. Rapoport JL, Wise SP. Obsessive-compulsive disorder: evidence for basal ganglia dysfunction. *Psychopharmacol Bull* 1988;24:380.
93. Trautner RJ, Cummings JL, Read SL, et al. Idiopathic basal ganglia calcification and organic mood disorder. *Am J Psychiatry* 1988;145:350–353.
94. Bowen FP. Behavioral alterations in patients with basal ganglia lesions. In: Yahr MD, ed. *The basal ganglia*. New York: Raven Press, 1975:169–180.
95. Buchwald NA, Hull CD, Levine MS, et al. The basal ganglia and the regulation of response and cognitive sets. In: Brazier MAB, ed. *Growth and development of the brain*. New York: Raven Press, 1975:171–189.
96. Hassler R. Striatal control of locomotion, intentional actions and of integrating and perceptive activity. *J Neurol Sci* 1978;36:187–224.
97. Teuber H, Proctor F. Some effects of basal ganglia lesions in subhuman primates and man. *Neuropsychologia* 1964;2:85–93.
98. Divac I. Functions of the caudate nucleus. *Acta Biol Exp* 1968;2:107–120.
99. Villablanca JR, Olmstead CE. The striatum: a fine tuner of the brain. *Acta Neurobiol Exp* 1982;42:227–299.
100. Rosvold HE, Mishkin M, Swarcbart MK. Effects of subcortical lesions in monkeys on visual- discrimination and single-alternation performance. *J Comp Physiol Psychol* 1958;51:437–444.
101. Rosvold HE, Szwarcbart MK. Neural structures involved in delayed response performance. In: Warren JM, Abert K, eds. *The frontal granular cortex and behavior*. New York: McGraw-Hill, 1964:1–15.
102. Delgado JMR. Inhibitory functions of the neostriatum. In: Divac I, Oberg RGE, eds. *The neostriatum*. Oxford: Pergamon Press,1979:241–262.
103. Iversen SD. Behavior after neostriatal lesions in animals. In: Divac I, Oberg RGE, eds. *The neostriatum*. Oxford: Pergamon Press, 1979:195–210.
104. Oberg RGE, Divac I. "Cognitive" functions of the neostriatum. In: Divac I, Oberg RGE, eds. *The neostriatum*. Oxford: Pergamon Press, 1979:291–313.
105. Walker-Batson D, Unwin H, Curtis S, et al. Use of amphetamine in the treatment of aphasia. *Restor Neurol Neurosci* 1992;4:47–50.
106. Hruska RE, Silbbergeld EK. Increased dopamine receptor sensitivity after estrogen treatment using the rat rotation model. *Science* 1980;208:1466–1468.
107. Yassa R, Lal S, Korpassy A, et al. Nicotine exposure and tardive dyskinesia. *Biol Psychiatry* 1987;22:67–72.
108. Olivera AA. Tardive dyskinesia in psychiatric patients with substance use disorders. *Am J Alcohol Abuse* 1990;16:57–66.
109. Zaretsky A, Rector NA, Seeman MV, et al. Current cannibus use and tardive dyskinesia. *Schizophr Res* 1993;11:3–8.
110. Gardos G, Casey DE. *Clinical insights monograph: tardive dyskinesia and affective disorders*. Washington, DC: American Psychiatric Press, 1984.
111. Gualtieri CT. Pharmacotherapy and the neurobehavioral sequelae of closed head injury. *Brain Inj* 1988;2: 101–129.

112. Kane JM, Woerner M, Weinhold P, et al. Incidence of tardive dyskinesia: five year data from a prospective study. *Psychopharmacol Bull* 1984;20:39–40.
113. Jeste D, Karlson CN, Wyatt RJ. Movement disorders and psychopathology. In: DV JESTE, Wyatt RJ, eds. *Neuropsychiatric movement disorders*. Washington, DC: APA Press, 1984.
114. Gualtieri CT, Sprague RL, Cole JO, et al. Tardive dyskinesia litigation and the dilemmas of neuroleptic treatment. *J Psychiatry Law* 1986;14:187–216.
115. Munyon WH, Salo R, Briones DF. Cytotoxic effects of neuroleptic drugs. *Psychopharmacology* 1987;91: 182–188.
116. Tkacz C, Hawkins DR. A preventive measure for tardive dyskinesia. *J Orthomol Psychol* 1981;10:119–123.
117. Lohr JB, Kuczenski R, Bracha HS, et al. Increased indices of free radical activity in the cerebrospinal fluid of patients with tardive dyskinesia. *Biol Psychiatry* 1990;28:535–539.
118. Peet M, Laugharne J, Rangarajan N, et al. Tardive dyskinesia, lipid peroxidation, and sustained amelioration with vitamin E treatment. *Int Clin Psychopharmacol* 1993;8:151–153.
119. Gattaz WF, Emrich A, Behrens S. Vitamin E attenuates the development of haloperidol-induced dopaminergic hypersensitivity in rats: possible implications for tardive dyskinesia. *J Neural Transm* 1993;92:197–201.
120. Tariq M, al-Deeb S, al-Moutairy K, et al. Effect of selenium and vitamin E on iminodipropionitrile induced dyskinesia in rats. *Int J Neurosci* 1994;78:185–192.
121. Adler LA, Peselow E, Duncan E, et al. Vitamin E in tardive dyskinesia: time course of effect after placebo substitution. *Psychopharmacol Bull* 1993;29: 371–374.
122. Akhtar S, Jajor TR, Kumar S. Vitamin E in the treatment of tardive dyskinesia. *J Postgrad Med* 1993;39: 124–126.
123. Dabiri LM, Pasta D, Darby JK, et al. Effectiveness of vitamin E for treatment of long-term tardive dyskinesia. *Am J Psychiatry* 1994;151:925–926.
124. Lohr JB, Caligiuri MP. A double-blind placebo-controlled study of vitamin E treatment of tardive dyskinesia. *J Clin Psychiatry* 1996;57:167–173.
125. Ananth J. Current psychopathological theories of tardive dyskinesia and their implications for future research. *Neuropsychobiology* 1982;8:210–222.
126. Creese I, Burt DR. Dopamine receptor binding enhancement accompanies lesion-induced behavioral supersensitivity. *Science* 1977;197:596–598.
127. Fjalland B, Nielson IM. Enhancement of methylphenidate-induced stereotypies by repeated administration of neuroleptics. *Psychopharmacologia* 1974; 34:105–109.
128. Weiss B, Santelli S. Dyskinesias evoked in monkeys by weekly administration of haloperidol. *Science* 1978;200:799–801.
129. Stahl SM, Davis KL, Berger PA. The neuropharmacology of tardive dyskinesia, spontaneous dyskinesia, and other dystonias. *J Clin Psychopharmacol* 1982;2: 321–328.
130. Casey DE, Povisen UJ, Meidahl B, et al. Neuroleptic-induced tardive dyskinesia and parkinsonism: changes during several years of continuing treatment. *Psychopharmacol Bull* 1986;22:250–253.
131. Waddington JL. Tardive dyskinesia: a critical re-evaluation of the causal role of neuroleptics and of the dopamine receptor supersensitivity hypothesis. In: Callaghan N, Galvin R, eds. *Recent research in neurology*. London: Pitman Books, 1984.
132. Tarsy D, Baldessarini RJ. The pathophysiologic basis of tardive dyskinesia. *Biol Psychiatry* 1977;12:431–450.
133. Fahn S. Therapeutic approach to tardive dyskinesia. *J Clin Psychiatry* 1985;46:19–24.
134. Hershey T, Bhargava N, Sadler M, et al. Conventional versus intensive diabetes therapy in children with type 1 diabetes: effects on memory and motor speed. *Diabetes Care* 1999;22:1318–1324.
135. Feeney DM, Gonzalez A, Law WA. Amphetamine, haloperidol and experience interact to affect rate of recovery after motor cortex surgery. *Science* 1982;217: 855–857.
136. Tsai G, Goff DC, Chang RW, et al. Markers of glutamatergic neurotransmission and oxidative stress associated with tardive dyskinesia. *Am J Psychiatry* 1998; 155:1207–1213.
137. Pandurangi AK, Devi V, Channabasavanna SM. Caudate atrophy in irreversible tardive dyskinesia. *J Clin Psychiatry* 1980;41:229–231.
138. Nielson EB, Lyon M. Evidence for cell loss in corpus striatum after long-term treatment with a neuroleptic drug flupenthixol in rats. *Psychopharmacology* 1978; 59:85–90.
139. Chadwick DREH, Marsden CD. Anticonvulsant-induced dyskinesias: a comparison with dyskinesias induced by neuroleptics. *J Neurol Neurosurg Psychiatry* 1976;39:1210–1218.
140. Jacome D. Carbamazepine-induced dystonia. *JAMA* 1979;241:2263.
141. Muenter MD, Whisnant JP. Basal ganglia calcification, hypoparathyroidism, and extrapyramidal motor manifestations. *Neurology* 1968;18:1075–1083.
142. Cummings JL, Gosenfeld LF, Houlihan JP, et al. Neuropsychiatric disturbances associated with idiopathic calcification of the basal ganglia. *Biol Psychiatry* 1983;18:591–599.
143. Burke RE, Fahn S, Jankovic J, et al. Tardive dystonia: late-onset & persistent dystonia caused by antipsychotic drugs. *Neurology* 1982;32:1335–1346.
144. Fahn S. Drug treatment of hyperkinetic movement disorders. *J Clin Psychiatry* 1987;7:192–207.
145. Fahn S. Treatment of tardive dyskinesia: use of dopamine depleting agents. *Clin Neuropharmacol* 1983; 6:151–158.
146. Asher SW, Aminoff MJ. Tetrabenzamine and movement disorders. *Neurology* 1981;31:1051–1054.
147. Casey DE, Denney D. Pharmacologic characterization of tardive dyskinesia. *Psychopharmacology* 1977; 54:1–8.
148. Moore DC, Bowers MB. Identification of a subgroup of tardive dyskinesia by pharmacological probes. *Am J Psychiatry* 1980;137:1202–1205.
149. Gelenberg AJ, Doller-Wojcik JC, Growden JH. Choline and lecithin in the treatment of tardive dyskinesia. *Am J Psychiatry* 1979;136:772–775.
150. Kang UJ, Burke RE, Fahn S. Natural history and treatment of tardive dyskinesia. *Mov Disord* 1986;1: 193–208.
151. Gualtieri CT, Hicks RE, Patrick K, et al. Clinical correlates of methylphenidate blood levels. *Ther Drug Monit* 1984;6:379–392.

152. Gualtieri CT, Keppel JM, Schroeder SR. Tardive dyskinesia: new facts and new recommendations. *Psychiatr Aspects Ment Retard Rev* 1986;5:1–6.
153. Glazor W, Moore DC, Schooler NR, et al. Tardive dyskinesia: a discontinuation study. *Arch Gen Psychiatry* 1984;41:623–627.
154. Yassa R, Nair V, Schwartz G. Tardive dyskinesia: a two-year follow-up study. *Psychosomatics* 1984;25.
155. Chouinard G, Annable L, Mercier P, et al. A five-year follow-up study of tardive dyskinesia. *Psychopharmacol Bull* 1986;22:259–263.
156. Casey DE. Tardive dyskinesia: reversible and irreversible. In: Casey DE, Chase TN, Christensen AV, et al., eds. *Dyskinesia—research and treatment*. Berlin/Heidelberg: Springer-Verlag, 1985.
157. Yagi G, Itoh H. Follow-up study of 11 patients with potentially reversible tardive dyskinesia. *Am J Psychiatry* 1987;144:1496–1498.
158. Quitkin F, Rifkin A, Gochfeld L, et al. Tardive dyskinesia: are first signs reversible? *Am J Psychiatry* 1977;134:84–87.
159. Kane JM, Weinhold P, Kinon B, et al. Prevalence of abnormal involuntary movements ("spontaneous dyskinesias") in the normal elderly. *Psychopharmacology* 1982;77:105–108.
160. Chaffin DS. Phenothiazine-induced acute psychotic reaction: the "psychotoxicity" of a drug. *Am J Psychiatry* 1964;121:26–32.
161. Singh MM, Kay SR. Dysphoric response to neuroleptic treatment in schizophrenia: its relationship to autonomic arousal and prognosis. *Biol Psychiatry* 1979;14:277–294.
162. Bachmann KM, Modestin J. Neuroleptic-induced panic attacks in a patient with delusional depression. *J Nerv Ment Dis* 1987;175:373–375.
163. Mikkelsen EJ, Detlor J, Cohen DJ. School avoidance and social phobia triggered by haloperidol in patients with Tourette's syndrome. *Am J Psychiatry* 1981;138:1572–1576.
164. Moller H, von Zerssen D. Depressive states occurring during the neuroleptic treatment of schizophrenia. *Schizophr Bull* 1982;8:109–117.

24
Extraterritorial Psychotropics

SUMMARY

During the late 1970s and early 1980s, new drug development in psychiatry was comparatively stagnant. There was nothing like the efflorescence of new drugs that began with the introduction of fluoxetine in 1986. In those years, neuropsychiatrists were eager to find drugs that were not tricyclic antidepressants, benzodiazepines, or neuroleptics. They turned to drugs that were being used in general medicine: the beta-blockers, calcium channel antagonists, and the α_2 agonists.

Since then, the new antidepressants, mood stabilizers, and antipsychotics have largely supplanted those extraterritorial psychotropics. Nevertheless, they continue to have at least a degree of clinical utility. There are some interesting theoretical issues behind them as well. The calcium blockers, for example, may be neuroprotective or possibly neurotoxic. In animal experiments, nimodipine enhances learning and prevents the cognitive deterioration associated with aging. Other studies have indicated accelerated aging-related cognitive decline in patients on calcium blockers.

Not every psychotropic is a drug. Cranial electrostimulation therapy (EST), a relatively innocuous treatment that can act like a mild antidepressant/anxiolytic, is used here to illustrate this point. It is sometimes helpful for chronic pain, insomnia, and anxiety in patients with brain injury. It is not a potent antidepressant, such as electroconvulsive therapy or vagal nerve stimulation, but it may be useful when one is reluctant to add one more drug to a complicated treatment regimen. How it compares with transcranial magnetic stimulation remains to be seen.

NOT EVERY PSYCHOTROPIC IS A PSYCHIATRIC DRUG

Effective psychopharmacology is not limited to drugs from the conventional categories. There are several interesting drugs that also have psychotropic effects but are not classified among the psychotropics. Clinical research interest in the beta-blockers, calcium channel blockers, and α_2 agonists has been eclipsed in recent years by the extraordinary wave of new antidepressants, atypical antipsychotics, and anticonvulsants, and clinical prescription has probably diminished as well. Nevertheless, they have a role to play, especially for patients with unusual conditions that are refractory to the usual treatments. Their occasional success in treatment is complemented by some interesting theoretical perspectives.

β-ADRENERGIC BLOCKERS

The beta-blockers are indicated for hypertension, angina pectoris, cardiac arrhythmia, essential tremor, and migraine prophylaxis. They have also been an important class of drugs for patients with neuropsychiatric disorders, and the list of indications is almost as diverse.

The beta-blockers are classified in the following ways:

1. By selectivity, i.e., selective affinity for the B_1 receptor. Atenolol, for example, is cardioselective, whereas propanolol and nadolol have mixed selectivity because they block both the B_1 and B_2 receptors.
2. By relative degree of lipophilia/hydrophilia. A lipophilic beta-blocker such as propanolol crosses the blood-brain barrier quite readily, and a hydrophilic drug such as nadolol crosses very

slowly, if at all. There is some disagreement on the importance of this point. Some maintain that the psychotropic effects of hydrophilic beta-blockers such as nadolol are entirely peripheral, whereas others maintain that its actions are explicable in terms of a central effect, which may be slower in onset, but central nevertheless.

3. By intrinsic sympathomimetic activity, i.e., the capacity to act as a partial agonist at the beta receptor. Pindolol, a drug with intrinsic sympathomimetic activity, does not cause the same degree of bradycardia and hypotension that the other beta-blockers do. Conversely, it has behavioral toxicity, such as excitement and agitation; this is unusual for beta-blockers, which are more often associated with depression. In fact, pindolol has been put forth as an antidepressant augmenter. For some reason, beta-blockers with high intrinsic sympathomimetic activity are the only ones with no proclivity to raise blood lipid levels (1).
4. By elimination half-life. Propanolol, for example, has a very short half-life, and unless the long-acting form is used, the patient with anxiety or akathisia may experience a disconcerting "on-off" phenomenon. Nadolol, in contrast, is a very long acting drug, so once-daily dosing is feasible.

In 1966, Granville-Grossman and Turner (2) reported relief of the somatic symptoms of anxiety in patients who were treated with propanolol and the first studies of propanolol as a psychotropic drug concentrated on the treatment of anxiety. It was thought that propanolol might be a superior anxiolytic for patients whose symptoms were mainly somatic, for example, tremor, tachycardia, palpitations, diaphoresis, and the urge to micturate (3). The preferential effect for somatic anxiety is arguable, but the beta-blockers have become the drugs of choice for performance anxiety. Performers like them because symptoms such as nervous tremor or diaphoresis are relieved with no detectable effect on memory or motor performance (4). Beta-blockers are banned for Olympic target shooters because they promote motor steadiness in the face of the anxiety of competition.

The next indication, historically at least, was schizophrenia. There was even a time when propanolol was advanced as an antipsychotic drug (5). It may only raise plasma concentrations of neuroleptics administered concomitantly (6,7). Beta-blockers may have a specific effect on aggressive behavior in patients with chronic psychotic disorders, just as they do in other classes of patients (8,9). They are also effective for neuroleptic-induced akathisia, but they are not antipsychotics.

Beta-blockers have been recommended for treatment of withdrawal symptoms from alcohol (10), benzodiazepines (11), and opiates (10).

Elliot (12,13) was the first to cite the effectiveness of propanolol for belligerence during coma recovery in patients with brain injury, and his findings have been extended to a wide range of patients with episodic rage and aggressive behavior owing to a number of organic disorders including infectious encephalopathy (14), temporal lobe epilepsy, Wilson's disease, mental retardation (15), the late sequelae of closed head injury (16), and dementia (17). These findings have been reiterated in large-scale surveys (18), and it is said that beta-blockers may be effective when more conventional therapies have failed (19). The usual dose of propanolol is approximately 160 mg per day, but the range of effective doses is quite broad, from 50 to 960 mg per day (18). It may also be necessary to wait for 2 or 3 months before the therapeutic effects of a beta-blocker are felt. This may be problematic in the treatment of the aggressive patient.

Propanolol has been successfully prescribed to treat temper outbursts in patients with attention deficit/hyperactivity disorder (ADHD) (20). In patients with ADHD who are only partially controlled with stimulants or antidepressants, beta-blockers may augment the therapeutic effect (21).

In 1967, Strang described success in treating restless legs syndrome (or Ekbom's syndrome) with propanolol (21a). In fact, it was not Ekbom who first described restless legs syndrome, it was Joseph Babinski [which rhymes with Lipinski, who first described the treatment of neuroleptic-induced akathisia with propanolol (22)]. The latter was a signal contribution because there have been several subsequent studies of beta-blockers in the treatment of neuroleptic-induced akathisia, and they tend to be favorable, even for the hydrophilic beta-blockers (23). Clonidine, another drug that diminished adrenergic outflow, has been effective in reducing symptoms of neuroleptic-induced akathisia (24,25). This is interesting because it suggests that adrenergic mechanisms may be involved in the development of akathisia (23).

Treatment with beta-blockers should be undertaken only with a clear understanding of their influence on peripheral β receptors. Beta-blockers are contraindicated in patients with asthma, sinus bradycardia, conduction defects, and brittle diabetes (because they may mask the symptoms of hypoglycemia), and in patients on concomitant adrenergic drugs such as the monoamine oxidase inhibitors.

The psychological side effect that is most commonly associated with beta-blockers is depression

(26). This significant factor has diminished their utility in general medicine. Conversely, the hyperaroused patients with neuropsychiatric disorders who are most likely to respond to beta-blockers are relatively inured to this effect.

Other negative effects include acute delirium with or without psychotic features (27–30), hallucinations (31), and vivid nightmares. Propanolol has been reported to cause transient spatial orientation disorder (32) and amnesia (33). It is not entirely clear whether beta-blockers that are highly lipophilic are more likely to cause neuropsychiatric impairment than the less lipophilic compounds (34,35).

The efficacy of the beta-blocking drugs for patients with neuropathic disorders, for example, victims of traumatic brain injury or mentally handicapped individuals, has elicited a number of speculations concerning the mechanism of action of this drug class. Several hypotheses have been offered, including central beta-blockade, nonspecific membrane stabilization effects, presynaptic noradrenergic effects, serotonergic effects, and attenuation of peripheral feedback via a number of different possible routes.

The last idea has given rise to an interesting hypothesis about the mechanism of drug action, apart from the obvious one that has to do with central adrenergic blockade at the β receptor. It is raised by the interesting observation that β antagonists that do not cross the blood-brain barrier, such as nadolol, are often as effective, and sometimes more effective, than β antagonists, such as propanolol, that enter the central nervous system (CNS) quite readily. As mentioned previously, the premise is shaky, but the argument is interesting.

The concept of noise, in this regard, refers to the relative inability of the patient with a neuropathic disorder to filter or screen out irrelevant signals from their internal or external environment. The stimuli that all of us receive are necessarily composed of signal (useful information) and noise (meaningless information). The patient with diffuse brain injury, congenital or acquired, is postulated to process information with a low signal-to-noise ratio. In response to a given stimulus, the patient receives a signal that is less clear than a normal person does and more noise or clutter as well (36).

A normal person who is exposed to severe static in a telephone conversation or to a channel of distracting information in a dichotic listening task is likely to experience annoyance, frustration, and irritability. A patient who receives such a noisy stimulus and then has to decode it with mental apparatus that is already compromised by injury experiences double the frustration. The attention deficit of the patient with schizophrenia, for example, may be attributable to a defective filter that allows irrelevant intrusions to overwhelm normal cognition (37,38).

The result of experiencing a signal that can neither be intelligibly perceived nor correctly integrated may produce stimulus overload and then internal chaos, personal distortions, impulsivity, hypervigilance, increased physiologic stress, and aggression (36,39,40). When the stimuli one receives over a long period of time, from the external environment as well as from one's own body, are chaotic and uncontrollable, one may be reduced to responding rigidly and sometimes very intensely in an attempt to organize the stimuli (41). To such a patient, novel stimuli are perceived as threatening, and the response is stereotyped (42).

The CNS seems to react to any overwhelming threatening and uncontrollable experience in a consistent pattern. Regardless of the precipitating event, traumatized people continue to have a poor tolerance for arousal. They tend to respond to stress in an all-or-nothing way: either unmodulated anxiety, often accompanied by motoric discharge that includes acts of aggression against the self and others, or social and emotional withdrawal (43).

Theoretically, at least, treatment with peripheral beta-blockers can reduce the noise level in a patient's incoming stimuli. Nadolol, for example, can reduce anxiety in the patient by relaxing the skeletal and striate musculature. This would decrease the somatic contribution to the noise level that a patient experiences and increase the signal-to-noise ratio, thus alleviating the chaotic internal environment and allowing the patient to tolerate a greater degree of external disorganization (44).

This is an attractive theory that allows the reader to contemplate, with sympathy, the psychology of the patient with brain damage. With respect to the specific issue at hand, however, it is posited on two requirements: (i) that peripherally active beta-blockers do not cross the blood-brain barrier (11) and (ii) that they are equally effective, or more effective, with a more benign side-effects profile than the centrally active beta-blockers (45–47). There is reason to believe that both these requirements have been met. Conversely, there is also reason to think that a combination of central and peripheral actions may account for the unique clinical utility of the β antagonists, even the ones that are supposed to stay outside the blood-brain barrier.

The beta-blockers were especially important in neuropsychiatry 10 years ago, before the atypical antipsychotics, new mood stabilizers, and new antidepressants were introduced. When the only reasonable alternatives were the conventional neuroleptics or lithium, they were an attractive choice. They are less attractive now, not because they were ineffective, but because they are less effective, in general, than the available alternatives.

α_2 AGONISTS

Clonidine is the prototypic α_2 agonist, an antihypertensive drug that causes sedation. Although it is counterintuitive that an α-mimetic drug can cause sedation and decrease the blood pressure, the central action of clonidine and of the less sedating α_2 agonist guanfacine is presumably at the presynaptic α_2 receptor (48). The effect of presynaptic receptor stimulation is to diminish the release of norepinephrine across the synaptic junction, lower the concentration of norepinephrine in the brain, and diminish sympathetic outflow—thus, its antihypertensive effect and the sedation and its purported effect in patients with neuropsychiatric disorders, mostly children with ADHD, in diminishing arousal, anxiety, aggression, and hyperactivity. It is also possible that α_2 agonists, by virtue of their negative effect on the adrenergic system, are also serotonin inhibitors (48).

The other interesting chemical effect is that, at high doses, clonidine and related drugs act as postsynaptic stimulants of the α_2 receptor. At high doses, then, they stimulate the adrenergic system, and this may account for their positive effects on memory and attention.

The α_2 agonists seem to have an oval effect in the treatment of children with ADHD, in which they do a good job in diminishing stimulant side effects such as irritability, insomnia, and tics and, at the same time, augment their positive cognitive and behavioral effects (49). It is impossible to attribute this to simultaneous and opposite effects on central sympathetic tone. Reducing noradrenergic tone does diminish hyperarousal, but it also tends to increase distractibility. One possible explanation is that α_2 agonists attenuate noradrenergic outflow from the locus ceruleus, but only when it is firing at increased rates in times of stress or when the organism is distracted by novel stimuli. Under such circumstances, they may reasonably be expected to attenuate the deleterious effects of stress or distracters on task performance (50). Thus, clonidine and guanfacine may only be indirect cognitive enhancers.

Clonidine seems to have some positive effects on cognition. It has been found to ameliorate the cognitive deficits of aged primates (51) and of patients with Korsakoff's psychosis (52). Presumably, this is because it is an adrenergic stimulant at certain doses and particularly at the α_2 receptors of the prefrontal cortex that mediate attention and resistance to distraction (53). Clonidine treatment has also been associated with functional restoration of the traumatically injured spinal cord in laboratory animals. This effect may have to do with the protective action of α_2 agonists against the occurrence of *N*-methyl-D-aspartate neurotoxicity (54). There is preliminary evidence that clonidine reduces spasticity in humans resulting from cervical or thoracic transverse myelopathy, perhaps by stimulating α_2 receptors in the cord and thus inhibiting γ and α motor neurons (55).

Conversely, clonidine has had a detrimental effect on cortical recovery in experimental brain injury paradigms (56,57), and treatment of patients with stroke with clonidine (for hypertension) seems to retard motor recovery (58). Clonidine and guanfacine have been promoted as treatments for dementia, especially in Europe, but the results of clinical trials have not been encouraging (59).

The positive cognitive effects of α_2 agonists remain a theoretical issue. Even in the treatment of ADHD, their main clinical application in psychiatry, the behavioral effects of the drugs are more prominent than their cognitive effects.

Clonidine and the related drug guanfacine seem to be partially effective for a wide range of neuropsychiatric conditions. (Partially effective means partial response in most patients, good therapeutic response for only some patients, or effective, but only for a while.) The list includes anxiety disorders (48), obsessive-compulsive disorder (60,61), bipolar disorder (62), tardive dyskinesia (63), Tourette's syndrome (64,65), posttraumatic stress disorder (66), posttraumatic stress disorder nightmares (67), and ADHD (49,68). In mentally retarded people, guanfacine is reported to reduce the problems of behavioral deterioration on neuroleptic withdrawal (69).

Clonidine was reported to raise the seizure threshold in one patient who was treated with electroconvulsive therapy for depression (70). In fact, clonidine is capable of a suppressant effect on seizures induced by a variety of stimuli including electric shock, sound, and decapitation (sic) and convulsant compounds such as picrotoxin, strychnine, pentylenetetrazol, and glycine (70). The effect can be blocked by yohimbine and idazoxin, α_2-adrenergic antagonists (71).

The syndrome of hypervigilance/hyperreactivity is sometimes seen in patients with brain injury with severe orbitofrontal lesions (72,73). This posttraumatic syndrome may be reflected in patients with developmental handicap, particularly patients with autism who can also be hypervigilant/hyperreactive and given to stereotypies, compulsive rituals, perseverative behavior, and motor and phonic tics. In both clinical conditions, the therapeutic effect of clonidine is probably mediated by its net effect in reducing adrenergic stimulation from brainstem nuclei. It may be augmented, if necessary, by concomitant therapy with β-adrenergic blockers. It may take several weeks for the full therapeutic effect to mature, however, so one should go very slowly before adding a second drug to a clonidine regime.

The recent reports of successful treatment with clonidine of children with Cornelia de Lange syndrome is particularly interesting in this regard because their behavioral problems are certainly characterized by a state of chronic hyperarousal and hyperreactivity. The case reports are only beginning to appear in the literature; even as they do, it is necessary to point out that, like every other treatment for children with Cornelia de Lange syndrome, the effects of clonidine are inconsistent.

Patients on α_2 agonists must be observed for signs of hypotension and bradycardia, especially when they are used in conjunction with beta-blockers. In fact, the toxicity profile of clonidine is hardly favorable, and there are several other things to look for. The common side effects of clonidine in patients with psychiatric disorders include sedation or, conversely, sleep disturbance, dry mouth, inattention, irritability, decreased sexual interest, impotence (48), dizziness, light-headedness, depression, delirium (74), hyperactivity, mania, and paranoia (75). Abrupt withdrawal from clonidine is known to cause hypertensive crisis; it may also lead to severe psychiatric decompensation, even to a state of acute psychosis in vulnerable patients (76). Guanfacine is less sedating than clonidine, and it is less likely to cause hypertensive rebound after abrupt withdrawal.

Three sudden deaths have been reported in children with ADHD treated with clonidine in combination with methylphenidate. Naturally, this caused quite a stir. The fatal cases were confounded by a number of other factors, however, such as general anesthesia, cardiac disease, and other drugs (77,78). Child psychiatrists have not given up on the combination of a psychostimulant and clonidine, and no further fatalities have been reported. The combination of two very short-acting drugs, both with a proclivity to acute withdrawal symptoms, may be unwise. When a stimulant is combined with an α_2 agonist, one or the other should be a long-acting drug.

The therapeutic utility of an α_2 antagonist such as clonidine may, in theory at least, be limited by the reciprocal association of α and β adrenoreceptors. For example, drugs that lower the synaptic availability of norepinephrine and serotonin (e.g., clonidine) may cause supersensitivity in the β receptor, whereas increased responsiveness in the α receptors may lead to β receptor down-regulation (79). The net effect on adrenergic neurotransmission may be zero, if alpha-blockade leads to beta-supersensitivity, whereas beta-blockade does the reverse. It is a theoretical concern, but it may explain why the beneficial effects of clonidine or the beta-blockers are only partial or transient and may predict that some patients with behavioral conditions characterized by diffuse adrenergic hyperactivity require cotreatment with clonidine and a beta-blocker.

In such cases, a beta-blocker with intrinsic sympathomimetic activity may be required to preserve cardiovascular integrity as the central effects of noradrenergic hyperactivity are managed. On the other hand, the combination of beta-blockers and α_2 agonists has been used in the treatment of refractory hypertension with no increased risk of cardiovascular side effects (80,81), although there are individual case reports of hypertensive crisis when clonidine was abruptly discontinued while treatment with beta-blockers continued (82).

If there is a moral to this story, it is that manipulating adrenergic overactivity may be a useful strategy in a number of different neuropsychiatric conditions. Neither beta-blockade nor central alpha-blockade at the presynaptic receptor is sufficiently reliable, at least with existing agents, to guide one's clinical practice with confidence of a favorable outcome. Aside from the unique case of ADHD, clonidine and guanfacine are uncertain agents, with only a small chance of success in the treatment of brain injury, stroke, autism, or mental retardation. The α_2 agonists, like the beta-blockers, are second- or third-line drugs. Their wide range of potential utility is, if anything, emblematic of their failure to secure reliable indications as first-line agents.

CALCIUM ANTAGONISTS

Calcium channel blockers were discovered in 1967 and have since occupied an important position in the treatment of cardiovascular disease, including hypertension, cardiac arrhythmias, and angina pectoris. They also play a role in neurology, stroke, vertigo, migraine, and epilepsy. They may have at least some usefulness in the treatment of various psychiatric disorders, especially manic depression. The first report of successful calcium antagonist therapy for a patient with bipolar disorder appeared in 1982; this interesting class of drugs has yet to find a regular place among the psychotropics.

Calcium channel blockers are an established tool in the management of acute stroke and severe brain injury. They are believed to be neuroprotective by virtue of their effect on calcium homeostasis and excitotoxicity. They are also thought to improve learning and cognitive performance, especially in the elderly.

Ionic calcium plays a critical role in regulating the function of excitable cells. In neurons and muscles at rest, the intracellular free calcium concentration is maintained at a level that is 10,000 times lower than that in the extracellular space. The concentration of intracellular calcium increases when the cell membrane is depolarized, as calcium ions move through pores in the cell membrane. These functional pores are glycoproteins and are called calcium channels. They are also called voltage-dependent channels because they only open in response to membrane depolarization. An agonist stimulates a membrane receptor, the membrane begins to depolarize, and calcium rushes in through the voltage-dependent calcium channel.

There is a dynamic balance of calcium influx and efflux through the calcium channels, and thus a state of calcium homeostasis is maintained. The calcium ion is a second messenger that couples receptor stimulation in various kinds of excitable cells with diverse physiologic responses including neurotransmitter release, secretion of circulating hormones, or muscle contraction. Drugs that block calcium channels block the entry of extracellular calcium into the target cell and thus diminish their excitability and alter their physiologic response (83,84).

Here it gets a little complicated. There are several different types of calcium channels. Each subtype has a narrow range of membrane potential at which it is most likely to be open. They are transient opening (T type), long-opening (L type), neuronal (N type), and Purkinje (P type) (85). Only the L channels (slow channels) are inactivated by calcium antagonists.

Within the L-type calcium channel, there is a protein complex, which has at least four distinct recognition sites. Each of these sites binds preferentially to different calcium channel blocker drugs. Therefore, there are four major classes of calcium channel blockers: the dihydropyridines (e.g., nimodipine, nifedipine, nicardipine, amlodipine), the phenyalkylamines (e.g., verapamil), the benzothiazepines (e.g., diltiazem), and the diphenylalkylamines (e.g., flunarizine).

Binding-site affinity on this protein complex is associated with tissue selectivity and different physiologic effects. The dihydropyridines and diphenylalkylamines are cerebroselective calcium antagonists. They have preferential effects on calcium channels located in the smooth muscle of cerebral blood vessels. They have potent vasodilatory effects on cerebral blood vessels. Because they increase cerebral blood flow, investigators explored their use in the treatment of poststroke ischemia.

The dihydropyridine nimodipine has been proven effective in improving neurologic outcome in patients who have had a subarachnoid hemorrhage. It is highly lipophilic, crosses the blood-brain barrier quite readily, and is selective for vascular smooth muscle. It is capable of reducing cerebral arterial spasm, which is one of the primary causes of neurologic deficits in patients who survive a subarachnoid hemorrhage. It is a delayed effect that occurs within 4 to 21 days after the initial hemorrhagic event. Because nimodipine can prevent or reverse arterial spasm, it can improve the survival rate and prevent neurologic deficits in patients with stroke and even in patients with TBI (86–88).

The beneficial effects of nimodipine are not necessarily the result of cerebral vasodilation. Rather, the drug appears to exercise a neuroprotective effect. It does so by preventing the accumulation of intracellular calcium that usually occurs in stroke and brain injury (89,90).

After some German neurologists noted that patients with stroke who were treated with nimodipine seemed to recover some earlier learning losses, neuroscientists investigated the effect of the drug for cognitive impairment in other conditions, most notably, aging. In theory, brain aging is owing to the accumulation of intraneuronal calcium, an ossification of the brain, as it were. It is said that cell death occurs because the aged neuron loses its ability to regulate calcium uptake properly (91).

In elderly rabbits, nimodipine treatment improves learning in a variety of cognitive tasks to the point that their performance equals that of young rabbits (92,93). Similar effects have been noted in rats (94) and primates (95). The results of several trials of nimodipine in patients with dementia have been equivocal but were sufficiently encouraging to permit the marketing of nimodipine in several European countries for the indication of impaired brain function in old age (96,97). This is the kind of information that elicits the interest of neuropsychiatrists, aging patients, or any person, for that matter, who wakes up in the morning to find a white crust on the inner lining of his or her neurons. However, the retail cost of nimodipine (in excess of $400 a week) militates against its common use in the United States, at least as a cerebral tonic or an antiaging formula.

Many other drugs also block the calcium channel, including reserpine, the benzodiazepines diazepam and flurazepam, morphine, and valproate (98). The neuroleptic pimozide is a diphenylbutylpiperidine calcium blocker. The phenothiazine and butyrophenone neuroleptics are very weak as calcium antagonists, but the atypical neuroleptic thioridazine has calcium-blocking activity at blood levels that occur during clinical treatment. In fact, this may account for the cardiotoxic effects of thioridazine and pimozide (83).

In a similar vein, drugs that are calcium antagonists may also exert other neurochemical effects. For example, some calcium channel blockers can block norepinephrine competitively at the α receptor (83). They also have varying effects on dopamine and serotonin (99,100). The caudate nucleus, for example, is a brain region with the highest density of specific binding sites for the calcium antagonists (101). The calcium channel blocker flunarizine is antihistaminic, antidopaminergic, and antiserotonergic (102).

Psychiatric interest in the calcium channel blockers was originally stimulated by the facts that several psychoactive drugs, most notably lithium, are calcium agonists (103) and that altered calcium metabolism seems to characterize particular psychiatric disorders (84). There have been several reports to suggest that calcium blockers are effective in bipolar affective disorders (103,104), alone or in combination with other mood-stabilizing drugs (105). Nimodipine was effective alone or with carbamazepine in approximately 50% of patients with refractory bipolar disorder (106). In a controlled study, nimodipine proved to be an effective antidepressant augmenter for elderly patients with vascular dementia (107). Verapamil, in particular, is well tolerated by patients with dementia with bipolar disorder (103) or depression (108). Calcium blockers are also effective in depression (109), panic disorder (110), and refractory schizophrenia (111), although the evidence is not strong (112). Childs (unpublished, 1986) described two severely disturbed individuals who responded very well to verapamil. One had severe aggression and self-injurious behavior; he had had traumatic brain injury. The other was an impulsive, aggressive adolescent.

The calcium blockers may be used to treat Tourette's syndrome (113,114) but have also been known to induce extrapyramidal side effects, such as oculogyric crisis and akathisia (115). Flunarizine is said to have a neuroleptic-like action (101). If it does, however, that attribute has been lost on the physicians who have used it safely for years for migraine, vertigo, and epilepsy. It is not prone to lower the blood pressure, and its cerebroprotective effects are thought to be superior (102,116,117). It is also widely used in Europe as a supplemental treatment for cases of refractory epilepsy (118).

In fact, the inhibition of neuronal calcium entry during abnormal electrical activity in the brain has been a major target in the development of novel antiepileptic drugs. It has even been suggested that the action of several established antiepileptic drugs is at least in part owing to their effects on calcium influx into neurons (119). Because patients with depression are also found to have an exaggerated pattern of calcium influx in response to certain stimuli (120), it is possible that calcium blockade is the common thread that unites the common anticonvulsant and mood-stabilizing effects of certain drugs. Verapamil and nimodipine inhibit amygdaloid kindling, another mechanism that is theoretically active in major depression (121).

The calcium channel blockers have a relatively favorable side-effect profile and may be even better tolerated by some patients than lithium (103). They are not sedating; the major effect is that they are somewhat stimulating. It might be appropriate to explore their clinical usefulness for problems related to severe affective disorders, especially in patients with encephalopathic conditions.

By 1996, the calcium channel blockers had become so popular that their prescription for hypertension equaled that of diuretics and angiotensin-converting enzyme inhibitors and exceeded that of the beta-blockers. However, concerns were raised about the relative safety of these drugs, especially the short-acting dihydropyridine derivatives. In overdose, the calcium channel blockers can cause hypotension and heart failure, and even at conventional doses, it was suggested that the long-term risk of myocardial infarction, gastrointestinal hemorrhage, or cancer may be increased (122). Even more disquieting is the proposal that reduced levels of cytosolic calcium in neurons may induce the synthesis of proteins associated with programmed cell death (apoptosis). The Canadian Study of Health and Aging reported that calcium channel blocker treatment seemed to be associated with cognitive decline (123). Even in patients with brain trauma, the results of controlled studies are actually quite uncertain (124).

The neuroprotective effects of calcium antagonists must thus be set against the potential danger of long-term neurotoxicity and other problems (125). Although the risks of long-term treatment with calcium channel blockers are probably small, they have yet to be fully appraised. It is not clear how this information will influence their prescription for neuropsychiatric disorders. In terms of cognitive enhancement, the evidence is not sufficiently solid to support any degree of risk.

The use of calcium channel blockers by psychiatrists illustrates a pattern that is characteristic of the extracurricular psychotropics. They are still used, but not very much. They are probably effective, but less reliably so than the established drugs, whether the condition is bipolar affective disorder, depression, or epilepsy. The introduction of a host of new antidepressant, antipsychotic, and anticonvulsant drugs in recent years has relegated interest in the calcium channel blockers and the other occasional psychotropics to a lower position. It is probably not the long-term dangers of calcium channel blockers that have limited their use; it is simply the availability of new and better drugs.

OPIATE ANTAGONISTS

The neuropsychiatric uses for opiate antagonists are limited. This is disappointing, in light of extensive literature and excursions into virtually every clinical and preclinical domain.

For example, there is preclinical evidence that some aspect of memory is mediated by opioid peptides. Opiate antagonists cause memory facilitation, and opiate agonists, in particular opioid peptides, cause amnesia (126). It was natural, therefore, to try opiate antagonists in the treatment of memory disorders, such as Alzheimer's disease. There were preliminary reports of improvement in patients with dementia with intravenous naloxone but subsequent experience has not corroborated the result, either with naloxone or oral naltrexone (127).

Opiate antagonists have interesting effects in experimental brain injury and brain injury preparations. Neurotrauma is usually associated with an increased concentration of endogenous opioids in the cerebrospinal fluid (128). Acute treatment with opiate antagonists has produced some amazing short-term results, including the reversal of coma in a child with necrotizing encephalomyelopathy (129) and the reversal of hemiplegia secondary to cerebral ischemia in two patients (130). In a variety of animal preparations, naloxone has been found to improve blood flow, blood gas, electrophysiologic activity, cell energetics, and neurologic outcome after traumatic brain injury or spinal cord injury (128,131). The mechanism is unclear. It may be the result of improved perfusion of damaged tissue, inhibition of excitatory neurotoxicity, or correction of an imbalance in calcium or magnesium homeostasis. In the CNS, opioids interact with most of the governing neurotransmitters (132).

The preclinical model is robust and far ranging. It is replicated in a model of ischemic stroke (130) and fetal asphyxia (133). The effect on long-term neurobehavioral outcome is positive (134). The various opioids appear to have a protective effect against seizure activity (135). In infant rats, naloxone increases brain size and cellular development (136).

In light of this body of evidence, one is naturally disappointed to learn that so little has been accomplished in the treatment for patients. There are occasional reports of naltrexone for postconcussion syndrome (137), in which it has helped neurocognitive, somatic, and emotional symptoms. There is also a report of improvement with naltrexone in four patients with bulimia and head injury (138). Clinical experience has not led to many published reports and to no clinical trials. There is a clear disparity, then, between the preclinical literature and clinical experience that remains to be reconciled.

The rationale for the treatment of organic bulimia with naltrexone was derived from early reports of patients with Prader-Willi syndrome who have compulsive hyperphagia, food stealing, and extreme obesity and who were once said to respond to opiate antagonists. The endogenous opioid system is supposed to have a robust effect on the control of food intake, and antagonists have reduced food intake in normal subjects, obese patients, and binge eaters (139,140). In my opinion, the effect is less than robust.

Naltrexone is presently used in psychiatry for opioid detoxification (141) and to prevent heroin reabuse after detoxification (142). It is also used for some appetitive disorders such as anorexia and bulimia nervosa (143), tobacco and alcohol addiction (144), and the opiate addictions. It is rarely used for compulsive hyperphagia or obesity or patients with Prader-Willi syndrome.

Modest results have characterized the research on naltrexone for children with autism (145,146). The only remaining indication in developmental medicine is for self-injurious behavior, as described in Chapter 15. It is recommended for acral lick dermatitis in dogs, but the sample size is small (147).

Naltrexone is expensive but is easy to take. There are few acute problems and the long-term side-effect profile is favorable (148). It is a shame that such an interesting compound should be so futile in the clinical arena. Perhaps nothing has been proved as yet; maybe time is needed to learn the full effects of naltrexone, as demonstrated in self-injurious behavior. The development of opiate antagonists with more specific effects on the different opiate receptors may change the situation.

NICOTINE

Years ago when I was just out of medical school, I was moonlighting in the emergency department of a small country hospital. It was a hot and humid July evening, and the patient was a 10-year old with sudden onset of nausea, weakness, and diaphoresis. I supposed it was some sort of toxic reaction.

In fact, it was, and his father told me exactly what. The child had been working on his grandfather's farm, "topping" tobacco, that is, clipping off the budding tops of tobacco plants to make the leaves grow better. He had green tobacco sickness, an illness they never taught me about in medical school in New York City, but a common problem, at least in those days, in rural North Carolina. On a hot day, workers absorb quite a lot of nicotine from the leaves of the tobacco plant as they work with bare hands and arms. Unless they have developed a tolerance to the drug, by smoking, chewing, or dipping snuff, handling the tobacco plant with warm, sweaty skin will have quite a reaction.

So, you see, nothing in God's creation is all bad. Smoking, chewing tobacco, or dipping snuff actually prevents the development of green tobacco sickness. That may not mean much to you, but around where I live, it is something. Or, at least, it used to be.

Is there anything else that tobacco is good for? It may be a negative risk factor for two prototypical neurodegenerative diseases, Parkinson's disease and Alzheimer's disease. A long train of epidemiologic studies, extending over more than 30 years, has indicated that regular tobacco consumption slows the onset of Parkinson's disease or prevents it entirely (149). Support for a protective effect against Alzheimer's disease is less well established and more controversial (150,151). The key element is nicotine, which has the properties of both an acetylcholine agonist and antagonist (152). Nicotinic receptors are widely distributed in brain; nicotine induces the release of dopamine and, like the psychostimulants, affects the other monoamine neurotransmitters (153–155). The dopaminergic effect of nicotine probably accounts for the fact that cigarette smoking aggravates tardive dyskinesia, which is, in contrast to Parkinson's disease, a hyperdopaminergic state (156).

This is not idle information presented to distract the reader but rather is given for his or her edification. At issue is not a provincial loyalty to the tobacco farmer, but, rather, the impact of drugs that act on the nicotinic acetylcholine receptor, including the nicotine patch itself, in patients with neuropsychiatric conditions. The physiologic effects of the CNS nicotinic acetylcholine receptor have not been well defined, although behavioral studies indicate that they participate in complex functions such as attention, memory, and cognition and are involved in the pathogenesis of Parkinson's disease, Alzheimer's disease, Tourette's syndrome, and other neuropsychiatric conditions (157).

Acetylcholine systems have long been appreciated in terms of their role in cognitive functioning, especially attention and memory. Most attention, however, has been directed to the muscarinic acetylcholine receptor, and one of the most replicated findings in behavioral pharmacology has been the negative effect of the muscarinic blocker scopolamine on memory performance. More recently, however, pharmacologists have established that blocking the nicotinic receptor has similar effects. Conversely, nicotine has been shown in many studies to improve performance on tasks of attention, learning, and memory (158).

Clinical trials of the nicotine patch are more interesting for their theoretical rather than practical importance. One is hardly likely to prescribe the nicotine patch to children with attention problems, but preliminary trials have demonstrated neuropsychological improvement in adults with ADHD, smokers, normal, nonsmoking adults, and patients with Alzheimer's disease and Parkinson's disease (159–162). The conclusion drawn from this line of investigation is not that nicotine has therapeutic potential but that pharmacologic manipulation of the nicotinic acetylcholine receptor by a less noxious avenue might have therapeutic potential, perhaps as a cognitive enhancer or a neuroprotective or antiaging drug. The ganglion-blocker mecamylamine may be interesting to investigate.

Ganglion-blocking drugs such as mecamylamine block transmission in autonomic ganglia by occupying receptor sites and stabilizing the postsynaptic membrane against the actions of acetylcholine. Mecamylamine is a relatively old drug, originally used, based on its peripheral effect, as an antihypertensive agent. Centrally, it is a reversible antagonist at the nicotinic acetylcholine receptor.

Mecamylamine is a nicotine antagonist (when smokers are given mecamylamine, they immediately begin to smoke more heavily), but it has been studied in clinical disorders in the same way as the nicotine patch (163–165). Theoretically, continuous nicotine exposure, through the nicotine patch, inactivates acetylcholinergic nicotine receptors in the brain. Therapeutically, then, mecamylamine should have effects similar to those of the nicotine patch. In one retrospective study, mecamylamine relieved tics, mood instability, and behavior disorders in 24 patients with Tourette's syndrome (166).

Reflections on the cognitive benefits of nicotine arise frequently when I consult with patients with head injuries who had been smokers and resumed the habit after the injury. The issue is pertinent to the operation of head injury rehabilitation centers, when assiduous directors seek to ban smoking on the premises. It is always the physician's responsibility to speak out against dangerous habits, and smoking is a dangerous habit. When addressing the problem among head-injury patients, however, one is contending not only with their loneliness and lack of safety awareness but also the likelihood of self-treatment that is not entirely misdirected.

The issue of smoking is relevant to the lives of mentally retarded people, but in a different vein. Community placement in least restrictive settings may compromise the success of an antismoking policy; indeed, government policy in the United States is supportive of age-appropriate recreation, and a strict antismoking policy may sometimes be viewed by regulators as unduly restrictive. Retarded people are as vulnerable as anyone else to the addictive properties of nicotine. Pica for cigarette butts is one of the more formidable behavioral problems one ever has to deal with.

CRANIAL ELECTROSTIMULATION

People have been experimenting with electricity for centuries to cure disease, to raise the dead, and for other gainful purposes. In fact, the first recorded experiments with electricity were by the Egyptians, and their source was the electric catfish (*Malopterurus electricus*). The Greeks knew that the torpedo fish and some other fish with electric organs could deliver a stinging sensation, and their name for those fish was *narke*, which was also their word for numbness, thus the derivation of two words (torpedo and narcotic) in current usage (167).

The ancient Greeks understood that the numbing force of the electric fish had a biologic purpose, for example, for defense or predation, but the nature of the force was not understood until Averroes (in the twelfth century) compared it with the effect of a lodestone on iron. This, of course, is remarkably close to the truth of the matter.

The use of electric fish for medicinal purposes was a contribution of Roman physicians who recommended the torpedo fish for several purposes including headache, gout, excess of venery, or, alternatively, as an aphrodisiac. Scribonius, who may be considered the father of the transcutaneous electrical nerve stimulation unit, applied the electrical discharge of the black torpedo fish as a form of galvanic headache therapy. His contemporary, Galen, had his doubts.

The people of ancient Nigeria and Abyssinia continued to use the discharge of electric fish as a remedy for various purposes, but electric fish therapy fell out of favor in the West, at least until people in Europe began to experiment with the Leyden jar circa 1745. The similarity between the shock it delivered and the discharge of the electric fish was soon pointed out, and there was renewed clinical interest in electric fish. In 1761, Frans van der Lott performed one of the first preclinical trials of a therapeutic agent when he threw a chicken into a barrel containing a live conger eel (*Gymnotus*). He thus cured a problem that the bird had with cramps in the feet (an animal model for writers' cramp or the "yips").

Then van der Lott took an inferential leap that was no less than breathtaking. He repeated the experiment with an Indian slave who was paraparetic and affected a dramatic cure. Barrel immersion with a conger eel became an established treatment thereafter, at least for slaves, for the treatment of paresis, headache, and other neurologic disorders.

With this sort of background, therefore, one can only wonder why electrotherapy is currently limited to the few psychiatrists who treat refractory depressive disorders (electroconvulsive therapy) and physical therapists who treat nonspecific pain syndromes (transcutaneous electrical nerve stimulation). The answer no doubt lies in the checkered history of electrotherapy in Western medicine since the days of the Leyden jar, a topic that has been described on numerous occasions in monographs more discursive even than this (168,169).

Many of us are dismayed, if not surprised, by the reintroduction of electrical stimulation therapy (EST) for several neuropsychiatric conditions. When we read of cranial EST, we tend to greet the news with a mixture of skepticism, *dèjà vu*, and morbid curiosity. Before we have even had a chance to digest the latest galvanic novelty, we are warned that magnetic stimulation of the CNS is useful for cases of multiple sclerosis, amyotrophic lateral sclerosis, and degenerative ataxia (170).

Cranial EST refers to the delivery of very small doses of alternating current (0.001 A), approximately 100 times per second in a sine wave burst. The devices marketed today in North America are small and inexpensive and use current generated by two 9-V flashlight batteries. The idea is to deliver a subthreshold current to the brain via electrodes placed on the mastoid processes for 20 to 40 minutes. The procedure is not painful at all; treatments may be self-administered safely several times daily.

The treatment was first recommended by Russian investigators during the 1950s, and they coined the term electrosleep or electronarcosis. That is a misnomer because whatever the beneficial effects that EST may have, they are not mediated by the induction of sleep (171). Of course, what it is precisely on a physiologic level that does mediate the effect of EST is not known, that is, assuming that the treatment has any effect. Not surprisingly, there have been speculations that EST stimulates alpha-wave production, increases the secretion of endogenous opiate neurotransmitters or biogenic amines, alters CNS reactivity, or is no more than an active placebo (172–174).

There is not much of an evidence base to support cranial EST, but little harm comes from its occasional use. It has been suggested as a way to reduce anxiety and tension, for example, in patients with mild anxiety disorders (175 [unpublished]), people who are being withdrawn from addicting drugs (176,177), as a treatment for insomnia (178), as a way to improve memory performance in patients who are alcoholics (179), and in patients with posttraumatic amnesia (180). There is little harm in a trial of EST for such patients.

Nor is it unreasonable to propose that EST may be a useful nonpharmacologic alternative for a variety of patients, especially people with symptoms of the postconcussion syndrome who are anxious, depressed, and insomniac and have headaches or deficits in attention and memory. I have found the treatment occasionally helpful in precisely such circumstances. Perhaps it is nothing more than an active placebo, but it may have a biologic spectrum of activity similar to that of the antidepressants, stimulants, minor tranquilizers, and mild analgesics, which are also active placebos sometimes. It is essentially free of untoward side effects, and its clinical utility is well worth exploring. It is certainly less expensive than referral to a pain clinic, a masseur, or a psychotherapist, it is not addicting, and there is no risk of rebound headache. If the effects of EST are, in fact, mediated by specific effects on neurotransmission or neuromodulation, and there is evidence that it might be (181), so much the better. Controlled, double-blind studies of cranial EST have been done and are mildly encouraging. Even if it is just an active placebo, however, it works sometimes and may be less problematic than some of the pharmacologic alternatives.

REFERENCES

1. Roberts WC. Recent studies on the effects of beta blockers on blood lipid levels. *Am Heart J* 1989;117: 709–714.
2. Granville-Grossman KL, Turner P. The effect of propranolol on anxiety. *Lancet* 1966;1:788–790.
3. Noyes R, Kathol R, Claney J. Antianxiety effects of propranolol: a review of clinical studies. In: Klein DF, Rabkin J, eds. *Anxiety—new research and changing concepts*. New York: Raven Press, 1981:81–93.
4. Lockwood AH. Medical problems of musicians. *N Engl J Med* 1989;320:221–227.
5. Atsmon A, Blum I, Steiner M, et al. Further studies with propranolol in psychotic patients. *Psychopharmacologia* 1972;27:249–254.
6. Peet M, Bethell MS, Coates A, et al. Propranolol in schizophrenia: I. Comparison of propranolol, chlorpromazine, and placebo. *Br J Psychiatry* 1981;139A: 105–111.
7. Peet M, Middlemiss DN, Yates RA. Propranolol in schizophrenia: II. Clinical and biochemical aspects of combining propranolol with chlorpromazine. *Br J Psychiatry* 1981;139B:112–117.
8. Sorji PJ, Ratey JJ, Polakoff S. B-adrenergic blockers for the control of aggressive behaviors in patients with chronic schizophrenia. *Am J of Psychiatry* 1986;143: 775–776.
9. Haspel T. Beta-blockers and the treatment of aggression. *Harv Rev Psychiatry* 1995;2:274–281.
10. Jefferson JW. Beta-adrenergic receptor blocking drugs in psychiatry. *Arch Gen Psychiatry* 1974;31: 681–691.
11. Tyrer P, Rutherford D, Huggett T. Benzodiazepine withdrawal symptoms and propranolol. *Lancet* 1981;1: 520–522.
12. Elliot FA. The neurology of explosive rage. *Practitioner* 1976;217:51–60.
13. Elliot FA. Propranolol for the control of the belligerent behavior following acute brain damage. *Ann Neurol* 1977;489–491.
14. Schreier HA. Use of propranolol in the treatment of post-encephalitic psychosis. *Am J Psychiatry* 1979;136: 840–841.
15. Yufodfsky S, Williams D, Gorman J. Propranolol in the treatment of patients with chronic brain syndrome. *Am J Psychiatry* 1981;138:218–330.
16. Mansheim P. Treatment with propranolol of the behavioral sequelae of brain damage. *J Clin Psychiatry* 1981; 42:132.
17. Petrie WM, Ban TA. Propranolol in organic agitation. *Lancet* 1981;1:324.
18. Williams DT, Mehl R, Yudofsky S, et al. The effect of propranolol on uncontrolled rage outbursts in children and adolescents with organic brain dysfunction. *JAm Acad Child Psychiatry* 1982;21:129–135.
19. Volavka J. Can aggressive behavior in humans be modified by beta blockers? *Postgrad Med* 1988;163–168.
20. Mattes JA. Propranolol for adults with temper outbursts and residual attention deficit disorder. *J Clin Psychopharmacol* 1986;6:299–302.
21. Ratey JJ, Greenberg MS, Linden KJ. Combination of treatments for attention deficit hyperactivity disorder in adults. *J Nerv Ment Dis* 1991;179:699–701.

21a. Strang RR. The symptom of restless legs. *Med J Austr* 1967;24:1211–1213.

22. Lipinski JF, Zubenko GS, Cohen BM, et al. Propranolol in the treatment of neuroleptic-induced akathisia. *Am J Psychiatry* 1984;141:412.
23. Adler L, Angrist B, Peselow E, et al. Noradrenergic mechanisms in akathisia: treatment with propranolol and clonidine. *Psychopharmacol Bull* 1987;23:21–23.
24. Zubenko GS, Cohen BM, Lipinski JF, et al. Use of clonidine in the treatment of akathisia. *Psychiatry Res* 1984;13:253–259.
25. Adler L, Angrist B, Peselow E, et al. Clonidine in neuroleptic-induced akathisia. *Am J Psychiatry* 1987;144: 235–236.

26. Petrie WM, Maffucci RJ, Woosley RL. Propranolol and depression. *Am J Psychiatry* 1982;139:92–94.
27. Peters NL, Anderson KC, Reid PR, et al. Acute mental status changes caused by propranolol. *Johns Hopkins Med J* 1978;143:163–164.
28. Fraser HS, Carr AC. Propranolol psychosis. *Br J Psychiatry* 1976;129:508–509.
29. Gershon ES, Goldstein RE, Moss AJ, et al. Psychosis with ordinary doses of propranolol. *Ann Intern Med* 1979;90:938–939.
30. Voltolina EJ, Thompson SI, Tisue J. Acute organic brain syndrome with propranolol. *Clin Toxicol* 1971;4: 357–359.
31. Shopsin B, Hirsch J, Gershon S. Visual hallucinations and propranolol. *Biol Psychiatry* 1975;10:105–107.
32. Belin C, Larmande P. Transitory spatial disorder with propranolol. *N Engl J Med* 1985;312:790–791.
33. Fisher CM. Amnestic syndrome associated with propranolol toxicity: a case report. *Clin Neuropharmacol* 1992;15:397–403.
34. McNeil GN, Shaw PK, Dock DS. Substitution of atenolol for propranolol in a case of propranolol-related depression. *Am J Psychiatry* 1982;139:9.
35. Gengo FM, Huntoon L, McHugh WB. Lipid-soluble and water-soluble B-blockers: comparison of the central nervous system depressant effect. *Arch Intern Med* 1987;147:39–43.
36. Sands S, Ratey J. The concept of noise. *Psychiatry* 1986;49:290–297.
37. Maher BA. *Principles of psychopathology*. New York: McGraw-Hill, 1966.
38. Rappaport M. Attention to competing voice messages by nonacute schizophrenic patients: effects of message load, drugs, dosage levels and patient background. *J Nerv Ment Dis* 1968;146:404–411.
39. Glass GV, Singer JE. *Urban stress: experiments on noise and social stressors*. New York: Academic Press, 1972.
40. Miller H. Accident neurosis. *BMJ* 1961;1:919–925.
41. Goldstein K. *After effects of brain injuries in war*. New York: Grune & Stratton, 1948.
42. Krystal H. Trauma and affects. *Psychoanal Study Child* 1978;33:81–116.
43. van der Kolk BA, Greenber MS. The psychobiology of the trauma response: hyperarousal, constriction and addiction to traumatic response. In: van der Kolk BA, ed. *Psychological trauma*. Washington, DC: American Psychiatric Press, 1987:63–78.
44. Ratey JJ, Gualtieri CT. Neuropsychiatry and mental retardation. In: Ratey JJ, ed. *Mental retardation: developing pharmacotherapies* . Washington, DC: American Psychiatric Press, 1991:1–18.
45. El-Mallakh H. Use of beta-blockers in neurology. *Resident Staff Phys* 1986;32:68–73.
46. Lader M. B-adrenoceptor antagonists in neuropsychiatry: an update. *J Clin Psychiatry* 1988;49:213–223.
47. Ratey JJ, Mikkelsen EJ, Smith GB, et al. Beta-blockers in the severely and profoundly mentally retarded. *J Clin Psychopharmacol* 1986;6:103–107.
48. Hoehn-Saric R, Merchant AF, Keyser ML, et al. Effects of clonidine on anxiety disorders. *Arch Gen Psychiatry* 1981;38:1278–1282.
49. Cohn LM, Caliendo GC. Guanfacine use in children with attention deficit hyperactivity disorder. *Ann Pharmacother* 1997;31:918–919.
50. Coull JT. Pharmacological manipulations of the alpha 2-noradrenergic system. Effects on cognition. *Drugs Aging* 1994;5:116–126.
51. Arnsten AFT, Goldman-Rakic PS. Alpha2-adrenergic mechanisms in prefrontal cortex associated with cognitive decline in aged nonhuman primates. *Science* 1985;230:1273–1276.
52. McEntee WJ, Mair RG. Memory enhancement in Korsakoff's psychosis by clonidine: further evidence for a noradrenergic deficit. *Ann Neurol* 1980;7:466–470.
53. Arnsten AF, Steere JC, Hunt RD. The contribution of alpha 2-noradrenergic mechanisms of prefrontal cortical cognitive function. Potential significance for attention-deficit hyperactivity disorder. *Arch Gen Psychiatry* 1996;53:448–455.
54. Farber NB, Foster JBA, Duhan NLBS, et al. A2 adrenergic agonists prevent MK-801 neurotoxicity. *Neuropsychopharmacology* 1995;12:347–349.
55. Naftchi NE. Functional restoration of the traumatically injured spinal cord in cats by clonidine. *Science* 1982; 217:1042–1044.
56. Goldstein LB, Davis JN. Clonidine impairs recovery of beam walking after a sensorimotor cortex lesion in the rat. *Brain Res* 1990;508:305–309.
57. Feeney DM, Westerberg VS. Norepinephrine and brain damage: alpha noradrenergic pharmacology alters functional recovery after cortical trauma. *Can J Psychol* 1990;44:233–252.
58. Goldstein LB. Common drugs may influence motor recovery after stroke. The Sygen in acute stroke study investigators. *Neurology* 1995;45:865–871.
59. Crook T, Wilner E, Rothwell A, et al. Noradrenergic intervention in Alzheimer's disease. *Psychopharmacol Bull* 1992;28:67–70.
60. Knesevich JW. Successful treatment of obsessive-compulsive disorder with clonidine hydrochloride. *Am J Psychiatry* 1982;139:364.
61. Jenike MA. Augmentation strategies for treatment-resistant obsessive-compulsive disorder. *Harv Rev Psychiatry* 1993;1:17–26.
62. Zubenko GS, Cohen BM, Lipinski JF, et al. Clonidine in the treatment of mania and mixed bipolar disorder. *Am J Psychiatry* 1984;141:1617.
63. Nishikawa T, Tanaka M, Tsuda A, et al. Clonidine therapy for tardive dyskinesia and related syndromes. *Clin Neuropharmacol* 1984;7:239–245.
64. Bruun RD. Clonidine treatment of Tourette syndrome. In: Friedhoff AJ, ed. *Gilles de la Tourette syndrome*. New York: Raven Press, 1982.
65. Chappell PB, Riddle MA, Scahill L, et al. Guanfacine treatment of comorbid attention-deficit hyperactivity disorder and Tourette's syndrome: preliminary clinical experience. *J Am Acad Child Adolesc Psychiatry* 1995; 34:1140–1146.
66. Viola J, Ditzler T, Batzer W, et al. Pharmacological management of post-traumatic stress disorder: clinical summary of a five-year retrospective study, 1990–1995. *Milit Med* 1997;162:616–619.
67. Horrigan JP. Guanfacine for PTSD nightmares. *J Am Acad Child Psychiatry* 1996;35:975–976.
68. Hunt RD, Minderaa RB, Cohen DJ. Clonidine benefits children with attention deficit disorder and hyperactivity: report of a double-blind placebo-crossover therapeutic trial. *J Am Acad Child Psychiatry* 1985;24: 617–629.

69. Sovner R. Thioridazine withdrawal-induced behavioral deterioration treated with clonidine: two case reports. *Ment Retard* 1995;33:221–225.
70. Elliot RL. Case report of a potential interaction between clonidine and electroconvulsive therapy. *Am J Psychiatry* 1983;140:1237–1238.
71. Shouse MN, Bier M, Langer J, et al. The alpha 2-agonist clonidine suppresses seizures, whereas the alpha 2-antagonist idazoxan promotes seizures—a microinfusion study in amygdala-kindled kittens. *Brain Res* 1994;648:352–356.
72. Bakchine S, Lacomblez L, Benoit N, et al. Manic-like state after bilateral orbitofrontal and right temporoparietal injury: efficacy of clonidine. *Neurology* 1989;39:777–781.
73. Bougousslavsky J, Ferrazzini M, Regli F, et al. Manic delirium and frontal-like syndrome with paramedian infarction of the right thalamus. *J Neurol Neurosurg Psychiatry* 1988;51:116–119.
74. Schaut J, Schnoll SH. Four cases of clonidine abuse. *Am J Psychiatry* 1983;140:1625.
75. Ahsanuddin K. Side effects of clonidine. *Am J Psychiatry* 1982;139:1083.
76. Adler LE, Bell J, Kirch D, et al. Psychosis associated with clonidine withdrawal. *Am J Psychiatry* 1982;139: 110.
77. Fenichel RR. Combining methylphenidate and clonidine: the role of post-marketing surveillance. *J Child Adolesc Psychopharmacol* 1997;5:155–156.
78. Popper CW. Combining methylphenidate and clonidine: pharmacologic questions and news reports about sudden death. *J Child Adolesc Psychopharmacol* 1997; 5:157–166.
79. Janowsky A, Sulser F. Alpha and beta adrenoceptors in brain. In: Meltzer HY, ed. *Psychopharmacology: the third generation of progress*, 2nd ed. New York: Raven Press, 1987:249–256.
80. Weber MA, Drayer JIM, Laragh JH. The effects of clonidine and propranolol, separately and in combination, on blood pressure and plasma renin activity in essential hypertension. *J Clin Pharmacol* 1978;233–240.
81. Vanholder R, Lamieire N, Ringoir S. Long-term experience with the combination of clonidine and beta-adrenoceptor blocking agents in hypertension. *Eur J Clin Pharmacol* 1985;28:125–130.
82. Jounela AJ, Lilja M. Interactions between beta-blockers and clonidine. *Ann Clin Res* 1984;16:181–182.
83. Snyder SH, Reynolds IJ. Calcium-antagonist drugs: receptor interactions that clarify therapeutic effects. *N Engl J Med* 1985;313:995–1001.
84. Dubovsky SL. Calcium antagonists: a new class of psychiatric drugs. *Psychiatr Ann* 1986;16:724–728.
85. Silverstone PH, Grahame-Smith DG. Effects of chronic lithium, amitriptyline, and electroconvulsive shock, on calcium channel binding in a rat brain homogenate. *Psychopharmacology (Berl)* 1991;105:132–133.
86. Gelmers HJ. Nimodipine in ischemic stroke. *Clin Neuropharmacol* 1987;10:412–422.
87. Pickard JD, Murray GD, Illingworth R, et al. Effect of oral nimodipine on cerebral infarction and outcome after subarachnoid haemorrhage: British Aneurysm Nimodipine Trial. *BMJ* 1989;298:636–642.
88. European Study Group on Nimodipine in Severe Head Injury. A multicenter trial of the efficacy of nimodipine on outcome after severe head injury. The European Study Group on Nimodipine in Severe Head Injury. *J Neurosurg* 1994;80:797–804.
89. Wong MCW, Haley EC Jr. Calcium antagonists: stroke therapy coming of age. *Stroke* 1989;24:31–36.
90. Zornow MH, Prough DS. Neuroprotective properties of calcium-channel blockers. *New Horiz* 1996;4:107–114.
91. Kirischuk S, Verkhratsky A. Calcium homeostasis in aged neurones. *Life Sci* 1996;59:451–459.
92. Deyo RA, Straube KT, Disterhoft JF. Nimodipine facilitates associative learning in aging rabbits. *Science* 1989;243:809–811.
93. Fanelli RJ, McCarthy RT, Chisholm J. Neuropharmacology of nimodipine: from single channels to behavior. *Ann N Y Acad Sci* 1994;747:336–350.
94. Levere TE, Walker A. Old age and cognition: enhancement of recent memory in aged rats by the calcium channel blocker nimodipine. *Neurobiol Aging* 1991; 13:63–66.
95. Sandin M, Jasmin S, Levere TE. Aging and cognition: facilitation of recent memory in aged nonhuman primates by nimodipine. *Neurobiol Aging* 1990;11:573–575.
96. Fritze J, Walden J. Clinical findings with nimodipine in dementia: test of the calcium hypothesis. *J Neural Transm* 1995;46:439–453.
97. Pantoni L, Carosi M, Amigoni S, et al. A preliminary open trial with nimodipine in patients with cognitive impairment and leukoaraiosis. *Clin Neuropharmacol* 1996;19:497–506.
98. Miranda HF, Paeile C. Interactions between analgesics and calcium channel blockers. *Gen Pharmacol* 1990; 21:171–174.
99. Hill NS, Lee S-L, Fanburg BL. Effect of calcium channel blockers on serotonin uptake. *Proc Soc Exp Biol Med* 1990;193:326–330.
100. Bagchi SP. Antidopaminergic action of verapamil and several other drugs: inactivation of vesicular dopamine. *Life Sci* 1990;46:857.
101. Fadda F, Gessa GL, Mosca E, et al. Different effects of the calcium antagonists nimodipine and flunarizine on dopamine metabolism in the rat brain. *J Neural Transm* 1989;75:195–200.
102. Olesen J. Calcium antagonists in migraine and vertigo. *Eur Neurol* 1990;39:31–34
103. Giannini AJ, Houser WL, Louiselle RH, et al. Antimanic effects of verapamil. *Am J Psychiatry* 1984;141: 1602–1603.
104. Gitlin MJ, Weiss J. Verapamil as maintenance treatment in bipolar illness: a case report. *J Clin Psychopharmacol* 1984;4:341–343.
105. Freeman MP, Stoll AL. Mood stabilizer combinations: a review of safety and efficacy. *Am J Psychiatry* 1998; 155:12–21.
106. Pazzaglia P, Post R, Ketter T. Nimodipine monotherapy and carbamazepine augmentation in patients with refractory recurrent affective illness. *J Clin Psychopharmacol* 1998;18:404–413.
107. Taragano F, Allegri R, Vicario A, et al. A double blind, randomized clinical trial assessing the efficacy and safety of augmenting standard antidepressant therapy with nimodipine in the treatment of vascular depression. *Int J Geriatr Psychiatry* 2001;16:254–260.
108. De Vry J, Fritze J, Post RM. The management of coexisting depression in patients with dementia: potential of calcium channel antagonists. *Clin Neuropharmacol* 1997;20:22–35.

109. Hoschl C. Verapamil for depression? *Am J Psychiatry* 1983;140:1100.
110. Klein E, Uhde TW. Controlled study of verapamil for treatment of panic disorder. *Am J Psychiatry* 1988; 145:431–434.
111. Bloom DM, Tourjman SV, Vasavan Nair NP. Verapamil in refractory schizophrenia: a case report. *Prog Neuropsychopharmacol Biol Psychiatry* 1987;11:185–188.
112. Hollister L, Trevino ES. Calcium channel blockers in psychiatric disorders: a review of the literature. *Can J Psychiatry* 1999;44:658–664.
113. Berg R. A case of Tourette's syndrome treated with nifedipine. *Acta Psychiatr Scand* 1985;72:400–401.
114. Walsh TL, Lavenstein B, Licamele WL, et al. Calcium antagonists in the treatment of Tourette's disorder. *Am J Psychiatry* 1986;143:1467–1468.
115. Singh I. Prolonged oculogyric crisis on addition of nifedipine to neuroleptic medication regime. *Br J Psychiatry* 1987;150:127–128.
116. Cohan SL. Pharmacology of calcium antagonists: clinical relevance in neurology. *Eur Neurol* 1990;30:28–30.
117. Hulser P-J, Kornhuber AW, Kornhuber HH. Treatment of acute stroke with calcium antagonists. *Eur Neurol* 1990;30:35–38.
118. Caers LI, De Beikelaar F, Amery WK. Flunarizine, a calcium-entry blocker, in childhood migraine, epilepsy, and alternating hemiplegia. *Clin Neuropharmacol* 1987; 10:162–168.
119. Sills GJ, Carswell A, Brodie MJ. Dose-response relationships with nimodipine against electroshock seizures in mice. *Epilepsia* 1994;35:437–442.
120. Konopka LM, Cooper R, Crayton JW. Serotonin-induced increases in platelet cytosolic calcium concentration in depressed, schizophrenic and substance abuse patients. *Biol Psychiatry* 1996;39:708–713.
121. Wurpel JND, Iyer SN. Calcium channel blockers verapamil and nimodipine inhibit kindling in adult and immature rats. *Epilepsia* 1994;35:443–449.
122. Chobanian AV. Calcium channel blockers: lessons learned from MIDAS and other clinical trials. *JAMA* 1996;276:829–830.
123. Maxwell CJ, Hogan DB, Ebly EM. Calcium-channel blockers and cognitive function in elderly people: results from the Canadian Study of Health and Aging. *CMAJ* 1999;161:501–506.
124. Langham J, Goldfrad C, Teasdale G, et al. Calcium channel blockers for acute traumatic brain injury. *Cochrane Database Sys Rev* 2000;2:CD000565.
125. Koh J-Y, Cotman CW. Programmed cell death: its possible contribution to neurotoxicity mediated by calcium channel antagonists. *Brain Res* 1992;587: 233–240.
126. Izquierdo I, Eias RD, Souza DO, et al. Review article: the role of opioid peptides in memory and learning. *Behav Brain Res* 1980;1:451–468.
127. Serby M, Resnick R, Jordan B, et al. Naltrexone and Alzheimer's disease. *Prog Neuropsychol Biol Psychiatry* 1986;10:587–590.
128. Armstead WM, Kurth CD. The role of opioids in newborn pig fluid percussion brain injury. *Brain Res* 1994;660:19–26.
129. Brandt NJ, Terenius L, Jacobsen BB, et al. Hyper-endorphin syndrome in a child with necrotizing encephalomyelopathy. *N Engl J Med* 1980;303:914–916.
130. Hosobuchi Y, Baskin DS. Reversal of induced ischemic neurologic deficit in gerbils by the opiate antagonist naloxone. *Science* 1982;215:69–71.
131. Vink R, Portoghese S, Faden AI. K-Opioid antagonist improves cellular bioenergetics and recovery after traumatic brain injury. *Am J Physiol* 1991;30:1527–1532.
132. Vink R, McIntosh TK, Rhomhanyi R, et al. Opiate antagonist nalmefene improves intracellular free Mg2+ bioenergic state, and neurologic outcome following traumatic brain injury in rats. *J Neurosci* 1990;10:3524–3530.
133. Chernick V, Craig RJ. Naloxone reverses neonatal depression caused by fetal asphyxia. *Science* 1982;216: 1252–1253.
134. McIntosh TK, Fernyak S, Hayes RL, et al. Beneficial effect of the nonselective opiate antagonist naloxone hydrochloride and the thyrotropin-releasing hormone (TRH) analog YM-14673 on long-term neurobehavioral outcome following experimental brain injury in the rat. *J Neurotrauma* 1993;10:373–384.
135. Hayes RL, Lyeth BG, Jenkins LW, et al. Possible protective effect of endogenous opioids in traumatic brain injury. *J Neurosurg* 1990;72:252–261.
136. Zagon IS, McLaughlin P. Increased brain size and cellular content in infant rats treated with an opiate antagonist. *Science* 1983;221:1179–1180.
137. Tennant FS, Wild J. Naltrexone treatment for post-concussional syndrome. *Am J Psychiatry* 1987;144: 813–814.
138. Childs A. Naltrexone in organic bulimia: a preliminary report. *Brain Inj* 1987;1:49–55.
139. deZwaan M, Mitchell JE. Opiate antagonists and eating behavior in humans: a review. *J Clin Pharmacol* 1992;32:1060–1072.
140. Drewnowski A, Krahn DD, Demitrack MA, et al. Naloxone, an opiate blocker, reduces the consumption of sweet high-fat foods in obese and lean female binge eaters. *Am J Clin Nutr* 1995;61:1206–1212.
141. O'Connor PG, Kosten TR. Rapid and ultrarapid opioid detoxification techniques. *JAMA* 1998;279:229–234.
142. Shufman EN, Porat S, Witztum E, et al. The efficacy of naltrexone in preventing reabuse of heroin after detoxification. *Biol Psychiatry* 1994;35:935–345.
143. Marrazzi MA, Bacon JP, Kinzie J, et al. Naltrexone use in the treatment of anorexia nervosa and bulimia nervosa. *Int Clin Psychopharmacol* 1995;10:163–172.
144. Volpicelli JR, Clay KL, Watson NT, et al. Naltrexone in the treatment of alcoholism: predicting response to naltrexone. *J Clin Psychiatry* 1995;56:39–44.
145. Campbell M, Adams P, Small AM, et al. Naltrexone in infantile autism. *Psychopharmacol Bull* 1988;24: 135–139.
146. Kolmen BK, Feldman HM, Handen BL, et al. Naltrexone in young autistic children: replication study and learning measure. *J Am Acad Child Psychiatry* 1997; 36:1570–1578.
147. Dodman NH, Shuster L, White SD, et al. Use of narcotic antagonists to modify stereotypic self-licking, self-chewing, and scratching behavior in dogs. *J Am Vet Med Assoc* 1988;193:815–819.
148. Kleber HD. Clinical aspects of the use of narcotic antagonists: the state of the art. *Int J Addict* 1977;12: 857–861.
149. Kessler II, Diamond EL. Epidemiologic studies of Parkinson's disease. I. Smoking and Parkinson's disease: a survey and explanatory hypothesis. *Am J Epidemiol* 1971;94:16–25.

150. Barclay L, Kheyfets S. Tobacco use in Alzheimer's disease. *Prog Clin Biol Res* 1989;317:189–194.
151. Merchant C, Tang MX, Albert S, et al. The influence of smoking on the risk of Alzheimer's disease. *Neurology* 1999;52:1408–1412.
152. Whitehouse PJ, Martino AM, Marcus KA, et al. Reductions in acetylcholine and nicotine binding in several degenerative diseases. *Arch Neurol* 1988;45:722–724.
153. Giorguieff-Chesselet MF, Kemel ML, Wandscheer D, et al. Regulation of dopamine release by presynaptic nicotinic receptors in rat striatal slices: effect of nicotine in a low concentration. *Life Sci* 1979;25:1257–1262.
154. Schwartz JM, Ksir C, Koob GF, et al. Changes in locomotor response to beta-endorphin microinfusion during and after opiate abstinence syndrome—a proposal for a model of the onset of mania. *Psychiatry Res* 1982;7:153–161.
155. Hall SM, Tunstall CD, Ginsberg D, et al. Nicotine gum and behavioral treatment: a placebo controlled trial. *J Consult Clin Psychol* 1987;55:603–605.
156. Yassa R, Lal S, Korpassy A, et al. Nicotine exposure and tardive dyskinesia. *Biol Psychiatry* 1987;22:67–72.
157. Mihailescu S, Drucker-Colin R. Nicotine and brain disorders. *Acta Pharmacol Sinai* 2000;21:97–104.
158. Levin ED. Nicotinic systems and cognitive function. *Psychopharmacology* 1992;108:417–431.
159. Fagerstrom KO, Pomerleau O, Giodani B, et al. Nicotine may relieve symptoms of Parkinson's disease. *Psychopharmacology (Berl)* 1994;116:117–119.
160. Levin ED, Conners CK, Sparrow E, et al. Nicotine effects on adults with attention-deficit/hyperactivity disorder. *Psychopharmacology* 1996;123:55–63.
161. Levin ED, Conners CK, Silva D, et al. Transdermal nicotine effects on attention. *Psychopharmacology (Berl)* 1998;140:135–141.
162. White HK, Levin ED. Four-week nicotine skin patch treatment effects on cognitive performance in Alzheimer's disease. *Psychopharmacology (Berl)* 1999;143:158–165.
163. Sanberg PR, Silver AA, Shytle RD, et al. Nicotine for the treatment of Tourette's syndrome. *Pharmacol Ther* 1997;74:21–25.
164. Dursun SM, Reveley MA. Differential effects of transdermal nicotine on microstructured analyses of tics in Tourette's syndrome: an open study. *Psychol Med* 1997;27:483–487.
165. Tizabi Y, Copeland RL, Brus R, et al. Nicotine blocks quinpirole-induced behavior in rats: psychiatric implications. *Psychopharmacology (Berl)* 1999;145:433–441.
166. Silver AA, Shytle RD, Sanberg PR. Mecamylamine in Tourette's syndrome: a two-year retrospective case study. *J Child Adolesc Psychopharmacol* 2000;10:59–68.
167. Kellaway P. *The William Osler Medal essay. The part played by electric fish in the early history of bioelectricity and electrotherapy.* Montreal: McGill University, 1971.
168. Valenstein ES. *Great & desperate cures: the rise and decline of psychosurgery and other radical treatments for mental illness.* New York: Basic Books, 1986.
169. Ellenberger HF. *The discovery of the unconscious.* New York: Basic Books, 1970.
170. Hallett M, Cohen LG. Magnetism: a new method for stimulation of nerve and brain. *JAMA* 1989;262:538–541.
171. Ryan JJ, Souheaver GT. The role of sleep in electrosleep therapy for anxiety. *Dis Nerv Sys* 1977;38:515.
172. Briones DR, Rosenthal SH. Changes in urinary free catecholamines and 17-ketosteroids with cerebral electrotherapy (electrosleep). *Dis Nerv Sys* 1973;34:57.
173. Amassian VE, Stewart M, Quirk GJ, et al. Physiological basis of motor effects of a transient stimulus to cerebral cortex. *Neurosurgery* 1987;20:74–93.
174. Empson JAC. Does electrosleep induce natural sleep? *Electroencephalogr Clin Neurophysiol* 1973;35:663.
175. Matteson MT, Ivancevich JM. An exploratory investigation of CES as an employee stress management procedure. 1985.
176. Schmitt R, Capo T, Boyd E. Cranial electrotherapy stimulation as a treatment for anxiety in chemically dependent persons. *Alcohol Clin Exp Res* 1986;10:158–160.
177. Gomez E, Mikhail AR. Treatment of methadone withdrawal with cerebral electrotherapy (electrosleep). *Br J Psychiatry* 1979;134:111.
178. Weiss MF. The treatment of insomnia through the use of electrosleep: an EEG study. *J Nerv Ment Dis* 1973;157:108.
179. Smith RB, Day E. The effects of cerebral electrotherapy on short-term impairment in alcoholic patients. *Int J Addict* 1977;12:575.
180. Childs A, Crismon ML. The use of cranial electrotherapy stimulation in post-traumatic amnesia: a report of two cases. *Brain Inj* 1988;2:243–247.
181. Gleiter CH, Nutt DJ. Chronic electroconvulsive shock and neurotransmitter receptors—an update. *Life Sci* 1989;44:985–1006.

25

Cognitive Enhancers and Neuroprotectants

SUMMARY

It has taken 24 chapters to finally reach this point: the drugs and supplements that might actually enhance cognition or at least prevent cognitive deterioration. We have already dealt with the psychostimulants, which are troublesome drugs with many side effects. They are not drugs that one prefers to take, or to prescribe, unless they are absolutely necessary.

One reason that this issue was reserved for the penultimate chapter is that the evidence base to support cognitive enhancement is so weak. Clearly, the cholinesterase inhibitors have positive cognitive effects, but only in patients with dementia and only for a while. They do have stimulant-like effects in patients with brain injury. However, they are rarely, if ever, effective for people with mild learning disabilities or attention deficit/hyperactivity disorder (ADHD); this is usually a good test for whether a drug is a general cognitive enhancer.

Nicotine, the neuropeptides, and the glycinergic prodrugs have all been proposed as cognitive enhancers. They are all interesting compounds, theoretically, but their clinical utility is marginal. Piracetam and its congeners are also said to be nootropic drugs. Piracetam has little theoretical support and even less empirical support.

On several occasions, the issue of free-radical generation, oxidative stress, and the utility of antioxidant supplements has been raised. This chapter is an opportunity to amplify those remarks and examine the wider utility of the antioxidants. If they are protective against age-related cognitive decline and dementia, we all should consider taking them regularly. Patients with brain injury and mentally retarded people, who are more vulnerable to age-related cognitive decline and more likely to develop dementia, might be well advised to take antioxidant supplements.

For generations, general physicians have recommended B vitamins, especially vitamin B_{12}, for vague and nonspecific neuropsychiatric symptoms. This practice has been criticized in the past, but it does have a theoretical basis and some empirical support. We shall venture to propose a defensible regimen of neuroprotective vitamins and supplements that the reader should consider for his or her patients with neuropsychiatric disorders.

The omega-3 fatty acids (fish oil) have received a good deal of attention recently for their putative effects in depression and bipolar disorder. Less well appreciated is their role in brain development and recovery from brain injury. When I was a child, the old people in my neighborhood used to refer to fish as "brain food." How did they know?

COGNITIVE ENHANCEMENT AND NEUROPROTECTION

Should everyone over 40 be taking daily aspirin, ibuprofen, celecoxib, or *Ginkgo biloba* to prevent dementia? Should we recommend them to our patients?

Psychopharmacology is concerned almost exclusively with the treatment of mental illness, the alleviation of psychiatric symptoms, and the control of untoward and maladaptive behaviors. If improving cognition were at all at issue, it was a byproduct, as it were, of improving the patient's overall mental state. The thoughts of a patient with a psychotic disorder are disorganized and loosely connected, and the patient is highly distractible; distracted is a good old English word to describe a patient who is mentally ill. Treating such a patient with an antipsychotic drug usually corrects the patient's cognitive impairment, just as it alleviates the rest of his or her psychotic symptoms. No one, however, is going to suggest that antipsychotic drugs are cognitive enhancers.

Patients with depression or anxiety disorders frequently complain of cognitive impairment. Inability to focus or concentrate, distractibility, poor memory, cognitive slowing, and mental fatigue are common symptoms of these disorders. When patients who are depressed or anxious are given neuropsychological tests, the psychologist has to work hard to obtain a valid result; even so, test scores are frequently low. After the patient is treated successfully, test scores return to premorbid levels of function. Still, no one would suggest that antidepressants or anxiolytics are cognitive enhancers.

A cognitive enhancer is a neuroactive substance that elevates an individual's cognitive abilities in a meaningful and sustained way, beyond that individual's basal level of performance. Another term that is sometimes used, especially in Europe, is nootropic drug. In everyday life, normal people (those who do not have psychiatric disorders or cognitive disabilities) seek drugs, herbal remedies, or nutritional supplements to improve their memory, ability to concentrate, or clarity of thought. People concerned with the mild memory impairment that occurs in "benign senescence" are especially likely to seek out such treatments. *Panax ginseng* and *Ginkgo biloba* are two popular remedies, so-called nutraceuticals, that are quite popular for just such an effect.

Despite all the attention given to cognitive enhancers in the popular press and health food industry, in all of medicine, there are only two classes of drug that are proven cognitive enhancers and even they operate within sharply circumscribed boundaries. They are the psychostimulants and cholinesterase inhibitors. Their conventional indications are ADHD and dementia, respectively, but they are also given to patients with cognitive impairments from other causes. Stimulants and cholinergics are often prescribed for patients with brain injury, sometimes to good effect. Stimulants are cognitive enhancers for normal people, at least to a degree, but they are only occasionally helpful to patients who are mentally retarded or autistic. The cholinergics, on the other hand, do not improve memory performance in normal subjects but may have a role for some mentally retarded patients.

A neuroprotective substance is a drug, nutraceutical, or dietary supplement that protects nerve cells from damage, either from pathologic events such as the excitotoxicity that accompanies stroke or brain injury or from normal biologic stressors, e.g., the generation of oxygen free radicals. There are many substances with proven neuroprotectant ability, at least *in vitro*. Deprenyl, for example, is said to retard the progression of Parkinson's disease (PD). Vitamins C and E are protective against oxidant stress.

Research on neuroprotective agents frequently addresses to the problem of acute ischemic injury in animal models or in humans with stroke. A large number of new compounds have been developed and are under investigation; a minimum of 800 such trials are currently underway (1). The pharmacologic strategies are diverse and wide ranging: drugs that inhibit lipid peroxidation or apoptosis, glutamate antagonists, γ-aminobutyric acid (GABA) agonists, sodium and calcium channel blockers, and so on (1–4). None, so far, has worked its way into the pharmacopoeia or engaged the attention of practitioners. A drug that controlled the neurotoxic events that arise immediately after stroke or brain injury would be welcome indeed, but it would still be necessary to evaluate its effects over the longer term in chronic conditions associated with deterioration over time.

Of course, the best cognitive enhancer is a well-chosen treatment for a specific neuropsychiatric condition. The appropriate treatment of depression, organic affective disorders, anxiety states, psychosis, chronic pain, epilepsy, and psychosis is almost invariably associated with cognitive improvement because these disorders compromise intellectual functions, sometimes to a remarkable degree. The second best cognitive treatment is withdrawal from an unnecessary or inappropriate drug. Antidepressants, mood stabilizers, anxiolytics, antiepileptic drugs, analgesics, antipsychotics, and antispasticity drugs all have the potential for cognitive toxicity. Even the newer agents do. Neuroprotection is not an established property of any of the current psychotropics, but appropriate treatment of a psychiatric disorder will certainly prevent secondary deterioration. Conversely, some neuroactive drugs, such as phenytoin and neuroleptics, are known to be neurotoxic, at least in some circumstances, and should be avoided, if possible.

Patients with brain injuries or developmental handicaps are obvious candidates for cognitive enhancement. They are good candidates for neuroprotection because they are more vulnerable to mental deterioration and dementia. What, then, do we have for these purposes, beyond optimal psychopharmacology and the measured avoidance of potentially neurotoxic compounds? Is there anything more credible than the exaggerated claims of the "smart drug" set? There is not very much, if one is seeking evidence-based recommendations.

A few candidates already have been discussed: the psychostimulants, dopamine agonists, and the glutamate antagonist amantadine were discussed in Chapter 18, deprenyl with the antidepressants in Chapter 19, megavitamins and vitamin B_6 in Chapter 14. This chapter rounds out the discussion: the cholinergics, neuroactive peptides, nootropics, glycinergic prodrugs, a few more vitamins, fish oil, nonsteroidal anti-inflammatory drugs (NSAIDs), and *Ginkgo biloba*.

CHOLINERGIC DRUGS

Drugs that enhance acetylcholine neurotransmission have always been problematic as far as psychiatrists are concerned because they may be depressants and may aggravate parkinsonian symptoms. Those effects should still be kept in mind because cholinergic drugs are used more frequently for the treatment of memory disorders in people with dementia, stroke, or brain injury, or, more recently, with benign senescence and ADHD.

The earliest attempt to correlate recovery of cortical function with cholinergic stimulation was made in 1928 when Chavany (5) advocated the use of acetylcholine in the treatment of hemiplegia. Positive effects with acetylcholine injections in patients with hemiplegia, aphasia, and other neuropathic conditions were at first attributed to cerebral vasodilation. Subsequent research was conducted by Luria et al. (6) and by Ward and Kennard (7) at Yale during the Fulton era.

This venerable treatment is still current. Indeed, it is central to pharmacologic development for dementia in general and for Alzheimer's disease (AD) in particular. It is a rational treatment insofar as it mitigates the deficit in cholinergic neurotransmission that stems from deterioration of cholinergic neurons in the basal forebrain of Meynert (8). Because acetylcholine is an important neurotransmitter in the physiology of memory and attention and because deficits in acetylcholine systems are found in patients with amnesia and patients with attentional disorders, it was appropriate to explore the potential utility of cholinergic drugs in treatment (9). Because memory impairment is a major element of traumatic brain injury (TBI), cholinergic treatments have been brought to bear in that group as well, with positive effects in at least one study (10).

Luria, the great Russian neuropsychologist, used a cholinergic drug called galanthamine in some of his patients with brain injury (6). Galanthamine is a long-acting acetylcholinesterase inhibitor that was not available in North America until very recently. Clinical scientists who were interested in exploring the clinical utility of cholinergic drugs, for example, in AD, were forced to rely on short-acting parenteral acetylcholinesterase inhibitors, such as physostigmine, acetylcholine precursors (e.g., lecithin), and direct muscarinic receptor agonists. However, "despite several years of clinical attempts to improve geriatric cognition, no therapeutically useful results have been demonstrated with cholinergic agents" (11). Combined treatment with an acetylcholine precursor and a cholinesterase inhibitor had more utility than treatment with either compound by itself (12,13), but even that approach was more theoretical than practical before the oral acetylcholinesterase inhibitors were available.

Tetrahydro-9-aminoacridine (THA) was the first such drug to be used in North America. THA is a potent, central-acting anticholinesterase that can be administered orally. It has a longer duration of action and more favorable therapeutic index than physostigmine (14). It was the first cholinergic treatment ever to attain clinical utility. Long-term treatment of patients with dementia with THA led to significant improvement in the patients' general clinical status and learning ability. It was a palliative treatment that alleviated some of the symptoms of AD. It, however, did not alter the ultimate course of the disease (15); none of the cholinergic drugs does. The utility of THA was sharply limited by its expense, the risk of hepatotoxicity, the cost of monitoring, the severe nausea that often occurred, and the time required for titration to a therapeutic dose.

Virtually all the published THA research was been concerned with patients with dementia. Its effectiveness for other categories of patients with memory impairment was never tested systematically, but many clinicians (myself included) used it in the occasional patient with stroke or TBI. In clinical practice, the results of THA treatment were generally positive, although modest, just as they are for patients with dementia. Side effects, cost, and the time commitment necessary to evaluate the drug were as limiting for patients with TBI as they were for patients with dementia.

When a patient with TBI responded to THA, the effect resembled that of the psychostimulants. The patient seemed to be more activated and alert, cognitively faster, more attentive, and more energetic. There has never been a head-to-head comparison of THA, or any cholinesterase inhibitor, with a stimulant, in any class of patients, but it would not be surprising if their spectrum of activity overlapped.

THA was an important drug in its day, but it has been eclipsed by the recent development of alternative cholinesterase inhibitors that are just as effective, better tolerated, and easier to use. These include donepezil (DNP), rivastigmine, metrifonate, and galanthamine (16,17). DNP is also a reversible inhibitor of acetyl cholinesterase, with significant advantages over THA. It has a longer half-life; therefore, so once-daily dosing is possible. It has no serious toxicity except in extreme overdose. Its effects are manifest within weeks, rather than months, and it is at least as effective as THA (18). DNP may well prove to be the first cholinergic drug to achieve wide use, even among general practitioners. Indeed, the manufacturer has undertaken to market the drug directly to the public.

The newer cholinesterase inhibitors all share these advantages, and they are probably equally effective. They are used, of course, for demented patients, where they are often good for a year or two of stability (i.e., no deterioration), if not a degree of improvement. Some of the behavioral and emotional problems of patients with dementia also improve with these drugs. They are also used for stroke, multiple sclerosis, and patients with TBI, and even for patients with age-related memory decline (19–21). Small, open trials with DNP in Down's syndrome have been encouraging.

In the course of my clinical practice, I have had the opportunity to observe the effects of DNP and rivastigmine for some "off-off label" indications, such as ADHD and refractory depression. They are well tolerated, even by children, but not particularly impressive. They are not likely to be broad-spectrum psychotropics, such as valproate, oxcarbazine, lamotrigine, and the selective serotonin reuptake inhibitors. Down's syndrome and TBI are the most promising new arenas for the cholinesterase inhibitors; they may also be effective for dementia prevention and improvement in attention and executive functions. The latter effects may prove to be more impressive than their specific effect on memory.

NOOTROPICS

Nootropic was coined to describe a class of drugs that improves higher cognitive function. The term was invented by Guirgea, who developed piracetam, the alleged "memory drug," described as the first of a new class of nootropic psychoactive drugs. Indeed, there have been several related compounds introduced in the subsequent 20 years (e.g., pramiracetam, oxiracetam, aniracetam, nefiracetam). Their mechanism of action, if they have one, is unknown. They were originally thought to enhance cerebral energy metabolism and were referred to as antihypoxidotics. It is also possible that they are mildly cholinergic, anti-GABAergic, or protective against excitotoxicity or interact with a steroid-sensitive memory system (22–24).

Piracetam has been reported to facilitate learning in animals, to limit the decline in human performance associated with cerebral hypoxia, and to improve cognitive performance, alertness, fatigue, and psychomotor retardation in aged subjects (25). It is said to improve verbal learning in normal individuals (26) and people with dyslexia (27). It may ameliorate memory deficits in 10% to 30% of patients with dementia or slow the progression of the disease (22,28,29). Clinical trials of piracetam for children with dyslexia were conducted in the United States, and although there were some indications of treatment success, the evidence was not very strong (30).

Pramiracetam is another cognition activator, which, in various behavioral models and electroencephalographic studies, is found superior to other drugs marketed for cognitive disorders in the elderly (31). Pharmacologically, it may be cholinergic and an indirect dopamine agonist. Like all the nootropics, it is well tolerated and apparently successful in improving the affective and behavioral symptoms of dementia: learning/memory, motivation, depression, anergia, and the ability to perform activities of daily living (32). It is important to emphasize that it was apparently successful.

Piracetam and its congeners are not available in the United States, and there are no plans to market them anytime soon. It has always been my opinion that they will not be missed. They remain favorites, however, of the "smart drug" set—people who buy cognitive enhancers from pharmacies abroad to improve their day-to-day intellectual performance. One continues to read of successful trials of piracetam in the wide range of neuropsychiatric conditions including myoclonus (33), epilepsy (34), aphasia (35), and stroke (36,37).

A recent meta-analysis of piracetam in 1,002 patients with stroke indicated that there was no benefit whatever (38).

NEUROPEPTIDES

Twenty years ago, there was intense interest in the therapeutic potential of various neuroactive peptides, driven by the discovery that the pituitary peptide hormones corticotropin (ACTH) and melanocyte-stimulating hormone (MSH) exerted a trophic influence enhancing the metabolic activity and viability of their target cells. These effects include enhanced blood flow in the target region and stimulation of macromolecular (RNA/protein) synthesis (39). The brain and behavior effects of the melanocortins (ACTH, MSH) were thought to result from peptide effects on neurons and/or glial cells, similar to the peptide-target cell interactions that are known to occur in peripheral tissues. The idea that the melanocortins might enhance adaptive neural responses to injury was tested and received some support in preclinical studies employing the following preparations: peripheral nerve damage, hippocampal plasticity, recovery from brain injury, and behavioral plasticity (39).

Some neuropeptides, notably ACTH, MSH, and vasopressin, were shown to affect the learning process, particularly in animals (40). Subsequent work demonstrated that the heptapeptide ACTH 4-10, a peptide fragment common to both the ACTH and the MSH molecular structures, was responsible for the learning effects of these compounds (41,42). In human volunteers a synthetic fraction of ACTH (ACTH 4-10) seemed to improve visual memory, enhance alertness, and increase motivation—all without the hormone's usual endocrine effects (43). Yet, in another such study, the effects of ACTH 4-10 were negative (44), and clinical studies have been inconclusive (45–47).

There were also studies of vasopressin and other posterior pituitary hormones. The idea was that vasopressin, like ACTH 4-10, might modulate some aspect of the learning/memory process (43,48). The long-term effects of vasopressin and oxytocin, another posterior pituitary hormone, indicated enhanced learning and memory consolidation in laboratory animals (49). However, it was not possible to extend the results of laboratory research to the clinical arena. Well-constructed clinical studies of patients with neuropsychiatric disorders, including cases of TBI, have not supported the idea that vasopressin improves memory performance (50). Conversely, elderly patients treated with vasopressin performed better in tests involving attention, concentration, motor speech, and memory (49). It is possible, however, that vasopressin peptides exercise positive effects on psychological performance, not through any direct nootropic effect, but indirectly by improving mood, motivation, or alertness (51). Intranasal vasopressin promotes sleep time and improves sleep architecture in elderly patients; that alone may explain its (putative) cognitive benefits (52).

The tripeptide thyrotropin-releasing hormone (TRH) has been shown to improve long-term neurologic outcome after experimental spinal cord injury in cats (53,54). TRH has also been successful in improving recovery from experimental brain injury in animals (55–57). DN-1417, a TRH analogue that is long acting and not as potent in stimulating the endocrine system, has been shown to promote recovery from concussive head injury in mice (58). In experimental animals, it is antiamnesic and proarousal (59). It has inhibitory and excitatory effects when applied to individual neurons and interacts with several neurotransmitters including norepinephrine, dopamine, serotonin, acetylcholine, GABA, and glutamate (59,60).

In Japan, TRH infusions are sometimes prescribed to enhance recovery in patients with TBI. TRH and its analogues have also been used in patients with AD (61,62), vascular dementia (63), alcoholism with cognitive impairment (64), and epilepsy (65) and in the post–electroconvulsive therapy state (66). Because TRH can only be given as continuous infusion, pharmacologic analogues with a longer half-life and the potential for oral administration will be required before clinical trials can be run (67). Indeed, little parenterally administered TRH ever reaches the brain because of its rapid metabolic clearance and its limited ability to cross the blood-brain barrier (60). My experience with TRH is limited. It is safe to try, however, with virtually no side effects and may conceivably exercise a degree of benefit. It may, for example, reverse glutamate-induced excitotoxicity (68) or stimulate nerve growth factor (NGF) (69).

NGF is a protein of known sequence and structure, a neurotrophic factor for central cholinergic neurons (but not for central catecholaminergic neurons). In animal studies, NGF preserves cholinergic neurons from lesion-induced degeneration and improves learning in rats with cholinergic septohippocampal lesions (70). NGF is difficult to test in humans with brain disorders associated with cholinergic deficits such as AD because the protein cannot cross the blood-brain barrier, but intraventricular infusions have been done, "with potentially beneficial effects" (71). The side effects outweighed whatever small benefit accrued, however. It is possible that compounds exercising NGF-like effects may at some point be a rational treatment, but their time has not yet arrived.

The neuroactive peptides are included in this chapter largely out of historical interest. Research on their neuropsychiatric effects has largely faded from the scene. Not because their effects are meaningless or that the preclinical studies are irrelevant; but probably because the technology does not yet exist to harness their effects in a clinically meaningful way.

GLYCINERGIC PRODRUGS

Vitamin B_{15}, or pangamic acid, is isolated from apricot kernels and other natural sources—a mixture of substances; its exact composition was never precisely defined, but it was said to be effective nevertheless for a host of diseases of the skin, respiratory tract, nerves, and joints. Or, at least, the people who sold it said that it was, and some credulous journalists did, too. In fact, it was first extracted by Ernst Krebs, the physician who gave us laetrile. Two of the constituents of this ersatz vitamin are glycine and *N,N*-dimethyl glycine (DMG) (72), and they deserve some attention here.

The amino acid glycine is an important inhibitory neurotransmitter in the brain. For example, it potentiates *N*-methyl-D- aspartate (NMDA) receptor neurotransmission and thus inhibits dopaminergic neurons in the substantia nigra and modulates dopamine release (73). In contrast, phencyclidine (angel dust) is an NMDA antagonist and a drug that causes psychosis. It is necessary to mention phencyclidine because a theoretical model has been based on its psychotomimetic effect, which inspired a series of NMDA augmentation strategies for the treatment of schizophrenia. This new avenue for treatment research is still quite active. Glycine, DMG, and D-cycloserine (a glycinergic agonist) have all been explored as potential treatments for schizophrenia because they are NMDA augmenters. The results have been mixed thus far.

Glycine exerts a profound inhibitory effect on nondopaminergic cells in the substantia nigra, possibly on interneurons that control the diffusion of generalized seizures (74). In fact, DMG, an analogue of glycine that is probably better able to penetrate the blood-brain barrier, was once claimed to be an effective treatment for refractory epilepsy (75). Subsequent studies, however, have been disappointing (75,76).

DMG is widely available in health food stores. It is supposed to stimulate the immune system and to improve athletic endurance (77,78). The autism community has embraced it for reducing behavioral problems and enhancing communication in autistic children. I have not been impressed with the results that I have seen.

D-Cycloserine is thought to be a nootropic drug, a cognitive enhancer, based on preclinical studies and clinical studies in patients with AD (79–82). It may also have antiseizure potential (83–85). D-Cycloserine was found to enhance recovery from experimental TBI in rats (86). A multicenter, controlled study of gavestinel, a selective glycine agonist, had no more effect than placebo in 1,367 patients with ischemic stroke (87).

D-Cycloserine is a prescription drug, but glycine and DMG are freely available over the counter. Physicians, then, are likely to encounter patients who are taking DMG or giving it to their children in the hope that it will correct a cognitive or a developmental weakness. It is probably a harmless drug, if one can call it a drug, and it is not an outlandish thing to try, but there is little scientific evidence to support its use. It is a good idea to pursue investigations of NMDA activators such as the glycinergic prodrugs, but there is no basis for recommending them to patients at this time.

THE THEORY OF OXIDANT STRESS

The uncontrolled production of free radicals is a primary cause of many pathophysiologic reactions, but because oxyradicals are difficult to study, their role as etiologic agents was viewed with some skepticism (88). However, the development of new experimental methods has generated evidence that oxidative damage does occur to tissue in the development of a number of pathologic states such as stroke (88), PD (89), brain injury (90), AD, and aging (91). Lipid peroxidation by free-radical reactions is now thought to be a basic deteriorative process in various pathologic conditions such as atherosclerosis, degenerative arthritis, cataracts, irradiation syndrome, and trauma (92).

There is agreement that oxidative stress is associated with neuronal degeneration under acute pathologic conditions, such as stroke and brain injury, and in brain aging. It is an intuitive concept because the life span in animals is inversely proportional to the basal metabolic rate, i.e., the rate of oxygen consumption, and is directly related to the extent of oxygen radical–scavenging systems (93). Tissue damage caused by oxidative stress accumulates with age (94). Because oxidation is a ubiquitous phenomenon in the aerobic environment of biologic systems and the damage that it may cause at a molecular level is so fundamental, there is no apparent limit to its potential relevance. Because oxidative stress may be attenuated, the theory opens avenues for pharmacologic manipulation.

The theory of oxidative stress has been related to the phenomenon of aging and the pathophysiologic conditions associated with aging such as atherosclerosis, dementia, PD, senile cataracts, and degenerative arthritis and to catastrophic events that are more likely to occur in older people such as cancer, stroke, and coronary artery disease. Relationships are usually drawn from preclinical studies that demonstrate oxidative events as a component of the pathologic process or suggest that oxidative stress may be a component. Epidemiologic studies indicate the favorable effects of a diet that is rich in antioxidant micronutrients. Treatment studies support the utility of antioxidant drugs or supplements in the prevention, treatment, or attenuation of the disorder. Oxidative stress, however, remains no more than a theory. Preclinical studies are only suggestive, and epidemiologic studies are never more than correlational. The treatment studies have never been conclusive. Therefore, no one can say that antioxidants are, in fact, therapeutic (or preventative) for anything. At least, no one can say that now.

Oxidative stress is a threshold reaction that occurs when antioxidant defenses are overwhelmed. The chain reactions that characterize oxidative stress stop when two free radicals react with each other or when they are quenched by reacting with an antioxidant. The major antioxidant defense systems include enzymes such as superoxide dismutase, catalase, and glutathione peroxidase and chemical reductants such as ascorbate (vitamin C), which is water soluble and present in the cytosol, and α-tocopherol (vitamin E), which is lipid soluble and localized to lipid membranes (94). The chemical antioxidants act by donating a hydrogen atom to the radical, and simultaneously a stable tocopherol or ascorbate radical is formed (89). They are referred to as free-radical scavengers, and vitamin E is the major chain-breaking lipid antioxidant.

Naturally, therapeutic attention has been directed to pharmacologic agents that also seem to function as free-radical scavengers or are integral to the function of antioxidant enzymes. These include vitamins C and E, retinoic acid (vitamin A, β-carotene), deprenyl or selegiline (a monoamine oxidase B inhibitor), *Ginkgo biloba* extract (95), selenium, zinc, and riboflavin (96). Regular intake of antioxidant vitamins and minerals is often recommended to ward off illnesses such as cancer, cardiovascular disease, and neurologic conditions associated with aging. For example, a scientific advisory group in the United States that works to advance medical research on human aging (but is not connected with the U.S. Food and Drug Administration or the National Institutes of Health) has already advised healthy adults to sharply increase their intake of selected antioxidant nutrients, suggesting a daily intake of 250 to 1,000 mg of vitamin C, 100 to 400 IU of vitamin E, and 10 to 30 mg of β-carotene (provitamin A), four to 16 times higher than current recommended daily allowances (97).

Brain Trauma and Ischemia

What happens to the brain after stroke or brain injury may be influenced by pro-oxidant/antioxidant status. Lipid peroxidation by free-radical chain reactions has been implicated in the pathophysiology of brain damage after ischemic stroke and brain trauma (98). When the flow of blood to brain tissue is interrupted, injury ensues from lack of oxygenation and then from subsequent reoxygenation (ischemia/reperfusion). It is during the reperfusion stage, however, that most of the tissue injury seems to occur, and this is believed to be a function of the generation of oxygen free radicals, especially in the presence of low molecular weight iron (88). The reintroduction of oxygen to ischemic tissue has been demonstrated to result in the explosive generation of oxygen free radicals (90,99).

The primary injury to brain tissue after trauma is mechanical in nature, but subsequent events amplify the pathologic process and lead to the death of additional tissue originally spared from the primary injury. Although not every aspect of this secondary process is understood, it is increasingly appreciated that a primary component is ischemia. Traumatic injury to the central nervous system (CNS) rapidly evolves into an ischemic insult.

Within brain, oxygen free radicals impair capillary endothelium that maintain water and electrolyte homeostasis, alter membrane fluidity characteristics, and contribute to synaptic damage. Because the brain has a high concentration of polyunsaturated fatty acids (PUFAs), it is very susceptible to injury by lipid peroxidation, and once peroxidative reactions have been set in motion, they are chain propagating in the presence of sufficient concentrations of oxygen (99).

After injury, astrocytes appear to exercise a neuroprotective effect by expressing antioxidant enzymes and recycling vitamin C (100). Intrinsic defense mechanisms may not be sufficient, however, to meet the acute demands of oxidant stress induced by ischemia/reperfusion. The idea, then, is to mitigate the process of secondary injury by increasing the availability of free-radical scavengers (101). In experimental models, pretreatment with α-tocopherol has been shown to attenuate lipid peroxidation during reperfusion. Another strategy has been to administer antioxidant enzymes such as superoxide dismutase or catalase, usually in modified forms (99). Novel free-radical scavengers and peroxidation antagonists have been developed, such as the so-called lazaroids (102).

Parkinson's Disease

In 1979, Stanley Fahn, a neurologist at Columbia University who specialized in the treatment of PD, began to recommend antioxidant vitamins to his patients. He was impressed with the antioxidant stress (endogenous toxin) theory of the disease. He recommended 3 g vitamin C and 3,200 IU of α-tocopherol per day, in divided doses. In 1992, he reported that his patients were able to delay the need for dopaminergic therapy by 2 to 3 years compared with a group of patients treated similarly by another neurologist but without the antioxidant vitamins (89). His contention that antioxidants might delay the progression of PD, led to the DATATOP study in 28 medical centers in the United States and Canada.

PD is the prototypic age-related neurodegenerative disease. It is especially attractive to the study of oxidative stress because the basal ganglia, of all the anatomic regions of the nervous system, may be particularly vulnerable to reactive oxygen species. For example, the catabolism of dopamine by monoamine oxidase is productive of hydroxyl radicals, especially in the presence of iron, and the basal ganglia contain the highest concentration of iron in the nervous system. Activity of monoamine oxidase is known to increase with age (103).

The results of DATATOP, however, were not supportive of the idea. End-point analysis (time to introduction of L-dopa treatment) indicated a positive effect for deprenyl but not for vitamin E (104). Neither treatment influenced mortality (105). The DATATOP study used a lower dose of vitamin E (2,000 IU per day) and no vitamin C. Other investigations have questioned the oxidant stress theory of PD (106), and epidemiologic studies of dietary antioxidants have had mixed results (107–109).

Aging, Dementia

The larger issue, going beyond the oversimplified view of PD as a disease of dopamine in the basal ganglia, is the fact of neurodegeneration itself in aging and dementia. If oxidant stress is relevant to PD, then it may also be relevant to AD.

The proposition that free radicals are an important factor in aging remains to be rigorously proven. We do know, however, that the damage caused by oxidative stress accumulates with age (94) and that aging systems have increased concentrations of oxidized proteins (110). We know that a relatively longer life expectancy within and between species is associated with a correspondingly lower accrual of oxidative damage. Aging itself is normally associated with an increase in the rate of generation of oxygen free radicals, a decline in the antioxidant defenses, and a decline in the efficiency of repair or removal of damaged molecules (111)

The brain is particularly vulnerable to oxidative stress owing to a relatively high rate of reactive oxygen species generation without commensurate levels of antioxidant defenses. In fact, there is a progressive increase in the steady-state concentration of oxidatively modified DNA and proteins in the brain during aging (112). Therefore, it is not surprising that preclinical and clinical studies show positive effects for various free-radical scavenger therapies, e.g., against age-related memory impairment (113–116).

AD is more than an exaggeration of the normal aging process, but oxidative stress is thought to play a role in both conditions. Perhaps it is only a secondary effect of the disease process, but it has opened new avenues for treatment. Direct and indirect indicators of free-radical injury in the patient with AD include increased iron, aluminum, and mercury, which stimulate free-radical generation, increased lipid peroxidation and decreased PUFAs, increased protein and DNA oxidation in the AD brain, diminished energy metabolism in the AD brain, increased concentration of oxidation byproducts in neurofibrillary tangles and senile plaques, and evidence that amyloid itself is capable of generating free radicals (117). The overall peroxidation activity of brain tissue from people with AD is elevated, and the levels of antioxidant enzymes are substantially reduced (118).

More to the point, treatment of patients with AD with 2,000 IU per day of vitamin E was found to retard the course of deterioration to a significant degree (119).

TREATMENT WITH ANTIOXIDANT SUPPLEMENTS

There is a substantial body of evidence, therefore, to support the theory that oxidative stress is a component of the aging process, in general, and of neurodegeneration, in particular. There is evidence—of varying degrees of cogency, but not to be ignored—that antioxidant supplementation in normal people reduces the incidence of cardiovascular events, cancer, cataracts, and degenerative joint disease. It may be recommended, then, to virtually any middle-aged person who is otherwise in good health but who wishes to attenuate physical and mental deterioration. It is arguably a universal cell protectant. Neuroprotection, then, would be a special case within that general rule. Granted, the evidence base for neuroprotection is shallow, but the theory base is deep.

Neuroprotectants are necessary and appropriate to consider as potential treatments during the acute stage of brain injury, be it injury caused by stroke or trauma or perinatal injury. They are appropriate for any middle-aged person to use if he or she is convinced that the oxidant stress theory of aging has merit. Do they have a specific role to play in the long-term management of people with brain injury or mental handicap? Oxidant stress, as we know, is implicated in the cascade of destructive events that follow acute stroke or brain injury, but is it a factor in the long-term, ongoing pathology that sometimes ensues?

With the exception of Down's syndrome, the evidence base is empty. One simply has nothing to go on, at least in terms of direct address to the question, except this syllogism:

1. Brain injury and mental handicap are neuropathic conditions characterized by significant reduction in the cerebral reserve.
2. That alone renders them more vulnerable to the normal biologic stressors that accompany aging and is sufficient to explain the substantial increase in the incidence of mental deterioration over time.
3. Other, specific mechanisms are at play in the development of posttraumatic or Down's syndrome dementia, for example, but oxidant stress is implicated in at least some of the purported mechanisms.
4. Antioxidant supplements, especially vitamins C and E, are efficient free-radical scavengers; they are inexpensive, safe, and well tolerated.
5. They are clearly neuroprotective in laboratory paradigms; in some clinical circumstances, they may be neuroprotective.
6. It is unlikely that definitive answers to the questions raised here, based on long-term clinical trials, will be forthcoming anytime soon.
7. Therefore, and as an interim measure, it is not unreasonable for physicians to recommend antioxidant supplements to patients at risk of cognitive deterioration or dementia because they are clearly safe and possibly effective.

To pose the question in a different way, is it not the physician's responsibility to set before the patient all the data that he or she needs to make an informed choice about a treatment that is clearly safe and possibly effective?

(Is antioxidant therapy clearly safe? Consider the massive population studies done by those in cardiovascular medicine, where seemingly innocent drugs that are cardioprotective in the short term are, in fact, associated with increased mortality over the long term. Could such a thing happen is this arena? Should we say clearly safe or probably safe?)

Psychiatrists have to contend with the possible value of antioxidant supplements when they care for patients who need long-term antipsychotic drug therapy. There is evidence that antioxidant supplements prevent the development of tardive dyskinesia, a particularly noxious side effect of those drugs. The evidence is not definitive, however. The physician is again dealing with a treatment that is probably safe and possibly effective.

Vitamin E

Two families of fat-soluble compounds, the tocopherols and the tocotrienols, constitute vitamin E. α-Tocopherol is the most biologically active of these compounds. Natural-occurring α-tocopherol is found only in the D isomer, whereas synthetic α-tocopherol is a racemic mixture of the D and L isomers, with approximately 75% of the biologic activity of the pure D-α-tocopherol. One milligram of the racemic form is the equivalent of 1 IU of vitamin E activity. The primary dietary source of vitamin E is vegetable oils, especially soybean, corn, safflower, and cottonseed oils. It is also found in wheat germ, nuts, and green leafy vegetables.

The neurologic problems associated with vitamin E deficiency respond to oral doses of 1,600 mg of synthetic α-tocopherol (120). Children with cystic fibrosis are advised to take 100 mg per day. The recommended daily allowance is 4 mg, and the average diet contains approximately 8 mg per day (121).

The Alliance for Aging Research recommends 250 to 1,000 mg per day of α-tocopherol. Fahn used 3,200 IU per day to treat his patients with PD (along with 3 g vitamin C) (89). He said that his treatment worked. According to DATATOP, it did not, but they used 2,000 mg per day of α-tocopherol and no vitamin C. Conversely, the Alzheimer's Disease Cooperative Study found substantial benefit from 2,000 IU per day without vitamin C. A dose of 800 mg per day may prevent tardive dyskinesia.

An ordinary multivitamin contains approximately 30 mg vitamin E, and an ordinary antioxidant formula contains 200 mg. What dose should one take for the purpose of neuroprotection? Should a patient with brain injury or a young person with Down's syndrome take more than a healthy 50-year-old person? They probably should, but how much more? No one can say; 400 to 2,000 mg per day of tocopherol is not unreasonable.

Vitamin C

Vitamin C is synergistic with vitamin E (122). One of its primary roles *in vivo* is the regeneration of oxidized tocopherols, recycling them to the reduced state that is essential for an antioxidant effect. This is one reason why DATATOP was not a fair test of Fahn's proposal that vitamin E (with vitamin C) delayed the progression of PD.

Linus Pauling's name is indelibly associated with the birth of "megavitaminism" since he proposed that high doses of vitamin C could prevent the common cold. The assumption was that the vitamin enhanced the immune response, and there is ample evidence to support that idea. For example, the concentration of vitamin C in leukocytes is quite high and decreases rapidly during phagocytosis and infection. Nevertheless, the metabolic function of vitamin C is not entirely understood, and its effect on human immunity continues to be a cause for debate. There have been innumerable studies on its effects against upper respiratory infections. The balance of the evidence is in favor of a small effect in reducing the severity and duration of the common cold (123).

The association between vitamin C intake and protection from cancer, heart disease, cataracts, and arthritis is based almost entirely on epidemiologic studies. Based on this research, it is virtually impossible to discern whether the protective effect is owing to vitamin C, to vitamin E, or β-carotene, to the combination thereof, or to some unmeasured constituent, such as the bioflavonoids. Nevertheless, the epidemiologic evidence does suggest a protective role for vitamin C (124).

Specific mental changes that occur in vitamin C deficiency (scurvy) include lassitude, depression, and personality change (125). Excluding scurvy, the health consequences of inadequate vitamin C are not well characterized (124).

The brain has the highest concentration of vitamin C in the body. Ascorbate in the CNS influences the actions and metabolism of dopamine, norepinephrine, serotonin, acetylcholine, NMDA, and glutamate (126). The clinical importance of these actions is not known. High doses of vitamin C have not been demonstrated to alter the course of neuropsychiatric disorders or the effects of neuroactive drugs.

Treatment of scurvy in adults requires 1 g per day of vitamin C for approximately a week, which is usually sufficient to replenish the body stores of 2 to 3 g. The recommended daily allowance for adults is 60 mg, and the average diet contains approximately 80 mg per day (121). Pauling recommended 1 to 5 g per day for the prevention of colds. The Alliance for Aging Research recommends daily intake of 250 to 1,000 mg. The ordinary multivitamin has approximately 60 mg, and the antioxidant formula has 250 mg.

You can probably take as much vitamin C as you can stand to swallow. After all, many people have been taking megadoses of vitamin C since the 1970s, and there is no fallout yet. A daily dose of 1 or 2 g is not an unreasonable dose.

THE B VITAMINS

Vitamin B_{12}

Folic acid and vitamin B_{12} (cobalamin) are essential in several metabolic pathways in the CNS, and a close relationship exists between them. Both are involved in single carbon transfer reactions necessary for the production of monoamine transmitters, phospholipids, and nucleotides. Deficiencies of either vitamin produce characteristic hematologic abnormalities and neuropsychiatric symptoms.

The recommended daily allowance for B_{12} is 6 μg, and the average diet contains approximately 20 μg per day. Because the vitamin is tightly conserved through the enterohepatic circulation, it takes 2 to 5 years to develop overt deficiency from malabsorption and 10 to 20 years from strict vegetarianism (vegans who do not eat eggs or dairy products) (127). Treatment of pernicious anemia usually begins with intramuscular injections of 100 to 1,000 μg B_{12} for 5 days and monthly thereafter (127). There is a prejudice against oral B_{12} among American physicians because it is poorly absorbed in the absence of gastric acid and intrinsic factor. In fact, a daily oral dose of 1,000 μg will allow absorption by passive diffusion (without hydrochloric acid or intrinsic factor) of 10 μg, which exceeds the recommended daily allowance (128). The ordinary B complex that one buys at the health food store or a high-potency multivitamin ordinarily contains only 25 to 75 μg B_{12}.

Cobalamin, pyridoxine, and folate are cofactors in the synthesis of methionine from homocysteine, which is the reason that homocystinemia is indicative of a B_{12}/B_6/folate deficiency. In the mitochondria, cobalamin catalyzes the conversion of methylmalonyl coenzyme A to succinyl coenzyme A, which is the reason that the elevated levels of methylmalonic acid are indicative of B_{12} deficiency.

Changes in mood and cognition may accompany low levels of B_{12} or folate, even in the absence of hematologic abnormalities. Such patients may present to neuropsychiatry clinics with undiagnosed deficiencies, and their conditions may improve dramatically with replacement therapy (129,130). Psychiatric abnormalities associated with cobalamin deficiency include depression, paranoia, organic psychosis, obsessive-compulsive disorder, personality, and mood changes (131). B_{12} deficiency is a reversible cause of dementia, and it is a subcortical dementia with processing-speed deficits and memory and visuospatial impairment. Not all the neurocognitive deficits improve after replacement therapy (132).

The common view is that the neurologic manifestations of cobalamin deficiency are a late manifestation that occurs only after the deficiency and its hematologic abnormalities are well established. In fact, neuropsychiatric abnormalities may occur even in the absence of low serum cobalamin levels, anemia, and macrocytosis (133). Neuropsychiatric symptoms in the absence of anemia "should not be considered rare" (129). Because the alleged neuropsychiatric manifestations of subclinical B_{12} may be nonspecific (weakness, fatigue, memory loss, irritability, mood, and personality disorders) and extremely common in the general population of clinic attenders, the issue of diagnosis is problematic. One can measure serum levels of the cobalamin metabolites methylmalonic acid and homocysteine (129), but the test is expensive and considerably more expensive than a therapeutic trial of weekly B_{12} injections.

Folate

Folate is a water-soluble vitamin of the vitamin B complex, and its function is closely related to vitamins B_{12} and B_6. It functions as an enzyme cosubstrate in the metabolism of amino acids and nucleotides. Nutritional deficiency results in impaired biosynthesis of DNA and RNA and thus in reduced cell division, which is manifested clinically as anemia, dermatologic lesions, and poor growth. Its status at the level of subclinical deficiency is difficult to assess (72,121).

Experimental folate deficiency has been shown to cause elevated plasma homocysteine concentrations, and the use of folate-containing multivitamin supplements is associated with low mean plasma homocysteine levels. Folate-responsive homocystinemia can be demonstrated in people who are apparently healthy, suggesting the prevalence of undiagnosed suboptimal vitamin status (72,134). Hyperhomocystinemia is especially prevalent in the elderly (as high as 29%) (135). This is important because homocystinemia is a risk factor for occlusive vascular disease, cancer, and birth defects. In fact, the U.S. Food and Drug Administration has recommended adding folate to foods to achieve a daily intake of 0.4 to 1.0 mg and thus reduce the occurrence of affected pregnancies. Fortification of the food supply may also reduce the occurrence of cardiovascular disease (136). Mandatory fortification of grain products with folate began in the United States in 1999.

Folate levels are often found to be low in psychiatric patients, e.g., in depression, dementia, schizophrenia, alcoholism, and anorexia. Experimentally induced folate deficiency in normal volunteers can cause sleeplessness, irritability, and memory deficits. The most common neuropsychiatric complication of severe folate deficiency is depression (137). Dietary intake may play a role, but the cause of folate deficiency in patients with psychiatric disorders, compared with normal controls, is unknown. The association of folate deficiency to neuropsychiatric disorders may be mediated by the metabolism of serotonin, phospholipid methylation in the neuronal membrane (138), or the neurotoxicity of homocysteine (139). Folate and B_{12} are both required for the methylation of homocysteine to methionine and in the synthesis of *S*-adenosyl-L-methionine, which is, in turn, involved in numerous methylation reactions involving proteins, phospholipids, DNA, and various neurotransmitters. *S*-adenosyl-L-methionine , by itself, is said to have antidepressant properties (137,139).

Folate therapy, however, does not always lead to clinical improvement, although patients with low baseline folic acid levels tend to respond less well to antidepressants (130,140), antipsychotic drugs (141,142), lithium (143), and anticonvulsants (144,145).

THE RATIONALE FOR TREATMENT WITH ANTIOXIDANTS AND B VITAMINS

Simply because a vitamin is essential to some aspect of metabolism in the CNS does not mean that supplemental vitamins will improve CNS function. Vitamins are taken up into the CNS by an active transport system that gives priority to the requirements of brain metabolism, and the synthetic steps in which the B vitamins participate are not usually rate-limiting steps in neurotransmitter synthesis. Nevertheless, it is arguable that some of the B vitamins, notably folate, enhance the response of patients to psychoactive drugs, and it does appear that a course of cobalamin may lead to nonspecific improvement in patients with a variety of neuropsychiatric conditions. The science is not well developed, and the controversies are not likely to be settled anytime soon. It is not unreasonable to offer patients with brain injury a course of B_{12} injections or to advise the patient on chronic psychotropic drug therapy to take a supplemental B complex tablet every day.

The science behind the theories of oxidative stress, however, is well developed. The patient with brain injury should be particularly interested in antioxidant supplementation, even if she or he is young and healthy and has made a good recovery from the trauma. Even mild brain injuries seem to be associated with at least a degree of compromise of the cerebral reserve; the young patient with brain injury has, for all practical purposes, a middle-aged brain. It is my custom to present this argument to patients who have sustained brain injuries, as we do to all our middle-aged patients, and to invite them to participate in a theoretical treatment that carries little, if any, risk and that may exercise at least a degree of benefit over the long term.

We do so with the caveat that large doses of vitamin supplements may induce a relative deficiency of other vitamins/minerals. Patients who choose to take high doses of C, E, or a B complex should also take a good multivitamin tablet as well.

OMEGA-3 FATTY ACIDS

The benefits of eating fish first came to the attention of the medical world in 1980, when Bang et al. suggested that the low rate of coronary artery disease in Greenland Eskimos might be attributable to their high consumption of seafood. Five years later, Kromhout and co-workers (146) showed that eating just one or two portions of fish every week was associated with a 50% reduction in coronary heart disease mortality. Since that time, more than 15 cohort studies have been done to address the topic, and the majority supported the cardioprotective role of the consumption of a small amount of fish (147).

Fish are high in n-3 fatty acids (omega-3 PUFAs), which experiments have indicated have antiarrhythmic properties. That may not be their only cardioprotective mechanism; they are also antihypertensive, decrease platelet aggregation, and sometimes lower serum triglycerides (148,149). In other areas, they also have been demonstrated to have anti-inflammatory effects and to be beneficial for ulcerative colitis, rheumatoid arthritis, asthma, and some types of cancer (150). Low levels of omega-3 fatty acids are associated with neuropathy and impairment of the immune system (151). Therefore, it is important to eat fish, but is it "brain food?"

Let us begin with mother's milk. The lipid fraction of human milk is the main energy source for the newborn infant and supplies essential nutrients including the PUFAs. The essential fatty acids in milk, linoleic, and linolenic acid have been known to be necessary for normal growth and development since 1930 (151). There is substantial transfer of omega-3 PUFAs from mothers to infants during pregnancy and lactation. In fact, mothers are found to have relative deficiencies of omega-3 PUFAs (152), which may influence the development of postpartum depression.

Linoleic and linolenic acid are precursors of the long-chain PUFAs, such as arachidonic acid (an omega-6 PUFA) and docosahexaenoic acid (DHA, an omega-3 PUFA). The long-chain PUFAs are indispensable structural components of all cellular membranes and are incorporated in relatively large amounts during early growth of the brain. Some long-chain PUFAs are precursors of eicosapentaenoic acid, an omega-3 PUFA with potent biologic activity (153). DHA and eicosapentaenoic acid together are referred to as omega-3 fatty acids or "fish oil" because they are found in high concentrations in fish, especially fatty fish such as salmon, tuna, and mackerel.

Several sources of information suggest that humans evolved on a diet with a ratio of omega-6 to omega-3 fatty acids of approximately 1:1, whereas today the ratio is 10:1 or 20:1. It would appear, then, that the conventional Western diet is deficient in omega-3 fatty acids compared with the diet on which humans evolved (149). In the general population, there is a wide range of omega-6:omega-3 proportions; some individuals are high in one and low in the other and vice versa. The two are not interconvertible, and their levels are inversely related in individuals and populations (149,151). It is tempting to think that the chronic diseases of modern humans are related to unnaturally low levels of omega-3 fatty acids in their diets; the composition of cell membranes is to a great extent dependent on dietary intake. In animals, for example, dietary restriction that decreases omega-3 fatty acids and raises levels of omega-6 fatty acids tends to accelerate age-related changes of dopamine and serotonin in the frontal cortex and the brainstem (154,155).

Omega-3 fatty acids are necessary for the normal growth and development of the brain and the maintenance of normal brain function in adults. The turnover of DHA in brain is very fast. Deficiencies of DHA are associated with learning deficits in infants and children, whereas including plenty of DHA in the diet improves learning ability. It is troubling to think that most infant formula diets lack omega-3 fatty acids (156).

Learning deficits are demonstrated in animals deficient in omega-3 fatty acids (157) and, in preliminary reports, in children with dyslexia (158), ADHD, and behavioral problems (159–162).

Studies of dementia are equally intriguing, although preliminary. Animal studies indicate a therapeutic role for DHA in rats subjected to transient forebrain ischemia (163) and in humans with dementia from cerebrovascular disease (164). Low serum DHA is said to be a significant risk factor for AD (165). There are lower levels of omega-3 fatty acids in the parahippocampal cortex of patients with AD (117,166). Dietary fatty acids may attenuate the neurotoxic effects of alcohol (167,168). Conversely, oxidative transformation of n-6 and n-3 fatty acids in the brain by free-radical species may adversely affect neuronal function (169). Oxidative products of essential fatty acids (isoprostanes or neuroprostanes) seem to be elevated in patients with dementia (170). For this reason, if a patient elects to take omega-3 supplements, he or she should take vitamins C and E as well.

The clinical relevance of long-chain fatty acids can be investigated by examining dietary intake, lipid fractions in serum, or the constitution of membrane phospholipids in tissue samples such as erythrocytes or fibroblasts; measuring light sensitivity because DHA is found in high concentrations in the photoreceptor cells of the retina; or measuring clinical response to dietary supplements of omega-3 fatty acids. This is a particularly fertile avenue for psychiatric investigation because even a modest abnormality in cell membrane metabolism would be greatly amplified in the brain, which requires the coordinated sequential and parallel activities of billions of neurons. The idea that schizophrenia, for example, may be a disorder of cell membrane phospholipid metabolism has been investigated with interesting results (171–173).

More pertinent to this discussion is the relationship between omega-3 fatty acids and affective disorders. There are a few reports of reduction in patients with depression (174–177); and one controlled study of omega-3 fatty acids for the treatment of patients with bipolar disorder (178). People who eat fish two or three times a week are less likely to be depressed or suicidal (178).

Low levels of serotonin and dopamine metabolites are inversely related to plasma DHA in patients with violent behavior (179). Omega-3 supplements are found to reduce stress-induced aggression in young adults (180). These observations may reflect on the problem of depression associated with low serum cholesterol. Serum cholesterol may simply be a surrogate marker for the long-chain PUFAs (181).

Dietary supplements of the two omega-3 fatty acids DHA and EHA are widely available and relatively inexpensive. A supplemental omega-3 fatty acid is attractive to consumers who are aware of its benefits as a putative cardioprotectant. It is sometimes promoted as an arthritis remedy. Neither indication is medically proven. Physicians are more likely to recommend a weekly serving or two of fish. It is possible that omega-3 fatty acids will be more interesting to psychiatrists for the adjunctive treatment of affective disorders and other mental conditions and for the prevention of cognitive deterioration in the elderly. Similarly, they may be included as part of a defensible neuroprotective regimen for patients with brain injury (Table 25.1). Paradoxically, patients taking omega-3 acids may become depressed or irritable. If this happens, the patient should stop taking the supplement immediately.

TABLE 25.1. *A defensible regime of neuroprotective supplements*

Vitamin E	400–800 units twice daily
Vitamin C	1,000–2,000 mg twice daily
B complex	1 tablet daily
Multivitamins	1 tablet daily
Omega-3 fatty acids	300–600 mg twice daily

ANTI-INFLAMMATORY DRUGS AND DEMENTIA

An interesting contribution of anti-inflammatory drugs, including dapsone, indomethacin, NSAIDs, and cyclooxygenase (COX)-2 inhibitors may be to inhibit the course of AD. [Aspirin, an antithrombotic drug and a selective COX-1 inhibitor, may not share this effect (182).] The idea originated with the pathologic demonstration of acute phase reactants and other markers of immune processes, absent or present at very low levels in normal brain, in the post-mortem brains of patients with AD. It was buttressed by a series of epidemiologic studies that consistently demonstrated lower rates of dementia in patients who take anti-inflammatory drugs for the usual medical indications (183–186). Several controlled studies have also demonstrated that AD occurs at a lower rate in patients who have received long-term NSAID treatment, for example, people with rheumatoid arthritis or osteoarthritis, and that a course of treatment with anti-inflammatory drugs may slow the progression of dementia in patients with AD. In the Rotterdam study of approximately 8,000 elderly people, the relative risk of AD among users of aspirin or NSAIDs was found to be 0.38 (187,188).

The weight of the evidence, therefore, is that drugs that limit inflammatory reactivity might reduce the risk of AD or slow its progression. How, precisely, does that happen, and how may it be relevant to the treatment of patients with brain injury?

The major mechanism of action of NSAIDs is the inhibition of COX activity and thus the synthesis of prostaglandins (189). Prostaglandins are potent mediators of the inflammatory response and are generated from arachidonic acid via the action of two distinct but related enzymes, COX-1 and COX-2. Both enzymes contribute to the inflammatory process, but COX-2 is of greater therapeutic interest because it is inducible (as opposed to constitutive). That is, its activity is induced by proinflammatory stimuli in migratory cells and inflamed tissues. This results in enhanced formation of prostaglandins (or prostanoids) during acute as well as chronic inflammation. The traditional NSAIDs are nonselective COX inhibitors, whereas the new ones, celecoxib and rofecoxib, are 100 to 1,000 times for selective for COX-2 than COX-1. Because COX-1 is mainly present in the gastric mucosa and kidney, the conventional NSAIDs are far more prone to gastrointestinal and renal side effects than the selective COX-2 inhibitors. Drugs with more COX-2 effect and less COX-1 effect have potent anti-inflammatory activity with fewer side effects (190,191).

The idea that inflammatory responses may be a component of the development of AD began with the observation in 1987 that plaques in the brains of patients with AD were filled with reactive microglial cells. The activity of microglial cells is not a harmless event, a form of neuronal housekeeping, as it were, and potentially toxic in its own right. Microglial cells are prone to secrete complement proteins and other biochemical weapons such as COX-2 that are by themselves potentially neurotoxic. In various experimental models, e.g., ischemia and neurotoxic injection, microglial cells can be induced to generate COX-2 and proinflammatory prostanoids. COX-2 induction is also a component of the cascade of events that surround neuronal excitotoxicity (192–195). Brain injury itself induces the expression of several genes including the gene for COX-2 (196).

Drugs that inhibit COX-2 activity are thus expected to interrupt or at least attenuate a series of inflammatory processes that are potentially neurotoxic in their own right and that aggravate the impact of the original pathogenic event, be it tau protein, ischemia, or traumatic injury. Thus, theories of pathogenesis complement the results of epidemiologic studies, and the COX-2 inhibitors, antioxidants, and omega-3 fatty acids are practical and potentially useful neuroprotectants. [The COX-2 inhibitors are also believed to prevent the development of some gastrointestinal cancers (197).]

Now, a familiar question arises: to what degree is a neuroprotectant NSAID useful for patients with brain injury or mental retardation? They are possibly effective in preventing some forms of late degeneration, but they are not inexpensive nor are they entirely free of side effects.

High doses of NSAIDs interfere with other biologic processes not dependent on prostaglandins: the activity of various enzymes and transmembrane ion fluxes (189). The inhibition of COX-2 is not inevitably beneficial for the health of one's brain; the expression of COX-2 is a normal component of brain development, and the basal production of prostaglandins through COX-2 may "participate in neuronal homeostasis" (182). Patients taking traditional NSAIDs, especially elderly patients, have had a variety of mental problems including depression, forgetfulness, difficulty concentrating, paranoia, mania, and frank psychosis; the COX-2 inhibitors are no different in this regard (198,199). Even young, healthy patients taking NSAIDs may experience mental slowing or "fuzziness" at high doses. Celecoxib has clinically significant interactions with fluconazole and lithium, as do other NSAIDs, and it is metabolized by CYP2C9 (200).

Just as one feels safe in encouraging patients to pursue an antioxidant/fish oil strategy to protect the health of his or her brain, one is hesitant to recommend routine daily dosing with a COX-2 inhibitor. Patients who are at high risk for dementia, however, should be considered for prophylactic treatment. This, at least, is an area where definitive studies will be done.

GINKGO BILOBA

Extracts from the leaves of the ginkgo tree (maidenhair tree) have been used for hundreds of years in Chinese medicine. *Ginkgo biloba* is now the most commonly prescribed drug in France and Germany. In the United States, it is not deemed a drug, but rather a dietary supplement and is one of the most popular herbal remedies.

In Europe, it is used for cerebral insufficiency, a term that covers a wide range of problems including absentmindedness, difficulties with concentration and memory, confusion, lack of energy, fatigue, impaired physical performance, depression, and anxiety, usually associated with aging. It is also used for intermittent claudication because it is said to decrease the viscosity of blood (201). In fact, health-conscious people who take daily aspirin and *Ginkgo biloba* may be given to nosebleeds; one of the components of ginkgo, ginkgolide B, is a potent platelet-activating factor antagonist (202).

There have been several controlled studies, published in respectable journals, that support the use of ginkgo extract for a number of neuropsychiatric problems such as neurasthenia (fatigue and tiredness) (201), age-associated memory impairment (203), cerebral insufficiency (204), and dementia (205). There are also preclinical studies that demonstrate a positive recovery effect for ginkgo in brain trauma and spinal cord injury (95,206,207).

Ginkgo extract is a potent antioxidant (208–210) and a reversible inhibitor of monoamine oxidase (211). It tends to reduce glucocorticoid synthesis, which may account for its purported antistress effect (212).

There is no apparent toxicity from *Ginkgo biloba*, aside from the interaction with aspirin, but there are no long-term safety/efficacy studies.

One might say this: patients deserve the opportunity to decide for themselves whether to take ginkgo, just as they have to decide about the antioxidants, B vitamins, and omega-3s. However, most people do not like to take a lot of pills, and the effects of these putative neuroprotectants is not something that the patient is likely to experience as immediately reinforcing (except possibly for the omega-3s). Even if each substance mentioned is, in fact, neuroprotective, we have no way of knowing whether, if they are taken together, their effects are additive, synergistic, or in some way, subtractive, or even dangerous.

I suppose that it falls to physicians to come to terms with this promising but woefully underdeveloped area as best he or she can do. Physicians have to decide whether to recommend this approach to long-term neuroprotection, how to educate patients about its pros and cons, and then how to keep after patients who must commit to a lifetime of treatment. In my practice, I tend to recommend the supplements listed in Table 25.1. As far as ginkgo is concerned, I am neutral, but do not take it with aspirin.

REFERENCES

1. Gagliardi RJ. Neuroprotection, excitotoxicity and NMDA antagonists. *Arq Neuropsiquitiatr* 2000;58: 583–588.
2. Chen XW, Yi Y, Qiu L, et al. Neuroprotective activity of tiagabine in a focal embolic model of cerebral ischemia. *Brain Res* 2000;874:75–77.
3. Green AR, Hainsworth AH, Jackson DM. GABA potentiation: a logical pharmacological approach for the treatment of acute ischaemic stroke. *Neuropharmacology* 2000;39:1483–1494.
4. Savitz SI, Erhardt JA, Anthony JV, et al. The novel beta-blocker, carvedilol, provides neuroprotection in transient focal stroke. *J Cereb Blood Flow Metab* 2000;20:1197–1204.
5. Chavany JA. Role des Causes Occasionelles dans le Determinisime du Ramolissement Cerebral (Reflections Therapeutiques a le Propos). *Pratique Med Francaise* 1928;7:285–295.
6. Luria A, Naydin V, Tsvetkova L, et al. Restoration of higher cortical function following local brain damage. In: Vinkin RJ, Bruyn GW, eds. *Handbook of clinical neurology*. Amsterdam: North Holland, 1968:368–433.
7. Ward AA, Kennard MA. Effect of cholinergic drugs on recovery of function following lesions of the central nervous system in monkeys. *Yale J Biol Med* 1942;15: 189–228.
8. Coyle JT, Price DL, DeLong MR. Alzheimer's disease: a disorder of cortical cholinergic innervation. *Science* 1983;219:1184–1190.
9. Sarter M, Bruno JP. Cognitive functions of cortical acetylcholine: toward a unifying hypotheses. *Brain Res Rev* 1997;23:28–46.
10. McLean A, Stanton KM, Cardenas DD, et al. Memory training combined with the use of oral physostigmine. *Brain Inj* 1987;1:145–159.
11. Bartus RT, Dean RL, Fisher SK. Cholinergic treatment for age-related memory disturbances: dead or barely coming of age? In: Crook T, Bratus RT, Ferris S, et al., eds. *Treatment development strategies for Alzheimer's disease*. Madison, WI: Mark Powley, 1986:421–450.
12. Jorm AF. Effects of cholinergic enhancement therapies on memory function in Alzheimer's disease: a meta-analysis of the literature. *Aust N Z J Psychiatry* 1986; 20:237–240.
13. Catsman-Berrevoets EC, van Harskamp F, Appelhof A. Beneficial effects of physostigmine on clinical amnesic behaviour and neropsychological test results in a patient with a post-encephalitic amnesic syndrome. *J Neurol Neurosurg Psychiatry* 1986;49:1088–1089.
14. Summers WK, Majovsky LV, Marsh GM, et al. Oral tetrahydroaminoacridine in long-term treatment of senile dementia, Alzheimer type. *N Engl J Med* 1986; 315:1241–1287.
15. Fitten LJ, Perryman KM, Gross PL, et al. Treatment of Alzheimer's disease with short- and long-term oral THA and lecithin: a double-blind study. *Am J Psychiatry* 1990;147:239–242.
16. Becker RE, Colliver JA, Markwell SJ, et al. Double-blind, placebo-controlled study of metrifonate, an acetylcholinesterase inhibitor, for Alzheimer's disease. *Alzheimer Dis Assoc Disord* 1996;10:124–131.
17. Pettigrew LC, Bieber F, Lettieri J, et al. Pharmacokinetics, pharmacodynamics, and safety of metrifonate in patients with Alzheimer's disease. *J Clin Pharmacol* 1998;38:236–245.
18. Rogers SL, Farlow MR, Doody RS, et al. A 24-week, double-blind, placebo-controlled trial of donepezil in patients with Alzheimer's disease. Donepezil Study Group. *Neurology* 1998;50:136–145.
19. Taverni J, Seliger G, Lichtman S. Donepezil medicated memory improvement in traumatic brain injury during post acute rehabilitation. *Brain Inj* 1998;12:77–80.
20. Greene YM, Tariot PN, Wishart H, et al. A 12-week, open trial of donepezil hydrochloride in patients with multiple sclerosis and associated cognitive impairments. *J Clin Psychopharmacol* 2000;20:350–356.
21. Whelan F, Walker M, Schultz S. Donepezil in the treatment of cognitive dysfunction associated with traumatic brain injury. *Ann Clin Psychiatry* 2000;12:131–135.
22. Mondadori C. The pharmacology of the nootropics;

new insights and new questions. *Behav Brain Res* 1993; 59:1–9.

23. Pizzi M, Consolandi O, Memo M, et al. *N*-Methyl-D-aspartate neurotoxicity in hippocampal slices: protection by aniracetam. *Eur J Pharmacol* 1995;275:311–314.
24. Galeotti N, Gherardini C, Bartolini A. Piracetam and aniracetam antagonism of centrally active drug- induced antinociception. *Pharmacol Biochem Behav* 1996;53:943–950.
25. Simeon JG, Volauka J, Trites R, et al. Electroencephalographic correlates in children with learning disorders treated with piracetam. *Psychopharmacol Bull* 1983;19:716–720.
26. Dimond SJ, Brouwers EYM. Increase in power of human memory in normal man through use of drugs. *Psychopharmacology* 1976;49:307–309.
27. Wilsher C, Melewski J. Effect of piracetam on dyslexics's verbal conceptualizing ability. *Psychopharmacol Bull* 1983;19:3–4.
28. Nicholson CD. Pharmacology of nootropics and metabolically active compounds in relation to their use in dementia. *Psychopharmacology* 1990;101:147–159.
29. Croisile B, Trillet M, Fondarai J, et al. Long-term and high-dose piracetam treatment of Alzheimer's disease. *Neurology* 1993;43:301–305.
30. Helfgott E, Rudel RG, Krieger J. Effect of piracetam on the single word and prose reading of dyslexic children. *Psychopharmacol Bull* 1984;20:688–690.
31. Shih YH, Pugsley TA. The effects of various cognition-enhancing drugs on in vitro rat hippocampal synaptosomal sodium dependent high affinity choline uptake. *Life Sci* 1985;36:2145–2152.
32. Branconnier RJ, Cole JD, Dessain EC, et al. The therapeutic efficacy of pramiracetam in Alzheimer's disease: preliminary observations. *Psychopharmacol Bull* 1983;19:726–730.
33. Ikeda A, Shibasaki H, Tashiro K, et al. Treatment of myoclonus with piracetam. *Mov Disord* 1996;11:691–700.
34. Koskiniemi M, Van Vleymen B, Hakamies L, et al. Piracetam relieves symptoms in progressive myoclonus epilepsy: a multicentre, randomised, double blind, crossover study comparing the efficacy and safety of three dosages of oral piracetam with placebo. *J Neurol Neurosurg Psychiatry* 1998;64:344–348.
35. Huber W, Willmes K, Poeck K, et al. Piracetam as an adjuvant to language therapy for aphasia: a randomized double-blind placebo-controlled pilot study. *Arch Phys Med Rehabil* 1994;78:245–250.
36. Enderby P, Broeckx J, Hospers W, et al. Effect of piracetam on recovery and rehabilitation after stroke: a double-blind, placebo-controlled study. *Clin Neuropharmacol* 1994;17:320–331.
37. De Deyn PP, Reuck JD, Deberdt W, et al. Treatment of acute ischemic stroke with piracetam. Members of the Piracetam in Acute Stroke Study (PASS) Group. *Stroke* 1997;28:2347–2352.
38. Ricci S, Celani MG, Cantisani AT, et al. Piracetam for acute ischaemic stroke. *Cochrane Database Sys Rev* 2000;2:CD000419.
39. Gispen WH, Isaacson RL, Spruijt BM, et al. Melanocortins, neural plasticity and ageing. *Prog Neuropsychol Biol Psychiatry* 1986;10:416–426.
40. Shen Y, Li R. The role of neuropeptides in learning and memory: possible mechanisms. *Med Hypotheses* 1995;45:529–538.
41. Reisberg B, Ferris SH, Gershon S. An overview of pharmacologic treatment of cognitive decline in the aged. *Am J Psychiatry* 1981;138:593–600.
42. Landfield PW, Baskin RK, Pitler TA. Brain aging correlates: retardation by hormonal-pharmacological treatments. *Science* 1981;214:581–584.
43. De Weid D. Hormonal influences on motivation learning and memory process. *Hosp Pract* 1976;11:123–131.
44. Smolnik R, Perras B, Molle M, et al. Event-related brain potentials and working memory function in healthy humans after single-dose and prolonged intranasal administration of adrenocorticotropin 4-10 and desacetyl-alpha-melanocyte stimulating hormone. *J Clin Psychopharmacol* 2000;20:145.
45. Rigter H, Van Riezen H. Hormones and memory. In: Lipton MA, Dimascib A, Killiam KF, eds. *Psychopharmacology: a generation of progress*. New York: Raven Press, 1978:677–689.
46. Frederiksen S, D'Elia G, Holsten R. Influence of ACTH-4-10 and unilateral ECT on primary and secondary memory in depressive patients. *Eur Arch Psychiatry Neurol Sci* 1985;234:291–294.
47. Heuser I, Heuser-Link M, Gotthardt U, et al. Behavioral effects of a synthetic corticotropin 4-9 analog in patients with depression and patients with Alzheimer's disease. *J Clin Psychopharmacol* 1993;13:171–174.
48. Jennekens-Schinkel A, Eintzen AR, Lanser BK. A clinical trial with desglycinamide arginine vasopressin for the treatment of memory disorders in man. *Prog Neuropsychopharmacol Biol Psychiatry* 1985;9:273–284.
49. Legros JJ, Gilot P, Seron X, et al. Influence on vasopressin on learning and memory. *Lancet* 1978;1:41–42.
50. Tinklenberg JR, Pigache R, Berger PA, et al. Desglycinamide-9-arginine-8-vasopressin in cognitively impaired patients. *Psychopharmacol Bull* 1982;18:202–204.
51. Koob GF, Lebrun C, Bluthe RM, et al. Role of neuropeptides in learning versus performance: focus on vasopressin. *Brain Res Bull* 1989;23:359–364.
52. Perras B, Pannenborg H, Marshall L, et al. Beneficial treatment of age-related sleep disturbances with prolonged intranasal vasopressin. *J Clin Psychopharmacol* 1999;19:28–36.
53. Faden AI, Jacobs TP. Effect of TRH analogs on neurologic recovery after experimental spinal trauma. *Neurology* 1985;35:1331–1334.
54. Faden AI. TRH analog YM-14673 improves outcome following traumatic brain and spinal cord injury in rats: dose-response studies. *Brain Res* 1989;486:228–235.
55. Fukuda N, Yoshiaki S, Nagaway J. Behavioral an EEG alterations with brain stem compression and effect of TRH in chronic cats. *Folia Pharmacol Jpn* 1979;75: 321–331.
56. Faden AI. Opiate antagonists and thyrotropin-releasing hormone. II. Potential role in the treatment of central nervous system injury. *JAMA* 1984;252:1452–1454.
57. Faden AI, Labroo VM, Cohen LA. Imidazole-substituted analogues of TRH limit behavioral deficits after experimental brain trauma. *J Neurotrauma* 1993;10: 101–108.
58. Miyamoto M, Fukuda N, Narumi S, et al. Gamma-butyrolactone-gamma-carbonyl-histidyl-prolinamide citrate (DN- 1417): a novel TRH analog with potent effects on the central nervous system. *Life Sci* 1981;28: 861–869.

59. Horita A. An update on the CNS actions of TRH and its analogs. *Life Sci* 1998;62:1443–1448.
60. Prange AJ Jr, Utiger RD. What does brain thyrotropin-releasing hormone do? *N Engl J Med* 1981;305: 1089–1090.
61. Mellow AM, Sunderland T, Cohen RM, et al. Acute effects of high-dose thyrotropin releasing hormone infusions in Alzheimer's disease. *Psychopharmacology (Berl)* 1989;98:403–407.
62. Bennett GW, Ballard TM, Watson CD, et al. Effect of neuropeptides on cognitive function. *Exp Gerontol* 1997;32:451–469.
63. Parnetti L, Ambrosoli L, Agliati G, et al. Posatirelin in the treatment of vascular dementia: a double-blind multicentre study vs placebo. *Acta Neurol Scand* 1996; 93:456–463.
64. Khan A, Mirolo MH, Claypoole K, et al. Low-dose thyrotropin-releasing hormone effects in cognitively impaired alcoholics. *Alcohol Clin Exp Res* 1993;17: 791–796.
65. Osonoe K, Osonoe M, Ariga K, et al. The effect of thyrotropin-releasing hormone (TRH) on limbic status epilepticus in rats. *Epilepsy Res* 1994;18:217–225.
66. Khan A, Mirolo MH, Claypoole K, et al. Effects of low-dose TRH on cognitive deficits in the ECT postictal state. *Am J Psychiatry* 1994;151:1694–1696.
67. Faden AI. Neuropeptides and central nervous system injury: clinical implications. *Arch Neurol* 1986;43: 501–503.
68. Renaud LP, Blume HW, Pittman QJ, et al. Thyrotropin-releasing hormone selectively depresses glutamate excitation of cerebral cortical neurons. *Science* 1979;205:1275–1277.
69. Walker P, Weichsel ME Jr, Fisher DA, et al. Thyroxine increases nerve growth factor concentration in adult mouse brain. *Science* 1979;204:427–429.
70. Hefti F, Weiner WJ. Nerve growth factor and Alzheimer's disease. *Ann Neurol* 1986;20:275–281.
71. Nabeshima T, Yamada K. Neurotrophic factor strategies for the treatment of Alzheimer disease. *Alzheimer Dis Assoc Disord* 2000;14:39–46.
72. Combs G. *The vitamins: fundamental aspects in nutrition and health*, 2nd ed. San Diego: Academic Press, 1998.
73. Leiderman E, Zylberman I, Zukin SR, et al. Preliminary investigation of high-dose oral glycine on serum levels and negative symptoms in schizophrenia: an open-label trial. *Biol Psychiatry* 1996;39:213–215.
74. Mercuri NB, Bonci A, Pisani A, et al. Actions of glycine on non-dopaminergic neurons of the rat substantia nigra. *Eur J Neurosci* 1995;7:2351–2354.
75. Roach ES, Gibson P. Failure of *N,N*-dimethylglycine in epilepsy. *Ann Neurol* 1983;14:347.
76. Gascon G, Patterson B, Yearwood K, et al. *N,N*-dimethylglycine and epilepsy. *Epilepsia* 1989;30:90–93.
77. Bishop PA, Smith JF, Young B. Effects of *N,N*-dimethylglycine on physiological response and performance in trained runners. *J Sports Med* 1987;27:53–56.
78. Reap EA, Lawson JW. Stimulation of the immune response by dimethylglycine, a nontoxic metabolite. *J Lab Clin Med* 1990;115:481–486.
79. Fishkin RJ, Ince ES, Carlezon WA Jr, et al. D-Cycloserine attenuates scopolamine-induced learning and memory deficits in rats. *Behav Neural Biol* 1993;59: 150–157.
80. Matsuoka N, Aigner TG. D-Cycloserine, a partial agonist at the glycine site coupled to *N*-methyl-D-aspartate receptors, improves visual recognition memory in rhesus monkeys. *J Pharmacol Exp Ther* 1996;278: 891–897.
81. Schwartz BL, Hashtroudi S, Herting RL, et al. D-Cycloserine enhances implicit memory in Alzheimer patients. *Neurology* 1996;46:420–424.
82. Tsai GEP, Falk WE, Gunther J, et al. Improved cognition in Alzheimer's disease with short-term D-cycloserine treatment. *Am J Psychiatry* 1999;156:467–469.
83. Norris DO, Mastropaolo J, O'Connor DA, et al. A glycinergic intervention potentiates the antiseizure efficacies of MK-801, flurazepam, and carbamazepine. *Neurochem Res* 1994;19:161–165.
84. Rolinski Z, Wlaz P, Czuczwar SJ. Influence of D-cycloserine on the anticonvulsant activity of phenytoin and carbamazepine against electroconvulsions in mice. *Epilepsia* 1996;37:617.
85. De Sarro G, Gratteri S, Naccari F, et al. Influence of D-cycloserine on the anticonvulsant activity of some antiepileptic drugs against audiogenic seizures in DBA/2 mice. *Epilepsy Res* 2000;40:109–121.
86. Temple M, Hamm R. Chronic, post-injury administration of D-cycloserine, an NMDA partial agonist, enhances cognitive performance following experimental brain injury. *Brain Res* 1996;741:246–251.
87. Sacco R, DeRosa J, Haley E, et al. Glycine antagonist in neuroprotection for patients with acute stroke. *JAMA* 2001;285:1719–1728.
88. Floyd RA. Role of oxygen free radicals in carcinogenesis and brain ischemia. *FASEB J* 1990;4:2587–2597.
89. Fahn S, Cohen G. The oxidant stress hypothesis in Parkinson's disease: evidence supporting it. *Ann Neurol* 1992;32:804–812.
90. Braughler JM, Hall ED. Central nervous system trauma and stroke. *Free Radic Biol Med* 1989;6: 289–301.
91. Penninx BW, Guralnik JM, Ferrucci L, et al. Depressive symptoms and physical decline in community-dwelling older persons. *JAMA* 1998;279:1720–1726.
92. Morrow JD, Frei B, Longmire AW, et al. Increase in circulating products of lipid peroxidation (F2-isoprostanes) in smokers. Smoking as a cause of oxidative damage. *N Engl J Med* 1995;332:1198–1203.
93. Wallace DC, Melov S. Radicals raging. *Nat Genet* 1998;19:105–106.
94. Frolich L, Riederer P. Free radical mechanisms in dementia of Alzheimer type and the potential for antioxidative treatment. *Arzneimittelforschung* 1995;45: 443–446.
95. Attella MJ, Hoffman SW, Stasio MJ, et al. *Ginkgo biloba* extract facilitates recovery from penetrating brain injury in adult male rats. *Exp Neurol* 1989;105: 62–71.
96. Hankinson S, Stampfer MJ. All that glitters is not beta carotene. *JAMA* 1994;272:1455–1456.
97. Voelker R. Recommendations for antioxidants: how much evidence is enough? *JAMA* 1994;271:1148–1149.
98. Yoshida S. Brain injury after ischemia and trauma. The role of vitamin E. *Ann N Y Acad Sci* 1989;570:219–236.
99. Traystman RJ, Kirsch JR, Koehler RC. Oxygen radical mechanisms of brain injury following ischemia and reperfusion. *J Appl Physiol* 1991;71:1185–1195.
100. Wilson JX. Antioxidant defense of the brain: a role

for astrocytes. *Can J Physiol Pharmacol* 1997;75: 1149–1163.

101. Shohami E, Beit-Yannai E, Horowitz M, et al. Oxidative stress in closed-head injury: brain antioxidant capacity as an indicator of functional outcome. *J Cereb Blood Flow Metab* 1997;17:1007–1019.
102. Hall ED, Braughler JM, McCall JM. Role of oxygen radicals in stroke: effects of the 21-aminosteroids (lazaroids). Novel class of antioxidants. *Prog Clin Biol Res* 1990;361:351–362.
103. Vatassery GT. Vitamin E. Neurochemistry and implications for neurodegeneration in Parkinson's disease. *Ann N Y Acad Sci* 1992;669:97–109.
104. DATATOP: a multicenter controlled clinical trial in early Parkinson's disease. Parkinson Study Group. *Arch Neurol* 1989;46:1052–1060.
105. Mortality in DATATOP: a multicenter trial in early Parkinson's disease. Parkinson Study Group. *Ann Neurol* 1998;43:318–325.
106. Ahlskog JE, Uitti RJ, Low PA, et al. No evidence for systemic oxidant stress in Parkinson's or Alzheimer's disease. *Mov Disord* 1995;10:566–573.
107. King D, Playfer JR, Roberts NB. Concentrations of vitamins A, C and E in elderly patients with Parkinson's disease. *Postgrad Med J* 1992;68:634–637.
108. de Rijk MC, Breteler MM, den Breeijen JH, et al. Dietary antioxidants and Parkinson disease. The Rotterdam Study. *Arch Neurol* 1997;54:762–765.
109. Scheider WL, Hershey LA, Vena JE, et al. Dietary antioxidants and other dietary factors in the etiology of Parkinson's disease. *Mov Disord* 1997;12:190–196.
110. Floyd RA. Oxidative damage to behavior during aging. *Science* 1991;254:1597.
111. Sohal RS, Weindruch R. Oxidative stress, caloric restriction, and aging. *Science* 1996;273:59–63.
112. Forster MJ, Dubey A, Dawson KM, et al. Age-related losses of cognitive function and motor skills in mice are associated with oxidative protein damage in the brain. *Proc Natl Acad Sci U S A* 1996;93:4765–4769.
113. Clausen J, Nielsen SA, Kristensen M. Biochemical and clinical effects of an antioxidative supplementation of geriatric patients. A double blind study. *Biol Trace Elem Res* 1989;20:135–151.
114. Stoll S, Hartmann H, Cohen SA, et al. The potent free radical scavenger alpha-lipoic acid improves memory in aged mice: putative relationship to NMDA receptor deficits. *Pharmacol Biochem Behav* 1993;46:799–805.
115. Socci DJ, Crandall BM, Arendash GW. Chronic antioxidant treatment improves the cognitive performance of aged rats. *Brain Res* 1995;693:88–94.
116. Gale CR, Martyn CN, Cooper C. Cognitive impairment and mortality in a cohort of elderly people. *BMJ* 1996;312:608–611.
117. Prasad MR, Lovell MA, Yatin M, et al. Regional membrane phospholipid alterations in Alzheimer's disease. *Neurochem Res* 1998;23:81–88.
118. Marcus DL, Thomas C, Rodriguez C, et al. Increased peroxidation and reduced antioxidant enzyme activity in Alzheimer's disease. *Exp Neurol* 1998;150:40–44.
119. Sano M, Ernesto C, Thomas RG, et al. A controlled trial of selegiline, alpha-tocopherol, or both as treatment for Alzheimer's disease. The Alzheimer's Disease Cooperative Study. *N Engl J Med* 1997;336:1216–1222.
120. Harding AE, Muller DP, Thomas PK, et al. Spinocerebellar degeneration secondary to chronic intestinal malabsorption: a vitamin E deficiency syndrome. *Ann Neurol* 1982;12:419–424.
121. Mason P. *Handbook of dietary supplements*. Oxford: Blackwell Science, 1998.
122. Ho CT, Chan AC. Regeneration of vitamin E in rat polymorphonuclear leucocytes. *FEBS Lett* 1992;306: 269–272.
123. Hemila H. Vitamin C intake and susceptibility to the common cold. *Br J Nutr* 1997;77:59–72.
124. Sauberlich HE. Pharmacology of vitamin C. *Annu Rev Nutr* 1994;14:371–391.
125. Carney MW. Vitamin deficiency and mental symptoms. *Br J Psychiatry* 1990;156:878–882.
126. Goldstein J. *Betrayal by the brain*. New York: Haworth Press, 1996.
127. Green R, Kinsella LJ. Current concepts in the diagnosis of cobalamin deficiency. *Neurology* 1995;45: 1435–1440.
128. Lederle FA. Oral cobalamin for pernicious anemia. Medicine's best kept secret? *JAMA* 1991;265:94–95.
129. Lindenbaum J, Healton EB, Savage DG, et al. Neuropsychiatric disorders caused by cobalamin deficiency in the absence of anemia or macrocytosis. *N Engl J Med* 1988;318:1720–1728.
130. Wesson VA, Levitt AJ, Joffe RT. Change in folate status with antidepressant treatment. *Psychiatry Res* 1994;53:313–322.
131. Miller DR, Specker BL, Ho ML, et al. Vitamin B-12 status in a macrobiotic community. *Am J Clin Nutr* 1991;53:524–529.
132. Meadows ME, Kaplan RF, Bromfield EB. Cognitive recovery with vitamin B12 therapy: a longitudinal neuropsychological assessment. *Neurology* 1994;44: 1764–1765.
133. Karnaze DS, Carmel R. Neurologic and evoked potential abnormalities in subtle cobalamin deficiency states, including deficiency without anemia and with normal absorption of free cobalamin. *Arch Neurol* 1990;47:1008–1012.
134. Nilsson K, Gustafson L, Faldt R, et al. Hyperhomocysteinaemia—a common finding in a psychogeriatric population. *Eur J Clin Invest* 1996;26:853–859.
135. Tucker KL, Mahnken B, Wilson PW, et al. Folic acid fortification of the food supply. Potential benefits and risks for the elderly population. *JAMA* 1996;276: 1879–1885.
136. Stampfer MJ, Rimm EB. Folate and cardiovascular disease. Why we need a trial now. *JAMA* 1996;275: 1929–1930.
137. Reynolds EH, Carney MW, Toone BK. Methylation and mood. *Lancet* 1984;2:196–198.
138. Young SN, Ghadirian AM. Folic acid and psychopathology. *Prog Neuropsychopharmacol Biol Psychiatry* 1989;13:841–863.
139. Bottiglieri T. Folate, vitamin B12, and neuropsychiatric disorders. *Nutr Rev* 1996;54:382–390.
140. Fava M, Borus JS, Alpert JE, et al. Folate, vitamin B12, and homocysteine in major depressive disorder. *Am J Psychiatry* 1997;154:426–428.
141. Godfrey PS, Toone BK, Carney MW, et al. Enhancement of recovery from psychiatric illness by methylfolate. *Lancet* 1990;336:392–395.
142. Procter A. Enhancement of recovery from psychiatric illness by methylfolate. *Br J Psychiatry* 1991;159: 271–272.

143. Lee S, Chow CC, Shek CC, et al. Folate concentration in Chinese psychiatric outpatients on long-term lithium treatment. *J Affect Disord* 1992;24:265–270.
144. Edeh J, Toone BK. Antiepileptic therapy, folate deficiency, and psychiatric morbidity: a general practice survey. *Epilepsia* 1985;26:434–440.
145. Froscher W, Maier V, Laage M, et al. Folate deficiency, anticonvulsant drugs, and psychiatric morbidity. *Clin Neuropharmacol* 1995;18:165–182.
146. Kromhout D, Bosschieter EB, Coulander CD. Potassium, calcium, alcohol intake and blood pressure: the Zutphen study. *Am J Clin Nutr* 1985;41:1299–1304.
147. Kromhout D. Fish consumption and sudden cardiac death. *JAMA* 1998;279:65–66.
148. Beilin LJ. Dietary fats, fish, and blood pressure. *Ann N Y Acad Sci* 1993;683:35–45.
149. Simopoulos AP. Omega-3 fatty acids in health and disease and in growth and development. *Am J Clin Nutr* 1991;54:438–463.
150. Albert CM, Hennekens CH, O'Donnell CJ, et al. Fish consumption and risk of sudden cardiac death. *JAMA* 1998;279:23–28.
151. Holman RT. The slow discovery of the importance of omega 3 essential fatty acids in human health. *J Nutr* 1998;128:427–433.
152. Holman RT, Johnson SB, Ogburn PL. Deficiency of essential fatty acids and membrane fluidity during pregnancy and lactation. *Proc Natl Acad Sci U S A* 1991;88:4835–4839.
153. Koletzko B, Rodriguez-Palmero M. Polyunsaturated fatty acids in human milk and their role in early infant development. *J Mammary Gland Biol Neoplasia* 1999; 4:269–284.
154. Delion S, Chalon S, Guilloteau D, et al. Alpha-linolenic acid dietary deficiency alters age-related changes of dopaminergic and serotoninergic neurotransmission in the rat frontal cortex. *J Neurochem* 1996;66:1582–1591.
155. Zimmer L, Delion-Vancassel S, Durand G, et al. Modification of dopamine neurotransmission in the nucleus accumbens of rats deficient in n-3 polyunsaturated fatty acids. *J Lipid Res* 2000;41:32–40.
156. Horrocks LA, Yeo YK. Health benefits of docosahexaenoic acid. *Pharmacol Res* 1999;40:211–225.
157. Carrie I, Clement M, De Javel D, et al. Learning deficits in first generation OF1 mice deficient in (n-3) polyunsaturated fatty acids do not result from visual alteration. *Neurosci Lett* 1999;266:69–72.
158. Stordy BJ. Dark adaptation, motor skills, docosahexaenoic acid, and dyslexia. *Am J Clin Nutr* 2000; 71:323–326.
159. Stevens LJ, Zentall SS, Deck JL, et al. Essential fatty acid metabolism in boys with attention-deficit hyperactivity disorder. *Am J Clin Nutr* 1995;62:761–768.
160. Stevens LJ, Zentall SS, Abate ML, et al. Omega-3 fatty acids in boys with behavior, learning, and health problems. *Physiol Behav* 1996;59:915–920.
161. Bekaroglu M, Aslan Y, Gedik Y, et al. Relationships between serum free fatty acids and zinc, and attention deficit hyperactivity disorder: a research note. *J Child Psychol Psychiatry* 1996;37:225–227.
162. Burgess JR, Stevens L, Zhang W, et al. Long-chain polyunsaturated fatty acids in children with attention-deficit hyperactivity disorder. *Am J Clin Nutr* 2000;71: 327–330.
163. Okada T, Amamoto T, Tomonaga M, et al. The chronic administration of docosahexaenoic acid reduces the spatial cognitive deficit following transient forebrain ischemia in rats. *Neuroscience* 1996;71:17–25.
164. Terano T, Fujishiro S, Ban T, et al. Docosahexaenoic acid supplementation improves the moderately severe dementia from thrombotic cerebrovascular diseases. *Lipids* 1999;34:345–346.
165. Kyle DJ, Schaefer E, Patton G, et al. Low serum docosahexaenoic acid is a significant risk factor for Alzheimer's dementia. *Lipids* 1999;34:245.
166. Corrigan FM, Horrobin DF, Skinner ER, et al. Abnormal content of n-6 and n-3 long-chain unsaturated fatty acids in the phosphoglycerides and cholesterol esters of parahippocampal cortex from Alzheimer's disease patients and its relationship to acetyl CoA content. *Int J Biochem Cell Biol* 1998;30:197–207.
167. Reitz RC. Dietary fatty acids and alcohol: effects on cellular membranes. *Alcohol Alcohol* 1993;28:59–71.
168. Hibbeln JR, Linnoila M, Umhau JC, et al. Essential fatty acids predict metabolites of serotonin and dopamine in cerebrospinal fluid among healthy control subjects, and early- and late-onset alcoholics. *Biol Psychiatry* 1998;44:235–242.
169. Roberts LJ 2nd, Montine TJ, Markesbery WR, et al. Formation of isoprostane-like compounds (neuroprostanes) in vivo from docosahexaenoic acid. *J Biol Chem* 1998;273:13605–13612.
170. Nourooz-Zadeh J, Liu EH, Yhlen B, et al. F4-isoprostanes as specific marker of docosahexaenoic acid peroxidation in Alzheimer's disease. *J Neurochem* 1999;72:734–740.
171. Horrobin DF. Schizophrenia as a membrane lipid disorder which is expressed throughout the body. *Prostaglandins Leukot Essent Fatty Acids* 1996;55: 3–7.
172. Warner R, Laugharne J, Peet M, et al. Retinal function as a marker for cell membrane omega-3 fatty acid depletion in schizophrenia: a pilot study. *Biol Psychiatry* 1999;45:1138–1142.
173. Richardson AJ, Easton T, Gruzelier JH, et al. Laterality changes accompanying symptom remission in schizophrenia following treatment with eicosapentaenoic acid. *Int J Psychophysiol* 1999;34:333–339.
174. Maes M, Smith R, Christophe A, et al. Fatty acid composition in major depression: decreased omega 3 fractions in cholesteryl esters and increased C20: 4 omega 6/C20:5 omega 3 ratio in cholesteryl esters and phospholipids. *J Affect Disord* 1996;38:35–46.
175. Adams PB, Lawson S, Sanigorski A, et al. Arachidonic acid to eicosapentaenoic acid ratio in blood correlates positively with clinical symptoms of depression. *Lipids* 1996;31:157–161.
176. Peet M, Murphy B, Shay J, et al. Depletion of omega 3 fatty acid levels in red blood cell membranes of depressive patients. *Biol Psychiatry* 1998;43:315–319.
177. Maes M, Christophe A, Delanghe J, et al. Lowered omega 3 polyunsaturated fatty acids in serum phospholipids and cholesteryl esters of depressed patients. *Psychiatry Res* 1999;85:275–291.
178. Stoll AL Severus WE, Freeman MP, et al. Omega 3 fatty acids in bipolar disorder: a preliminary double-blind, placebo-controlled trial. *Arch Gen Psychiatry* 1999;56:407–412.
179. Hibbeln JR, Umhau JC, Linnoila M, et al. A replica-

tion study of violent and nonviolent subjects: cerebrospinal fluid metabolites of serotonin and dopamine are predicted by plasma essential fatty acids. *Biol Psychiatry* 1998;44:243–249.
180. Hamazaki T, Sawazaki S, Itomura M, et al. The effect of docosahexaenoic acid on aggression in young adults. A placebo-controlled double-blind study. *J Clin Psychiatry* 1996;97:1129–1133.
181. Tanskanen A, Vartiainen E, Tuomilehto J, et al. High serum cholesterol and risk of suicide. *Am J Psychiatry* 2000;157:648–650.
182. Blain H, Jouzeau JY, Blain A, et al. Non-steroidal anti-inflammatory drugs with selectivity for cyclooxygenase-2 in Alzheimer's disease. Rationale and perspectives. *Presse Med* 2000;29:267–273.
183. McGeer PL, Harada N, Kimura H, et al. Prevalence of dementia amongst elderly Japanese with leprosy: apparent effect of chronic drug therapy. *Dementia* 1992; 3:146–149.
184. McGeer P, McGeer EG. The inflammatory response system of brain: implications for therapy of Alzheimer and other neurodegenerative diseases. *Brain Res Rev* 1995;21:195–218.
185. Beard CM, Waring SC, O'Brien PC, et al. Nonsteroidal anti-inflammatory drug use and Alzheimer's disease: a case-control study in Rochester, Minnesota, 1980 through 1984. *Mayo Clin Proc* 1998;73:951–955.
186. Anthony JC, Breitner JC, Zandi PP, et al. Reduced prevalence of AD in users of NSAIDs and H2 receptor antagonists: the Cache County study. *Neurology* 2000;54:2066–2071.
187. Andersen K, Launer LJ, Ott A, et al. Do Nonsteroidal anti-inflammatory drugs decrease the risk for Alzheimer's disease? *Neurology* 1995;45:8:1441–1445.
188. Rich JB, Rasmusson DX, Folstein MF, et al. Nonsteroidal anti-inflammatory drugs in Alzheimer's disease. *Neurology* 1995;45:51–55.
189. Brooks P, Day RO. Nonsteroidal antiinflammatory drugs—differences and similarities. *N Engl J Med* 1991;324:1716–1725.
190. Vane JR, Botting RM. Mechanism of action of antiinflammatory drugs. *Int J Tissue React* 1998;20:3–15.
191. Everts B, Wahrborg P, Hedner T. COX-2–specific inhibitors—the emergence of a new class of analgesic and anti-inflammatory drugs. *Clin Rheumatol* 2000; 19:331–343.
192. Tocco G, Freire-Moar J, Schreiber SS, et al. Maturational regulation and regional induction of cyclooxygenase-2 in rat brain: implications for Alzheimer's disease. *Exp Neurol* 1997;144:339–349.
193. Nogawa S, Forster C, Zhang F, et al. Interaction between inducible nitric oxide synthase and cyclooxygenase-2 after cerebral ischemia. *Proc Natl Acad Sci U S A* 1998;95:10966–10971.
194. Dash PK, Mach SA, Moore AN. Regional expression and role of cyclooxygenase-2 following experimental traumatic brain injury. *J Neurotrauma* 2000;17:69–81.
195. Scali C, Prosperi C, Vannucchi MG, et al. Brain inflammatory reaction in an animal model of neuronal degeneration and its modulation by an anti-inflammatory drug: implication in Alzheimer's disease. *Eur J Neurosci* 2000;12:1900–1912.
196. Koistinaho J, Chan PH. Spreading depression-induced cyclooxygenase-2 expression in the cortex. *Neurochem Res* 2000;25:645–651.
197. Sheehan KM, Sheahan K, O'Donoghue DP, et al. The relationship between cyclooxygenase-2 expression and colorectal cancer. *JAMA* 1999;282:1254–1257.
198. Browning CH. Nonsteroidal anti-inflammatory drugs and severe psychiatric side effects. *Int J Psychiatry Med* 1996;26:25–34.
199. Karplus TMSKG. Nonsteroidal anti-inflammatory drugs and cognitive function: do they have a beneficial or deleterious effect? *Drug Saf* 1998;19:427–433.
200. Davies NM, McLachlan AJ, Day RO, et al. Clinical pharmacokinetics and pharmacodynamics of celecoxib: a selective cyclo-oxygenase-2 inhibitor. *Clin Pharmacokinet* 2000;38:225–242.
201. Wesnes KA, Faleni RA, Hefting NR. The cognitive, subjective, and physical effects of a *Ginkgo biloba/Panax ginseng* combination in healthy volunteers with neurasthenic complaints. *Psychopharmacol Bull* 1997;33:677–683.
202. Smith PF, Maclennan K, Darlington CL. The neuroprotective properties of the *Ginkgo biloba* leaf: a review of the possible relationship to platelet-activating factor (PAF). *J Ethnopharmacol* 1996;50:131–139.
203. Semlitsch HV, Anderer P, Saletu B, et al. Cognitive psychophysiology in nootropic drug research: effects of *Ginkgo biloba* on event-related potentials (P300) in age-associated memory impairment. *Pharmacopsychiatry* 1995;28:134–142.
204. Kleijnen J, Knipschild P. *Ginkgo biloba* for cerebral insufficiency. *Br J Clin Pharmacol* 1992;34:352–358.
205. Le Bars PL, Katz MM, Berman N, et al. A placebo-controlled, double-blind, randomized trial of an extract of *Ginkgo biloba* for dementia. North American EGb Study Group. *JAMA* 1997;278:1327–1332.
206. Koc RK, Akdemir H, Kurtsoy A, et al. Lipid peroxidation in experimental spinal cord injury. Comparison of treatment with *Ginkgo biloba*, TRH and methylprednisolone. *Res Exp Med (Berl)* 1995;195:117–123.
207. Brailowsky S, Montiel T. Motor function in young and aged hemiplegic rats: effects of a *Ginkgo biloba* extract. *Neurobiol Aging* 1997;18:219–227.
208. Oyama Y, Chikahisa L, Ueha T, et al. *Ginkgo biloba* extract protects brain neurons against oxidative stress induced by hydrogen peroxide. *Brain Res* 1996;712: 349–352.
209. Noda Y, Anzai K, Mori A, et al. Hydroxyl and superoxide anion radical scavenging activities of natural source antioxidants using the computerized JES-FR30 ESR spectrometer system. *Biochem Mol Biol Int* 1997;42:35–44.
210. Sastre J, Millan A, Garcia A, et al. A *Ginkgo biloba* extract (EGb 761) prevents mitochondrial aging by protecting against oxidative stress. *Free Radic Biol Med* 1998;24:298–304.
211. White HL, Scates PW, Cooper BR. Extracts of *Ginkgo biloba* leaves inhibit monoamine oxidase. *Life Sci* 1996;58:1315–1321.
212. Amri H, Ogwuegbu SO, Boujrad N, et al. In vivo regulation of peripheral-type benzodiazepine receptor and glucocorticoid synthesis by *Ginkgo biloba* extract EGb 761 and isolated ginkgolides. *Endocrinology* 1996; 137:5707–5718.

26

The Problem of Drug Treatment in Neuropsychiatry

SUMMARY

If there is a conventional theory of psychopharmacology, it is based on two assumptions: on a molecular level, that drugs affect synaptic neurotransmission (SNT) and on a clinical level, that they exercise categorical effects on discretely defined psychiatric disorders. Drug treatment in neuropsychiatry, however, only makes sense within an expanded theory of psychopharmacology. An expanded theory must address the broad spectrum of psychotropic drug effects and the diversity of conditions that respond to drug treatment. It must also address influences that drugs can have, not just on overt symptoms, but also on adaptive functions such as cognition and brain plasticity.

SNT is only one form of interneuronal communication. It is complemented by a phylogenetically older form of neuronal communication: nonsynaptic diffusion neurotransmission (NDNT). The latter is slower, more energy efficient, and more likely to mediate mass-sustained actions such as mood, appetite, arousal, and pain. Diffusion neurotransmission is also a mediator of neuromodulation and glial communication and participates in several of the biological mechanisms of neuronal plasticity. The governing neurotransmitters dopamine (DA), norepinephrine (NE), and serotonin (5-HT) are both synaptic and nonsynaptic to varying degrees. The actions of the psychotropic drugs are equally well understood in terms of their actions on synaptic and nonsynaptic connectivity.

The second premise of the conventional theory is kraepelinian diagnosis: that drugs exert categorical effects on specific psychiatric disorders. It, too, is sound but insufficient and needs to be amplified by addressing the dimensional effects of drugs on underlying psychophysical functions. Drugs change the behavior of complex functional systems that mediate arousal, affective regulation, attention, and sensory integration. It is only by doing so that they are able to change the adaptive capacity of the organism.

The kraepelinian contribution to the theory of psychopharmacology should be complemented by contributions from the meyerian school, which stresses adaptation, and the freudian school, which stresses individual psychology and the dynamic interactions of complex functional systems. We may be taking liberties with Meyer and Freud, but their contributions are pertinent to an expanded theory of psychopharmacology.

The behavior of complex systems, such as the central nervous system (CNS), is not always given to classical analysis. So-called "fuzzy logic" is an alternative way to understand how complex systems operate. According to this view, complex systems function as "centroid averagers," integrating and summating dimensional inputs from myriad sources. By this line of reasoning, psychotropic drugs are dimensional inputs that participate in the organism's computation of a new and perhaps more adaptive "centroid average."

PSYCHOPARMACOLOGY IN NEUROPSYCHIATRY

Neuropsychiatry is a special branch of psychiatry. Like all of psychiatry, it is concerned with behavioral and emotional problems; in patients with neuropsychiatric disorders, these are superimposed on and are strongly influenced by an underlying encephalopathic condition. Most patients with neuropsychiatric disorders also have some degree of cognitive impairment that either causes or contributes to their unique patterns of behavioral and emotional reactivity. Although this monograph has dealt with only two groups of patients with neuropsychiatric disorders, one is necessarily impressed by the diversity of their problems and the complexity of the mechanisms that give rise to them. In their behavioral and emotional problems and their response to treatment, they resemble the "conventional" patients with neuropsychiatric disorders to some degree. There are also important differences, and for this reason, conventional psychiatric approaches, especially drug treatment, must be modified accordingly.

- *The diversity of their problems*. The immense range of behavioral and emotional problems in patients with neuropsychiatric disorders can only sometimes be expressed in conventional psychiatric terms. Most of the time, diagnosis requires a special approach.
- *The complexity of the mechanisms that give rise to them*. Diagnosis, prognosis, and drug treatment in patients with neuropsychiatric disorders require an understanding of the encephalopathic mechanisms that have brought the patient to his or her present state and may still be active.
- *Their cognitive impairments*. For this reason, the neurocognitive effects of drug treatment and the potential effects of drugs on brain plasticity have special importance.

I have tried to address these three points as they bear on the practice of psychopharmacology. Perhaps, now, I can suggest how they bear on the theory of psychopharmacology.

IS THERE A THEORY OF PSYCHOPHARMACOLOGY?

Is there a theory of psychopharmacology? It is arguable. One can aver that psychopharmacology is nothing more than an empirical exercise. It is an impressive technology, but one that has been engaged for 50 years with only a shallow conception of how and why it works. A skeptic can point to the serendipitous origins of the first psychotherapeutic drugs. The pioneering psychopharmacologists simply gave every drug that came along to every patient they had and waited to see what happened. Some say that psychiatrists today do the same thing.

Psychiatrists in general and psychopharmacologists in particular are always vulnerable to criticisms of this sort. Rather than remark the signal accomplishments of the field (50 years ago, the most hospital beds in this country were occupied by psychiatric inpatients), they dwell on our foibles and idiosyncrasies. Sometimes, we are taken to task for being atheoretical and unscientific. Sometimes, we are taken to task because our theories are odd, unduly complex, or simply outlandish.

In Chapter 19, I presented an oversimplified version of the theory of depression and antidepression. To simplify it even further, it was this: one disorder—one neurotransmitter—one drug. Stated thus, the theory is absurd. The device was entirely rhetorical, however. It was to make a point that the broad spectrum of antidepressant activity was more concordant with the known functions of the NE and 5-HT systems than with even an expanded view of the mood disorders. The point was also made that antidepressant treatment for patients with neuropsychiatric disorders was better understood in terms of the effects on functional systems rather than the action against depression.

There is a theory of psychopharmacology that is built on two foundations. One is SNT. The other is the kraepelinian view that psychiatric disorders are discrete conditions. Based on these two working assumptions, psychiatrists propose that psychoactive drugs work because they alter the behavior of neurotransmitters at synaptic junctions, thus correcting aberrations in neuronal activity. In so doing, drugs exercise a categorical effect on the psychiatric disorder, which is thus cured or at least controlled.

Both premises, SNT and kraepelinian diagnosis, are correct but only partially. The former speaks to only one aspect of brain connectivity and is ill-equipped to address important issues, such as neuromodulation, mass action, brain plasticity, and even the activity of the two most important governing neurotransmitters NE and 5-HT. The latter speaks to a taxonomic ideal that is only occasionally met with in conventional psychiatry and hardly ever in neuropsychiatry. The idea that drug effects are categorical suffuses the theory of psychopharmacology. Drugs act at synapses, which are on-off switches, such as transistors. Action potentials are generated or not. A psychiatric disorder is present or not. A treatment is effective if it is evidence based; if not, it is "clinical experience," a lesser order of being.

Categorical thinking is a valid approach to some problems, but it is not universally applicable. The behavior of highly complex systems such as the CNS does not always obey *a priori* categories. Categories are useful conventions. They facilitate communication among professionals in the field and render what we do understandable to patients. They may or may not capture what is really happening to patients when we give them a drug. It is equally plausible that psychotropic drug effects are dimensional in nature—that what they do is to enhance functions rather than cure diseases.

HARD NEUROSCIENCE, FUZZY LOGIC

Information technology is classically binary: on or off, 0 or 1. So is the synapse; an action potential is generated or it is not. Ever since Aristotle, a dominant theme in Western thinking has been the law of the excluded middle: that everything is, in principle at least, either A or not A.

Fuzzy logic is different. Fuzzy logicians grapple, in mathematical terms, with the behavior of complex systems in which, in reality, things may be a bit A and a bit not A. Fuzzy set theory allows something to be partly a member of one set and partly a member of another. It is not simply a theoretical exercise. Applications of fuzzy set theory allow the digital computer to run complex systems (such as climate-control systems in large buildings or mass transportation networks) with a high degree of precision.

The founder of fuzzy set theory, Lofti Zadeh, was preoccupied with applying mathematical principles to the study of biologic systems. His basic rule for dealing with complexity was to simplify. Not all available information needs to be used and an increased amount of uncertainty is accepted to create robust summary concepts. The rules of fuzzy logic are clearly applicable to the study of the nervous system, a system of inordinate complexity and in which the guiding principles of structure-function interactions are obscure, to say the least. In the CNS, the idea of organization by serial and hierarchical control modules has been abandoned in favor of the idea of functional assemblies or syncytia of cells, whose aggregate behavior may vary in nature and intensity in response to a host of internal and external constraints. Cells in one assembly are associated with cells in other assemblies; under some circumstances, they have a partial association with one behavioral action, and in other circumstances have different amounts of association with other behavioral actions (1). The boundaries of structures within the CNS are imprecise because they participate to varying degrees in many behavioral programs. CNS structures or cell assemblies are not well insulated one from another. They "leak" on "cross-talk."

Classical SNT has always found it problematic that an individual neuron can release multiple transmitters and contains receptors for many more, and for good reason. Crisp logic demands that a neuron be A or not A. In fact, the receptive properties of a neuron are partly A, partly B, partly C, and so on. The neuron responds to 5,000 to 25,000 synaptic connections, to an extracellular medium that is actively circulating and flush with neuroactive substances (NAS), and also to a glial matrix that is electrically and chemically active—the input from synapses, from the interstitium and from glial cells is partly A, partly B, partly C, and so on. Even the solitary neuron performs operations of inordinate complexity.

When a digital computer is programmed to operate by fuzzy logic, it uses an algorithm known as centroid averaging. The relative importance of a host of dimensional inputs is computed and translated into an intelligent action step. This process is iterated and reiterated by feedback from the environment until the desired result is attained. It is appropriate to suggest that the neuron, too, is a centroid averager, processing input from synapses and extrasynaptic receptors, from glia and the extracellular fluid; and that cell assemblies are centroid averagers, processing input from other cell assemblies with which they are associated in different ways. Complex functional systems compute dimensional inputs from multiple sources, and the organism itself is the final or ultimate centroid averager.

The diagnostic entities of kraepelinian psychiatry are categories by convention. In fact, they are centroid averages. They are the overt manifestation of a host of dimensional inputs. That is why their symptoms are so diverse and overlapping and why symptoms are mutable over time. All the psychiatric disorders have a well-defined center and fuzzy boundaries, i.e., pure types are readily diagnosable, but borderline conditions, with symptoms that are typical of different conditions, are very difficult to diagnose with precision.

The effects of a psychiatric drug, in the same vein, are categorical: it is effective or not, according to the conventions of evidence-based medicine. In reality, drugs are nothing more than dimensional inputs to a complex system. They are new and potent variables that are inserted into the organism's computation of a new, and perhaps more adaptive, centroid average.

The diagnoses and treatment approaches of conventional psychiatry are amenable to the categorical basis of the theory of psychopharmacology in the same way that principles of classical, newtonian physics are suitable to the understanding of the everyday world around us. Newtonian physics, however, is not universally applicable. At the extreme boundaries of the physical world, alternative physical principles are brought to bear. It is my belief that the extraordinary conditions with which we are concerned in neuropsychiatry defy the categorical basis of conventional psychiatry. If there is to be an effective theory of psychopharmacology, one that can embrace the expanding boundaries of the field, it will be necessary to think in terms, not of categories, but of the immense number of dimensional inputs that mediate the behavior of the organism.

We can do that in two places. First, we can examine the nature of neuronal communication and show how it must be amplified to incorporate non-SNT. Then, we examine the influence of kraepelinian diagnosis and propose that it has to be expanded to incorporate adaptationist and functionalist approaches.

NONSYNAPTIC DIFFUSION NEUROTRANSMISSION

The neuron theory was developed by Waldeyer and Cajal a century ago: that the neuron is a discrete cellular entity that communicates with other cells through a window, a "surface of separation," the synapse (2). The synaptic basis of neurotransmission has been the dominant conceptual model of information flow in the nervous system during most of the twentieth century (3,4).

At about the same time, however, Golgi had proposed a reticular or network theory of nerve cells as an anatomical and functional syncytium (5). The neuron theory, of course, was been proven correct and has dominated thinking in neuroscience ever since, but the neuronal and reticular theories, although once in competition, are not mutually exclusive. Neuronal communication also seems to occur by diffusion of electrochemical signals in the extracellular space. Neural operations of functional syncytia are an equally important feature of the organization of the CNS (5). It also is germane to the mechanism of psychotropic drug action.

Neuronal information flow is transsynaptic or junctional, but it is important to appreciate that it is not exclusively so. NDNT is an alternative form of interneuronal communication. It is relevant to several problems raised in this monograph: brain plasticity and the ways drugs may influence it, the actions of the governing neurotransmitters, especially NE and 5HT, the integration of complex functional systems, and the notion of an optimal monoamine environment.

The neuronal theory of Cajal addresses the structure of the brain. NDNT revisits the reticular doctrine of Golgi and addresses the function of the brain. Both views contribute to a holistic concept of the brain: neural information flowing along confluent pathways between relatively large, confluent territories, and not only at specific points between individual cells (6).

If SNT is wired, there is a wireless transmission of NAS, released from nonsynaptic sites to diffuse to nonsynaptic receptors on cells distant from the site of release. NDNT is interneuronal communication by diffusion of informational substances or NAS, which include the classical neurotransmitters as well as neuropeptides, amino acids, and free radical gases such as nitric oxide (NO) and carbon monoxide. NAS are released from nonsynaptic (or nonjunctional) sites into the extracellular space (7) and diffuse through the interstitial fluid to bind to extrasynaptic receptors on cells, which may be remote from the cells of origin. NAS can diffuse into the synaptic cleft to activate junctional receptors and can even diffuse through the cell membrane to activate cytoplasmic receptors (8).

In NDNT, receptor interactions with NAS do not require the preservation of impulse frequency coding offered by synaptic specialization; in other words, they do not necessarily generate an action potential in the target cell. They are, however, capable of modulating the membrane potential of the target neuron, its metabolism, or its structure (3). NDNT is also the basis of information flow between neurons and glial cells (9).

NDNT is a phylogenetically ancient form of neuronal communication (10), and its actions are preserved in the higher mammals, including humans. Its biologic function, relative to SNT, is still open to interpretation. There is reason to believe that it is the neurochemical basis of certain mass, sustained actions of the brain, such as sleep, vigilance, hunger, brain "tone" and mood, that it subserves the action of psychoactive drugs, and that it plays a role in mechanisms of brain plasticity, such as long-term potentiation (LTP), kindling, and diaschisis (7).

Extrasynaptic diffusion as a mechanism of neurotransmission was initially described by Bach-y-Rita in 1964. In 1968, investigators demonstrated that monoamine neurotransmitters diffused into the extracellular space and were capable of moving freely there (11,12). Fuxe also demonstrated that DA transmission could be maintained in the striatum despite a massive disappearance of DA nerve terminals, as long as DA was capable of diffusing through the extracellular space to reach supersensitive receptors (13)—a process that may be clinically relevant to the action of dopaminergic cell autografts. To describe this phenomenon, Fuxe et al. (5) coined the term volume transmission, a synonym for NDNT.

In 1967, Florey introduced the idea of modulator substances that originated in nerve cells, gland cells, neurosecretory cells, or glial cells and that reached effector cells by humoral pathways, (14). In contrast to electrical neurotransmitters, chemical modulators were capable of generating only local potentials to influence the excitability of target cells. The concept of neuromodulation was further developed by Barchas et al. (15), who defined neuroregulators to include neurotransmitters and neuromodulators, which behave in a hormonal-like manner.

The concept of parasynaptic information transmission in the brain was formulated by Schmitt et al. (10,16), who proposed that neuronal communication was mediated not only by the classical neurotransmitters but also by neuropeptides, neurohormones (such as vasopressin), factors (such as nerve growth factor), proteins, ion fluxes, and many other kinds of informational substances or NAS in the ambient extracellular fluid. Specificity of action could be attained not only through the synaptic circuitry but also by the equally specific binding of NAS to receptors, "arrayed not only at synaptic regions but over the entire neuronal surface" (10). Parasynaptic transmission, another term for NDNT, was said to possess a domain of versatility and plasticity lacking in hard-wired circuitry.

Evidence for Nonsynaptic Diffusion Neurotransmission

If nerve cells were incapable of responding to circulating substances that bind to receptors on their surface, they would be unique among cells in the body. The development of synaptic specialization in nervous tissue is an evolutionary advance that permits rapid and highly specific communication, but the principle of conservation favors the retention of less specialized forms of communication as well. If one thinks of synaptic function as "the light play of high notes in an organ recitation," then diffusion neurotransmission might represent "the sustained structure of base notes" (17–19). The model of SNT is the digital computer, with synapses for transistors. The model for NDNT is an analog system that allows signals to be broadcast and picked up by any properly equipped receiver, that is, cells equipped with the proper receptors (20).

The intuitive appeal of NDNT resides in its accommodation of an extraordinary number of NAS and receptor subtypes, the cohabitation of different neurotransmitters and different receptors in a given neuron and the metabolic complexity of the cellular interstitium. The evidence for NDNT is summarized in this section:

- NDNT is demonstrated in lower organisms and the peripheral nervous system. Ontogenetically, neurotransmitters were synthesized within cells before the appearance of neurons, and NDNT is widely represented among the invertebrates. The diffusion of transmitters over distances to bind to nonjunctional receptors has been documented in several invertebrate and submammalian species (10). It also is characteristic of neurotransmission in the vertebrate peripheral nervous system (3).
- NDNT occurs in nonneuronal structures of the CNS. Receptors for classical neurotransmitters and other NAS have been demonstrated on the cerebral vasculature, glial and ependymal cells, and choroid plexus. These receptors are not junctional (i.e., synaptic), but they are physiologically active. They are activated, one presumes, by NAS that diffuse through the extracellular space (3).
- The volume of the extracellular space is sufficient to support widespread diffusion. The relative obscurity of NDNT may be the result of artifacts in research methodology. Experimental techniques such as homogenization of brain tissue with selective centrifugation are not likely to lend an appreciation of the importance of the extracellular space. An electron micrograph of the brain demonstrates beautiful cross sections of structures interlocked like pieces of a jigsaw puzzle (21). A tight, interlocking cross section, however, conveys the erroneous impression that substances cannot move freely in the tight spaces between the cellular membranes (22). In fact, an electron micrograph is not necessarily a true representation of the brain *in vivo*. Recent studies confirm that no less than 20% of the brain is extracellular space (22), ample indeed for the dynamic interplay of many kinds of informational substances to diffuse from release points to receptors on or within neurons (10). It has been known since the late 1960s that transmitters could readily move in the extracellular space (21), and microdialysis studies indicate that virtually all the known neurotransmitters are found in the extracellular fluid (23).
- The problem of neurotransmitter/receptor mismatch. If neurochemical communication between

neurons were confined to synaptic junctions, a logical expectation would be that for each neurotransmitter/receptor system, the distribution of receptors, mapped by autoradiography, should closely resemble the locations of transmitter release, as inferred by immunohistochemistry of nerve terminal distributions. In the recent literature, many such mapping studies have appeared (for reviews, see refs. 3 and 24). In fact, close correspondence between receptors and transmitters are the exception rather than the rule. For example, the neuroactive peptides (e.g., opiates, neurotensin, somatostatin, thyrotropin-releasing hormone) and their receptors are not anatomically related and, instead, seem to be independently distributed in the brain.

The same pattern is true for other neurotransmitters. Indeed, it is likely that every neurotransmitter is given to at least some degree of receptor mismatch. For example, acetylcholine (ACh), a classical neurotransmitter and neuromodulator, is active at muscarinic and nicotinic receptors in the CNS. However, markers for nicotinic receptors in the brain are variably associated with sites of cholinergic terminals. Many nuclei in the brainstem have dense concentrations of muscarinic receptors but no documented cholinergic terminals. In the forebrain, there are areas that are selectively dense with terminals but with no corresponding receptor enrichment (3).

In 1978, Beaudet and Descarries presented electron microscopic evidence that neuronal varicosities containing NE and 5-HT could be either synaptic or nonsynaptic. They proposed that nonjunctional varicosities were equally capable of releasing the biogenic amines. Thus released into the extracellular space, the neurotransmitters acted not only on adjacent surfaces but also more diffusely on distant receptor elements. Nonjunctional release was hypothesized to exert action at a distance in the form of desynchronized and sustained influences on vast neuronal ensembles (25).

Although these findings sparked a major controversy at the time, numerous cytochemical, radioautographic, and immunocytochemical studies have since disclosed similar features on different monoamine innervations in other parts of the rat, cat, and monkey brain; the studies have been summarized (25). Electron microscopic studies have confirmed that NE, 5-HT, and even DA are, in some regions, "contained in varicosities that have no synaptic specialization associated with them" (26). Other NAS, such as substance P, histamine, somatostatin, neuropeptide Y, and vasoactive intestinal peptide are also found in neuronal vesicles that have no synaptic specialization (3).

Similarly, it has also been demonstrated that receptors are not always synaptically localized (27). For example, in some preparations, opiate receptors are found in cell membranes that are not synaptic (28,29). Substance P receptors are expressed on the surface of certain neurons, but only seldom in opposition to substance P release sites, suggesting that they "can be targeted by substance P that diffuses a considerable distance from its site of release" (30). As a rule, receptors that are located far from their presynaptic counterparts have affinities similar to those of receptors located closer by. The failure of remote receptors to demonstrate supersensitivity suggests that they, too, are reached by endogenous ligands (31).

The Problem of the Biogenic Amines

The biogenic amines have always represented a conceptual challenge to classical transmission, for reasons that are amplified below. They also demonstrate significant mismatches between neurotransmitters and receptors, although they differ in the degree to which their innervation is predominantly junctional or nonjunctional. DA innervation, for example, is predominantly junctional. Localization of D_2 receptors by tritiated spiperone seems to be restricted to areas of the striatum and prefrontal cortex where there is dopaminergic innervation. Conversely, even in the case of a comparatively targeted amine such as DA, when other ligands to the D_2 receptor are studied, receptor binding is discovered in areas where there are no known DA afferents. Areas with measurable D_1 receptors but no DA innervation are found in the hippocampus, thalamus, superior colliculus, and cerebellum (3).

The cortical NE system, in contrast, appears to be mostly nonjunctional. NE receptors are far more widely distributed than their nerve terminals, and the pattern of adrenergic receptor distributions do not resemble the patterns of adrenergic fiber distributions (3). The proportion of NE varicosities engaged in synaptic contact is 17% to 26% (compared with 56% to 93% for DA) (7,25).

The innervation of 5-HT also appears to be predominantly nonjunctional, 26% to 46% synaptic incidence in the brain (25) and as little as 4% in the dorsal spinal cord (7).

The differing synaptic incidences of DA, NE, and 5-HT may be related to the degree of spatial convergence of the corresponding pathways. There seems to be a principle of convergence involved, whereby highly divergent and dispersed afferent systems (NE and 5-HT) tend to establish mostly loose relationships at the ultrastructural level as well, whereas a more focused or restricted input (DA) is also the one showing a more punctate and perhaps a more stable, structurally differentiated synaptic connectivity (7).

A Gaseous Neurotransmitter, Nitric Oxide

If the classical neurotransmitters and other NAS have the potential for NDNT in some circumstances, diffusion is the natural state for NO. This "highly unorthodox messenger molecule" (32) produces its effects by diffusion, out of one cell and into another, without exocytosis or membrane binding (33).

The biologic activities of this "small, simple and highly toxic" molecule have been summarized by Bredt and Snyder (33). They developed a technique to measure the activity of the enzyme NO synthetase, which forms NO, determined that it is made in neurons and that inhibiting its manufacture could inhibit nerve stimulation.

NO fulfills all the classical criteria for a neurotransmitter. In fact, Snyder (34) has called NO "one of the main neurotransmitters in the brain." However, it is not stored in vesicles but is probably synthesized on demand, diffuses out of the neuron and then across the cell membrane of an adjacent neuron or a glial cell, where its action is to activate soluble guanylate cyclase (35).

The activation of NO is extremely fast and short-lived (decay by 50% within 4 seconds), and so its action differs from the sustained effects of NDNT by other NAS. Nevertheless, the discovery of NO, the first representative of a completely new concept of neurotransmission affirms an old concept that neuronal communication does indeed occur by extrasynaptic diffusion.

Diffusion vs. Synaptic Neurotransmission

The weight of the evidence, therefore, is in support of (at least) two kinds of information flow in the CNS. SNT and NDNT coexist as vehicles for neuronal communication. They exhibit profound differences but also a high degree of complementarity:

- The characteristics of SNT are necessary only for cellular responses that require short latencies, brief duration of action, and tight stimulus-response coupling. NDNT is a form of transmitter-receptor interaction not requiring preservation of frequency coding offered by synaptic specialization (3).
- In SNT, neurons summate excitatory and inhibitory inputs and transmit information in all-or-nothing impulses along axons whose terminals release chemical substances. In NDNT, neurons and glial cells receive information from NAS and encode it as a change in charge, structure, or metabolism. In SNT, digital information is coded; in NDNT, analog information is coded.
- The activation of neurons by SNT is fast, concisely targeted to individual cells, and quickly reversed. In contrast, NDNT is associated with activation of groups of neurons and glial cells. It is slower and more sustained. (The action of NO is so fast that it is almost ephemeral; it is not only a novel form of neurotransmission but also a novel form of diffusion neurotransmission.)
- NDNT is probably more energy efficient than SNT. Analog systems are, as a rule, more energy efficient than digital systems. NDNT is likely to consume smaller quantities of neurotransmitter over time. Whereas the synapse has a full complement of degradation enzymes and reuptake mechanisms, the nonjunctional receptor sites possess few, if any, of these inactivating devices (7). As described below, NDNT also confers spatial efficiency to the organization of the CNS.
- In SNT, the lines of transmission are discrete tracts, capable of transmitting impulses over long distances. In NDNT, transmission is less circumscribed. The propagation of information usually occurs locally, via passive diffusion, to subsume local cellular elements into functional syncytia (5), although NDNT may also occur over long distances, along preferential pathways (21,36).

NDNT is a primitive form of neuronal communication that is conserved from the invertebrate nervous system. It is an analog complement to synaptic information flow and confers a degree of subtlety that is lacking in the point-to-point transistor model of transsynaptic transmission. If NDNT is nothing more than a synonym for neuromodulation, then it is only an adjunct to SNT, and its obscurity is well deserved. However, careful consideration of the evidence at hand should incline the reader to accept NDNT as the general case and neuromodulation as a particular case. The theory of NDNT goes well beyond the concept of neuromodulation.

For example, it leads to a reexamination of the roles of governing neurotransmitters such as NE, 5-HT, DA, ACh, and the opiate peptides. Their roles in neuronal plasticity and in the generation and maintenance of mass-sustained actions (8) such as mood and arousal are open to new understanding. If SNT provides the vectors of neuronal communication, then NDNT provides the matrix. The image of neurons and synapses embedded in a matrix of inert substance is untenable. It is through NDNT that the extracellular space and the glial cells participate in the ebb and flow of information.

Neuromodulation

The concept of neuromodulation represented an early modification of synaptic theory to accommodate some of the early evidence of NDNT (37). It was driven by the discovery of NAS that did not have synaptic specialization and did not meet criteria for inclusion among the classical neurotransmitters but that seemed to alter the responsiveness of neurons (15). In contrast to neurotransmitters, compounds that convey information between nerve cells, neuromodulators serve to amplify or dampen neuronal activity. The former have a transsynaptic action, whereas the latter have a hormone-like or paracrine action (15).

Neuromodulation has always been an attractive idea, not only because it embraces a series of observations that are incompatible with simple point-to-point synaptic information flow, but also because it lends a degree of intricacy to the process of neuronal communication that is commensurate with the functions it serves. Neuromodulation is an essential element of neuronal information flow: "virtually every neuronal pathway is modulated and virtually every endogenous neuroactive agent has been shown, in one preparation or another, to be capable of modifying synaptic transmission, conduction of nerve impulses and cellular excitability" (38).

From the very beginning, when Florey (37) introduced the concept of neuromodulation, it was believed that modulator substances could be released at specialized or unspecialized regions of cells, or even by glial cells, which do not, obviously, establish synaptic connections (39). Neuromodulators may be released by another nerve terminal (interneuronal modulation); they may be released from the postsynaptic side (transsynaptic modulation), the presynaptic terminal itself (autoinhibition), or astrocytes (glial modulation) (40,41). The common morphologic feature of all these modulating mechanisms is the lack of close apposition characteristic of classical neurotransmitters (40).

The biogenic amines, NE, 5-HT, and even DA have been assigned roles as both neurotransmitters and neuromodulators (42,43) as have ACh, NO, and the opiate peptides. The profile of a particular NAS is probably defined by its degree of synaptic specialization relative to its action on receptors via diffusion through the extracellular space.

It is likely that neuromodulation and neurotransmission, rather than functional opposites, are in fact, poles on a continuum of neurotransmitter action; NE acting as a modulator, for example, should not be regarded as belonging to a separate category (44) from NE acting as a neurotransmitter. In each case, the chemical is released from one cell to interact with a receptor molecule on another cell; the result is greater or lesser alteration in permeability, conductance or resistance, and voltage across the membrane (45).

Monoaminergic Neurotransmission

The amine systems, with their unique cellular morphology (highly divergent axonal arborizations) and their unique physiologic actions, require considerable conceptual expansion of the concept of how neuronal communication comprises neurotransmission and neuromodulation, SNT and NDNT. The DA systems, for example, are tight clusters with specific targets and a relatively high degree of synaptic specialization. In contrast, the NE system spreads an axonal net widely throughout the cortex, with diffuse targeting and an extremely low incidence of synaptic specialization. The NE system is far from nonspecific in its pattern of innervations. It achieves a high degree of anatomic specificity, although not through specialized synaptic contacts but rather by virtue of target cell specificity (46). As NE diffuses through the interstitial fluid, its effects are felt by the mass activation of target cell receptors.

The arithmetic is telling. It is calculated that only approximately one in 10,000 nerve terminals in the cortex contains NE (47), but no fewer that 12% of cortical synaptosomes are immunoreactive to the β-adrenergic receptor (48). This percentage is curiously high in light of the very sparse adrenergic innervation that the cortex receives.

The source of NE is in the locus ceruleus (LC), a small pontine nucleus with 13,000 neurons/hemisphere in humans (49). The LC spreads hundreds of millions of axons and terminal branches throughout every layer and region of the cortex. The LC innervates the cerebral cortex in a continuous sheet of fibers overlying the white matter. NE-containing varicosities on these fibers, are, as described above, primarily nonsynaptic. Thus, the LC must function primarily by NDNT mechanisms. Even the afferents to the LC are largely nonsynaptic; it apparently only has two sources of direct neural inputs, yet it has a high density of numerous kinds of receptors (3).

The LC also exemplifies the comparative efficiency of NDNT. It is capable of activating over a long period of time and at a relatively low energy cost. Because NE varicosities are mainly nonjunctional, released transmitter must necessarily take time to diffuse through the extracellular fluid to extrasynaptic receptors. Activity induced in the distant dendritic tree takes considerable time to reach the soma, where the influence is sustained over time. In the absence of a synapse, inactivation of NE is comparatively slow.

NDNT also confers a degree of spatial efficiency in the organization of the cortex. If the LC, containing few cells, were to innervate every individual neuron of the cortex by synaptic transmission, the number of fibers required would be much greater than actually exist and would create a severe "packing" problem (7). As Mitchison (50) suggested, the cortex seems to be organized to minimize "wiring" (i.e., axons and dendrites) and to maximize space available for cell bodies.

The functions of the LC typify the kind of mass-sustained activity that characterizes NDNT. It is implicated in numerous functions, such as arousal, attention, sensory perception, memory, and mood. In the most general terms, it is an agent of what may be termed cortical "tone," the overall orientation of behavior or mode of sensorimotor activities to favor either automatic or vegetative behavioral programs or phasic adaptive responses to salient environmental stimuli (49).

The clinical concerns of psychiatry are largely oriented toward functions that may be described as mass-sustained actions. Mood, arousal, and "brain tone" are mediated by NAS such as NE and 5-HT that act largely by diffusion and influence the tone of large syncytia or functional assemblies of neurons. Disorders of mood, for example, may be conceptualized in terms of reduced activation of NE and 5-HT in the cellular interstitium, and the treatment of mood disorders may be a function of enhancing the activation of interstitial NAS such as NE and 5-HT. The slow onset of the psychotropic drug effect in depression is entirely consistent with this model.

NONSYNAPTIC DIFFUSION NEUROTRANSMISSION AND MECHANISMS OF NEURONAL PLASTICITY

Four processes, LTP, long-term depression (LTD), diaschisis, and kindling, are regarded as candidate substrates for at least some aspects of brain plasticity and memory formation in normal development and neuropsychopathology (51). Although the mechanisms responsible for the development and persistence of LTP, LTD, diaschisis, and kindling are unknown, consideration is usually given to changes in synaptic strength, neosynaptogenesis, and use-dependent sprouting. The diffusion of NAS such as NO and NE and of neuronotropic compounds such as nerve growth factor probably play a role in the mechanisms of plasticity.

Although the induction of LTP requires a postsynaptic event (i.e., activation of the *N*-methyl-D-aspartate receptor), the maintenance of LTP requires a change in presynaptic behavior. Siegelbaum and Kandel (52), among others, consider that "some message must be sent from the postsynaptic to the presynaptic neurons." They suggest that a retrograde plasticity factor is released from the postsynaptic dendritic spines, which then diffuses to the presynaptic neuron to activate second messengers, which in turn enhance transmitter release and thereby maintain LTP. This retrograde factor can recruit other parallel synaptic fibers in addition to those that synapse on the active postsynaptic cell. The diffusion of a retrograde presynaptic factor outside the synaptic cleft implies extrasynaptic transmission via the extracellular fluid.

LTD is a mechanism of synaptic plasticity that has been demonstrated in neurons of the cerebellum. The opposite of LTP, it represents a lowering of synaptic efficiency or a depression in synaptic transmission after low-frequency repetitive stimulation (53). LTD appears to be mediated by a reduction in sensitivity of postsynaptic glutamate receptors and lasts for hours or days (53). Just as NO, a diffusable molecule, diffuses antidromically to cause LTP expression (54,55), the expression of LTD also appears to be mediated by retrograde diffusion of a messenger substance, perhaps NO (56,57).

Traumatic brain injuries and strokes are known to cause dysfunction in brain areas remote from the primary insult. The resulting impaired regional blood flow and cerebral metabolism in these distant areas is referred to as cerebral diaschisis (58) or temporary functional deactivation of intact brain regions remote from the area of primary injury (59).

In the phenomena of LTP, LTD, diaschisis, and kindling, a considerable body of evidence points to a link to the central catecholamines, especially NE. For example, depletion of central NE or destruction of noradrenergic fibers by 6-hydroxydopamine results in a dramatic acceleration in the rate of kindling with electrical stimulation of limbic or cortical sites. Depletion of NE does not affect established seizures, suggesting that the suppressive action of NE is limited to seizure development *per se*. Depletion of DA, a neurotransmitter with more synaptic specialization than NE, appears to have no such effect (60). In the case of 5-HT, intermediate between NE and DA in its degree of synaptic specialization, the effect of depletion is ambiguous (61).

If LTP, LTD, diaschisis, and kindling are mediated, at least in part, by NDNT, the mechanism may not be only a function of sprouting or synaptogenesis, but perhaps also a change in the dynamics of the interstitial flow of NAS, such as NO or NE. The study of NDNT, therefore, may be key to understanding the various processes associated with brain plasticity, in particular what we have referred to as an optimal monoamine environment.

Glial Communication

Astrocytes have been known to guide neuronal development, metabolize neurotransmitters, and regulate the CNS vasculature, but the critically important role of glia in neuronal communication has only been recognized in recent years. Astrocytes display rapid electrical responses to neuronal activity, and intense neuronal activity can trigger slowly propagating astrocytic calcium (Ca^{2+}) waves. Recent evidence has been advanced to show that Ca^{2+} signals can propagate from astrocytes to neurons and thereby directly modulate neuronal activity. In fact, astrocyte-neuron signaling is found to be nonsynaptic (41).

Astrocytes contain receptors for transmitters and for neuroactive peptides (62). Sommer et al. (63) suggest that glutamate released from excitatory synapses may spill over from the synaptic cleft to activate ion channels on glial cells. The recent discovery that astrocytes possess ion channels that are opened on a millisecond time scale by glutamate suggests that they also play a role in rapid signal transmission (9). NAS, like glutamate, diffusing through the extracellular space, bind target receptors on glial cells, increase cytoplasmic free calcium, and propagate waves within the cytoplasm of individual astrocytes and even between astrocytes in confluent cultures (9). Diffusion of K^+ or glutamate in the interstitial space has been proposed as the mechanism for spreading depression, a slow-moving wave of tissue depolarization, possibly mediated by astrocytic signaling (41).

Glial profiles are discovered in apposition to serotonergic and noradrenergic varicosities devoid of synaptic specialization, suggesting that neurotransmitters other than glutamate may activate glial responses (64). It would appear, then, that glial cells activated by NDNT and acting by NDNT, are a component of a dynamic system of cell-to-cell molecular interactions with neurons. It is arguable that glia-neuron interactions provide a favorable microenvironment for neuronal plasticity. The contribution of glia to neuromodulation, LTP, synaptogenesis, and plasticity mechanisms are another manifestation of NDNT.

CLINICAL IMPORTANCE OF NONSYNAPTIC DIFFUSION NEUROTRANSMISSION

Individual movements or functions, such as playing the piano or a game of tennis, require great selectivity, rapid initiation, and rapid ending; for such functions, synaptic action is essential. In contrast, NDNT is likely to be more important to mass-sustained functions such as mood, arousal, appetite, and pain, which require sustained, widespread neural activity rather than activity that is fast and selective (4).

In ergonomic terms, it makes sense to use an energy-efficient analog process such as NDNT to mediate essential background functions such as arousal, attention, and mood and thus lower the "fixed cost" of brain metabolism. In ontogenetic terms, a primitive process such as NDNT should be expected to mediate vital functions such as brain tone, appetite, and the perception of pain.

In cybernetic terms, one may suggest that the conceptual preoccupation with SNT represented a necessary stage in the development of neuropharmacology, analogous to computational models that proposed a relationship between brain structure and complex behavior in terms of serial processing of information along a hierarchy of dedicated centers. That view has been supplanted by current concepts of complex behavior subserved by neural networks or syncytia with more versatile computational architecture (65). The problem with serial processing is that it becomes increasingly inefficient as the number of constraints increases, as it inevitably does in a natural system confronted with a complex task. Parallel distributed processing, conversely, allows acceleration of the process as additional constraints become exploited (66). There is increasing evidence that complex behavioral domains are mapped at the level of multifocal networks and that these networks contain an internal structure, including cell syncytia or assemblies, commensurate with parallel distributive processing (65).

The computational architecture of such a model includes projection channels that are "anatomically addressed" and others that are "chemically addressed" (65). The former represent established neuroanatomic projections that are targeted and reciprocal and respect cytoarchitectonic boundaries. One presumes that SNT is the predominant mechanism for information flow within such channels. Chemically addressed channels refer to projections from small, discrete brainstem nuclei that are widely dispersed to all the cortical areas and that contain neurotransmitters that are largely given to NDNT, such as ACh, NE, 5-HT, and, to a degree, DA. These chemically addressed projections are in a much better position to alter the tone and coloring of behavior rather than its specific content. Their access to all areas of cortical information processing enables them to influence emotional-motivational perspectives directed toward the environment. The anatomically addressed channels provide the vectors of information transfer, whereas chemically addressed systems provide a matrix that influences the state of information processing (65).

The chemical address of a functional syncytium is probably defined by the specific sensitivity of target cell receptors to NAS diffusing in the extracellular medium. These "grids of connectivity," both localized and distributed, are the probable basis for mass-sustained actions such as mood, arousal, attention, motivation, and learning. These grids may also represent the chemical basis for the diffuse functional systems spoken about earlier.

The therapeutic manipulation of mass-sustained actions is one of the foundations of biologic psychiatry, by using psychopharmaceuticals that influence DA, NE, 5-HT, and ACh. Indeed, the contributions of chemically addressed pathways are much more accessible to pharmacologic intervention than the contributions of anatomically addressed pathways (65).

Although SNT has long been considered the functional locus of psychopharmacologic treatments, it is likely that drug effects are mediated, at least in part, through NDNT. Centrally acting drugs are taken up from the circulation into the extracellular space, where they diffuse to reach target receptors. The chemical systems that they affect, NE, 5-HT, ACh, DA, γ-aminobutyric acid, opiates, are synaptic or nonsynaptic in varying degrees. It has been proposed that neuroactive drugs have more difficulty reaching intrasynaptic receptors than nonsynaptic receptors and that nonsynaptic receptors are more sensitive than synaptic receptors to the effects of low concentrations of drugs (20).

The treatment of mood disorders with agents that block reuptake of NE or 5-HT or with agents that inhibit the degradation of monoamines allows the transmitter to remain active and extracellular for longer. The relative importance of extracellular NAS in the synaptic cleft compared with the cellular interstitium is, at present, unknown. That drug action is felt only in the synapse is an unwarranted assumption.

The therapeutic actions of the lithium ion are a good example of pharmacologic action through NDNT. With chronic administration, its distribution in tissue is relatively uniform, with some degree of variation in different organs, or comparing the extracellular to the intracellular compartments (67). Although the mechanism of action of lithium is unknown [at least 36 possible mechanisms have been proposed (67)], recent attention has focused on the effect of the lithium ion on second messenger systems. At the most fundamental level, however, the biologic activity of lithium is necessarily a function of the physicochemical properties of the lithium ion, which allow it to subserve the actions of other ions, sodium, potassium, calcium, and magnesium. As lithium, a small monovalent cation, diffuses through the interstitial space, it appears to be capable of acting, alone or with other NAS, to stabilize membrane receptors (68). Lithium is also known to exercise a selective effect on astrocytes, which can in turn influence the traffic of impulses in neurons (68).

The action of some drugs on presynaptic receptors in the terminal axon is usually explained in terms of synaptic theory. If the presynaptic receptor, however, were designed to be activated by SNT, one would expect to find axonal terminals synapsing on it. After all, the presynaptic receptors are not there simply to await the effects of an exogenous compound. They exist to mediate the action of an endogenous compound. The occurrence of axo-axonal synapses between nerve terminals has hardly ever been observed (3).

For example, in the striatum, there is abundant evidence of presynaptic control of DA release from nerve terminals by drugs that mimic the effects of endogenous opiates, 5-HT, NE, and ACh. It is reasonable to assume that observed pharmacologic effects reflect the potential activity of endogenous neurotransmitter systems. If that activity were mediated by SNT, there would have to be evidence at the synaptic level for axon terminals making synapses with DA-containing terminals. Numerous ultrastructural studies, however, have demonstrated that there are no axo-axonal synapses in the striatum (3).

It is only reasonable to propose that some aspect of the mechanism of drug action on presynaptic receptors, reuptake mechanisms, catabolic enzymes, and target cell receptors occurs in the dynamic medium of the extracellular space. As the drug diffuses through the interstitium, it follows paths that have been laid down for the diffusion of endogenous NAS, and it interacts with receptors in ways that mimic the action of endogenous compounds. The ultimate effect is to augment or inhibit SNT, but the setting event is, to some degree at least, extrasynaptic.

The attributes of SNT conform to a categorical view of neuronal communication and the actions of psychotropic drugs. NDNT, conversely, is consistent with the view that psychotropic drugs behave as dimensional inputs in a dynamic matrix of NAS and that they affect mass-sustained actions of the brain. Both views need to be incorporated into a modern theory of psychopharmacology.

NEUROPSYCHIATRY AND THE KRAEPELINIAN TRADITION

In 1950, when psychopharmacology was about to burst on the scene, three intellectual traditions were current in psychiatry. They were all identified with their founders. The first, identified with the German psychiatrist Emil Kraepelin was primarily nosologic. Kraepelin developed the first modern descriptions of the major mental illnesses. He gave us recognizable descriptions of dementia praecox and manic depression, indicated major and minor symptoms, and discussed the natural history of the disorders. The descriptions were empirical and based on data collected in systematic fashion. Kraepelin was a naturalist—a taxonomist. Of the three schools, his is the most recognizably medical, at least by today's standards. At the time, it was influential in Europe, but not in the United States.

The second was the adaptationist tradition, identified with the Swiss-American psychiatrist Adolf Meyer. Meyer asserted that mental disorders should be understood as reactions of the organism to its environment as a function of its history and inborn proclivities. Meyer's approach was, in today's terms, holistic. His tradition was influenced by prevailing theories of organismic homeostasis. It was an open system and quite tolerant of other theoretical schools such as psychoanalysis. The great German-American neuropsychiatrist Kurt Goldstein was arguably a meyerian.

The third great intellectual tradition in psychiatry at the time was identified with the Viennese neurologist Sigmund Freud. Freud's intellectual activities were so broad and far-reaching that they defy simple description. One may argue, however, that Freud never abandoned his biologic roots. His ambition was to develop a psychology rooted in biologic drives and what he called mental structures. He hardly ever spoke about the conventional mental disorders, unless it was to examine their roots in the interactions of their underlying components: mental drives and structures, early learning, and their dynamic interactions.

Psychopharmacology could have found a home, conceptually, within any of these three traditions. It might even have been possible for psychopharmacology to bridge the theoretical gaps that separated them, but that did not happen. What happened was one tradition was chosen. Among academic psychopharmacologists, the kraepelinian tradition became the dominant school.

Indeed, the clinical behavior of psychotropic drugs seemed to validate the nosologic categories that Kraepelin had put forth. It was discovered that the drugs could be classified in terms of their nosologic pertinence, e.g., antidepressants for depression and antipsychotics for schizophrenia. Practitioners knew, of course, that the connections were not nearly as tight; the tricyclic antidepressants were, for example, good for anxiety as were the neuroleptics. Combinations of drugs from different "diagnostic" categories were often necessary. Lithium stabilized the emotional reactivity of individuals with numerous conditions and so on. These facts were never allowed to intrude on the purity of the model. The intellectual discourse was conducted in kraepelinian terms. It became the dominant force.

The nosologic specificity of the psychotropic drugs is characterized by a main effect (e.g., antidepressants for depression). Conceptually, it is a categorical effect. The broad spectrum of activity of the psychotropic drugs, however, across diagnostic categories is conceptually a dimensional effect. The behavior of the psychotropic drugs is amenable to both interpretations, but as a theory of psychopharmacology developed, it incorporated the former and largely ignored the latter.

It was certainly convenient to do so, if only for the dissemination of scientific articles and development of new drugs. The early drug literature was, indeed, hard to interpret because one was seldom sure exactly what was wrong with the patients who were being studied. If the field was to advance at all, it had to define its terms more carefully. Thus, kraepelinian psychiatry was resurrected in the United States. It was a sound decision. It did more than create a lucrative cottage industry for psychiatric associations that promulgated diagnostic manuals. It made psychiatrists think a little more strictly about what disorders they were treating and why, and it made the field more congenial to the rest of medicine. These were signal accomplishments.

Although the link between psychopharmacology and kraepelinian psychiatry was a fruitful partnership, it was never more than a "marriage of convenience." It was able to strengthen the core of psychiatry, but on the periphery, its limitations were always obvious. On several occasions, I have mentioned that conventional psychiatric categories are inappropriate for understanding or treating the behavioral and emotional problems of patients with neuropsychiatric disorders. In neuropsychiatry, kraepelinian categories have always been a Procrustean bed.

Marriages of convenience seldom last very long. As time went by, the accumulated weight of new experience forced psychiatry to move away from categorical thinking about drugs and their actions and move toward a more dimensional position. One influential factor has been the introduction of an extraordinary panoply of new drugs. In Chapter 19, the new antidepressants as broad-spectrum psychoactive drugs were described. Their wide range of therapeutic activity is largely coincident with the activity of the serotonergic and noradrenergic systems, but those systems, as we have seen, govern a host of disparate functions. One can also describe the new mood stabilizers and the atypical antipsychotics as broad-spectrum agents.

Drugs are still classified in terms of their main effects, but their wide spectrum of therapeutic activity is increasingly demonstrated even in controlled studies. Psychotropic drugs do have categorical effects, but the categories are remarkably permeable. One way that conventional psychiatry has dealt with this problem is by positing comorbidity, that is, the coexistence of more than one mental illness in the same patient. It is a clever stratagem, but it grows increasingly complex. The average patient with a mental illness can easily accumulate five or six categorical diagnoses. It has come to look more and more like the ptolemaic stratagem of cycles and epicycles to preserve the geocentric theory of the universe.

Another influence that has moved psychiatry away from the categorical is an expanded number of minor conditions that are being treated, intelligently and effectively, with psychoactive drugs. They are conditions that are hardly recognizable as mental illness at all. When antidepressants are prescribed for people who want to stop smoking, women who get grumpy around their periods, or people with migraine headaches and when stimulants and antidepressants are given to help students at school or older people who are inattentive in meetings, it is hard to maintain that the drugs are having anything more than a dimensional effect. As Meyer would have suggested, they are just enhancing the organism's capacity to adapt to internal and/or external stress.

The last nail in the coffin of categorical psychopharmacology is from the core of kraepelinian psychiatry itself. When antidepressants are given to patients with recurrent depression, antipsychotics to patients with schizophrenia, or mood stabilizers to patients with bipolar disorders, the effects are marvelous indeed. The therapeutic effects of the drugs, however, are only to control symptom expression. They do not change the underlying biology of the disorder. We know that because after the drugs are withdrawn, even after years of treatment, patients relapse.

Psychiatry will never abandon kraepelinian traditions of concise description, careful definition, and statistical analysis, but kraepelinian diagnosis is only one component of a proper theory of psychopharmacology. Psychotropic drugs have main effects, or categorical effects, but they also have dimensional effects, and both components deserve to be incorporated into the theory. We concede that point whenever a new antidepressant is brought to market. A drug can be approved as long as it shows a decrease in patient scores on a rating scale such as the Hamilton. The drug is not required to cure depression; it is simply required to make patients feel less depressed.

The dimensions that are affected by psychotropic drugs may be as simple and overt as the symptom lists that comprise rating scales such as the Hamilton, or they may be some of the dimensions alluded to in the foregoing chapters as complex functional systems. In fact, the dimensional effects of drugs were presaged in the intellectual traditions of Meyer and Freud.

The Meyerian Model: Drug Effects on the Organism

We have ascribed to Meyer the idea that mental illness represents a failure in adaptation. Premorbid personality traits, or proclivities, interact with events in the patient's environment. The dynamic process thus engendered results in varying degrees of successful adaptation or maladaptation. In the years of meyerian ascendancy, psychiatric disorders were known as "reactions."

Meyer proposed that by understanding the dialectic relationship that existed between inherent traits and external stressors, one was better positioned to understand the individual patient. It was the psychiatrist's business to appreciate the various dimensions, biologic, personal, and social, that were at play in the life of the mentally ill patient. A mentally ill patient might be given diagnoses, in the kraepelinian sense, but that was only one aspect of the patient's condition. The diagnostic process, in the etymologic sense of diagnosis as thorough understanding, required a unique, individual formulation of the case.

From the time of Kurt Goldstein, neuropsychiatry has acknowledged this adaptationist tradition. A specific cognitive deficit may be the direct consequence of a lesion or a particular genotype. Psychopathology or, as Goldstein would say, the personality of the patient with brain injury is the result of an interaction between the patient's biotype and a host of pre- and postmorbid factors. The relationship is categorical in one sense but also dimensional.

In my treatment of the relevant literature, I have demonstrated that this dynamic interaction is not only amenable to individual case study, in the tradition of Meyer and Goldstein, but that lawful and predictable relationships exist and can be defined for patients in general. Adaptation to injury is a unique process for the individual. It follows lawful rules, however, that apply to everyone.

In Chapter 1, the impact of patient-related variables on the outcome of traumatic brain injury (TBI) was examined and in Chapter 4, the development of Alzheimer's disease. In both instances, the patient's premorbid level of intelligence is found to have an inverse relationship to pathologic outcome. High premorbid intelligence predicts good outcome after TBI; it also forestalls the onset of dementia, even in people who are genetically predisposed. Intelligence itself, as described in Chapter 4, is a function of neuronal efficiency, the capacity of the brain to muster vast neuronal syncytia in the service of a complex task and to do so quickly and reliably and with a minimal expenditure of energy.

Elements that contribute to cerebral efficiency participate in the metaconcept of cerebral reserve. This concept is important for understanding the impact of successive brain traumas and why elderly people do poorly after a simple concussion. The connectivity of neuronal assemblies and the bioenergetics of neurons are well maintained in the healthy brain but are compromised in injured or aged brains. Brains exposed to chronic toxins such as alcohol, lead, or carbon monoxide or compromised by the vasculitides induced by diabetes, hypertension, or hyperlipidemia gradually lose their cerebral reserve. Chronic, subclinical encephalopathies generate oxidative stress, excitotoxicity, and local inflammatory response. As the patient's reserve is gradually spent down, neuronal connectivity and bioenergetics are diminished. A brain thus compromised loses its ability to adapt to sudden trauma. Recovery is prolonged and usually incomplete.

The relationship between external stressors and brain response is quantitative. This principle is embedded in the continuum of casualty, one of the fundamental principles of developmental medicine (Chapter 2). It is also central to the understanding of closed head injury in general and diffuse axonal injury in particular: some neurons are damaged, some are not, some recover, others do not. The severity of outcome is directly related to the relative proportion of nonsurviving neurons.

The relationship between Down's syndrome and dementia is also quantitative. In trisomy 21, extra genes on a supernumerary chromosome are responsible for overproducing amyloid precursor protein and generating free radicals. In the mosaic form of the condition, fewer cells are aneuploid, the rate of production of toxic substrates is lower, and dementia is less likely to occur.

The complexity of the relationship between stressors and pathologic result is also captured in the study of acquired and congenital brain injury. The relationship is quantitative but not necessarily linear. There are threshold effects; for example, the perinatal brain is tolerant of a certain level of hypoxia; as long as the threshold is not exceeded, no damage will ensue. The adult brain, of course, is much less tolerant of any degree of hypoxia. Alternatively, the relationship may be exponential. This is typified by the association between low birth weight and developmental delay and by the incidence of epilepsy relative to the level of mental handicap.

The study of brain trauma also demonstrates that stressors have primary and secondary effects and that secondary effects are sometimes more damaging than the primary trauma (Chapter 4). Drug treatment for acute stroke and TBI has been directed, with some success, at mitigating secondary damage.

Severe brain injuries sometimes have delayed effects, such as epilepsy, psychosis, and dementia. One presumes that mechanisms such as excitotoxicity, oxidative stress, and inflammatory response mediate the evolution of delayed sequelae of brain injury. Another potential mechanism is kindling. Here again, drug treatment may be directed at preventing delayed sequelae.

Drugs themselves have primary and secondary effects. The immediate action of an antidepressant is to elevate levels of synaptic NE and/or 5-HT. This action is sufficient to account for the utility of antidepressant drugs for attention deficit/hyperactivity disorder, chronic pain, and headache. It is not sufficient to explain their effect in depression, which is thought to be mediated by signal transduction, activation of immediate-early response genes, protein synthesis, and modification of receptor dynamics. Even the psychostimulants, which are prototypical immediate-acting drugs, modify genomic expression. This may explain their beneficial effects on brain plasticity as well as their positive long-term effects in patients with attention deficit/hyperactivity disorder, even after drug treatment has been stopped.

Brain injuries have local and remote effects. Diaschisis is an example of the latter. This peculiar event is thought to be a manifestation of NE depletion, insofar as it is abetted by NE blockers and attenuated by NE agonists. NE plays a role in neuronal plasticity, learning, and memory, as exemplified in LTP studies. Drugs that enhance the activity of the governing neurotransmitters, especially NE, enhance the recovery of patients with stroke and brain injury just as they improve the academic performance of children with learning disabilities.

No issue is more complex in terms of the adaptation of the organism to stress than the study of brain plasticity. As seen in Chapters 2 and 4, the Kenard principle, that plasticity inheres to the young brain, continues to be appealing but is only partially correct. Plasticity is an enduring characteristic of a healthy brain. The capacity for collateral sprouting, vicariation, behavioral compensation, and even neurononeogenesis persists throughout life, at least in the healthy brain.

Brain plasticity requires an optimal monoamine environment. This principle is amply supported by research in experimental animals during early development and adult animals after experimental trauma. It is relevant to the intellectual and neurobehavioral problems of phenylketonuria (Chapter 11). The same principle is probably active in the natural course of affective disorders, which appear to be associated with subtle long-term changes in cognition and symptom severity that can be induced by a chronically suboptimal monoamine environment (Chapter 19). Some components of an optimal monoamine environment are suggested in the above discussion of non-SNT and the active properties of the cellular interstitium.

Virtually every stage of the adaptive response to brain injury is equally given to positive and negative results. In brain injury and stroke, the ischemic cell generates unusual amounts of excitatory amino acids, which leads to excitotoxic cell damage. Reperfusion should alleviate the problem. In fact, when damaged tissue is reexposed to oxygen, the level of oxidative stress increases, and further tissue damage ensues. When the brain is injured, the blood-brain barrier breaks down, and macrophages and inflammatory substances migrate into the brain. As they do, they aggravate the process of inflammatory cell death. Later, exogenous and endogenous macrophages clear the damaged area of cellular debris and noxious substances.

Mechanisms of plasticity can be ameliorative or destructive. Neurons adjust to the death of a neighbor through collateral sprouting. This may permit restoration of function. Sprouting, however, can generate inappropriate connectivity and thus compromise functional restoration. Excessive sprouting increases the metabolic load on surviving neurons and reduces their adaptability to future stress. This is probably the mechanism of the postpolio syndrome.

A meyerian theory of psychopharmacology would focus on how drugs affect adaptive processes. Neuroactive drugs would be thought of as agents that normalize basic neurobiologic functions, enhance recovery, and prevent secondary injury and delayed sequelae. The conventional theory proposes that psychopathology is the result of a disease process and that drugs eliminate or at least dampen that process. An organismic theory would propose that psychopathology is the result of abnormal or deficient adaptation to a stressor. Drugs work by improving the organism's adaptive capacity. Understanding how drugs work and developing a theory of how they work demand an appreciation of the processes of neuronal adaptation.

Nowhere is the meyerian model more cogent than in the problem of self-injurious behavior (SIB), addressed in Chapters 15 and 16. As discussed, a disease model of SIB originated with a series of studies of the biochemical basis of Lesch-Nyhan syndrome. The underlying pathologic process, a common final pathway, was posited to reside in the D_1 dopamine receptor. The model was fruitful and even generated an interesting approach to treatment, but it failed to solve the problem of SIB. At the same time, however, SIB has diminished considerably as a severe, persistent, and virtually epidemic problem among mentally retarded people. Why did this occur? Because of something that Meyer would call "mental hygiene"—improved living and learning for retarded people, an end to oppressive treatment in inhumane environments, an end to drug treatment that induced dysphoria and akathisia and thwarted cognitive development, improved medical diagnosis and treatment, and the use of better drugs to reduce feelings of pain, stress, anxiety, and depression. SIB, as pointed out, was not a "unitary disorder," a category. It was the behavioral expression of various dimensional inputs, turned in on themselves, jarring, and chaotic. Solving the problem of SIB has been to turn them outward, in the service of development, maturation, and adaptation.

The Freudian Model: Drug Effects on Complex Functional Systems

Freud was relatively disinterested in psychiatric diagnosis in the kraepelinian sense. He was more concerned with the dynamics of the patient's individual psychology. Trying to understand mental illness in terms of individual psychology, he emphasized the dynamic interaction of early experience and instinctual drives and posited the existence of mental structures. To Freud, as to Meyer, mental disorders were not reified entities. They were the summation of internal and external influences, interacting in unique ways in every individual. In the terminology of fuzzy logic, what Freud and Meyer were concerned with were dimensional inputs that were summated by the organism.

The freudian model of mental illness was one of dynamic interaction between drives and experience and among three mental structures in particular: the ego, id, and superego. The old terminology is no longer pertinent, but the principle of dynamic interaction is. If we substitute for mental structures the term complex functional systems, we can appreciate the salience of this model.

Complex Functional Systems

A complex functional system includes the following elements: a psychological function, its anatomic address, its mediating neurohumors, and its potential for interacting with other systems. The arousal system, for example, is a complex functional system. It is defined in terms of its functional properties; it resides in a reticulated neural syncytium based in the brainstem and ramifies widely as it projects rostrally to the convexity of the frontal lobes. The monoamines, especially NE, are central to its function. It is an active participant in all the higher cortical functions.

Every nervous system, even the invertebrate nervous system, possesses functional systems, such as perception, motor behavioral, and homeostatic regulation. In higher organisms, functional systems are more complex, occupy many anatomic addresses, and incorporate the behavior of multiple neurohumors. Their capacity for interaction increases exponentially as one ascends the evolutionary ladder.

The higher cortical functions are complex functional systems that are identified with the cerebral cortex and subcortical structures such as the cerebellum and basal ganglia. In Chapter 7, for example, the executive functions of the frontal lobes were described: attention, motivation, planning, self-regulation, self-awareness, and other awareness. They reside in the frontal cortex, but their elements are also distributed among other cortical regions: the subcortical nuclei, the brainstem, and cerebellum. Every higher function has roots in more simple functions. Functional systems that occupy the frontal and temporal lobes are also represented in the subcortical nuclei, brainstem, and cerebellum.

Consider the motor system. It is cortically localized but also represented at many different levels of the neuraxis. Voluntary movement is not localized to the motor strip. Rather, the motor cortex participates in the generation of voluntary movement along with the prefrontal cortex, basal ganglia, and cerebellum. Voluntary movement is mediated at different levels of the neuraxis.

Voluntary movement is not usually deemed a higher cortical function. In Chapter 7, however, I described how the prefrontal cortex participates in motor behavior through corollary discharge and the generation of a kinesthetic guidance set. This represents an evolutionary adumbration of the frontal lobe capacity for abstract reasoning. It illustrates how a higher cortical function such as abstract thinking originates in a phylogenetically more primitive function. It also illustrates how contiguity, in this case between the motor strip and prefrontal cortex, leads to activation of a neighboring region through corollary discharge. The capacity of cell assemblies in the motor cortex to activate cell assemblies in the neighboring frontal lobe was adaptive because it led to more refined control of motor activity. It was a selective advantage for the organism to incorporate kinesthetic guidance sets into its behavioral repertoire. The evolutionary development of association areas in the cerebral cortex was thus the result of amplifying and refining simpler functions and integrating them into complex functional systems.

Perception is a simple functional system that is discrete and localized, but the integration and analysis of sensory input are complex functional systems, concentrated in the temporal lobes but also widely dispersed. Speech is a simple, localized function, language is more complex, and communication is even more so. Language is a lateralized function; communication, conversely, is bihemispheric. Deficits in social communication, such as observed in those with autism, are not localized but involve structures in the limbic cortex, cerebellum, and elsewhere.

Withdrawal from a noxious stimulus is a simple behavioral system. Emotional reactivity is more complex but can be modified in lower mammals by making a small lesion in the midbrain. Affective regulation is a complex system that is mediated by the orbitofrontal cortex, limbic cortex, and brainstem.

The higher cortical functions, therefore, have two important characteristics. They are neocortical and reside in the expanse of uncommitted or association cortex. Their evolutionary derivation is from simple, subcortical functions. Their phylogenetic origins, therefore, are represented by the continuing participation of subcortical structures.

The relationship between neocortical structures and subcortical structures in the maintenance of complex functional systems is typified by the functional anatomy of the monoamine neurotransmitters. The monoamines originate in the brainstem, whence they disperse to a broad swath of cortical and subcortical tissue, occupying more complex functions as they advance into the cerebral and cerebellar cortex. The structure of the monoamine systems, the major governing neurotransmitters, reflects the phylogeny of complex systems: tightly bound to specific nuclei in the brainstem, then ramifying widely throughout the cortex. In their wide-ranging influence, the governing neurotransmitters use communication that is junctional or synaptic. SNT is a phylogenetically more recent form of neuronal communication, but the monoamines also preserve the phylogenetically more ancient form of nonjunctional communication.

The phylogeny of complex behavioral systems is reiterated during development. In children, complex social and cognitive behaviors are mediated by subcortical structures, as demonstrated by the description of the delayed response paradigm in Chapter 7. During adolescence, functional systems that had been subserved by the basal ganglia begin to occupy the frontal cortex. Where would the lesion that disrupted a very simple cognitive task such as the delayed response experiment be located? At one stage of development, it would be in the striatum, at a later stage, in the frontal cortex.

In Chapter 7, Luria's view that lesion studies never prove that a complex psychological function is localized but rather that the structure that is lesioned participates, with other structures at other levels of the neuraxis, in an integrated system was presented. To complicate matters, the degree of participation varies during development was discussed. Transitional phases of the life cycle, such as puberty, climacteric, and senium, are times when the anatomic and chemical balance among functional systems is in a state of transition. These are also times when the manifestations of psychopathology are likely to change.

Psychiatry and the Complex Functional Systems

In the past, medical students learned that the difference between psychiatry and neurology was that psychiatric disorders were functional and neurologic disorders were organic. That view is no longer politically correct. Now we say that the psychiatric disorders are brain based. If we cannot say exactly where in the brain they reside, it is simply because we have not yet found the right spot.

In fact, "functional" is not such a bad word. The psychiatric disorders are functional—not in the sense that they are artificial, neurotic, or learned behaviors, but in the sense that they represent derangements of complex functional systems. The reason that psychiatric disorders are not localized is that they are derangements of complex functional systems. The reason that complex functional systems are not localized is that they are dispersed throughout the neuraxis. They have evolved from simpler functional systems. Thus, components of every such system are represented at many different levels of the neuraxis, with an increasing degree of complexity as one moves rostrally.

When psychiatrists or neurologists say that a patient's condition is one of hypoarousal, they are describing a symptom. Like all symptoms, it has a differential diagnosis. Whatever the diagnosis, however, the symptom itself is an expression of dysfunction in a complex functional system that mediates arousal. Similarly, inattention and distractibility are symptoms; whatever their cause, they are derangements of the attentional system. A kraepelinian psychiatrist is interested in symptoms and their differential diagnosis. The freudian/meyerian tradition is interested in the underlying physiology, the status of the underlying functional systems, and their interactions.

Complex functional systems interact in various ways. Systems with overlapping functions interact on a functional level. Memory and attention are higher cortical functions that are dissociable but also highly interactive. In diaschisis, a functional region that is damaged tends to shut down remote areas that are functionally related, but dynamic interactions also occur between brain regions and functional assemblies that are not functionally related. Brain systems can interact simply by virtue of contiguity. Corollary discharge and prefrontal participation in refined motor behavior are an example in the neocortex. Interaction by contiguity is even more important in the brainstem.

Reciprocal connections up and down the neuraxis create a severe packing problem in the lower brainstem. The proximity of cells within this narrow and circumscribed region creates a potential problem of cross-talk between functional systems. Neural tracts are not particularly well insulated from each other. Assemblies of neurons are stimulated by the activity of nearby assemblies, although they are components of different functional systems. Combining the problem of insulation with the problem of packing in the brainstem, one is hardly surprised when functional systems overlap or when derangements in one system recruit another into a pattern of aberrant activity.

If the genesis of a psychiatric disorder resides in a complex behavioral system, it may be impossible to localize because functional systems are comprised of structures up and down the neuraxis. The genesis of a condition such as schizophrenia may begin with a deficit in the integration and analysis of sensory information. The lesion that is responsible may be frontal, temporal, thalamic, and cerebellar or even lower, or it may reside in the aberrant resonance of an integrated circuit. An important system that functions in an aberrant way is likely to influence other systems that are nearby and from which it is poorly insulated. In a small structure such as the thalamus, the excessive activation of sensory integration systems can induce activity in systems that mediate communication or memory. This is ultimately represented on a clinical level by the manifestation of new behavioral symptoms that are hard to localize to a conventional topographic map of brain function.

The dynamic interaction among complex functional systems is a much more cogent model for the protean manifestations of mental illness than an approach based on a topographic brain map. Psychiatric disorders are functional in the sense that they are functionally rather than anatomically addressed.

Psychopharmacology and Complex Functional Systems

Psychopharmacology operates on a brain map that is functional, diffuse, and dynamic and better understood in terms of processes rather than locations. Psychoactive drugs act on functional systems, not on brain regions or psychiatric disorders. The pathologic conditions that have been the subject of this book, syndromes associated with brain injury and mental handicap, are good examples.

The frontal lobe syndromes were discussed in depth because they are the best documented of all the static cortical syndromes. Their gratifying response to treatment with stimulants, amantadine, and the dopamine agonists raises interesting questions about how the drugs really work. In Chapter 18, I proposed that the drugs operate on functional systems. They activate an arousal system that originates in the reticular complex of the brainstem and terminates in the convexity of the frontal cortex. They enhance a regulatory system in the orbitomedial cortex that is the apex of the homeostatic mechanisms of the autonomic nervous system. They affect the attentional system and consolidation of long-term memory. They enhance recovery from stroke and TBI by reversing diaschisis and enhancing new learning in the process of LTP.

The neuropsychological deficits of patients with frontal lobe injury are described in terms of the executive functions. When one treats a patient with frontal lobe damage with a stimulant drug or amantadine, one does not expect the drug to influence, directly and immediately, higher cortical functions such as cognitive flexibility, motivation, planning, or empathy. Rather, the drugs affect more fundamental systems such as arousal, attention, and affective regulation. Direct drug effects on these systems are ultimately reflected in improvements in the higher cortical functions, but the effects on the latter are indirect or secondary. One may even think of the higher cortical functions as the neuropsychological equivalents of psychiatric disorders. They are affected by drugs but at a lower level on the hierarchy of functional systems.

On several occasions, the problem of affective dysregulation in patients with brain injury and stroke and in the mentally retarded was discussed. In Chapter 19, I suggested that the clinical manifestation of depression should be understood in terms of the functional systems that participate in its generation and expression. I demonstrated that the activity of antidepressant and mood-stabilizing drugs is on the fundamental processes that participate in affective regulation. Because these same processes are involved in other psychopathologic conditions, the antidepressants are also effective. They are broad-spectrum psychotropic drugs because the systems that they affect are involved in many pathologic conditions.

SIB was also one of the major subjects of this book. It is a primitive, undifferentiated behavior that can be evoked in the lowest mammals through simple pharmacologic manipulations, for example, of the DA system. In its clinical expression, however, SIB is by no means simple. Its expression is extraordinarily varied, and the clinical approach to it, with various classes of drugs, is quite diverse and unpredictable. SIB may be rooted in very simple animal behaviors, such as grooming, but its diverse clinical manifestations are the result of the involvement of other systems that govern habit, affective regulation, and the experience of pain. The primary lesion may reside in any of these systems but with time will influence the activity of other systems and incorporate them into the clinical manifestation of the problem.

In Cornelia de Lange syndrome, I proposed that the genesis of SIB is the child's experience of painful physical states, such as gastroesophageal reflux, peripheral neuropathy, and dysautonomia. In other cases, SIB begins as way to deal with hypoarousal through self-stimulation. With time, however, the expression of SIB occupies a role in the child's social communication and affective self-regulation. What begins as a stereotypy becomes a habit and then a compulsion.

The treatment of SIB can be directed against one system or another, depending on where one thinks the primary lesion resides. Stereotyped grooming behavior can be addressed with dopamine blockers. Habit and compulsion are more complex forms of stereotyped behavior; they are amenable to treatment by dopamine blockers or serotonin agonists. Opiate antagonists such as naltrexone might be affecting functional systems that mediate the experience of pain, motivation, reinforcement, or new learning. SIB in patients with TBI occurs in a state of confused hyperarousal and can be treated with α_2 agonists such as clonidine. When affective dysregulation is an important component of SIB, one may rely on antidepressant or mood-stabilizing drugs. The relationship here is between the symptom , SIB, and the functional system that is posited to have led to its genesis.

This is pure Freud. The symptom, SIB, is related to an underlying dynamic relationship among functional systems. Kraepelinian diagnosis is irrelevant.

Psychoactive drugs act by affecting complex functional systems whose interactions summate to generate neurobehavioral syndromes. We identify the activity of drugs with their effects on specific neurotransmitters, receptors, and transporters, especially NE, DA, 5-HT, ACh, and γ-aminobutyric acid, but we also know that the organization of these governing neurotransmitters is largely based on functional systems, not anatomic areas. That is why the theory of NDNT is so important for understanding how drugs work. Drugs deliver their influence to functional addresses, not anatomic addresses. Psychoactive drugs, altering as they do the behavior of these NAS, exert their effects not on specific brain regions, but on functional systems. NDNT mediates mass-sustained functions such as mood, arousal, appetite, and pain. It mediates the cerebral tone and bioenergetics of the neuron. The psychoactive drugs, operating on nonjunctional receptors on neurons and glial cells, slowly correct the derangements in neural assemblies and diminish the cross-talk that recruits other systems into a pathologic network. In the cellular interstitium, they reestablish an optimal environment of NAS. At least, when they work, they do.

That, of course, is the irony of the psychotropic drugs. Drugs that are ostensibly similar can have divergent and unpredictable effects in individuals. This small but important point, so rarely dealt with in the psychiatric literature, merits at least a passing explanation.

There may well be a theory of psychopharmacology, but practice is always empirical. That is nowhere so true as it is for patients with neuropsychiatric disorders whose response to drugs is so unpredictable that it seems idiosyncratic. Amantadine is effective for agitation during coma recovery, but no more than half the time. Naltrexone works in SIB, perhaps for one patient in four. Carbamazepine is an anticonvulsant that can cause seizures. Fluoxetine can cause hypersomnia or insomnia, hyperphagia or anorexia, akathisia or anergia, hypo- or hypersexuality, and so on.

Psychoactive drugs are "dirty," in the sense that they have affinities for many different receptors and affect different functional systems. They operate on NAS, commonly known as neurotransmitters and neuromodulators; they work on second messenger systems and activate the immediate early genes to modify the sensitivity of receptors. They work on receptors in synapses on neurons and on nonsynaptic receptors on neurons and glial cells. They have specific effects, for example, to block a particular receptor, but every drug in psychiatric practice also has nonspecific effects, an affinity to other receptors. The complexity of drug activity is paralleled by the complexity of the organism on the receiving end. The strength that a particular drug has on a particular population of receptors varies from one person to another, and every other process in the cascade of drug action is subject to interindividual variation. People vary in the rate at which they metabolize drugs, in the degree to which metabolites are active or not, and in the degree to which drug interactions are likely to be clinically important.

No brain region is excited by only one transmitter or excited/inhibited by only two. Every area of the brain is comprised of many different kinds of cells, and every cell possesses receptors for several NAS. Even glial tissue is responsive to NAS and contributes to neuromodulation. No transmitter functions in a narrowly circumscribed area. The effects of transmitters are not even confined to the synapse. No drug in the current pharmacopoeia is a "clean" drug that affects only one NAS or only one receptor in a particular way.

We know that drugs have a greater or lesser affinity for some receptors and that some receptors are more or less localized, such as the DA receptors, and some are not, such as the glutamate and NE receptors. The distribution of drug within the brain, however, is dispersed in the cellular interstitium of the CNS. Drug effects cannot be said to be localized, at least in the way Broca localized the speech center in the prefrontal cortex. That is all right because none of the psychiatric disorders and few of the neuropsychiatric disorders can be localized either.

The alternative to localizationism is not mass action, an old concept that is associated with Karl Lashley, but the theory of complex functional systems. What we understand as psychiatric disorders are, in fact, derangements of functional systems. Complex functional systems are dispersed in the neuraxis. They interact with other systems based on functional relationships and based on mere proximity. It is possible that the origins of some forms of mental illness resemble what happens after brain injury. After brain injury, even mild brain injury, axonal sprouting and ingrowth can lead to inappropriate connectivity (Chapter 2). Immature patterns of neuronal communication that would ordinarily be lost are stabilized and preserved. Neuronal connections that would ordinarily be quiescent are unmasked. Events such as this can disrupt, in subtle ways, the behavior of the functional systems and the manner in which they interact with other systems.

Into this tangled nest, a drug is proffered. It is not delivered, surgically, to a specific site. It is broadcast into the cellular interstitium, one more dimensional input into mix of NAS. What happens next is sometimes hard to predict.

THE ECOLOGY OF DRUG TREATMENT

Finally, a successful theory of psychopharmacology needs to address the ecology of the patient, the system in which the patient resides—its weaknesses and its resources. There is a personal economy to consider—the resources a patient brings to bear—and a wider economy, the resources and limitations of the patient's environment.

A patient may not have the personal strength to tolerate the effects of a drug. Some patients are exquisitely sensitive to toxic effects. In psychiatry, many patients with anxiety disorders are extremely vulnerable to the activating effects of selective 5-HT reuptake inhibitors. Patients with bipolar disorder detest the cognitive blunting that sometimes accompanies treatment with mood stabilizers. In neuropsychiatry, patients with TBI are very sensitive to drug-induced neurotoxicity during the coma-recovery phase. Very young children with developmental disabilities are also sensitive to drug side effects. That is what makes the severe behavioral problems of young children with developmental handicaps so difficult to treat with drugs. The real problem of tardive dyskinesia is that some patients are exquisitely sensitive to the neurotoxic effects of DA-blocking drugs.

Drugs enhance the activity of complex functional systems in the brain, but there has to be sufficient substrate for drugs to exert their effects. Patients with severe dementia and patients with advanced Parkinson's disease reach a point where they no longer respond favorably to pharmacotherapy. The same is true of patients with schizophrenia, especially when they "burn out" late in the course of the illness. When a patient reaches end state and deficit symptoms predominate, he or she is not likely to respond to the specific effects of drug treatment. In patients with TBI, DA agonists may enhance recovery from coma. If the damage is profound, the drugs induce nothing more than agitation. It is extraordinary to see coma coexist with agitation, but it happens if you administer a DA agonist, and there is no substrate for the drug to work properly.

This is also true of mentally retarded people. Drug treatment may eliminate a negative behavior; if there is not a repertoire of positive behaviors to fill the void, however, the behavioral problem will recur or another kind of maladaptive behavior. The patient's repertoire of positive behaviors is an important predictor of the success of pharmacotherapy. There is a behavioral reserve just as there is a cerebral reserve.

Drug treatment affects an individual, but it also affects an ecologic system. How much can caretakers abide in the way of difficult behavior as one experiments with drug-free baselines and slow titrations to the optimal dose or as one tries to eschew polypharmacy to get a clear picture of the effect of one drug? Is it possible to have one-to-one or two-to-one supervision during this period of experimentation? Do the regulations tolerate physical restraint or isolation? Can such interventions be applied humanely and intelligently? Is the staff skilled in behavioral management in times of crisis? If they are not and the patient has to be maintained on one or two nonspecific (i.e., sedating) drugs, how can we get a clear idea of how a new, specific drug intervention is working?

These issues first arose years ago, when we were trying to withdraw large numbers of institutionalized retarded patients from neuroleptics. The practice quickly lost its appeal when it became clear that most facilities could not abide the behavioral instability that accompanied neuroleptic withdrawal, especially when a few especially troublesome patients were being withdrawn at the same time. The trial withdrawals were perfunctory and meaningless because the economy of the unit could not sustain the additional programming that was necessary. Even today, it is unwise to attempt a trial medication withdrawal unless there are resources available to cope with withdrawal-related difficulties. Issues such as this, related to the ecology of a residential unit, influence drug decisions by practitioners far more than anyone likes to admit.

In residential facilities, there is an admonition to the effect that drugs are not a substitute for programming and should never be used as such. What is missing from this old maxim is the fact that clinical decisions are not made based on a one-time choice between drugs and programming. The choice is never quite as stark. A psychoactive drug can compensate for the programmatic deficiencies of a residential unit. It can be the means to raise the threshold to overstimulation by a noisy disruptive environment. It may be an adjunct during a period of difficult transition. It may allow a resident to adjust to a community setting, when his or her drug-free behavior, although difficult, is entirely manageable within a residential setting.

Another aspect of the ecology of drug treatment is the old belief that behaviors that are a reaction to an inappropriate or toxic environment should not be handled pharmacologically. This, of course, is a dualistic fallacy; etiology is biologic or psychological but never both and never the product of an interaction. A biochemical imbalance should be treated with drugs, and a psychological problem should be treated behaviorally or psychotherapeutically. However, it is a matter of relative proportions, not of absolute choices. The degree to which a behavioral problem is an appropriate reaction to a disturbed environment, then to that degree the physician should try to address the patient's environment. That does not mean drug treatment is altogether inappropriate. It is not an either/or thing. Sometimes we have to help a patient cope with a suboptimal environment.

Regulators, who preside over the quality of treatment in public facilities, are driven by this categorical approach to psychopharmacology, e.g., drugs versus programming. Physicians who treat patients and who are responsible for the quality of life in the facility are motivated by the dimensional effects of drugs. The right drug at the right time can make things a little better for the patient and for everybody around.

In the day-to-day practice of psychopharmacology, drugs such as the selective 5-HT reuptake inhibitors are frequently used for purely psychologic problems, such as grieving. In neuropsychiatry, family caretakers sometimes get exhausted, frustrated, and demoralized. Parents of severely retarded children or children with severe TBI and spouses of patients with TBI or stroke are all vulnerable to this reaction. They want to feel good about what they are doing because they are doing the right thing, but they get tired. They become irritable, short, and unpleasant and are ashamed of themselves for being so. They are not so much depressed as they are demoralized. An activating antidepressant can go a long way toward improving their attitude and giving them the strength to carry on.

The conventional theory of psychopharmacology proposes that drugs have specific effects for specific disorders, and they do sometimes, but drug treatment, especially in patients with chronic conditions, is not nearly as specific or targeted. Initiating treatment, choosing a particular drug, combining drugs, evaluating the success of the intervention, and withdrawing a drug that may not be necessary are all steps influenced by patient-related factors and environmental factors that are external to kraepelinian diagnosis or the theory of complex functional systems. Drug treatment has to be adapted to the patient's ecology.

REFERENCES

1. Isaacson RL. A fuzzy limbic system. *Behav Brain Res* 1992;52:129–131.
2. Kandel ER. Neurobiology and molecular biology: the second encounter. *Cold Spring Harb Symp Quant Biol* 1983;48:891–908.
3. Herkenham M. Mismatches between neurotransmitter and receptor localizations in brain: observations and implications. *Neuroscience* 1987;23:1–38.
4. Bach-y-Rita P. The brain beyond the synapse: a review. *Neuroreport* 1994;5:1553–1557.
5. Agnati LF, Tiengo M, Ferraguti F, et al. Pain, analgesia, and stress: an integrated view. *Clin J Pain* 1991;7:23–37.
6. Zoli M, Guidolin D, Agnati LF. Morphometric evaluation of populations of neuronal profiles (cell bodies, dendrites, and nerve terminals) in the central nervous system. *Microsc Res Tech* 1992;21:315–337.
7. Bach-y-Rita P, Smith CU. Comparative efficiency of volume and synaptic transmission in the coerulean system: relevance to neurologic rehabilitation. *Scand J Rehabil Med* 1993;25:3–5.
8. Bach-y-Rita P, Bjelke B. Lasting recovery of motor function, following brain damage, with a single dose of amphetamine combined with physical therapy; changes in gene expression. *Scand J Rehabil Med* 1991;23:219–220.
9. Cornell-Bell AH, Finkbeiner SM, Cooper MS, et al. Glutamate induces calcium waves in cultured astrocytes: long-range glial signaling. *Science* 1990;247: 470–473.
10. Schmitt FO. Molecular regulators of brain function: a new view. *Neuroscience* 1984;13:991–1001.
11. Fuxe K, Hokfelt T, Ungerstedt U. Localization of indolealkylamines in CNS. *Adv Pharmacol* 1968;6: 235–251.
12. Routtenberg A, Sladek J, Bondareff W. Histochemical fluorescence after application of neurochemicals to caudate nucleus and septal area in vivo. *Science* 1968;161: 272–274.
13. Fuxe K, Goldstein M, Hokfelt T, et al. Immunohistochemical localization of dopamine- -hydroxylase in the

peripheral and central nervous system. *Res Commun Chem Pathol Pharmacol* 1970;1:627–636.
14. Florey E. Neurotransmitters and modulators in the animal kingdom. *Fed Prac Fed Am Soc Exp Biol* 1967;26: 1164–1178.
15. Barchas JD, Akil H, Elliott GR, et al. Behavioral neurochemistry: neuroregulators and behavioral states. *Science* 1978;200:964–973.
16. Schmitt R, Capo T, Boyd E. Cranial electrotherapy stimulation as a treatment for anxiety in chemically dependent persons. *Alcohol Clin Exp Res* 1986;10:158–160.
17. Freeman TB, Spence MS, Boss BD, et al. Development of dopaminergic neurons in the human substantia nigra. *Exp Neurol* 1991;113:344–353.
18. Freeman AJ, Cunningham KT, Tyers MB. Selectivity of 5-HT3 receptor antagonists and anti-emetic mechanisms of action. *Anticancer Drugs* 1992;3:79–85.
19. Zhang J, Chiodo LA, Wettstein JG, et al. Acute effects of sigma ligands on the electrophysiological activity of rat nigrostriatal and mesoaccumbal dopaminergic neurons. *Synapse* 1992;11:267–278.
20. Vizi ES, Oberfrank F. Na+/K(+)-ATPase, its endogenous ligands and neurotransmitter release. *Neurochem Int* 1992;20:11–17.
21. Meberg PJ, Routtenberg A. Selective expression of protein F1/(GAP-43) mRNA in pyramidal but not granule cells of the hippocampus. *Neuroscience* 1991; 45:721–733.
22. Rice ME, Nicholson C. Diffusion characteristics and extracellular volume fraction during normoxia and hypoxia in slices of rat neostriatum. *J Neurophysiol* 1991; 65:264–272.
23. Zetterstrom T, Ungerstedt U. Effects of apomorphine on the in vivo release of dopamine and its metabolites, studied by brain dialysis. *Eur J Pharmacol* 1984;97:29–36.
24. Herkenham M. Characterization and localization of cannabinoid receptors in brain: an in vitro technique using slide-mounted tissue sections. *NIDA Res Monogr* 1991;112:129–145.
25. Beaudet A, Descarries L. The monoamine innervation of rat cerebral cortex: synaptic and nonsynaptic axon terminals. *Neuroscience* 1978;3:851–860.
26. Holtman JR Jr, Vascik DS, Maley BE. Ultrastructural evidence for serotonin-immunoreactive terminals contacting phrenic motoneurons in the cat. *Exp Neurol* 1990;109:269–272.
27. Inoue Y, Wagner HN Jr, Wong DF, et al. Atlas of dopamine receptor images (PET) of the human brain. *J Comput Assist Tomogr* 1985;9:129–140.
28. Hamel E, Beaudet A. Electron microscopic autoradiographic localization of opioid receptors in rat neostriatum. *Nature* 1984;312:155–157.
29. Hamel E, Beaudet A. Opioid receptors in rat neostriatum: radioautographic distribution at the electron microscopic level. *Brain Res* 1987;401:239–257.
30. Feuerstein GZ, Liu T, Barone FC. Cytokines, inflammation, and brain injury: role of tumor necrosis factor-α. *Cerebrovasc Brain Metab Rev* 1994;6:341–360.
31. Agnati LF, Fuxe K, Zoli M, et al. A correlation analysis of the regional distribution of central enkephalin and beta-endorphin immunoreactive terminals and of opiate receptors in adult and old male rats. Evidence for the existence of two main types of communication in the central nervous system: the volume transmission and the wiring transmission. *Acta Psychiatr Scand* 1986;128:201–207.
32. Southam E, Garthwaite J. Intercellular action of nitric oxide in adult rat cerebellar slices. *Neuroreport* 1991;2: 658–660.
33. Bredt DS, Snyder SH. Nitric oxide, a novel neuronal messenger. *Neuron* 1992;8:3–11.
34. Snyder SH. Janus faces of nitric oxide. *Nature* 1993; 364:577.
35. Snyder SH, Bredt DS. Biological roles of nitric oxide. *Sci Am* 1992;266:68–71.
36. Bjelke B, England R, Nicholson C, et al. Long distance pathways of diffusion for dextran along fibre bundles in brain. Relevance for volume transmission. *Neuroreport* 1995;6:1005–1009.
37. Florey E. Neurotransmitters and modulators in the animal kingdom. *Fed Proc* 1967;26:1164–1178.
38. Cooper JR, Pearce LB, Benishin CG. Isolation of a factor that reverses presynaptic inhibition of acetylcholine release. *J Physiol Paris* 1986;81:266–269.
39. Florey E, Rathmayer M. Is glutamate the transmitter of crustacean motoneurons? *J Physiol Paris* 1979;75: 629–634.
40. Vizi ES. Modulation of cortical release of acetylcholine by noradrenaline released from nerves arising from the rat locus coeruleus. *Neuroscience* 1980;5:2139–2144.
41. Nedergaard M. Direct signaling from astrocytes to neurons in cultures of mammalian brain cells. *Science* 1994;263:1768–1771.
42. Woodward DJ, Moises HC, Waterhouse BD, et al. Modulatory actions of norepinephrine in the central nervous system. *Fed Proc* 1979;38:2109–2116.
43. Waszcak BL, Walters JR. Dopamine modulation of the effects of gamma-aminobutyric acid on substantia nigra pars reticulata neurons. *Science* 1983;220:218–221.
44. Iversen SD. Behavior after neostriatal lesions in animals. In: Divac I, Oberg RGE, eds. *The neostriatum* Oxford: Pergamon Press, 1979:195–210.
45. Chan-Palay V, Palay SL, Wu JY. Gamma-aminobutyric acid pathways in the cerebellum studied by retrograde and anterograde transport of glutamic acid decarboxylase antibody after in vivo injections. *Anat Embryol (Berl)* 1979;157:1–14.
46. Bloom FE. Whither neuropeptides? *Res Publ Assoc Res Nerv Ment Dis* 1986;64:335–349.
47. Lapierre Y, Beaudet A, Demianczuk N, et al. Noradrenergic axon terminals in the cerebral cortex of rat. II. Quantitative data revealed by light and electron microscope radioautography of the frontal cortex. *Brain Res* 1973;63:175–182.
48. Aoki C, Joh TH, Pickel VM. Ultrastructural localization of beta-adrenergic receptor-like immunoreactivity in the cortex and neostriatum of rat brain. *Brain Res* 1987; 437:264–282.
49. Foote SL, Morrison JH. Development of the noradrenergic, serotonergic, and dopaminergic innervation of neocortex. *Curr Top Dev Biol* 1987;21:391–423.
50. Mitchison G. Axonal trees and cortical architecture. *Trends Neurosci* 1992;15:122–126.
51. Brinton RE. Neuromodulation: associative & nonlinear adaptation. *Brain Res Bull* 1990;24:651–658.
52. Siegelbaum SA, Kandel ER. Learning-related synaptic plasticity: LTP and LTD. *Curr Opin Neurobiol* 1991; 1:113–120.
53. Oguro K, Ito M, Tsuda H, et al. Interactions of thyroid hormones with L-(3H) glutamate binding sites, with special reference to *N*-methyl-D-aspartate receptors.

Res Commun Chem Pathol Pharmacol 1989;65: 181–196.

54. Bon L, Lucchetti C. The dorsomedial frontal cortex of the Macaca monkey: fixation and saccade-related activity. *Exp Brain Res* 1992;89:571–580.
55. Madison DV, Schuman EM. LTP, post or pre? A look at the evidence for the locus of long-term potentiation. *New Biol* 1991;3:549–557.
56. Shibuki K, Okada D. Endogenous nitric oxide release required for long-term synaptic depression in the cerebellum. *Nature* 1991;349:326–328.
57. Bolshakov VY, Siegelbaum SA. Postsynaptic induction and presynaptic expression of hippocampal long- term depression. *Science* 1994;264:1148–1152.
58. von Monakow C. "Diaschisis," localization in the cerebrum and functional impairment by cortical loci (1914). In: Pribram KH, ed. *Brain and behavior, vol. I.* Baltimore: Penguin, 1969:27–36.
59. Feeney DM, Baron JC. Diaschisis. *Stroke* 1986;17: 817–830.
60. Lewis J, Westerberg V, Corcoran M. Monoaminergic correlates of kindling. *Brain Res* 1987;403:205–212.
61. Wada Y, Nakamura M, Hasegawa H, et al. Effect of serotonin update inhibiting antidepressants on hippocampal kindled seizures in cats. *Neurosci Res Commun* 1993;12:119–124.
62. Hanson GR, Singh N, Bush L, et al. Role of NMDA receptors in methamphetamine-induced changes in extrapyramidal and limbic neuropeptide systems. *NIDA Res Monogr* 1991;105:439.
63. Sommer B, Monyer H, Wisden W, et al. Glutamate-gated ion channels in the brain. Genetic mechanism for generating molecular and functional diversity. *Arzneimittelforschung* 1992;42:209–210.
64. Ridet JL, Rajaofetra N, Teilhac JR, et al. Evidence for nonsynaptic serotonergic and noradrenergic innervation of the rat dorsal horn and possible involvement of neuron-glia interactions. *Neuroscience* 1993;52: 143–157.
65. Mesulam MM. Large-scale neurocognitive networks and distributed processing for attention, language, and memory. *Ann Neurol* 1990;28:597–613.
66. McClelland JL, McNaughton BL, O'Reilly RC. Why there are complementary learning systems in the hippocampus and neocortex: insights from the successes and failures of connectionist models of learning and memory. *Psychol Rev* 1995;102:419–457.
67. Klemfuss H. Diminishing toxic effects of lithium administration. *Am J Psychiatry* 1992;149:846.
68. Pert A, Rosenblatt J, Sivit C, et al. Long-term treatment with lithium prevents the development of dopamine receptor supersensitivity. *Science* 1978;201:171–173.

Appendices

A Few Useful Questionnaires

In Chapter 5, we alluded to a number of rating scales, psychological tests, and questionnaires that can make the evaluation process more efficient. Most are proprietary instruments, protected by copyright, but available from the usual purveyors of psychological materials. The following are instruments that we have developed ourselves, and refined over the years.

My colleagues and I developed these scales years ago, because there were no alternative instruments to use for our patients. As far as I am aware, there still aren't.

These are evaluative tools, not diagnostic instruments. They do not have impeccable pedigrees, or any at all, from the psychometric standpoint. But they are easy to use by patients, family members, or caregivers; even people with limited training. They generate a lot of information in a short period of time. They are useful for initial or for serial evaluation. They address symptoms that are germane to neuropsychiatric diagnosis and drug treatment.

The author will not make any proprietary claims on these instruments, and the reader is invited to use them, as he or she deems appropriate. Hard copies are available on request. Cyber-copies are available on **www.ncneuropsych.com**.

APPENDIX 1

Head Injury Questionnaire

We give this questionnaire to all our patients with brain injury and stroke who are capable of reading and writing. Usually, patients complete the form. Sometimes, a family member has to help. It is simply a list of the most common symptoms.

Patient's Name: ______________________________ Date: ______________

Instructions: The items listed below are symptoms that may occur after a head injury. Please check the appropriate box if you have experienced the problem over the past couple of weeks. If the answer is yes, check the appropriate box indicating the degree of your problem.

	No	Mild problem	Moderate problem	Severe problem
Headache	0	1	2	3
Neck pain	0	1	2	3
Back pain	0	1	2	3
Insomnia	0	1	2	3
Fatigue	0	1	2	3
Low energy	0	1	2	3
Lack of initiative	0	1	2	3
Low motivation	0	1	2	3
Problems with memory	0	1	2	3
Forgetting where you have put things	0	1	2	3
Finding a television story hard to follow	0	1	2	3
Forgetting when something happened	0	1	2	3
Forgetting names	0	1	2	3
Problems remembering what you've read	0	1	2	3
Getting lost while driving or walking	0	1	2	3
Difficulty concentrating	0	1	2	3
Short attention span	0	1	2	3
Distractibility	0	1	2	3
Letter reversals	0	1	2	3
Number reversals	0	1	2	3
Word-finding difficulty	0	1	2	3
Alcohol intolerance	0	1	2	3
Problems starting projects	0	1	2	3
Problems planning activities	0	1	2	3
Problems getting things done	0	1	2	3
Blurred vision	0	1	2	3
Nausea, vomiting	0	1	2	3
Drowsiness	0	1	2	3
Forgetting things that happened when you were very young	0	1	2	3
Not recognizing people you know very well	0	1	2	3
Feeling confused, disoriented	0	1	2	3

continued

	No	Mild problem	Moderate problem	Severe problem
Depression	0	1	2	3
Disinterest in your usual activities	0	1	2	3
Crying spells	0	1	2	3
Extreme emotional reaction	0	1	2	3
Poor appetite/weight loss	0	1	2	3
Sleeping too much	0	1	2	3
Thoughts of ending your life	0	1	2	3
Feeling worthless	0	1	2	3
Feeling bored	0	1	2	3
Loss of affection for people close to you	0	1	2	3
Mood swings	0	1	2	3
Less control over your anger	0	1	2	3
Angry outbursts	0	1	2	3
Irritability	0	1	2	3
Interpersonal problems	0	1	2	3
Impulsiveness	0	1	2	3
Low frustration tolerance	0	1	2	3
Verbal aggression	0	1	2	3
Physical aggression	0	1	2	3
Impatience	0	1	2	3
Restlessness	0	1	2	3
Suspiciousness	0	1	2	3
Mistrust of others	0	1	2	3
Thoughts that people are talking about you	0	1	2	3
Hearing things that are not really there	0	1	2	3
Seeing things that are not really there	0	1	2	3
Loss of your sense of taste	0	1	2	3
Loss of your sense of smell	0	1	2	3
Smelling peculiar odors	0	1	2	3
Feeling dizzy	0	1	2	3
Seeing double	0	1	2	3
Hearing loss	0	1	2	3
Ringing in your ears	0	1	2	3
Sensitivity to bright light	0	1	2	3
Sensitivity to loud noise	0	1	2	3
Anxiety	0	1	2	3
Nightmares	0	1	2	3
Recurrent dreams of the accident	0	1	2	3
Recurrent thoughts of the accident	0	1	2	3
Lapses of attention	0	1	2	3
Spells, blackouts	0	1	2	3
Increased activity levels	0	1	2	3
Increased talkativeness	0	1	2	3
Racing thoughts	0	1	2	3
Increased self-esteem	0	1	2	3
Decreased need for sleep	0	1	2	3
Reckless behavior	0	1	2	3
Socially inappropriate behavior	0	1	2	3
Less interest in sex	0	1	2	3
More interest in sex	0	1	2	3
More likely to talk about sex	0	1	2	3
Weakness	0	1	2	3
Tremors	0	1	2	3
Poor coordination	0	1	2	3
Poor balance	0	1	2	3

	No	Mild problem	Moderate problem	Severe problem
Feelings of déjà vu	0	1	2	3
Feeling strange	0	1	2	3
Out-of-body experience	0	1	2	3
A sense of floating	0	1	2	3
Things look larger than they are	0	1	2	3
Things look smaller than they are	0	1	2	3
Extremely vivid memories	0	1	2	3
Hearing music that is not really there	0	1	2	3
Profound thoughts of God and the universe	0	1	2	3
Inner voices guiding you through the day	0	1	2	3

Number of "moderate" problems: ____________

Number of "severe" problems: ____________

Head injuries effect people in different ways. Please give us any additional information you think may reflect on your problem or how you deal with it.

List the medicine you take and the doctors/therapists you are consistently seeing.

Have you ever had a head injury before? If so, give some details.

Habits:

Alcohol: ____________

Tobacco: ____________

Other: ____________

APPENDIX 2
Neurobehavioral Rating Scale

We use this instrument for patients with brain injury who are severely compromised. Family members or caregivers fill it out. It addresses not only symptoms but also the patient's functional status.

Patient's Name: ______________________ Date: __________

Rater's Name: ______________________

Instructions: Consider the individual's behavior in settings you are familiar with, over the past week. Circle the appropriate number for each item. Answer all items.

RATING SCALE SCORES

0	NA	Not a functional deficit or a problem
1	Mild	Behavior inappropriate, does not interrupt treatment or prevent community/family activities, can be redirected
2	Moderate	Behavior interrupts activities, requires intervention, not potentially harmful, requires close monitoring
3	Severe	Behavior interrupts all activities and is potentially harmful to self, others or property, requires close supervision

	NA	Mild	Moderate	Severe
Cognitive				
1 Disoriented, confused about person, place, or time	0	1	2	3
2. Short attention span, distractible	0	1	2	3
3. Low arousal, hard to arouse	0	1	2	3
4. Memory deficit	0	1	2	3
5. Disorganized thinking, confused, disconnected, loose, tangential	0	1	2	3
		Subtotal: __________		
Performance				
6. Speech articulation deficit	0	1	2	3
7. Expressive language deficit	0	1	2	3
8. Comprehension deficit	0	1	2	3
9. Motor coordination deficit	0	1	2	3
10. Low energy level, easily fatigued	0	1	2	3
		Subtotal: __________		
Social interactions				
11. Withdrawn, socially isolated	0	1	2	3
12. Noncompliant, uncooperative	0	1	2	3
13. Hostile	0	1	2	3
14. Disinhibited, inappropriate comments or actions	0	1	2	3
		Subtotal: __________		

	NA	Mild	Moderate	Severe
Emotional state				
15. Decreased initiative/motivation	0	1	2	3
16. Depressed mood	0	1	2	3
17. Anxiety/tension	0	1	2	3
18. Excitable	0	1	2	3
19. Lability of mood	0	1	2	3
20. Emotional incontinence	0	1	2	3
21. Irritability	0	1	2	3
22. Low frustration tolerance	0	1	2	3
23. Agitation	0	1	2	3
		Subtotal: ______		
Behavior				
24. Restless, overly active, fidgety	0	1	2	3
25. Impulsive	0	1	2	3
26. Temper outbursts, explosive behavior	0	1	2	3
27. Destructive	0	1	2	3
28. Aggressive	0	1	2	3
		Subtotal: ______		
		Total Score: ______		

Comments:

APPENDIX 3
Memory Questionnaire

This is an essential instrument for evaluating neuropsychiatric patients. It addresses two important questions: is the patient cognizant of memory problems? If so, in what functional domains are they manifest? If you were to take the test yourself, your mean item score would be less than 1.5. Patients with memory problems usually score between 1.5 and 3.0. A score higher than 3.0 is suspicious; if the patient's memory is that bad, how can he or she remember how bad it is.

Patient's Name: ______________________________ Date: ______________

Instructions: We want to know if you have any memory or concentration difficulties. Please circle the following numbered columns where appropriate.

Situation	None or a little of the time	Some of the time	A good part of the time	Most or all the time
1. Forgetting where you have put something, losing things around the house	1	2	3	4
2. Failing to recognize places that you have been before	1	2	3	4
3. Finding a television story difficult to follow	1	2	3	4
4. Not remembering a change in your daily routine, such as a change in the place where something is kept or a change in the time something happens; following your old routine by mistake	1	2	3	4
5. Having to go back to check whether you have done something that you meant to do	1	2	3	4
6. Forgetting when it was that something happened	1	2	3	4
7. Completely forgetting to take things with you or leaving things behind and having to go back and fetch them	1	2	3	4
8. Forgetting that you were told something yesterday or a few days ago and having to be reminded about it	1	2	3	4
9. Starting to read something (book, newspaper, magazine) without realizing you have already read it before	1	2	3	4
10. Letting yourself ramble on about unimportant or irrelevant things	1	2	3	4
11. Failing to recognize by sight close relatives or friends that you meet frequently	1	2	3	4
12. Having difficulty picking up a new skill, for example, finding it hard to learn a new game or to work a new gadget after you have practiced it once or twice	1	2	3	4
13. Finding that a word is "on the tip of your tongue"; you know what it is but you cannot quite find it	1	2	3	4
14. Completely forgetting to do things that you said you would do or things you planned to do	1	2	3	4

continued

Situation	None or a little of the time	Some of the time	A good part of the time	Most or all the time
15. Forgetting important details of what you did or what happened to you the day before	1	2	3	4
16. When talking to someone, forgetting what you have just said; maybe saying "what was I talking about?"	1	2	3	4
17. When reading a newspaper or magazine, being unable to follow the thread of a story, losing track of what it is about	1	2	3	4
18. Forgetting to tell somebody something; perhaps forgetting to pass on a message or to remind someone of something	1	2	3	4
19. Forgetting important details about yourself like your birthday or where you live	1	2	3	4
20. Getting the details of what someone has told you mixed up and confused	1	2	3	4
21. Telling someone a story or joke that you have told them already	1	2	3	4
22. Forgetting details of things you do regularly, whether at home or work, for example, forgetting details of what to do or what time it is	1	2	3	4
23. Finding that the faces of famous people seen on television or in photographs look unfamiliar	1	2	3	4
24. Forgetting where things are normally kept or looking for them in the wrong place	1	2	3	4
25. Getting lost or turning in the wrong direction on a journey, on a walk, or in a building where you have been before	1	2	3	4
26. Repeating to someone what you have just told them or asking them the same question twice	1	2	3	4
27. Doing some routine thing twice by mistake, for example, putting two bags of tea in the teapot, or going to brush/comb your hair when you have just done so	1	2	3	4

Mean item score: ____________________

Total score: ____________________

APPENDIX 4

Attention Deficit/Hyperactivity Disorder Checklist

There are a number of rating scales in use for attention deficit/hyperactivity disorder (ADHD) in children and adults. Why do we use this one? We use it because it addresses four symptom domains that are central to ADHD (inattention, hyperactivity) or associated with it (instability of mood, oppositional behavior). Each domain is scored independently, and this gives you a pretty good idea where the patient's most troublesome symptoms lie.

We use this scale routinely for ADHD evaluations. Parents and teachers find it easy to use. We also use it routinely when we evaluate patients with mild brain injury. These are the symptoms that they are most likely to complain about. The patient or someone who knows the patient well can fill it out.

Patient's Name: ______________________ Date: __________

Rater's Name: ______________________

Instructions: This scale rates four prominent symptom clusters associated with ADHD: inattention, hyperactivity, instability of mood, and oppositional behavior. Please rate the following on the basis of your observation on a scale of 1 (not a problem) to 5 (a serious problem).

	Rating				
Inattention					
Inattentive, short attention span	1	2	3	4	5
Cannot concentrate	1	2	3	4	5
Easily distracted	1	2	3	4	5
Fails to complete tasks	1	2	3	4	5
Forgetful, needs constant reminding	1	2	3	4	5
		Subtotal: ______			
Hyperactivity					
Restless, overactive	1	2	3	4	5
Fidgeting, cannot sit still	1	2	3	4	5
Cannot play quietly	1	2	3	4	5
Impulsive, acts without thinking	1	2	3	4	5
Impatient, talks out of turn	1	2	3	4	5
		Subtotal: ______			
Instability of mood					
Moods change quickly	1	2	3	4	5
Easily frustrated	1	2	3	4	5
Excitable nature	1	2	3	4	5
Explosive behavior	1	2	3	4	5
Nervous, high-strung, tense	1	2	3	4	5
		Subtotal: ______			
Oppositional behavior					
Stubborn, sullen, irritable	1	2	3	4	5
Defiant, argumentative	1	2	3	4	5
Temper tantrums	1	2	3	4	5
Blames others for mistakes	1	2	3	4	5
Hostile, negative, oppositional	1	2	3	4	5
		Subtotal: ______			

Mean item score: ______________

Total score: ______________

APPENDIX 5

Self-injurious Behavior Questionnaire

Patient's Name: ________________________ Date: __________

Rater's Name: ________________________

Instructions: Please consider the individual's behavior in settings you are familiar with over the past week. Circle the appropriate number for each item. Answer all items.

	Not a problem	Minimal problem	Mild problem	Moderate problem	Severe problem
Self-injurious behavior (SIB)					
1. Frequency of SIB	0	1	2	3	4
2. Severity of SIB	0	1	2	3	4
3. Restraints used for SIB	0	1	2	3	4
4. Presence of self-inflicted bruises	0	1	2	3	4
5. Presence of self-inflicted wounds or tissue damage	0	1	2	3	4
			Subtotal: ______		
Behavioral problems					
6. Physical aggression toward others	0	1	2	3	4
7. Difficulty sleeping	0	1	2	3	4
8. Stereotypic, repetitive movements	0	1	2	3	4
9. Excessive yelling or screaming	0	1	2	3	4
10. Overactive	0	1	2	3	4
11. Destructive to property or objects	0	1	2	3	4
12. Eating nonfood items (pica)	0	1	2	3	4
13. Tantrums	0	1	2	3	4
14. Peculiar or bizarre behavior	0	1	2	3	4
			Subtotal: ______		
Performance					
15. Does not follow directions	0	1	2	3	4
16. Difficulty paying attention	0	1	2	3	4
17. Poor motor coordination	0	1	2	3	4
18. Poor performance in class/workshop	0	1	2	3	4
			Subtotal: ______		
Emotional problems					
19. Withdrawn, isolated	0	1	2	3	4
20. Mood changes quickly, emotionally labile	0	1	2	3	4
21. Hostile, angry	0	1	2	3	4

Comments: ________________________

APPENDIX 6

Tardive Dyskinesia and Tardive Akathisia: Examination

The acronym TDAK is taken from tardive dyskinesia and akathisia and is pronounced tee-dak. It is an Abnormal Involuntary Movement Scale (AIMS) examination, with three additional clusters of symptoms.

The AIMS was developed at the National Institute of Mental Health and is the most widely used instrument for tardive dyskinesia evaluation. It is not a rating scale so much as a structured examination. We used the AIMS for years in studies of tardive dyskinesia in retarded people. We developed an expanded AIMS because it was necessary to record symptoms and signs of akathisia, stereotypy, and locomotor hyperactivity, in addition to the abnormal movements of tardive dyskinesia.

Patient's Name: ______________________ Date: __________

Rater's Name: ______________________ Location: __________

AIMS examination: Rate involuntary movements and rate the highest severity observed. Rate movements that occur on activation one less than those observed spontaneously.

Stereotypies examination: Rate the severity of persistent and stereotyped repetition of words, posture, or movements based on your global impression. Each item indicates the general location from which the behaviors originate. Do not rate self-injurious behavior.

TDAK examination: Rate voluntary movements and affective behavior. Rate the severity of each item based on your global impression. Do not rate involuntary or dyskinetic movements.

Hyperactivity examination: Rate the severity of hyperactivity and motor actions based on your global impression. Do not rate dyskinetic movements or stereotypies.

DYSKINESIA AND TARDIVE AKATHISIA: RATING INSTRUCTIONS

Rating Scale Scores

NA	Not applicable	Item cannot be rated owing to physical handicaps, restraints, or inability to comply with examination procedures
0	Absent	Not present or not abnormal
1	Minimal	Questionably present or normal variant
2	Mild	Present: infrequent, low intensity
3	Moderate	Present: frequent, not constant
4	Severe	Present: persistent, extremely intense, debilitating

Rating Rules

1. Please rate the individual's movements and behaviors by circling one of the numbers beside each item listed.
2. Circle NA when an item cannot be rated.
3. Rate movements and behavior that are observed during the clinical examination period. Items should be rated based on global impressions during the examination period.
4. Please consider a number of variables when judging the severity of the movement or behavior such as frequency of occurrence, persistence, intensity, degree of debilitation.
5. Avoid rating between two scores by always choosing the lower score. For example, a mild to moderate rating (2–3) should be rated as 2.

continued

6. Items in which no score has been circled will be scored as 0.
7. Movements that are initially dyskinetic and then become more "voluntary, organized, directed, and complete" should be rated in the following way:
   a Rate the dyskinesia in the AIMS section
   b. Rate the voluntary motion in the TDAK section under the fidgety item.

AIMS examination						
1. Muscles of facial expression	NA	0	1	2	3	4
2. Lips and perioral area	NA	0	1	2	3	4
3. Jaw	NA	0	1	2	3	4
4. Tongue	NA	0	1	2	3	4
5. Upper extremities	NA	0	1	2	3	4
6. Lower extremities	NA	0	1	2	3	4
7. Neck, shoulders, and hips	NA	0	1	2	3	4
			Total: ______			
Stereotypies examination						
1. Upper extremities	NA	0	1	2	3	4
2. Lower extremities	NA	0	1	2	3	4
3. Trunk	NA	0	1	2	3	4
4. Neck, shoulders, and head	NA	0	1	2	3	4
5. Oral (verbal)	NA	0	1	2	3	4
			Total: ______			
Akathisia examination						
1. Rocking from foot to foot	NA	0	1	2	3	4
2. Walking on the spot	NA	0	1	2	3	4
3. Pacing	NA	0	1	2	3	4
4. Restlessness	NA	0	1	2	3	4
5. Dysphoria	NA	0	1	2	3	4
			Total: ______			
Hyperactivity examination						
1. Hyperactivity	NA	0	1	2	3	4
2. Fidgeting (exclude stereotypies)	NA	0	1	2	3	4
3. Self-injurious behavior	NA	0	1	2	3	4
			Total: ______			

Subject Index

Note: Page numbers followed by "t" indicate tabular material.

O

Q